# FITZPATRICK'S
# COLOR ATLAS AND SYNOPSIS OF CLINICAL DERMATOLOGY

## FIFTH EDITION

### Klaus Wolff
*Professor and Chairman Emeritus*
Department of Dermatology,
Medical University of Vienna
Chief Emeritus Dermatology Service,
General Hospital of Vienna
Vienna, Austria

### Richard Allen Johnson
*Clinical Instructor and Associate in Dermatology*
Massachusetts General Hospital
Harvard Medical School
Boston, Massachusetts

### Dick Suurmond
*Professor and Chairman Emeritus*
Department of Dermatology, University Hospital
Leiden, The Netherlands

## McGraw-Hill
### MEDICAL PUBLISHING DIVISION
New York / Chicago / San Francisco / Lisbon / London / Madrid
Mexico City / Milan / New Delhi / San Juan / Seoul /Singapore / Sydney / Toronto

Available Translations of *Color Atlas and Synopsis of Clinical Dermatology*, *Fourth edition*

| | |
|---|---|
| Chinese (Short Form) | McGraw-Hill Education (Asia), Jurong, Singapore |
| Chinese (Long Form) | McGraw-Hill International Enterprises, Inc., Taipei, Taiwan |
| Greek | Paschalidis Medical Publications, Athens, Greece |
| Indonesian | Penerbit Salemba Medika, Jakarta, Indonesia |
| Italian | McGraw-Hill, s.r.l., Milan, Italy |
| Portuguese | McGraw-Hill Interamericana Editores, S.A. de C.V., Mexico City |
| Spanish | McGraw-Hill Interamericana de Espana. S.A., Madrid |

# FITZPATRICK'S COLOR ATLAS AND SYNOPSIS OF CLINICAL DERMATOLOGY, FIFTH EDITION

1234567890   DOC DOC 098765

ISBN 0-07-144019-4

This book was set in Times Roman by TechBooks Inc. The editors were Andrea Seils and Mariapaz Ramos Englis. The production supervisor was Phil Galea. The text designer was Marsha Cohen of Parallelogram. The index was prepared by Barbara Littlewood.
RR Donnelley was printer and binder.

This book is printed on acid-free paper.

Library of Congress Cataloging-in-Publication Data
Fitzpatrick's color atlas and synopsis of clinical dermatology.—5th ed. / Klaus Wolff,
   Richard Allen Johnson ; Dick Suurmond.
      p. ; cm.
   Rev. ed. of: Color atlas and synopsis of clinical dermatology / Thomas B. Fitzpatrick,
   Richard Allen Johnson, Klaus Wolff. 4th ed. c2001.
   Includes bibliographical references and index.
   ISBN 0-07-144019-4 (alk. paper)
      1. Dermatology—Atlases. I. Title: Color atlas and synopsis of clinical dermatology. II.
   Fitzpatrick, Thomas B. (Thomas Bernard); III. Wolff, Klaus; IV. Johnson,
   Richard Allen; V. Suurmond, Dick. VI. Fitzpatrick, Thomas B. (Thomas Bernard),
   Color atlas and synopsis of clinical dermatology.
      [DNLM: 1. Skin Diseases—Atlases, WR 17 F5594 2005]
   RL81.C65 2005
   616.5—dc22
                                                                    2004065649

This *Fifth Edition* is dedicated to the memory of

**Thomas B. Fitzpatrick** and **Beatrice D. Fitzpatrick**

# NOTICE

Medicine is an ever-changing science. As new research and clinical experience broaden our knowledge, changes in treatment and drug therapy are required. The authors and the publisher of this work have checked with sources believed to be reliable in their efforts to provide information that is complete and generally in accord with the standards accepted at the time of publication. However, in view of the possibility of human error or changes in medical sciences, neither the authors nor the publisher nor any other party who has been involved in the preparation or publication of this work warrants that the information contained herein is in every respect accurate or complete, and they disclaim all responsibility for any errors or omissions or for the results obtained from use of the information contained in this work. Readers are encouraged to confirm the information contained herein with other sources. For example and in particular, readers are advised to check the product information sheet included in the package of each drug they plan to administer to be certain that the information contained in this work is accurate and that changes have not been made in the recommended dose or in the contraindications for administration. This recommendation is of particular importance in connection with new or infrequently used drugs.

# CONTENTS

## PART I
## DISORDERS PRESENTING IN THE SKIN AND MUCOUS MEMBRANES

### SECTION 1
### DISORDERS OF SEBACEOUS AND APOCRINE GLANDS    2

### SECTION 2
### ECZEMA/DERMATITIS    18

## SECTION 8

## ERYTHRODERMA AND RASHES IN THE ACUTELY ILL PATIENT                           158

## SECTION 9

## BENIGN NEOPLASMS AND HYPERPLASIAS                                            166

## SECTION 10

## PHOTOSENSITIVITY, PHOTO-INDUCED DISORDERS, AND DISORDERS BY IONIZING RADIATION      226

## SECTION 11

## PRECANCEROUS LESIONS AND CUTANEOUS CARCINOMAS      270

# PART II
## DERMATOLOGY AND INTERNAL MEDICINE

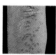

**S E C T I O N    1 5**

## ENDOCRINE, METABOLIC, NUTRITIONAL, AND GENETIC DISEASES   432

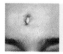

# P A R T    I I I
## DISEASES DUE TO MICROBIAL AGENTS

## SECTION 23
## CUTANEOUS FUNGAL INFECTIONS    686

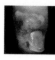
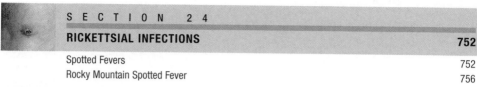
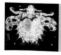
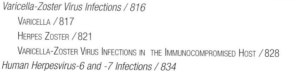

## S E C T I O N 2 7
### SEXUALLY TRANSMITTED INFECTIONS 882

## S E C T I O N 2 8
### MUCOCUTANEOUS MANIFESTATIONS OF HUMAN IMUNODEFICIENCY VIRUS DISEASE 936

# P A R T    I V
## SKIN SIGNS OF HAIR, NAIL, AND MUCOSAL DISORDERS

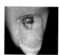

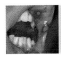

## S E C T I O N   3 1
## DISORDERS OF OROPHARYNX — 1016

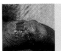

## S E C T I O N   3 2
## DISORDERS OF THE GENITALIA, PERINEUM, AND ANUS — 1034

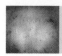

S E C T I O N   3 3
## GENERALIZED PRURITUS WITHOUT SKIN LESIONS                          1052

A  P  P  E  N  D  I  C  E  S                                          1056

I  N  D  E  X                                                         1061

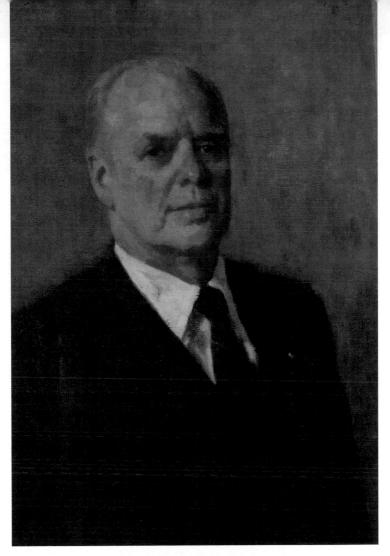

**THOMAS BERNARD FITZPATRICK**
**19 December 1919–16 August 2003**

This Fifth Edition of *Fitzpatrick's Color Atlas and Synopsis of Clinical Dermatology* is dedicated to Thomas B. Fitzpatrick, the founding Editor and Editor-in-Chief for the first four editions. On August 16, 2003, Thomas B. Fitzpatrick succumbed to a disease he had fought patiently and courageously. One of the giants of dermatology had gone—a man who had moved the world of dermatology had left the scene.

The name Thomas B. Fitzpatrick is associated with many milestones: the melanosome and tyrosinase, the epidermal melanin unit, skin phototypes, melanoma, PUVA photochemotherapy, sun protection factors, vitiligo, and many others; the landmark books *Fitzpatrick's Dermatology in General Medicine* and this *Color Atlas and Synopsis of Clinical Dermatology* are milestones in themselves. Thomas B. Fitzpatrick was a towering personality—what he created in the twentieth century is a challenge for the dermatosciences of the future.

Thomas B. Fitzpatrick was born on December 19, 1919, in Madison, Wisconsin. After undergraduate studies at the University of Wisconsin, where he obtained a Bachelor of Arts degree with honors, he graduated from Harvard Medical School in 1945, obtained a Ph.D. at the University of Minnesota in 1952, and was certified the same year by the American Board of Dermatology. At the age of 32 Fitzpatrick was named Professor and Head of the Division of Dermatology of the University of Oregon, and at the age of 39 he was named Edward Wigglesworth Professor and Chairman of the Department of Dermatology at Harvard Medical School and Chief of Dermatology at Massachusetts General Hospital and Harvard Medical School—positions he held until he became emeritus in 1990. He was a member of a large number of scientific societies, among them the prestigious American Academy of Arts and Sciences and the National Academy of Sciences, Institute of Medicine; 17 scientific societies conferred an honorary membership on him. He was the founder of the Dermatology Foundation where he served as President from 1971 to 1973 and was President of the Society for Investigative Dermatology (1959–1960). Among the appointments to important national and international organizations were memberships of the World Health Organization Melanoma Program and the Committee on Impacts of Stratospheric Change of the National Academy of Sciences, and he was Chairman of the Panel on Effects on Human Health, National Academy of Sciences. He served on the Science Advisory Boards of the Environmental Protection Agency and the American Skin Association and was a member of the Editorial Board of The New England Journal of Medicine from 1961 to 1969. Among a long list of awards and honors Dr. Fitzpatrick received were the Myron Gordon Award for Distinguished Contributions; the Dohi International Exchange Lectureship; the Stephen Rothman Award (Gold Medal); the Order of the Rising Sun with Gold Rays, conferred upon him in 1986 by the Emperor of Japan; honorary membership of the Society for Investigative Dermatology; and the Award for Distinguished Career in Dermatology by The New England Dermatological Society. He was also named Master of Dermatology by the American Academy of Dermatology in 1990 and received the Melanoma Program Award for outstanding achievements in the field of cutaneous melanoma by the World Health Organization. The International League of Dermatological Societies awarded him the Certificate of Appreciation for Lifelong Commitment to Academic Dermatology and Seminal Scientific Contributions. As an example of the impact Dr. Fitzpatrick had even on the nondermatologic and nonmedical community, it should be mentioned that the Governor of the Commonwealth of Massachusetts proclaimed May 2, 1994, as the Dr. Thomas Bernard Fitzpatrick Day.

Thomas B. Fitzpatrick was a creative scientist and prolific writer. Breakthrough discoveries were

- The identification of the essential elements of melanin pigmentation: the first demonstration of tyrosinase in humans; the isolation and characterization of the metabolic unit of melanin pigmentation, which he called the melanosome; the development of the concept of the epidermal melanin unit, which recognizes a partnership of melanocytes and keratinocytes in the process of pigmentation.
- The development of clinical criteria for the early detection of cutaneous malignant melanoma; the application of scientific methods to a rational development of topical sunscreens, which led to the definition and use of sun protection factors that changed the attitudes of both industry and consumers; the concept of skin phototypes, which is now used worldwide for the assessment of sunlight-induced cancer risk and the role of sunlight in the etiology of melanoma.
- The identification of delineation of white leaf-shaped macules as the earliest sign of tuberous sclerosis.
- The demonstration of β-carotene as a photoprotective agent in erythropoetic protoporphyria, which was the first application of an in vivo systemic photoprotective biologic principle to the treatment of human disease.
- Last, but not least, the introduction of psoralens into twentieth century medicine, with the use as pigmenting agents with UVA and their application to vitiligo—the development of the concept of photochemotherapy. PUVA became the single most effective treatment of psoriasis and mycosis fungoides in the 1970s and 1980s and is still widely used worldwide.

Tom Fitzpatrick, TBF or Fitz, was not only a great scientist but was also a brilliant clinical dermatologist and a warm-hearted and compassionate physician, and these are traits known not only to those who have had the privilege of being closely associated with him but also to a wider, in fact a worldwide, community. He was a compassionate and cherished teacher. Tom was witty, understanding, and exceedingly curious, and since curiosity is the source of creativity we now understand the level of excellence he achieved. Tom Fitzpatrick's curiosity was infectious, and it was coupled with compassion and a deep interest in people. For him the individual patient was always center stage.

Thomas B. Fitzpatrick has become an icon in dermatology not only in the United States but worldwide and also inspired admiration coupled with affection, something that few people do successfully. This does not come as surprise because Fitz was a true renaissance man, an *uomo universale* as scientist, teacher, compassionate physician, and philosopher—sharing quotations from himself and his wife, Bea, with *Boston Globe* readers through the small vignette called "Reflection of the day." He loved music, particularly Bach and Brahms, and rarely ever traveled without tapes or discs of Brahms' chamber music. Thus it does not come as a surprise that he was chosen to sit on the Board of Governors of the Boston Symphony.

Tom Fitzpatrick was a devoted husband and father. He loved his children but Bea was the center of his life. Tom married Beatrice Devaney, in 1944, and she provided the climate of a family life that represented the haven to which Tom returned from his hectic professional work. "Bea became his wife, lover, best friend, sustainer, and social grace," according to a close friend and colleague—she was his sun, radiating warmth and light and love. It is to the memory of this great physician, scientist, and teacher whose life and work have so inspired us and of his wonderful wife Beatrice, whom we admired and loved and who followed him a year after his death, that this Fifth Edition of *Fitzpatrick's Color Atlas and Synopsis of Clinical Dermatology* is dedicated.

# PREFACE

**"Time is change; we measure its passage by how much things alter."**
*Nadine Gordimer*

The *First Edition* of this book appeared 21 years ago (1983) and has been expanded *pari passu* with the major developments that have occurred in dermatology over the past two decades. Dermatology is now one of the most sought after medical specialties because the burden of skin disease has become enormous and the many new innovative therapies available today attract large patient populations.

The *Color Atlas and Synopsis of Clinical Dermatology* has been used by thousands of primary care physicians, dermatologists, internists, and other health care providers principally because it facilitates dermatologic diagnosis by providing large color photographs of skin lesions and, juxtaposed, a succinct summary outline of skin disorders as well as the skin signs of systemic diseases.

The Fifth Edition has been extensively revised and more than 50% have been rewritten with 857 photographs and an updating and expansion of the text relating to management and therapy. The previous editions of the *Atlas* have been translated into many languages.

# ACKNOWLEDGMENTS

Our secretary, Renate Kosma, worked hard to meet the demands of the writers. Looking back, it was the Dutch Professor M. Polano's initial superb "picture only" Atlas that was the stimulus that led Thomas B. Fitzpatrick to write the text for the First Edition, with the present editors joining in in the subsequent editions. In the present McGraw-Hill team, we appreciated the counsel of Martin Wonsiewicz, Vice President and Publisher; Darlene Cooke, Executive Editor; Andrea Seils, Senior Editor; Eileen Scott, the Development Editor for this edition; Marsha Cohen, who has been the text designer of CASD since the third edition; and Phil Galea, the Senior Production Manager who expertly managed the production process. But the major force behind this edition and previous editions was Mariapaz Ramos Englis, Senior Managing Editor, whose good nature, good judgment, loyalty to the authors, and most of all, patience, guided the authors to make an even better book.

# INTRODUCTION

The *Color Atlas and Synopsis of Clinical Dermatology* is proposed as a "field guide" to the recognition of skin disorders and their management. The skin is a treasury of important lesions that can usually be recognized clinically. Gross morphology in the form of skin lesions remains the hard core of dermatologic diagnosis, and therefore this text is accompanied by 857 color photographs illustrating skin diseases, skin manifestations of internal diseases, infections, tumors, and incidental skin findings in otherwise-well individuals. We have endeavored to include information relevant to gender dermatology and a large number of images showing skin disease in different ethnic populations. This *Atlas* covers the entire field of clinical dermatology but does not include very rare syndromes or conditions. With respect to these the reader is referred to another McGraw-Hill Publication: *Dermatology in General Medicine*, 6th ed., 2003, edited by IM Freedberg et al.

This text is intended for all physicians and other health care providers, including medical students, dermatology residents, internists, oncologists, and infectious disease specialists dealing with diseases with skin manifestations. For non-dermatologists, it is advisable to start with "Approach to Dermatologic Diagnosis" and "Outline of Dermatologic Diagnosis," below, to familiarize themselves with the principles of dermatologic nomenclature and lines of thought.

The *Atlas* is organized in 4 Parts, subdivided into 33 Sections, and there are 3 short Appendices. Each section has a color label that is reflected by the bar on the top of each page. This is to help the reader to find his or her bearings rapidly when leafing through the book. Also, the first page of each section carries an "icon," i.e., a small photograph of a condition that is representative for that particular section.

Each disease is labeled with little symbols to provide first-glance information on incidence (squares) and morbidity (circles).

| | |
|---|---|
| ❑ rare | ○ low morbidity |
| ◪ not so common | ◑ considerable morbidity |
| ■ common | ● serious |

For instance, the symbols ■ ● for melanoma are meant to indicate that melanoma is common and serious. There are also some variations in this symbology. For instance, ❑ → ■ means that the disease is rare but may be common in specific populations or in endemic regions or in epidemics. Another example ◑ → ● indicates that the disease causes considerable morbidity and may become serious.

## APPROACH TO DERMATOLOGIC DIAGNOSIS

There are two distinct clinical situations regarding the nature of skin changes:

I. The skin changes are *incidental* findings in *well* individuals noted during the routine general physical examination
   A. *"Bumps and blemishes"*: many asymptomatic lesions that are medically inconsequential may be present in well persons and are not the reason for the visit to the physician; every general physician should be able to recognize these lesions to differentiate them from asymptomatic important, e.g., malignant, lesions.

B. *Important skin lesions not* noted by the patient but that must not be overlooked by the physician: e.g., atypical nevi, melanoma, basal cell carcinoma, squamous cell carcinoma, café-au-lait macules in von Recklinghausen's disease, xanthomas.

II. The skin changes are the *chief complaint* of the patient

A. "Minor" problems: e.g., localized itchy rash, "rash," rash in groin, nodules such as common moles, seborrheic keratoses.

B. "4-S": *serious skin signs in sick patients*
1. Generalized red rash with fever
   a. Viral exanthems
   b. Rickettsial exanthems
   c. Drug eruptions
   d. Bacterial infections with toxin production.
2. Generalized red rash with blisters and prominent mouth lesions
   a. Erythema multiforme (major)
   b. Toxic epidermal necrolysis
   c. Bullous pemphigoid
   d. Drug eruptions
3. Generalized rash without redness with blisters, erosions, and mouth lesions
   a. Pemphigus
4. Generalized red rash with pustules
   a. Pustular psoriasis (von Zumbusch)
   b. Drug eruptions
5. Generalized rash with vesicles
   a. Disseminated herpes simplex
   b. Generalized herpes zoster
   c. Varicella
   d. Drug eruptions
6. Generalized red rash with scaling over whole body
   a. Exfoliative erythroderma
7. Generalized wheals and soft tissue swelling
   a. Urticaria and angioedema
8. Generalized purpura
   a. Thrombocytopenia
   b. Purpura fulminans
   c. Drug eruptions
9. Generalized purpura that can be palpated
   a. Vasculitis
   b. Bacterial endocarditis
10. Multiple skin infarcts
    a. Meningococcemia
    b. Gonococcemia
    c. Disseminated intravascular coagulopathy
11. Localized skin infarcts
    a. Calciphylaxis
    b. Atherosclerosis obliterans
    c. Atheroembolization
    d. Warfarin necrosis
    e. Antiphospholipid antibody syndrome
12. Facial inflammatory edema with fever
    a. Erysipelas
    b. Lupus erythematosus

## OUTLINE OF DERMATOLOGIC DIAGNOSIS

In contrast to other fields of clinical medicine, patients should be examined before a detailed history is taken because patients can see their lesions and thus often present with a history that is flawed with their own interpretation of the origin or causes of the skin eruption. Also, diagnostic accuracy is higher when objective examination is approached without preconceived ideas. Many skin eruptions are so characteristic that they don't require a history initially. However, a history should always be obtained but if taken during or after the visual and physical examination, it can be shaped according to the objective findings.

## PHYSICAL EXAMINATION

### Appearance
Uncomfortable, "toxic," well

### Vital Signs
Pulse, respiration, temperature

## Skin: "Learning to Read"

The entire skin should be inspected and this should include mucous membranes, genital and anal regions, as well as hair and nails and peripheral lymph nodes. Reading the skin is like reading a text. The basic skin lesions are like the letters of the alphabet: their shape, color, margination, and other features combined will lead to words, and their localization and distribution to a sentence or paragraph. The prerequisite of dermatologic diagnosis is thus the recognition of (1) the type of skin lesion, (2) the color, (3) margination, (4) consistency, (5) shape, (6) arrangement, and (7) distribution of lesions.

### Recognizing Letters: Types of Skin Lesions

- *Macule* (Latin: *macula*, "spot")  A macule is a circumscribed area of change in skin color without elevation or depression. It is thus not palpable. Macules can be well- and ill-defined. Macules may be of any size or color (Image I-1). White, as in vitiligo, brown, as in café-au-lait spots (A); blue, as in Mongolian spots (B); or red, as in permanent vascular abnormalities such as port-wine stains (C) or capillary dilatation due to inflammation (erythema, D). Pressure of a glass slide (*diascopy*) on the border of a red lesion is a simple and reliable method for detecting the extravasation of red blood cells. If the redness remains under pressure from the slide, the lesion is purpuric; if the redness disappears, the lesion is due to vascular dilatation. A rash consisting of macules is called a *macular exanthem.*

- *Papule* (Latin: *papula*, "pimple")  A papule is a superficial, solid lesion, generally considered <0.5 cm in diameter. Most of it is elevated above, rather than deep within, the plane of the surrounding skin (Image I-2). A papule is palpable. It may be well- or ill-defined. In papules the elevation is caused by metabolic or locally produced deposits (A), by localized cellular infiltrates (B), or by hyperplasia of local cellular elements (C). Superficial papules are sharply defined. Deeper dermal papules resulting from cellular infiltrates have indistinct borders. Papules with distinct borders are seen when the lesion is the result of an increase in the number of epidermal cells (C) or a very superficial inflammatory infiltrate. Papules may be dome-shaped, cone-shaped or flat-topped (as in lichen planus) or consist of multiple, small, closely packed, projected elevations that are known as a *vegetation* (C). A rash consisting of papules is called a *papular exanthem.* Papular exanthems may be

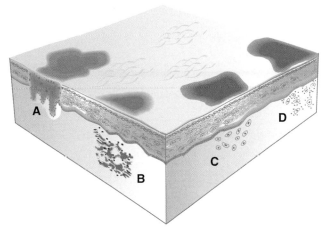

**IMAGE I-1**

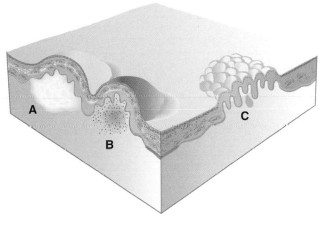

**IMAGE I-2**

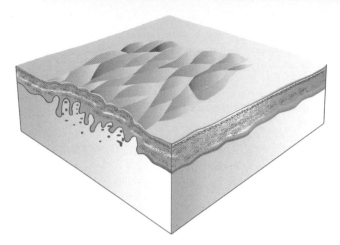

**IMAGE I-3**

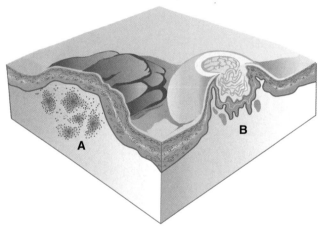

**IMAGE I-4**

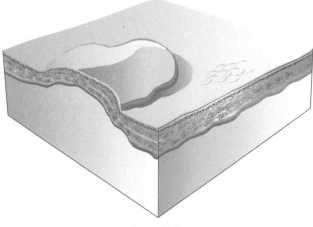

**IMAGE I-5**

grouped ("lichenoid") or disseminated (dispersed). Confluence of papules leads to the development of larger, usually flat-topped, circumscribed, plateau-like elevations known as plaques (French: *plaque,* "plate"). See below.

- *Plaque* A plaque is a plateau-like elevation above the skin surface that occupies a relatively large surface area in comparison with its height above the skin (Image I-3). It is usually well defined. Frequently it is formed by a confluence of papules, as in psoriasis. Lichenification is a less well-defined, large plaque where the skin appears thickened and the skin markings are accentuated (as shown in Image I-3). Lichenification occurs in atopic dermatitis, eczematous dermatitis, psoriasis, and mycosis fungoides.

- *Nodule* (Latin: *nodulus,* "small knot") A nodule is a palpable, solid, round or ellipsoidal lesion that is longer than a papule (Image I-4) and may involve the epidermis (*B*), dermis (*A*), or subcutaneous tissue. The depth of involvement and the size differentiate a nodule from a papule. Nodules result from inflammatory infiltrates (*A*), neoplasms (*B*), or metabolic deposits in the dermis or subcutaneous tissue. Nodules may be well-defined (superficial, *B*) or ill-defined (deep); if localized in the subcutaneous tissue, they can often be better felt than seen. Nodules can be hard or soft upon palpation. They may be dome-shaped and smooth or may have a warty surface or crater-like central depression.

- *Wheal*  A wheal is a rounded or flat-topped, pale red papule or plaque that is characteristically evanescent, disappearing within 24 to 48 h (Image I-5). It is due to edema in the papillary body of the dermis. Wheals may be round, gyrate, or irregular with pseudopods—changing rapidly in size and shape due to shifting papillary edema. A rash consisting of wheals is called an *urticarial exanthem* or *urticaria.*

- *Vesicle-Bulla (Blister)* (Latin: *vesicula*, "little bladder"; *bulla*, "bubble")  A vesicle (<0.5 cm) or a bulla (>0.5 cm) is a circumscribed, elevated, superficial cavity containing fluid (Image I-6). Often the roof of a vesicle/bulla is so thin that it is transparent, and the serum or blood in the cavity can be seen. Vesicles containing serum are yellowish; those containing blood from red to black. Vesicles and bullae arise from a cleavage at various levels of the superficial skin; the cleavage may be subcorneal or within the visible epidermis (i.e., intraepidermal vesication) or at the epidermal-dermal interface (i.e., subepidermal), as in Image I-6. A rash consisting of vesicles is called a *vesicular exanthem*; a rash consisting of bullae a *bullous exanthem.*

- *Pustule* (Latin: *pustula*, "pustule")  A pustule is a circumscribed, superficial cavity of the skin that contains a purulent exudate (Image I-7), which may be white, yellow, greenish-yellow, or hemorrhagic. This process may arise in a hair follicle or independently. Pustules may vary in size and shape. Pustules are usually dome-shaped or can be multicentric. Follicular pustules, however, are always conical and usually contain a hair in the center. The vesicular lesions of herpes simplex and varicella zoster virus infections may become pustular. A rash consisting of pustules is called a *pustular exanthem.*

- *Crusts* (Latin: *crusta*, "rind, bark, shell")  Crusts develop when serum, blood, or purulent exudate dries on the skin surface (Image I-8). Crusts may be thin, delicate, and friable (*A*) or thick and adherent (*B*). Crusts are yellow when formed from dried serum; green or yellow-green when formed from purulent exudate; or brown, dark red, or black when formed from blood. Superficial crusts occur as honey-colored, delicate, glistening particulates on the surface (*A*) and are typically found in impetigo. When the exudate involves the entire epidermis, the crusts may be thick and adherent (*B*), and if it is accompanied by necrosis of the deeper tissues (e.g., the

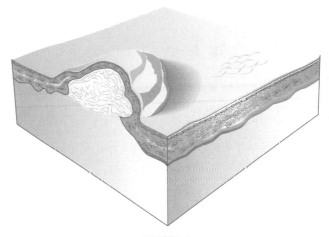

**IMAGE I-6**

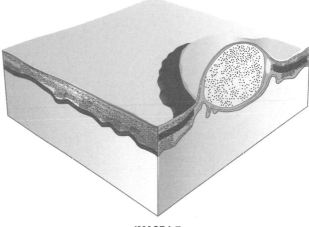

**IMAGE I-7**

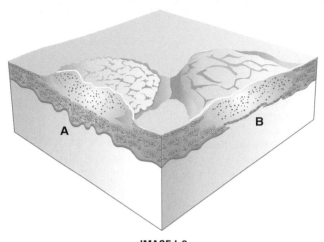

**IMAGE I-8**

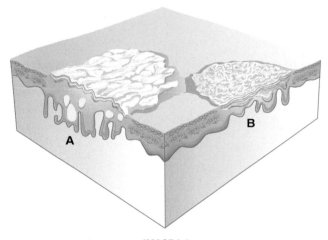

**IMAGE I-9**

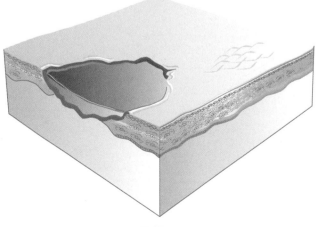

**IMAGE I-10**

dermis), the condition is known as *ecthyma*.

• *Scales (squames)* (Latin: *squama*, "scale") Epidermal cells are replaced every 27 days. The end product of this holocrine process is the stratum corneum, the outermost layer of skin, which is normally lost imperceptibly. With an increased rate of proliferation of epidermal cells (e.g., as in psoriasis), the stratum corneum is not formed normally, and the outermost desquamating layers of skin are seen clinically as scales (Image I-9). Scales are thus flakes of stratum corneum. They may be large (like membranes, *A*), tiny (like dust), pityriasiform (Greek: *pityron*, "bran"), adherent, or loose. Densely adherent scales that have a gritty feel (like sandpaper) result from a localized increase in the stratum corneum and are a characteristic of solar keratosis (*B*). A rash consisting of papules with scales is called a *papulosquamous exanthem*.

• *Erosion* An erosion is a defect only of the epidermis, not involving the dermis (Image I-10); in contrast to an ulcer, which always heals with scar formation (see below), an erosion heals without a scar. An erosion is sharply defined and is red and oozes. There are superficial erosions, which are subcorneal or run through the epidermis, and deep erosions, the base of which is the papillary body (Image I-10). Except for physical abrasions, erosions are always the result of intraepidermal or subepidermal cleavage and thus of vesicles or bullae.

- *Ulcer* (Latin: *ulcus,* "sore") An ulcer is a skin defect that extends into the dermis or deeper (Image I-11) into the subcutis and always occurs within pathologically altered tissue. An ulcer is therefore always a secondary phenomenon. The pathologically altered tissue giving rise to an ulcer is usually seen at the border or the base of the ulcer and is helpful in determining its cause. Other features helpful in this respect are whether borders are elevated (Image I-11), undermined, hard, or soggy; location of the ulcer; discharge; and any associated topographic features, such as nodules, exoriations, varicosities, hair distribution, presence or absence of sweating, and arterial pulses. Ulcers always heal with scar formation.

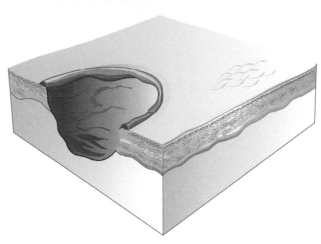

IMAGE I-11

- *Scar* A scar is the fibrous tissue replacement of the tissue defect by previous ulcer or a wound. Scars can be hypertrophic and hard (Image I-12, *A*) or atrophic and soft with a thinning or loss of all tissue compartments of the skin (Image I-12, *B*).

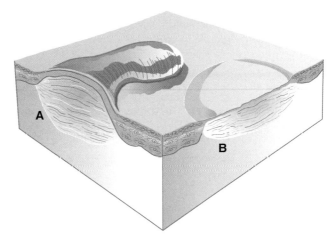

IMAGE I-12

- *Atrophy* This refers to a diminution of some or all layers of the skin (Image I-13). Epidermal atrophy is manifested by a thinning of the epidermis, which becomes transparent, revealing the papillary and subpapillary vessels (*B*); there are loss of skin texture and cigarette paper–like wrinkling. In dermal atrophy there are loss of connective tissue of the dermis and depression of the lesion (*A*).

- *Cyst* A cyst is a cavity containing liquid or solid or

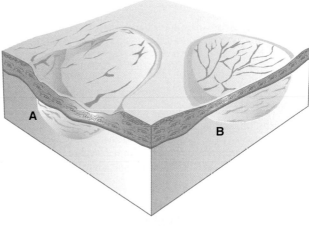

IMAGE I-13

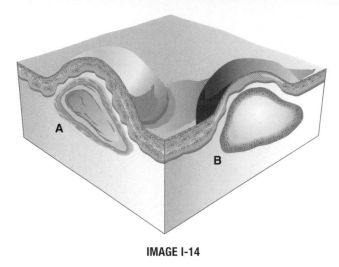

**IMAGE I-14**

semisolid (Image I-14) materials and may be superficial or deep. Visually it appears like a spherical, most often dome-shaped papule or nodule, but upon palpation it is resilient. It is lined by an epithelium and often has a fibrous capsule; depending on its contents it may be skin colored, yellow, red, or blue. An epidermal cyst producing keratinaceous material (*A*) and a pilar cyst that is lined by a multilayered epithelium (*B*) are shown in Image I-14.

### Shaping Letters into Words: Further Characterization of Identified Lesions

- *Color*    Pink, red, purple [purpuric lesions do not blanch with pressure with a glass slide (diascopy)], white, tan, brown, black, blue, grey, yellow. The color can be uniform or variegated.
- *Margination*    Well-defined (can be traced with the tip of a pencil), ill-defined.
- *Shape*    Round, oval, polygonal, polycyclic, annular (ring-shaped), iris, serpiginous (snakelike), umbilicated.
- *Palpation*    Consider (1) *consistency* (soft, firm, hard, fluctuant, boardlike); (2) *deviation in temperature* (hot, cold); and (3) *mobility*. Note presence of *tenderness,* and estimate the *depth* of the lesion (i.e., dermal or subcutaneous).

### Forming Sentences and Understanding the Text: Evaluation of Arrangement, Patterns, and Distribution

- *Number*    Single or multiple lesions.
- *Arrangement*    Multiple lesions may be (1) *grouped*: herpetiform, arciform, annular, reticulated (net-shaped), linear, serpiginous (snakelike); or (2) *disseminated*: scattered discrete lesions.
- *Confluence*    Yes or no.
- *Distribution*    Consider (1) *extent*: isolated (single lesions), localized, regional, generalized, universal, and (2) *pattern*: symmetric, exposed areas, sites of pressure, intertriginous area, follicular localization, random, following dermatomes or Blaschko's lines.

Table I-1 provides an algorithm showing how to proceed.

## HISTORY

**Demographics**    Age, race, sex, etiology, occupation.
**History**

1. Constitutional symptoms
    a. "Acute illness" syndrome: headaches, chills, feverishness, weakness
    b. "Chronic illness" syndrome: fatigue, weakness, anorexia, weight loss, malaise
2. History of skin lesions. Seven key questions:
    a. When? Onset
    b. Where? Site of onset
    c. Does it itch or hurt? Symptoms
    d. How has it spread (pattern of spread)? Evolution
    e. How have individual lesions changed? Evolution

# TABLE I-1  Algorithm for Evaluating Skin Lesions

**Identify lesions**

**Is lesion solitary or are there multiple lesions?**

## Solitary

**Macule**
- portwine stain*
- fixed drug eruption
- erythema migrans

**Papule/nodule**
- dermal nevus
- basal cell carcinoma
- nodular melanoma

**Plaque**
- lichen simplex chronicus
- Bowen's disease
- superficial spreading melanoma

**Ulcer**
- basal cell carcinoma
- diabetic ulcer
- primary chancre of syphilis

## Multiple

### Localized

**Macular**
- solar lentigines
- fixed drug eruption

**Papular**
- condylomata accuminata
- syringomas
- lichen planus

**Plaque**
- psoriasis
- mycosis fungoides

**Nodular**
- metastatic cancer

**Vesicular/bullous**
- herpes zoster
- herpes simplex

**Pustular**
- folliculitis barbae
- herpes zoster
- impetigo

### Generalized

**Macular**
- viral exanthem
- drug eruption

**Papular**
- psoriasis
- lichen planus
- secondary syphilis
- neurofibromatosis

**Vesicular/bullous**
- varicella
- bullous pemphigoid

**Pustular**
- pustular psoriasis
- smallpox

**Nodular**
- metastatic melanoma
- lipomas

*Conditions labeled with dots (•) are examples.

f. Provocative factors? Heat, cold, sun, exercise, travel history, drug ingestion, pregnancy, season
g. Previous treatment (s)? Topical and systemic,
3. General history of present illness as indicated by clinical situation, with particular attention to constitutional and prodromal symptoms
4. Past medical history
   a. Operations
   b. Illnesses (hospitalized?)
   c. Allergies, especially drug allergies
   d. Medications (present and past)
   e. Habits (smoking, alcohol intake, drug abuse)
   f. Atopic history (asthma, hay fever, eczema)
5. Family medical history (particularly of psoriasis, atopy, melanoma, xanthomas, tuberous sclerosis)
6. Social history, with particular reference to occupation, hobbies, exposures, travel, injecting drug use
7. Sexual history: history of risk factors of HIV: blood transfusions, IV drugs, sexually active, multiple partners, sexually transmitted disease?

## REVIEW OF SYMPTOMS

This should be done as indicated by the clinical situation, with particular attention to possible connections between signs and disease of other organ systems (e.g., rheumatic complaints, myalgias, arthralgias, Raynaud's phenomenon, sicca symptoms).

## SPECIAL CLINICAL AND LABORATORY AIDS TO DERMATOLOGIC DIAGNOSIS

### SPECIAL TECHNIQUES USED IN CLINICAL EXAMINATION

*Magnification with hand lens.* To examine lesions for fine morphologic detail, it is necessary to use a magnifying glass (hand lens) (7×) or a binocular microscope (5× to 40×). Magnification is especially helpful in the diagnosis of lupus erythematosus (follicular plugging), lichen planus (Wickham's striae), basal cell carcinomas (translucence and telangiectasia), and melanoma (subtle changes in color, especially gray or blue); this is best visualized after application of a drop of mineral oil. Use of the dermatoscope is discussed below (see "Dermoscopy").

*Oblique lighting* of the skin lesion, done in a darkened room, is often required to detect slight degrees of elevation or depression, and it is useful in the visualization of the surface configuration of lesions and in estimating the extent of the eruption.

*Subdued lighting* in the examining room enhances the contrast between circumscribed hypopigmented or hyperpigmented lesions and normal skin.

*Wood's lamp* (ultraviolet long-wave light, "black" light) is valuable in the diagnosis of certain skin and hair diseases and of porphyria. With the Wood's lamp (360 nm), fluorescent pigments and subtle color differences of melanin pigmentation can be visualized. Wood's lamp is particularly useful in the detection of the fluorescence of dermatophytosis in the hair shaft (green to yellow) and of erythrasma (coral red). A presumptive diagnosis of porphyria can be made if a pinkish-red fluorescence is demonstrated in urine examined with the Wood's lamp; addition of dilute hydrochloric acid intensifies the fluorescence. Wood's lamp also helps to estimate variation in the lightness of lesions in relation to the normal skin color in both dark-skinned and fair-skinned persons; e.g., the lesions seen in tuberous sclerosis and tinea versicolor are hypomelanotic and are not as white as the lesions seen in vitiligo, which are amelanotic. Circumscribed hypermelanosis, such as a freckle and melasma, is much more evident (darker) under Wood's lamp. By contrast, dermal melanin, as in a Mongolian sacral spot, does not become accentuated under Wood's lamp. Therefore, it is possible to localize the site of melanin by use of the Wood's lamp; *however, this is more difficult or not possible in patients with brown or black skin.*

*Diascopy* consists of firmly pressing a microscopic slide or a glass spatula over a skin lesion. The examiner will find this procedure of special value in determining whether the red color of a macule or papule is due to capillary dilatation (erythema) or to extravasation of blood (purpura) that does not blanch. Diascopy is also useful for the detection of the glassy yellow-brown appearance of papules in sarcoidosis, tuberculosis of the skin, lymphoma, and granuloma annulare.

*Dermoscopy* (also called *epiluminescence microscopy*). A hand lens with built-in lighting and a magnification of $10\times$ to $30\times$ is called a *dermatoscope* and permits the noninvasive inspection of deeper layers of the skin (dermal-epidermal junction and beyond). This is particularly useful in the distinction of benign and malignant growth patterns in pigmented lesions. *Digital dermoscopy* is particularly useful in the monitoring of pigmented skin lesions because images can be retrieved and examined at a later date to permit comparison quantitatively and qualitatively and to detect changes over time. Digital dermoscopy uses computer image analysis programs that provide (1) objective measurements of changes; (2) rapid storage, retrieval, and transmission of images to experts for further discussion (teledermatology); and (3) extraction of morphologic features for numerical analysis. Dermoscopy and digital dermoscopy require special training.

## CLINICAL SIGNS

*Darier's sign* is "positive" when a brown macular or a slightly papular lesion of urticaria pigmentosa (mastocytosis) becomes a palpable wheal after being vigorously rubbed with an instrument such as the blunt end of a pen. The wheal may not appear for 5 to 10 min.

*Auspitz's sign* is "positive" when slight scratching or curetting of a scaly lesion reveals punctate bleeding points within the lesion. This suggests psoriasis, but it is not specific.

The *Nikolsky phenomenon* is positive when the epidermis is dislodged from the dermis by lateral, shearing pressure with a finger, resulting in an erosion. It is an important diagnostic sign in acantholytic disorders such as pemphigus or the staphylococcal scalded skin (SSS) syndrome or other blistering or epidermonecrotic disorders, such as toxic epidermal necrolysis.

## CLINICAL TESTS

*Patch testing* is used to document and validate a diagnosis of allergic contact sensitization and identify the causative agent. Substances to be tested are applied to the skin in shallow cups (Finn chambers), affixed with a tape and left in place for 24 to 48 h. Contact hypersensitivity will show as a papular vesicular reaction that develops within 48 to 72 h when the test is read. It is a unique means of in vivo reproduction of disease in diminutive proportions, for sensitization affects all the skin and may therefore be elicited at any cutaneous site. The patch test is easier and safer than a "use test" with a questionable allergen, for test items can be applied in low concentrations in small areas of skin for short periods of time (see Section 2).

*Photopatch testing* is a combination of patch testing and UV irradiation of the test site and is used to document photoallergy (see Section 10).

*Prick testing* is used to determine type I allergies. A drop of a solution containing a minute concentration of the allergen is placed on the skin and the skin is pierced through this drop with a needle. Piercing should not go beyond the papillary body. A positive reaction will appear as a wheal within 20 min. The patient has to be under observation for possible anaphylaxis.

*Acetowhitening* facilitates detection of subclinical penile or vulvar warts. Gauze saturated with 5% acetic acid (white vinegar) is wrapped around the glans penis or used on the cervix and anus. After 5 to 10 min, the penis or vulva is inspected with a $10\times$ hand lens. Warts appear as small white papules.

## LABORATORY TESTS

### Microscopic Examination of Scales, Crusts, Serum, and Hair

*Gram's stains* and *cultures of exudates and of tissue minces* should be made in lesions suspected of being bacterial or yeast (*Candida albicans*) infections. Ulcers and nodules require a scalpel biopsy in which a wedge of tissue consisting of all three layers of skin is obtained; the biopsy specimen is minced in a sterile mortar and is then cultured for bacteria (including typical and atypical mycobacteria) and fungi.

*Microscopic examination* for mycelia should be made of the roofs of vesicles or of the scales (the advancing borders are preferable) or of the hair in dermatophytoses. The tissue is cleared with 10 to 30% KOH and warmed gently (Fig. 23-2). Fungal cultures with Sabouraud's medium should be made (see Section 23).

*Microscopic examination of cells obtained from the base of vesicles* (Tzanck preparation) may reveal the presence of acantholytic cells in the acantholytic diseases (e.g., pemphigus or SSS syndrome) or of giant epithelial cells and multinucleated giant cells (containing 10 to 12 nuclei) in herpes simplex, herpes zoster, and varicella. Material from the base of a vesicle obtained by *gentle* curettage with a scalpel is smeared on a glass slide, stained with either Giemsa's or Wright's stain or methylene blue, and examined to determine whether there are acantholytic or giant epithelial cells, which are diagnostic (Fig. 25-23). In addition, culture, immunofluorescent tests, or polymerase chain reaction for herpes have to be ordered.

*Laboratory diagnosis of scabies.* The diagnosis of scabies is usually considered immediately in a patient with intractable generalized pruritus and with papules and excoriations distributed in characteristic locations. The diagnosis is established by identification of the mite, or ova or feces, in skin scrapings removed from the papules or burrows (see Section 26). Using a sterile scalpel blade on which a drop of sterile mineral oil has been placed, apply oil to the surface of the burrow or papule. Scrape the papule or burrow vigorously to remove the entire top of the papule; tiny flecks of blood will appear in the oil. Transfer the oil to a microscopic slide and examine for mites, ova, and feces. The mites are 0.2 to 0.4 mm in size and have four pairs of legs (Fig. 26-23).

### Biopsy of the Skin

Biopsy of the skin is one of the simplest, most rewarding diagnostic techniques because of the easy accessibility of the skin and the variety of techniques for study of the excised specimen (e.g., histopathology, immunopathology, electron microscopy).

Selection of the site of the biopsy is based primarily on the stage of the eruption, and early lesions are usually more typical; this is especially important in vesiculobullous eruptions (e.g., pemphigus, herpes simplex), in which the lesion should be no more than 24 h old. However, older lesions (2 to 6 weeks) are often more characteristic in discoid lupus erythematosus.

A common technique for diagnostic biopsy is the use of a 3- to 4-mm punch, a small tubular knife much like a corkscrew, which by rotating movements between the thumb and index finger cuts through the epidermis, dermis, and subcutaneous tissue; the base is cut off with scissors. If immunofluorescence is indicated (e.g., as in bullous diseases or lupus erythematosus), a special medium for transport to the laboratory is required.

For nodules, however, a large wedge should be removed by excision including subcutaneous tissue. Furthermore, when indicated, lesions should be bisected, one-half for histology and the other half sent in a sterile container for bacterial and fungal cultures or in special fixatives or cell culture media, or frozen for immunopathologic examination.

Specimens for light microscopy should be fixed immediately in buffered neutral formalin. A brief but detailed summary of the clinical history and description of the lesions should accompany the specimen. Biopsy is indicated in *all* skin lesions that are suspected of being neoplasms, in all bullous disorders with immunofluoresence used simultaneously, and in all dermatologic disorders in which a specific diagnosis is not possible by clinical examination alone.

# PART

## I

# DISORDERS PRESENTING IN THE SKIN AND MUCOUS MEMBRANES

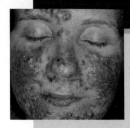

# DISORDERS OF SEBACEOUS AND APOCRINE GLANDS

## ACNE VULGARIS (COMMON ACNE) AND CYSTIC ACNE ■ ○ → ◑

Acne is an inflammation of the pilosebaceous units of certain body areas (face and trunk, rarely buttocks) that occurs most frequently in adolescence and mainfests itself as comedones (*comedonal acne*), papulopustules (*papulopustular acne*), or nodules and cysts (*nodulocystic acne* and *acne conglobata*). Pitted, depressed, or hypertrophic scars may follow all types but especially nodulocystic acne and acne conglobata.

### EPIDEMIOLOGY

**Occurrence** Very common, affecting approximately 85% of young people.

**Age of Onset** Puberty—10 to 17 years in females, 14 to 19 in males; however, may appear first at 25 years or older.

**Sex** More severe in males than in females.

**Race** Lower incidence in Asians and Africans.

**Genetic Aspects** Multifactorial genetic background. Majority of individuals with cystic acne have parent(s) with a history of severe acne. Severe acne may be associated with XYY syndrome.

### PATHOGENESIS

*Key factors* are follicular keratinization, androgens, and *Propionibacterium acnes* (Image 1-1).

Acne results from a change in the keratinization pattern in the pilosebaceous unit, with the keratinous material becoming more dense and blocking secretion of sebum. These keratin plugs are called *comedones* and represent the "time bombs" of acne. Comedonal plugging and a complex interaction between androgens and bacteria (*P. acnes*) in the plugged pilosebaceous units lead to inflammation. Androgens (qualitatively and quantitatively normal in the serum) stimulate sebaceous glands to produce larger amounts of sebum. Bacteria contain lipase, which converts lipid into fatty acids, and produce proinflammatory mediators, (interteukin 1, tumor necrosis factor α). Fatty acids and proinflammatory mediators cause a sterile inflammatory response to the pilosebaceous unit. The distended follicle walls break, and the contents (sebum, lipids, fatty acids, keratin, bacteria) enter the dermis, provoking an inflammatory and foreign-body response (papule, pustule, nodule). Rupture plus intense inflammation lead to scars.

**Contributory Factors** Acnegenic mineral oils, rarely dioxin and others.

***Drugs*** Lithium, hydantoin, isoniazid, glucocorticoids, oral contraceptives, iodides, bromides and androgens (e.g., testosterone), danazol.

***Others*** *Emotional stress* can definitely cause exacerbations. *Occlusion* and *pressure* on the skin, such as by leaning face on hands, *very important* and often unrecognized exacerbating factor (*acne mechanica*). Acne is not caused by chocolate or fatty foods or, in fact, by any kind of food.

### HISTORY

**Duration of Lesions** Weeks to months.

**Season** Often worse in fall and winter.

**Symptoms** Pain in lesions (especially nodulocystic type).

### PHYSICAL EXAMINATION

#### Skin Lesions

*Comedones*—open (blackheads) or closed (whiteheads) (Fig. 1-1). *Papules* and *papulopustules*—i.e., a papule topped by a pustule

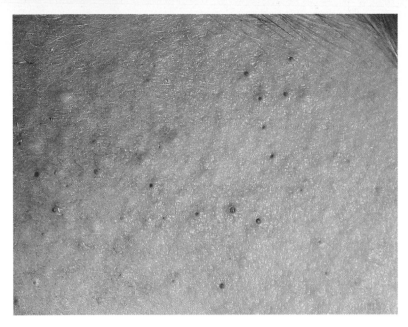

**FIGURE 1-1   Acne vulgaris: comedones**   *Are keratin plugs that form within follicular ostia, frequently associated with surrounding erythema and pustule formation. Comedones associated with small ostia are referred to as closed comedones or "white heads"; those associated with large ostia, are referred to as open comedones or "black heads." Comedones are best treated with topical retinoids.*

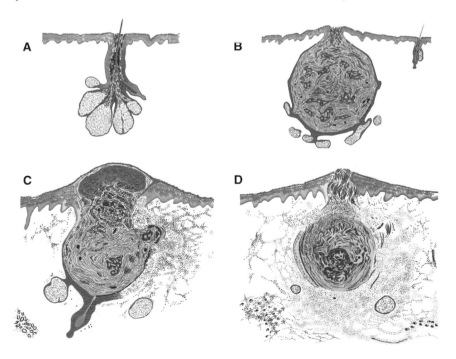

**IMAGE 1-1   Acne**   *The evolution of a sebaceous follicle (A) to a comedo (B), to a papulo pustule (C), and an inflammatory cyst (D). See text for pathogenuis. (From G Plewig, AM Kligman: Acne and Rosacea, 2d ed. Berlin, New york, Springer, p 153, 2000; with permission.)*

(Fig. 1-2). *Nodules* or *cysts*—1 to 4 cm in diameter (Fig. 1-3). Soft nodules result from repeated follicular ruptures and reencapsulations with inflammation, abscess formation, and foreign-body reaction. Cysts are actually pseudocysts as they are not lined by epithelium but represent fluctuating abscesses. Round isolated single nodules and cysts coalesce to linear mounds and sinus tracts (Fig. 1-3). *Sinuses*: draining epithelial-lined tracts, usually with nodular acne. *Scars*: atrophic depressed (often pitted) or hypertrophic (at times, keloidal). *Seborrhea* of the face and scalp often present and sometimes severe.

*Sites of Predilection* Face, neck, trunk, upper arms, buttocks.

### Special Forms

**Acne Conglobata** Severe cystic acne (Fig. 1-4) with more involvement of the trunk than the face. Coalescing nodules, cysts, abscesses, and ulceration. Spontaneous remission is long delayed. Rarely, acne conglobata seen in XYY genotype (tall males, slightly mentally retarded, with aggressive behavior) or in the polycystic ovary syndrome.

**Acne Fulminans** Teenage boys (ages 13 to 17). *Acute onset*, severe cystic acne with concomitant suppuration and always *ulceration*; also present are malaise, fatigue, fever, generalized arthralgias, leukocytosis, and elevated erythrocyte sedimentation rate.

**Tropical Acne** Flare of acne, usually with severe folliculitis, inflammatory nodules, and draining cysts on trunk and buttocks in tropical climates; secondary infection with *Staphylococcus aureus*.

**Acne with Facial Edema** Associated with recalcitrant, disfiguring midline facial edema. Woody induration with and without erythema.

**Acne in the Adult Woman** Persistent acne in an (often) hirsute female with or without *irregular* menses needs an evaluation for hypersecretion of adrenal and ovarian androgens: total testosterone, free testosterone, and/or dehydroepiandrosterone sulfate (DHEAS) (e.g., in the polycystic ovary syndrome).

**Recalcitrant Acne** Can be related to congenital adrenal hyperplasia (11β- or 21β-hydroxylase deficiencies).

**Acne Excoriée** Mild acne, usually in young women, associated with extensive excoriations and scarring due to emotional and psychological problems (obsessive compulsive disorder).

**Neonatal Acne** On nose and cheeks in newborns or infants, related to glandular development; transient.

**Occupational Acne** Due to exposure to tar derivatives, cutting oils, chlorinated hydrocarbons (see "Chloracne," below). Large comedones, inflammatory papules and cysts; not restricted to predilection sites of acne but can appear on other (covered) body sites.

**Chloracne** Due to exposure to chlorinated aromatic hydrocarbons in electrical conductors, insecticides, and herbicides. Sometimes very severe due to industrial accidents (e.g., dioxin).

**Acne Cosmetica** Due to comedogenic cosmetics.

**Pomade Acne** On the forehead, usually in Africans applying pomade to hair.

**Acne Mechanica** Flares of preexisting acne in face, because of leaning face on hands, or on forehead, from pressure of football helmet.

### Acne-Like Conditions

**Steroid Acne** Following systemic or topical glucocorticoids. Monomorphous folliculitis—small erythematous papules and pustules *without* comedones.

**Drug-Induced Acne** Monomorphous acne-like eruption due to phenytoin, lithium, isoniazid, and others. No comedones.

**Acne Aestivalis** Papular eruption after sun exposure ("Mallorca acne"). Usually on shoulders, arms, neck, and chest. No comedones. Pathogenesis unknown; may be polymorphous light eruption (see Section 10).

**Gram-Negative Folliculitis** Multiple tiny yellow pustules develop on top of acne vulgaris as a result of long-term antibiotic administration.

## DIAGNOSIS AND DIFFERENTIAL DIAGNOSIS

*Note*: Comedones are required for diagnosis of any type of acne. Comedones are not a feature of the conditions listed below.

**Face** *S. aureus* folliculitis, pseudofolliculitis barbae, rosacea, perioral dermatitis, and acne-like conditions (see above).

**Trunk** *Malassezia* folliculitis, "hot-tub" pseudomonas folliculitis, *S. aureus* folliculitis, and acne-like conditions (see above).

## LABORATORY EXAMINATION

No laboratory examinations required. If there is a suspicion of endocrine disorder, free testosterone, follicle-stimulating hormone, luteinizing hormone, and DHEAS should be determined to exclude hyperandrogenism and

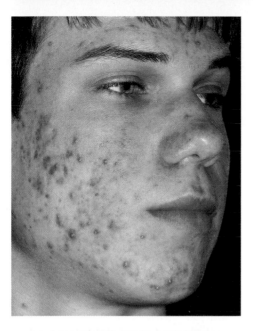

**FIGURE 1-2   Acne vulgaris: papulopustular**   *A spectrum of lesions is seen on the face of a 17-year-old male: comedones, papules, pustules, and erythematous macules and scars at site of resolving lesions. The patient was successfully treated with a 4-month course of isotretinoin; there was no recurrence over the next 5 years.*

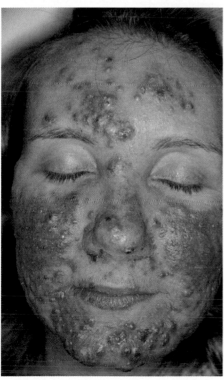

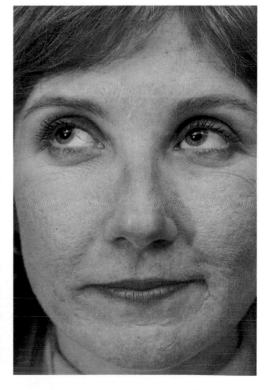

**FIGURE 1-3   Acne vulgaris: nodulocystic**   *Inflammatory nodules, cysts, and pustules (left). Ruptured cysts have coalesced and have led to painful disfiguring inflammatory nodules. This 23-year-old female was resistant to oral and topical treatment and has developed some scarring. The photograph on the right exhibits a remarkable remission of the disfiguring acne following a course of oral isotretinoin, 1 mg/kg, over a period of 4 months.*

polycystic ovary syndrome. *Note*: In the overwhelming majority of acne patients, hormone levels are normal.

Laboratory examinations [transaminases (ALT, AST), triglycerides, and cholesterol levels] may be required if systemic treatment is planned (see below).

## COURSE

Acne most often clears spontaneously by the early twenties but can persist to the fourth decade or older. Flares occur in the winter and with the onset of menses. The sequela is scarring, which should be avoided by proper treatment, *especially with oral isotretinoin early in the course of the disease* (see below).

## MANAGEMENT

The psychological impact of acne (perceived cosmetic disfigurement) should be assessed individually in each patient and therapy modified accordingly. The goal of therapy is to remove the plugging of the pilar drainage, reduce sebum production, and treat bacterial colonization.

### Mild Acne

Topical antibiotics (clindamycin and erythromycin)

Benzoyl peroxide gels (2%, 5%, or 10%)

Topical retinoids (tretinoin, adapalene) require detailed instructions regarding gradual increases in concentration from 0.01% to 0.025% to 0.05% cream/gel or liquid. After improvement, medication is reduced to the lowest effective maintenance.

Improvement occurs over a period of months (2 to 5) but may take even longer for noninflamed comedones. Topical retinoids are applied in the evening; topical antibiotics and benzoyl peroxide gels are applied during the day.

Combination therapy is best, using benzoyl peroxide–erythromycin gels *plus* topical retinoids (tretinoin *or* tazarotene gel, adapalene).

### Moderate Acne

Oral antibiotics are added to the above regimen. Most effective antibiotic is minocycline, 50 to 100 mg bid, or doxycycline, 50 to 100 mg bid, and this is tapered to 50 mg/d as acne lessens. In females, moderate acne can be controlled with high doses of oral estrogens combined with progesterone or antiandrogens, but recurrences are the rule after cessation of treatment. Cerebrovascular accidents are a serious risk.

### Severe Acne

In addition to the topical treatment outlined above, systemic treatment with isotretinoin is indicated for cystic or conglobate acne or for acne refractory to treatment. Isotretinoin is a retinoid that inhibits sebaceous gland function and keratinization and is very effective in acne. Oral isotretinoin leads to complete remission in almost all cases, which last for months to years in the majority of patients (Fig. 1-3).

*Indications for Oral Isotretinoin* For moderate and severe, recalcitrant, nodular acne. The patient must have been resistant to other acne therapies, including systemic antibiotics.

*Contraindications* Isotretinoin is teratogenic. Therefore, pregnancy must be prevented and effective contraception is necessary, i.e., oral. Both tetracycline and isotretinoin may cause pseudotumor cerebri (benign intracranial swelling); therefore, the two medications should *never* be used together.

*Warnings* Blood lipids and transaminases (ALT, AST) should be determined before therapy. About 25% of patients can develop *increased plasma triglycerides*; 15% of patients a decrease in *high-density lipoproteins*, and about 7% an *increase in cholesterol levels*. This may increase the cardiovascular risk. When levels of serum triglycerides rise above 800 mg/$\mu$L, the patient may develop acute pancreatitis. Patients should not take vitamin supplements containing vitamin A. *Hepatotoxicity* has been very rarely reported in the form of clinical hepatitis, but patients may develop mild to moderate elevation of transaminase levels that normalize with reduction of the dose of the drug. *Eyes*: *night blindness* has been reported, and patients should be warned about driving at night. Also, patients may have *decreased tolerance to contact lenses* during and after therapy. *Skin*: An eczema-like rash due to drug-induced dryness often appears, and this responds dramatically to low potency (class III) topical glucocorticoids. Dry lips and cheilitis occur in practically all patients and must be treated. Reversible thinning of hair may occur very rarely, as may paronychia. *Nose*: dryness of nasal mucosa and nose bleeds (rare). *Other systems*: Rarely, depression, headaches, arthritis, and muscular pain. For additional rare possible complications, consult the package insert.

*Dosage* Isotretinoin, 0.5 to 1 mg/kg given in divided doses with food. Most patients improve and clear within 20 weeks with 1 mg/kg. For severe disease, especially on the trunk, 2 mg/kg and longer treatment may be required. As many

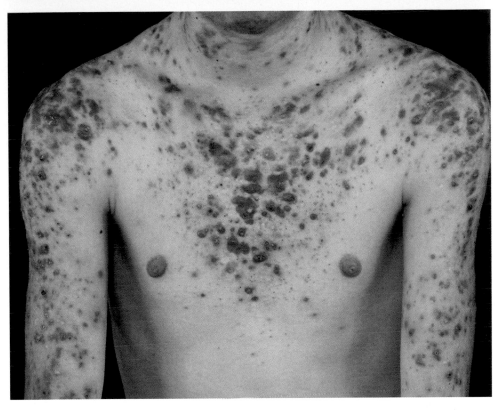

**FIGURE 1-4   Acne vulgaris: acne conglobata**   *Inflammatory nodules and cysts have coalesced forming abscesses and even leading to ulceration. There are multiple comedones and many recent red scars following resolution of inflammatory lesions on the upper chest, neck, and arms.*

as three or more courses of isotretinoin have been given in refractory cases, but in most cases a single course is sufficient to induce lasting remission.

*Note*: For inflammatory cysts and nodules, intralesional triamcinolone (0.05 mL of a 3 to 5 mg/mL) is indicated.

Website: *http://www.aad.org/pamphlets/acnepamp.html*

## ROSACEA    ■  ○ → ◐

This is a common chronic inflammatory acneiform disorder of the facial pilosebaceous units, coupled with an increased reactivity of capillaries leading to flushing and telangiectasia.

### EPIDEMIOLOGY

**Occurrence**  Common, affecting approximately 10% of fair-skinned people.
**Age of Onset**  30 to 50 years; peak incidence between 40 and 50 years.
**Sex**  Females predominantly, but rhinophyma occurs mostly in males.
**Race**  Celtic persons (skin phototypes I and II) but also southern Mediterraneans; less frequent or rare in pigmented persons (skin phototypes V and VI, i.e., brown and black)

### STAGES OF EVOLUTION (PLEWIG AND KLIGMAN CLASSIFICATION)

*The rosacea diathesis*: episodic erythema, "flushing and blushing"
*Stage I:* Persistent erythema with telangiectases.
*Stage II:* Persistent erythema, telangiectases, papules, tiny pustules.
*Stage III:* Persistent deep erythema, dense telangiectases, papules, pustules, nodules; rarely persistent "solid" edema of the central part of the face

### HISTORY

Usually a history of episodic reddening of the face (flushing) with increases in skin temperature in response to heat stimuli in the mouth (hot liquids); spicy foods; alcohol, possibly because it causes flushing. Exposure to sun—rosacea is often associated with solar elastosis—and heat (such as chefs working near a hot stove) may cause exacerbations. Acne may have preceded the onset of rosacea by years; nevertheless, rosacea may and usually does arise de novo without any preceding history of acne or seborrhea.
**Duration of Lesions**  Days, weeks, months.
**Skin Symptoms**  Concern about cosmetic facial appearance; patients are often perceived as being alcoholic—which, of course, is not true.

### PHYSICAL EXAMINATION

Skin Lesions
*Early*  Pathognomonic flushing; tiny papules and papulopustules (2 to 3 mm), pustule often small (<1 mm) and on the apex of the papule (Figs. 1-5 and 1-6). *No comedones.*
*Late*  Red facies and dusky-red papules and nodules (Figs. 1-5, 1-6, and 1-7) Scattered, discrete lesions. Telangiectases. Marked sebaceous hyperplasia and lymphedema in chronic rosacea, causing disfigurement of the nose, forehead, eyelids, ears, and chin.
*Distribution*  Characteristic is the symmetric localization on the face (Fig. 1-7). Rarely, neck, chest (V-shaped area), back, and scalp.

Special Lesions
*Rhinophyma* (enlarged nose, Fig. 1-8), *metophyma* (enlarged cushion-like swelling of the forehead), *blepharophyma* (swelling of the eyelids), *otophyma* (cauliflower-like swelling of the earlobes), and *gnathophyma* (swelling of the chin) result from marked sebaceous gland hyperplasia and fibrosis. Upon palpation: soft, rubber-like.

Eye Involvement
"Red" eyes as a result of chronic blepharitis, conjunctivitis, and episcleritis. Rosacea keratitis, albeit rare, is a serious problem because corneal ulcers may develop.

### LABORATORY EXAMINATIONS

**Bacterial Culture**  Rule out *S. aureus* infection. Scrapings may reveal massive concurrent *Demodex folliculorum* infestation.
**Dermatopathology**  Nonspecific perifollicular and pericapillary inflammation with occasional foci of "tuberculoid" granulomatous areas; dilated capillaries. Foci of neutrophils high and within the follicle. *Later stages*: diffuse hypertrophy of the connective tissue, sebaceous gland hyperplasia, epithelioid granuloma without caseation, and foreign-body giant cells.
**Rhinophyma**  Very marked lobular sebaceous hyperplasia (*glandular type*) and/or marked

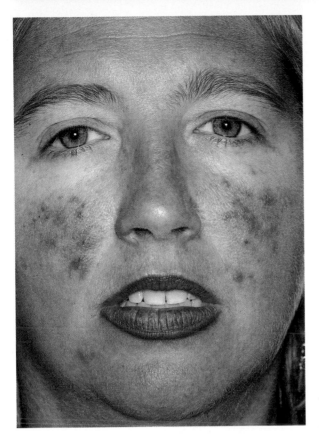

**FIGURE 1-5    Rosacea**    *Moderately severe rosacea in a 29-year-old female in stage II with persistent erythema, telangiectasia, red papules, and tiny pustules.*

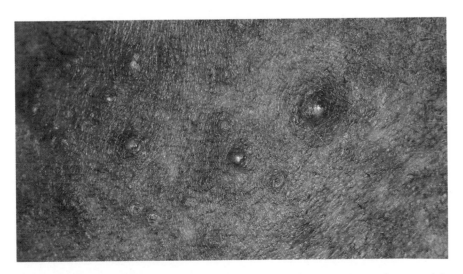

**FIGURE 1-6    Rosacea**    *Closeup of tiny 1- to 3-mm pustules, often occurring at the apex of the papules. Note multiple, tiny telangiectasias imparting a red color to the otherwise noninvolved skin → "red face."*

increase in connective tissue (*fibrous type*) with large ectatic veins (*fibroangiomatous type*).

## DIFFERENTIAL DIAGNOSIS

**Facial Papules/Pustules**   Acne (in rosacea there are no comedones), perioral dermatitis, *S. aureus* folliculitis, gram-negative folliculitis, *D. folliculorum* infestation.

**Facial Flushing/Erythema**   Seborrheic dermatitis, prolonged use of topical glucocorticoids, systemic lupus erythematosus; dermatomyositis.

## COURSE

**Prolonged**   Recurrences are common. After a few years, the disease may disappear spontaneously. Men and very rarely women may develop rhinophyma.

## MANAGEMENT

**Prevention**   Marked reduction or elimination of alcoholic and hot beverages may be helpful in some patients.

**Topical**

  *Metronidazole gel* or *cream*, 0.75%, twice daily—very effective

  *Metronidazole cream*, 1%, once daily

  *Sodium sulfacetamide*, *sulfur lotions* 10% and 5%

  *Topical antibiotics* (e.g., erythromycin gel) are less effective.

**Systemic**   Oral antibiotics are more effective than topical treatment.

  *Minocycline or doxycycline*, 50 to 100 mg twice daily, first-line antibiotics; very effective (doxycycline is a phototoxic drug and its use limits exposure to sunlight in summer).

  *Tetracycline*, 1 to 1.5 g/d in divided doses until clear; then gradually reduce to once-daily doses of 250 to 500 mg.

  A dose of 50 mg minocycline or doxycycline **or** 250 to 500 g tetracycline is given as maintenance.

**Oral Isotretinoin**   For individuals with severe disease (especially stage III) not responding to antibiotics and topical treatments. A low-dose regimen of 0.1 to 0.5 mg/kg body weight per day is effective in most patients, but occasionally 1 mg/kg may be required. (For side effects and precautions see p. 6.)

**Rhinophyma and Telangiectasia**   Treated by surgery or laser surgery with excellent cosmetic results.

Website *http://www.aad.org/pamphlets/rosacea.html*

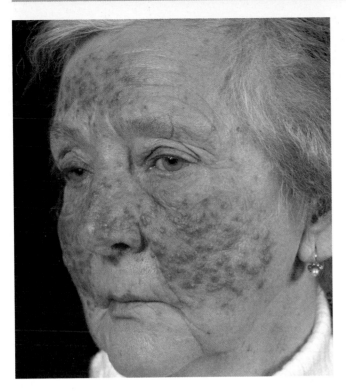

**FIGURE 1-7   Rosacea: Stage III** *Typical moderately severe involvement with confluent erythematous papules and pustules on the forehead, cheeks, and nose. Note the absence of comedones that are typically seen with acne vulgaris.*

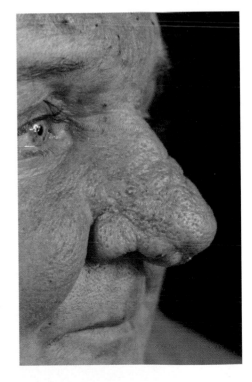

**FIGURE 1-8   Rosacea with rhinophyma** *Mild involvement with few erythematous papules and striking erythema, edema, and telangiectasias on the nose (early rhinophyma). Note dilated follicles and "orange peel skin" appearance of enlarged nose which appears soft and rubbery upon palpation.*

## PERIORAL DERMATITIS   ■  ○ → ◑*

Perioral dermatitis occurs mainly in young women, characterized by discrete erythematous micropapules and micropapulovesicles that often become confluent on the perioral and periorbital skin. *Synonym*: Rosacea-like dermatitis.

### EPIDEMIOLOGY AND ETIOLOGY

**Age of Onset**   16 to 45 years; can occur in children.
**Sex**   Females predominantly.
**Etiology**   Unknown but may be markedly aggravated by potent topical (fluorinated) glucocorticoids.

### HISTORY

**Duration of Lesions**   Weeks to months. Skin symptoms perceived as cosmetic disfigurement; occasional itching or burning, feeling of tightness.

### PHYSICAL EXAMINATION

**Skin Lesions**
1- to 2-mm erythematous papulopustules on an erythematous background (Fig. 1-9) irregularly grouped, symmetric. Lesions increase in number with central confluence and satellites; confluent plaques may appear eczematous with tiny scales. There are no comedones.
*Distribution*   Initially perioral. Rim of sparing around the vermilion border of lips. At times, in the periorbital area (Fig. 1-10). Uncommonly, only periorbital involvement; occasionally, glabella and forehead.

### LABORATORY EXAMINATIONS

**Culture**   Rule out *S. aureus* infection.

### DIFFERENTIAL DIAGNOSIS

Allergic contact dermatitis, atopic dermatitis, seborrheic dermatitis, rosacea, acne vulgaris, steroid acne.

### COURSE

Appearance of lesions usually subacute over weeks to months. At times, misdiagnosed as an eczematous or a seborrheic dermatitis and treated with a potent topical glucocorticoid preparation, aggravating perioral dermatitis or inducing steroid acne. Untreated, perioral dermatitis fluctuates in activity over months to years but is not nearly as chronic as rosacea.

### MANAGEMENT

**Topical**
   Avoid topical glucocorticoids!
   *Metronidazole*, 0.75% gel two times daily **or** 1% once daily
   *Erythromycin*, 2% gel applied twice daily
**Systemic**
   *Minocycline* or *doxycycline*, 100 mg daily until clear, then 50 mg daily for another 2 months (caution, doxycycline is a photosensitizing drug) **or**
   *Tetracycline*, 500 mg bid until clear, then 500 mg daily for 1 month, then 250 mg daily for an additional month.

---

* Rarely.

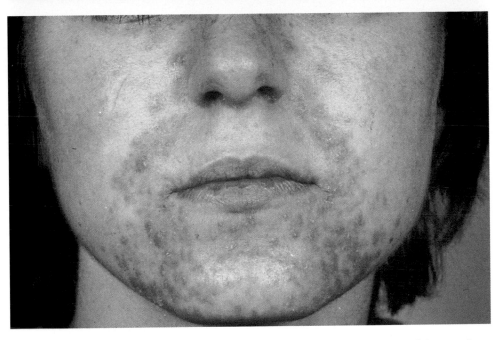

**FIGURE 1-9 Perioral dermatitis** *Moderately severe involvement with confluence of tiny papules and a few pustules in a perioral and nasolabial distribution. Note typical sparing of the vermilion border (mucocutaneous junction).*

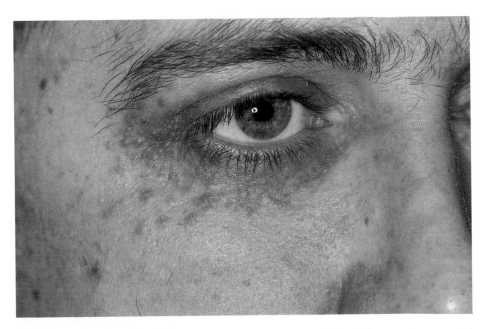

**FIGURE 1-10 Periorbital dermatitis** *Note presence of tiny papules and a few pustules around the eye. This is a much less common site than the lesions around the mouth.*

## HIDRADENITIS SUPPURATIVA

Hidradenitis suppurativa is a chronic, suppurative, often cicatricial disease of apocrine gland–bearing skin in the axillae, the anogenital region, and rarely, the scalp (called *cicatrizing perifolliculitis*). May be associated with severe nodulocystic acne and pilonidal sinuses (termed *follicular occlusion syndrome*).
*Synonyms*: Apocrinitis, hidradenitis axillaris, abscess of the apocrine sweat glands.

### EPIDEMIOLOGY

**Age of Onset**    From puberty to climacteric.
**Sex**    Affects more females than males; estimated to be 4% of female population. Males more often have anogenital and females axillary involvement.
**Race**    All races.
**Heredity**    Mother-daughter transmission has been observed repeatedly. Families give a history of nodulocystic acne and hidradenitis suppurativa occurring separately or together in blood relatives.

### ETIOLOGY AND PATHOGENESIS

Unknown. Predisposing factors: obesity, genetic predisposition to acne, apocrine duct obstruction, secondary bacterial infection.

### PATHOGENESIS

The following sequence may be the mechanism of the development of the lesions: keratinous plugging of the apocrine duct and hair follicle → dilatation of the apocrine duct and hair follicle → inflammatory changes limited to a single apocrine gland → bacterial growth in dilated duct → ruptured duct/gland resulting in extension of inflammation/infection → extension of suppuration/tissue destruction → ulceration and fibrosis, sinus tract formation.

### HISTORY

*Symptoms*: Intermittent pain and marked point tenderness related to abscess formation in axilla(e) and/or anogenital area.

### PHYSICAL EXAMINATION

**Skin Lesions**
Initial lesion: *very tender*, red inflammatory nodule/abscess (Fig. 1-11) that may resolve or drain purulent/seropurulent material. The same lesion may appear repeatedly in the same location. Open comedones, and at times unique *double* comedones, are highly characteristic of the disease (Fig. 1-11) and may be present even when active nodules are absent. Eventually, sinus tracts may form lesions moderately to exquisitely tender. Pus drains from opening of abscess and sinus tracts (Fig. 1-12). Fibrosis, "bridge" scars, hypertrophic and keloidal scars, contractures. Rarely, lymphedema of the associated limb may develop.
**Distribution**    Axillae, breasts, anogenital area, groin. Often bilateral in axillae and/or anogenital area; may extend over entire back, buttocks (Fig. 1-12), and scalp.
**Associated Findings**    Cystic acne, pilonidal sinus. Often obesity.

### LABORATORY EXAMINATIONS

**Bacteriology**    Various pathogens may secondarily colonize or "infect" lesions. These include *S. aureus*, streptococci, *Escherichia coli*, *Proteus mirabilis*, and *Pseudomonas aeruginosa*.
**Dermatopathology**    *Early*: keratin occlusion of apocrine duct and hair follicle, ductal/tubular dilatation, inflammatory changes limited to a single apocrine gland. *Late*: destruction of apocrine/eccrine/pilosebaceous apparatus, fibrosis, pseudoepitheliomatous hyperplasia in sinuses.

### DIFFERENTIAL DIAGNOSIS

Painful papule, nodule, abscess in groin and axilla. *Early*: furuncle, carbuncle, lymphadenitis, ruptured inclusion cyst, cat-scratch disease. *Late*: lymphogranuloma venereum, donovanosis, scrofuloderma, actinomycosis, sinus tracts and fistulas associated with ulcerative colitis and regional enteritis.

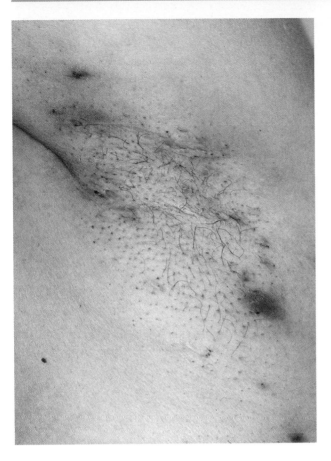

**FIGURE 1-11   Hidradenitis suppurativa**   *Many black comedones, some of which are paired, are a characteristic finding, associated with deep exquisitely painful abscesses and old scars in the axilla.*

## COURSE AND PROGNOSIS

The severity of the disease varies considerably. Many patients have only mild involvement with recurrent, self-healing, tender red nodules and do not seek therapy. The disease usually undergoes a spontaneous remission with age (>35 years). In some individuals, the course can be relentlessly progressive, with marked morbidity related to chronic pain, draining sinuses, and scarring, with restricted mobility. Complications (rare): fistulas to urethra, bladder, and/or rectum; anemia, amyloidosis.

## MANAGEMENT

Hidradenitis suppurativa is *not* simply an infection, and systemic antibiotics are only part of the treatment program. Combinations of (1) intralesional glucocorticoids, (2) surgery, (3) oral antibiotics, and (4) isotretinoin are used.

### Medical Management
**Acute Painful Lesions** *Nodule* Intralesional triamcinolone (3 to 5 mg/mL).
*Abscess* Intralesional triamcinolone (3 to 5 mg/mL) into the wall followed by incision and drainage of abscess fluid.
**Chronic Low-Grade Disease** Oral antibiotics: erythromycin (250 to 500 mg qid), tetracycline (250 to 500 mg qid), or minocycline (100 mg

bid) until lesions resolve; may take weeks. Intralesional triamcinolone (3 to 5 mg/mL) into early inflammatory lesions helpful in hastening resolution of individual lesions.
**Prednisone**   May be given concurrently if pain and inflammation are severe: 70 mg daily for 2 to 3 days, tapered over 14 days.
**Oral Isotretinoin**   Not useful in severe disease, but it appears to be useful in early disease and when combined with surgical excision of individual lesions.

### Surgical Management
- Incise and drain acute abscesses.
- Excise chronic recurrent, fibrotic nodules or sinus tracts. If one or two nodules can be pinpointed with recurrent disease, they can be excised with a good result.
- With extensive, chronic disease, complete excision of axilla or involved anogenital area may be required. Excision should extend down to fascia and requires split skin grafting.

### Psychologic Management
These patients need constant reassurance, as they become very depressed because of the nature of the illness, e.g., pain, soiling of clothing by draining pus, odor, and the site of occurrence (anogenital area). Therefore, every effort should be made to deal with the disease, using every modality possible.

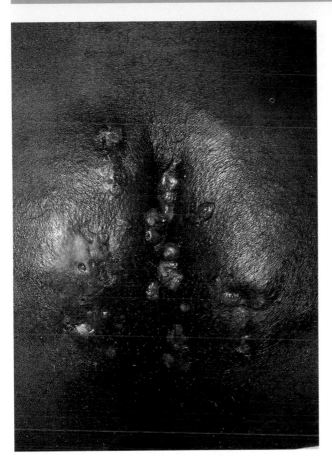

**FIGURE 1-12    Hidradenitis sup-
purativa**    *Severe scarring on the
buttocks, inflammatory painful
nodules with fistulas and draining sinuses. When the patient
sits down, pus will squirt from
the sinus openings.*

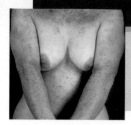

# ECZEMA/DERMATITIS

The terms *eczema* and *dermatitis* are used interchangeably, denoting a polymorphic inflammatory reaction pattern involving the epidermis and dermis. There are many etiologies and a wide range of clinical findings. Acute eczema/dermatitis is characterized by pruritus, erythema, and vesiculation; chronic eczema/dermatitis, by pruritus, xerosis, lichenification, hyperkeratosis, ± fissuring.

## CONTACT DERMATITIS

*Contact dermatitis* is a generic term applied to acute or chronic inflammatory reactions to substances that come in contact with the skin. Irritant contact dermatitis (ICD) is caused by a chemical irritant; allergic contact dermatitis (ACD) by an antigen (allergen) that elicits a type IV (cell-mediated or delayed) hypersensitivity reaction.

The acute form of ICD, which in severe cases may even lead to necrosis, occurs after a single exposure to the offending agent that is toxic to the skin (e.g., croton oil, phenols, kerosene, organic solvents, sodium and potassium hydroxide, lime acids). It is dependent on concentration of the offending agent and occurs in everyone, depending on the penetrability and thickness of the stratum corneum. There is a threshold concentration for these substances above which they cause acute dermatitis and below which they do not. This sets acute ICD apart from acute ACD, which is dependent on sensitization and thus occurs only in sensitized individuals. Depending on the degree of sensitization, minute amounts of the offending agents may elicit a reaction. Since ICD is a toxic phenomenon, it is confined to the area of exposure and is therefore always sharply marginated and never spreads. ACD is an immunologic reaction that tends to involve the surrounding skin (spreading phenomenon) and may even spread beyond affected sites. Generalization may occur.

## IRRITANT CONTACT DERMATITIS ■ ◐

ICD is caused by exposure of the skin to chemical or other physical agents that are capable of irritating the skin, acutely or chronically. Severe irritants can cause toxic reactions even after a short exposure. Most cases, however, are caused by chronic cumulative exposure to one or more irritants. The hands are the most commonly affected area. In addition to dermatitis, irritant contact responses of the skin include: subjective irritancy, transient irritant reactions, persistent irritant reactions, toxic (caustic) burn. Irritant contact responses of skin appendages and pigmentary system include: follicular and acneform eruptions, miliaria, pigmentary changes (hypo- and hyperpigmentation), granulomatous reactions, and alopecia.

### EPIDEMIOLOGY

ICD is the most common form of occupational skin disease, accounting for up to 80% of all oc-cupational skin disorders. However, ICD need not be occupational and can occur in anyone being exposed to a substance irritant or toxic to the skin.

**Occupational Exposure**  Individuals engaged in the following occupations/activities are at risk for ICD: housekeeping; hairdressing; medical, dental, and veterinary services; cleaning; floral arranging; agriculture; horticulture; forestry; food preparation and catering; printing; painting; metal work; mechanical engineering; car maintenance; construction; fishing.

## ETIOLOGY

**Etiologic Agents**  (Table 2-1) Abrasives, cleaning agents, oxidizing agents (e.g., sodium hypochlorite); reducing agents (e.g., phenols, hydrazine, aldehydes, thiophosphates), plants (e.g., spurge, Boracinaceae, Ranunculaceae), animal enzymes, secretions; dessicant powders, dust, soils; excessive exposure to water. **Predisposing Factors**  Atopics with a history of atopic dermatitis are at highest risk for ICD; the majority of workers with significant occupational ICD are atopics. Others: white skin, temperature (low), climate (low humidity), occlusion, mechanical irritation. Cement ICD tends to flare in summer in hot humid climates.

## PATHOGENESIS

Both chemical and physical agents can be irritants, causing cell damage if applied for sufficient time and in adequate concentration. ICD occurs when defense or repair capacity of the skin is unable to maintain normal skin integrity and function or when penetration of chemical(s) induces an inflammatory response. Lesser irritants cause reaction only after prolonged exposure. The initial reaction is usually limited to the site of contact with the irritant; the concentration of irritant diffusing outside the area of contact almost always falls below the critical threshold necessary to provoke a reaction.

Mechanisms involved in acute and chronic phases of ICD are fundamentally different. Acute reactions involve direct cytotoxic damage to keratinocytes. Chronic ICD results from repeated exposures to solvents and surfactants that cause slow damage to cell membranes, disrupting the skin barrier and leading to protein denaturation and cellular toxicity.

---

## ACUTE IRRITANT CONTACT DERMATITIS

### SYMPTOMS

In some individuals, subjective symptoms (burning, stinging, smarting) may be the only manifestations. Painful sensations can occur within seconds after exposure (immediate-type stinging), e.g., to acids, chloroform, and methanol. Delayed-type stinging occurs within 1 to 2 min, peaking at 5 to 10 min, fading by 30 min, and is caused by agents such as aluminum chloride, phenol, propylene glycol, and others. In acute delayed ICD, objective skin symptoms do not start until 8 to 24 after exposure (e.g., anthralin, ethylene oxide, benzalconium chloride) and are accompanied by burning rather then itching.

---

### TABLE 2-1    Most Common Irritant/Toxic Agents

- Soaps, detergents, waterless hand cleaners
- Acids and alkalis*: hydrofluoric acid, cement, chromic acid, phosphorus, ethylene oxide, phenol, metal salts.
- Industrial solvents: coal tar solvents, petroleum, chlorinated hydrocarbons, alcohol solvents, ethylene glycol ether, turpentine, ethyl ether, acetone, carbon dioxide, DMSO, dioxane, styrene.
- Plants: Euphorbiaceae (spurges, crotons, poinsettias, machneel tree). Racunculaceae (buttercup), Cruciferae (black mustard), Urticaceae (nettles), Solanaceae (pepper, capsaicin), Opuntia (prickly pear).
- Others: fiberglass, wool, rough synthetic clothing, fire-retardant fabrics, "NCR" paper.

* Lead to chemical burns and necrosis, if concentrated.

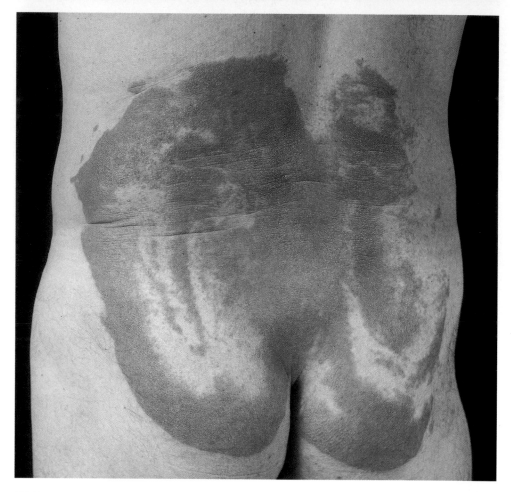

**FIGURE 2-1   Irritant contact dermatitis of back, acute: croton oil**   *Erythema and edema on the back at sites in contact with the irritant in 30-year-old male. Croton oil was mistakenly used as a remedy for back pain and rubbed into skin. Note spared areas where contact with the irritant had not occurred.*

## PHYSICAL EXAMINATION

### Skin Findings

May occur minutes after exposure or may be delayed up to ≥24 h. The spectrum of changes ranges from erythema to vesiculation (Figs. 2-1 and 2-2) and caustic burn with necrosis. Acute ICD represents sharply demarcated erythema and superficial edema, corresponding to the application site of the toxic substance (Fig. 2-1). Lesions do not spread beyond the site of contact. In more severe reactions vesicles and blisters arise within the erythematous lesions (Fig. 2-2), followed by erosions and/or even frank necrosis, as with acids or alkline solutions. No papules. Configuration often bizarre or linear ("outside job" or dripping effect).

**Evolution of Lesions**   Erythema with a dull, nonglistening surface (Fig. 2-1) → vesiculation (or blister formation) (Fig. 2-2) → erosion → crusting → shedding of crusts and scaling or (in chemical burn) erythema → necrosis → shedding of necrotic tissue → ulceration → healing.

***Distribution***   Isolated, localized to one region or generalized (plant dermatitis), depending on contact with toxic agent.

***Duration***   Days, weeks depending on tissue damage.

### Constitutional Symptoms

Usually none, but in widespread acute ICD "acute illness" syndrome, including fever.

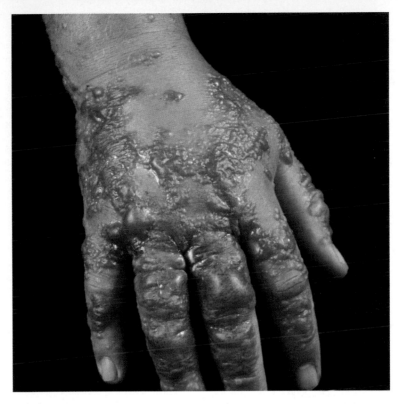

**FIGURE 2-2   Irritant contact dermatitis of hand, acute: kerosene**   *This airport worker had repeatedly spilled kerosene over his hands and developed acute bullous and extremely painful ICD 24 h later.*

# CHRONIC IRRITANT CONTACT DERMATITIS

## TYPES

**Cumulative ICD**   Most common; develops slowly after repeated additive exposure to mild irritants (water, soap, detergents etc.), usually on hands. Repeated exposures to toxic or subtoxic concentrations of offending agents usually associated with a chronic disturbance of the barrier function that allows even subtoxic concentrations of offending agents to penetrate into the skin and elicit a chronic inflammatory response; e.g., after repeated exposure to alkaline detergents and organic solvents, which, if applied only once to normal skin, do not elicit a reaction. Injury (e.g., repeated rubbing of the skin), prolonged soaking in water, or chronic contact after repeated, cumulative physical trauma — friction, pressure, abrasions in individuals engaged in manual work (*traumatic ICD*).

**Irritant Reaction ICD**   Early, subclinical dermatitis on hands of individuals exposed to wet work. Usually during first months of training of hair dressers or of metal workers.

## SYMPTOMS

Stinging *and* itching, pain as fissures develop.

## PHYSICAL EXAMINATION

### Skin Findings
Dryness → chapping → erythema → hyperkeratosis and scaling → fissures and crusting (Fig. 2-3). Sharp margination gives way to ill-defined borders, lichenification. In irritant reaction ICD also vesicles, pustules, and erosions.

*Distribution*   Usually on hands (Fig. 2-3). In cumulative ICD usually starting at finger web spaces, spreading to sides and dorsal surface of hands and then to palms. In housewives often starting on finger tips (*pulpitis*). Rarely in other locations exposed to irritants and/or trauma, e.g., in violinists on mandible or neck, or on exposed sites as in airborne ICD (see below).

*Duration*   Chronic, months to years.

### Constitutional Symptoms
None, except when infection occurs. Chronic ICD (e.g., hand dermatitis; see below) can become a severe occupational and emotional problem.

## LABORATORY EXAMINATION

**Histopathology**   In acute ICD, epidermal cell necrosis, neutrophils, vesiculation, and necrosis. In chronic ICD, acanthosis, hyperkeratosis, lymphocytic infiltrate.

**Patch Tests**   These are negative in ICD unless allergic contact dermatitis is also present (see below).

# SPECIAL FORMS OF ICD

### Hand Dermatitis
Most cases of chronic ICD occur on the hands and are occupational. Often sensitization to allergens (such as nickel or chromate salts) occurs, and then ACD (acute and/or chronic) is superimposed on ICD. A typical example is hand dermatitis in construction and cement workers. Cement is alkaline and corrosive, leading to chronic ICD; chromates in cement sensitize and lead to ACD. In such cases the eruption may spread beyond the hands and may even generalize.

### Airborne ICD
Characteristically face, neck, anterior chest, and arms are involved. Most frequent causes are irritating dust and volatile chemicals (ammonia, solvents, formaldehyde, epoxy resins, cement, fiberglass, sawdust from toxic woods). This has to be distinguished from photoallergic contact dermatitis (see p. 238).

### Pustular and Acneiform ICD
ICD may target follicles and become pustular and papulopustular. It may result from metals, mineral oils, greases, cutting fluids, naphthalenes.

## DIAGNOSIS AND DIFFERENTIAL DIAGNOSIS

Diagnosis is by history and clinical examination (lesions, pattern, site). Most important differential diagnosis is ACD (see Table 2-3, p. 27). On palms and soles: palmoplantar psoriasis; in exposed sites: photoallergic contact dermatitis.

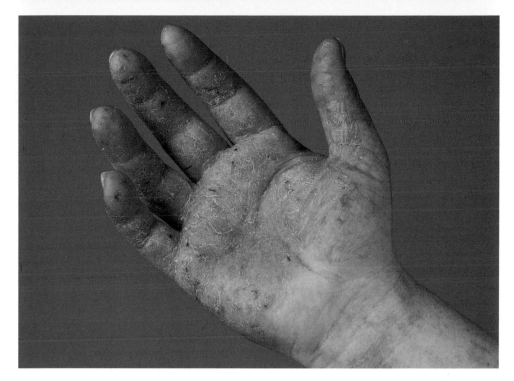

**FIGURE 2-3   Irritant contact dermatitis of hand: subacute/chronic**   *Erythema, edema, scaling, fissuring, crusting of the palmar aspect of the hand and wrist; the other hand had similar involvement. The patient, a housewife, is atopic and has ignored instructions to wear gloves during work in the kitchen and to use lubricating creams.*

## COURSE AND PROGNOSIS

Healing usually occurs within 2 weeks of removal of noxious stimuli; in more chronic cases, 6 weeks or longer may be required. In the setting of occupational ICD, only one-third of individuals have complete remission and may require allocation to another job; atopic individuals have a worse prognosis. In cases of chronic subcritical levels or irritant, some workers develop tolerance or "hardening."

## MANAGEMENT

### Prevention

- Avoid irritant or caustic chemical(s) by wearing protective clothing (i.e., goggles, shields, gloves).
- If contact does occur, wash with water or weak neutralizing solution.
- Barrier creams.
- In occupational ICD that persists in spite of

adherence to the above measures, change of job may be necessary.

**TREATMENT**   *Acute*   Identify and remove the etiologic agent. Wet dressings with gauze soaked in Burow's solution, changed every 2 to 3 h. Larger vesicles may be drained, but tops should *not* be removed. Topical class I glucocorticoid preparations. In severe cases, systemic glucocorticoids may be indicated. Prednisone: 2-week course, 60 mg initially, tapering by steps of 10 mg.
*Subacute and Chronic*   Identify and remove etiologic/pathogenic agent. Employ a potent topical glucocorticoid preparation, betamethasone dipropionate or clobetasol propionate, and provide adequate lubrication. As healing occurs, continue with lubricating/protective creams or ointments.

In chronic ICD of hands a "hardening effect" can be achieved in most cases with topical (soak or bath)-PUVA therapy (see page 69). The newer topical anti-inflammatory agents (pimecrolimus and tacrolimus) are being evaluated.

## ALLERGIC CONTACT DERMATITIS   ■   ◗

One of the most frequent, vexing, and costly skin problems. An eczematous (papules, vesicles, pruritic) dermatitis due to reexposure to a substance to which the individual is sensitized.

### EPIDEMIOLOGY

Frequent. Accounts for 7% of occupationally related illnesses in the United States. However, there are data suggesting that the actual indicence rate is 10 to 50 times greater than reported in the U.S. Bureau of Labor Statistics data. In addition, nonoccupational ACD is estimated to be three times greater than occupational ACD.

**Age of Onset**   No influence on capacity for sensitization; however, allergic contact dermatitis is uncommon in young children and in individuals older than 70 years.

**Occupation**   One of the most important causes of disability in industry.

### PATHOGENESIS

ACD is a classic, delayed, cell-mediated hypersensitivity reaction. Exposure to a strong sensitizer such as poison ivy resin results in sensitization in a week or so, while exposure to a weak allergen may take months to years for sensitization. The antigen is taken up by Langerhans cells in the epidermis, which process the antigen and migrate from the epidermis to the draining lymph nodes, where they present the processed antigen in association with MHC class II molecules to T cells that then proliferate. Sensitized T cells leave the lymph node, enter the blood circulation, home to the skin, and, after being presented by Langerhans cells with the same specific antigen, produce and mediate the release by other cells of a variety of cytokines. Thus, all the skin becomes hypersensitive to the contact allergen and will react wherever the specific allergen is represented.

### ALLERGENS

Contact allergens are diverse and range from metal salts to antibiotics, dyes to plant products. Thus, allergens are found in jewelry, personal care products, topical medications, plants, house remedies, and chemicals the individual may come in contact with at work. The most common allergens in the United States are listed in Table 2-2.

### HISTORY

The eruption starts in a sensitized individual 48 h or days after contact with the allergen; repeated exposures lead to a crescendo reaction, i.e., the eruption worsens. Site of the eruption is confined to site of exposure.

**Symptoms**   Subjective symptoms are intense pruritus; in severe reactions also stinging and pain.

**Constitutional Symptoms**   "Acute illness" syndrome, including fever, but only in severe allergic contact dermatitis (e.g., poison ivy).

### PHYSICAL EXAMINATION

Skin Lesions
The appearance of ACD depends on severity, location, and duration.

**Type**   *Acute*   Well-demarcated erythema and edema on which are superimposed closely spaced, nonumbilicated vesicles, and/or papules (Figs. 2-4 and 2-5); in severe reactions, bullae, confluent erosions exuding serum, and crusts (Fig. 2-6).

*Subacute*   Plaques of mild erythema showing small, dry scales, sometimes associated with small, red, pointed or rounded, firm papules.

*Chronic*   Plaques of lichenification (thickening of the epidermis with deepening of the skin lines in parallel or rhomboidal pattern), scaling with satellite, small, firm, rounded or flat-topped papules, excoriations, erythema, and pigmentation.

**Arrangement**   Initially, confined to area of contact with allergen [e.g., earlobe (earrings), dorsum of foot (shoes), wrist (watch or watchband), collar-like (necklace), lips (lipstick)]. Often linear, with artificial patterns, an "outside job." Plant contact often results in linear lesions (e.g., *Rhus* dermatitis). Initially confined to site of contact, later spreading beyond.

**Distribution**   *Extent*   Isolated, localized to one region (e.g., shoe dermatitis), or generalized (e.g., plant dermatitis).

*Pattern*   Random or on exposed areas (as in airborne ACD).

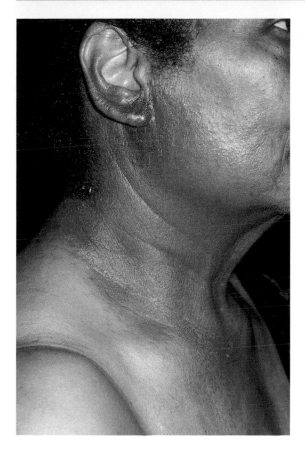

**FIGURE 2-4   Allergic contact dermatitis of ear and neck: neomycin** *Erythema, edema microvesiculation. Most severe on the ear and adjacent neck associated with severe pruritus in a 64-year-old female. The patient was allergic to neomycin and had applied neomycin-containing otic drops for 2 weeks.*

## COURSE

**Evolution of ACD**   The duration of ACD varies among individuals, resolving in some in 1 to 2 weeks. ACD continues to get worse as long as allergen continues to come into contact with the skin.

*Acute*   Erythema → papules → vesicles → erosions → crusts → scaling.

*Note*: In the acute forms of contact dermatitis, papules occur only in ACD, not in ICD.

*Chronic*   Papules → scaling → lichenification –› excoriations. Chronic inflammation with thickening, fissuring, scaling, and crusting results.

*Note*: Contact dermatitis is always confined to the site of exposure to the allergen. Margination is originally sharp in ACD; however, it spreads in the periphery beyond the actual site

of exposure. If strong sensitization has occurred, spreading to other parts of the body and generalization occur. The main differences between toxic irritant and allergic contact dermatitis are summarized in Table 2-3.

## LABORATORY EXAMINATIONS

**Dermatopathology**   *Acute* Prototype of spongiotic dermatitis. Inflammation with intraepidermal intercellular edema (*spongiosis*), lymphocytes and eosinophils in the epidermis, and monocyte and histiocyte infiltration in the dermis.

*Chronic*   In chronic ACD there are also spongiosis plus acanthosis, elongation of rete ridges, and elongation and broadening of papillae; hyperkeratosis; and a lymphocytic infiltrate.

**Table 2-2   Top Ten Contact Allergens (North American Contact Dermatitis Group) and Other Common Contact Allergens**

| Allergen | Principal Sources of Contact |
|---|---|
| Nickel sulfate | Metals, metals in clothing, jewelry, catalyzing agents |
| Neomycin sulfate | Usually contained in creams, ointments |
| Balsam of Peru | Topical medications |
| Fragrance mix | Fragrances, cosmetics |
| Thimerosal | Antiseptics |
| Sodium gold thiosulfate | Medication |
| Formaldehyde | Disinfectant, curing agents, plastics |
| Quaternium-15 | Disinfectant |
| Cobalt chloride | Cement, galvanization, industrial oils, cooling agents, eyeshades |
| Bacitracin | Ointments, powder |
| Methyldibromoglutaronitrile, phenoxylethanol | Preservatives, cosmetics |
| Carba mix | Rubber, latex |
| Ethyleneurea melamine-formaldehyde resin | Textile additives |
| Thiuram | Rubber |
| p-Phenylene diamine | Black or dark dyes of textiles, printer's ink |
| Parahydroxybenzoic acid ester | Conserving agent in foodstuffs |
| Propylene glycol | Preservatives, cosmetics |
| Procaine, benzocaine | Local anesthetics |
| Sulfonamides | Medication |
| Turpentine | Solvents, shoe polish, printer's ink |
| Mercury salts | Disinfectant, impregnation |
| Chromates | Cement, antioxidants, industrial oils, matches, leather |
| Cinnamic aldehyde | Fragrance, perfume |

**Patch Tests**   In ACD sensitization is present on every part of the skin; therefore, application of the allergen to any area of normal skin provokes an eczematous reaction. A positive patch test shows erythema and papules, as well as possibly vesicles confined to the test site. Patch tests should be delayed until the dermatitis has subsided for at least 2 weeks and should be performed on a previously uninvolved site. (See Appendix A.)

## DIAGNOSIS AND DIFFERENTIAL DIAGNOSIS

By history and clinical findings including evaluation of site and distribution. Histopathology may be helpful; verification of offending agent (allergen) by patch test. Exclude ICD (Table 2-3), atopic dermatitis, seborrheic dermatitis (face), psoriasis (palms and soles), epidermal dermatophytosis (KOH), fixed drug eruption, erysipelas phytophotodermatitis.

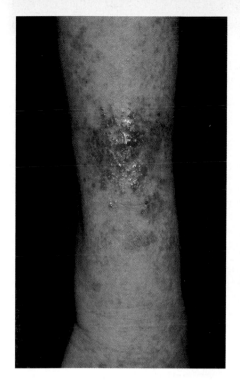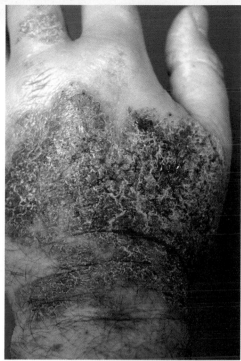

**FIGURE 2-5 (Left) Allergic contact dermatitis of lower leg, acute: neomycin.** *Erythema, papules, vesicles, and erosions with oozing on the pretibial skin. Note spreading of lesions in the periphery. This woman was allergic to neomycin and had used a neomycin-containing cream to treat an insect bite.*

**FIGURE 2-6 (Right) Allergic contact dermatitis of hands: chromates** *Confluent papules, vesicles, erosions and crusts on the dorsum of the left hand in a construction worker who was allergic to chromates.*

**Table 2-3 Differences Between Irritant and Allergic Contact Dermatitis\***

|  |  | Irritant CD | Allergic CD |
|---|---|---|---|
| Symptoms | Acute | **Stinging, smarting → itching** | **Itching → pain** |
|  | Chronic | Itching/pain | Itching/pain |
| Lesions | Acute | Erythema → vesicle → erosion → crust → scaling | Erythema → **papules** → vesicles → erosions → crust → scaling |
|  | Chronic | Papules, plaques, fissures, scaling, crusts | Papules, plaques, scaling, crusts |
| Margination and site | Acute | **Sharp, strictly confined to site of exposure** | Sharp, confined to site of exposure **but spreading in the periphery; usually tiny papules; may become generalized** |
|  | Chronic | Ill-defined | Ill-defined, **spreads** |
| Evolution | Acute | **Rapid** (few hours after exposure) | **Not so rapid** (12 to 72 h after exposure) |
|  | Chronic | Months to years of repeated exposure | Months or longer; exacerbation after every reexposure |
| Causative agents |  | **Dependent on concentration of agent and state of skin barrier; occurs only above threshold level** | **Relatively independent of amount applied, usually very low concentrations sufficient but depends on degree of sensitization** |
| Incidence |  | **May occur in practically everyone** | **Occurs only in the sensitized** |

\* Differences are printed in bold.

# SPECIAL FORMS OF ACD

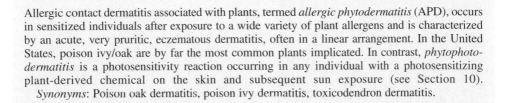

ALLERGIC CONTACT DERMATITIS
DUE TO PLANTS

Allergic contact dermatitis associated with plants, termed *allergic phytodermatitis* (APD), occurs in sensitized individuals after exposure to a wide variety of plant allergens and is characterized by an acute, very pruritic, eczematous dermatitis, often in a linear arrangement. In the United States, poison ivy/oak are by far the most common plants implicated. In contrast, *phytophotodermatitis* is a photosensitivity reaction occurring in any individual with a photosensitizing plant-derived chemical on the skin and subsequent sun exposure (see Section 10).

*Synonyms*: Poison oak dermatitis, poison ivy dermatitis, toxicodendron dermatitis.

## EPIDEMIOLOGY AND ETIOLOGY

**Age of Onset**  Occurs in individuals of all ages. Very young and very old are less likely to be sensitized to plants. Sensitization is lifelong.

**Etiology**  Pentadecylcatechols, present in the Anacardiaceae plant family, are the most common sensitizers in the United States. Pentadecylcatechols cross-react with other phenolic compounds such as resorcinol, hexylresorcinol, and hydroxyquinones.

**Plants** *Anacardiaceae Family*  Poison ivy (*Toxicodendron radicans*) and poison oak (*T. querifolium*, *T. diversilobum*). Also poison sumac (*T. vernix*). Plants related to poison ivy group: Brazilian pepper, cashew nut tree, ginkgo tree, Indian marker nut tree, lacquer tree, mango tree, rengas tree.

**Geography**  Poison ivy occurs throughout the United States (except extreme southwest) and southern Canada; poison oak on the west coast. Poison sumac and poison dogwood grow only in woody, swampy areas.

**Exposure**  Telephone and electrical workers working outdoors. Leaves, stems, seeds, flowers, berries, and roots contain milky sap that turns to a black resin on exposure to air. Cashew oil: unroasted cashew nuts (heat destroys hapten); cashew oil in wood (Haitian voodoo dolls, swizzle sticks), resins, printer's ink. Mango rind. Marking nut tree of India: laundry marker (dhobi itch). Furniture lacquer from Japanese lacquer tree.

**Season**  APD usually occurs in the spring, summer, and fall; can occur year-round if exposed to stems or roots. In southwest of the United States, occurs year-round.

## PATHOGENESIS

All *Toxicodendron* plants contain identical allergens. Hapten is present in milky sap in leaves, stems, seeds, flowers, berries, and roots. The oleoresins are referred to as *urushiol*. The haptens are the pentadecylcatechols (1,2-hydroxybenzenes with a 15-carbon side chain in position three). Washing with soap and water removes oleoresins.

More than 70% of individuals can be sensitized to *Toxicodendron* haptens. Dark-skinned individuals are less susceptible to APD. After first exposure (sensitization) dermatitis occurs 7 to 12 days later. In a previously sensitized person (may be many decades before), dermatitis occurs (especially on face or genitalia) in <12 h after reexposure. Difference in clinical course varies with individual reactivity, inoculum of hapten on skin, and regional variation.

*Note*: Blister fluid does not contain hapten and cannot spread the dermatitis; exposure to smoke from the burning plant is harmless, but dermatitis can occur from particulate matter in the smoke.

## HISTORY

**Exposure** *Poison Ivy/Oak Dermatitis*  Direct plant exposure: plant brushes against exposed skin giving rise to linear lesions (Fig. 2-7); resin usually is not able to penetrate the thick stratum

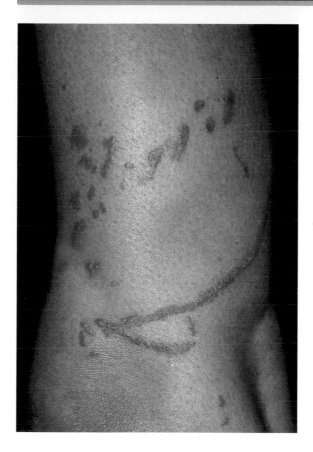

**FIGURE 2-7    Allergic phytodermatitis of leg: poison ivy** *Linear vesicular lesions with erythema and edema on the calf at sites of direct contact of the skin 5 days after exposure with the poison ivy leaf.*

corneum of palms/soles. Clothing: wearing clothing previously contaminated with resin can reexpose the skin.

*Food Containing Urushiol* Eating unpeeled mango or unroasted cashew nuts can expose lips to oleoresin. Mucous membranes uncommonly experience APD but ingestion of urushiol can produce allergic contact dermatitis of the anus and perineum.

**Skin Symptoms**   Pruritus mild to severe. Often sensed before any detectable skin changes. Pain in some cases. Secondary infection associated with local tenderness.

**Constitutional Symptoms**   Sleep deprivation due to pruritus.

## PHYSICAL EXAMINATION

### Skin Lesions

Initially, well-demarcated patches of erythema, characteristic linear lesions (Fig. 2-7); rapidly evolve into papules and edematous plaques; may be severe especially on face and/or genitals, resembling cellulitis (Fig. 2-8). Microvesiculation may evolve to vesicles and/or bullae. Erosions, crusts. With resolution, erythematous plaques ±scale, ±erosion, ±crusting. Postinflammatory hyperpigmentation common in darker skinned individuals.

*Distribution* Most commonly on exposed extremities, where contact with the plant occurs; blotting can transfer to any exposed site; palms/soles are usually spared; however, lateral fingers can be involved.

*Clothing-Protected Sites* Oleoresin can penetrate damp clothing onto covered skin.

*Nonexposed Sites* "Id"-like reaction or some systemic absorption can be associated with disseminated urticarial, erythema multiforme-like, or scarlatiniform lesions away from sites of exposure in some individuals with well-established APD.

## LABORATORY EXAMINATIONS

**Dermatopathology**   See ACD, above.

**Patch Tests with Pentadecylcatechols**   Contraindicated. Can sensitize the individual to hapten.

## DIAGNOSIS

By history and clinical findings.

## DIFFERENTIAL DIAGNOSIS

ACD to other allergens, phytophotodermatitis, soft-tissue infection (cellulitis, erysipelas), atopic dermatitis, inflammatory dermatophytosis, early herpes zoster, fixed drug eruption.

## SYSTEMIC ACD (SACD)

After systemic exposure to an allergen to which the individual had prior ACD. A delayed T cell–mediated reaction. Examples: ACD to ethylenediamine → subsequent reaction to aminophylline (which contains ethylene diamine); poison ivy dermatitis → subsequent reaction to ingestion of cashew nuts; also antibiotics, sulfonamides, propylene glycol, metal ions, sorbic acid, fragrances.

## AIRBORNE ACD

Contact with airborne allergens in exposed body sites, notably the face (Fig. 2-9); also including eyelids, "V" of the neck, arms, and legs. In contrast to airborne ICD, papular from the beginning, extremely itchy. Prolonged repetitive exposure leads to dry, lichenified ACD with erosions and crusting (Fig. 2-9). Due to plant allergens, especially from compositae, natural resins, woods, essential oils volatizing from aroma therapy.

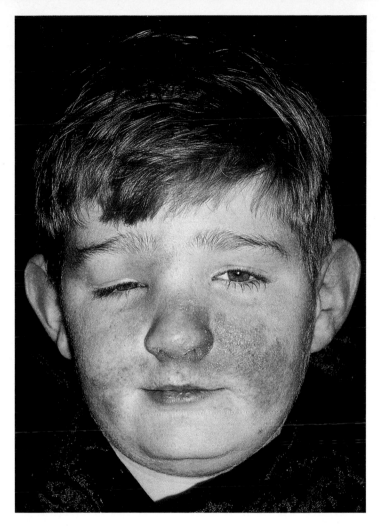

**FIGURE 2-8    Allergic phytodermatitis of face: poison ivy**    *Very pruritic erythema, edema, microvesiculation of the cheeks and periorbital area in a previously sensitized 7-year-old boy, occurring 3 days after exposure.*

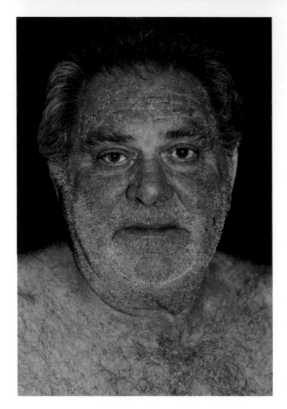

**FIGURE 2-9    Airborne allergic contact dermatitis on the face.**   *Extremely itchy, confluent papular, erosive, and crusted/scaly lesions with lichenification on the forehead, following exposure to pinewood dust.*

## MANAGEMENT OF ACD

**Termination of Exposure**   Identify and remove the etiologic agent.

**Topical Therapy**   Topical glucocorticoid ointments/gels (classes I to III) are effective for early nonbullous lesions. Larger vesicles may be drained, but tops should not be removed. Wet dressings with cloths soaked in Burow's solution changed every 2 to 3 h. Since treatment with glucocorticoids is usually short-term in ACD, there is usually no danger of glucocorticoid side effects. An exception is airborne ACD, which may require systemic treatment. The newer immunomodulating topicals pimecrolimus and tacrolimus are effective in ACD but are still being evaluated.

**Systemic Therapy**   Glucocorticoids are indicated if severe (i.e., if patient cannot perform usual daily functions, cannot sleep) for exudative lesions. Prednisone beginning at 70 mg (adults), tapering by 5 to 10 mg/d over a 1- to 2-week period.

In airborne ACD where complete avoidance of allergen may be impossible, immunosuppression with oral cyclosporine may become necessary.

## ATOPIC DERMATITIS ■ ◐

Atopic dermatitis (AD) is an acute, subacute, or chronic relapsing skin disorder that usually begins in infancy and is characterized principally by dry skin and pruritus; consequent rubbing and scratching lead to lichenification and hence to further itching and scratching (*itch-scratch cycle*). The diagnosis is based on clinical findings, although the serum IgE level is usually (85%) elevated. AD is often associated with a personal or family history of AD, allergic rhinitis, and asthma; 35% of infants with AD develop asthma later in life.

*Synonyms*: IgE dermatitis, "eczema," atopic eczema.

### EPIDEMIOLOGY

**Age of Onset** First 2 months of life and by the first years in 60% of patients. 30% are seen for the first time by age 5, and only 10% develop AD between 6 and 20 years of age. Rarely AD has an adult onset.

**Gender** Slightly more common in males than females.

**Prevalence** Between 7 and 15% reported in population studies in Scandinavia and Germany.

**Genetic Aspects** The inheritance pattern has not been ascertained. However, in one series, 60% of adults with AD had children with AD. The prevalence in children was higher (81%) when both parents had AD.

**Eliciting Factors** *Inhalants* Specific aeroallergens, especially dust mites and pollens, have been shown to cause exacerbations of AD.

**Microbial Agents** Exotoxins of *Staphylococcus aureus* may act as superantigens and stimulate activation of T cells and macrophages.

**Autoallergens** Sera of patients with AD contain IgE antibodies directed at human proteins. The release of these autoallergens from damaged tissue could trigger IgE or T cell responses, suggesting maintenance of allergic inflammation by endogenous antigens.

**Foods** Subset of infants and children have flares of AD with eggs, milk, peanuts, soybeans, fish, and wheat.

### Other Exacerbating Factors

*Skin Barrier Disruption:* decrease of barrier function associated with reduced ceramide levels and increased transepidermal water loss by frequent bathing and hand washing; dehydration is an important exacerbating factor.

*Infections:* S. *aureus* is almost always present in severe cases; group A streptococcus; rarely fungus (dermatophytosis, candidiasis).

*Season:* in temperate climates, AD usually improves in summer, flares in winter.

*Clothing:* pruritus flares *after* taking off clothing. Wool is an important trigger; wool clothing or blankets directly in contact with skin (also wool clothing of parents, fur of pets, carpets).

*Emotional Stress:* results from the disease or is itself an exacerbating factor in flares of the disease.

### PATHOGENESIS

Complex interaction of skin barrier, genetic, environmental, pharmacologic, and immunologic factors. Type I (IgE-mediated) hypersensitivity reaction occurring as a result of the release of vasoactive substances from both mast cells and basophils that have been sensitized by the interaction of the antigen with IgE (reaginic or skin-sensitizing antibody). The role of IgE in AD is still not fully clarified, but epidermal Langerhans cells possess high-affinity IgE receptors through which an eczema-like reaction can be mediated. $T_H2$ and $T_H1$ both contribute to skin inflammation in AD. Acute T cell infiltration in AD is associated with a predominance of interleukin (IL) 4 and IL-13 expression, and chronic inflammation in AD with increased IL-5, granulocyte-macrophage colony-stimulating factor (GM-CSF), IL-12, and interferon (IFN) γ. Thus, skin inflammation in AD shows a biphasic pattern of T cell activation.

### HISTORY

**Skin Symptoms** Patients have dry skin. Pruritus is the sine qua non of atopic dermatitis—

"eczema is the itch that rashes." The constant scratching leads to a vicious cycle of itch → scratch → rash → itch.

**Other Symptoms of Atopy** Allergic rhinitis, characterized by sneezing, rhinorrhea, obstruction of nasal passages, conjuctival and pharyngeal itching, and lacrimation; may be seasonal when associated with pollen.

## PHYSICAL EXAMINATION

### Skin Lesions

*Acute* Poorly defined erythematous patches, papules, and plaques with or without scale. Edema with widespread involvement; skin appears "puffy" and edematous (Fig. 2-10). Erosions: moist, crusted. Linear or punctate, resulting from scratching. Secondarily infected sites: *S. aureus.* Oozing erosions (Figs. 2-11 and 2-12) and/or pustules (usually follicular). Crusts.

*Chronic* Lichenification (thickening of the skin with accentuation of skin markings): results from repeated rubbing or scratching (Fig. 2-13); follicular lichenification (especially in brown

and black persons) (Fig. 2-14). Fissures: painful, especially in flexures (Fig. 2-15), on palms, fingers, and soles. Alopecia: lateral one-third of the eyebrows as a result of rubbing. Periorbital pigmentation: also as a result of compulsively rubbing. Characteristic infraorbital fold in the eyelids (Dennie-Morgan sign).

*Distribution* Predilection for the flexures, front and sides of the neck, eyelids, forehead, face, wrists, and dorsa of the feet and hands (Image 2-1). Generalized in severe disease.

### Special Features Related to Ethnicity

In blacks, so-called follicular eczema is common and is characterized by discrete follicular papules (Fig. 2-14) involving all hair follicles of the involved site.

### Special Features Related to Age

*Infantile AD* The lesions present as red skin, tiny vesicles on "puffy" surface. Scaling, exudation with wet crusts and cracks (fissures) (Figs. 2-10 to 2-12). Skin lesions seem to be a reaction to itching and rubbing.

*Childhood-type AD* The lesions are papular, lichenified plaques, erosions, crusts, especially

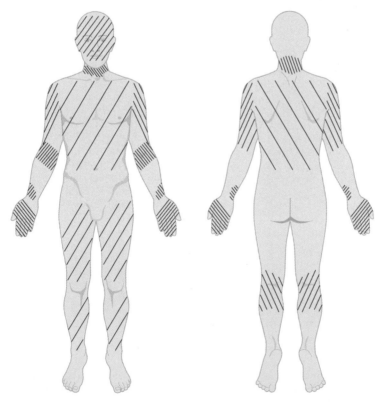

**IMAGE 2-1** *Predilection sites of atopic dermatitis.*

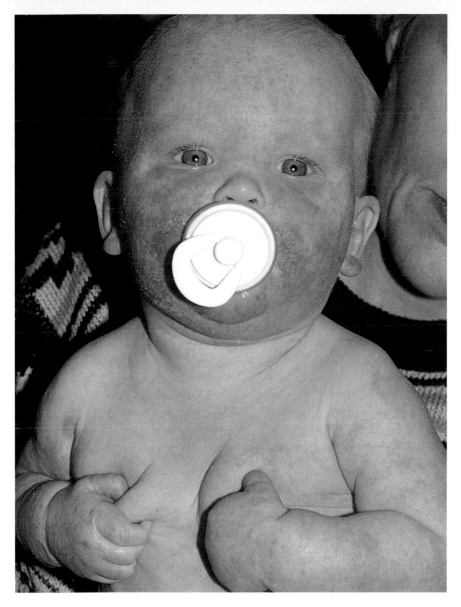

**FIGURE 2-10   Atopic dermatitis: infantile** *Confluent erythema, papules, microvesiculation, scaling, and crusting on the face, with similar involvement (to a lesser degree) of the trunk and arms. The facial involvement is more severe due to easier access to scratching. The baby is squeezing the breast skin to relieve the intense pruritus.*

on the antecubital and popliteal fossae (Figs. 2-13 to 2-16), the neck and face.

***Adult-type AD*** There is a similar distribution, with lichenification and exoriations being the most conspicuous symptoms (Fig. 2-17).

### Associated Findings

"White" dermatographism is a special and unique feature of involved skin: stroking will not lead to redness as in normal skin but to blanching; delayed blanch to cholinergic agents. Ichthyosis vulgaris and keratosis pilaris occur in 10% of patients. Vernal conjuctivitis with papillary hypertrophy or cobblestoning of upper eyelid conjuctiva. Atopic keratoconjunctivitis is disabling, may result in corneal scarring. Keratoconus rare. Cataracts in a small percentage.

### DIAGNOSIS

History in infancy, clinical findings (typical distribution sites, morphology of lesions, white dermatographism).

### DIFFERENTIAL DIAGNOSIS

Seborrheic dermatitis, ICD, ACD, psoriasis, nummular eczema, dermatophytosis, early stages of mycosis fungoides. Rarely, acrodermatitis enteropathica, glucagonoma syndrome, histidinemia, phenylketonuria; also, some immunologic disorders including Wiskott-Aldrich syndrome, X-linked agammaglobulinemia, hyper-IgE syndrome, Letterer-Siwe disease, and selective IgA deficiency.

### LABORATORY EXAMINATIONS

**Bacterial Culture**   Colonization with *S. aureus* is very common in the nares and in the involved skin; almost 90% of patients with severe AD are secondarily colonized/infected. Look out for MRSA.

**Viral Culture**   Rule out herpes simplex virus (HSV) infection in crusted lesions (eczema herpeticum; see Section 25).

**Blood Studies**   Increased IgE in serum, eosinophilia.

**Dermatopathology**   Various degrees of acanthosis with rare intraepidermal intercellular edema (spongiosis). The dermal infiltrate is composed of lymphocytes, monocytes, and mast cells with few or no eosinophils.

### SPECIAL FORMS OF AD

***Hand Dermatitis*** Aggravated by wetting and washing with detergents, harsh soaps, and *disinfectants*; leads to ICD in the atopic. Clinically indistinguishable from "normal ICD" (see p. 22).

***Exfoliative Dermatitis*** (See Section 8) Erythroderma in patients with extensive skin involvement. Generalized redness, scaling, weeping, crusting, lymphadenopathy, fever, and systemic toxicity.

### COURSE AND PROGNOSIS

Untreated involved sites persist for months or years. Spontaneous, more or less complete remission during childhood occurs in >40% with occasional, more severe recurrences during adolescence. In many patients, the disease persists for 15 to 20 years, but is less severe. From 30 to 50% of patients develop asthma and/or hay fever. Adult-onset AD often runs a severe course. *S. aureus* infection leads to extensive erosions and crusting, and herpes simplex infection to eczema herpeticum, which may be life-threatening (see Section 25).

### MANAGEMENT

Education of the patient to avoid rubbing and scratching is most important. Topical antipruritic (menthol/camphor) lotions are helpful in controlling the pruritus but are useless if emollients are not used and the patient continues to scratch and rub the plaques.

An allergic workup is rarely helpful in uncovering an allergen; however, in patients who are hypersensitive to house dust, mites, various pollens, and animal hair proteins, exposure to the appropriate allergen may cause flares. Atopic dermatitis is considered by many to be related, at least in part, to emotional stress.

Patients should be warned of their special problems with herpes simplex and the frequency of superimposed staphylococcal infection, for which oral antibiotics are indicated. Antiviral drugs for herpes simplex are indicated if HSV infection is suspected.

**Acute**

1.  Wet dressings and topical glucocorticoids; topical antibiotics (mupirocin ointment) when indicated.
2.  Hydroxyzine, 10 to 100 mg qid for pruritus.
3.  Oral antibiotics (dicloxacillin, erythromy-

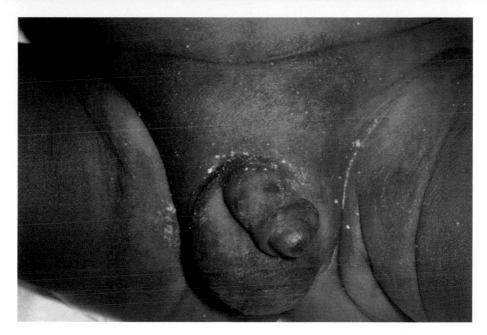

**FIGURE 2-11 Atopic dermatitis: infantile-type** *Confluent papules, microvesiculation and erosions in the diaper area of a 4-month-old infant.*

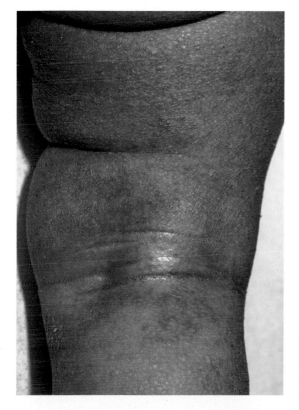

**FIGURE 2-12 Atopic dermatitis: infantile-type** *Papular lesions on the lower extremity with oozing erosions in the popliteal fossa.*

cin) to eliminate *S. aureus* and treat MRSA according to sensitivity as shown by culture.

## Subacute and Chronic

1. Hydration (oilated baths or baths with oatmeal powder) followed by application of unscented emollients (e.g., hydrated petrolatum) form the basic daily treatment needed to prevent xerosis. Soap showers are permissible to wash the body folds, but soap should seldom be used on the other parts of the skin surface. 12% ammonium lactate or 10% α-hydroxy acid lotion is very effective for the xerosis seen in AD.

2. Topical anti-inflammatory agents such as glucocorticoids, hydroxyquinoline preparations, and tar are the mainstays of treatment. Of these, glucocorticoids are the most effective. However, topical glucocorticoids may lead to skin atrophy if used for prolonged periods of time and if used excessively will lead to suppression of the pituitary-adrenal axis, osteoporosis, growth retardation. Another problem is "glucocorticoidophobia." Patients or their parents are increasingly aware of glucocorticoid side effects and refuse their use, no matter how beneficial they may be.

3. New nonsteroidal anti-inflammatory agents are now available and will probably replace glucocorticoids for most patients in the future. These are topical tacrolimus and pimecrolimus. They potently suppress itching and inflammation and do not lead to skin atrophy. The only problem with tacrolimus is that some patients cannot tolerate the immediate (but transient) burning on application. Burning is less of a problem with pimecrolimus.

4. Oral $H_1$ antihistamines are useful in reducing itching.

5. Systemic glucocorticoids should be avoided, except in rare instances in adults for only short courses (rescue treatment). They are widely overused. Osteopenia and cataracts are complications. For severe intractable disease, prednisone, 60 to 80 mg daily for 2 days, then halving the dose each 2 days for the next 6 days. Patients with AD tend to become dependent on oral glucocorticoids. Often, small doses (5 to 10 mg) make the difference in control and can be reduced gradually to even 2.5 mg/d, as is often used for the control of asthma. Intramuscular glucocorticoids are risky and should be avoided.

6. UVA-UVB phototherapy (combination of UVA plus UVB and increasing the radiation dose each treatment, with a frequency of two to three times weekly). Narrow band UV (311 nm), PUVA photochemotherapy also effective.

7. In severe cases of adult AD and in normotensive healthy persons without renal disease cyclosporin treatment (starting dose 5 mg/kg per day) is indicated when all other treatments fail, but should be monitored closely. Treatment is limited to 3 to 6 months because of potential side effects, including hypertension and reduced renal function. Blood pressure should be checked weekly and chemistry panels biweekly. Nifedipine can be used for moderate increases in blood pressure.

8. Patients should learn and use stress management techniques.

9. A suggested algorithm of AD management is as follows:

   - Baseline therapy of dryness with emollients
   - Suppression of mild to moderate AD by prolonged topical pimecrolimus or tacrolimus and continued emollients
   - Supression of severe flares with topical glucocorticoids followed by pimecrolimus or tacrolimus and emollients
   - Oral and topical antibiotics to eliminate *S. aureus*
   - Hydroxyzine to suppress pruritus

Website: *http://www.aad.org/pamphlets/eczema.html.*

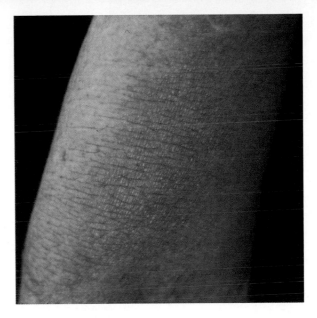

**FIGURE 2-13   Atopic dermatitis: childhood-type**   *Erythematous lichenification with accentuation of skin markings in the antecubital fossa of a 9-year-old girl. These lesions are extremely pruritic.*

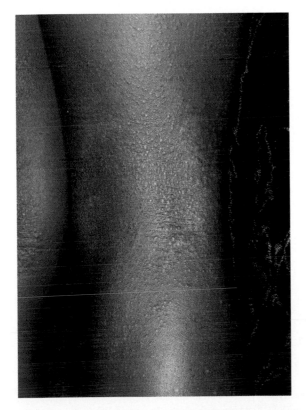

**FIGURE 2-14   Atopic dermatitis in black child: follicular**   *Pruritic follicular papules on the posterior leg. Follicular eczema is a reaction pattern that occurs more commonly in African and Asian children.*

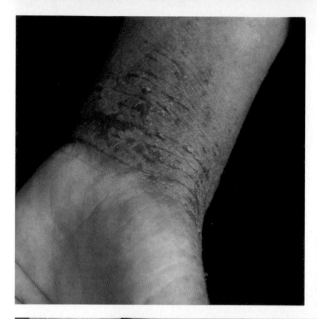

**FIGURE 2-15  Atopic dermatitis: childhood-type**  *Massive lichenification in the wrist region with linear, oozing erosions due to infection with Staphylococcus aureus.*

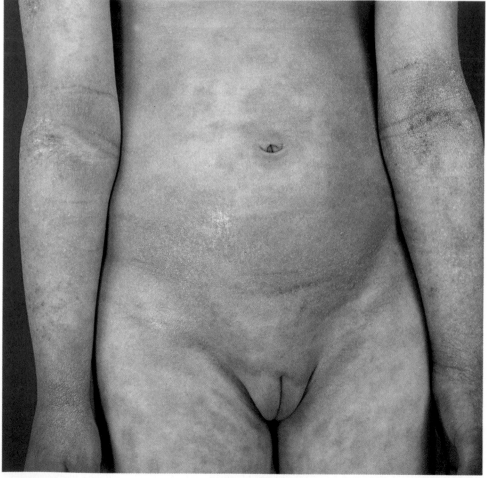

**FIGURE 2-16  Atopic dermatitis: childhood-type**  *Ill-defined erythema, papules, excoriations, lichenification in the antecubital fossae, with less severe changes on the trunk and thighs.*

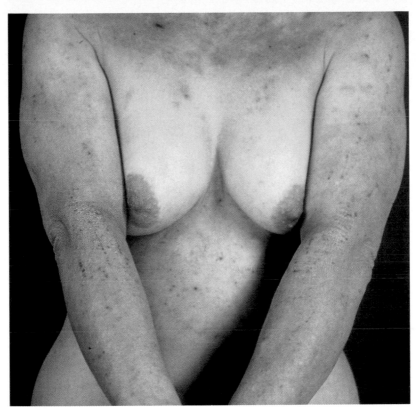

**FIGURE 2-17   Atopic dermatitis: chronic, adult-type**   *Chronic eczematous dermatitis with sparing under the bra. Note lichenification and numerous long excoriations. One does not have to take a history to realize that this condition itches severely.*

# LICHEN SIMPLEX CHRONICUS  

Lichen simplex chronicus (LSC) is a special localized form of lichenification, occurring in circumscribed plaques; it results from repetitive rubbing and scratching. Lichenification is a characteristic feature of atopic dermatitis, whether generalized or localized. Lichen simplex can last for decades unless the rubbing and scratching are stopped by treatment. It occurs in individuals older than 20 years, is more frequent in women, and possibly more frequent in Asians.

## PATHOGENESIS

A special predilection of the skin to respond to physical trauma by epidermal hyperplasia; skin becomes highly sensitive to touch. The very abnormal itching hyperexcitability of lichenified skin arises in response to minimal external stimuli that would not elicit an itch response in normal skin. Emotional stress in some cases. It becomes a habit and may persist for months to years, with resulting marked lichenification.

Skin symptoms mainly consist of pruritus, often in paroxysms. The lichenified skin is like an erogenous zone—it becomes a pleasure (orgiastic) to scratch. Often the areas on the feet are rubbed at night with the heel and the toes. The rubbing becomes automatic and reflexive and an unconscious habit. Most patients with LSC give a history of itch attacks starting from minor stimuli: putting on clothes, removing ointments, clothes rubbing the skin; in bed, the skin becomes warmer and the warmth precipitates itching. Many patients have AD or an atopic background.

## PHYSICAL EXAMINATION

### Skin Lesions

A solid plaque of lichenification, arising from the confluence of small papules; scaling is minimal except on lower extremities (Fig. 2-18). Lichenified skin is palpably thickened; skin markings (barely visible in normal skin) are accentuated and can be seen readily. Excoriations are often present. Usually dull red, later brown or black hyperpigmentation, especially in skin phototypes IV, V, and VI. Round, oval, linear (following path of scratching). Usually sharply defined. Isolated single lesion or several randomly scattered plaques. Nuchal area (female) (Fig. 2-18), scalp, ankles, lower legs, upper thighs, exterior forearms, vulva, pubis, anal area, scrotum, and groin.

In black skin, lichenification may assume a special type of pattern—there is not a solid plaque, but the lichenification consists instead of a multitude of small (2- to 3-mm) closely set papules—i.e., a "follicular" pattern (as in Fig. 2-14).

## DIFFERENTIAL DIAGNOSIS

Includes a chronic pruritic plaque of psoriasis vulgaris, early stages of mycosis fungoides, ICD, ACD, epidermal dermatophytosis.

## LABORATORY EXAMINATION

**Dermatopathology** Hyperplasia of all components of epidermis: hyperkeratosis, acanthosis, and elongated and broad rete ridges. Spongiosis is infrequent. In the dermis there is a chronic inflammatory infiltrate.

## MANAGEMENT

Difficult. Repeatedly explain to the patient that the rubbing and scratching must be stopped. It is important to apply occlusive bandages at night to prevent rubbing. Topical glucocorticoid preparations or tar preparations such as combinations of 5% crude coal tar in zinc oxide paste plus class II glucocorticoids all covered by occlusive cloth dry dressings are effective for body areas where this approach is feasible (e.g., legs, arms). Occlusive dressings: glucocorticoid preparations are usually applied first, followed by an occlusive (plastic) dressing (like saran wrap). Glucocorticoids incorporated in adhesive plastic tape are very effective and can be left on for 24 h. Unna Boot: a gauze roll dressing impregnated with zinc oxide paste is wrapped around a large lichenified area such as the calf. The dressing can be left on for up to 1 week.

Intralesional triamcinolone is often highly effective in smaller lesions (3 mg/mL; higher concentrations may cause atrophy). Oral hydroxyzine, 25 to 50 g at night, may be helpful.

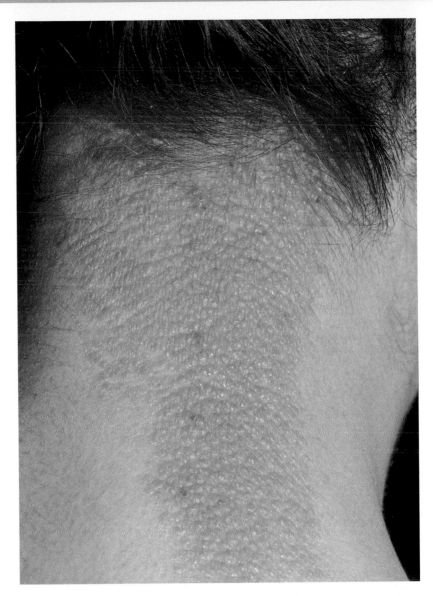

**FIGURE 2-18   Lichen simplex chronicus**   *Confluent, papular, follicular eczema, creating a plaque of lichen simplex chronicus of the posterior neck and occipital scalp. Condition had been present for many years as a result of chronic rubbing of the area.*

## PRURIGO NODULARIS (PN)    ▢▮   ◑

Is often associated with AD or occurs without AD. PN patients with AD are younger and have reactivity to environmental allergens, nonatopic PN patients are older and lack hypersensitivities to environmental allergens. As in LSC the underlying stimulus is pruritus. Dome-shaped nodules — several millimeters to 2 cm — develop on sites in which persistent itching and scratching occur (Fig. 2-19). They are often eroded, excoriated, and sometimes even ulcerated as patients dig into them with their nails. Usually multiple on the extremities. PN usually occurs in younger or middle-age females, who often exhibit signs of neurotic stigmatization. PN starts with piercing pruritus that leads to picking and scratching. Lesions persist for months after the trauma has been discontinued.

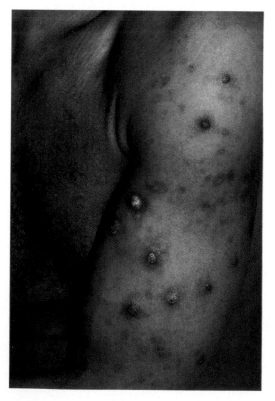

FIGURE 2-19   Prurigo nodularis   *Multiple, firm, excoriated nodules arising at sites of chronically picked or excoriated skin. Often occurring in patients with atopy but also without it. This is a 36-year-old male with HIV disease. He had MRSA secondary infection of prurigo nodules. Cellulitis originated in prurigo nodules requiring multiple hospitalizations.*

# DYSHIDROTIC ECZEMATOUS DERMATITIS ■ ◑

Dyshidrotic eczema is a special vesicular type of hand and foot dermatitis. It is an acute, chronic, or recurrent dermatosis of the fingers, palms, and soles, characterized by a sudden onset of many deep-seated pruritic, clear "tapioca-like" vesicles; later, scaling fissures and lichenification occur.

*Synonyms*: Pompholyx, vesicular palmar eczema.

## LABORATORY EXAMINATIONS

**Bacterial Culture** Rule out *S. aureus* infection.
**KOH Preparation** Rule out epidermal dermatophytosis.
**Dermatopathology** Eczematous inflammation (spongiosis and intraepidermal edema) with intraepidermal vesicles.

## COURSE AND PROGNOSIS

Recurrent attacks are the rule. Spontaneous remissions in 2 to 3 weeks. Interval between attacks is weeks to months. Secondary infection may complicate the course: pustules, crusts, cellulitis, lymphangitis, and painful lymphadenopathy. Disabling because of severe, frequently recurring outbreaks.

## MANAGEMENT

**Wet Dressing** For vesicular stage: Burow's wet dressings. Large bullae drained with a puncture but not unroofed.
**Fissures** Topical application of flexible collodion.
**Glucocorticoids**
*Topical* High-potency glucocorticoids with plastic occlusive dressings for 1 to 2 weeks.
*Intralesional Injection* Triamcinolone, 3 mg/mL. Very effective for small areas of involvement.
*Systemic* In severe cases, a short, tapered course of prednisone can be given: 70 mg/d, tapering by 10 or 5 mg/d over 7 or 14 days.
**Systemic Antibiotic** For suspected (localized pain) or documented secondarily infected lesions (usually *S. aureus*; less commonly group A streptococcus).
**PUVA** (See page 70) Oral or topical as "soaks." Successful in many patients if given over prolonged periods of time and worth trying, especially in severe cases.

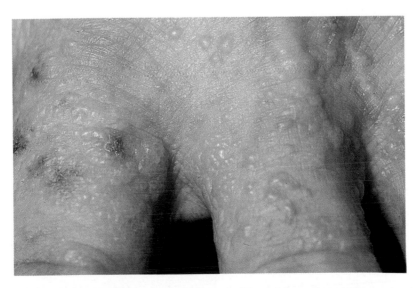

**FIGURE 2-20 Dyshidrotic eczema** *Confluent tapioca-like vesicles and crusted (excoriated) erosions on the dorsum of fingers and finger webs.*

## NUMMULAR ECZEMA

Nummular eczema is a chronic, pruritic, inflammatory dermatitis occurring in the form of coin-shaped plaques composed of grouped small papules and vesicles on an erythematous base, especially common on the lower legs of older males during winter months; often seen in atopic individuals.

*Synonym*: Discoid eczema, microbial eczema.

### EPIDEMIOLOGY

Two peaks in incidence: young adulthood and old age. Fall and winter.

### PATHOGENESIS

Unknown. Unrelated to atopic diathesis; IgE levels normal. Incidence peaks in winter, when xerosis is maximal. *S. aureus* often present.

### HISTORY

**Skin Symptoms**   Pruritus, often intense.

### PHYSICAL EXAMINATION

Skin Lesions
Closely grouped, small vesicles and papules that coalesce into plaques (Fig. 2-21A), often more than 4 to 5 cm in diameter, with an erythematous base with distinct borders. Plaques may become exudative and crust (Fig. 2-21B). Excoriations secondary to scratching. Dry scaly plaques that may be lichenified. Round or *coin-shaped* (Fig. 2-21A) hence the adjective *nummular* (Latin: *nummularis*, "like a coin"). Margins often more pronounced than center.
*Distribution* Regional clusters of lesions (e.g., on legs or trunk) or generalized, scattered. Lower legs (older men), trunk, hands and fingers (younger females).

### DIFFERENTIAL DIAGNOSIS

**Scaling Plaques** Epidermal dermatophytosis, ICD or ACD, psoriasis, early stages of mycosis fungoides, impetigo, familial pemphigus.

### LABORATORY EXAMINATIONS

**Bacterial Culture**   Rule out *S. aureus* infection.
**Dermatopathology**   Subacute   inflammation with acanthosis and spongiosis.

### COURSE AND PROGNOSIS

Chronic. Lesions last from weeks to months. Often difficult to control even with potent topical glucocorticoid preparations.

### MANAGEMENT

**Skin Hydration**   "Moisturize" involved skin after bath or shower with hydrated petrolatum or other moisturizing cream.
**Glucocorticoids**   *Topical Preparations* Classes I and II applied bid until lesions have resolved. Steroid impregnated tape. *Intralesional* triamcinolone, 3 mg/mL.
**Crude Coal Tar**   2 to 5% crude coal tar ointment daily. May be combined with glucocorticoid preparation. Tar baths are useful in patients with refractory lesions.
**Systemic Therapy**   Systemic antibiotics if *S. aureus* is present.
**PUVA or UVB 311-nm Therapy**   Very effective.

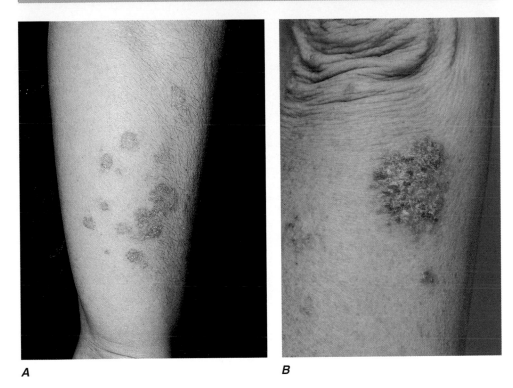

*A*                                                        *B*

**FIGURE 2-21   Nummular eczema**   *A. Pruritic, round, nummular (coin-shaped) plaques with erythema, scales, and crusts on the forearm.* ***B.*** *Closeup of nummular lesion on the forearm of another patient showing papular component with crusts and erosions. It is obvious that this lesion is highly pruritic.*

## AUTOSENSITIZATION DERMATITIS

This term refers to an often unrecognized generalized pruritic dermatitis directly related to a primary dermatitis elsewhere. For example, a patient with venous stasis dermatitis on the lower legs may develop pruritic, symmetric, scattered, erythematous, maculopapular, or papulovesicular lesions on the trunk, forearms, thighs, or legs, which persist and spread until the basic underlying primary dermatitis is controlled. Similarly, autosensitization may occur as an "id" reaction in inflammatory tinea pedis and manifests as a dyshidrosiform, vesicular eruption on the feet and hands (Fig. 2-22) and papulovesicular eczematoid lesions on the trunk.

The phenomenon results from the release of cytokines in the primary dermatitis, as a result of sensitization. These cytokines circulate in the blood and heighten the sensitivity of the distant skin areas. The diagnosis of autosensitization dermatitis is often *post hoc*, i.e., the distant eruption disappears when the primary dermatitis is controlled. Oral glucocorticoids hasten the disappearance of the lesions.

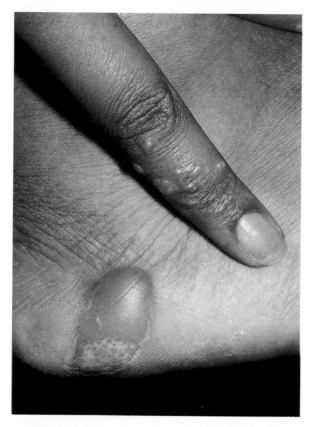

**FIGURE 2-22    Autosensitization dermatitis ("id" reaction): dermatophytid**   *Vesicles and bullae on the finger and the lateral foot of a 21-year-old female. Bullous (inflammatory) tinea pedis was present and was associated with dermatophytid reaction. Prednisone was given for 2 weeks; pruritus and vesiculation resolved.*

# SEBORRHEIC DERMATITIS

Seborrheic dermatitis (SD) is a very common chronic dermatosis characterized by redness and scaling and occurring in regions where the sebaceous glands are most active, such as the face and scalp, the presternal area, and in the body folds. Mild scalp SD causes flaking, i.e., dandruff. Generalized SD, failure to thrive, and diarrhea in an infant should bring to mind Leiner's disease with a variety of immunodeficiency disorders.

*Synonyms*: "Cradle cap" (infants), pityriasis sicca (dandruff).

## EPIDEMIOLOGY AND ETIOLOGY

**Age of Onset** Infancy (within the first months), puberty, most between 20 and 50 years or older.

**Sex** More common in males.

**Incidence** 2 to 5% of the population.

**Predisposing and Exacerbating Factors** In immunocompetent patients there is often a hereditary diathesis, the so-called seborrheic state, with marked seborrhea and marginal blepharitis. May be associated with psoriasis as a pre-psoriasis state in which the patient later develops psoriasis; in some patients a mix of lesions (superficial scales on the scalp and eyebrows and polycyclic scaling patches on the trunk) suggests the use of the term *seborrhiasis*. There is reputedly an increased incidence in Parkinson's disease and facial paralysis. Also, some neuroleptic drugs are possibly a factor, but the disease is so common that this has not been proved. Emotional stress is a putative factor in flares. HIV-infected individuals have an increased incidence, and severe intractable SD should be a clue to the existence of HIV disease.

## PATHOGENESIS

*Malassezia furfur* is said to play a role in the pathogenesis, and the response to topical ketoconazole and selenium sulfide is some indication that this yeast may be pathogenic; also the frequency of SD in immunosuppressed patients (HIV, cardiac transplants). SD-like lesions are seen in nutritional deficiencies such as zinc deficiency (as a result of IV alimentation) and experimental niacin deficiency and in Parkinson's disease (including drug-induced). SD develops in experimental pyridoxine deficiency in humans.

## HISTORY

**Duration of Lesions** Gradual onset.

**Seasonal Variations** Some patients are worse in winter in a dry, indoor environment. Sunlight exposure causes SD to flare in a few patients and promotes improvement of the condition in others.

**Skin Symptoms** Pruritus is variable, often increased by perspiration.

## PHYSICAL EXAMINATION

### Skin Lesions

Orange-red or gray-white skin, often with "greasy" or white dry scaling macules and papules of varying size (5 to 20 mm) (Fig. 2-23), rather sharply marginated (Fig. 2-24). Sticky crusts and fissures are common in the folds behind the external ear. On the scalp there is mostly marked scaling ("dandruff"). Scattered, discrete on the face and trunk. Nummular, polycyclic, and even annular on the trunk; diffuse involvement of scalp.

**Distribution and Major Types of Lesions (Based on Localization and Age)** *Hairy Areas of Head* Scalp, eyebrows, eyelashes (blepharitis), beard (follicular orifices); cradle cap (Fig. 2-23).

*Face* The flush ("butterfly") areas, on forehead ("corona seborrhoica"), nasolabial folds, eyebrows, glabella (Fig. 2-24). Ears: retroauricular, meatus.

*Trunk* Simulating lesions of pityriasis rosea or pityriasis versicolor; yellowish-brown patches over the sternum common.

*Body Folds* Axillae, groins, anogenital area, submammary areas, umbilicus—presents as a diffuse, exudative, sharply marginated, brightly erythematous eruption; erosions and fissures common.

*Genitalia* Often with yellow crusts and psoriasiform lesions.

## DIAGNOSIS/DIFFERENTIAL DIAGNOSIS

Usually made on clinical criteria.

### Red Scaly Plaques

*Common* Mild psoriasis vulgaris (the two diseases can sometimes be indistinguishable), impetigo (rule out by smears for bacteria), dermatophytosis (tinea capitis, tinea facialis, tinea corporis), pityriasis versicolor, intertriginous candidiasis (KOH: rule out dermatophytes and yeasts), subacute lupus erythematosus, "seborrheic" papules in secondary syphilis (darkfield: rule out *Treponema pallidum*).

*Rare* Langerhans cell histiocytosis (occurs in infants, often associated with purpura), acrodermatitis enteropathica, zinc deficiency, pemphigus foliaceus, glucagonoma syndrome.

## LABORATORY STUDIES

**Dermatopathology** Focal parakeratosis, with few neutrophils, moderate acanthosis, spongiosis (intercellular edema), nonspecific inflammation of the dermis. The most characteristic feature is neutrophils at the tips of the dilated follicular openings, which appear as crusts/scales.

## COURSE AND PROGNOSIS

SD is very common, affecting the majority of individuals at some time during life. The condition improves in the summer and flares in the fall. Recurrences and remissions, especially on the scalp, may be associated with alopecia in severe cases. Infantile and adolescent SD disappears with age. Seborrheic erythroderma may occur. *Seborrheic erythroderma with diarrhea and failure to thrive (Leiner's disease) is associated with a variety of immunodeficiency disorders including defective yeast opsonization, C3 deficiency, severe combined immunodeficiency, hypogammaglobulinemia, and hyperimmunoglobulinemia.*

## MANAGEMENT

This chronic disorder requires initial therapy followed by chronic maintenance therapy. Topical glucocorticoid preparations are effective but can cause atrophy and erythema and telangiectasia, especially on the face, or initiation/exacerbation of perioral dermatitis or rosacea. UV radiation is beneficial for many individuals.

### Initial Topical Therapy

**Scalp** *Adults* Effective over-the-counter (OTC) *shampoos* containing selenium sulfide, zinc pyrithione, are helpful. By prescription (U.S.), 2% ketoconazole shampoo, used initially to treat and subsequently to control the symptoms; lather can be used on face and chest during shower. Tar shampoos (OTC) are equally effective in many patients.

Low-potency *glucocorticoid* solution, lotion, or gels following a medicated shampoo (ketoconazole or tar) for more severe cases. Pimecrolimus, 1% cream, is beneficial.

*Infants* For cradle cap, removal of crusts with warm olive oil compresses, followed by baby shampoo, 2% ketoconazole shampoo, and application of 1 to 2.5% hydrocortisone cream, 2% ketoconazole cream, 1% pimecrolimus cream.

**Face and Trunk** *Ketoconazole shampoo, 2%.* Glucocorticoid cream and lotions: initially 1 or 2.5% hydrocortisone cream, 2% ketoconazole cream, 1% pimecrolimus cream, 0.03 or 0.1 tacrolimus ointment.

*More potent glucocorticoid lotions* (e.g., clobetasol propionate) may be used for *initial* control and are used along with the medicated shampoos.

**Eyelids** Gentle removal of the crusts in the morning with a cotton ball dipped in diluted baby shampoo. Apply 10% sodium sulfacetamide in a suspension containing 0.2% prednisolone and 0.12% phenylephrine (use cautiously because it contains glucocorticoids). Sodium sulfacetamide ointment alone is also effective, as is 2% ketoconazole cream, 1% pimecrolimus cream, or 0.03% tacrolimus ointment.

**Intertriginous Areas** *Ketoconazole, 2%*; if uncontrolled with these treatments, Castellani's paint for dermatitis of the body folds is often very effective, but staining is a problem. Pimecrolimus cream, 1%; tacrolimus ointment, 0.03%.

### Systemic Therapy

In severe cases, 13-*cis* retinoic acid orally, 1 mg/kg, is highly effective. Contraception should be used in females of child-bearing age.

### Maintenance Therapy

Ketoconazole 2% shampoo; tar shampoos may be equally effective; ketoconazole cream. If these do not work, then the old "standard," 3% sulfur precipitate and 2% salicylic acid in an oil-in-water base is effective; this must be properly compounded. Also, 1 to 2.5% hydrocortisone cream qd will work, but patients should be monitored for signs of atrophy. 1% pimecrolimus cream and 0.03% tacrolimus ointment are effective.

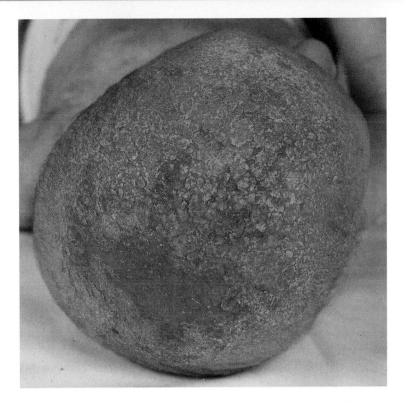

**FIGURE 2-23  Seborrheic dermatitis of scalp: infantile-type**  *Erythema and yellow-orange scales and crust on the scalp of an infant ("cradle cap"). Eczematous lesions are also present on the arms and trunk.*

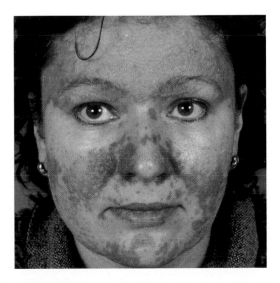

**FIGURE 2-24  Seborrheic dermatitis of face: adult-type**  *Erythema and yellow-orange scaling of the forehead, cheeks, nasolabial folds, and chin. Scalp and retroauricular areas were also involved.*

## ASTEATOTIC DERMATITIS    ■  ○ → ◐

*Synonym:* Eczema craquelé (French *craquelé*, "marred with cracks," such as in old china and ceramic tile).

A common pruritic dermatitis that occurs especially in older persons, in the winter in temperate climates—related to the low humidity of heated houses. The sites of predilection are the legs (Fig. 2-25), arms, and hands but also the trunk. The eruption is characterized by dry, "cracked," superficially fissured skin with slight scaling. The incessant pruritus can lead to lichenification, which can even persist when the environmental conditions have been corrected. The disorder results from too frequent bathing in hot soapy baths or showers and/or in older persons living in rooms with a high environmental temperature and low relative humidity. The disorder is managed by avoiding overbathing with soap, especially tub baths, and increasing the ambient humidity to >50%, by using room humidifiers; also using tepid water baths containing bath oils for hydration, followed by immediate liberal application of emollient ointments, such as hydrated petolatum. If skin is inflamed, use medium-potency glucocorticoid ointments, applied twice daily until the eczematous component has resolved.

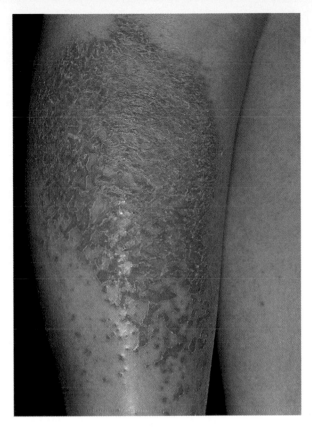

**FIGURE 2-25    Asteatotic dermatitis (eczema craquelé)**   *Erythema with a tessellated (tilelike) pattern arising in fissures on an area of xerosis of the lower leg of a 46-year-old female. Occurred in midwinter.*

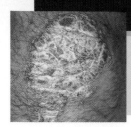

# PSORIASIS

Psoriasis is a challenge for the physician, because chronic generalized psoriasis is one of the "miseries that beset mankind," causing shame and embarrassment and a compromised lifestyle. The "heartbreak of psoriasis" is no joke. As the writer John Updike (who himself has psoriasis) so poignantly said about being a person with psoriasis, "I am silvery, scaly. Puddles of flakes form wherever I rest my flesh. Lusty, though we are loathsome to love. Keen-sighted, though we hate to look upon ourselves. The name of the disease, spiritually speaking, is Humiliation."

Psoriasis, which affects 1.5 to 2% of the population in western countries, is a hereditary disorder of skin with several clinical expressions. The most frequent type is *psoriasis vulgaris*, which occurs as chronic, recurring, scaling papules and plaques. Clinical presentation varies in individuals, from those with only a few localized plaques to those with generalized skin involvement.

## CLASSIFICATION

**Psoriasis vulgaris**
  Acute guttate
  Chronic plaque
  Inverse
  Palmoplantar

**Psoriatic erythroderma**
**Pustular psoriasis**
  Pustular psoriasis of von Zumbusch
  Palmoplantar pustulosis
  Acrodermatitis continua

## PSORIASIS VULGARIS

### EPIDEMIOLOGY

**Age of Onset** *Early*: Peak incidence occurs at 22.5 years of age (in children, the mean age of onset is 8 years). *Late*: Presents about age 55. *Early onset* predicts a more severe and long-lasting disease, and there is usually a positive family history of psoriasis.

**Incidence** In the United States, there are 3 to 5 million persons with psoriasis. Most have localized psoriasis, but approximately 300,000 persons have generalized psoriasis.

**Sex** Equal incidence in males and females.

**Race** Low incidence in West Africans, Japanese, and Inuits; very low incidence or absence in North and South American Indians.

**Heredity** Polygenic trait. When one parent has psoriasis, 8% of offspring develop psoriasis; when both parents have psoriasis, 41% of children develop psoriasis. HLA types most frequently associated with psoriasis are HLA-B13, -B17, -Bw57, and, most importantly, HLA-Cw6.

**Trigger Factors** *Physical trauma* (Koebner's phenomenon) is a major factor in eliciting lesions; rubbing and scratching stimulate the psoriatic proliferative process. *Infections*: acute streptococcal infection precipitates guttate psoriasis. *Stress*: a factor in flares of psoriasis is said to be as high as 40% in adults and higher in children. *Drugs*: systemic glucocorticoids, oral lithium, antimalarial drugs, interferon, and

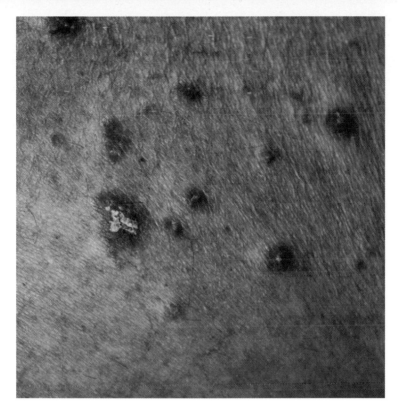

**FIGURE 3-1   Psoriasis vulgaris**   *Primary lesions are well-defined, reddish or salmon-pink papules, drop-like, with a loosely adherent silvery-white lamellar scale.*

β-adrenergic blockers can cause flares in existing psoriasis and cause a psoriasiform drug eruption. *Alcohol ingestion* is a putative trigger factor.

## PATHOGENESIS

The most obvious abnormality in psoriasis is an alteration of the cell kinetics of keratinocytes with a shortening of the cell cycle from 311 to 36 h, resulting in 28 times the normal production of epidermal cells. The epidermis and dermis react as an integrated system: the described changes in the germinative layer of the epidermis and inflammatory changes in the dermis, which trigger the epidermal changes. Psoriasis is a T cell–driven disease. There are many T cells present in psoriatic lesions surrounding the upper dermal blood vessels, and the cytokine spectrum is that of a $T_H1$ response.

Maintenance of psoriatic lesions is considered an ongoing autoreactive immune response.

## HISTORY

There are two types:

1.  *Eruptive, inflammatory type* with multiple small (guttate or nummular) lesions and a greater tendency toward spontaneous resolution (Figs. 3-1 and 3-3); relatively rare (<2.0% of all psoriasis); similar to an exanthem: a shower of lesions appears rather rapidly and in young adults, often but not always following streptococcal pharyngitis.
2.  *Chronic stable (plaque) psoriasis* (Figs. 3-2; 3-4): Majority of patients, with chronic indolent lesions present for months and years, changing only slowly.

**Skin Symptoms**　Pruritus is reasonably common, especially in scalp and anogenital psoriasis.

## PHYSICAL EXAMINATION

### Skin Lesions

The classic lesion of psoriasis is a sharply marginated erythematous papule with a silvery-white scale (Fig. 3-1). Scales are lamellar, loose, and easily removed by scratching. Removal of scale results in the appearance of minute blood droplets (*Auspitz' sign*). Papules grow to sharply marginated plaques with lamellar scaling (Fig. 3-2) that coalesce to form polycyclic or serpiginous patterns (Fig. 3-4). May occur anywhere on the body but there are classic predilection sites (see Image 3-1).

*Acute Guttate Type* Salmon-pink papules (guttate: Latin *gutta*, "drop"), 2.0 mm to 1.0 cm with or without scales (Figs. 3-1; 3-3) scales may not be visible but become apparent upon scraping. Scattered discrete lesions, like a rash; generally concentrated on the trunk (Fig. 3-3), less on the face and scalp, and usually sparing palms and soles. Guttate lesions may resolve spontaneously within a few weeks but usually become recurrent and may evolve into chronic, stable psoriasis.

*Chronic Stable Type* Sharply marginated, dull-red plaques with loosely adherent, lamellar, silvery-white scales (Fig. 3-2). Plaques coalesce to form polycyclic, geographic lesions (Fig. 3-4) and may partially regress, resulting in annular, serpiginous, and arciform patterns. Lamellar scaling can easily be removed, or, when the lesion is extremely chronic, it adheres tightly to the underlying inflammatory and infiltrated skin, resulting in hyperkeratosis that looks like asbestos or the shell of an oyster (Fig. 3-2).

### Distribution and Predilection Sites

*Acute Guttate* Disseminated, generalized, mainly trunk (Fig. 3-3).

*Chronic Stable* Single lesion or lesions localized to one or more predilection sites: elbows, knees, sacral-gluteal region, scalp, palm/soles (Graph 3-1). Sometimes only regional involvement (scalp), often generalized.

*Pattern* Bilateral, often symmetric (predilection sites); often spares exposed areas; facial region is *uncommonly* involved, and when involved, it is usually associated with a refractory type of psoriasis.

### Special Sites

**Palms and Soles**　May be the only areas involved. There is massive silvery white or yellowish hyperkeratosis and scaling, which in contrast to lesions on the trunk, is not easily removed (Figs. 3-5 and 3-6). Desquamation of hyperkeratosis will, however, reveal an inflammatory plaque at the base that is always sharply demarcated (Fig. 3-5). There may be cracking and painful fissures and bleeding.

**Scalp**　Plaques, sharply marginated, with thick adherent scales (Fig. 3-7). Scattered discrete or diffuse involvement of entire scalp. Often very pruritic. *Note*: psoriasis of the scalp does not lead to hair loss, even after years of thick plaque-type involvement. Scalp psoriasis may be part of generalized psoriasis or coexist with isolated plaques, or the scalp may be only site involved.

**Chronic Psoriasis of the Perianal and Genital Regions and of the Body Folds—Inverse Psoriasis**　Due to the warm and moist environment in these regions psoriatic plaques are usually not scaly but are bright red and fissured (Fig. 3-8). The sharp demarcation permits distinction from intertrigo, candidiasis, contact dermatitis, tinea cruris.

**Nails**　Fingernails and toenails frequently (25%) involved, especially with concomitant arthritis (Fig. 3-9). Nail changes include pitting, subungual hyperkeratosis, onycholysis, and yellowish-brown spots under the nail plate—the *oil spot* (pathognomonic) (see Fig. 30-9).

## LABORATORY EXAMINATIONS

### Dermatopathology

- Marked overall thickening of the epidermis (acanthosis) and thinning of epidermis over elongated dermal papillae
- Increased mitosis of keratinocytes, fibroblasts, and endothelial cells
- Parakeratotic hyperkeratosis (nuclei retained in the stratum corneum)
- Inflammatory cells in the dermis (lymphocytes and monocytes) and in the epidermis (polymorphonuclear cells), forming microabscesses of Munro in the stratum corneum.

**Serology**　Increased antistreptolysin titer in acute guttate psoriasis with antecedent streptococcal infection. Sudden onset of psoriasis may be associated with HIV infection. Determination of HIV serostatus is indicated in at-risk individuals. Serum uric acid is increased in 50%

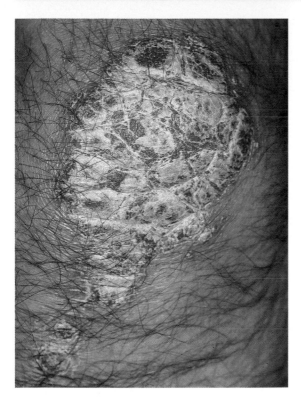

**FIGURE 3-2    Psoriasis vulgaris:
elbow**   *Well-demarcated, dull-red
plaque with a thick whitish scale, which
has arisen from the coalescence of
smaller papular lesions.*

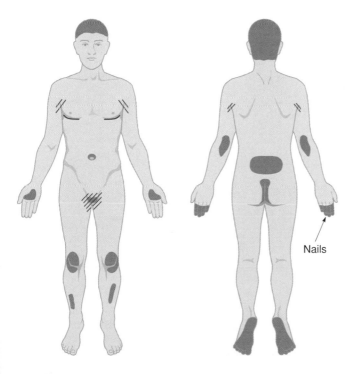

Nails

**IMAGE 3-1**   *Predilection
sites of psoriasis.*

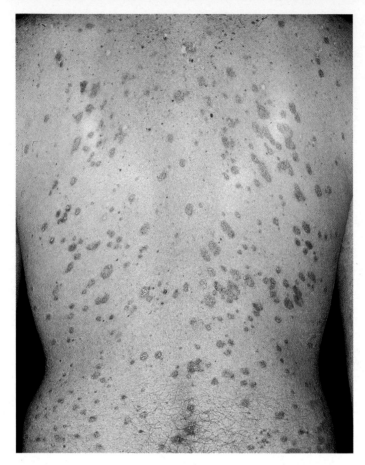

**FIGURE 3-3    Psoriasis vulgaris: trunk (guttate type)**    *Discrete, erythematous scaling, small papules and plaques on the trunk, appearing after a group A streptococcal pharyngitis. There was a family history of psoriasis.*

of patients, usually correlated with the extent of the disease; there is an increased risk of gouty arthritis. The levels of uric acid decrease as therapy is effective.

**Culture**    Throat culture for group A β-hemolytic streptococcus infection.

## DIAGNOSIS AND DIFFERENTIAL DIAGNOSIS

Diagnosis is made on clinical grounds.

**Acute Guttate Psoriasis**    Any maculopapular drug eruption, secondary syphilis, pityriasis rosea.

**Small Scaling Plaques**    *Seborrheic dermatitis*—may be indistinguishable in sites involved and morphology; sometimes termed *seborrhiasis*. *Lichen simplex chronicus*—may complicate psoriasis as a result of pruritus. *Psoriasiform drug eruptions*—especially beta blockers, gold, and methyldopa. *Tinea corporis*—KOH examination is mandatory, particularly in single lesions. *Mycosis fungoides*—scaling plaques can be an initial stage of mycosis fungoides.

**Large Geographic Plaques**    Tinea corporis, mycosis fungoides.

**Scalp Psoriasis**    Seborrheic dermatitis, tinea capitis.

**Inverse Psoriasis**    Tinea, candidiasis, intertrigo, extramammary Paget's disease. *Glucagonoma syndrome*—an important differential because this is a serious disease; the lesions  look like intertriginous psoriasis (see Section 17). Langerhans cell histiocytosis, Hailey-Hailey disease.

**Nails**    Onychomycosis. KOH is mandatory.

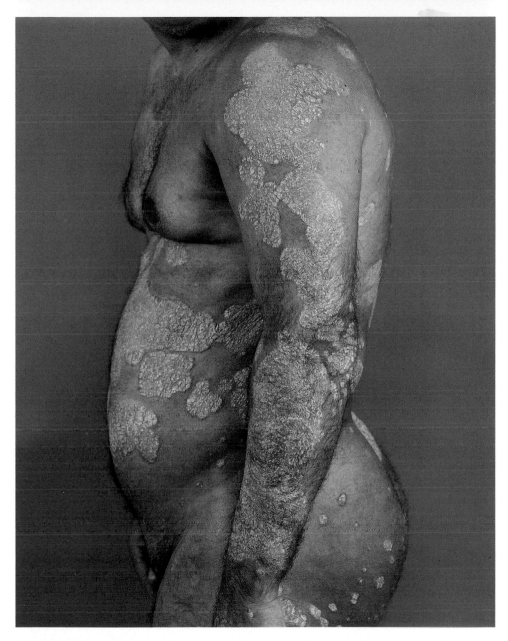

**FIGURE 3-4   Psoriasis vulgaris: chronic stable type**   *Multiple large scaling plaques on the trunk, arm, buttocks, and abdomen. Lesions are polycyclic and confluent forming geographic patterns. This patient was cleared by acitretin/PUVA combination treatment within 4 weeks.*

## COURSE AND PROGNOSIS

Acute guttate psoriasis appears rapidly, a generalized "rash." Sometimes this type of psoriasis disappears spontaneously in a few weeks without any treatment. More often, guttate psoriasis evolves into chronic plaque psoriasis. This is stable and may undergo remission after months or years, recur, and be a lifelong companion.

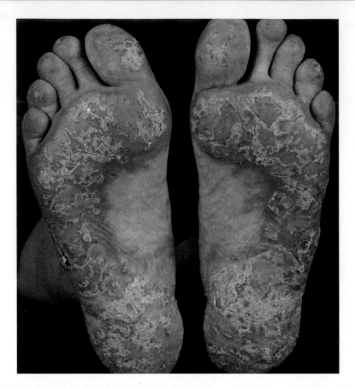

**FIGURE 3-5    Psoriasis vulgaris: soles**  *Well-demarcated, erythematous plaques with thick, yellowish lamellar scale and desquamation on sites of pressure arising on the plantar feet; similar lesions were present on the palms.*

**FIGURE 3-6 (Opposite page, top)    Psoriasis vulgaris: palm**  *Silvery-white scaly plaque, sharply demarcated, of irregular configuration. On palms and soles the lamellar scales are more adherent than on other parts of the body and only their removal will reveal the reddish inflammatory base.*

**FIGURE 3-7 (Opposite page, bottom)    Psoriasis vulgaris: scalp**  *Only the margin of this hyperkeratotic plaque on the scalp reveals the red, inflammatory nature of this extremely pruritic lesion. Right above the ear the lamellar scales bound down by hair have been removed by scratching revealing beefy-red base of the lesion.*

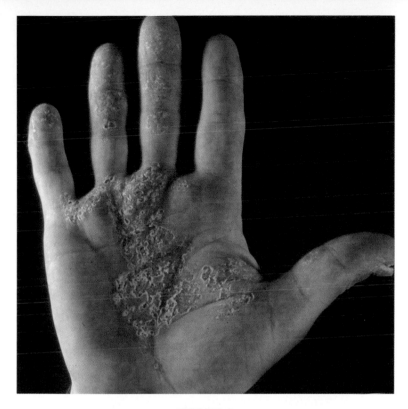

FIGURE 3-6

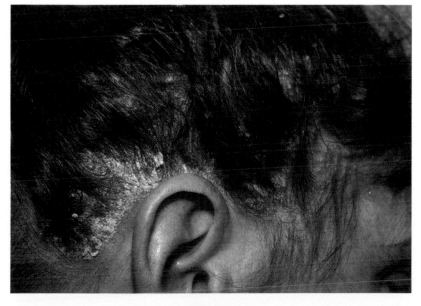

FIGURE 3-7

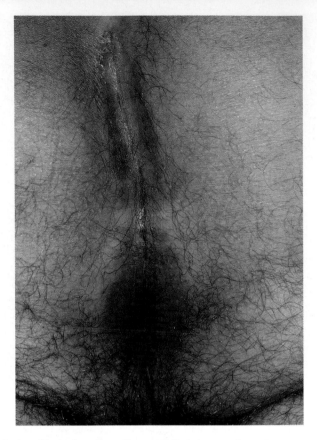

**FIGURE 3-8    Psoriasis vulgaris: inverse pattern**    *Well-demarcated, erythematous plaque (so-called "pinking") of the intergluteal fold (may be only skin manifestation), perianal area, and medial raphe of a 30-year-old male with psoriasis of elbows, knees, and fingernails. So-called inverse pattern psoriasis occurs in moist intertriginous sites (skin touching skin): in the axillae, inframammary region, umbilicus, and intergluteal/inguinal folds and is commonly mistaken for candidiasis or tinea corporis, seborrheic and intertriginous dermatitis.*

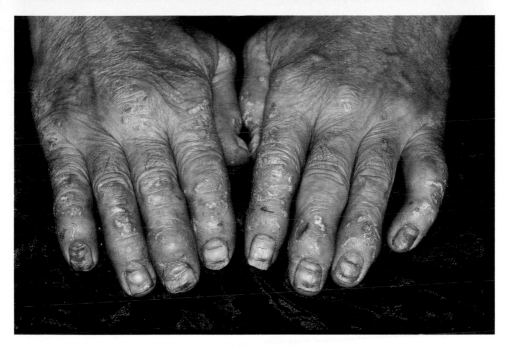

**FIGURE 3-9   Psoriasis vulgaris: hands with nail involvement; and psoriatic arthritis**   *Striking joint swelling of the distal interphalangeal and several metacarpophalangeal joints with associated severe nail dystrophy. The transverse nail ridges are associated with psoriatic involvement of the nail matrix.*

# PUSTULAR PSORIASIS

Characterized by pustules, not papules, arising on normal or inflamed, erythematous skin. Two types.

## PALMOPLANTAR PUSTULOSIS    ▢ ◑

Palmoplantar pustulosis is a chronic, relapsing eruption limited to the palms and soles. Numerous very typical sterile, yellow, deep-seated pustules that evolve into dusky-red crusts. It is considered by some as a localized form of pustular psoriasis (Barber type) and by others as a separate entity.

## EPIDEMIOLOGY

**Incidence**  Low as compared to psoriasis vulgaris.
**Age of Onset**  50 to 60 years. More common in females (4:1).

## HISTORY

**Symptoms**  Stinging, burning → itching. Eruptions come and go, in waves.

## PHYSICAL EXAMINATION

**Skin Lesions**  Pustules in stages of evolution, 2 to 5 mm, deep-seated, yellow, develop into dusky-red macules and crusts; present in areas of erythema and scaling or normal skin (Fig. 3-10). Limited to palms and soles, may be only a localized patch on the sole or hand, or involve both hands and feet with a predilection of thenar and hypothenar, flexor aspects of fingers, heels, and insteps; acral portions of the fingers and toes usually spared.

## DIFFERENTIAL DIAGNOSIS

Conditions confined to palms and soles. Epidermal dermatophytosis (tinea manus, tinea pedis), dyshidrotic eczematous dermatitis, irritant or allergic contact dermatitis, herpes simplex virus (HSV) infection (if localized to one site).

## LABORATORY EXAMINATIONS

**KOH Preparations**  To exclude dermatophytosis.
**Bacterial or Viral Culture**  To exclude *Staphylococcus aureus* infection and HSV infection.
**Dermatopathology**  Edema and exocytosis of mononuclear cells that appear first to form a vesicle, and later myriads of neutrophils, which form a unilocular spongiform pustule. Acanthosis.

## COURSE AND PROGNOSIS

Persistent for years and characterized by unexplained remissions and exacerbations; rarely psoriasis vulgaris may develop elsewhere.

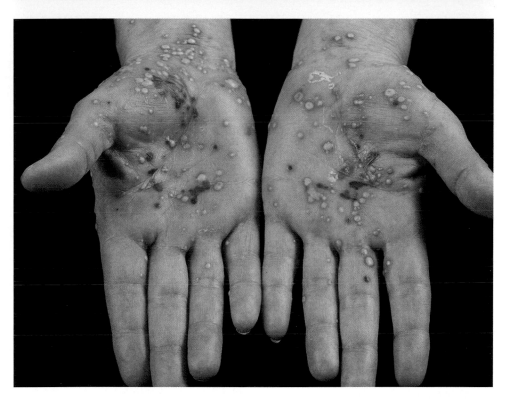

**FIGURE 3-10 Palmar pustulosis** *Deep-seated, dusky-red macules and creamy-yellow pustules progress to hyperkeratotic/crusted papules. Lesions are confined to the palms and/or soles and hardly extend over the wrist line. Because of the pustules, the disorder is commonly mistaken for a bacterial or, if confined to a single digit, for herpetic infection.*

## GENERALIZED ACUTE PUSTULAR PSORIASIS (VON ZUMBUSCH)   □  ●

This disorder can be a life-threatening medical problem with an abrupt onset. The skin involvement is distinctive and starts with a burning fiery-red erythema that spreads in hours with pinpoint pustules appearing in clusters. Fever, generalized weakness, severe malaise, and leukocytosis are prominent features in almost every patient.

## EPIDEMIOLOGY

Rare, occurs in adults, rarely in children.

## PATHOGENESIS

Unknown. The fever and leukocytosis result from the release of cytokines and chemokines from the skin into the circulation. There are no known precipitating factors, and the patient may or may not have had a stable plaque-type psoriasis in the past.

## HISTORY

**Onset of Lesions**    The constellation of fiery-red erythema followed by formation of pustules occurs over a period of less than 1 day. Waves of pustules may follow each other; as one set dries, another appears.
**Skin Symptoms**    Marked burning, tenderness.
**Constitutional Symptoms**    Headache, chills, feverishness, marked fatigue, severe malaise.

## PHYSICAL EXAMINATION

**Appearance of Patient**    Frightened, "toxic."
**Vital Signs**    Fast pulse, rapid breathing, fever that may be high.
**Skin Lesions**    There is a sequence of burning, diffuse erythema followed by the appearance of clusters of tiny, nonfollicular, and very superficial yellowish to whitish pustules that usually become confluent, forming circinate lesions and "lakes" of pus (Figs. 3-11 and 3-12), Nikolsky's phenomenon is positive. Removal of the tops of pustules yields superficial, oozing erosions. Crusting. Once crusts are shed, new crops of pustules may appear in the same site. The eruption is generalized.
**Hair and Nails**    Nails become thickened, and there is onycholysis; subungual "lakes" of pus lead to shedding of nails; hair loss of the telogen defluvium type may develop in 2 or 3 months.
**Mucous Membranes**    Circinate desquamation of the tongue. This is the only form of psoriasis that involves mucous membranes.

## DIFFERENTIAL DIAGNOSIS

**Widespread Erythema with Pustules**    The abrupt onset and the typical evolution of erythema followed by pustulation are highly characteristic. Nevertheless, blood cultures should always be obtained because of possible superinfection and bacteremia, especially with *S. aureus*. Generalized HSV infection has umbilicated pustules, and the Tzanck tests and viral cultures establish the diagnosis. Generalized pustular drug eruptions [e.g., after furosemide, amoxicillin/clavulanic acid, and other drugs (see Fig. 20-2)] may be clinically indistinguishable, but patients are less toxic.

## LABORATORY EXAMINATIONS

**Dermatopathology**    Large spongiform pustules resulting from the migration of neutrophils to the upper stratum malpighi, where they aggregate within the interstices between the degenerated and thinned keratinocytes.
**Bacterial Culture of Tissue**    Rule out *S. aureus* infection.
**Hematologic**    Polymorphonuclear leukocytosis —white blood cell count as high as 20,000/$\mu$L.

## COURSE AND PROGNOSIS

These patients are often brought to the emergency rooms of hospitals, and there is the question of overwhelming bacteremia until a dermatologist is consulted and the blood cultures are shown to be negative. Relapses and remissions may occur over a period of years. In the elderly prognosis is guarded if not treated. May follow, evolve into, or be followed by psoriasis vulgaris.

## SPECIAL TYPES

**Impetigo Herpetiformis**    This is von Zumbusch pustular psoriasis in a pregnant woman with hypocalcemia, leading to tetanic seizures.

  **Annular Type** of pustular psoriasis this occurs in children with less consitutional symptoms.
**Acrodermatitis Continua of Hallopeau**    This is a chronic recurrent pustulation of nail folds, nail bed, and distal fingers leading to loss of nails. It can occur alone or in association with pustular psoriasis of Zumbusch.

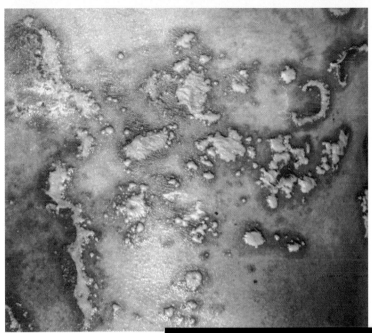

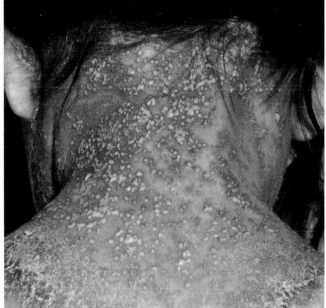

**FIGURE 3-11 (Top)    Generalized acute pustular psoriasis (von Zumbusch)**    *Multiple, creamy-white pustules on an erythematous base coalesce to form lakes of pus. These primary lesions rupture, resulting in large areas of secondary erosion.*

**FIGURE 3-12 (Bottom)    Generalized acute pustular psoriasis (von Zumbusch)**    *In a female patient who was toxic, had fever, and peripheral leukocytosis. Only the neck is shown but the entire body was covered with showers of creamy-white coalescing pustules on a fiery-red base. Since these pustules are very superficial they can be literally whipped off, which results in red oozing erosions.*

## PSORIATIC ERYTHRODERMA   

This is a condition in which psoriasis involves practically the entire skin and leads to constitutional symptoms. It is a serious condition and is discussed in Section 8.

## PSORIATIC ARTHRITIS   

Psoriatic arthritis is included among the seronegative spondyloarthropathies, which include ankylosing spondylitis, enteropathic arthritis, and Reiter's syndrome. Asymmetric peripheral joint involvement of upper extremities and especially smaller joints. Associated with MHC class I antigens, while rheumatoid arthritis is associated with MHC class II antigens. Incidence is 5 to 8%. Rare before age 20. *May be present (in 10% of individuals) without any visible psoriasis; if so, search for a family history.*

### TYPES

1. "Distal"—seronegative, without subcutaneous nodules, and involving, asymmetrically, a few distal interphalangeal joints of the hands and feet: an asymmetric oligoarthritis (see Fig. 3-9).
2. Enthesitis—inflammation of ligament insertion into bone.
3. Multilating psoriatic arthritis with bone erosion and ultimately leading to osteolysis or ankylosis.
4. "Axial"—especially involving the sacroiliac, hip, and cervical areas with ankylosing spondylitis.

### SKIN SYMPTOMS AND SIGNS

Swelling, redness, tenderness of involved joints or site of enthesitis (e.g., insertion of Achilles tendon in calcaneus). Dactylitis—sausage fingers. May or may not be associated with psoriasis elsewhere. Often psoriatic involvement of fingertips and periungual skin (see Fig. 3-9). Massive nail involvement by psoriasis is frequent.

## MANAGEMENT OF PSORIASIS

### Factors Influencing Selection of Treatment

1. Age: childhood, adolescence, young adulthood, middle age, >60 years.
2. Type of psoriasis: guttate, plaque, palmar and palmopustular, generalized pustular psoriasis, erythrodermic psoriasis.
3. Site and extent of involvement: *localized* to palms and soles, scalp, anogenital area, scattered plaques but <5% involvement; *generalized* and >30% involvement.
4. Previous treatment: ionizing radiation, systemic glucocorticoids, photochemotherapy (PUVA), cyclosporine (CS), methotrexate (MTX).
5. Associated medical disorders (e.g., HIV disease).

Ideally all patients with suspected psoriasis should be seen at least once by a dermatologist to establish the diagnosis and select the best available treatment regimen. Localized psoriasis (covering <5% of the body surface) can be managed by the primary care physician if a proper regimen is selected. Psoriasis of all other types, especially generalized psoriasis, should be managed by a dermatologist who has access to and knowledge of all therapies, as combinations and "rotational" therapy shifting from ultraviolet to PUVA to MTX or the "biologicals."

In the following pages management of psoriasis is discussed in the context of types of psoriasis, sites, and extent of involvement.

## LOCALIZED PSORIASIS

This consists of a limited number of chronic stable psoriasis plaques (see Fig. 3-2) on the predilection sites or elsewhere. Here, first-line therapies are topical treatments.

### Trunk and Extremities

- Topical fluorinated glucocorticoids (betamethasone valerate, fluocinolone acetonide, betamethasone propionate, clobetasol propionate) in *ointment* base applied after the scales are removed by soaking in water. Ointment applied to wet skin, covered with plastic wrap, left on overnight. Glucocorticoid-impregnated tape useful for small plaques.
- Hydrocolloid dressing, left on for 24 to 48 h, is effective and prevents scratching. During the day, classes I and II fluorinated glucocorticoid creams can be used without occlusion. Patients develop tolerance (tachyphylaxis) after long periods. *Caveat*: Prolonged application of the fluorinated glucocorticoids leads to atrophy of the skin, permanent striae, and unsightly telangiectasia. Clobetasol-17-propionate is stronger and active even without occlusion. To avoid systemic effects of this class I glucocorticoid: maximum of 50 g ointment per week.
- For small plaques ($\leq$4cm), triamcinolone acetonide aqueous suspension 3 mg/mL diluted with normal saline is injected into the lesion. Must be *intradermal*. *Warning*: Hypopigmentation at the injection site can result; this is more apparent in brown and black skin but is reversible.
- Topical anthralin preparations are excellent when used properly. Can be very irritant; therefore follow directions on the package insert with attention to details.
- Vitamin D analogues (calcipotriene, 0.005%, ointment and cream) are good nonsteroidal antipsoriatic topical agents and are not associated with cutaneous atrophy. Not as potent as class I glucocorticoids (e.g., clobetasol propionate) but can be combined with them. Calcipotriene should not be applied to more than 40% of the body surface and not more than 100 g per week to avoid hypercalcemia. Topical tacrolimus, 0.1%, has efficacy similar to that of vitamin D analogues.
- Tazarotene (a topical retinoid, 0.05 and 0.1% gel) is another alternative to topical glucocorticoids but can best be combined with class II (medium strength) topical glucocorticoids, as tazarotene can cause irritation.
- When there is >10% (palm of the hand =1%) involvement with psoriatic plaques, it is preferable to combine these topical treatments with 311-nm UVB phototherapy or PUVA photochemotherapy.

**Scalp**   *Mild* Superficial scaling and lacking thick plaques: Tar or ketoconazole shampoos *followed by* betamethasone valerate, 1% lotion; if refractory, clobetasol propionate, 0.05% scalp application.
*Severe* Thick, adherent plaques (Fig. 3-7): Removal of scales from plaques before active treatment by 10% salicylic acid in mineral oil, covered with a plastic cap and left on overnight. After shedding of scales, fluocinolone cream or lotion with the scalp covered with plastic or a shower cap, left on overnight or for 6 h. When the thickness of the plaques is reduced, clobetasol propionate, 0.05% lotion, or calcipotriene lotion can be used for maintenance. If unsuccessful or rapid recurrence or if associated with generalized psoriasis, consider systemic treatment (see below).

**Palms and Soles** (Figs. 3-5 and 3-6)   Occlusive dressings with class I topical *glucocorticoids* in petrolatum. If ineffective, *PUVA photochemotherapy*, administered in specially designed hand-and-foot lighting cabinets that deliver UVA. *PUVA "soaks"*: In this treatment the hands and feet are immersed in a solution of 8-methoxypsoralen (10 mg/L of warm water) for 15 min and then exposed to hand and foot UVA phototherapy units. Retinoids (acitretin > isotretinoin) given orally are effective in removing the thick hyperkeratosis of the palms and soles; however, combination with topical glucocorticoids or PUVA (Re-PUVA) is much more efficacious. Systemic treatments should be considered.

**Palmoplantar Pustulosis** (Fig. 3-10)   The condition is recalcitrant to treatment, but persistence in treatment can be rewarding.
*PUVA "Soaks" of Hands and Feet* (See above) Ideal for this condition. Re-PUVA (see below) is highly efficacious.
*Topical Glucocorticoids, Dithranol, and Coal Tar* Ineffective. Strong glucocorticoids under plastic occlusion (e.g., for the night) may be effective but do not prevent recurrences. MTX or CS for recalcitrant cases.

**Inverse Psoriasis** (Fig. 3-8)   Initiate therapy with *topical glucocorticoids* (caution: these are atrophy-prone regions, steroids should be applied for only limited periods of time); switch to topical vitamin D derivatives or tazarotene or topical tacrolimus or pimecrolimus. Tar baths or Castellani's paint sometimes useful. If resistant or recurrent, consider systemic therapy.

**Nails** (Figs. 3-9, 30-6)   Topical treatments of the fingernails are unsatisfactory. Note also that nail psoriasis may disappear spontaneously or pari passu with successful treatment of psoriasis. Injection of the nail fold with intradermal triamcinolone acetonide (3 mg/mL) effective but painful and impractical when all nails are involved. PUVA photochemotherapy somewhat effective when administered in special hand-and-foot lighting units providing high-intensity UVA. Long-term systemic retinoids (acitretin, 0.5 mg/kg) are also effective, as are systemic MTX and CS therapy. Since a diseased nail (plate) cannot be cured, therapy of nails aims at securing *regrowth* of a normal nail plate. It therefore depends on the speed of nail growth, which is slow and thus requires a long time; this should be taken into account when considering treatment that may cause side effects when administered over a prolonged period of time.

## GENERALIZED PSORIASIS

**Acute, Guttate Psoriasis** (Fig. 3-3)
Treat streptococcal infection with antibiotics. Topical treatment as for localized psoriasis. Narrow-band UVB irradiation most effective. If it fails, oral PUVA photochemotherapy (see below).

**Generalized Plaque-Type Psoriasis** (Fig. 3-4)
Performed either by office-based dermatologist or in a psoriasis center where all major options are available: phototherapy, PUVA, or systemic treatments which are given as either mono- or combined or rotational therapy. Combination therapy denotes the combination of two or more modalities (as in chemotherapy); rotational therapy denotes switching the patient after clearing and a subsequent relapse to another different treatment. This is done to prevent cumulative long-term side effects.

**Narrow-Band UVB Phototherapy**   (311 nm) Effective only in psoriasis with very thin plaques; effectiveness is increased by combination with topical glucocorticoids, vitamin D analogues, tazarotene, or topical tacrolimus.

**Oral PUVA Photochemotherapy**   Treatment consists of oral ingestion of 8-methoxypsoralen (8-MOP) (0.6 mg 8-MOP per kilogram body weight) or, in some European countries, 5-MOP (1.2 mg/kg body weight) and exposure to doses of UVA that are adjusted to the sensitivity of the patient. UVA is given 1 h (8-MOP) or 2 h (5-MOP) after ingestion of the psoralen, starting at a dose of 0.5 to 1 $J/cm^2$, adjusted upward for skin phototype. Alternatively, phototoxicity testing is done prior to treatment, which permits a better adjustment of the UVA dose to the individual's sensitivity to PUVA. The UVA dose is increased at successive treatment sessions. Treatments are performed two or three times a week or, with a more aggresive protocol, four times a week. Most patients clear after 19 to 25 treatments, and the amount of UVA needed ranges from 100 to 245 $J/cm^2$. *Long-term side effects*: PUVA keratoses and squamous cell carcinomas in some patients who receive an excessive number of treatments. Re-PUVA (see below) reduces the total number of treatments.

In patients with recalcitrant plaque-type psoriasis, acitretin (in males) or isotretinoin (in females) may be combined with other antipsoriatic therapy, e.g., PUVA, UVB (311 nm), topical glucocorticoids, or anthralin. These combination modalities reduce the length of treatments as well as the total amount of antipsoriatic drug necessary for clearing. Topical glucocorticoids, calcipotriene ointments, anthralin, oral MTX, and oral acitretin, combined with either PUVA or 311-nm UVB, are all effective in reducing the dose of one another.

**Oral Retinoids**   Acitretin, and isotretinoin are very effective in inducing desquamation but only moderately effective in suppressing psoriatic plaques (an exception is pustular psoriasis—see below). They are highly effective when combined according to established protocols with narrow-band UVB and PUVA photochemotherapy (called Re-PUVA). The latter is in fact the most effective therapy to date for generalized plaque psoriasis. A combination of PUVA with acitretin (25 to 50 mg/d) is used for males; for females, PUVA is combined with isotretinoin (1 mg/kg body weight). Contraception is mandatory during treatment and for 2 months after it is completed. Combinations of oral retinoids and PUVA improve the efficacy of each and permit a reduction of the dose and duration of each if refractory to treatment. For side effects of retinoids, see page 6.

**Methotrexate Therapy[1]**   Oral MTX is one of the most effective treatments and certainly the most convenient treatment for generalized plaque-

---

[1] For details regarding MTX therapy of psoriasis, see HH Roenigk Jr et al: Methotrexate in psoriasis: Revised guidelines. J Am Acad Dermatol 19:145, 1988.

type psoriasis. Nevertheless, MTX is a potentially dangerous drug, principally because of liver toxicity that can occur after prolonged use. Hepatic toxicity may occur after cumulative doses in normal persons (1.5 g), but additional risk factors include a history of or actual alcohol intake, abnormal liver chemistries, IV drug use, and obesity. Inasmuch as hepatic toxicity is related to total life dose, this therapy should, in general, not be given to young patients who may face many years of therapy.

***Schedule of Methotrexate Therapy with the Triple-Dose (Weinstein) Regimen*** Preferred by most over the single-dose MTX once weekly. Begin with a test dose of 5 mg (2.5-mg tablet followed 24 h later with a second 2.5-mg tablet); this dose will ascertain whether there is a special sensitivity to MTX. A complete blood count (CBC), liver function tests, and serum creatinine levels are obtained before start of treatment, after 1 week, and every week thereafter as the dose of MTX is increased. One tablet (2.5 mg) is given every 12 h for a total of three doses, i.e., 7.5 mg/week (1/1/1 tablet schedule). Some patients respond to this dose; if not, the dose is increased after 2 weeks to 2/2/2, or 15 mg/week total dose. This regimen achieves an 80% improvement but total clearing only in some, and higher doses increase the risk of toxicity. The dose of MTX can be reduced by one or two tablets periodically.

***CBC, Liver Function, and Creatinine*** These have to be monitored every 3 months. In patients with normal liver chemistries and no risk factors present, a liver biopsy should be done after a cumulative dose of approximately 1500 mg MTX; if the post-MTX liver biopsy is normal, repeat liver biopsy should be done after further therapy with an additional 1000 to 1500 mg MTX. Be aware of the various drug interactions with MTX.

**Cyclosporine[2]** CS treatment is highly effective at a dose of 3 to 5 mg/kg per day. As the patient responds, the dose is tapered to the lowest effective maintenance dose. Monitoring blood pressure and serum creatinine is mandatory because of the known nephrotoxicity of the drug. *CS should be employed only in patients without risk factors.*

**Monoclonal Antibodies and Fusion Proteins** Some of these proteins, specifically targeted to pathogenically relevant receptors on T cells or cytokines, have been recently approved and more are being developed. They should be employed only by specifically trained dermatologists who are familiar with the dosage schedules, drug interactions, and short- or long-term side effects. *Alefacept* targets CD45RO-positive memory T cells, is given intramuscularly, and is only moderately effective but induces long periods of remission. *Infliximab*, a monoclonal antibody that targets tumor necrosis factor α (TNF-α), is highly effective for plaque psoriasis and psoriatic arthritis but may reactivate latent tuberculosis. *Etanercept*, a fusion protein of the TNF-α receptor with the Fc of IgG1, is highly effective for psoriatic arthritis but less so for plaque psoriasis. *Efalizumab* targets CD11α on T cells and is also effective but there are rebounds. Long-term safety of these "biologicals" has yet to be determined. For doses, warnings, and side effects, see package.

## GENERALIZED PUSTULAR PSORIASIS
(Figs. 3-11, 3-12)

These ill patients with generalized rash should be hospitalized and treated in the same manner as patients with extensive burns, toxic epidermal necrolysis, or exfoliative erythroderma—in a specialized unit: isolation, fluid replacement, and repeated blood cultures are necessary. Rapid suppression and resolution of lesions is achieved by oral retinoids (acitretin, 50 mg/d). Supportive measures should include fluid intake, IV antibiotics to prevent septicemia, cardiac support, temperature control, topical lubricants, and antiseptic baths. Systemic glucocorticoids to be used only as rescue intervention as rapid tachyphylaxis occurs. Oral PUVA photochemotherapy is effective, but logistics are usually prohibitive in a toxic patient with fever.

## ACRODERMATITIS CONTINUA HALLOPEAU

Oral retinoids as in von Zumbusch pustular psoriasis; MTX, once-a-week schedule, is the second-line choice.

## PSORIATIC ARTHRITIS

Should be recognized early in order to prevent bony destruction. MTX, once-a-week schedule as outlined above; infliximab or etanercept are highly effective.

---

[2] For details and drug interactions see MJ Mihatsch, K Wolff: Consensus Conference on Cyclosporin A for Psoriasis. Br J Dermatol 126:621, 1992.

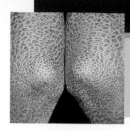

# S E C T I O N 4

# ICHTHYOSES

A group of hereditary disorders characterized by an excess accumulation of cutaneous scale, varying from very mild and asymptomatic to life-threatening. A relatively large number of types of ichthyoses exist; most are extremely rare and often part of multiorgan syndromes. The four most common and important types are discussed here plus a brief discussion of two types affecting newborns. Support groups such as Foundation for Ichthyosis and Related Skin Types (FIRST) exist.

## CLASSIFICATION

Dominant ichthyosis vulgaris (DIV)
X-linked ichthyosis (XLI)
Lamellar ichthyosis (LI)
Epidermolytic hyperkeratosis (EH)

## ETIOLOGY AND PATHOGENESIS

Individual keratin genes may not be expressed or may result in the formation of abnormal keratins. In DIV and XLI, formation of thickened stratum corneum is caused by increased adhesiveness of the stratum corneum cells and/or failure of normal cell separation. Abnormal stratum corneum formation results in variable increases in transepidermal water loss. The etiology of the most common ichthyosis, DIV, is unknown; in XLI, there is a

steroid sulfatase deficiency. LI shows increased germinative cell hyperplasia and increased transit rate through the epidermis, and there is a transglutaminase deficiency. In EH, there are mutations in the genes encoding keratins 1 or 10; here the disturbance of epidermal differentiation and the expression of abnormal keratin genes result in vacuolization of the upper epidermal layers, blistering, and hyperkeratosis.

## HISTORY

All four types of ichthyosis tend to be worse during the dry, cold winter months and improve during the hot, humid summer. Patients living in tropical climates may remain symptom-free but may experience appearance or worsening of symptoms on moving to a temperate climate.

## ICHTHYOSIS VULGARIS   ■

Ichthyosis vulgaris is characterized by usually mild generalized xerosis with scaling, most pronounced on the lower legs, and by perifollicular hyperkeratosis (keratosis pilaris); frequently associated with atopy.

## EPIDEMIOLOGY

**Age of Onset**   3 to 12 months.
**Sex**   Equal incidence in males and females.
Autosomal dominant inheritance
**Incidence**   Common (1 in 250).

## PATHOGENESIS

Etiology unknown. There is reduced or absent filaggrin. Epidermis proliferates normally, but keratin is retained with a resultant thickened stratum corneum.

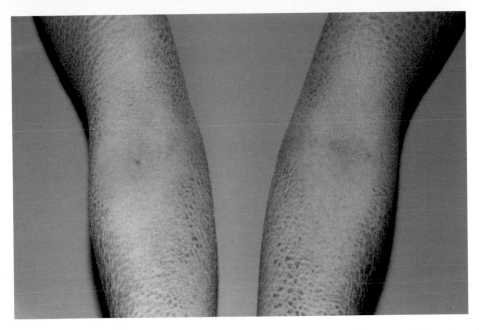

**FIGURE 4-1   Ichthyosis vulgaris: arms**   *Fish scale-like hyperkeratosis of the arms with sparing of the antecubital fossae.*

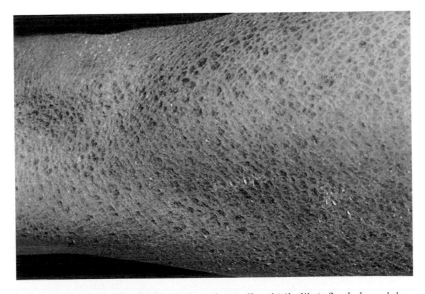

**FIGURE 4-2   Ichthyosis vulgaris: thigh**   *Brownish tessellated (tile-like), firmly bound down scales. The similarity to fish-skin or the skin of an amphibian is quite obvious.*

## HISTORY

Very commonly associated with atopy. Xerosis and pruritus worse in winter months. Cosmetic concern to many patients, particularly when hyperkeratosis is severe.

## PHYSICAL EXAMINATION

### Skin Lesions

Xerosis (dry skin) with fine, powdery scaling but also larger, firmly adherent tacked-down scales in a fish-scale pattern (Figs. 4-1 and 4-2). Diffuse general involvement, accentuated on the shins, arms, and back but also on the buttocks and lateral thighs; axillae and the anticubital and popliteal fossae spared (Fig. 4-1; Image 4-1); face usually also spared but cheeks and forehead may be involved. *Keratosis pilaris* is perifollicular hyperkeratosis with little, spiny hyperkeratotic follicular papules of normal skin color, either grouped or disseminated, mostly on the extensor surfaces of the extremities (Fig. 4-3); in childhood, also on cheeks. Hands and feet usually spared, but palmoplantar markings are more accentuated (hyperlinear).

**Associated Diseases**   More than 50% of individuals with DIV also have atopic dermatitis; rarely, keratopathy can occur.

## DIFFERENTIAL DIAGNOSIS

**Xerosis/Hyperkeratosis**   Xerosis; acquired ichthyosis (may be a paraneoplastic syndrome; drug-induced ichthyosis (triparanol); all other forms of ichthyosis.

## LABORATORY EXAMINATION

**Dermatopathology**   Compact hyperkeratosis; reduced or absent granular layer; germinative layer flattened. Electron microscopy: small, poorly formed keratohyalin granules.

## DIAGNOSIS

Usually by clinical findings; abnormal keratohyalin granules in electron microscopy.

## COURSE AND PROGNOSIS

Improvement in the summer, in humid climates, and in adulthood. Keratosis pilaris occurring on the cheeks during childhood usually improves during adulthood.

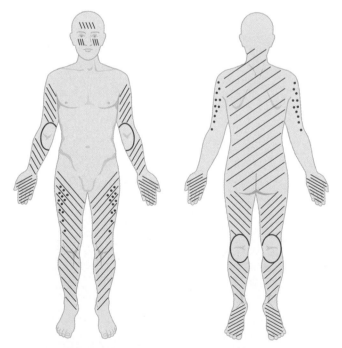

**IMAGE 4-1**   *Distribution of ichthyosis vulgaris. Dots indicate keratosis pilaris.*

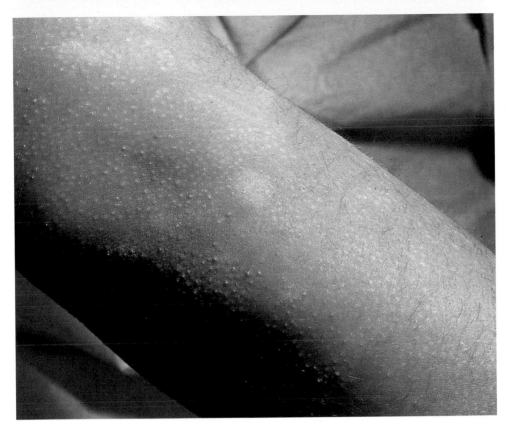

**FIGURE 4-3   Ichthyosis vulgaris. Keratosis pilaris: arm**   *Small, follicular, horny spines occur as a manifestation of mild ichthyosis vulgaris; arising mostly on the shoulders, upper arms and thighs. Desquamation of the nonfollicular skin results in hypomelanotic (less pigmented) spots similar to pityriasis alba (compare with Fig. 13-14).*

## MANAGEMENT

**Hydration of Stratum Corneum**  Pliability of stratum corneum is a function of its water content. Hydration best accomplished by immersion in a bath followed by the application of petrolatum. Urea-containing creams bind water in the stratum corneum.

**Keratolytic Agents**  Propylene glycol–glycerin– lactic acid mixtures. 6% salicylic acid in propylene glycol and alcohol, which is used under plastic occlusion. α-Hydroxy acids (lactic acid or glycolic acid) control scaling. Urea-containing preparations (2 to 10%) are effective.

**Systemic Retinoids**  Isotretinoin and acitretin are very effective, but careful monitoring for toxicity is required. Only severe cases may require intermittent therapy.

# X-LINKED ICHTHYOSIS ▯ ◐

X-linked ichthyosis (XLI) occurs only in males and is characterized by prominent, dirty brown scales occurring on the neck, extremities, trunk, and buttocks, with onset soon after birth.

## EPIDEMIOLOGY

**Age of Onset**   Birth or infancy. Males.
**Incidence**   1:2000 to 1:6000.

## ETIOLOGY AND PATHOGENESIS

X-linked recessive; gene locus Xp22.32.
**Genetic Defect**   Steroid sulfatase deficiency, which is associated with failure to shed senescent keratinocytes normally, resulting clinically in retention hyperkeratosis associated with normal epidermal proliferation.

## HISTORY

Onset of skin abnormality at 2 to 6 weeks of age; corneal opacities develop during the second to third week. Usually asymptomatic; may also be present in female carriers of XLI. Discomfort due to xerosis. Cosmetic disfigurement due to the dirty brown scales.

## PHYSICAL EXAMINATION

### Skin Lesions
Large adherent scales that appear brown or dirty (Fig. 4-4); most pronounced on posterior neck, extensor arms, antecubital and popliteal fossae, and trunk. Absence of palm/sole and face involvement (Image 4-2).
**Eye Lesions**   Comma-shaped stromal corneal opacities in 50% of adult males. Present in some female carriers. Asymptomatic.
**Genitourinary Abnormality**   Cryptorchidism in 20% of individuals.

## DIFFERENTIAL DIAGNOSIS

All forms of ichthyosis, contiguous gene syndromes.

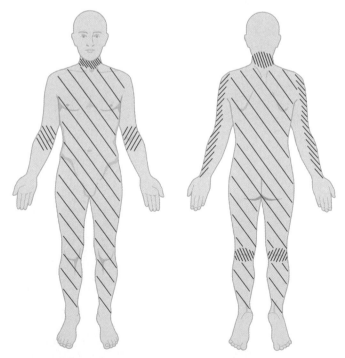

**IMAGE 4-2**   *Distribution of X-linked ichthyosis.*

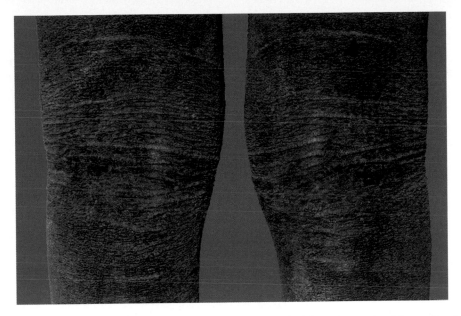

**FIGURE 4-4   X-linked ichthyosis: popliteal fossae**   *Almost black hyperkeratosis of the popliteal fossae gives a dirty, elephant skin-like appearance to the area.*

## LABORATORY EXAMINATIONS

**Chemistry**   Cholesterol sulfate level elevated. Increased mobility of β-lipoproteins in electrophoresis. Steroid sulfatase decreased or absent.
**Dermatopathology**   Hyperkeratosis; granular layer present, sometimes hypergranulosis.

## DIAGNOSIS

By family history and clinical findings.
**Prenatal Diagnosis**   Via amniocentesis and chorionic villus sampling; steroid sulfatase assay detects enzyme deficiency.

## COURSE AND PROGNOSIS

No improvement with age. Usually worse in temperate climates and in winter season. With placental sulfatase deficiency, failure of labor to begin or progress in mother carrying affected fetus.

## MANAGEMENT

### Topical Therapy
**Emollients**   Hydrated petrolatum.
**Keratolytics**   *Propylene glycol*, 44 to 60% in water, applied half strength after bath and occluded with a plastic suit worn as pajamas. When excess scaling has been removed, repeat once weekly as necessary.
**Other Agents**   Salicylic acid (beware of hypersalicism), urea, and α-hydroxy acids (glycolic acid, lactic acid) in various vehicles.

### Systemic Treatment
*Acitretin*, 0.5 to 1 mg/kg orally until marked improvement, then taper dose to maintenance level. Continuous laboratory monitoring and, in long-term regimens, x-rays for calcifications and diffuse idiopathic skeletal hyperostosis (DISH) syndrome mandatory.

# LAMELLAR ICHTHYOSIS   □  

Lamellar ichthyosis (LI) often presents at birth with the infant encased in a collodion–like membrane (collodion baby) (page 85) that is soon shed, with subsequent formation of large, coarse scales involving the entire body, including all flexural areas as well as the palms and soles. During childhood and adulthood, the skin is encased in this platelike scale, which causes significant cosmetic disfigurement.

## EPIDEMIOLOGY

**Age of Onset**   At birth, usually as collodion baby.
**Sex**   Presents equally in both sexes.
**Incidence**   ≤ 1:300,000.

## ETIOLOGY AND PATHOGENESIS

**Mode of Inheritance**   Autosomal recessive; gene locus is 14q11 in some families. Mutation in the gene encoding transglutaminase 1, an enzyme that catalyzes the cross-linking of proteins during the formation of cornified envelopes of corneocytes.

## HISTORY

Heat intolerance, usually during exercise and hot weather because of inability to sweat. Water loss (excess)/dehydration due to fissuring of stratum corneum. Increased nutritional requirements for young children due to rapid growth and shedding of stratum corneum. Painful palmar/plantar fissures.

## PHYSICAL EXAMINATION

### Skin Lesions
*Newborn* Collodion baby, encased in a translucent collodion-like membrane (see Fig. 4-8); shed in a few weeks. Ectropion; eclabion. Generalized erythroderma.
*Child/Adult* Large parchment–like hyperkeratosis (Fig. 4-5) over entire body; fracturing of the hyperkeratotic plate results in a tessellated (tilelike) pattern (Fig. 4-6). Scales are large and very thick and brown, over most of the body (Fig. 4-6), accentuated on lower extremities, and involving the flexural areas. Hyperkeratosis around joints may be verrucous. Hands/feet: keratoderma; accentuation of palmar/plantar

creases (Image 4-3). Erythroderma may develop.
**Hair**   Bound down by scales; frequent infections may result in scarring alopecia (Fig. 4-5).
**Nails**   Dystrophy secondary to nail fold inflammation.
**Mucous Membranes**   Usually spared.
**Eye Lesions**   Ectropion (Fig. 4-5).

## DIFFERENTIAL DIAGNOSIS

X-linked ichthyosis, epidermolytic hyperkeratosis, congenital ichthyosiform erythroderma, Netherton's syndrome, trichothiodystrophy.

## LABORATORY EXAMINATIONS

**Culture**   Rule out secondary infection and sepsis, especially in newborns.
**Dermatopathology**   Hyperkeratosis; granular layer present; acanthosis. Epidermal transglutaminase ↓.

## COURSE AND PROGNOSIS

Collodion membrane present at birth is shed within first few days to weeks (see Fig. 4-8). Newborns are at risk for hypernatremic dehydration, secondary infection, and sepsis. Disorder persists throughout life. No improvement with age. Obstruction of eccrine sweat glands with resultant impairment of sweating.

## MANAGEMENT

**Newborn**   Care in neonatal intensive care unit. High-humidity chamber. Emolliation. Monitor electrolytes, fluids. Follow for signs of local or systemic infection.
**Child/Adult**   *Emollients* Hydrated petrolatum.
*Keratolytics* As in XLI.

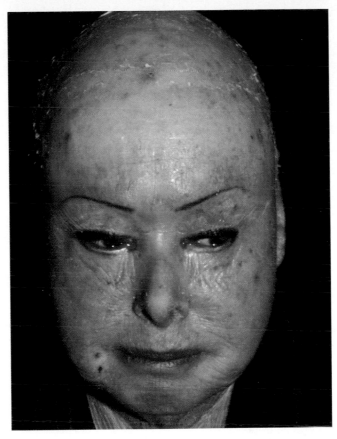

**FIGURE 4-5   Lamellar ichthyosis**   *Parchment-like hyperkeratosis gives the impression of the skin being too tight on the face of this woman. She has lost all hairs and there is pronounced ectropium.*

**Overheating**   Parents and affected individuals should be instructed about overheating and heat prostration that can follow exercise, high environmental temperatures, and fever. Repeated application of water to skin can somewhat replace function of sweating, cooling the body.

**Retinoids**   Acitretin, and, to a lesser degree, isotretinoin (0.5 to 1 mg/kg) are effective. Monitor continuously for serum triglycerides, transaminases, and bony toxicities if given over prolonged period of time. Teratogenicity requires effective contraception.

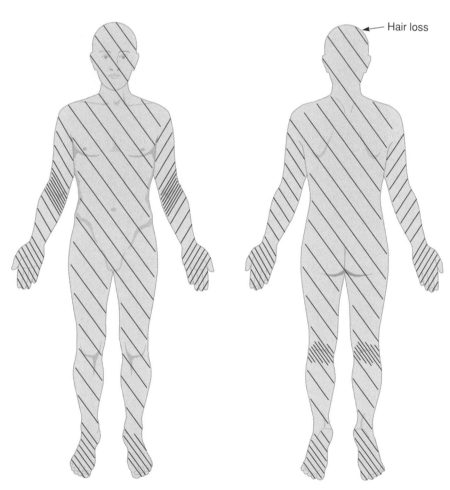

Hair loss

**IMAGE 4-3**   *Distribution of lamellar ichthyosis.*

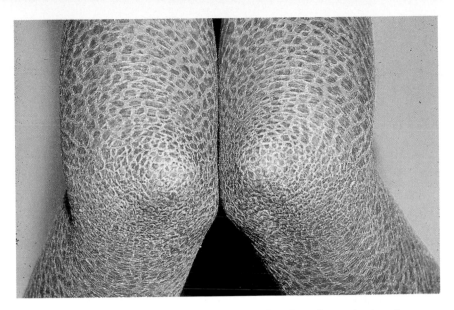

**FIGURE 4-6    Lamellar ichthyosis: arms**    *Tesselated (tile-like) hyperkeratosis gives the appearance of reptilian scales on the arms around the elbows. The entire body was involved and there was ectropium.*

# EPIDERMOLYTIC HYPERKERATOSIS

Epidermolytic hyperkeratosis (EH) presents at or shortly after birth with blistering. With time, the skin becomes keratotic and even verrucous, particularly in the flexural areas, knees, and elbows.

## EPIDEMIOLOGY

**Age of Onset**   Birth or shortly thereafter.
**Sex**   Equal incidence in males and females.
**Incidence:**   very rare.

## ETIOLOGY AND PATHOGENESIS

**Mode of Inheritance**   Autosomal dominant. Mutations of genes that encode the epidermal differentiation keratins, keratin 1 and 10.

## HISTORY

Blistering may recur periodically, leading to denuded areas, secondary infection, and sepsis. Hyperkeratotic lesions become verrucous, particularly in the flexural areas, and are associated with an unpleasant odor.

## PHYSICAL EXAMINATION

### Skin Lesions
Blistering at birth or shortly thereafter. Generalized or localized. Denuded areas heal with normal-appearing skin. With time, the skin becomes keratotic and verrucous (Fig. 4-7), particularly in the flexural areas, knees, and elbows. Hyperkeratotic scales adhere to underlying skin, often in a mountain range–like appearance; may be quite dark in color and associated with an unpleasant odor (like rancid butter). Recurrent blisters in hyperkeratotic areas (Fig. 4-7) and also shedding of hyperkeratotic masses result in circumscribed areas of skin that are relatively normal in appearance. A valuable diagnostic sign. Secondary pyogenic infections, especially impetigo.

Generalized distribution with prominent involvement of flexural areas (Image 4-4).

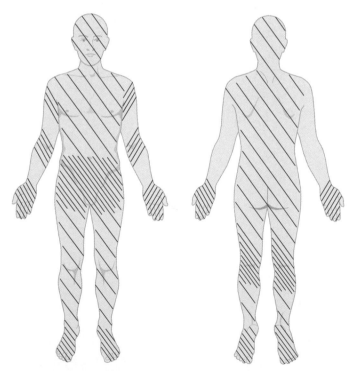

**IMAGE 4-4**   *Distribution of epidermolytic hyperkeratosis.*

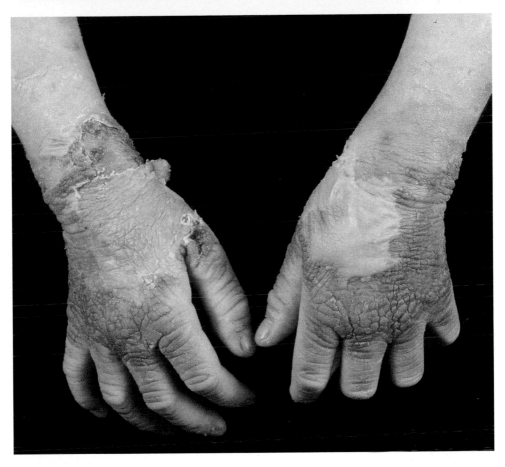

**FIGURE 4-7    Epidermolytic hyperkeratosis: arms and hands**    *Mountain range-like hyperkeratosis of the dorsum of hands with blistering that results in erosions and shedding of large sheets of keratin.*

Palmar and plantar involvement (hyperkeratosis). (*Note*: A variant of epidermolytic hyper-ker-atosis is localized to palms and soles and is genetically distinct from the generalized form.)

**Hair and Nails**    Hair normal, but involvement of the nails may produce abnormal nail plates.

**Mucous Membranes**    Spared.

### LABORATORY EXAMINATION

**Dermatopathology**    Giant, coarse keratohyalin granules and vacuolization of the granular layer, resulting in cell lysis and subcorneal multiloculated blisters. Papillomatosis, acanthosis, and hyperkeratosis.

### COURSE AND PROGNOSIS

Blister formation and massive hyperkeratosis are prone to bacterial superinfection, which is probably also responsible for the unpleasant odor. Palmar involvement can adversely affect manual dexterity.

### MANAGEMENT

Topical application of α-hydroxy acids. Antimicrobial therapy. Systemic retinoids (isotretinoin and acitretin) may transiently lead to a worsening of the condition because of increased blister formation but later improve the skin dramatically owing to a relative normalization of epidermal differentiation. Predisposes to impetigo. Determine dose carefully, and monitor for side effects.

# ICHTHYOSIS IN THE NEWBORN

## COLLODION BABY

Encasement of entire baby in a transparent parchment-like membrane (Fig. 4-8) impairs respiration and sucking. Breaking and shedding of the collodion membrane initially leads to difficulties in thermoregulation and increased risk of infection. Skin is bright red and moist. After healing, skin appears normal for some time until signs of ichthyosis develop. Collodion baby may be the initial presentation of lamellar ichthyosis or some less common forms of ichthyosis not discussed here. Collodion baby also may be a condition which, after the collodion membrane is shed and the resultant erythema has cleared, will progress to normal skin for the rest of the child's life (Fig. 4-8).

### MANAGEMENT

Newborns should be kept in an incubator in which the air is saturated with water. Careful monitoring of temperature and parenteral fluids and nutrient replacement may be necessary for some time. Infection of the skin and lungs is an important problem, and aggressive antibiotic therapy may be indicated.

## HARLEQUIN FETUS

Harlequin fetus is an extremely rare condition in which the child is born with very thick plates of stratum corneum separated by deep cracks and fissures. Eclabium, ectropion, and absence of or rudimentary ears result in a grotesque appearance. These babies usually die shortly after birth, but there are reports of survival for weeks to several months. This condition is different from collodion baby and the other forms of ichthyosis, with an unusual fibrous protein within the epidermis.

**FIGURE 4-8 (Opposite page)    Ichthyosis in the newborn**  *A.  "Collodion baby" shortly after birth with a parchment-like membrane covering the entire skin. The eyes and lips pucker outward, i.e., ectropion and eclabion.*  ***B.*** *At 6 months of age, the same infant is a beautiful baby with minimal residual scale and erythema on the cheeks.*

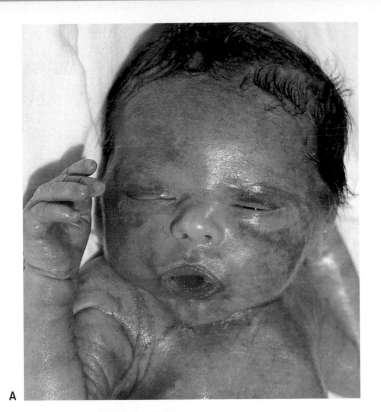

A

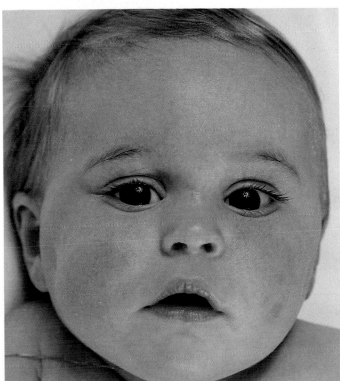

B

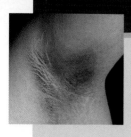

# MISCELLANEOUS EPIDERMAL DISORDERS

## ACANTHOSIS NIGRICANS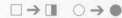

Acanthosis nigricans (AN) is a velvety thickening and hyperpigmentation of the skin, chiefly in axillae and other body folds, the etiology of which may be related to factors of heredity, associated endocrine disorders, obesity, drug administration, and malignancy (see Section 17, "Skin Signs of Systemic Cancers").

### CLASSIFICATION

**Type 1: Hereditary Benign AN**   No associated endocrine disorder.

**Type 2: Benign AN**   Endocrine disorders associated with insulin resistance: insulin-resistant diabetes mellitus, hyperandrogenic states, acromegaly/gigantism, Cushing's disease, hypogonadal syndromes with insulin resistance, Addison's disease, hypothyroidism.

**Type 3: Pseudo-AN**   Associated with obesity; more common in patients with darker pigmentation. Obesity produces insulin resistance.

**Type 4: Drug-induced AN**   Nicotinic acid in high dosage, stilbestrol in young males, glucocorticoid therapy, diethylstilbestrol/oral contraceptive, growth hormone therapy.

**Type 5: Malignant AN**   Paraneoplastic, usually adenocarcinoma of gastrointestinal or genitourinary tract; less commonly, lymphoma (see Section 17).

### EPIDEMIOLOGY

**Age of Onset**   Type 1: during childhood or puberty; other types dependent on associated conditions.

### ETIOLOGY AND PATHOGENESIS

Dependent on associated disorder. Epidermal changes may be caused by hypersecretion of pituitary peptide or nonspecific growth-promoting effect of hyperinsulinemia. Type 5: associated with transforming growth factor α and epidermal growth factor receptors in skin.

### HISTORY

Insidious onset; first visible change is darkening of pigmentation.

### PHYSICAL EXAMINATION

#### Skin Lesions
*All types of AN*: Darkening of pigmentation, skin appears dirty (Fig. 5-1). As skin thickens, appears velvety; skin lines accentuated; surface becomes rugose, mammillated. *Type 3*: velvety patch on inner, upper thigh at site of chafing; often has many skin tags in body folds and neck. *Type 5*: hyperkeratosis and hyperpigmentation more pronounced (see Fig. 17-14). Hyperkeratosis of palms/soles, with accentuation of papillary markings: "Tripe hands" (see Fig. 17-16), involvement of oral mucosa and vermilion border of lips (see Fig. 17-15).

**Distribution**   Most commonly, axillae, neck (back, sides) (Fig. 5-1); also, groins (see Fig. 17-14), anogenitalia, antecubital fossae, knuckles, submammary, umbilicus.

**Mucous Membranes**   Oral mucosa: velvety texture with delicate furrows. *Type 5*: Mucous membranes and mucocutaneous junctions commonly involved; warty papillomatous thickenings periorally (see Fig. 17-15).

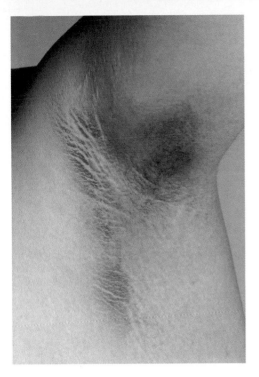

**FIGURE 5-1  Acanthosis nigricans**  *Velvety, dark-brown epidermal thickening of the armpit with prominent skin fold and feathered edges in a 25-year-old obese woman with a family history of acanthosis nigricans. Changes had been stable for more than 5 years. There were similar changes on the neck, in the antecubital fossae, and dorsum of the knuckles.*

**General Examination**
Examine for underlying endocrine disorder and malignancy.

## DIAGNOSIS AND DIFFERENTIAL DIAGNOSIS

**Clinical Findings**  Dark thickened flexural skin: Confluent and reticulated papillomatosis (Gougerot-Carteaud syndrome), pityriasis versicolor, X-linked ichthyosis, retention hyperkeratosis, nicotinic acid ingestion.

## LABORATORY EXAMINATIONS

**Chemistry**  Rule out diabetes mellitus.
**Dermatopathology**  Papillomatosis, hyperkeratosis; epidermis thrown into irregular folds, showing various degrees of acanthosis.

**Imaging and Endoscopy**  Rule out associated carcinoma.

## COURSE AND PROGNOSIS

*Type 1*: Accentuated at puberty and, at times, regresses when older. *Type 2*: Depends on underlying disturbance. *Type 3*: May regress after significant weight loss. *Type 4*: Resolves when causative drug is discontinued. *Type 5*: AN may precede other symptoms of malignancy by 5 years; removal of malignancy may be followed by regression of AN.

## MANAGEMENT

Symptomatic. Treat associated disorder.

# DARIER'S DISEASE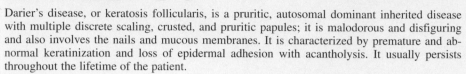

Darier's disease, or keratosis follicularis, is a pruritic, autosomal dominant inherited disease with multiple discrete scaling, crusted, and pruritic papules; it is malodorous and disfiguring and also involves the nails and mucous membranes. It is characterized by premature and abnormal keratinization and loss of epidermal adhesion with acantholysis. It usually persists throughout the lifetime of the patient.

## EPIDEMIOLOGY AND ETIOLOGY

Rare.

**Age of Onset**   Usually in the first or second decade, males and females equally affected.

**Genetics**   Autosomal dominant trait, new mutations common, penetrance >95%. A diverse set of mutations in $Ca^{2+}$-ATPase isoform-2 (SERCA-2).

**Precipitating Factors**   Frequently worse in summer with heat and humidity as major factors; can be exacerbated by UVB, mechanical trauma, bacterial infections. Often associated with affective disorders and rarely with decreased intelligence.

## HISTORY

Usually insidious; onset is abrupt after precipitating factors; associated with severe pruritus and often pain.

## PHYSICAL EXAMINATION

### Skin Lesions
Multiple discrete scaling of crusted, pruritic papules (Fig. 5-2); when scaling crust is removed, a slitlike opening becomes visible. Confluence to large plaques covered by hypertrophic warty masses (Fig. 5-3) that are foul smelling, particularly in intertriginous areas.

*Distribution* Corresponding to the "seborrheic areas": chest (Fig. 5-3), back, ears, nasolabial folds, forehead, scalp, and groin.

**Appendages**   Hair not involved, but permanent alopecia may result from extensive scalp involvement. Nails thin, splitting distally and showing characteristic V-shaped scalloping (see Fig. 30-9).

**Mucous Membranes**   White, centrally depressed papules on mucosa of cheeks, hard and soft palate, and gums, "cobblestone" lesions.

## LABORATORY EXAMINATION

**Dermatopathology**   Eosinophilic dyskeratotic cells in the spinous layer (corps ronds) and stratum corneum (grains), suprabasal acantholysis and clefts (lacunae), papillary overgrowth of the epidermis and hyperkeratosis.

## DIAGNOSIS AND DIFFERENTIAL DIAGNOSIS

Diagnosis based on history of familiar involvement, clinical appearance, and histopathology. May be confused with seborrheic dermatitis, Grover's disease, benign familial pemphigus (Hailey-Hailey disease), and pemphigus foliaceus.

## COURSE AND PROGNOSIS

Persisting throughout life, not associated with cutaneous malignancies.

## MANAGEMENT

Sunscreens to avoid UV-induced exacerbations, avoidance of friction and rubbing (turtle neck sweaters), antibiotic therapy (systemic and topical) to suppress bacterial infection, topical retinoids (tazarotene and adaptalene) or systemic retinoids (isotretinoin or acitretin). Systemic therapy can be modified according to seasonal variation of the disease.

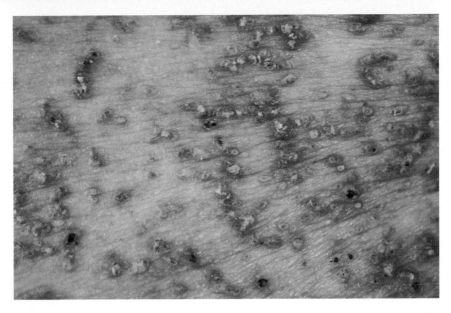

**FIGURE 5-2   Darier's disease**   *Primary lesions are reddish, scaling and crusted papules that, when stroked, feel warty. Where crusts have been removed there are slit-like erosions that are later covered by hemorrhagic crusts.*

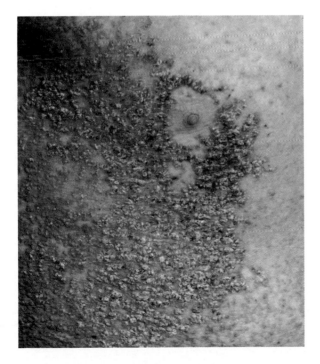

**FIGURE 5-3   Darier's disease: chest**   *Papules have coalesced to a large warty plaque sparing the areola. These lesions, particularly when they are in body folds, are often foul smelling.*

# GROVER'S DISEASE   ☐ ◑

Grover's disease (GD), or transient acantholytic dermatosis, is a pruritic dermatosis primarily affecting middle-aged men, located principally on the trunk, and occurring as crops of discrete papular and papulovesicular lesions, sparse or numerous. Pruritus can be a major problem. Principal histopathologic feature of the lesions is the presence of acantholysis.

## EPIDEMIOLOGY

**Age of Onset**  Middle age and older, mean age 50 years.
**Sex**  Males > females.
**Precipitating Factors**  Heavy, sweat-inducing exercise, excessive solar exposure, exposure to heat, and persistent fever; may also occur in bedridden patients, with heat and sweating as factors.

## HISTORY

Usually abrupt onset of pruritus and simultaneous appearance of crops of lesions

## PHYSICAL EXAMINATION

### Skin Lesions
Skin-colored or reddish papules (small, 3 to 5 mm, some with slight scale or smooth) (Fig. 5-4), papulovesicles, and erosions. Very similar to Darier's disease. Upon palpation, smooth or warty. Scattered, discrete on central trunk (Fig. 5-4) and proximal extremities.

## LABORATORY EXAMINATION

**Dermatopathology**  Acantholysis and spongiosis, focal acantholytic dyskeratosis occurring at the same time and simulating Darier's disease, pemphigus foliaceus, and Hailey-Hailey dis-

ease; in the dermis there is a superficial infiltrate of eosinophils, lymphocytes, and histiocytes.

## DIAGNOSIS AND DIFFERENTIAL DIAGNOSIS

Often difficult.
**Small Discrete Pruritic Papules on Chest**  Darier's disease, heat rash (miliaria rubra), papular urticaria, scabies, dermatitis herpetiformis (here there is grouping and the lesions are symmetric), *Pityrosporum* or eosinophilic folliculitis, insect bites, and drug eruptions.

## COURSE AND PROGNOSIS

The disease is by no means always transient, and there appear to be two types: acute ("transient") and chronic relapsing. The mean duration in one series was 47 weeks.

## MANAGEMENT

**Topical**  Class I topical glucocorticoids under plastic (e.g., dry-cleaning plastic suit bags with holes cut for arms) are used for 4 h.
**Systemic**  Oral glucocorticoids and dapsone have been used with success, but relapses occur after withdrawal.
**Phototherapy**  UVB or PUVA photochemotherapy may be useful for patients who do not respond to topical glucocorticoids under occlusion.

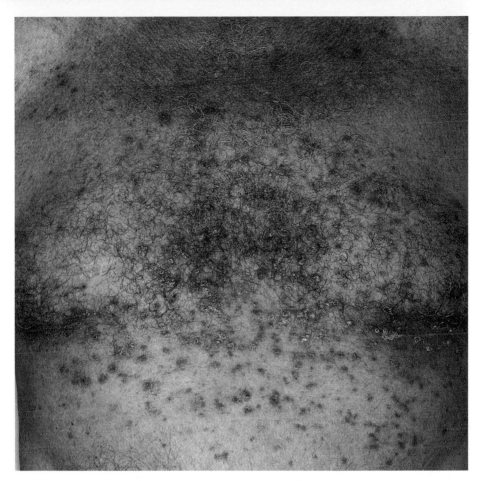

**FIGURE 5-4   Grover's disease**   *A rash consisting of reddish hyperkeratotic scaling and/or crusted papules with a sandpaper feel upon palpation. Papules are discrete, scattered on the central trunk and are extremely pruritic.*

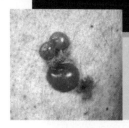

# S E C T I O N 6

# BULLOUS DISEASES

## HEREDITARY EPIDERMOLYSIS BULLOSA (EB)

A spectrum of rare genodermatoses in which a disturbed coherence of the epidermis and/or dermis leads to blister formation following trauma. Hence, the designation *mechano-bullous dermatoses*; there are more than 20 different types. Disease manifestations range from very mild to severely mutilating and even lethal forms that differ in mode of inheritance, clinical manifestations, and associated findings. Classification is best based on the site of blister formation distinguishing among three main groups: epidermolytic or EB simplex (EBS), junctional EB (JEB), and dermolytic or dystrophic EB (DEB) (Table 6-1). In each of these groups there are several distinct types of EB based on clinical, genetic, histologic, and biochemical evaluation (Table 6-2). Image 6-1 shows the cleavage planes in the major forms of EB.

### EPIDEMIOLOGY

The overall incidence of hereditary EB is placed at 19.6 live births per one million births in the United States. Stratified by subtype, the incidences are 11 for EBS, 2 for JEB, and 5 for DEB. The estimated prevalence in the United States is 8.2 per million, but this figure represents only the most severe cases as it does not include the majority of very mild disease going unreported.

### CLINICAL PHENOTYPES

#### EB Simplex

A trauma-induced, intraepidermal blistering, based in most cases on mutations of the genes for keratins 5 and 14 resulting in a disturbance of the stability of the keratin filament network (Table 6-3). This causes cytolysis of basal keratinocytes and a cleft in the basal cell layer (Image 6-1). Different subgroups have considerable phenotypic variations (Tables 6-2 and 6-3), and there are 10 distinct forms, most of which are dominantly inherited. The two most common are described below.

*Generalized EBS* (Table 6-2) The so-called Koebner variant is dominantly inherited, with onset at birth to early infancy. There is generalized blistering following trauma with a predilection for traumatized body sites such as feet, hands; elbows, knees. Blisters are tense or flaccid at first and lead to erosions (Fig. 6-1). There is rapid healing and only minimal scarring at sites of repeated blistering. Palmoplantar hyperkeratoses may be present. Nails, teeth, and oral mucosa are usually spared.

*Localized EBS* Weber-Cockayne subtype (Table 6-2). This is the most common form of EBS. Onset in childhood or later. The disease may not present itself until adulthood when thick-walled blisters on the feet and hands occur after excessive exercise, manual work, or military training. Increased ambient temperature facilitates lesions. Hyperhydrosis of palms and soles is associated, and secondary infection of blistered lesions often occurs.

#### Junctional EB

All forms of JEB share the pathologic feature of blister formation within the lamina lucida of the basement membrane (Image 6-1). Mutations are in the gene for bullous pemphigoid antigen 2 and laminin 5 (Table 6-3). This trait is autosomal recessive and comprises clinical phenotypes depending on the type of genetic lesion and environmental factors. The three principal subtypes (see Table 6-2) are described below.

*JEB Gravis (Herlitz EB)* Patients often do not survive infancy; the mortality rate is 40% during the first year of life. There is generalized blistering at birth (Fig. 6-2) or clinically distinctive and severe periorificial granulation, loss of nails, and involvement of most mucosal surfaces. The skin of these children may be

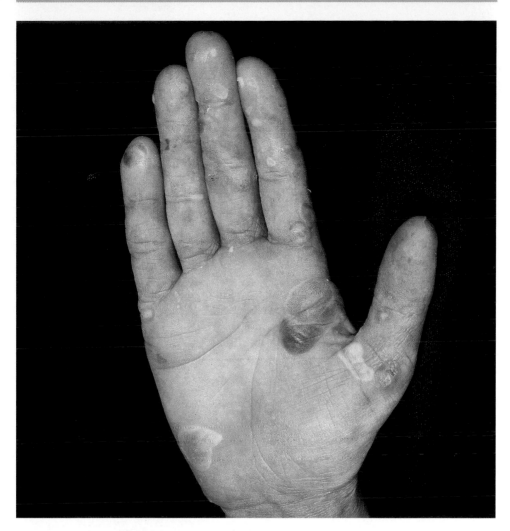

**FIGURE 6-1   Generalized EBS**   *This 22-year-old male has had blistering since early infancy with a predilection for traumatized body sites such as the palms and soles, but also the elbows and knees. Blistering also occurs on the trunk. His initial aspiration to become a mechanic had to be dropped because severe blistering on the palms occurred every time he handled tools. The present eruption occurred after the patient helped his mother in the garden using a shovel. Note that despite multiple blistering episodes, there is hardly any evidence of scarring on his palm.*

**TABLE 6-1    Classification of Epidermolysis Bullosa (EB)**

| Blister Location | Disease Group | Inheritance |
|---|---|---|
| Intraepidermal | EB simplex | Autosomal dominant[*] |
| | | Autosomal recessive |
| Basement membrane zone | Junctional EB | Autosomal recessive |
| Sublamina densa | Dystrophic EB | Autosomal recessive |
| | | Autosomal dominant |

[*]Most EB simplex patients are from autosomal dominant kindreds.

SOURCE: From MP Marinkovich et al, Inherited epidermolysis bullosa in IM Freedberg, AZ Eisen, K Wolff, KF Austen, LA Goldsmith, SI Katz (eds): *Fitzpatrick's Dermatology in General Medicine*, 6th ed. New York, McGraw-Hill, 2003.

completely denuded, representing oozing painful erosion. Associated findings include all symptoms resulting from generalized epithelial blistering with respiratory, gastrointestinal, and genitourinary organ systems involved.

***JEB Mitis*** These children may have moderate or severe JEB at birth but survive infancy and clinically improve with age. Periorificial nonhealing erosions during childhood.

***Generalized Atrophic Benign Epidermolysis Bullosa (GABEB)*** GABEB is a separate JEB that presents at birth with generalized cutaneous blistering and erosions not only on the extremities but also on the trunk, face, and scalp. Sur-

vival to adulthood is the rule, but blistering on traumatized areas continues (Fig. 6-3). It is particularly pronounced with increased ambient temperature, and there is atrophic healing of the lesions. Nail dystrophy, nonscarring or scarring alopecia, mild oral mucous membrane involvement; enamel defects may occur. Mutations are in the gene for bullous pemphigoid antigen 2 and laminin 5 (Table 6-3).

## Dystrophic Epidermolysis Bullosa

A spectrum of dermolytic diseases where blistering occurs below the basal lamina (Image 6-1); healing is therefore usually accompanied

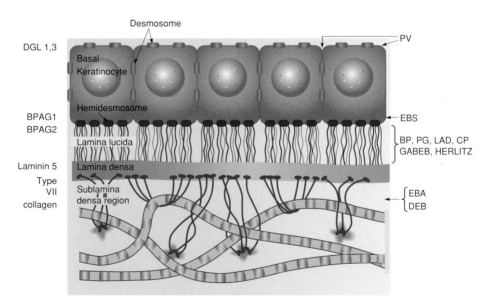

**IMAGE 6-1**    *Localization of target adhesion sites and cleft formation in selected hereditary and autoimmune bullous diseases. (Modified from Fig. 30-5 in JL Bolognia et al:* Dermatology; *Mosby, London, Philadelphia, 2003; with permission.)*

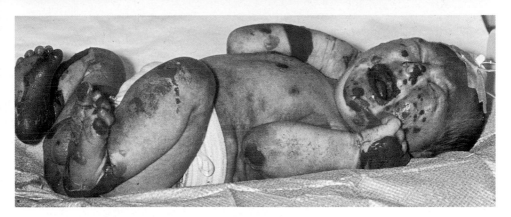

**FIGURE 6-2   Junctional epidermolysis bullosa (Herlitz variant)**   *There are large eroded, oozing and bleeding areas that occurred intrapartum. When this newborn is lifted up, dislodgment of epidermis as well as erosions occur due to manual handling.*

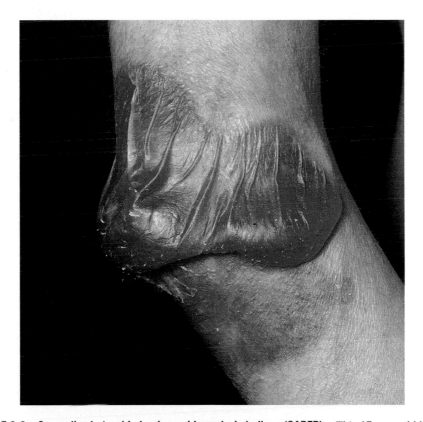

**FIGURE 6-3   Generalized atrophic benign epidermolysis bullosa (GABEB)**   *This 17-year-old boy has had generalized cutaneous blistering since birth, with blisters and erosions arising on the elbows and knees but also on the trunk and face. Note large flaccid bulla in an area of atrophy over the elbow; milia were also seen on the trunk.*

**STABLE 6-2   Clinical Heterogeneity of Epidermolysis Bullosa (EB)**

| Epidermolytic | Junctional | Dermolytic |
|---|---|---|
| Generalized EBS (Koebner) | JEB gravis (Herlitz) | Generalized RDEB (Hallopeau-Siemens) |
| Localized EBS (Weber-Cockayne) | JEB mitis | Localized RDEB |
| EB herpetiformis (Dowling-Meara) | JEB—pyloric atresia | Dominant DEB (Cockayne-Touraine) |
| EBS (Ogna) | GABEB | Dominant DEB albopapuloid (Pasini) |
| Muscular dystrophy-EBS | Localized JEB | |

NOTE: EBS, EB simplex; JEB, junctional EB; RDEB, recessive DEB; GABEB, generalized atrophic benign EB.

SOURCE: From MP Marinkovich et al, Inherited epidermolysis bullosa in IM Freedberg, AZ Eisen, K Wolff, KF Austen, LA Goldsmith, SI Katz (eds): *Fitzpatrick's Dermatology in General Medicine*, 6th ed. New York, McGraw-Hill, 2003.

by scarring and milia formation—hence, the name dystrophic. There are four principal subtypes, and all are due to mutations in anchoring fibril type 7 collagen (Table 6-3). Anchoring fibrils are therefore only rudimentary or absent. The four main types of DEB are shown in Table 6-2, but only two of these are described below.

***Dominant DEB*** Cockayne-Touraine's disease. Onset in infancy or early childhood with acral blistering and nail dystrophy; milia and scar formation, which may be hypertrophic or hyperplastic. Oral lesions are uncommon, and teeth are usually normal.

***Recessive DEB (RDEB)*** Comprises a larger spectrum of clinical phenotypes. The localized, less severe form (RDEB mitis) occurs at birth, shows acral blistering, atrophic scarring, and little or no mucosal involvement. Generalized, severe RDEB, the Hallopeau-Siemens variant, is mutilating. There is generalized blistering at birth, and progression and repeated blistering at the same sites (Fig. 6-4) result in remarkable scarring, syndactyly with mitten-like deformities of hands and feet (Fig. 6-5), flexion contractures. These are enamel defects with caries and parodontitis, strictures and scarring in the oral mucous membrane and esophagus, urethral and anal stenosis, and ocular surface scarring; also malnutrition, growth retardation, and anemia. The most serious complication is squamous cell carcinoma in chronic recurrent erosions.

## DIAGNOSIS

Based on clinical appearance and history. Histopathology determines the level of cleavage, which is further defined by electron microscopy and/or immunohistochemical mapping. Western blot, Northern blot, restriction fragment length polymorphism (RFLP) analysis, and DNA sequences may then identify the mutated gene.

## MANAGEMENT

There is as yet no causal therapy for EB. Management is tailored to the severity and extent of skin involvement and consists of supportive skin care, supportive care for other organ systems, and systemic therapies for complications. Wound management, nutritional support, and infection control are key to the management of all EB patients.

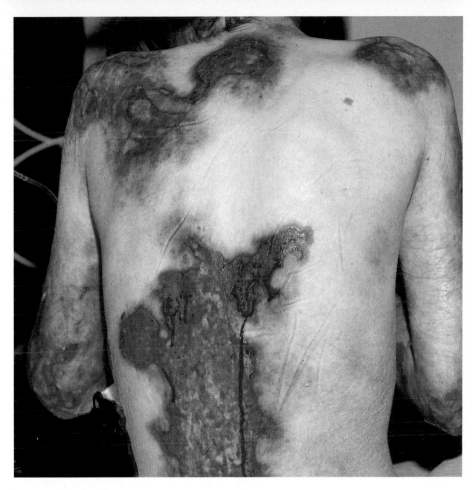

**FIGURE 6-4   Generalized recessive dystrophic epidermolysis bullosa (RDEB)**   *This is a severe disease with generalized blistering, often in the same sites, as in this 14-year-old girl. Erosions have become ulcers that have a low tendency to heal; and when healing occurs, it results in scarring. This girl also has enamel defects with caries, strictures in the esophagus, growth retardation and severe anemia. Any time the skin is even slightly traumatized, new blisters will appear. It is obvious that these large wounds are portal entries for systemic infection.*

In EBS, maintenance of a cool environment and use of soft, well-ventilated shoes, are important. Blistered skin is treated by saline compresses and topical antibiotics or, in the case of inflammation, with topical steroids. More severely affected JEB and DEB patients are treated like patients in a burn unit. Gentle bathing and cleansing are followed by protective emollients and nonadherent dressings.

Management of cutaneous infection is important, and surgical treatment is often required in DEB for the release of fused digits and correction of limb contractures.

Although rare, EB and, in particular, JEB and DEB pose a major health and socioeconomic problem. Organizations such as the Dystrophic Epidermolysis Bullosa Research Association (DEBRA) offer assistance that includes patient education and support.

### TABLE 6-3   Clinical Phenotype—Molecular Defect Correlations in Epidermolysis Bullosa

| Disease[*] | Genes[†] | Proteins |
|---|---|---|
| EBS-DM | KRT5, 14 | Keratins 5, 14 |
| EBS-WC | KRT5, 14 | Keratins 5, 14 |
| EBS-K | KRT5, 14 | Keratins 5, 14 |
| Recessive EBS-K | KRT 14 | Keratins 14 |
| Recessive EBS-MD | PLEC1 | Plectin |
| JEB-lethal | LAMA3, B3, C2 | Laminin $5\alpha_3$, $\beta_3$, $\gamma_2$ |
| JEB-PA | ITGA6, B4 | Integrin $\alpha_6$, $\beta_4$ |
| GABEB | COL17A1, LAMB3 | BP180, laminin |
| DDEB | COL7A1 | Type VII collagen |
| RDEB | COL7A1 | Type VII collagen |

[*]Disease categories reflect clinical phenotypes of individual EB patients studied.

[†]Genes indicated represent candidate genes identified by DNA mutation analysis as correlating with disease phenotype. Examples of genetic defects include: KRT5 or 14 heterozygous missense or in-frame deletions in dominant forms of EBS; KRT5 or 14 homozygous missense or premature termination codons (PTC) in recessive EBS; PLEC1 homozygous in-frame deletion or PT in EBS-MD; LAMA3, B3, C2 homozygous PTC in Herlitz JEB; ITGA6 or B4 heterozygous PTC/in-frame deletion or homozygous PTC in JEB-PA; COL17A1 heterozygous PTC/missense or homozygous PT in GABEB; COL7A1 heterozygous gly substitution in DDEB; COL7A1 homozygous PT or gly substitution in RDEB-HS; COL7A1 homozygous missense or gly substitution or heterozygous PTC/gly substitution in RDEB mitis.

NOTE: EBS-DM, EB simplex, Dowling-Meara type; EBS-WC, EB simplex, Weber-Cockayne type; EBS-K, EB simplex, Koebner type; recessive EBS-MD, EB simplex associated with muscular dystrophy; JEB-lethal, junctional EB, Herlitz type; JEB-PA, JEB associated with pyloric atresia; GABEB, generalized atrophic benign EB; DDEB, dominant dystrophic EB; RDEB, recessive dystrophic EB.

SOURCE: From MP Marinkovich et al, Hereditary epidermolysis bullosa in IM Freedberg, AZ Eisen, K Wolff, KF Austen, LA Goldsmith, SI Katz, TR Fitzpatrick (eds): *Fitzpatrick's Dermatology in General Medicine*, 6th ed. New York, McGraw-Hill, 2003, p. 599.

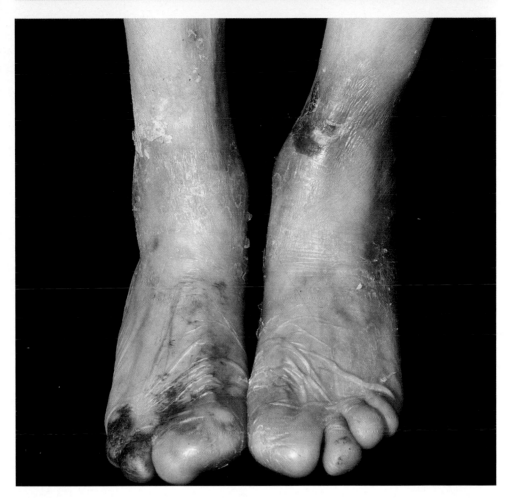

**FIGURE 6-5 Generalized recessive dystrophic epidermolysis bullosa** *Loss of toenails and mitten-like deformities of the feet due to repeated blistering, reepithelialization and scarring. This is the same patient as shown in Fig. 6-4.*

## FAMILIAL BENIGN PEMPHIGUS   □ ◑

Familial benign pemphigus, or Hailey-Hailey disease, is a rare genodermatosis with dominant inheritance that is classically described as a blistering disorder but actually presents as an erythematous, erosive, oozing condition with cracks and fissures localized to the nape of the neck, axillae (Fig. 6-6), submammary regions, unguinal folds, and scrotum. The underlying pathologic process is acantholysis whereby the fragility of the epidermis is due to a defect in the adhesion complex between desmosomal proteins and tonofilaments. The genetic abnormality lies in *ATP2CI*, which encodes an ATP-powered calcium pump. Onset is usually between the third and fourth decade, and the disease is often mistaken for intertrigo, candidiasis, or frictional or contact dermatitis. Individual lesions consist of microscopically small flaccid vesicles on an erythematous background that soon turn into eroded plaques with the described, highly characteristic, fissured appearance (Fig. 6-6). Crusting, scaling, and hypertrophic vegetative growths may occur. Histology explains the clinical appearance as epidermal cells lose their coherence with acantholysis throughout the epithelium, giving the appearance of a dilapidated brick wall.

Colonization of the lesions, particularly by *Staphylococcus aureus* is a trigger for further acantholysis and maintenance of the pathologic process. Secondary colonization by *Candida* has a similar effect.

Treatment rests on anti-infective agents, administered both topically and systemically; systemically, the tetracyclines seem to work better than most. Topical glucocorticoids depress the anti-inflammatory response and accelerate healing. In severe cases, dermabrasion or carbon dioxide laser vaporization leads to healing with scars, which are resistant to recurrences. The condition becomes less troublesome with age.

## PEMPHIGUS VULGARIS   □ ●

Pemphigus vulgaris (PV) is a serious, acute or chronic, bullous, autoimmune disease of skin and mucous membranes that is often fatal unless treated with immunosuppressive agents. It is the prototype of the pemphigus family, a group of autoimmune acantholytic blistering diseases (Table 6-4).

### EPIDEMIOLOGY

More common in Jews and people of Mediterranean descent. In Jerusalem the incidence is estimated at 1.6 per 100,000, whereas in France it is 1.3 per million.
**Age of Onset**   40 to 60 years.
**Sex**   Equal incidence in males and females.

### ETIOLOGY AND PATHOGENESIS

An autoimmune disorder. Loss of the normal cell-to-cell adhesion in the epidermis (*acantholysis*) occurs as a result of circulating antibodies of the IgG class; these antibodies bind to cell surface glycoproteins (pemphigus antigens;

most important: desmoglein 3, a member of the cadherin superfamily) of the epidermis and induce acantholysis (Image 6-1).

### TABLE 6-4   Classification of Pemphigus

Pemphigus vulgaris
   Pemphigus vegetans: localized
   Drug-induced
Pemphigus foliaceus
   Pemphigus erythematosus: localized
   Fogo selvagem: endemic
   Drug-induced
Paraneoplastic pemphigus

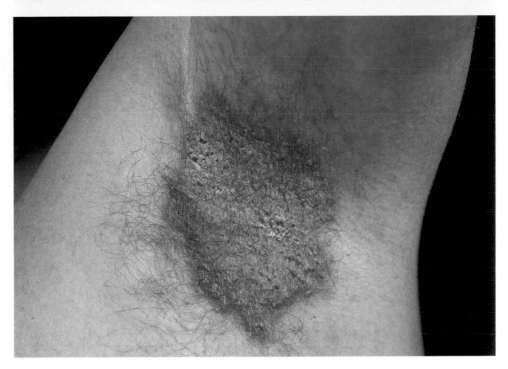

**FIGURE 6-6  Familial benign pemphigus**  *This 46-year-old male has had oozing lesions in both axillae, occasionally in the groins and sometimes also on the nape of the neck, for several years. Eruptions worsen during the summer months. The father and sister have similar lesions that wax and wane. Lesions are painful and show typical cracks and fissures within an erosive erythematous plaque. Although classified among the blistering diseases, familial benign pemphigus hardly ever shows intact vesicles and is often mistaken for intertrigo.*

## HISTORY

PV usually starts in the oral mucosa, and months may elapse before skin lesions occur; lesions may be localized for months, after which generalized bullae occur. Less frequently there may be a generalized, acute eruption of bullae from the beginning. No pruritus, but considerable burning and pain. Painful and tender mouth lesions may prevent adequate food intake. Epistaxis, hoarseness, dysphagia. Weakness, malaise, weight loss.

## PHYSICAL EXAMINATION

### Skin Lesions

Round or oval vesicles and bullae with serous content, flaccid (flabby) (Fig. 6-7), easily ruptured, and weeping (Fig. 6-8), arising on *normal* skin, randomly scattered, discrete. Localized (e.g., to mouth or circumscribed skin area Fig. 6-8), or generalized with a random pattern. Extensive erosions that bleed easily (Fig. 6-9), crusts (Fig. 6-8) particularly on scalp. Since blisters rupture so easily, only erosions are seen in many patients. These are very painful (Fig. 6-9).

*Nikolsky Sign* Dislodging of epidermis by lateral finger pressure in the vicinity of lesions, which leads to an erosion. Pressure on bulla leads to lateral extension of blister.

*Sites of Predilection* Scalp, face, chest, axillae, groin, umbilicus. In bedridden patients, there is extensive involvement of back (Fig. 6-9).

**Mucous Membranes** Bullae rarely seen, erosions of mouth (see Fig. 31-12) and nose, pharynx and larynx, vagina.

## LABORATORY EXAMINATIONS

**Dermatopathology** Light microscopy (select early small bulla or, if not present, margin of larger bulla or erosion): Separation of keratinocytes, suprabasally, leading to split just *above* the basal cell layer and vesicles containing separated, rounded-up (acantholytic) keratinocytes.

**Immunopathology** Direct immunofluorescence (IF) staining reveals IgG and often C3 deposited in lesional and paralesional skin in *the intercellular substance of the epidermis.*

**Serum** Autoantibodies (IgG) detected by indirect IF (IIF) or enzyme-linked immunosorbent assay (ELISA). Titer usually correlates with activity of disease process. Autoantibodies are directed against a 130-kDa glycoprotein designated desmoglein 3 and located in desmosomes (Image 6-1).

## DIAGNOSIS AND DIFFERENTIAL DIAGNOSIS

Can be a difficult problem if only mouth lesions are present. Differential diagnosis includes all forms of acquired bullous diseases (Table 6-5). Biopsy of the skin and mucous membrane, direct IF, and demonstration of circulating autoantibodies confirm a high index of suspicion.

## COURSE

In most cases the disease inexorably progresses to death unless treated aggressively with immunosuppressive agents. The mortality rate has been markedly reduced since treatment has become available.

## VARIANTS (See Table 6-4)

*Pemphigus Vegetans (PVeg)* Usually confined to intertriginous regions, perioral area, neck, and scalp. Granulomatous vegetating purulent plaques that extend centrifugally. Suprabasal acantholysis with intraepidermal abscesses containing mostly eosinophils and acantholytic cells. Pseudoepitheliomatous hyperplasia of the epidermis, exuberant granulation tissue with abscess formation. IgG autoantibodies as in PV. PV may evolve into PVeg and vice versa.

*Pemphigus Foliaceus (PF)* Most commonly on face, scalp, upper chest, and abdomen but may involve entire skin, presenting as exfoliative erythroderma. Superficial form of pemphigus with acantholysis in the granular layer of the epidermis. Bullae hardly ever present; lesions consist of erythematous patches and erosions covered with crusts. PF is mediated by circulating autoantibodies to a 160-kDa intercellular (cell surface) antigen, desmoglein 1, in the desmosomes of keratinocytes. PV (130 kDa) and PF (160 kDa) antigens differ. This explains the different sites of acantholysis and thus the different clinical appearances of the two conditions.

*Brazilian Pemphigus (Fogo Selvagem)* A distinctive form of PF endemic to south central Brazil. Clinically, histologically, and immunopathologically identical to PF. Patients improve when moved to urban areas but relapse after returning to endemic regions. It is speculated that the disease is somehow related to an

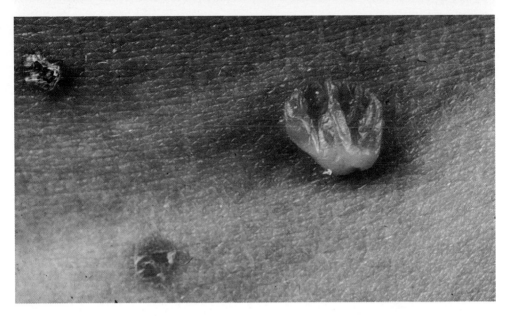

**FIGURE 6-7  Pemphigus vulgaris**  *These are the classic initial lesions: flaccid, easily ruptured vesicles and bullae on normal appearing skin. Ruptured vesicles lead to erosions that subsequently crust.*

arthropod-borne infectious agent. More than 1000 new cases per year are estimated to occur in the endemic regions.

***Pemphigus Erythematosus (PE)*** *Synonym:* Senear-Usher syndrome. A localized variety of PF largely confined to seborrheic sites. Erythematous, crusted, and erosive lesions in the "butterfly" area of the face, forehead, and presternal and interscapular regions. Despite clinical, histopathologic, and immunopathologic similarity to PF, PE may be unique, since patients have immunoglobulin and complement deposits at the dermal-epidermal junction, in addition to intercellular pemphigus antibody in the epidermis and antinuclear antibodies, as is the case in lupus erythematosus.

***Drug-Induced Pemphigus*** A PV- and PF/PE-like syndrome can be induced by D-penicillamine and less frequently by captopril and other drugs. In most, but not all, instances the eruption resolves after termination of therapy with the offending drug.

***Paraneoplastic Pemphigus (PNP)*** Mucous membranes primarily and most severely involved. Lesions combine features of pemphigus vulgaris and erythema multiforme, clinically and histologically (see Section 17).

## MANAGEMENT

**Glucocorticoids**  2 to 3 mg/kg body weight of prednisone until cessation of new blister formation and disappearance of Nikolsky sign. Then rapid reduction to about half the initial dose until patient is almost clear, followed by very slow tapering of dose to minimal effective maintenance dose.

**Concomitant Immunosuppressive Therapy**  Immunosuppressive agents are given concomitantly for their glucocorticoid-sparing effect:

  *Azathioprine*, 2 to 3 mg/kg body weight until complete clearing; tapering of dose to 1 mg/kg. Azathioprine alone is continued even after cessation of glucocorticoid treatment and may have to be continued for many months.

  *Methotrexate*, either orally (PO) or IM at doses of 25 to 35 mg/week. Dose adjustments are made as with azathioprine.

  *Cyclophosphamide*, 100 to 200 mg daily, with reduction to maintenance doses of 50 to 100 mg/d. Alternatively, cyclophosphamide "bolus" therapy with 1000 mg IV once a week or every 2 weeks in the initial phases, followed by 50 to 100 mg/d PO as maintenance.

*Plasmapheresis*, in conjunction with glucocorticoids and immunosuppressive agents in poorly controlled patients, in the initial phases of treatment to reduce antibody titers.

*Gold therapy*, for milder cases. After an initial test dose of 10 mg IM, 25 to 50 mg of gold sodium thiomalate is given IM at

weekly intervals to a maximum cumulative dose of 1 g.

*Mycophenolate mofetil* (1 g bid) has been reported to be beneficial, and clinical studies are ongoing.

*High-dose intravenous immunoglobulin (HIVIg)* (2 g/kg body weight every 3 to 4 weeks) has been reported to have a glucocorticoid-sparing effect.

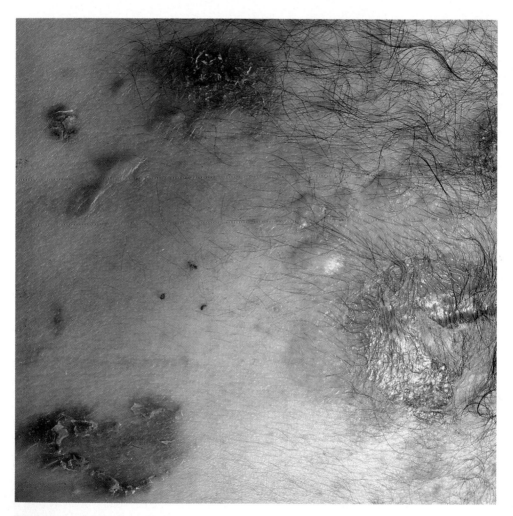

**FIGURE 6-8   Pemphigus vulgaris**   *This 56-year-old male patient noticed areas of increased skin fragility on his trunk; and only when examined more closely, were flaccid bullae seen on normal appearing skin that easily ruptured and turned into erosions. The patient previously had erosive and very painful stomatitis for over 6 months and was treated unsuccessfully with topical remedies by his dentist. When skin lesions as shown in this picture appeared, he consulted a dermatologist who made the correct diagnosis.*

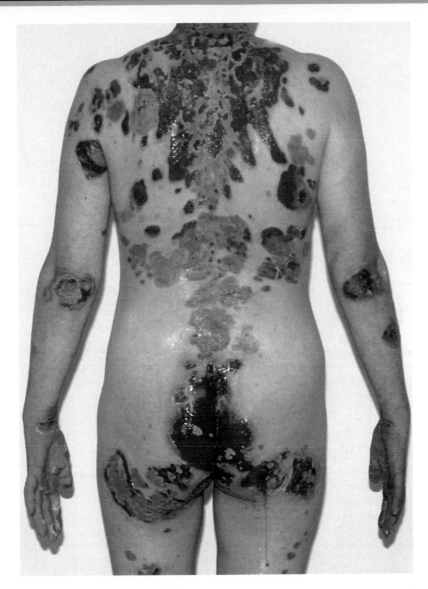

**FIGURE 6-9   Pemphigus vulgaris**   *Widespread, confluent erosions on the back of a female patient who has a generalized eruption including the scalp and the mucous membranes. Due to the fragility of the blisters, pemphigus vulgaris presents as erosions which are extremely painful and tend to bleed with minimal trauma.*

**Other Measures**   Cleansing baths, wet dressings, topical and intralesional glucocorticoids, antibiotics to combat bacterial infections. Correction of fluid and electrolyte imbalance.

**Monitoring**   Clinical, for improvement of skin lesions and development of drug-related side effects. Laboratory monitoring of pemphigus antibody titers and for hematologic and metabolic indicators of glucocorticoid- and/or immunosuppressive-induced adverse effects.

## BULLOUS PEMPHIGOID

Bullous pemphigoid is an autoimmune disorder presenting as a chronic bullous eruption, mostly in patients over 60 years of age.

### EPIDEMIOLOGY

**Age of Onset**   60 to 80 years.
**Sex**   Equal incidence in males and females.
**Incidence**   The most common bullous autoimmune disease.

### PATHOGENESIS

Interaction of autoantibody with bullous pemphigoid antigen (BPAG1e and BPAG2) in hemidesmosomes of basal keratinocytes (Image 6-1) is followed by complement activation and attraction of neutrophils and eosinophils. Bullous lesion results from interaction of multiple bioactive molecules released from inflammatory cells.

### HISTORY

Often starts with a prodromal eruption (urticarial, papular lesions) and evolves in weeks to months to bullae that may appear suddenly as a generalized eruption. Initially no symptoms except moderate or severe pruritus; later, tenderness of eroded lesions. No constitutional symptoms, except in widespread, severe disease.

### PHYSICAL EXAMINATION

#### Skin Lesions
Erythematous, papular or urticarial-type lesions (Fig. 6-10) may precede bullae formation by months. Bullae: large, tense, firm-topped, oval or round (Figs. 6-10 and 6-11); may arise in normal or erythematous skin and contain serous or hemorrhagic fluid. The eruption may be localized or generalized, usually scattered but also grouped in arciform and serpiginous patterns. Bullae rupture less easily than in pemphigus, but sometimes large, bright red, oozing, and bleeding erosions become a major problem. Usually, however, the originally tense bullae collapse and transform into crusts (Fig. 6-11).
*Sites of Predilection* Axillae; medial aspects of thighs, groins, abdomen; flexor aspects of forearms; lower legs (often first manifestation).

**Mucous Membranes** Practically only in the mouth (10 to 35%); less severe and painful and less easily ruptured than in pemphigus.

### LABORATORY EXAMINATIONS

**Dermatopathology** *Light Microscopy* Neutrophils in "Indian-file" alignment at dermal-epidermal junction; neutrophils, eosinophils, and lymphocytes in papillary dermis; *subepidermal* bullae.
*Electron Microscopy* Junctional cleavage, i.e., split occurs in lamina lucida of basement membrane.
**Immunopathology** Linear IgG deposits along the basement membrane zone. Also, C3, which may occur in the absence of IgG.
**Serum** Circulating antibasement membrane IgG antibodies detected by IIF in 70% of patients. Titers do not correlate with course of disease. Autoantibodies in bullous pemphigoid recognize two types of antigens. BPAG1e is a 230-kDa glycoprotein that has high homology with desmoplakin I/II and is part of hemidesmosomes. BPAG2 is a transmembranous 180-kDa polypeptide (type XVII collagen).
**Hematology** Eosinophilia (not always).

### DIAGNOSIS AND DIFFERENTIAL DIAGNOSIS

Clinical appearance, histopathology, and immunology permit a differentiation from other bullous diseases (see Table 6-5).

### MANAGEMENT

Systemic prednisone with starting doses of 50 to 100 mg/d continued until clear, either alone or combined with azathioprine, 150 mg daily, for remission induction and 50 to 100 mg for maintenance; in milder cases, sulfones (dapsone), 100 to 150 mg/d. In very mild cases and for local recurrences, topical glucocorticoid

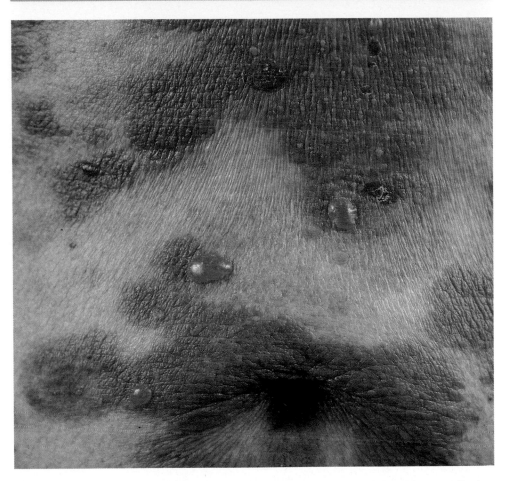

**FIGURE 6-10   Bullous pemphigoid**   *This 70-year-old female had a severely pruritic generalized eruption that consisted of urticarial, inflammatory plaques, papules and crusted lesions. Originally diagnosed as generalized eczema by the family doctor, the patient was eventually referred to us; upon close inspection, small vesicles and occasional bullae were seen arising not only in normal skin but also, and most prominently, in the inflammatory plaques. The diagnosis of bullous pemphigoid, was verified by biopsy and immunofluorescence studies. Note that in contrast to pemphigus vulgaris (Fig. 6-8), where blisters arise exclusively in normal-appearing skin, bullous pemphigoid shows blistering in inflamed areas as well; and these blisters are tense.*

therapy may be beneficial. Tetracycline $\pm$ nicotinamide has been reported to be effective in some cases.

Patients often go into a permanent remission and do not require therapy; local recurrences can sometimes be controlled with topical gluco-corticoids.

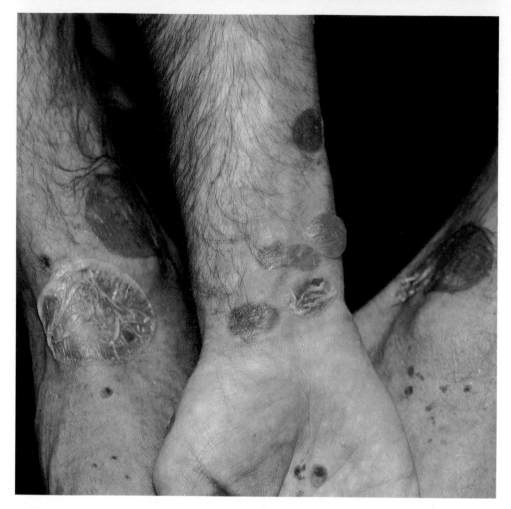

**FIGURE 6-11    Bullous pemphigoid**    *Multiple tense serous bullae are seen on the legs and arm of this 38-year-old-male with HIV infection. The initial diagnoses was bullous drug eruption. As a bulla ruptures it collapses and the blister roof then appears like a crinkled sheet covering an erosion as seen on the right lower leg and wrist. Removal of this epidermal sheet then reveals a bright red circular erosion and this will be subsequently covered by a crust.*

## CICATRICIAL PEMPHIGOID  □ ●

Cicatricial pemphigoid is a rare disease, largely of the elderly, that leads to blisters that rupture easily and also to primary erosions resulting from epithelial fragility in the mouth, oropharynx, and, more rarely, the nasopharyngeal, esophageal, genital, and rectal mucosae. Ocular involvement may initially manifest as unilateral or bilateral conjunctivitis with burning, dryness, and foreign body sensation as the first symptoms. Chronic involvement results in scarring, symblepharon (Fig. 6-12), and, in severe disease, fusing of the bulbar and palpebral conjunctiva. Entropion and trichiasis result in corneal irritation, superficial punctate keratinopathy, corneal neovascularization, ulceration, and blindness. Scarring also in the larynx; esophageal involvement results in stricture formation leading to dysphagia or dynophagia. The skin is involved in roughly 30% of patients. *Brunsting-Perry pemphigoid* describes a subset of patients whose skin lesions recur at the same sites, mainly on the head and neck, and also lead to scarring. Autoantigens in patients with cicatricial pemphigoid include bullous pemphigoid antigen BPAG2, type VII collagen, integrin subunit β4, M168 antigen, and laminin-5.

*Management*: Most patients respond to dapsone in combination with low-dose prednisone. Some patients may require more aggressive immunosuppressive treatment with cyclophosphamide or azathioprine, in combination with glucocorticoids. In addition, surgical intervention for scarring and supportive measures.

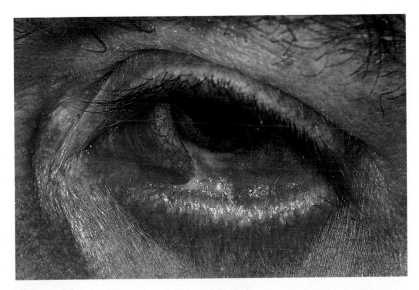

**FIGURE 6-12  Cicatricial pemphigoid**  *This severely scarring condition with symblepharon and fusion of the bulbar and palpebral conjunctiva in a 75-year-old female started as bilateral conjunctivitis with foreign body sensation as the first symptom. The conjunctiva then became erosive with scarring and fibrous tracts between the eyelids and the eye. The patient also had esophageal involvement with strictures and dysphagia.*

## PEMPHIGOID GESTATIONIS    □    ◑

Pemphigoid gestationis (PG) is a rare pruritic and polymorphic inflammatory bullous dermatosis of pregnancy and the postpartum period. The estimated incidence is from 1 in 1700 to 1 in 10,000 deliveries. It is an extremely pruritic vesicular eruption mainly on the abdomen but also on other areas, with sparing of the mucous membranes. Lesions vary from erythematous, edematous papules to urticarial plaques to vesicles and large tense bullae (Fig. 6-13). PG usually begins from the fourth to the seventh month of pregnancy but can also occur in the first trimester and in the immediate postpartum period. It may recur in subsequent pregnancies; if it does, it is likely to begin earlier. PG can be exacerbated by the use of estrogen- and progesterone-containing medications. Histopathologically it is a subepidermal blistering condition, and there is a heavy linear deposition of C3 along the basement membrane zone with concomitant IgG deposition in roughly 30% of patients. Serum contains IgG antibasal membrane antibodies, but these are detected in only 20% of patients by IIF. ELISA and immunoblotting assays detect antibodies in >70%, with presence of a serum complement-fixing factor (HG factor) in many patients. HG factor is an avid complement-fixing IgG antibody that binds to amniotic epithelial basement membrane. It can also be detected in the blood of some infants.

Some 5% of babies born to mothers with PG have urticarial, vesicular, or bullous lesions, which resolve spontaneously during the first several weeks. Some reports of fetal prognosis have revealed significant fetal death and premature deliveries, whereas others have suggested no increase in fetal mortality.

*Management* is geared to suppressing blister formation and relieving the intense pruritus. Prednisone, 20 to 40 mg/d, is given but sometimes higher doses are required. Prednisone is tapered gradually during the postpartum period. Only a few patients do not require systemic prednisone and can be managed with antihistamines and topical glucocorticoids.

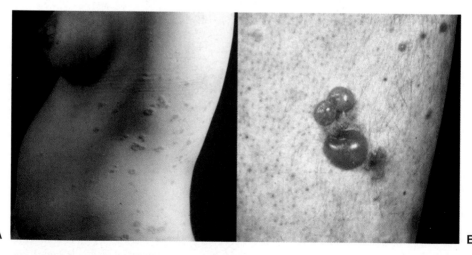

**A**                                                                                                              **B**

**FIGURE 6-13   Pemphigoid gestationis**   *A. Erythematous papules and small plaques that were highly pruritic and had appeared on the trunk and abdomen of this 33-year-old pregnant female (third trimester) were a cause of great concern. At this time there were no blisters and diagnosis was established by biopsy and immunopathology.* **B.** *Grouped blisters on the leg of another patient who had similar eruptions in a previous pregnancy. She responded rapidly to systemic corticosteroids; the delivery was uneventful and the baby was healthy.*

# DERMATITIS HERPETIFORMIS

Dermatitis herpetiformis (DH) is a chronic, recurrent, intensely pruritic eruption occurring symmetrically on the extremities and the trunk and comprising tiny vesicles, papules, and urticarial plaques that are arranged in groups. It is associated with gluten-sensitive enteropathy (GSE) and IgA deposits in skin.

## EPIDEMIOLOGY

Prevalence in Caucasians varies from 10 to 39 per 100,000 persons.

**Age of Onset**  20 to 60 years, but most common at 30 to 40 years; may occur in children.

**Sex**  Male:female ratio is 2:1.

## ETIOLOGY AND PATHOGENESIS

The GSE probably relates to IgA deposits in the skin. Patients have antibodies to transglutaminases (TGs) that may be the major autoantigens in this disease. Epidermal TG autoantibody probably binds to TG in the gut and circulates as immune complexes and deposits in skin. With additional factors IgA activates complement via the alternative pathway, with subsequent chemotaxis of neutrophils releasing their enzymes and producing tissue injury.

## HISTORY

Pruritus, intense, episodic; burning or stinging of the skin; rarely, pruritus may be absent. Symptoms often precede the appearance of skin lesions by 8 to 12 h. Ingestion of iodides and overload of gluten are exacerbating factors.

**Systems Review**  Laboratory evidence of small-bowel malabsorption is detected in 10 to 20%. GSE occurs in nearly all patients and is demonstrated by small-bowel biopsy. There are usually no systemic symptoms.

## PHYSICAL EXAMINATION

### Skin Lesions

Lesions consist of erythematous papules or wheal-like plaques; tiny firm-topped vesicles, sometimes hemorrhagic (Fig. 6-14); occasionally bullae. Lesions are arranged in groups (hence the

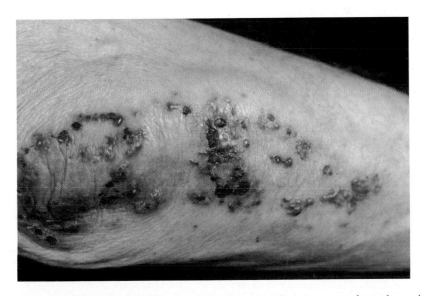

**FIGURE 6-14  Dermatitis herpetiformis**  *These are the classic lesions: grouped papules and vesicles, erosions, excoriations and crusting on the elbow.*

name herpertiformis); the distribution is strikingly symmetric. Scratching results in excoriations, crusts (Fig. 6-15). Postinflammatory hyper- and hypopigmentation at sites of healed lesions. *Sites of Predilection* Typical and almost diagnostic: extensor areas—elbows, knees. Buttocks, scapular and sacral areas (Fig. 6-15). Scalp, face, and hairline.

## LABORATORY EXAMINATIONS

**Immunogenetics**   Association with HLA-B8, HLA-DR, and HLA-DQ.
**Dermatopathology**   Biopsy is best from early erythematous papule. Microabscesses (polymorphonuclear cells and eosinophils) at the tips of the dermal papillae. Dermal infiltration of neutrophils and eosinophils. *Subepidermal vesicle.*
**Immunofluorescence**   Of perilesional skin, best on the buttocks. Granular IgA deposits in tips of papillae that correlate well with small-bowel disease. Granular IgA is found in most patients and is diagnostic.
**Circulating Autoantibodies**   Antireticulin antibodies of the IgA and IgG types, thyroid antimicrosomal antibodies, and antinuclear antibodies can be present. Putative immune complexes in 20 to 40% of patients. IgA antibodies binding to the intermyofibril substance of smooth muscles (*antiendomysial antibodies*) are present in most patients and have specificity for TGs.
**Other Studies**   Steatorrhea (20 to 30%) and abnormal D-xylose absorption (10 to 73%). Anemia secondary to iron or folate deficiency. *Endoscopy of small bowel*: blunting and flattening of the villi (80 to 90%) in the small bowel as in celiac disease. Lesions are focal; verification is by small-bowel biopsy.

## DIAGNOSIS AND DIFFERENTIAL DIAGNOSIS

Grouped papulovesicles at predilection sites accompanied by severe pruritus are highly suggestive. Biopsy of early lesions usually diagnostic, but IgA deposits in perilesional skin detected by IF are the best confirming evidence. Differential diagnosis is to allergic contact dermatitis, atopic dermatitis, scabies, neurotic excoriations, papular urticaria, bullous pemphigoid, pemphigoid gestationis (Table 6-5).

## COURSE

Prolonged, for many years, with a third of the patients eventually having a spontaneous remission.

## MANAGEMENT

**Systemic Therapy**   *Dapsone* 100 to 150 mg daily, with gradual reduction to 50 to 25 mg and often as low as 50 mg twice a week. There is a dramatic response, often within hours. Obtain a glucose-6-phosphate dehydrogenase level before starting sulfones; obtain methemoglobine levels in the initial 2 weeks, and follow blood counts carefully for the first few months.
*Sulfapyridine* 1 to 1.5 g/d, with plenty of fluids, if dapsone contraindicated or not tolerated. Monitor for casts in urine and kidney function.
**Diet**   A gluten-free diet *may* suppress the disease or allow reduction of the dosage of dapsone or sulfapyridine, but response is very slow.

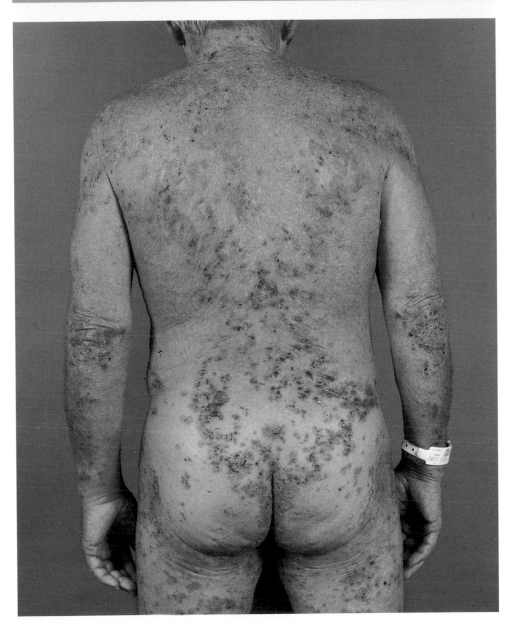

**FIGURE 6-15   Dermatitis herpetiformis**   *In this 56-year-old male patient with a generalized highly pruritic eruption, the diagnosis can be made upon first sight by the distribution of the lesions. Most heavily involved are the elbows, the scapular, sacral, and gluteal areas and (not seen in this picture) the knees. Upon close inspection there are grouped papules, small vesicles, crusts and erosions on an erythematous base and there is postinflammatory hypo- and hyperpigmentation. The patient had previously been diagnosed as having atopic dermatitis, scabies, and allergic contact dermatitis and had responded only poorly to topical glucocorticoids. This particular eruption occurred after he had spent a vacation on the Dalmation coast (having been told that sunbathing would be good for his condition) where his meals consisted of seafood (iodides) and white bread (gluten).*

**TABLE 6-5    Differential Diagnosis of Important Acquired Bullous Diseases**

| Disease | Skin Lesions | Mucous Membranes | Distribution |
|---------|--------------|------------------|--------------|
| PV | Flaccid bullae on normal skin, erosions | Almost always involved, erosions | Anywhere, localized or generalized |
| PF | Crusted erosions, occasionally flaccid vesicles | Rarely involved | Exposed, seborrheic regions or generalized |
| PVeg | Granulating plaques, occasionally vesicles at margin | As in PV | Intertriginous regions, scalp |
| Bullous pemphigoid | Tense bullae on normal and erythematous skin; urticarial plaques and papules | Mouth involved in 10–35% | Anywhere, localized or generalized |
| EBA | Tense bullae and erosions, non-inflammatory or BP-, DH- or LAD-like presentation | May be severely involved (oral esophagus, vagina) | Traumatized regions or random |
| Dermatitis herpetiformis | Grouped papules, vesicles, urticarial plaques, crusted | None | Predilection sites: elbows, knees, gluteal, sacral, and scapular areas |
| Linear IgA dermatosis | Annular, grouped papules, vesicles, and bullae | Oral erosions and ulcers, conjunctival erosions and scarring | Anywhere |

NOTE: AB, antibody; BMZ, basement membrane zone; BP, bullous pemphigoid; DH, dermatitis herpetiformis; EB, epidermolysis bullosa acquisita; ELISA, enzyme-linked immunosorbent assay; IIF, indirect immunofluorescence; LAD, linear IgA dermatosis; PF, pemphigus foliaceus; PV, pemphigus vulgaris; PVeg, pemphigus vegetans.

## TABLE 6-5  (Continued)

| Disease | Histopathology | Immunopathology/ Skin | Serum |
|---|---|---|---|
| PV | Suprabasal acantholysis | IgG intercellular pattern | IgA AB to intercellular substance of epidermis (IIF) ELISA : AB to desmoglein 3 >>desmoglein 1 |
| PF | Acantholysis in granular layer | IgG, intracellular pattern | IgG AB to intercellular substance of epidermis (IIF) ELISA: AB to desmoglein 1 only |
| PVeg | Acantholysis Intraepidermal neutrophilic abscesses epidermal hyperplasia | As in PV | As in PV |
| Bullous pemphigoid | Subepidermal blister | IgG and C3 linear at BMZ | IgG AB to BMZ (IIF); directed to BPAG1e and BPAG2 |
| EBA | Subepidermal blister | Linear IgG at BMZ | IgG AB to BMZ (IIF) directed to type VII collagen (ELISA, Western blot) |
| Dermatitis herpetiformis | Papillary microabscesses, subepidermal vesicle | Granular IgA in tips of papillae | Antiendomysial antibodies |
| Linear IgA dermatosis | Subepidermal blister with neutrophils | Linear IgA at BMZ | Low titers of IgA AB against BMZ |

NOTE: AB, antibody; BMZ, basement membrane zone; BP, bullous pemphigoid; DH, dermatitis herpetiformis; EB, epidermolysis bullosa acquisita; ELISA, enzyme-linked immunosorbent assay; IIF, indirect immunofluorescence; LAD, linear IgA dermatosis; PF, pemphigus foliaceus; PV, pemphigus vulgaris; PVeg, pemphigus vegetans.

## LINEAR IgA DERMATOSIS    □  

Linear IgA dermatosis (LAD) is a rare, immune-mediated, subepidermal blistering skin disease defined by the presence of homogeneous linear deposits of IgA at the cutaneous basement membrane zone (Image 6-1). It is clearly separate from dermatitis herpetiformis (DH) on the basis of immunopathology, immunogenetics, and lack of association with GSE. It is probably identical with chronic bullous disease of childhood (CBDC), which is a rare blistering disease that occurs predominantly in children <5 years and has an identical pattern of homogeneous linear IgA deposits at the epidermal basement membrane. LAD most often occurs after puberty. Clinical manifestations are very similar to those of DH, but there is more blistering. Patients present with combinations of annular or grouped papules, vesicles, and bullae (Fig. 6-16) that are distributed symmetrically on extensor surfaces including elbows, knees, and buttocks. The lesions are very pruritic but less severe than those of DH. Mucosal involvement is important and ranges from large asymptomatic oral erosions and ulceration to severe oral disease alone, or severe generalized cutaneous involvement and oral disease similar to that in cicatricial pemphigoid. Circulating autoantibodies against various epidermal basement membrane antigens have been found.

*Management*: Patients respond to dapsone or sulfapyridine but in addition, most may require low-dose prednisone. Patients do not respond to a gluten-free diet.

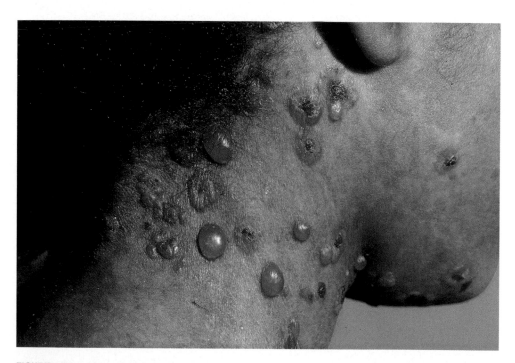

**FIGURE 6-16   Linear IgA dermatosis**   *Annular and grouped vesicles, bullae. Initially, they are tense, but become flaccid after they have ruptured.*

**FIGURE 6-17 (Opposite page)   Epidermolysis bullosa acquisita**   *This is the bullous pemphigoid-like presentation with (initially) tense bullae, erythematous papular and urticarial lesions, erosions, and crusting.*

# EPIDERMOLYSIS BULLOSA ACQUISITA

Epidermolysis bullosa acquisita (EBA) is a chronic subepidermal bullous disease associated with autoimmunity to the type VII collagen within the anchoring fibrils in the basement membrane zone. In the *classic mechano-bullous presentation* it is a noninflammatory, blistering eruption with acral distribution that heals with scarring and milia formation. It is a mechano-bullous disease marked by skin fragility, and patients have tense blisters within noninflamed skin, erosions, and scars in traumatized regions such as the dorsa of the hands, knuckles, elbows, knees, sacral area, and toes. This presentation thus resembles porphyria cutanea tarda (see Section 10) or hereditary epidermolysis bullosa. In the *bullous pemphigoid–like presentation* there is a widespread inflammatory vesiculo-bullous eruption where erythematous or even urticarial skin lesions are associated with tense bullae involving the trunk, central body, and skin folds in addition to the extremities (Fig. 6-17). The *cicatricial pemphigoid–like presentation* has prominent mucosal involvement—erosions and scarring in the mouth, esophagus, conjunctiva, anus, and vagina. In the *IgA bullous dermatosis–like presentation* vesicles arranged in an annular fashion are reminiscent of linear IgA bullous dermatosis, DH, or CBDC. Histopathology of lesional skin shows, subepidermal blisters with a clean separation between the epidermis and dermis, and immunopathology reveals linear IgG (plus IgA, IgM, factor B, and properdin) at the dermal-epidermal junction. If salt split-skin IIF is performed, circulating antibasement membrane zone antibodies bind the floor of the blister, in contrast to bullous pemphigoid where antibodies are bound to the roof. Antibodies in EBA sera will bind to a 290-kD band in Western blots containing type VII collagen. An ELISA that is very specific for antibodies to type VII collagen is now available.

*Treatment* of EBA is difficult, particularly in patients with the classic mechano-bullous presentation. Patients are refractory to high doses of systemic glucocorticoids, azathioprine, methotrexate, and cyclophosphamide, which are somewhat helpful in the inflammatory BP-like form of the disease. Some EBA patients improve on dapsone and high doses of colchicine. Supportive therapy is warranted in all patients with EBA.

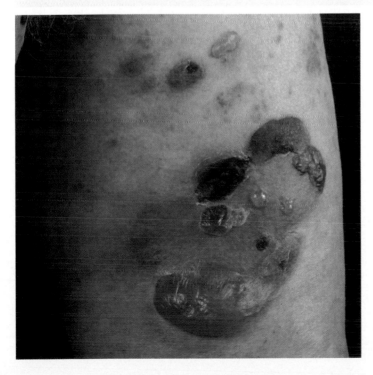

**FIGURE 6-17**

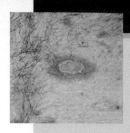

# MISCELLANEOUS INFLAMMATORY DISORDERS

## PITYRIASIS ROSEA

Pityriasis rosea is an acute exanthematous eruption with a distinctive morphology and often with a characteristic self-limited course. First, a single (primary, or "herald") plaque lesion develops, usually on the trunk, and 1 or 2 weeks later a generalized secondary eruption develops in a typical distribution pattern; the entire process remits spontaneously in 6 weeks.

### EPIDEMIOLOGY AND ETIOLOGY

**Age of Onset**  10 to 43 years, but can occur rarely in infants and old persons.
**Season**  Spring and fall.
**Etiology**  Herpes virus type 7 is suspected.

### HISTORY

**Duration of Lesions**  A single herald patch precedes the exanthematous phase; which develops over a period of 1 to 2 weeks. Pruritus—absent (25%), mild (50%), or severe (25%).

### PHYSICAL EXAMINATION

#### Skin Lesions
*Herald Patch*  80% of patients. Oval, slightly raised plaque 2 to 5 cm, salmon-red, fine collarette scale at periphery; may be multiple (inset in Fig. 7-1).
*Exanthem*  Fine scaling papules and plaques with marginal collarette (Fig. 7-1). Dull pink or tawny. Oval, scattered, with characteristic distribution with the long axes of the oval lesions following the lines of cleavage in a "Christmas tree" pattern (Graph 7-1). Lesions usually confined to trunk and proximal aspects of the arms and legs. Rarely on face.
*Atypical Pityriasis Rosea*  Lesions may be present only on the face and neck. The primary plaque may be absent, may be the sole manifestation of the disease, or may be multiple. Most confusing are the examples of pityriasis rosea with vesicles or simulating erythema multiforme.

This usually results from irritation and sweating, often as a consequence of inadequate treatment (*pityriasis rosea irritata*).

### DIFFERENTIAL DIAGNOSIS

**Multiple Small Scaling Plaques**  *Drug eruptions* (e.g., captopril, barbiturates); *secondary syphilis* (obtain serology); *guttate psoriasis* (no marginal collarette); *erythema migrans* with secondary lesions; *erythema multiforme;* and *tinea corporis.*

### LABORATORY EXAMINATION

**Dermatopathology**  Patchy or diffuse parakeratosis, absence of granular layer, slight acanthosis, focal spongiosis, microscopic vesicles. Occasional dyskeratotic cells with an eosinophilic homogeneous appearance. Edema of dermis, homogenization of the collagen. Perivascular infiltrate mononuclear cells.

### COURSE

Spontaneous remission in 6 to 12 weeks or less. Recurrences are uncommon.

### MANAGEMENT

**Symptomatic**  Oral antihistamines and/or topical antipruritic lotions for relief of pruritus. Topical glucocorticoids. May be improved by UVB phototherapy or natural sunlight exposure if treatment is begun in the first week of eruption. Short course of systemic glucocorticoids.

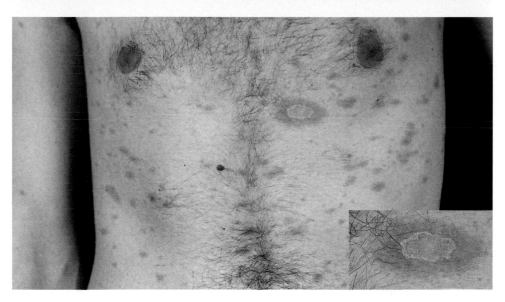

**FIGURE 7-1   Pityriasis rosea**   *Overview of exanthem of pityriasis rosea with the herald patch shown in the inset. There are papules and small plaques with oval configuration that follow the lines of cleavage. The fine scaling of the salmon-red papules cannot be seen at this magnification, while the collarette of the herald patch is quite obvious. Inset: Herald patch. An erythematous (salmon-red) plaque with a collarette scale on the trailing edge of the advancing border. Collarette means that scale is attached at periphery and loose toward the center of the lesion.*

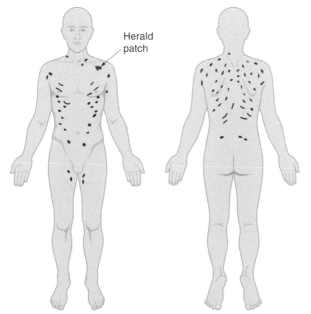

Herald patch

**IMAGE 7-1   Pityriasis rosea:** *distribution "Christmas Tree" pattern on the back.*

# PARAPSORIASIS EN PLAQUES

Two types are now generally recognized: (1) *Small-plaque parapsoriasis* (also known as digitate dermatosis, or chronic superficial dermatitis); it is not regarded as a lesion that can turn into mycosis fungoides [cutaneous T cell lymphoma (CTCL)]. (2) *Large-plaque parapsoriasis* is an important disorder to follow carefully with repeated biopsies to rule out early mycosis fungoides.

## SMALL-PLAQUE PARAPSORIASIS (DIGITATE DERMATOSIS)    □  ○

### HISTORY

Gradual development over months. Rare pruritus. Middle age.

### PHYSICAL EXAMINATION

#### Skin Lesions
Round, oval, erythematous, yellowish, only slightly elevated plaques, <5 cm in diameter (Fig. 7-2). Slight scale and wrinkled surface with cigarette-paper appearance. Finger-like (digitate) shapes on trunk, proximal extremities, and buttocks, following lines of cleavage, giving appearance of a hug that left finger-prints.

### DIFFERENTIAL DIAGNOSIS

Pityriasis rosea, large-plaque parapsoriasis.

### LABORATORY EXAMINATION

**Dermatopathology**   Spongiform dermatitis with focal areas of hyperkeratosis, parakeratosis, and exocytosis. In the dermis there are a mild super-ficial vascular lymphohistiocytic infiltrate and dermal edema.

### MANAGEMENT

No treatment necessary, but patients should be reassured. Disease may be treated with lubricant or topical steroids. Broad-band phototherapy; UVB (311 nm) and PUVA are highly effective.

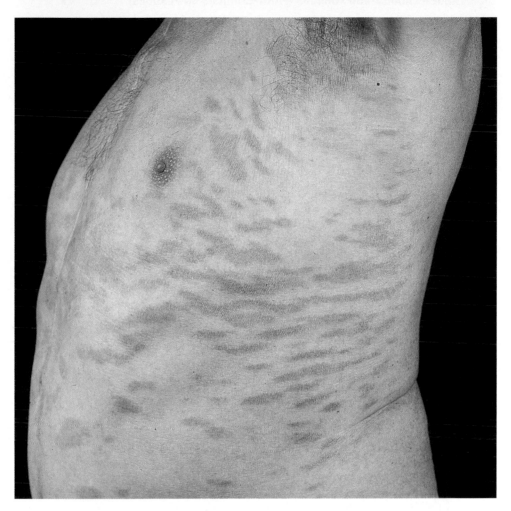

**FIGURE 7-2   Digitate dermatosis (small plaque parapsoriasis)**   *The lesions are asymptomatic, yellowish or fawn-colored, very thin, well defined, slightly scaly plaques. They are oval and follow the lines of cleavage of the skin, giving the appearance of a "hug" that left fingerprints on the trunk. The long axis of these lesions often reaches more than 5 cm.*

## HISTORY

Gradual development over months and years, starting with one or two plaques. Pruritus is rare; the lesions may disappear after exposure to sun in the summer to recur in the fall and winter. Middle age.

## PHYSICAL EXAMINATION

### Skin Lesions

Barely elevated, erythematous, dusky-red, sometimes yellowish plaques (Fig. 7-3), with or without slight atrophy and smooth or slightly scaling surface. Circular, >10 cm in diameter and well defined, and randomly scattered on trunk, buttocks, breasts, or extremities.

## DIFFERENTIAL DIAGNOSIS

**Scaling Plaques**   "Early" stages of CTCL (mycosis fungoides). The development of *infiltration* in the lesions, *atrophy*, and *poikilodermatous changes* are clues to early mycosis fungoides.

## LABORATORY EXAMINATIONS

**Dermatopathology**   Nonspecific or, later, a bandlike mononuclear cell infiltrate ($CD4^+$) with atrophy of the epidermis, vacuolization of the basal cell layer, capillary dilatation. There are no atypical lymphocytes. Mild exocytosis.
**Peripheral Blood**   Monoclonal T helper cells with skin-homing specificity can be detected.

## COURSE AND PROGNOSIS

The lesions persist for life and can progress to CTCL.

## MANAGEMENT

**Topical**   Temporary remission with topical glucocorticoids.
**Phototherapy**   Good responses to narrow-band 311-nm UVB or PUVA photochemotherapy.

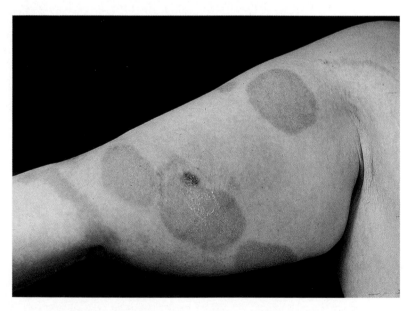

**FIGURE 7-3   Large plaque parapsoriasis (parapsoriasis en plaques)**   *The lesions are asymptomatic, well defined, rounded, slightly scaly, thin plaques. The lesions are most often larger than 10 cm and are light red-brown or salmon-pink. There may be atrophy in some areas. The lesions here are located on the extremities but they are more commonly noted on the trunk. These lesions must be carefully followed and repeated biopsies are necessary to detect mycosis fungoides. Some regard this entity as a prestage of mycosis fungoides.*

# LICHEN PLANUS   ▢▮  ◐

Lichen planus (LP) is an acute or chronic inflammatory dermatosis involving skin and/or mucous membranes, characterized by flat-topped (Latin *planus*, "flat"), pink to violaceous, shiny, pruritic polygonal papules on the skin and milky white reticulated papules in the mouth. The features of the lesions have been designated as the four P's—papule, purple, polygonal, pruritic.

## EPIDEMIOLOGY AND ETIOLOGY

**Age of Onset**   30 to 60 years.
**Sex**  Females > males.
**Race**   Hypertrophic LP more common in blacks.
**Etiology**   Idiopathic in most cases but it is evident that cell-mediated immunity plays a major role. Majority of lymphocytes in the infiltrate are $CD8^+$ and $CD45Ro^+$ (memory) cells. Drugs, metals (gold, mercury), or infection [hepatitis C virus (HCV)] result in alteration in cell-mediated immunity. There could be HLA-associated genetic susceptibility that would explain a predisposition in certain persons. Lichenoid lesions of chronic graft-versus-host disease (GVHD) of skin are indistinguishable from those of LP.

## HISTORY

**Onset**   Acute (days) or insidious (over weeks). Lesions last months to years, asymptomatic or pruritic; sometimes severe pruritus. Mucous membrane lesions are painful, especially when ulcerated.

## PHYSICAL EXAMINATION

### Skin Lesions
Papules, flat-topped, 1 to 10 mm, sharply defined, shiny (Figs. 7-4 and 7-5). Violaceous, with white lines (Wickham's striae) (Fig. 7-4), seen best with hand lens after application of mineral oil. Polygonal or oval. Grouped (Figs. 7-4 and 7-5), linear (isomorphic phenomenon), annular, or disseminated scattered discrete lesions when generalized (Fig. 7-6). In dark-skinned individuals, postinflammatory hyperpigmentation is common.
*Sites of Predilection*   Wrists (flexor), lumbar region, shins (thicker, hyperkeratotic lesions), scalp, glans penis, mouth (Graph 7-2).

### Variants
*Hypertrophic*   Large thick plaques arise on the foot (Fig. 7-5A) and shins (Fig. 7-5B); more common in black males. Although typical LP papule is smooth, hypertrophic lesions may become hyperkeratotic.
*Follicular*   Individual keratotic-follicular papules and plaques that lead to cicatricial alopecia. Spinous follicular lesions, typical skin and mucous membrane LP, and cicatricial alopecia of the scalp are called *Graham Little syndrome*. (See Section 29.)
*Vesicular*   Vesicular or bullous lesions may develop within LP patches or independent of them within normal-appearing skin. There are direct immunofluorescence findings consistent with bullous pemphigoid, and the sera of these patients contain bullous pemphigoid IgG autoantibodies (see Section 6).
*Actinicus*   Papular LP lesions arise in sun-exposed sites, especially the dorsa of hands and arms.
*Ulcerative*   LP may lead to therapy-resistant ulcers, particularly on the soles, requiring skin grafting.
### Mucous Membranes   Some 40 to 60% of individuals with LP have oropharyngeal involvement.
*Reticular LP*   Reticulate (netlike) pattern of lacy white hyperkeratosis on buccal mucosa (see Fig. 31-13), lips (Fig. 7-7), tongue, gingiva; the most common pattern of oral LP.
*Erosive or ulcerative LP*   Superficial erosion with/without overlying fibrin clot; occurs on tongue and buccal mucosa (see Fig. 31-14); shiny red painful erosion of gingiva (desquamative gingivitis) (see Fig. 31-14) or lips (Fig. 7-7). Carcinoma may very rarely develop in mouth lesions.
### Genitalia   Papular (see Fig. 32-8), annular, or erosive lesions arise on penis (especially glans), scrotum, labia majora, labia minora, vagina.
### Hair and Nails
*Scalp*   Atrophic scalp skin with scarring alopecia.
*Nails*   Destruction of nail fold and nail bed with longitudinal splintering (see Fig. 30-8).

## LICHEN PLANUS–LIKE ERUPTIONS

Lichen planus–like eruptions closely mimic typical LP, both clinically and histologically. They occur as a clinical manifestation of chronic GVHD; in dermatomyositis, and as cutaneous manifestations of malignant lymphoma but may also develop as the result of therapy with certain drugs and after industrial use of certain compounds (Table 7-1).

## DIAGNOSIS AND DIFFERENTIAL DIAGNOSIS

Clinical findings confirmed by histopathology.
### Skin Lesions
*Papular LP* Chronic cutaneous lupus erythematosus, psoriasis, pityriasis rosea, eczematous dermatitis, lichenoid GVHD; superficial basal cell carcinoma, Bowen's disease (in situ squamous cell carcinoma).
*Hypertrophic LP* Psoriasis vulgaris, lichen simplex chronicus, prurigo nodularis, stasis dermatitis, Kaposi's sarcoma.
*Drug-Induced LP* See Table 7-1.

**Mucous Membranes** Leukoplakia, pseudomembranous candidiasis (thrush), HIV-associated hairy leukoplakia, lupus erythematosus, bite trauma, mucous patches of secondary syphilis, pemphigus vulgaris, bullous pemphigoid.

## LABORATORY EXAMINATION

**Dermatopathology** Inflammation with hyperkeratosis, increased granular layer, irregular acanthosis, liquefaction degeneration of the basal cell layer, and bandlike mononuclear infiltrate that hugs the epidermis. Degenerate keratinocytes (colloid, Civatte bodies) are found at the dermal-epidermal junction. Direct immunofluorescence reveals heavy deposits of fibrin at the junction and IgM and, less frequently, IgA, IgG, and C3 in the colloid bodies.

## COURSE

Cutaneous LP usually persists for months, but in some cases, for years; hypertrophic LP on the shins and oral LP often for decades. The incidence of oral cancer (squamous cell carcinoma)

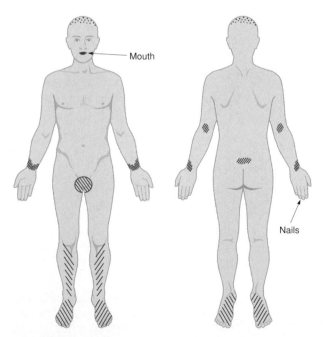

Mouth

Nails

**IMAGE 7-2   Lichen planus:** *predilection sites.*

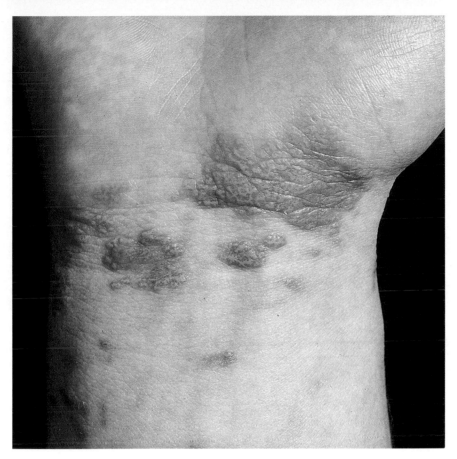

**FIGURE 7-4    Lichen planus**    *Flat-topped, polygonal, sharply defined papules of violaceous color, grouped and confluent. Surface is shiny and upon close inspection or a hand lens, reveals fine white lines (Wickham's striae), which can be further enhanced by applying a drop of mineral oil to the lesions.*

in individuals with oral LP is increased by 5%; patients should be followed at regular intervals.

## MANAGEMENT

### Topical Therapy
***Glucocorticoids*** Topical glucocorticoids with occlusion for cutaneous lesions. Intralesional triamcinolone (3 mg/mL) is helpful for symptomatic cutaneous or oral mucosal lesions and lips.
***Cyclosporine and Tacrolimus Solutions*** Retention "mouthwash" for severely symptomatic oral LP.

### Systemic Therapy
***Cyclosporine*** In very resistant and generalized cases, 5 mg/kg per day will induce rapid remission, quite often not followed by recurrence.

***Glucocorticoids*** Oral prednisone is effective for individuals with symptomatic pruritus, painful erosions, dysphagia, or cosmetic disfigurement. A short, tapered course is preferred: 70 mg initially, tapered by 5 mg.
***Systemic Retinoids (Acitretin)*** 1 mg/kg per day is helpful as adjunctive measure in severe (oral, hypertrophic) cases, but usually additional topical treatment is required.

### PUVA Photochemotherapy
In individuals with generalized LP or cases resistant to topical therapy.

### Reports of Other Successful Treatment
Mycophenolate mofetil, heparin analogues (enoxaparin) in low doses have antiproliferative and immunomodulatory properties; azathioprine.

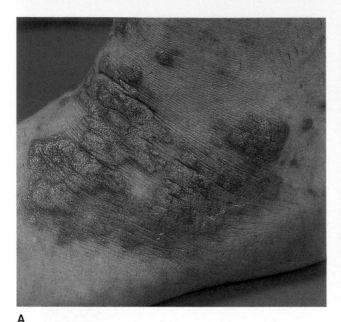
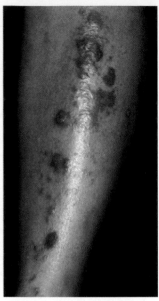

A                                                                                          B

**FIGURE 7-5    Lichen planus    *A. Violaceous color of flat-topped, confluent papules that form
plaques. This color is highly characteristic and Wickham's striae are also present. Note also that
lesions are thicker than in Fig. 7-4, which is due to their location on a dependent site (foot). These
lesions will later evolve into hypertrophic lichen planus. B. Hypertrophic lichen planus in the
pretibial region in a dark-skinned individual. Lesions are almost nodular and very dark with the
characteristic violaceous sheen on the surface. These lesions may later become hyperkeratotic
that will obscure the typical color.***

**TABLE 7-1    Agents Inducing Lichen Planus and Lichenoid Reactions**

|  | Less-common Inducers | |
| --- | --- | --- |
| **Common Inducers** | **Commonly Prescribed Drugs** | **Uncommonly Prescribed Drugs** |
| Gold salts | ACE inhibitors | Methyldopa |
| Beta blockers | Calcium channel | Antitubercular |
| Antimalarials | blockers | Sulfasalazine |
| Thiazide diuretics | Sulfonylurea | Heavy metals |
| Furosemide | hypoglycemic agents | (arsenic, mercury) |
| Spironolactone | Nonsteroidal anti- | Lithium |
| Penicillamine | inflammatory drugs | Iodides and radiocontrast |
|  | Ketoconazole | media |
|  | Tetracycline | Antimony |
|  | Phenothiazine | Carbamazepine |
|  | derivatives |  |

SOURCE: From MS Daoud, M Pittelkow, Lichen planus, in IM Freedberg, AZ Eisen, K Wolff, KF Austen, LA Goldsmith, SI
  Katz (eds). *Fitzpatrick's Dermatology in General Medicine*, 6th ed. New York, McGraw-Hill, 2003.

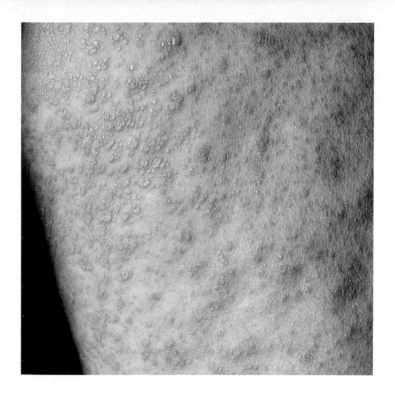

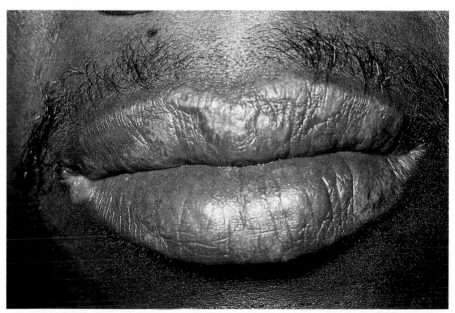

**FIGURE 7-6 (Top)   Generalized lichen planus**   *Small, flat-topped, violaceous papules, some grouped and some disseminated, becoming confluent on the trunk.*

**FIGURE 7-7 (Bottom)   Lichen planus**   *Silvery white flat-topped papules on the lips. Note Wickham's striae. In Africans these lesions can lead to considerable disfigurement.*

## GRANULOMA ANNULARE    ■  ○ → ◑

Granuloma annulare (GA) is a self-limited, asymptomatic, chronic dermatosis of the dermis that exhibits papules in an annular arrangement, commonly arising on the dorsa of the hands and feet, elbows, and knees, and which sometimes becomes generalized in distribution.

### EPIDEMIOLOGY

Common.
**Age of Onset**  Children and young adults.
**Sex**  Female:male ratio 2:1.

### ETIOLOGY AND PATHOGENESIS

Unknown. An immunologically mediated necrotizing inflammation that surrounds blood vessels, altering collagen and elastic tissue. Generalized GA may be associated with diabetes mellitus.

### HISTORY

Duration months to years. Usually asymptomatic and only cosmetic disfigurement.

### PHYSICAL EXAMINATION

**Skin Lesions**
Firm, smooth, shiny dermal papules and plaques, 1 to 5 cm (Fig. 7-8). Annular, arciform plaques with central depression (Fig. 7-9), skin-colored, violaceous, erythematous. *Subcutaneous GA* (rare): painless, skin-colored, deep dermal or subcutaneous, solitary or multiple nodules.
***Distribution***  Isolated lesion, particularly on dorsum of hand (Fig. 7-8), multiple lesions on extremities and trunk (Fig. 7-9), or generalized (papular; older patients). Subcutaneous lesions are located near joints, palms and soles, buttocks.

**Variants**

• *Perforating* lesions are very rare and mostly on the hands; central umbilication followed by crusting and ulceration; this type was associated with diabetes in one series.
• GA associated with necrobiosis lipoidica can be confusing, as some patients can have both diseases at the same time.
• May rarely involve fascia and tendons, causing sclerosis.
• Generalized GA: in this form a search for diabetes mellitus should be made.

### DIFFERENTIAL DIAGNOSIS

GA is important because of its differential diagnosis to more serious conditions.
**Papular Lesions and Plaques**  Necrobiosis lipoidica, papular sarcoid, lichen planus, lymphocytic infiltrate of Jessner.
**Subcutaneous Nodules**  Rheumatoid nodules: confusion can occur because of the same pathology of GA and rheumatic nodule or rheumatoid nodules.
**Annular Lesions**  Tinea, erythema migrans, sarcoid, lichen planus.

### LABORATORY EXAMINATION

**Dermatopathology**  Foci of chronic inflammatory and histiocytic infiltrations in superficial and mid-dermis, with necrobiosis of connective tissue surrounded by a wall of palisading histiocytes and multinucleated giant cells.

### COURSE

The disease disappears in 75% of patients in 2 years. Recurrences are common (40%), but they also disappear.

### MANAGEMENT

GA is a local skin disorder and not a marker for internal disease, and spontaneous remission is the rule. *No treatment is an option if the lesions are not disfiguring.*
**Topical Therapy**  *Topical Glucocorticoids*  Applied under plastic occlusion or hydrocolloid.
*Intralesional Triamcinolone*  3 mg/mL into lesions is effective.
*Cryospray*  Superficial lesions respond to liquid nitrogen, but atrophy may occur.
**PUVA Photochemotherapy**  Effective in generalized GA.

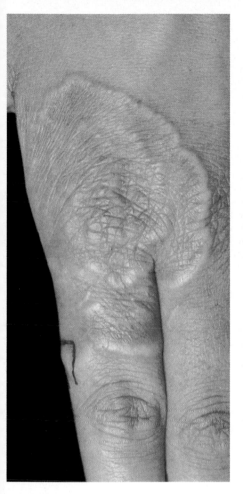 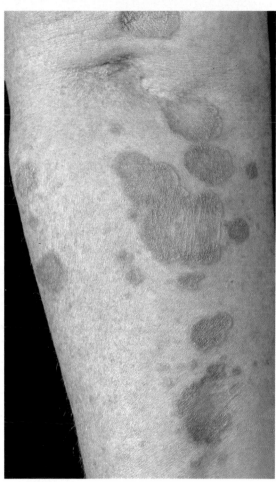

**FIGURE 7-8 (Left)   Granuloma annulare**   *Confluent, pearly white, firm papules forming two rings, 1 cm and 5 cm in diameter on the dorsum of hand that is a site of predilection. Lesions are firm and asymptomatic. Note there is no scaling.*

**FIGURE 7-9 (Right)   Granuloma annulare**   *Multiple annular and semicircular plaques with central regression on the arm. When located in sites other than the dorsa of the hands, granuloma annulare may acquire a reddish or brownish color and is then very difficult to distinguish from sarcoidosis.*

## MORPHEA　☐　◐

Morphea is a localized and circumscribed cutaneous sclerosis characterized by early violaceous, later ivory-colored, hardened skin; may be solitary, linear, generalized, and, rarely, accompanied by atrophy of underlying structures. It is unrelated to systemic scleroderma.
*Synonyms*: Localized scleroderma, circumscribed scleroderma.

### EPIDEMIOLOGY AND ETIOLOGY

**Incidence** Rare between the ages of 20 and 50; in linear morphea, earlier. Pansclerotic morphea, a disabling disorder, usually starts before age 14.
**Sex** Females are affected about three times as often as males, including children. Linear scleroderma is the same in males and females
**Etiology** Unknown. At least some patients (predominantly in Europe) with classic morphea have sclerosis due to *Borrelia burgdorferi* infection, and, if not too sclerotic, the lesions can disappear with prolonged courses of oral antibiotics. Pigmentation, however, persists. Morphea has been noted after x-irradiation for breast cancer. Morphea is not related to systemic scleroderma.

### CLASSIFICATION OF VARIOUS TYPES OF LOCALIZED SCLERODERMA

*Circumscribed*: plaques or bands
*Linear scleroderma*: upper or lower extremity
*Frontoparietal (en coup de sabre)*
*Generalized morphea*
*Pansclerotic*: involvement of dermis, fat, fascia, muscle, bone.

### HISTORY

**Symptoms** Usually none. No history of Raynaud's phenomenon. Pansclerotic morphea can result in major facial or limb asymmetry, flexion contractures, and disability.

### PHYSICAL EXAMINATION

**Skin Findings**
*Plaques*—circumscribed, indurated, hard, but poorly defined areas of skin; 2 to 15 cm in diameter, round or oval, often better felt than seen. Initially, purplish or mauve. In time, surface becomes smooth and shiny (Fig. 7-10) after months to years, ivory with lilac-colored edge "lilac ring" (Fig. 7-11). May have hyperpigmentation in involved sclerotic areas. Rarely, lesions become atrophic and hyperpigmented without going through a sclerotic stage (atrophoderma of Pasini and Pierini).

*Distribution*
*Circumscribed:* Trunk (Fig. 7-10), limbs, face, genitalia; less commonly, axillae, perineum, areolae.
*Linear:* Usually on extremity (Fig. 7-12) or *frontoparietal*—scalp and face (Fig. 7-13); here it may resemble a scar from a strike with a saber (en coup de sabre).
*Generalized:* Initially on trunk (upper, breasts, abdomen) (Fig. 7-11) thighs.
*Pansclerotic:* On trunk (Fig. 7-14) or extremities.

**Mouth** With linear morphea of head, may have associated hemiatrophy of tongue.
**Hair and Nails** Scarring alopecia with scalp plaque. Nail dystrophy in linear lesions of extremity or in pansclerotic morphea.

**FIGURE 7-10 (Opposite page)　Morphea** *This is an indurated, ivory-colored plaque with a lilac-colored, ill-defined border. Typically localized on the trunk, below the breast, this lesion is better felt than seen and since it is hard and close to the breast, it is of considerable concern to the patient.*

**FIGURE 7-11 (Opposite page)　Morphea** *Generalized lesions on trunk. Ill-defined, indurated; some being ivory-colored, some hypo- or hyperpigmented. If the hyperpigmented lesions are just atrophic and cannot be felt, they are called atrophoderma of Pasini and Pierini.*

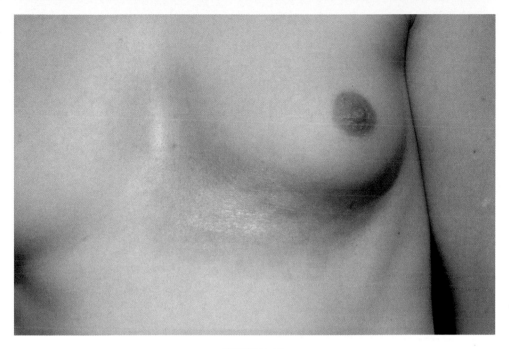

FIGURE 7-10

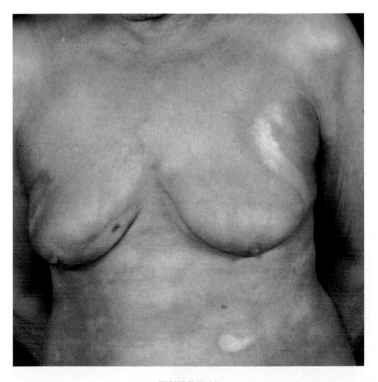

FIGURE 7-11

## General Examination

Morphea around joints may lead to flexion contractures. Pansclerotic morphea is associated with atrophy and fibrosis of muscle (Fig. 7-14). Extensive involvement of trunk may result in restricted respiration. With linear morphea of the head (Fig. 7-13), there may be associated atrophy of ocular structures and atrophy of bone.

## DIAGNOSIS AND DIFFERENTIAL DIAGNOSIS

Clinical, confirmed by biopsy. Sclerotic plaque associated with *B. burgdorferi* infection, acrodermatitis chronica atrophicans, progressive systemic sclerosis, lichen sclerosus et atrophicus, eosinophilic fasciitis, toxic oil syndrome, eosinophilia-myalgia syndrome associated with L-tryptophan ingestion, scleredema, Parry-Romberg syndrome (hemiatrophy).

## LABORATORY EXAMINATIONS

**Serology**   Appropriate serologic testing to rule out *B. burgdorferi* infection.

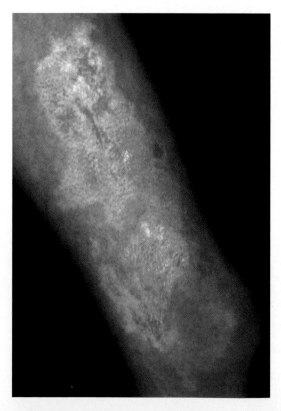

**Dermatopathology**   Epidermis appears normal to atrophic with loss of rete ridges. Dermis edematous with homogeneous and eosinophilic collagens. Slight infiltrate, perivascular or diffuse; lymphocytes, plasma cells, macrophages. Later, dermis thickened with few fibroblasts and dense collagen; inflammatory infiltrate at dermal-subcutis junction; dermal appendages disappear progressively. Pansclerotic lesions show fibrosis and disappearance of subcutaneous tissue, with fibrosis involving fascia. Silver stains should be performed to rule out *B. burgdorferi* infection.

## DIAGNOSIS

Clinical diagnosis, usually confirmed by skin biopsy.

## COURSE

May be slowly progressive; "burn out" and spontaneous remissions can rarely occur.

## MANAGEMENT

There is no effective treatment for morphea, but some reports of treatment are as follows:
**Morphea-Like Lesions Associated with Lyme Borreliosis**   In patients with early involvement, there may be a reversal of sclerosis with high-dose parenteral penicillin or ceftriaxone; treatment given in several courses over a time span of several months. Best response if combined with oral glucocorticoids.
**Phototherapy with UVA-1 (340 to 400 nm).** In our experience, the treatment is not easy or very successful because of the prolonged irradiation times and the disfiguring hyperpigmentation of the irradiated areas.

**FIGURE 7-12   Linear morphea**   *Indurated, ivory-white lesion extending from upper thigh to dorsum of foot. If induration is pronounced and extends to fascia (pansclerotic morphea), it will severely limit movements of joints.*

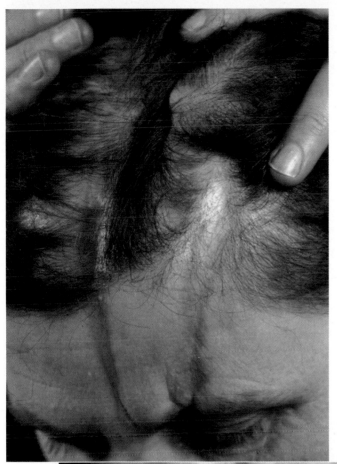

**FIGURE 7-13   Linear morphea, "en coup de sabre"**   *Two linear, partially ivory-white and/or hyperpigmented lesions extending from the crown of the head over the forehead to the orbita. They look like scars after strikes with a saber, hence the French designation. These lesions can extend to the bone and, rarely, to the dura mater.*

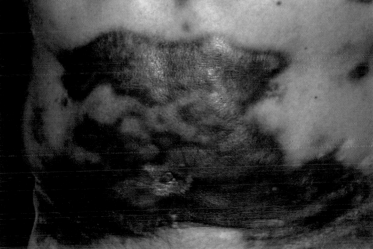

**FIGURE 7-14   Pansclerotic morphea**   *This type affects all layers of the skin and includes the fascia and even muscle. Skin is glistening, hyperpigmented, and hard as wood. It is obvious that pansclerotic morphea leads to considerable functional impairment, particularly when it occurs around joints or on the hands. These lesions impaired breathing.*

# LICHEN SCLEROSUS      □  ◐

Lichen sclerosus et atrophicus (LSA) is a chronic atrophic disorder mainly of the anogenital skin of females but also of males and of the general skin. A disease of adults, but also occurring in children 1 to 13 years of age. Females are ten times more often affected than males. Whitish, ivory or porcelain-white, sharply demarcated, individual papules may become confluent, forming *plaques* (Fig. 7-15). Surface of lesions may be elevated or in the same plane as normal skin; older lesions may be depressed. Dilated pilosebaceous or sweat duct orifices filled with keratin plugs (dells); if plugging is marked, surface appears verrucous. *Bullae* and *erosions* occur and *purpura* is often a characteristic and identifying feature (Fig. 7-15); *telangiectasia.* Lesions occur on general skin or on the genitalia. On vulva, hyperkeratotic plaques may become erosive, macerated; vulva may become atrophic, shrunken, especially clitoris and labia minora, with vaginal introitus reduced in size (see Fig. 32-10). Fusion of labia minora and majora. In uncircumcised males, prepuce first shows ivory white confluent papules (see Fig. 32-9) but then becomes sclerotic and cannot be retracted (*phimosis*). Glans appears ivory or porcelain-white, semitransparent, resembling mother-of-pearl with admixed purpuric hemorrhages. Nongenital LSA is usually asymptomatic; genital often asymptomatic, even with striking clinical changes. In females, vulvar lesions may be sensitive, especially while walking; pruritus; painful, especially if erosions are present; dysuria; dyspareunia. In males, recurrent balanitis acquired phimosis.

The histopathology is diagnostic with a dense lymphocytic infiltrate hugging the initially hypertrophic and later; atrophic epidermis and then sinking down into the dermis, being separated from the epidermis by an edematous, structureless subepidermal zone. The etiology of LS is unknown, but reports from Europe have documented an association of DNA of *Borrelia* spp. with LS in cases from Germany and Japan; DNA of the spirochetes detected in these patients was not found in any of the American samples.

The course of LS waxes and wanes. In girls it may undergo spontaneous resolution; in older women it leads to atrophy of the vulva and in men to phimosis. Patients should be checked for the occurrence of squamous cell carcinoma of the vulva and penis.

Management is very important, as this disease can cause a devastating atrophy of the labia minora and clitoral hood. Potent topical *glucocorticoid preparations* (clobetasol propionate) have proved effective for genital LS and should be used for 6 to 8 weeks only. Patients should be monitored for signs of glucocorticoid-induced atrophy. *Pimecrolimus* and *tacrolimus* are almost as effective. *Topical androgens* are less used now because they can sometimes cause a clitoral hypertrophy. *Systemic therapy*: hydrochloroquine, 125 to 150 mg/d, for weeks to a few months (monitor for ocular side effects).

In males, *circumcision* relieves symptoms of phimosis and in some cases can result in remission.

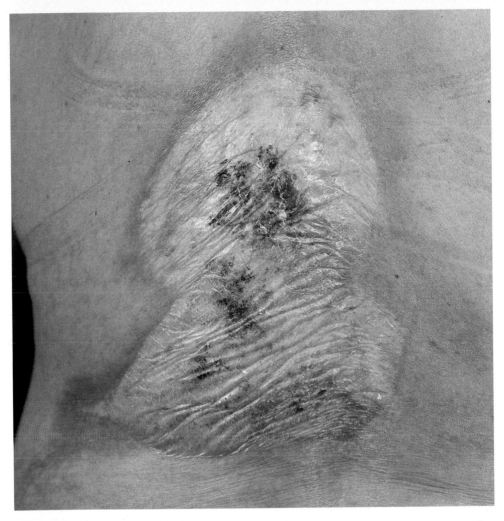

**FIGURE 7-15   Lichen sclerosus et atrophicus**   *An ivory-white, indurated but superficially atrophic plaque on the lower back that has arisen from the confluence of multiple whitish papules (best seen on left border). Initially these papules may show follicular hyperkeratosis and dry, hyperkeratotic scaling is also evident in the center of this glistening plaque where there is also superficial petechial hemorrhage. The border is surrounded by a hyperpigmented ring of otherwise normal-appearing skin.*

# PIGMENTED PURPURIC DERMATOSES    □   ○

Pigmented purpuric dermatoses are distinguished by their clinical characteristics, having identical dermatopathologic findings, and include:

- Schamberg's disease, also known as progressive pigmented purpuric dermatosis and progressive pigmentary purpura
- Majocchi's disease, also known as purpura annularis telangiectodes
- Gougerot-Blum disease, also known as pigmented purpuric lichenoid dermatitis and purpura pigmentosa chronica
- Lichen aureus, also known as lichen purpuricus

Clinically, each entity shows recent pinpoint cayenne pepper–colored hemorrhages associated with older hemorrhages and hemosiderin deposition. Capillaritis histologically. Pigmented purpuric dermatoses are significant only if they are a cosmetic concern to the patient; they are important because they are often mistaken as manifestations of vasculitis or thrombocytopenia. *Synonym*: Capillaritis of unknown cause.

## EPIDEMIOLOGY AND ETIOLOGY

**Age of Onset**   30 to 60 years; uncommon in children.

**Sex**   More common in males.

**Etiology**   Unknown. Primary process believed to be cell-mediated immune injury with subsequent vascular damage and erythrocyte extravasation. Other etiologic factors: pressure, trauma, drugs (acetaminophen, ampicillin–carbromal, diuretics, meprobamate, nonsteroidal anti-inflammatory drugs, zomepirac sodium).

**Onset and Duration**   Insidious, slow to evolve—except drug-induced variant, which may develop rapidly and be more generalized in distribution. Persists for months to years. Most drug-induced purpuras resolve more quickly after discontinuation of the drug. Usually asymptomatic but may be mildly pruritic.

## PHYSICAL EXAMINATION

**Schamberg's Disease**   Discrete clusters of pinhead-sized red macules and barely palpable papules become confluent, coalescing into patches (Fig. 7-16). Diascopy reveals pinpoint hemorrhages (hence the term *purpura*). New lesions are red, representing pinpoint hemorrhages; older lesions tan to brown, representing degradation of extravasated erythrocytes with the formation of hemosiderin. Overall color impression: reddish brown, "cayenne pepper" (Fig. 7-16). Lower extremities (especially pretibial and on ankles) but may extend proximally to lower trunk and to upper extremities. Usually bilateral but may be unilateral. Uncommonly, generalized.

**Majocchi's Disease**   Essentially an annular form of Schamberg's disease with telangiectasias (Fig. 7-17). An arciform variant has also been described.

**Gougerot-Blum Disease**   Lichenoid papules, plaques, macules in association with lesions of Schamberg's disease.

**Lichen Aureus**   Solitary or few patches or plaques, rust-colored, purple, or golden, arising on the extremities or trunk.

## LABORATORY EXAMINATIONS

**Dermatopathology**   Epidermal involvement varies, but dermal pathology (capillaritis) with extravasation of erythrocytes, hemosiderin pigment–laden macrophages (more extensive in lichen aureus), mild perivascular and interstitial lymphohistiocytic infiltrate in reticular dermis is common to all. Immunofluorescence is variable and nonspecific.

## DIAGNOSIS AND DIFFERENTIAL DIAGNOSIS

**Nonpalpable Purpura**   Chronic venous insufficiency with clotting abnormalities, glucocorticoid usage, CTLC; dysproteinemias, nummular eczema, old fixed drug eruption, parapsoriasis, poikiloderma vasculare atrophicans, primary amyloidosis, scurvy, senile purpura, stasis dermatitis, thrombocytopenia, trauma.

**Palpable Purpura**   Leukocytoclastic vasculitis.

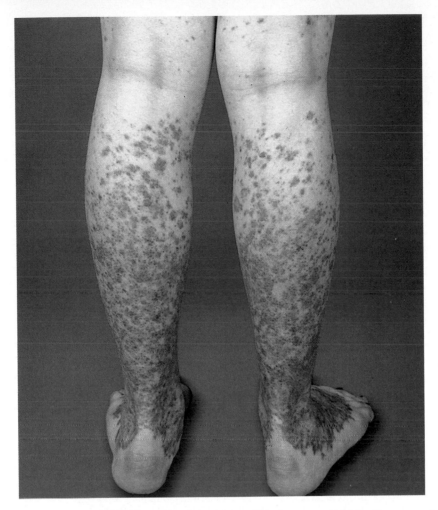

**FIGURE 7-16   Pigmented purpuric dermatosis: Schamberg's disease**   *Multiple, discrete, and confluent nonpalpable, nonblanching purpuric lesions of many months duration on the legs. Acute microhemorrhages resolve with deposition of hemosiderin, creating a disfiguring dark-brown peppered stain.*

## COURSE

Chronic (months to years), slow to evolve and resolve; spontaneous resolution has occurred. In lesions of long standing, hemosiderin deposits resolve very slowly (months to years). Almost all cases due to drugs clear within months after discontinuation of the offending agent.

## MANAGEMENT

**Symptomatic**   Long-standing lesions are cosmetically disfiguring, and patients may choose to treat these lesions. Topical low- and middle-potency glucocorticoid preparations may inhibit new purpuric lesions. Systemic tetracycline or minocycline (50 mg bid) are effective. PUVA is effective in severe forms. Supportive stockings required in all forms.

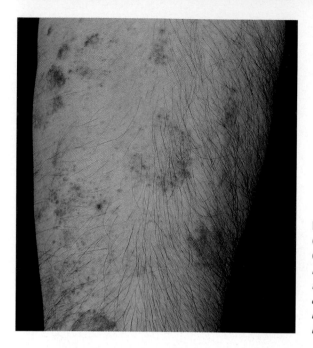

**FIGURE 7-17   Pigmented purpuric dermatosis: Majocchi's disease** *Multiple nonpalpable, nonblanching purpuric lesions arranged in annular configurations and associated with tiny telangiectasias. Note brownish discoloration of older lesions.*

# PITYRIASIS LICHENOIDES (ACUTE AND CHRONIC)    □   ○

Pityriasis lichenoides (PL) is an eruption of unknown etiology, characterized clinically by successive crops of a wide range of morphologic lesions. It is classified into an acute form, pityriasis lichenoides et varioliformis acuta (PLEVA, Mucha-Habermann disease), and a chronic form, pityriasis lichenoides chronica (PLC, guttate parapsoriasis of Juliusberg); however, most patients have lesions of PLEVA and PLC simultaneously. PLEVA is important because it can be mistaken for lymphomatoid papulosis (see Section 19).
*Synonym*: Guttate parapsoriasis.

## EPIDEMIOLOGY AND ETIOLOGY

**Age of Onset**   Adolescents and young adults.
**Sex**   More common in males than females.
**Etiology**   Unknown.

## HISTORY

Lesions tend to appear in crops over a period of weeks or months. Uncommonly, patients with an acute onset of the disorder may have symptoms of an acute infection with fever, malaise, and headache. Cutaneous lesions are usually asymptomatic but may be pruritic or sensitive to touch. Lesions may heal with significant scarring and postinflammatory pigmentation.

## PHYSICAL EXAMINATION

### Skin Lesions

Initially, randomly distributed, bright-red edematous papules (i.e., lichenoides), less commonly vesicles, which undergo central necrosis with hemorrhagic crusting (i.e., varioliformis, hence the designation *PLEVA*) (Fig. 7-18). In the chronic form (PLC), scaling papules of

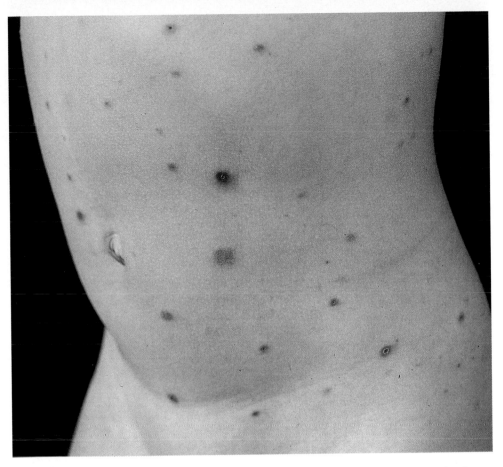

**FIGURE 7-18   Pityriasis lichenoides et varioliformis acuta (PLEVA)**   *Randomly distributed red papules of different size, some of which show central hemorrhagic crusting. In this 5-year-old child the eruption appeared in crops over a period of 10 days. Since individual lesions showed minimal signs of vesiculation and lesions were of different age, the eruption was mistaken for varicella.*

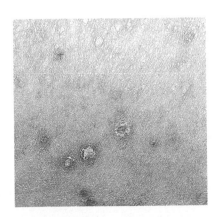

**FIGURE 7-19   Pityriasis lichenoides chronica (PLC)**   *Discrete papules with fine, mica-like scales that become better visible after slight scraping, on the trunk of a 19-year-old adolescent. Note, in contrast to PLEVA (Fig. 7-18), there is no hemorrhagic crusting.*

reddish-brown color and a central mica-like scale are seen (Fig. 7-19). Postinflammatory hypo- or hyperpigmentation often present after lesions resolve. PLEVA may heal with depressed or elevated scars.

**Distribution** Randomly arranged, most commonly on trunk, proximal extremities but also generalized, including palms and soles.

**Oral and Genital Mucosa** Inflammatory papules and necrotic lesions may occur.

## LABORATORY EXAMINATION

**Dermatopathology** *Epidermis*: spongiosis, keratinocyte necrosis, vesiculation, ulceration; exocytosis or erythrocytes within epidermis. *Dermis*: Edema, chronic inflammatory cell infiltrate in wedge shape extending to deep reticular dermis; hemorrhage; vessels congested with blood; endothelial cells swollen.

## DIAGNOSIS AND DIFFERENTIAL DIAGNOSIS

Clinical diagnosis is confirmed by skin biopsy. Differential diagnosis: varicella, guttate psoriasis, lymphomatoid papulosis.

## COURSE AND PROGNOSIS

New lesions appear in successive crops. PLC tends to resolve spontaneously after 6 to 12 months. In some cases, relapses after many months or years.

## MANAGEMENT

Most patients do not require any therapeutic intervention. Oral erythromycin and tetracycline are reported to be effective in some cases. Ultraviolet radiation (whether natural sunlight or broad-band UVB), 311-nm UVB, and PUVA are the treatments of choice if the oral antibiotics fail after a 2-week trial.

# ERYTHEMA MULTIFORME SYNDROME

This reaction pattern of blood vessels in the dermis with secondary epidermal changes manifests clinically as characteristic erythematous iris-shaped papular and vesiculobullous lesions typically involving the extremities (especially the palms and soles) and the mucous membranes.

## EPIDEMIOLOGY

**Age of Onset**   50% under 20 years.
**Sex**   More frequent in males than in females.

## ETIOLOGY

A cutaneous reaction to a variety of antigenic stimuli.
**Drugs**   Sulfonamides, phenytoin, barbiturates, phenylbutazone, penicillin, allopurinol.
**Infection**   Especially following herpes simplex, *Mycoplasma*.
**Idiopathic**   More than 50%.

## HISTORY

Evolution of lesions over several days. May have history of prior episode of erythema multiforme (EM). May be pruritic or painful, particularly mouth lesions. In severe forms constitutional symptoms such as fever, weakness, malaise.

## PHYSICAL EXAMINATION

### Skin Lesions

Lesions may develop over ≥10 days. Macule (48 h) → papule (1 to 2 cm; Fig. 7-20) → vesicles and bullae in the center of the papule; (Fig. 7-21). Dull red. *Iris* or *targetlike lesions* result and are typical (Figs. 7-20 and 7-21). Localized to hands and face or generalized (Fig. 7-22). Bilateral and often symmetric.

**Sites of Predilection** Dorsa of hands, palms (Fig. 7-20), and soles; forearms; feet; face (Fig. 7-21); elbows and knees; penis (50%) and vulva (Image 7-3).

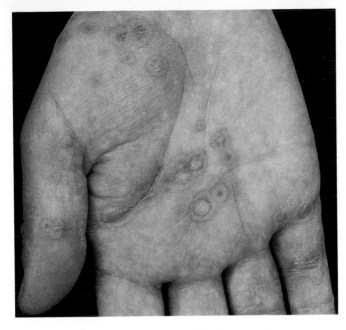

**FIGURE 7-20   Erythema multiforme**   *Iris and target-like lesions with concentric macules and papules on the palm.*

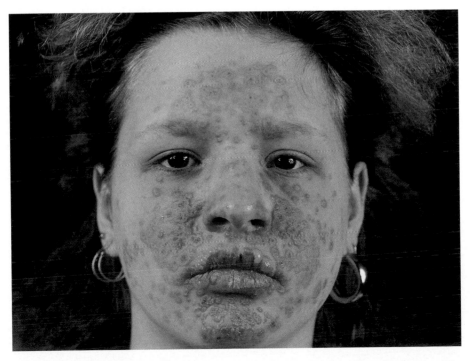

**FIGURE 7-21   Erythema multiforme**   *Multiple, confluent target-like papules and vesicles on the central facies. Bullae are seen on the lips and were also present on the buccal mucosa.*

**Mucous Membranes**   Erosions with fibrin membranes; occasionally ulcerations: lips (Fig. 7-22), oropharynx (see Fig. 31-15), nasal, conjunctival, vulvar, anal.

**Other Organs**   Eyes, with corneal ulcers, anterior uveitis.

## COURSE

**Mild Forms (EM Minor)**   Little or no mucous membrane involvement; vesicles but no bullae or systemic symptoms. Eruption usually confined to extremities, face, classic target lesions (Figs. 7-20, 7-21). Recurrent EM minor is usually associated with an outbreak of herpes simplex preceding it by several days.

**Severe Forms (EM Major)**   Most often occurs as a drug reaction, always with mucous membrane involvement; severe, extensive, tendency to become confluent and bullous, positive Nikolsky sign in erythematous lesions (Fig. 7-22). Systemic symptoms: fever, prostration. Cheilitis and stomatitis interfere with eating; vulvitis and balanitis with micturition. Conjunctivitis can lead to keratitis and ulceration; lesions also in pharynx, larynx, and trachea.

**Maximal Variant**   Life-threatening. In addition to the preceding, necrotizing tracheobronchitis, meningitis, renal tubular necrosis (Stevens-Johnson syndrome, see below).

## LABORATORY EXAMINATION

**Dermatopathology**   Inflammation characterized by perivascular mononuclear infiltrate, edema of the upper dermis; apoptosis of keratinocytes with focal epidermal necrosis and subepidermal bulla formation. In severe cases, complete necrosis of epidermis as in toxic epidermal necrolysis.

## DIAGNOSIS AND DIFFERENTIAL DIAGNOSIS

The target-like lesion and the symmetry are quite typical, and the diagnosis is not difficult.

**Acute Exanthematic Eruptions**   Drug eruption, psoriasis, secondary syphilis, urticaria, generalized Sweet's syndrome. Mucous membrane lesions may present a difficult differential diagnosis: bullous diseases, fixed drug eruption, acute lupus erythematosus, primary herpetic gingivostomatitis.

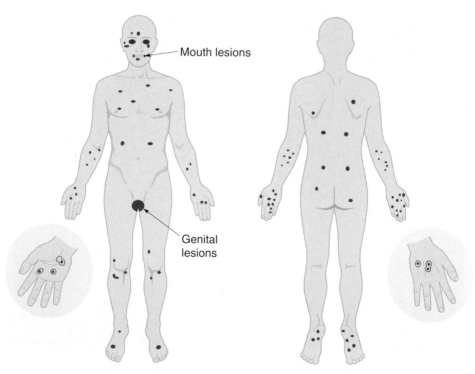

Mouth lesions

Genital lesions

**IMAGE 7-3   Erythema multiforme:** *predilection sites and distribution*

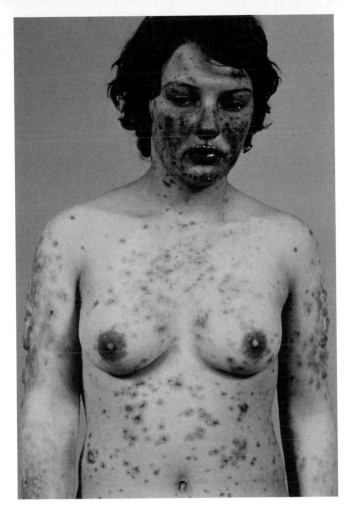

**FIGURE 7-22  Erythema multiforme: major** *Erythematous iris and target-like papules, plaques, bullae, and erosions on the trunk, arms, neck, and face. Facial lesions are erosive and crusted and mucosal involvement is manifested by erosive lip lesions and conjunctivitis.*

## MANAGEMENT

**Prevention** Control of herpes simplex using oral valacyclovir or penciclovir may prevent development of recurrent EM.

**Glucocorticoids** In severely ill patients, systemic glucocorticoids are usually given (prednisone, 50 to 80 mg/d in divided doses, quickly tapered), but their effectiveness has not been established by controlled studies.

# STEVENS-JOHNSON SYNDROME AND TOXIC EPIDERMAL NECROLYSIS □ ●

Stevens-Johnson syndrome (SJS) and toxic epidermal necrolysis (TEN) are mucocutaneous drug-induced or idiopathic reaction patterns characterized by skin tenderness and erythema of skin and mucosa, followed by extensive cutaneous and mucosal epidermal necrosis and sloughing. They are potentially life-threatening due to multisystem involvement.
*Synonym*: TEN: Lyell's syndrome.

## DEFINITION

Not clearly defined. SJS is considered by most a maximal variant of EM (major) and TEN a maximal variant of SJS. Both can start with target-like lesions; however, about 50% of TEN cases do not, and in these the condition evolves from diffuse erythema to immediate necrosis and epidermal detachment.

*SJS* <10% epidermal detachment
*SJS/TEN overlap* 10% to 30% epidermal detachment.
*TEN* >30% epidermal detachment.

## EPIDEMIOLOGY

**Age of Onset**   Any age, but most common in adults >40 years. Equal sex incidence.
**Overall Incidence**   *TEN*: 0.4 to 1.2 per million person-years. *SJS*: 1.2 to 6 per million person-years.
**Risk Factors**   Systemic lupus erythematosus, HLA-B12, HIV disease.

## ETIOLOGY AND PATHOGENESIS

Polyetiologic reaction pattern, but drugs are clearly the leading causative factor. *TEN*: 80% of cases have strong association with specific medication (Table 7-2); <5% of patients report no drug use. Also: chemicals, *Mycoplasma* pneumonia, viral infections, immunization. *SJS*: 50% are associated with drug exposure; etiology often not clear-cut.

Pathogenesis of SJS-TEN is only partially understood. It is viewed as a cytotoxic immune reaction aimed at the destruction of keratinocytes expressing foreign (drug-related) antigens. Epidermal injury is based on the induction of apoptosis. Drug-specific activation of T cells has been shown in vitro on peripheral blood mononuclear cells of patients with drug eruptions. The nature of the antigens that drive the cytotoxic cellular immune reaction is not well understood. Drugs or their metabolites act as haptens and render keratinocytes antigenic by binding to their surfaces. Cutaneous drug eruptions have been linked to a defect of the detoxification systems of liver and skin, which results in direct toxicity or alteration of antigenic properties of keratinocytes. Cytokines produced by activated mononuclear cells and keratinocytes probably contribute to local cell death, fever, and malaise.

## HISTORY

Time from first drug exposure to onset of symptoms: 1 to 3 weeks. Occurs more rapidly with rechallenge. Occurs after days of ingestion of the drug; newly added drug is most suspect. Prodromes: fever, influenza-like symptoms 1 to 3 days prior to mucocutaneous lesions. Mild to moderate skin tenderness, conjunctival burning or itching, then skin pain, burning sensation, tenderness, paresthesia. Mouth lesions are painful, tender. Impaired alimentation, photophobia, painful micturition, anxiety.

## PHYSICAL EXAMINATION

### Skin Lesions
***Prodromal Rash*** Is morbilliform, EM-like; diffuse erythema (Fig. 7-23).
***Early*** Necrotic epidermis first appears as macular areas with crinkled surface that enlarge and coalesce (Fig. 7-23). Sheetlike loss of epidermis. Raised flaccid blisters (Figs. 7-23 and 7-24) that spread with lateral pressure (Nikolsky sign) on erythematous areas. With trauma, full-thickness epidermal detachment yields exposed, red, oozing dermis (Fig. 7-24) resembling a second-degree thermal burn.
***Recovery*** Regrowth of epidermis begins within days; completed in ≥3 weeks. Pressure points and periorificial sites exhibit delayed healing. Skin that is not denuded acutely is shed in sheets, especially palms/soles. Nails and cilia may shed.

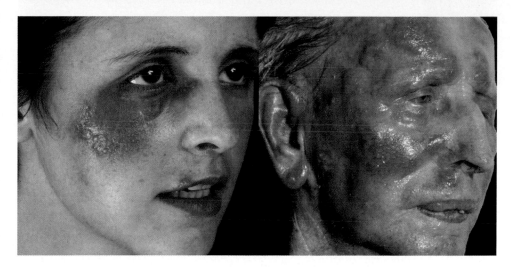

**FIGURE 7-32 Sweet's syndrome** *Left. Edematous, erythematous papules coalesce to form irregular, inflammatory plaques on the lower eyelid and cheek. Some of the papules look like vesicles (pseudovesiculation) and thus are similar to herpes simplex or erythema multiforme. The eruption occurred in a 28-year-old female following an upper respiratory infection. The patient also had fever and leukocytosis. Right. A similar eruption in a 68-year-old male, but here the lesions are more widespread and more edematous; they are bilateral and also occur on shoulders and chest. The patient was febrile, felt ill, and upon systemic review he turned out to have myelomonocytic leukemia.*

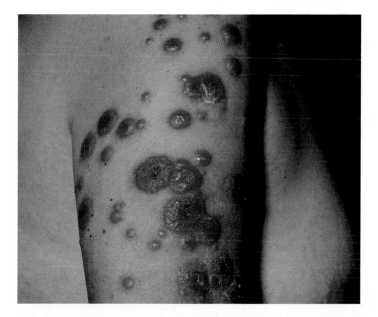

**FIGURE 7-33 Sweet's syndrome** *A sudden, painful eruption in a 50-year-old female who was febrile and had general malaise. There are multiple very edematous and erythematous papules and plaques, most of which upon first sight, appear as if they were vesicles or bullae but are firm upon palpation (pseudovesiculation). However, the confluent lesions in the lower part of the picture are indeed bullous and here there is also exudation and crusting. Systems review in this patient revealed myelocytic leukemia.*

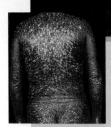

# ERYTHRODERMA AND RASHES IN THE ACUTELY ILL PATIENT

## EXFOLIATIVE ERYTHRODERMA SYNDROME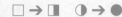

The exfoliative erythroderma syndrome (EES) is a serious, at times life-threatening reaction pattern of the skin characterized by generalized and uniform redness and scaling involving practically the entire skin and associated with systemic "toxicity," generalized lymphadenopathy, and fever. Two stages, acute and chronic, merge one into the other. In the acute and subacute phases, there is rapid onset of generalized vivid red erythema and fine branny scales; the patient feels hot and cold, shivers, and has fever. In chronic EES, the skin thickens, and scaling continues and becomes lamellar. There is a loss of scalp and body hair, the nails become thickened and separated from the nail bed (onycholysis), and there may be hyperpigmentation or patchy loss of pigment in patients whose normal skin color is brown or black. About 50% of the patients with EES have a history of a preexisting dermatosis, which is recognizable only in the acute or subacute stages. The most frequent preexisting skin disorders are (in order of frequency) psoriasis, atopic dermatitis, adverse cutaneous drug reaction, lymphoma, allergic contact dermatitis, and pityriasis rubra pilaris (Table 8-1). Drugs most commonly implicated in erythroderma are found in Table 8-2. In 10 to 20% of patients it is not possible to identify the cause by history or histology.
[See "Sézary's Syndrome" (Section 19) for a special consideration of this form of EES.]

### EPIDEMIOLOGY

**Age of Onset** Usually >50 years; in children, EES usually results from pityriasis rubra pilaris or atopic dermatitis.
**Sex** Males > females.

### PATHOGENESIS

The metabolic response to exfoliative dermatitis may be profound. Large amounts of warm blood are present in the skin due to the dilatation of capillaries, and there is considerable heat dissipation through insensible fluid loss and by convection. Also, there may be high-output cardiac failure; the loss of scales through exfoliation can be considerable, up to 9 g/m$^2$ of body surface per day, and this may contribute to the reduction in serum albumin and the edema of the lower extremities so often noted in these patients.

### HISTORY

Depending on the etiology, the acute phase may develop rapidly, as in a drug reaction, lymphoma, eczema, or psoriasis. At this early acute stage it is still possible to identify the preexisting dermatosis. There is pruritus, fatigue, weakness, anorexia, weight loss, malaise, feeling cold.

### PHYSICAL EXAMINATION

**Appearance of Patient** Frightened, red, "toxic."

#### Skin Lesions
Skin is red, thickened, scaly. Dermatitis is uniform involving the entire body surface (Figs. 8-1 to 8-3), except for pityriasis rubra pilaris, where EES spares sharply defined areas of normal skin. Thickening leads to exaggerated skin folds (Figs. 8-2 and 8-3); scaling

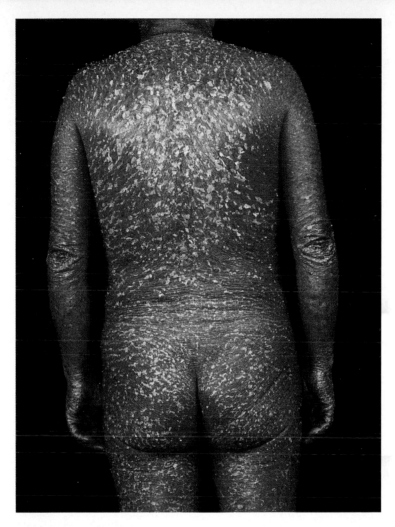

**FIGURE 8-1   Erythroderma psoriasis**   *There is universal erythema, thickening of the skin, and heavy scaling. This patient had psoriasis as suggested by the large silvery white scales and the scalp and nail involvement not seen in this illustration. The patient had fatigue, weakness, malaise, and was shivering. It is quite obvious that such massive scaling can lead to protein loss and the maximal dilatation of skin capillaries to considerable heat dissipation and high output cardiac failure.*

may be fine and branny and may be barely perceptible or large, up to 0.5 cm, and lamellar (Fig. 8-1).

*Palms and Soles* Usually involved, with massive hyperkeratosis and deep fissures in pityriasis rubra pilaris, Sézary's syndrome, and psoriasis.

**Hair**   Thinning of hair, even alopecia, except for EES arising in eczema or psoriasis.

**Nails**   Onycholysis, shedding of nails.

### General Examination

Lymph nodes generalized, rubbery, and usually small; enlarged in Sézary's syndrome. Edema of lower legs and ankles.

## LABORATORY EXAMINATIONS

**Chemistry**   Low serum albumin and increase in gammaglobulins; electrolyte imbalance; acute-phase proteins increased.

**Hematology**   Leukocytosis.

**Bacterial Culture**   *Skin*: rule out secondary *Staphylococcus aureus* infection. *Blood*: rule out sepsis.

**TABLE 8-1   Etiology of Exfoliative Dermatitis in Adults**

| Cause | Average Percent[*] |
|---|---|
| Undetermined or unclassified | 23 |
| Psoriasis | 23 |
| Atopic dermatitis, eczema | 16 |
| Drug allergy | 15 |
| Lymphoma, leukemia | 11 |
| Allergic contact dermatitis | 5 |
| Seborrheic dermatitis | 5 |
| Stasis dermatitis with "id" reaction | 3 |
| Pityriasis rubra pilaris | 2 |
| Pemphigus foliaceus | 1 |

[*] As collated from the literature.

Source: Abbreviated from IM Freedberg et al. (eds): *Fitzpatrick's Dermatology in General Medicine,* 5th ed. New York, McGraw-Hill, 1999.

**TABLE 8-2   Drugs that Cause Exfoliative Dermatitis**

| | | | |
|---|---|---|---|
| **Allopurinol**[*] | Codeine | Mercurials | Sulfasalazine |
| Aminoglycosides | Cyanamide | Mesna | Sulfonamide |
| Aminophylline | Dapsone | Methylprednisolone | antibiotics |
| Amiodarone | Dideoxyinosine | Minocycline | Sulfonylureas |
| Amonafide | Diflunisal | Mitomycin C | Tar preparations |
| Ampicillin | Diphenylhydantoin | Omeprazole | Terbinafine |
| Antimalarials | Ephedrine | Penicillin | Terbutaline |
| Arsenicals | Ethambutol | Pentostatin | Thalidomide |
| Aspirin | Ethylenediamine | Peritrate and | Thiacetazone |
| Aztreonam | Etretinate | glyceryl trinitrate | Thiazide diuretics |
| Bactrim | Fluorouracil | Pheneturide | Ticlopidine |
| Barbiturates | GM-CSF | Phenophthalein | Timolol maleate |
| Bromodeoxyuridine | **Gold** | Phenothiazines | eyedrops |
| Budenoside | Herbal medications | Phenylbutazone | Tobramycin |
| **Calcium channel** | Indeloxazine | **Phenytoin** | Tocainide |
| **blockers** | hydrochloride | Phototherapy | Trimetrexate |
| Captopril | Indinavir | Plaquenil | Trovafloxacin |
| **Carbamazepine** | Interleukin-2 | Practolol | Tumor necrosis |
| Carboplatin | Iodine | **Quinidine** | factor α |
| Cefoxitin | Isoniazid | Ranitidine | Vancomycin |
| Cephalosporins | Isosorbide dinitrate | Retinoids | Yohimbine |
| **Cimetidine** | Lansoprazole | Ribostamycin | Zidovudine |
| Cisplatin | Lidocaine | Rifampicin | Lidocaine |
| Clodronate | **Lithium** | St. John's wort | |
| Clofazamine | Mefloquine | Streptomycin | |

*The more commonly implicated agents are listed in bold.

Source: MH Jih, A Kimyai-Asadi, and IM Freedberg, in IM Freedberg et al. (eds): *Fitzpatrick's Dermatology in General Medicine,* 6th ed. New York, McGraw-Hill, 2003, p. 487.

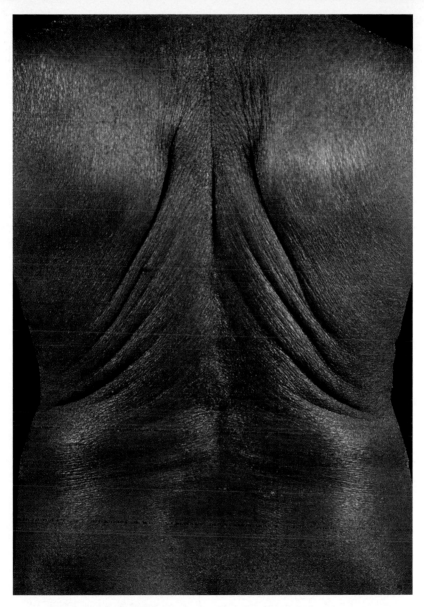

**FIGURE 8-2   Erythroderma: drug-induced**   *This is generalized erythroderma with thickening of skin resulting in increased skin folds, universal redness, a fine brawny scaling. This patient had developed erythroderma following the injection of gold salts for rheumatoid arthritis.*

**Dermatopathology** Depends on type of underlying disease. Parakeratosis, inter- and intracellular edema, acanthosis with elongation of the rete ridges, and exocytosis of cells. There is edema of the dermis and a chronic inflammatory infiltrate.

**Imaging** CT scans or MRI should be used to find evidence of lymphoma.

**Lymph Node Biopsy** When there is suspicion of lymphoma.

### DIAGNOSIS

Diagnosis is not easy, and the history of the pre-existing dermatosis may be the only clue. Also, pathognomonic signs and symptoms of the pre-existing dermatosis may help, e.g., dusky-red color in psoriasis and yellowish-red in pityriasis rubra pilaris; typical nail changes of psoriasis; lichenification, crosions, and excoriations in atopic dermatitis and eczema; diffuse, relatively nonscaling palmar hyperkeratoses with fissures in cutaneous T cell lymphoma (CTCL) and pityriasis rubra pilaris; sharply demarcated patches of noninvolved skin within the erythroderma in pityriasis rubra pilaris; massive hyperkeratotic scale of scalp, usually without hair loss in psoriasis and with hair loss in CTCL and pityriasis rubra pilaris; in the latter and in CTCL, ectropion may occur.

### COURSE AND PROGNOSIS

Guarded, depends on underlying etiology. Despite the best attention to all details, patients may succumb to infections or, if they have cardiac problems, to cardiac failure ("high-output" failure) or to the effects of prolonged glucocorticoid therapy.

### MANAGEMENT

This is an important medical problem that should be dealt with in a modern inpatient dermatology facility with experienced personnel. The patient should be hospitalized in a single room, at least for the beginning workup and during the development of a therapeutic program. The hospital room conditions (heat and cold) should be adjusted to the patient's needs; most often these patients need a warm room with many blankets.

**Topical** Water baths with added bath oils, followed by application of bland emollients.

**Systemic** Oral glucocorticoids for remission induction but not for maintenance; *systemic and topical therapy as required by underlying condition.*

**Supportive** Supportive cardiac, fluid, electrolyte, protein replacement therapy as required.

## RASHES IN THE ACUTELY ILL FEBRILE PATIENT

The sudden appearance of a rash and fever is frightening for the patient. Medical advice is sought immediately and often in the emergency units of hospitals; about 10% of all patients seeking emergency medical care have a dermatologic problem.

The diagnosis of an acute rash with a fever is a clinical challenge (see Fig. 25-11). Rarely do physicians have to "lean" on their eyes as much as when confronted by an acutely ill patient with fever and a skin eruption. If a diagnosis is not established promptly in certain patients [e.g., those having septicemia (see Fig. 22-36)], lifesaving treatment may be delayed.

The cutaneous findings alone may be diagnostic before confirmatory laboratory data are available. As in problems of the acute abdomen, the results of some laboratory tests, such as microbiologic cultures, may not be available immediately. On the basis of a differential diagnosis, appropriate therapy—whether antibiotics or glucocorticoids—may be started. Furthermore, prompt diagnosis and isolation of the patient with a contagious disease, which may have serious consequences, prevent spread to other persons. For example, varicella in adults (see Figs. 25-34 and 25-35) rarely can be fatal. Contagious diseases presenting with rash and fever as the major

## LABORATORY TESTS AVAILABLE FOR QUICK DIAGNOSIS

The physician should make use of the following laboratory tests immediately or within 8 h:

1. *Direct smear from the base of a vesicle.* This procedure, known as the *Tzanck test*, is performed by unroofing an intact vesicle, gently scraping the base with a curved scalpel blade, and smearing the contents on a slide. After air drying, the smear is stained with Wright's or Giemsa's stain and examined for acantholytic cells, giant acanthocytes, and/or multinucleated giant cells (see Fig. 25-19).

2. *Viral culture*, negative stain (electron microscopy), polymerase chain reaction for infections with herpes viruses.

3. *Gram stain of aspirates or scraping.* This is essential for proper diagnosis of pustules. Organisms can be seen in the lesions of acute meningococcemia, rarely in the skin lesions of gonococcemia and ecthyma gangrenosum.

4. *Touch preparation.* This is especially helpful in deep fungal infections and leishmaniasis. The dermal part of a skin biopsy specimen is touched repeatedly to a glass slide; the touch preparation is *immediately* fixed in 95% ethyl alcohol. Special stains are then performed, and the slide examined for organisms in the cytology laboratory.

5. *Biopsy of the skin lesion.* All purpuric lesions should be biopsied. Inflammatory dermal nodules and most ulcers should be biopsied and a portion of tissue minced and cultured for bacteria and fungi. A 3- to 4-mm trephine and local anesthesia are used. In many laboratories the biopsy specimen can be processed within 8 h if necessary.

6. *Blood and urine examinations.* Blood culture, rapid serologic tests for syphilis, and serology for lupus erythematosus require 24 h. Examination of urine sediment may reveal red cell casts in allergic vasculitis.

7. *Dark-field examination.* In the skin lesions of secondary syphilis, repeated examination of papules may show *Treponema pallidum*. The dark-field examination is not reliable in the mouth because nonpathogenic organisms are almost impossible to differentiate from *T. pallidum*, but a lymph node aspirate can be subjected to dark-field examination.

### TABLE 8-3   (Continued)

| Generalized Eruptions Manifested by Purpuric Macules, Purpuric Papules, or Purpuric Vesicles | Diseases Manifested by Widespread Erythema ± Papules Followed by Desquamation |
|---|---|
| Drug hypersensitivities | Drug hypersensitivities |
| Meningococcemia[*] (acute or chronic) | Staphylococcal scalded- |
| Gonococcemia[*] | skin syndrome |
| Staphylococcemia *Pseudomonas* | Toxic shock syndrome |
| bacteremia | Kawasaki's syndrome |
| Subacute bacterial endocarditis | Graft-versus-host reaction |
| Enterovirus infections (echovirus and | Erythroderma (exfoliative dermatitis) |
| Coxsackie) | |
| Rickettsial diseases: Rocky Mountain | |
| spotted fever | |
| Typhus, louse-borne (epidemic) | |
| "Allergic" vasculitis[*] | |
| Disseminated intravascular coagulation | |
| (purpura fulminans[§]) | |
| *Vibrio* infections | |

[§] Leading to large areas of black necrosis.

[*] Often present as infarcts.

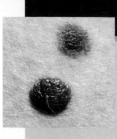

# BENIGN NEOPLASMS AND HYPERPLASIAS

## DISORDERS OF MELANOCYTES

### ACQUIRED NEVOMELANOCYTIC NEVI  ■ ○

Nevomelanocytic nevi (NMN), commonly called *moles*, are small (<1 cm), circumscribed, acquired pigmented macules, papules, or nodules composed of groups of melanocytic nevus cells located in the epidermis, dermis, and, rarely, subcutaneous tissue.

### EPIDEMIOLOGY AND ETIOLOGY

One of the most common acquired new growths in Caucasians (most adults have about 20 nevi), less common in blacks or pigmented persons, and sometimes absent in persons with red hair and marked freckling.

**Race**   Blacks and Asians have more nevi on the palms, soles, nail beds.

**Heredity**   Common acquired NMN occur in family clusters. Atypical melanocytic nevi (AMN, see Section 12), which are putative precursor lesions of malignant melanoma, occur in virtually every patient with familial cutaneous melanoma and in 30 to 50% of patients with sporadic nonfamilial primary melanoma.

**Sun Exposure**   A factor in the induction of nevi on the exposed areas.

**Significance**   Risk of melanoma is related to the numbers of NMN and to AMN, even if only a few lesions are present.

### HISTORY

**Duration and Evolution of Lesions**   NMN appear in early childhood and reach a maximum in young adulthood even though some NMN may arise in adulthood. Later on there is a grad-

ual involution and fibrosis of lesions, and most disappear after the age of 60. In contrast, AMN continue to appear throughout life and are believed not to involute (see Section 12).

**Skin Symptoms**   NMN are asymptomatic. If a lesion *persistently* itches or is tender, it should be followed carefully or excised, since *persistent* pruritus may be an early indication of malignant change.

### CLASSIFICATION

NMN can be classified according to their state of evolution and thus according to the site of the clusters of nevus cells.

1. *Junctional melanocytic NMN*: These arise at the dermal-epidermal junction, on the epidermal side of the basement membrane; in other words, they are intraepidermal (Fig. 9-1).

2. *Compound melanocytic NMN*: Nevus cells invade the papillary dermis, and nevus cell nests are now found both intraepidermally and dermally (Fig. 9-2).

3. *Dermal melanocytic NMN*: These represent the last stage of the evolution of NMN. "Dropping off" into the dermis is now completed, and the nevus grows or remains

**FIGURE 9-1   Junctional NMN**   *Two uniformly dark brown small macules, round in shape with smooth regular borders.*

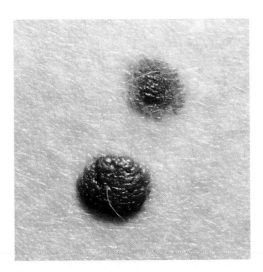

**FIGURE 9-2   Compound NMN**   *Uniformly pigmented papule and domed nodule; the upper lesion is flatter and tan with a more elevated, darker center; the larger (lower) lesion is older and choco-late brown; the upper lesion is younger and has a predominantly junctional component at the periphery.*

intradermal. With progressive age, there will be gradual fibrosis (Fig. 9-3).

Thus, melanocytic NMN undergo the evolution from junctional → compound → dermal NMN. Since the capacity of NMN cells to form melanin is greatest when they are located at the dermal-epidermal junction (intraepidermally) and since NMN cells lose their capacity for melanization, the further they penetrate into the dermis, the lesser is the intensity of pigmentation with the increase in the dermal proportion of the nevus. Purely dermal NMN are therefore almost always without pigment. In a simplified manner, the clinical appearance of NMN along this evolutionary path can be characterized as follows: junctional NMN is flat and dark, compound NMN is raised and dark, and dermal NMN is raised and light. This evolution also reflects the age at which the different types of NMN are found. Junctional and compound NMN are usually seen in childhood and through the teens, whereas dermal NMN start manifesting in the third and fourth decade.

### Junctional Melanocytic Nevocellular Nevi

**Lesions** Macule, or only very slightly raised (Fig. 9-1). Never >1 cm in diameter; if >1 cm, the "mole" is a congenital nevomelanocytic nevus, a atypical nevus, or a melanoma. Uniform tan, brown, dark brown, or even black. Round or oval with smooth, regular borders. Scattered discrete lesions.

### Compound Melanocytic Nevocellular Nevi

**Lesions** Papules or small nodules (Fig. 9-2). Dark brown, sometimes even black; dome-shaped, smooth or cobblestone-like surface, regular and sharply defined border, sometimes papillomatous or hyperkeratotic. Never >1 cm in diameter; if >1 cm, it is either a congenital NMN, atypical nevus, or a melanoma. Consistency either firm or soft. Color may become mottled as progressive conversion into dermal NMN occurs. May have hairs.

### Dermal Melanocytic Nevocellular Nevi

**Lesions** Sharply defined papule or nodule. Skin-colored, tan or flecks of brown, often with telangiectasia. Round, dome-shaped (Fig. 9-3), smooth surface, diameter <1 cm. Usually not present before the second or third decade. Older lesions, mostly on the trunk, may become pedunculated and do not disappear spontaneously. May be hairy.
*Distribution* Face, trunk, extremities, scalp. Random, but some predilection for sun-exposed

areas. Occasionally palmar and plantar, in which case these NMN usually have the appearance of junctional NMN.

## DIAGNOSIS AND DIFFERENTIAL DIAGNOSIS

**Diagnosis** Made clinically. As for all pigmented lesions the ABCD rule applies (see page 304). In cases of doubt apply dermoscopy (epiluminescence microscopy), and if malignancy cannot be excluded even by this procedure, excise lesions with a narrow margin.

**Differential Diagnosis** *Junctional NMN*: all flat, deeply pigmented lesions. Solar lentigo, flat atypical nevus, lentigo maligna. *Compound NMN*: all raised pigmented lesions. Seborrheic keratosis, atypical nevus, small superficial spreading melanoma, early nodular melanoma, pigmented basal cell carcinoma, dermatofibroma, Spitz nevus, blue nevus. *Dermal NMN*: all light tan or skin-colored papules. Basal cell carcinoma, neurofibroma, trichoepithelioma, dermatofibroma, sebaceous hyperplasia.

## MANAGEMENT

Indications for removal of acquired melanocytic NMN are the following:

*Site*: Lesions on the scalp (difficult to follow), mucous membranes, anogenital area.

*Growth*: If there is rapid change in size.

*Color*: If color becomes variegated.

*Border*: If irregular borders are present or develop.

*Erosions*: If lesion becomes eroded without major trauma.

*Symptoms*: If lesion begins to *persistently* itch, hurt, or bleed.

*Dermoscopy*: If criteria for melanoma or very atypical atypical nevus are present or appear de novo.

Melanocytic NMN never become malignant because of manipulation or trauma. In those cases where this was claimed, the lesion was initially a melanoma. If there is an indication for the removal of an NMN, the nevus should always be excised for histologic diagnosis and for definite treatment (particularly applicable to and decisive in ruling out congenital, dysplastic, or blue nevi). Removal of papillomatous, compound, or dermal NMN for cosmetic

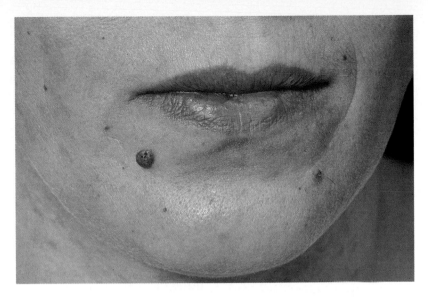

**FIGURE 9-3 Dermal NMN** *Dome-shaped, soft, tan papule on the left. A smaller dermal nevus with a single hair is seen on the right.*

reasons by electrocautery requires that a nevus be unequivocally diagnosed as benign NMN and histology be performed. If an early melanoma cannot be excluded with certainty, an excision for histologic examination is obligatory but can be performed with narrow margins.

## HALO NEVOMELANOCYTIC NEVUS    ■    ○

This lesion is an NMN that is encircled by a halo of leukoderma or depigmentation. The leukoderma is based on a decrease of melanin in melanocytes or disappearance of melanocytes at the dermal-epidermal junction. Halo nevi most often undergo spontaneous involution, often with regression of the centrally located pigmented nevus.
*Synonym*: Sutton's leukoderma acquisitum centrifugum.

### EPIDEMIOLOGY

Overall prevalence 1%. Onset in the first three decades. Occurs spontaneously and in patients with vitiligo (18 to 26%). Also in patients with metastatic melanoma (around metastatic lesions and around primary melanoma). May herald vitiligo. All races, both sexes. Halo nevi occur in siblings and in those with a family history of vitiligo.

### PATHOGENESIS

Immunologic phenomena, both humoral and cellular, are responsible for the dynamic changes that eventually lead to nevus involution.

### HISTORY

There are three stages: (1) Development (in months) of white halo around preexisting NMN; halo may be preceded by faint erythema; (2) disappearance (months to years) of NMN; and (3) repigmentation (months to years) of halo.

### PHYSICAL EXAMINATION

Skin Lesions
Papular brown NMN (<5 mm) with oval or round halo of sharply marginated hypomelanosis (Fig. 9-4). The NMN is *centrally* located. Scattered discrete lesions (1 to >30)

mostly on the trunk, but in general the same distribution as of NMN.

Special Forms
Congenital halo NMN occur rarely (Fig. 9-5).

### DIAGNOSIS AND DIFFERENTIAL DIAGNOSIS

If clinical findings atypical: the nevus has variegation of color and/or irregular borders, confirm histologically.
"Halo" Depigmentation around Other Lesions
Can occur around blue nevus, congenital NMN, Spitz's juvenile nevus, verruca plana, primary melanoma, melanoma metastases, dermatofibroma, neurofibroma.

### LABORATORY EXAMINATION

Dermatopathology    Junctional dermal or compound nevus surrounded by lymphocytic infiltrate (lymphocytes and histiocytes) around and between nevus cells. Nevus cells develop evidence of cell damage and disappear. Halo shows decrease or total absence of melanin and melanocytes.

### MANAGEMENT

Reassurance. Excision if the features of the nevus are atypical: variegation of color, irregular borders.

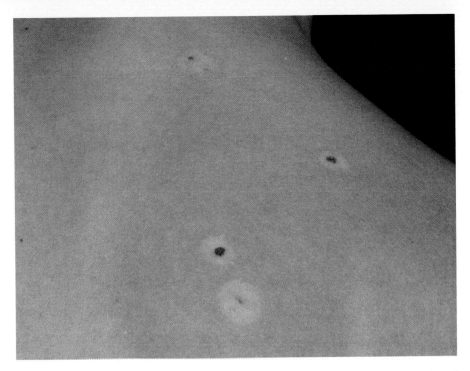

**FIGURE 9-4   Halo NMN**   *White depigmented halos surround several compound NMN nevi on the upper back; in time, the nevus may disappear leaving only the white macular portion, as is the case in the lowermost lesion.*

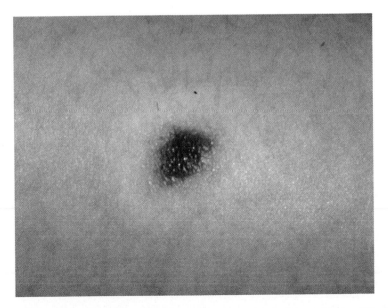

**FIGURE 9-5   Halo melanocytic NMN**   *This is a small congenital NMN (see Section 12) with a halo indicating incipient involution. This occurs only rarely.*

## BLUE NEVUS

A blue nevus is an acquired, benign, firm, dark-blue to gray-to-black, sharply defined papule or nodule representing a localized proliferation of melanin-producing dermal melanocytes. *Synonyms*: Blue neuronevus, dermal melanocytoma.

### EPIDEMIOLOGY

**Onset** In childhood and late adolescence. Equal sex distribution.
**Variants** Three types: common blue nevus, cellular blue nevus, combined blue nevus–nevomelanocytic nevus.

### PATHOGENESIS

Ectopic accumulations of melanin-producing melanocytes in the dermis derived from melanoblasts that became arrested during their migration from neural crest to sites in the skin.

### HISTORY

Nearly always asymptomatic, occasionally of cosmetic concern; often feared to be melanoma.

### PHYSICAL EXAMINATION

Skin Lesions
Papules to nodules, blue, blue-gray, blue-black, usually <10 mm in diameter (Fig. 9-6). *Cellular blue nevi* are larger (1 to 3 cm) (Fig. 9-7). Occasionally have target-like pattern of pigmentation. Usually round to oval. *Combined blue nevus–NMN*: blue-brown or blue-black with a lighter rim.
*Sites of Predilection* Most commonly located on the dorsa of hands or feet (50%); cellular blue nevi occur on the buttocks, lower back, scalp (Fig. 9-7), and face.

### LABORATORY EXAMINATION

**Dermatopathology** Melanin-containing wavy dermal melanocytes with long thin dendrites grouped in irregular bundles admixed with melanin-containing macrophages in the upper or middle dermis: excessive fibrous tissue production in upper reticular dermis. *Cellular blue nevus*: in addition to spindle-shaped melanocytes, epithelioid nevus cells in dermis and subcutaneous fat in nests and neuroid forms. *Combined blue nevus–NMN*: combination of blue nevus and compound NMN.

### DIAGNOSIS AND DIFFERENTIAL DIAGNOSIS

Usually made on clinical findings, at times confirmed by excision and dermatopathologic examination to rule out nodular melanoma.
**Blue/Gray Papule** Dermatofibroma, glomus tumor, primary (nodular) or metastatic melanoma, pigmented spindle cell (Spitz) nevus, traumatic tattoo, angiokeratoma, pigmented basal cell carcinoma.

### COURSE AND PROGNOSIS

Most remain unchanged. Malignant melanoma rarely develops in cellular blue nevi.

### MANAGEMENT

Blue nevi <10 mm in diameter and stable for many years usually do not need excision. Sudden appearance or change of an apparent blue nevus warrants surgical excision and dermatopathologic examination. Cellular blue nevi (≥1 to 3 cm; Fig. 9-7) are usually excised to rule out melanoma.

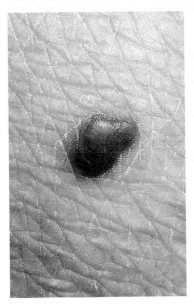

**FIGURE 9-6**

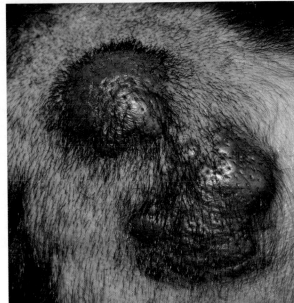

**FIGURE 9-7**

**FIGURE 9-6   Blue nevus**   *The blue nevus presented in the photograph has some irregular borders and is solidly blue-black in color. Therefore, the differential diagnosis must include nodular melanoma. If the lesion has been present for years, then biopsy is not necessary; if the lesion was noted only a few months ago, excision biopsy is required to rule out nodular melanoma. Dermoscopy greatly facilitates clinical differential diagnosis.*

**FIGURE 9-7   Cellular blue nevus**   *Two large, bluish-black nodules on the scalp. After excision histology showed that they were contiguous and thus represented one single lesion. Cellular blue nevi are much larger and should always be excised to rule out melanoma and because melanoma, albeit rarely, can develop in these lesions.*

## SPITZ NEVUS     ■   ○

*Synonyms*: Pigmented and epithelioid spindle cell nevus.

Spitz nevus is a benign, dome-shaped, hairless, small (<1 cm in diameter) nodule, most often pink or tan. There is often a history of recent rapid growth. However, the pathology of Spitz nevus is misleading, consisting of spindle and epithelioid nevus cells, some of which may be atypical. Differentiation from nodular malignant melanoma may thus require the help of a dermatopathologist who is familiar with pigment cell neoplasms.

Incidence is 1.4:100,000 (Australia). It occurs at all ages. A third of the patients are children <10 years, a third are 10 to 20 years old, and a third are > 20; rarely seen in persons ≥40 years. *Lesions* arise within months. They are papules or dome-shaped or relatively flat nodules, round, well-cirumscribed, smooth-topped, and hairless. They are a uniform pink (Fig. 9-8), tan, brown, dark brown, or even black (Fig. 9-9); are firm; and usually distributed on the head and neck.

*Differential diagnosis* includes all pink, tan, or darkly pigmented papules: pyogenic granuloma, hemangioma, molluscum contagiosum, juvenile xanthogranuloma, mastocytoma, dermatofibroma, NMN, AMN, nodular melanoma.

*Dermatopathology* consists of hyperplasia of the epidermis and of melanocytes, dilatation of capillaries. There are admixed large epithelioid cells, large spindle cells with abundant cytoplasm, and occasional mitotic figures. There are sometimes bizarre cytologic patterns: nests of large cells extend from the epidermis ("raining down") into the reticular dermis as fascicles of cells form an "inverted triangle," with the base lying at the dermal-epidermal junction and the apex in the reticular dermis.

Although the clinical appearance and recent growth are characteristic of a Spitz nevus, histologic examination must be done to confirm the clinical diagnosis. Excision in its entirety is important because the condition recurs in 10 to 15% of all cases in lesions that have not been excised completely. Spitz nevi are benign, but there can be a histologic similarity between Spitz nevi and melanoma and the histopathologic diagnosis may be difficult.

Spitz tumors probably do not usually involute, as do common acquired NMN nevi. However, some lesions have been observed to transform into common compound NMN, and some undergo fibrosis and in late stages may resemble dermatofibromas.

---

<sup>*</sup> In Asians.

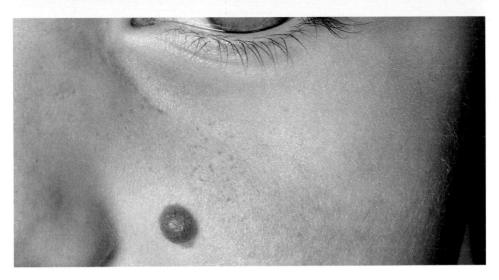

**FIGURE 9-8  Spitz nevus**  *Pink dome-shaped nodule on the cheek of a child, developing abruptly within the previous few months; the lesion can be mistaken for a hemangioma.*

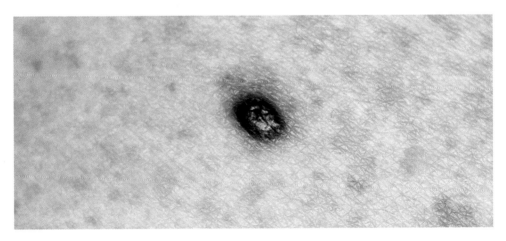

**FIGURE 9-9  Spitz nevus**  *Pigmented Spitz nevus. A black papule surrounded by a tan macular region (lentiginous) developed within a few months on the back of a young female; as such a lesion cannot be distinguished from a nodular melanoma. The lesion was excised and the diagnosis confirmed histologically.*

## NEVUS SPILUS     ■   ○

This is a rather common disorder of melanocytic lesion morphology that consists of a light brown pigmented macule varying from a few centimeters to a very large area (>15 cm); the distinctive feature of this lesion is the many dark brown small macules (2 to 3 mm) or papules scattered throughout the pigmented background (Fig. 9-10). The pathology of the background of the macular pigmented lesion is the same as lentigo simplex, i.e., increased numbers of melanocytes, while the flat or raised lesions scattered throughout are either junctional or compound nevi; rarely, these are atypical melanocytic nevi. The lesions are not as common as junctional or compound nevi but are not at all rare. In one series in a large dermatology practice, the nevus spilus was present in 3% of white patients. Malignant melanoma very rarely arises in these lesions.

## MONGOLIAN SPOT     □   ■   ○

These congenital gray-blue macular lesions are characteristically located on the lumbosacral area (Fig. 9-11) but can also occur on the scalp or anywhere on the skin. There is usually a single lesion, but rarely, several truncal lesions can be present at birth. The underlying pathology is dispersed spindle-shaped melanocytes within the dermis (dermal melanocytosis). Melanocytes are not normally present in the dermis, and it is believed that these ectopic melanocytes represent pigment cells that have been interrupted in their migration from the neural crest to the epidermis. Mongolian spots may disappear in early childhood, in contrast to nevus of Ota (see Fig. 9-12). As the term *Mongolian* implies, these lesions are found almost always (99 to 100%) in infants of Asiatic and Native American origin; however, they have been reported in black and, rarely, in white infants. No melanomas have been reported to occur in these lesions.

* In Asians.

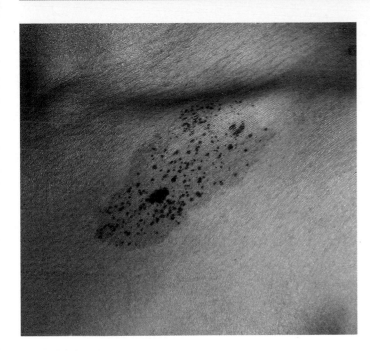

**FIGURE 9-10   Nevus spilus** *This light brown pigmented macule measuring about 10 cm along the long axis is peppered with many small, dark brown to black macules and papules.*

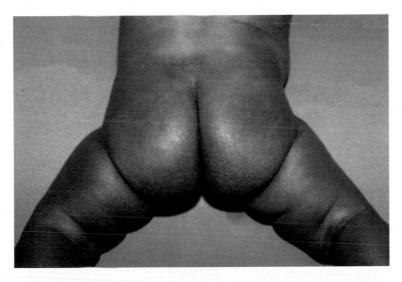

**FIGURE 9-11   Mongolian spot** *A large gray-blue macular lesion involving the entire lumbosacral and gluteal area and the left thigh in a baby from Sri Lanka. Although Mongolian spots are common in Asians, the parents of this baby were alarmed because the lesion was so large.*

## NEVUS OF OTA    ■*   ○

This pigmentary disorder is very common in Asian populations and is said to occur in 1% of dermatologic outpatients in Japan. It has been reported in East Indians, blacks, and, rarely, whites. The pigmentation, which can be quite subtle or markedly disfiguring, consists of a mottled, dusky admixture of blue and brown hyperpigmentation of the skin. The pigmentation mostly involves the skin and mucous membranes innervated by the first and second branches of the trigeminal nerve (Fig. 9-12). The blue hue results from the presence of ectopic melanocytes in the dermis. It can occur in the hard palate and in the conjunctivae, sclerae, and tympanic membranes. It may be bilateral. It may be congenital but is not hereditary; more often it appears in early childhood or during puberty and remains for life, in contrast to the Mongolian spot, which may disappear in early childhood. Treatment with lasers is an effective modality for this disfiguring disorder. Malignant melanoma can occur but is rare.

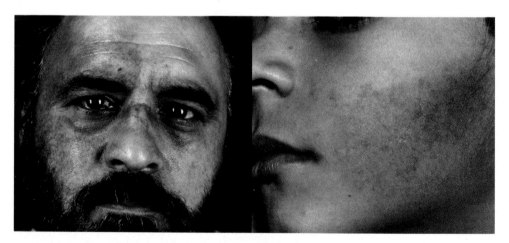

**FIGURE 9-12   Nevus of Ota   A.** *This pigmentary disorder is very common in Asian populations and is seen here in an East Indian involving the skin of the forehead, periorbital area and right cheek, as well as the sclera and conjunctiva of the right eye (regions supplied by the first and second branches of the trigeminal nerve). However, the mottled dusky, blue and brown hyperpigmentation also extended over the bridge of the nose to the left infraorbital region and is thus not completely unilateral.* **B.** *Nevus of Ota with the characteristic blue color in a Pakistani child. It is confined to an area supplied by the second and third branches of the trigeminal nerve. The parents were highly concerned about the cosmetic consequences.*

* In Asians.

## VASCULAR TUMORS AND MALFORMATIONS

The present binary biologic classification distinguishes between vascular tumors and vascular malformations. The latter are subclassified according to the structural components into capillary, venous, lymphatic, arterial, or combined forms. *Vascular tumors* (e.g., hemangiomas) show endothelial hyperplasia, whereas *malformations* have a normal endothelial turnover. Hemangiomas of infancy are not present at birth but appear postnatally; grow rapidly during the first year (proliferating phase), undergo slow spontaneous regression during childhood (involution phase), and remain stable thereafter. On the other hand, vascular malformations are errors of morphogenesis and are presumed to occur during intrauterine life. Most are present at birth, though some do not appear until years later. Once manifest they grow proportionally, but enlargement can occur as a result of various factors. Both vascular tumors and malformations can be separated into slow-flow or fast-flow types. The distinguishing features of vascular tumors and vascular malformations are shown in Table 9-1.

**TABLE 9-1   Distinguishing Features of Vascular Tumors (Hemangiomas) and Vascular Malformations**

|  | Tumors | Malformations |
|---|---|---|
| Presence at birth | Usually postnatal, 30% nascent, rarely full grown | 100% (presumably), not always obvious |
| Male:female ratio | 1:3–1:5 | 1:1 |
| Incidence | 1-12.6 percent at birth; 10-12 percent at 1 year | 0.3–0.5% port-wine stain |
| Natural history | Phases: proliferating, involuting, and involuted | Proportionate growth; can expand |
| Cellular | Endothelial hyperplasia | Normal endothelial turnover |
| Skeletal changes | Occasional mass effect on adjacent bone; rare hypertrophy | Slow-flow: distortion, hypertrophy, or hyperplasia<br>Fast-flow: destruction, distortion, or hypertrophy |

SOURCE: S Virnelli-Grevelink, JB Mulliken, Vascular anomalies and tumors of skin and subcutaneous tissues, in IM Freedberg, AZ Eisen, K Wolff, KF Austen, LA Goldsmith, SI Katz, (eds): *Fitzpatrick's Dermatology in General Medicine*, 6th ed. New York, McGraw-Hill, 2003, pp 1002–1019.

# VASCULAR TUMORS

## HEMANGIOMA OF INFANCY (HI)

(Formerly strawberry, cherry, capillary hemangioma.)

### EPIDEMIOLOGY

HI is the most common tumor of infancy. The incidence in newborns is between 1 and 2.5%; in white children by 1 year of age it is 10%. Females more affected than males by a 3 to 1 ratio.

### ETIOLOGY AND PATHOGENESIS

HI is a localized proliferative process of angioblastic mesenchyme. It represents a clonal expansion of endothelial cells that may result from somatic mutations of genes regulating endothelial cell proliferation.

### HISTORY AND NATURAL LIFE COURSE OF LESIONS

The initial proliferative phase lasts from 3 to 9 months, sometimes more. HIs usually enlarge rapidly during the first year. In a subsequent phase of involution the HI regresses, and this occurs gradually over 2 to 6 years and is usually complete by the age of 10. Involution varies greatly between individuals and is not correlated with size, location, or appearance of the lesion.

### PHYSICAL EXAMINATION

**Skin Lesions**
Soft, bright red to deep purple, compressible. On diascopy, does not blanch completely. Nodule or plaque, 1 to 8 cm (Figs. 9-13 to 9-15). With the onset of spontaneous regression, a white-to-gray area appears on the surface of the central part of the lesion (Fig. 9-14). Ulceration may occur.
***Distribution*** Lesions are usually solitary and localized or extend over an entire region. Head and neck 50%, trunk 25%. Face, trunk, legs, oral mucous membrane.

### SPECIAL PRESENTATIONS

**Deep Hemangioma**   (Formerly, cavernous hemangioma.) In the lower dermis and subcutaneous fat. Localized, firm rubbery mass of bluish color with telangiectases in overlying skin (Fig. 9-16). Can be combined with superficial hemangioma (Fig. 9-14). Does not involute as well as superficial type.
**Multiple HIs**   Multiple small (<2 cm), cherry-red papular lesions involving skin alone (*benign cutaneous hemangiomatosis*) or skin and internal organs (*diffuse neonatal hemangiomatosis*).
**Congenital Hemangiomas**   These develop in utero and are subdivided into rapidly involuting congenital hemangiomas (RICH) and noninvoluting congenital hemangiomas (NICH). They present as violaceous tumors with overlying telangiectasia with large veins in periphery or as red-violaceous plaques invading deeper tissues. NICH are fast-flow hemangiomas requiring surgery.

### LABORATORY EXAMINATION

**Dermatopathology**   Proliferation of endothelial cells in various amounts in the dermis and/or subcutaneous tissue; there is usually more endothelial proliferation in the superficial type and little in the deep angiomas. GLUT-1 immunoreactivity is found in all hemangiomas but not in vascular malformations.

### DIAGNOSIS

Made on clinical findings and MRI; Doppler and arteriography to demonstrate fast flow. Measure GLUT-1 immunoreactivity to rule out vascular malformation.

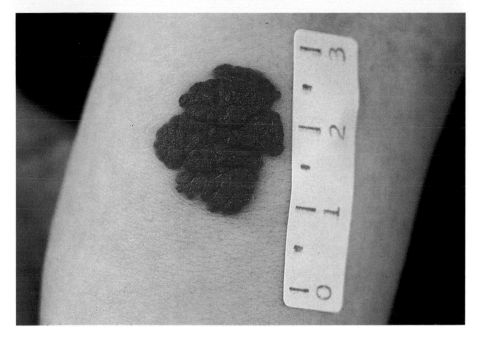

**FIGURE 9-13   Hemangioma of infancy**  *This bright red nodular plaque is frightening to the parents, and caution is needed to prevent scarring from the treatment itself. Since most of these lesions disappear spontaneously with only 20% showing residual atrophy or depigmentation, a wait and see strategy is recommended.*

## COURSE AND PROGNOSIS

HIs spontaneously involute by the fifth year, with some few percent disappearing only by age 10 (Fig. 9-14). There is virtually no residual skin change at the site in most lesions (80%); in the rest there is residual atrophy, depigmentation, telangiectasia, and scarring. HIs may, however, pose a considerable problem during the growth phase when they interfere with vital functions, such as obstruction of vision (Fig. 9-15) or of larynx, nose, or mouth. Deeper lesions, especially those involving mucous membranes, may not involute completely. Synovial involvement may be associated with hemophilia-like arthropathy. Large HIs, usually associated with deep hemangiomas, may have platelet entrapment, thrombocytopenia (Kasabach-Merritt syndrome), and even disseminated intravascular coagulation. Rarely, morbidity associated with HI occurs secondary to hemorrhage or high-output heart failure.

## MANAGEMENT

Each lesion must be judged individually regarding the decision to treat or not to treat and the selection of a treatment mode. Systemic treatment is difficult, requires experience, and should be performed by an expert. Surgical and medical interventions include continuous wave or pulsed dye laser, cryosurgery, intralesional and systemic high-dose glucocorticoids, and interferon-α (IFN-α). For the majority of HIs active nonintervention is the best approach because spontaneous resolution gives the best cosmetic results (Fig. 9-14). Treatment is indicated in about a quarter of HIs (5% that ulcerate; 20% that obstruct vital structures, i.e., eyes, ears, larynx) and in the <1% that are life threatening.

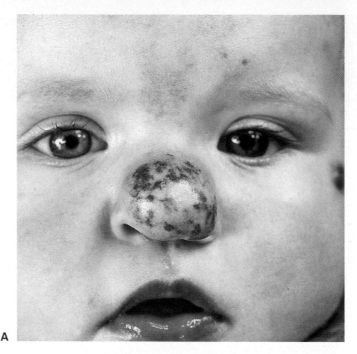

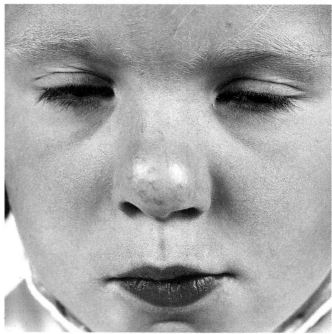

**FIGURE 9-14   Hemangioma of infancy**   *A. This lesion consists of a superficial and deep portion and incipient involution is already apparent for the superficial compartment. **B.** By the fifth year the hemangioma has almost disappeared.*

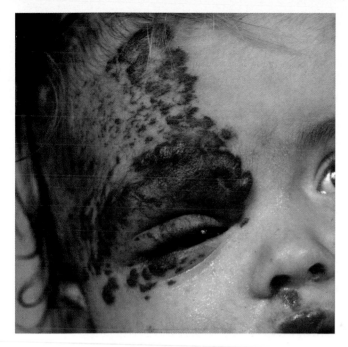

**FIGURE 9-15 Hemangioma of infancy** *Here it involves a large segment of skin. While involution is already apparent on the forehead, the lesion on the upper eyelid and the medial canthus is impairing proper function of the lid and this indicates that vision might be impaired in the future. In this patient, treatment was indicated.*

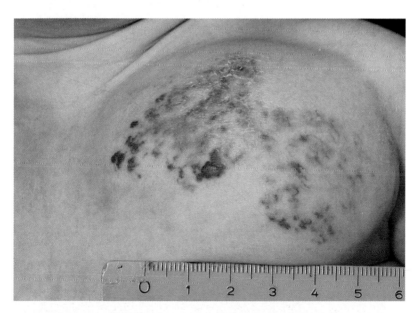

**FIGURE 9-16 Hemangioma of infancy** *Large subcutaneous mass with a bluish tinge, combined with superficial HI in the clavicular region of an infant. While the superficial HI involuted completely, the subcutaneous portion showed only minimal spontaneous regression and was surgically removed when the child was 10 years old.*

## PYOGENIC GRANULOMA   ■

Pyogenic granuloma is a rapidly developing vascular lesion usually following minor trauma. This is a very common solitary eroded vascular nodule that bleeds spontaneously or after minor trauma. The lesion has a smooth surface, with or without crusts, with or without erosion (Fig. 9-17). It appears as a bright red, dusky red, violaceous, or brown-black papule with a collar of hyperplastic epidermis at the base and occurs on the fingers, lips, mouth, trunk, and toes. Histopathologically there are lobular aggregates of proliferating capillaries with edema and numerous neutrophils. Treatment is surgical excision or curettage with electrodesiccation at the base. The importance of pyogenic granuloma is that it can be mistaken for amelanotic nodular melanoma, and vice versa.

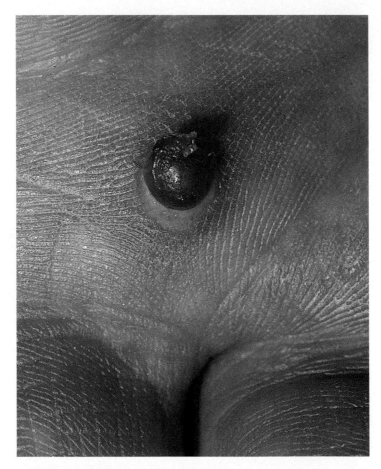

**FIGURE 9-17   Pyogenic granuloma**   *This is a solitary eroded vascular nodule that bleeds spontaneously or after minor trauma. The lesions have a smooth surface, with or without crusts, with or without erosion. They appear as bright red, dusky red, violaceous, brown-black, and occur on the fingers, lips, mouth, trunk, and toes. On palms and soles they have a typical collar of thickened stratum corneum at the base.*

## GLOMUS TUMOR    □    ◐

This is a tumor of the glomus body. The *glomus body* is an anatomic and functional unit composed of specialized smooth muscle, the *glomus cells* that surround thin-walled endothelial spaces; this anatomic unit functions as an arteriovenous shunt linking arterioles and venules. The glomus cells surround the narrow lumen of the Sucquet-Hoyer canal that branches from the arteriole and leads to the collecting venule segment that acts as a reservoir. Glomus bodies are present on the pads and nail beds of the fingers and toes and also on the volar aspect of hands and feet, in the skin of the ears, and in the center of the face.

The glomus tumor presents as an exquisitely tender subungual papule or nodule. Glomus tumors are characterized by paroxysmal painful attacks, especially elicited by exposure to cold. They are most often present as solitary subungual tumors (Fig. 9-18) but may rarely occur as multiple papules or nodules. These are noted, especially in children, as discrete papules or sometimes plaques anywhere on the skin surface. They are mostly vascular and not solid, as are the solitary glomus tumors. Therapy is by excision.

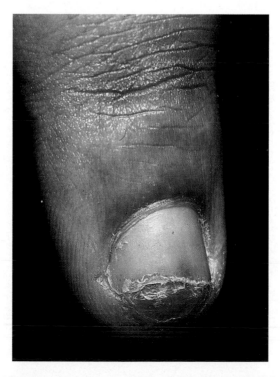

**FIGURE 9-18    Glomus tumor**    *This is an exquisitely painful subungual nodule of reddish color; pain becomes paroxysmal upon exposure to cold.*

## ANGIOSARCOMA　□　●

This is a rare, highly malignant proliferation of endothelial cells manifesting as purpuric macules and/or papules and nodules of bright red or violaceous and even black color (Fig. 9-19). Nodules are solid, bleed easily, and ulcerate and occur in normal skin, usually on the scalp and upper forehead or in localized lymphedema, for instance in postmastectomy lymphedema (*Stuart-Treves syndrome*) or postirradiation lymphedema (Fig. 9-19). Histologically: channels lined by pleomorphic endothelial cells with a high number of mitoses. Treatment is by surgery and/or chemotherapy (doxorubicin). The 5-year survival is just above 10%.

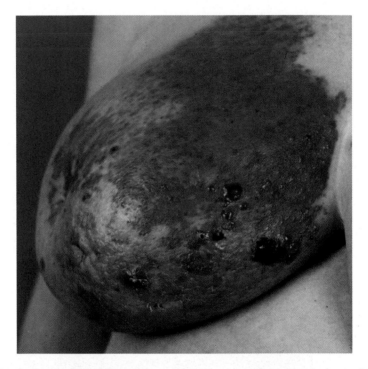

**FIGURE 9-19　Angiosarcoma**　*This lesion occurred in postirradiation lymphedema of the breast. There is a sharply marginated bright red plague studded with red and black papules and nodules that in part have become necrotic.*

**FIGURE 9-20 (Across)　Port-wine stain**　*Sharply marginated, port-wine red macule occurring in a distribution of the second branch of the trigeminal nerve in a young child.*

# VASCULAR MALFORMATIONS

These are *capillary malformations* (CMs) that do not undergo spontaneous involution (e.g., nevus flammeus, or portwine stain, according to the old nomenclature), *lymphatic malformation*, *capillary-lymphatic malformation* (CLM), *venous malformation* (VM), and *arteriovenous malformation* (AVM). Only the most common and important are being dealt with here.

## CAPILLARY MALFORMATIONS

### PORT-WINE STAIN      ■   ◑

*Synonym*: Nevus flammeus.
A port-wine stain (PWS) is an irregularly shaped, red or violaceous, macular CM of dermal blood vessels that is present at birth and never disappears spontaneously. It is common (0.3% of newborns); the malformation is usually confined to the skin but may be associated with vascular malformations in the eye and leptomeninges (Sturge-Weber syndrome).

#### Skin Lesions
These are macular (Fig. 9-20) with varying hues of pink to purple. Large lesions follow a dermatomal distribution and are usually unilateral (85%) though not always. Most commonly involve the face where the CM occurs in the distribution of the trigeminal nerve (Fig. 9-20), usually the superior and middle branches; mucosal involvement of conjunctiva and mouth may occur. CM may also involve other sites.

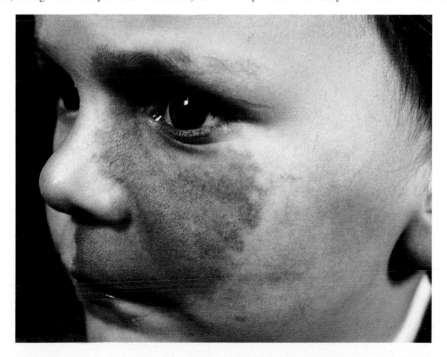

With increasing age of the patient, papules or rubbery nodules (Fig. 9-21) often develop, leading to significant disfigurement.

### Clinical Variant

*Nevus flammeus nuchae* ("stork bite," erythema nuchae, salmon patch) occurs in approximately one-third of infants on the nape of the neck and tends to regress spontaneously. Similar lesions may occur on eyelids and glabella. It is not really a CM but rather a transitory vasodilatation phenomenon.

## HISTOPATHOLOGY

Reveals ectasia of capillaries and no proliferation of endothelial cells. GLUT-1 immunoreactivity is negative.

## COURSE AND PROGNOSIS

PWSs are CMs that do not regress spontaneously. The area of involvement tends to increase in proportion to the size of the child. In adulthood, PWSs usually become raised with papular and nodular areas and are the cause of significant progressive cosmetic disfigurement (Fig. 9-21).

## MANAGEMENT

During the macular phase, PWS can be covered with makeup. Treatment with tunable dye or copper vapor lasers is highly effective.

## SYNDROMIC CM

*Sturge-Weber syndrome* (SWS) is the association of PWS in the trigeminal distribution with vascular malformations in the eye and leptomeninges and superficial calcifications of the brain. SWS may be associated with contralateral hemiparesis, muscular hemiatrophy, epilepsy, and mental retardation; glaucoma and ocular palsy may occur. Skull x-rays show characteristic calcifications of vascular malformations or localized linear calcification along cerebral convolutions. CT scan should be done. It should, however, be noted that PWS with trigeminal distribution is common and does not necessarily indicate the presence of SWS. *Klippel-Trénaunay-Weber syndrome* may have an associated PWS overlying the deeper vascular malformation of soft tissue and bone. *PWS on the midline back* may be associated with an underlying arteriovenous malformation of the spinal cord.

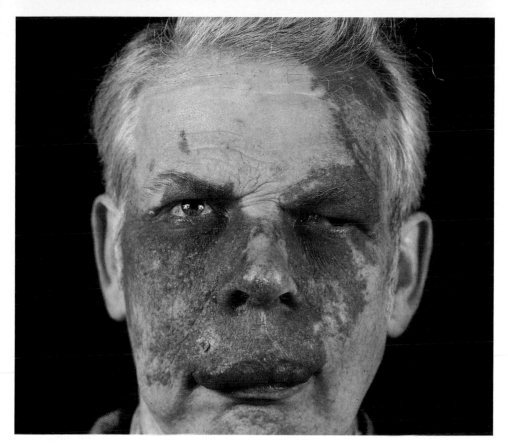

**FIGURE 9-21   Port-wine stain**   *With increasing age, the color deepens, papular and nodular hemangiomas develop within the previously macular lesion causing progressively increasing disfigurement.*

## SPIDER ANGIOMA    ■    ○

*Synonyms:* Nevus araneus, spider nevus, arterial spider, spider telangiectasia, vascular spider. Spider angioma is a very common red focal telangiectatic network of dilated capillaries radiating from a central arteriole (punctum) (Fig. 9-22A). The central papular punctum is the site of the feeding arteriole with macular radiating telangiectatic vessels. Up to 1.5 cm in diameter. Usually solitary. On diascopy, the radiating telangiectasia blanches and the central arteriole may pulsate. Most commonly occurs on the face, forearms, and hands. It frequently occurs in normal persons and is more common in females. It may be associated with hyperestrogenic states, such as pregnancy (one or more in two-thirds of pregnant women), or occurs in patients receiving estrogen therapy, e.g., oral contraceptives, or in those with hepatocellular disease such as subacute and chronic viral hepatitis and alcoholic cirrhosis (Fig. 9-22B). The lesion can occur in young children without any singnificance. Spider angioma arising in childhood and pregnancy may regress spontaneously. The lesion may be confused with *hereditary hemorrhagic telangiectasia*, *ataxia-telangiectasia*, or *telangiectasia* in systemic scleroderma. Lesions may be treated easily with electro- or laser surgery.

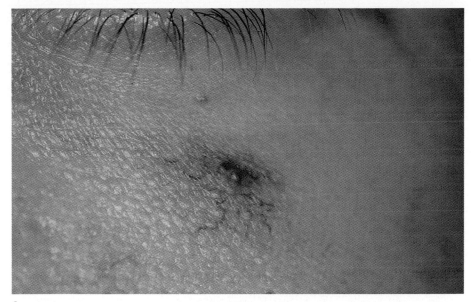

A

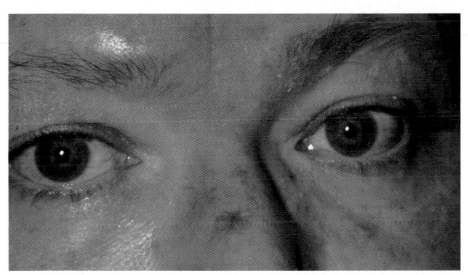

B

**FIGURE 9-22    Spider angioma**    *A. Two small red papules from which telangiectasias radiate. Upon compression the lesion blanches completely. **B.** Spider angioma on the bridge of the nose in a patient with cirrhosis. Note jaundice of sclerae.*

## VENOUS LAKE     ■   ○

A venous lake is a dark blue to violaceous, asymptomatic, soft papule resulting from a dilated venule, occurring on the face, lips, and ears of patients >50 years of age (Fig. 9-23). The etiology is unknown, although it has been thought to be related to solar exposure. These lesions are few in number and remain for years. The lesion results from a dilated cavity lined with a single layer of flattened endothelial cells and a thin wall of fibrous tissue filled with red blood cells. Due to its dark blue or sometimes even black color, the lesion may be confused with nodular melanoma or pyogenic granuloma. The lesion can be partially compressed and lightened up by diascopy, and the use of dermoscopy permits its easy diagnosis as a vascular lesion. Management is for cosmetic reasons and can be accomplished with electrosurgery, laser, or, rarely, with surgical excision.

## CHERRY ANGIOMA     ■   ○

*Synonyms*: Campbell de Morgan spots, senile (hem)angioma.

Cherry angiomas are exceedingly common, asymptomatic, bright red to violaceous, domed vascular lesions (~3 mm) (Fig. 9-24) or occurring as myriads of tiny red papular spots simulating petechiae. They are found principally on the trunk. The lesions appear first at about age 30 and increase in number over the years. There are hardly any elderly people who do not have at least a few lesions. The histology consists of numerous moderately dilated capillaries lined by flattened endothelial cells; stroma is edematous with homogenization of collagen. They are of no consequence other than their cosmetic appearance. Management is electro- or laser coagulation if indicated cosmetically. Cryosurgery is not effective.

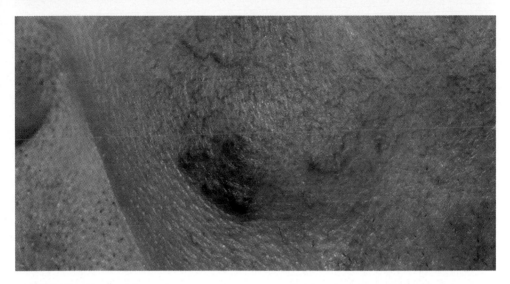

**FIGURE 9-23  Venous lake**  *On the cheek of a 70-year-old male. The lesion was almost black and became a matter of concern to the patient who feared he might have melanoma. However, it blanched completely after compression.*

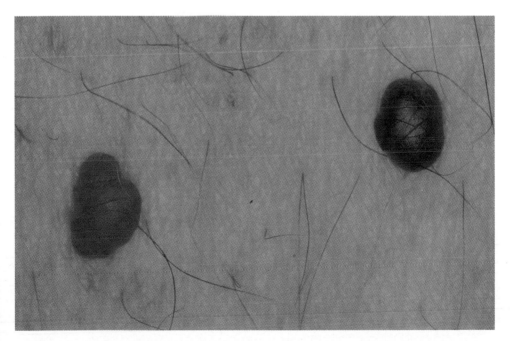

**FIGURE 9-24  Cherry angiomas**  *These bright red, violaceous or even black lesions appear progressively with advancing age.*

## ANGIOKERATOMA    ◨ ○ ●*

The term *angio* ("blood vessel") *keratoma* would imply a vascular tumor with keratotic elements. It is *not* a tumor. Capillaries and postcapillary venules are packed into the papillary body just beneath and bulging into the epidermis, leading to hyperkeratosis. This and the fact that the lumina are usually at least partially thrombosed impart a firm consistency to the lesions. Angiokeratoma has been used to describe several quite distinctive conditions, each with its own characteristic features. Angiokeratomas are dark violaceous to black, often keratotic papules or small plaques that are hard upon palpation and cannot be compressed by diascopy (Fig. 9-25). Angiokeratoma can appear as a solitary lesion (*solitary angiokeratoma*), and then the most important differential diagnosis is a small nodular or superficial spreading melanoma (Fig. 9-25). The most common is *angiokeratoma of Fordyce*; this disease involves the scrotum and vulva; the lesions are papules (≤4 mm) that are dark red in color and present in quite large numbers (Fig. 9-26); *Angiokeratoma of Mibelli* comprises pink to dark red papules that occur on the elbows, knees, and dorsa of the hands. This autosomal dominant disease is rare and occurs in young females. *Angiokeratoma corporis diffusum* (*Fabry's disease*), an x-linked recessive disease, is an inborn error of metabolism in which there is a deficiency of α-galactosidase A leading to an accumulation of neutral glycosphingolipid ceramide trihexoside in endothelial cells, fibrocytes, and pericytes in the dermis, heart, kidneys, and autonomic nervous system. Lesions are numerous dark red, punctate, and tiny (<1 mm), located on the lower half of the body: lower abdomen, genitalia, and buttocks, although lesions may also occur on the lips. The homozygous males have not only the skin lesions but also symptoms related to involvement of other organ systems: acroparesthesias, excruciating pain, transient ischemic attacks, and myocardial infarction. Heterozygous females may have corneal opacities. Fabry's disease is rare.

*Fabry disease.

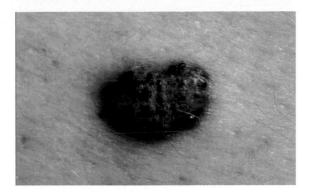

**FIGURE 9-25   Angiokeratoma: solitary**   *This black, firm lesion with a pebbled surface immediately sparks the suspicion of superficial spreading melanoma. It is noncompressible but dermoscopy reveals the typical lacunae of thrombosed vascular spaces. Nonetheless, such lesions should be excised.*

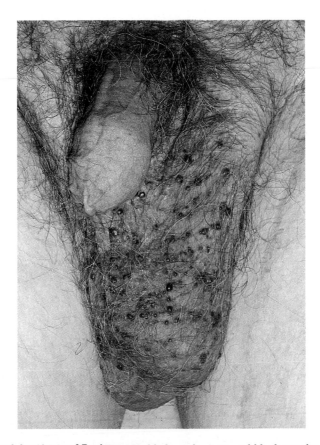

**FIGURE 9-26   Angiokeratoma of Fordyce**   *Reddish, violaceous and black papules on the scrotum. They blanch upon diascopy and this verifies the diagnosis. Note: Thrombosed angiokeratomas do not blanch.*

# LYMPHATIC MALFORMATION (LM)

## LYMPHANGIOMA ☐ ○

The term *lymphatic malformation* is the new terminology for what was formerly called "lymphangioma." These typical lesions comprise multiple, grouped, small macroscopic vesicles filled with clear or serosanguineous fluid ("frog-spawn") (Fig. 9-27). However, these are not true vesicles but microcystic lesions (lymphangioma) as opposed to a macrocystic lesion (cystic hygroma), which is located deep in the dermis and subcutis and appears as a large soft subcutaneous tumor often distorting the face or an extremity. The microcystic LM is present at birth or appears in infancy or even in childhood. It does not disappear spontaneously. Bacterial infection may occur. LM may occur as an isolated solitary lesion, as in Fig. 9-27, or cover large areas (up to 10 × 20 cm); it may be associated with a capillary venous lymphatic (CVL) malformation. The lesion can be excised, if feasible, or treated with sclerotherapy.

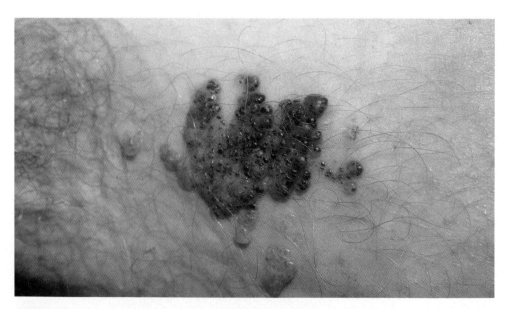

**FIGURE 9-27 Lymphatic malformation (lymphangioma)** *Frog-spawnike confluent grouped "vesicles" filled with a serosanguineous fluid.*

## CAPILLARY/VENOUS MALFORMATIONS (CVMs)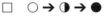

CVMs are deep vascular malformations characterized by soft, compressible deep-tissue swelling. Lesions are not apparent at birth but become so during childhood. They manifest as soft tissue swelling, dome-shaped or multinodular (Fig. 9-28), and are slow-flow lesions. When vascular malformation extends to the epidermis, the surface may be verrucous. The borders are poorly defined, and there is considerable variation in size. Often, CVMs are normal skin color, with the nodular portion blue to purple. They are easily compressed and fill promptly when pressure is released. Some types may be tender, and they may be associated with CMs.

CVMs may be complicated by ulceration and bleeding, scarring, and secondary infection; and, with large lesions, by high-output heart failure. Platelet sequestration and destruction may result in thrombocytopenia (Kasabach-Merritt syndrome), with petechiae in mucous membranes of the mouth, pharynx, and larynx. CVMs may interfere with food intake or breathing and, if located on the eyelids or in the vicinity of the eyes, will obstruct vision and may lead to blindness. There is no satisfactory treatment except compression. In larger lesions—if organ function is compromised—surgical procedures and intravascular coagulation should be performed. High-dose systemic glucocorticoids or IFN-α may be effective.

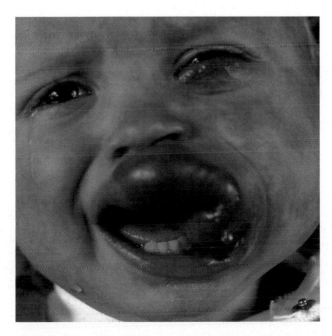

**FIGURE 9-28   Capillary-venous malformation**   *In an infant. There is a soft, compressible, bluish-red tissue swelling distorting the upper lip and lower eyelid. It is a slow flow lesion but requires therapeutic intervention.*

## VARIANTS

**Vascular Hamartomas**   CVLs with deep soft tissue involvement and resultant swelling or diffuse enlargement of an extremity. May involve skeletal muscle with muscle atrophy. Cutaneous changes include dilated tortuous veins and arteriovenous fistulas.

**Klippel-Trénaunay Syndrome**   A CVM or CVL malformation, slow-flow lesion. Local overgrowth of soft tissue and bone results in enlargement of an extremity. Associated cutaneous changes include phlebectasia, nevus flammeus–like cutaneous CM (Fig. 9-29), lymphatic hypoplasia, and lymphedema.

**Blue Rubber Bleb Nevus**   A venous malformation that is spontaneously painful and/or tender. It is a compressible, soft, blue swelling in the dermis and subcutaneous tissue. Size ranges from a few millimeters to several centimeters. The lesion may exhibit localized hyperhidrosis over CVL malformations and occurs, often multiply, on the trunk and upper arms. Similar vascular lesions can occur in the gastrointestinal tract and may be a source of hemorrhage.

**Marfucci's Syndrome**   A slow-flow venous or lymphatic/venous malformation associated with enchondromas and manifested as hard nodules on fingers or toes and as bony deformities. Patients may develop chondrosarcoma.

**Parkes-Weber Syndrome**   A fast-flow capillary arteriovenous malformation (CAVM) or CM, with soft tissue and skeletal hypertrophy.

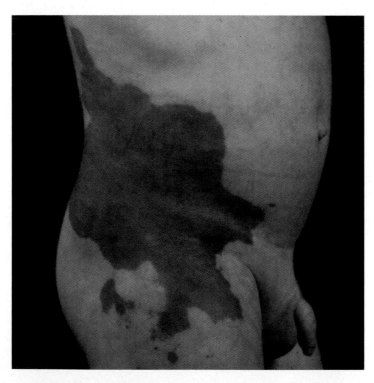

**FIGURE 9-29   Capillary-venous malformation**   *In a 7-year-old boy. This nevus flammeus-like lesion was associated with phlebectasia, lymphedema, and an enlarged right lower extremity (Klippel-Trénaunay syndrome).*

## MISCELLANEOUS CYSTS AND PSEUDOCYSTS

### EPIDERMOID CYST   ■   ○

*Synonyms*: Wen, sebaceous cyst, infundibular cyst, epidermal cyst.
An epidermal cyst is the most common cutaneous cyst, derived from epidermis or the epithelium of the hair follicle, and is formed by cystic enclosure of epithelium within the dermis that becomes filled with keratin and lipid-rich debris. Because of its thin wall, rupture is common and accompanied by a painful inflammatory mass. It occurs in young to middle-aged adults on the face, neck, upper trunk, and scrotum. The lesion, which is usually solitary but may be multiple, is a dermal-to-subcutaneous nodule, 0.5 to 5 cm, which often connects with the surface by keratin-filled pores (Fig. 9-30). The cyst has an epidermal-like wall (stratified squamous epithelium with well-formed granular layer); the content of the cyst is keratinaceous material—cream-colored with a pasty consistency and the odor of rancid cheese. Scrotal lesions may calcify. The cyst wall is relatively thin. Following rupture of the wall, the irritating cyst contents initiate an inflammatory reaction, enlarging the lesion manyfold; the lesion is now associated with a great deal of pain. Ruptured cysts (Fig. 9-31) are often misdiagnosed as being infected rather than ruptured.

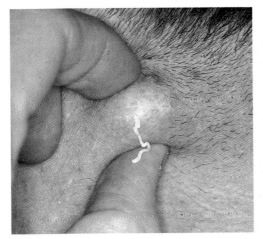

**FIGURE 9-30   Epidermoid cyst**   *A rounded nodule within the dermis. Not always is there an opening through which caseous keratinous material can be expressed.*

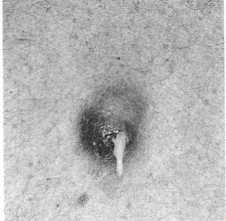

**FIGURE 9-31   Ruptured epidermoid cyst**   *These inflammatory lesions are often misdiagnosed as being infected.*

## TRICHILEMMAL CYST     ■  ○

*Synonyms*: Pilar cyst, isthmus catagen cyst. *Archaic* terms: Wen, sebaceous cyst.
A trichilemmal cyst is the second most common type of cutaneous cyst and is seen most often on the scalp and, in middle age, more frequently in females. It is often familial and occurs frequently as multiple lesions. These are smooth, firm, dome-shaped, 0.5- to 5-cm nodules to tumors; they lack the central punctum seen in epidermoid cysts. Over 90% occur on the scalp, and the overlying scalp hair is usually normal but may be thinned if the cyst is large (Fig. 9-32). It is not connected to the epidermis. The cyst wall is usually thick, and the cyst can be removed intact. The wall is a stratified squamous epithelium with a palisaded outer layer resembling that of the outer root sheath of hair follicles. The inner layer is corrugated without a granular layer. The cyst contains keratin—very dense, pink, and homogeneous; it is often calcified, with cholesterol clefts. If cyst ruptures, it may be inflamed and very painful.

## EPIDERMAL INCLUSION CYST     ◨  ○

*Synonym*: Traumatic epidermoid cyst.
An epidermal inclusion cyst occurs secondary to traumatic implantation of epidermis into the dermis. Traumatically grafted epidermis grows in the dermis, with accumulation of keratin within the cyst cavity, enclosed in a stratified squamous epithelium with a well-formed granular layer. The lesion appears as a dermal nodule (Fig. 9-33) and most commonly occurs on the palms, soles, and fingers. It should be excised.

## MILIUM     ■  ○

A milium is a 1- to 2-mm, superficial, white to yellow, keratin-containing epidermal cyst, occurring multiply, located on the eyelids, cheeks, and forehead in pilosebaceous follicles and at sites of trauma (Fig. 9-34). The lesions can occur at any age, even in infants. Milia arise either de novo, especially around the eye, or in association with various dermatoses with subepidermal bullae or vesicles (pemphigoid, porphyria cutanea tarda, bullous lichen planus, epidermolysis bullosa) and skin trauma (abrasion, burns, dermabrasion, radiation therapy). Incision and expression of contents are the method of treatment.

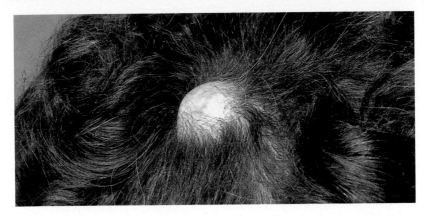

**FIGURE 9-32   Trichilemmal cyst**   *A firm, dome-shaped nodule on the scalp. Pressure by the cyst has caused atrophy of hair bulbs and it thus appears without hairs.*

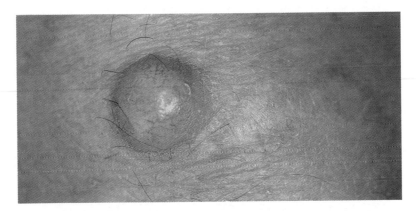

**FIGURE 9-33   Epidermal inclusion cyst**   *A small dermal nodule on the knee at the site of the laceration.*

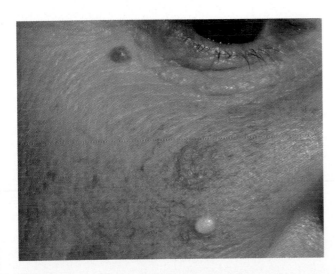

**FIGURE 9-34   Milium**   *A small chalk-white or yellowish papule which can be slit with a scalpel releasing a little ball of horny material.*

## DIGITAL MYXOID CYST ◧ ○

*Synonyms*: Mucous cyst, synovial cyst, myxoid pseudocyst.

A digital myxoid cyst is a pseudocyst occurring over the distal interphalangeal joint and the base of the nail of the finger (Fig: 9-35A) or toe, often associated with Heberden's (osteophytic) node. The lesion occurs in older patients, usually >60 years of age. It is usually a solitary cyst, rubbery, translucent. A clear gelatinous viscous fluid may be extruded from the opening (Fig. 9-35B). When the myxoid cyst is over the nail matrix, a nail plate dystrophy occurs in the form of a 1- to 2-mm groove that extends to the length of the nail (Fig. 9-35A). Various methods of management have been advocated, including surgical excision, incision and drainage, injection of sclerosing material, and injection of a triamcinolone suspension. A simple and most effective method is to make a small incision, express the gelatinous contents, and use a firm compression bandage over the lesion over a period of weeks.

## CUTANEOUS ODONTOGENIC (DENTAL) ABSCESS ☐ ◑

A bacterial infection involving a tooth can spread beyond the pulp of the tooth to become a periapical abscess and extend further to the bone, causing osteomyelitis and perforating into the overlying soft tissues. Such an abscess can make its way through the surface epithelium of the face, producing a cutaneous sinus. It usually presents as an inflammatory papule or nodule discharging pus upon pressure (Fig. 9-36). Patients may be asymptomatic, but without drainage there may be signs and symptoms of acute inflammation with pain. Always check the smear for grains, as *Actinomyces* may be involved, and culture for aerobic and anaerobic bacteria. The condition requires dental surgical intervention.

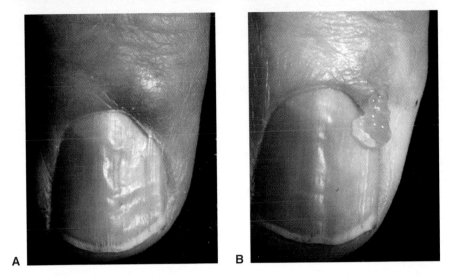

A B

**FIGURE 9-35    Digital myxoid cyst**    *A. The cyst has led to a 3-4 mm groove of the nail plate. **B.** Pressure releases a gelatinous viscous fluid.*

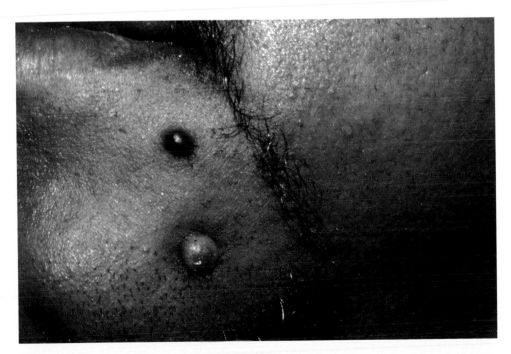

**FIGURE 9-36    Cutaneous odontogenic abscess**    *An inflammatory papule with a tiny central fistula that will release pus upon pressure. This is the typical site for such lesions. The black papule closer to the lower lip is a compound NMN.*

# MISCELLANEOUS BENIGN NEOPLASMS AND HYPERPLASIAS

## SEBORRHEIC KERATOSIS   ■  ○

The seborrheic keratosis is the most common of the benign epithelial tumors. These lesions, which are hereditary, do not appear until age 30 and continue to occur over a lifetime, varying in extent from a few scattered lesions to literally hundreds in some very elderly patients.

## EPIDEMIOLOGY

**Onset**   Rarely before 30 years.
**Sex**   Slightly more common and more extensive involvement in males.

## HISTORY

Evolve over months to years. Rarely pruritic; tender if secondarily infected.

## PHYSICAL EXAMINATION

### Skin Lesions
*Early* Small, 1- to 3-mm, barely elevated papule, later a larger plaque (Figs. 9-37 and 9-38) with or without pigment. The surface has a greasy feel and often shows, with a hand lens, fine stippling like the surface of a thimble.
*Late* plaque with warty surface and "stuck on" appearance (Fig. 9-39), "greasy". With a hand lens horn cysts can often be seen; with dermoscopy they can always be seen. Size from 1 to 6 cm. Flat nodule. Brown, gray, black, skin-colored, round or oval (Figs. 9-37 to 9-39).
*Distribution* Isolated lesion or generalized. Face, trunk (Fig. 9-40), upper extremities.

## LABORATORY EXAMINATION

**Dermatopathology**   Proliferation of monomorphous keratinocytes (with marked papillomatosis) and melanocytes, formation of horn cysts. Some lesions can exhibit atypia of keratinocytes, mimicking Bowen's disease or squamous cell carcinoma (SCC), and these should be excised.

## DIAGNOSIS AND DIFFERENTIAL DIAGNOSIS

Clinically, the diagnosis is made easily. Curettage may be helpful: seborrheic keratosis comes off easily after slight freezing and permits histopathologic examination.
**"Tan Macules"**   Early "flat" lesions may be confused with solar lentigo or spreading pigmented actinic keratosis (see Fig. 10-21).
**Skin-Colored/Tan/Black Verrucous Papules/Plaques**   Larger pigmented lesions are easily mistaken for pigmented basal cell carcinoma (BCC) or malignant melanoma (only biopsy will settle this, or dermoscopy will be of assistance); verruca vulgaris may be similar in clinical appearance, but thrombosed capillaries are present in verrucae.

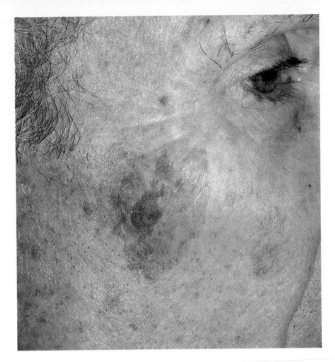

**FIGURE 9-37   Seborrheic keratosis, solitary**   *A slightly raised, keratotic, brown, flat plaque with a slightly more raised center on the zygomatic region in an older female. The differential diagnosis includes lentigo maligna and lentigo maligna melanoma.*

## COURSE AND PROGNOSIS

Lesions develop with increasing age; they are benign and do not become malignant.

## MANAGEMENT

Light electrocautery permits the whole lesion to be easily rubbed off. Then the base can be lightly cauterized to prevent recurrence. This, however, precludes histopathologic verification of diagnosis and should be done only by an experienced diagnostician. Cryosurgery with liquid nitrogen spray works only in flat lesions, and recurrences are possibly more frequent. The best approach is curettage after slight freezing with cryospray, which also permits histopathologic examination. In a solid black lesion without horn cysts, a punch biopsy is mandatory to rule out malignant melanoma; in this case a shave biopsy should not be performed as, in the case of melanoma, it will not permit evaluation of the level of invasion.

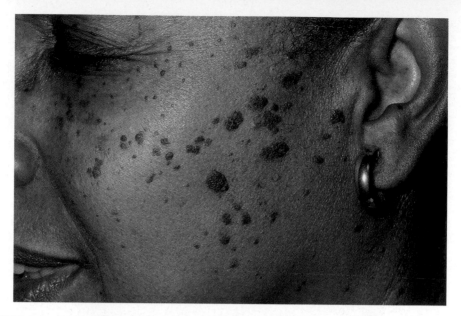

**FIGURE 9-38    Seborrheic keratosis (dermatosis papulosa nigra)**    *This consists of myriads of tiny black lesions, some enlarging to more than a centimeter. This is seen in Black Africans, African Americans, and deeply pigmented South East Asians. Treatment is a problem because hypopigmented spots can arise at sites where these seborrheic keratoses have been removed.*

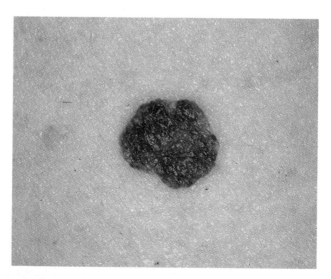

**FIGURE 9-39    Seborrheic keratosis**    *This has a "stuck on" appearance but is very dark and quite irregular and may pose a problem in the differential diagnosis of superficial spreading melanoma. The examination with dermoscopy reveals horn cysts that are virtually (not 100%) pathognomonic of seborrheic keratosis. If in doubt, a punch biopsy should be obtained for diagnosis.*

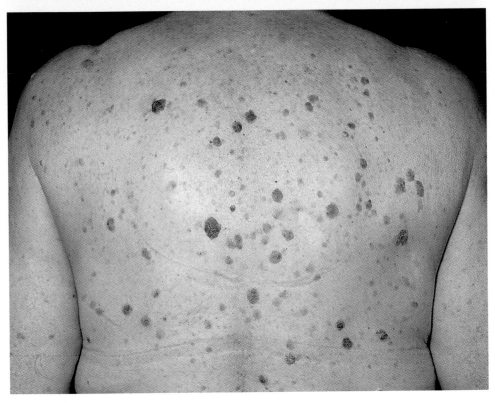

**FIGURE 9-40   Seborrheic keratoses, multiple** *Multiple brown, warty papules and nodules on the back, having a "greasy-feel" and "stuck on" appearance. This picture also shows the evolution of the lesions: from small only slightly tan, very thin papules or plaques to larger, darker nodular lesions with a verrucous surface. Practically all lesions on the back of this elderly patient are seborrheic keratoses; what they have in common is that they give the impression that they could be scraped off easily which, in fact, they can.*

# KERATOACANTHOMA

Keratoacanthoma (KA) is a special lesion, a pseudocancer, occurring as an isolated nodule, usually on the face, and mimicking squamous cell carcinoma. Unique features are its rapid growth rate, much faster than that of an SCC, and also its spontaneous remission over a period of several months.

## EPIDEMIOLOGY

**Age of Onset**   Over 50 years; rare below 20 years. Male:female ratio 2:1.

## PATHOGENESIS

Human papillomavirus (HPV) -9, -16, -19, -25, and -37 have been identified in KAs. Other possible etiologic factors include UV radiation and chemical carcinogens (industrial: pitch and tar).

## HISTORY

Rapid growth, achieving a size of 2.5 cm within a few weeks. No symptoms, but there are occasional tenderness and cosmetic disfigurement.

## PHYSICAL EXAMINATION

### Skin Lesions
Nodule, dome-shaped, often with a central keratotic plug (Figs. 9-41 and 9-42). Skin-colored or slightly red, tan/brown. Firm but not hard. 2.5 cm (range 1 to 10 cm), round. Keratotic plug may appear like a cutaneous horn (Fig. 9-42). Removal of plug results in a crater.
*Distribution* Isolated single lesion. Uncommonly, may be multiple, eruptive. On exposed skin: cheeks, nose, ears, hands (dorsa).

## LABORATORY EXAMINATION

**Dermatopathology**   A representative biopsy that extends through the entire lesion to preserve the architecture of the nodule or primary excision is required. Central, large, irregularly shaped crater filled with keratin. The surrounding epidermis extends in a liplike manner over the sides of the crater. The keratinocytes are atypical and many are dyskeratotic. Differentiation of KA from SCC may not always be possible.

## DIAGNOSIS AND DIFFERENTIAL DIAGNOSIS

Clinical findings confirmed by representative biopsy. SCC, hypertrophic actinic keratosis, verruca vulgaris.

## COURSE AND PROGNOSIS

Spontaneous regression in 2 to 6 months or sometimes >1 year.

## MANAGEMENT

**Surgery**   Surgical excision is recommended in that KA cannot be distinguished from SCC on clinical findings.
**Multiple KAs**   Systemic retinoids and methotrexate have been used. Imiquimod is being evaluated.

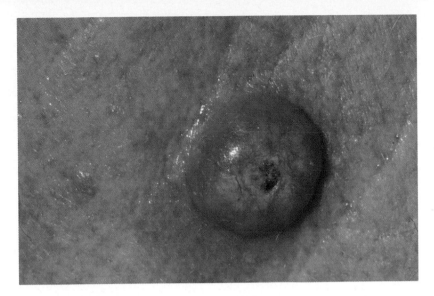

**FIGURE 9-41   Keratoacanthoma**   *Erythematous, dome-shaped tumor, 1 cm in diameter, smooth with a reddish color and teleangiectasias and with a keratinaceous plug in the center, developing on facial skin exhibiting moderate dermatoheliosis.*

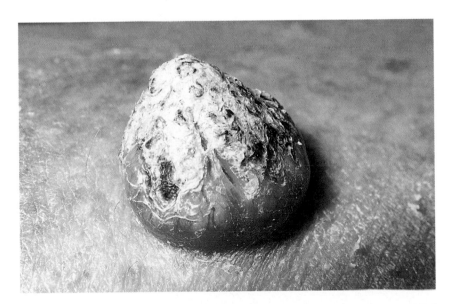

**FIGURE 9-42   Keratoacanthoma**   *Erythematous, dome-shaped tumor with a large, central, keratotic plug of 6-weeks duration. The lesion cannot be distinguished clinically from squamous cell carcinoma.*

## BECKER'S NEVUS ☐ ○

Becker's nevus (BN) is a distinctive asymptomatic clinical lesion that is a pigmented hamartoma— i. e., a developmental anomaly consisting of changes in pigmentation, hair growth, and, most important, a slightly elevated smooth verrucous surface (Fig. 9-43). It occurs mostly in males and in all races. It appears not at birth but usually before 15 years of age and sometimes after this age. The lesion is predominantly a macule but with a papular verrucous surface not unlike the lesion of acanthosis nigricans. It is light brown in color and has a geographic pattern (like the coast of Maine) with sharply demarcated borders (Fig. 9-43). Commonest locations are the shoulders and the back. The increased hair growth follows the onset of the pigmentation and is localized to the areas that are pigmented. The pigmentation is related to increased melanin in basal cells and not to an increased number of melanocytes. It is differentiated from a hairy congenital melanocytic nevus, because BN is not usually present at birth, and from Albright's pigmentation, which is also present at birth and there is no increased hair growth. The lesion extends for a year or two and then remains stable, only rarely fading. There is very rarely hypoplasia of underlying structures, e.g., shortening of the arm or reduced breast development in areas under the lesion.

## TRICHOEPITHELIOMA ☐ ◑

Trichoepitheliomas are benign appendage tumors with hair bulb differentiation. The lesions, which appear at puberty, occur on the face and less often on the scalp, neck, and upper trunk (Fig. 9-44). The lesions, which may be only a few small pink or skin-colored papules at first, gradually increase in number and may become quite large and be confused with BCC (Fig. 9-44). Trichoepitheliomas can also appear as solitary tumors, which may be nodular, or appear as ill-defined plaques like sclerosing BCC.

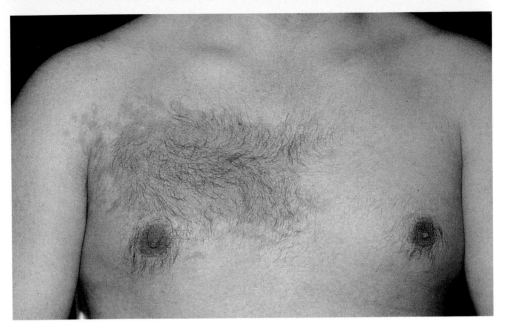

**FIGURE 9-43  Becker's nevus**  *A slightly raised light-tan plaque with sharply defined and highly irregular border and hypertrichosis on the chest of a 35-year-old male patient.*

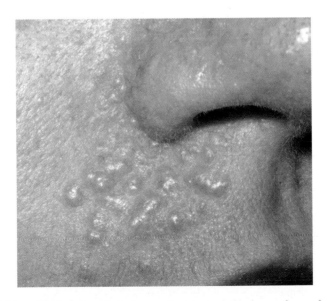

**FIGURE 9-44  Trichoepitheliomas**  *Multiple, small, sharply defined smooth papules that look like early BCCs.*

## SYRINGOMA

Syringomas are benign adenomas of the eccrine ducts. They are 1- to 2-mm, skin-colored or yellow, firm papules that occur mostly in women, beginning at puberty; they may be familial. The lesions, most often multiple rather than solitary, occur most frequently around the eyelids (Fig. 9-45) and on the face, axillae, umbilicus, upper chest, and vulva. The lesions have a specific histologic pattern: many small ducts in the dermis with comma-like tails with the appearance of "tadpoles." The lesions can be disfiguring, and most patients want them removed; this can be done easily with electrosurgery.

## SEBACEOUS HYPERPLASIA

These are very common lesions in older persons and are confused with small BCCs. The lesions are 1 to 3 mm in diameter and have both telangiectasia and central umbilication (Fig. 9-46). Two features distinguish sebaceous hyperplasia from BCC: (1) sebaceous hyperplasia is soft to palpation, not firm as in BCC; and (2) with firm lateral compression it is often possible to elicit a very small globule of sebum in the valley of the umbilicated portion of the lesion. Sebaceous hyperplasias can be destroyed with light electrocautery.

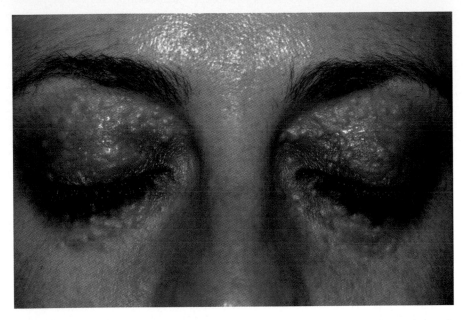

**FIGURE 9-45   Syringomas**   *Symmetric eruption of 1-2 mm skin-colored, smooth papules on the upper and lower eylids.*

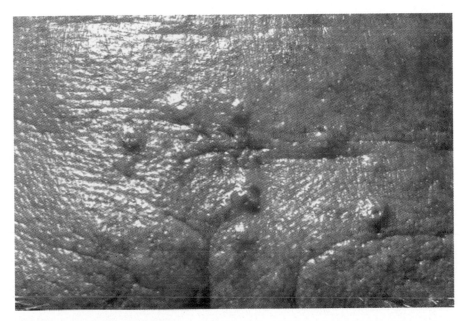

**FIGURE 9-46   Sebaceous hyperplasia**   *1-3 mm smooth papules with central umbilication on the forehead.*

## NEVUS SEBACEOUS    □  ◑

*Synonym*: Organoid nevus.

This congenital malformation of sebaceous differentiation occurs on the scalp or, rarely, on the face (Fig. 9-47). The lesion appears on the scalp and has a distinctive morphology: a hairless, thin, elevated, 1- to 2-cm plaque with a characteristic orange color and a pebbly or warty surface. About 10% of patients can be expected to develop BCC in the lesion. Excision is recommended at around puberty for cosmetic reasons and to prevent the occurrence of BCC.

## EPIDERMAL NEVUS    □  ○ → ◑

As the name *nevus* implies this is a developmental (hamartomatous) disorder characterized by hyperplasia of epidermal structures (epidermis and adnexa). There are no nevocellular nevus cells (melanocytes). Epidermal nevus is usually present at birth or occurs in infancy; rarely, it develops in puberty. All epidermal nevi on the head are present at birth.

There are several variants of epidermal nevi. The *verrucous epidermal nevus* may be localized or multiple. The lesions are skin-colored, brown, or grayish-brown (Fig. 9-48) and are composed of closely set verrucous papules, well circumscribed; they are often in a linear arrangement—especially on the leg—or they may appear in Blaschko's lines on the trunk. Excision is the best treatment, if feasible. Biopsy of the lesions should be considered to rule out BCC.

When the lesions are extensive they are termed *systematized epidermal nevus*, and when they are located on half the body they are termed *nevus unius lateris*. The lesions can exhibit erythema, scaling, and crusting and are then called *inflammatory linear verrucous epidermal nevus* (ILVEN). The lesions gradually enlarge and become stable in adolescence. *There is also a noninflammatory linear verrucous epidermal nevus* (NILVEN).

Extensive epidermal nevi (*epidermal nevus syndrome*) may be multisystem disorders and may be associated with developmental abnormalities (bone cysts, hyperplasia of bone, scoliosis, spina bifida, kyphosis), vitamin D–resistant rickets, and neurologic problems (mental retardation, seizures, cortical atrophy, hydrocephalus). These patients require a complete examination, including the eyes (cataracts, optic nerve hypoplasia), and cardiac studies to rule out aneurysms, patent ductus arteriosus.

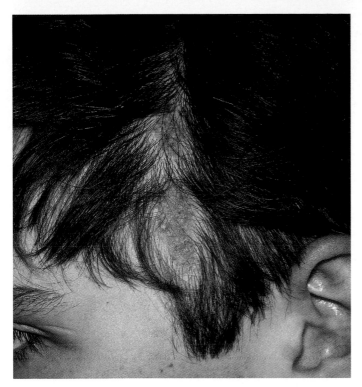

**FIGURE 9-47  Nevus sebaceous**  *Two hairless, barely elevated plaques of orange color and pebbly surface.*

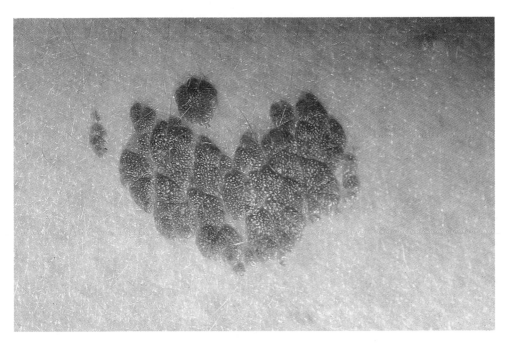

**FIGURE 9-48  Epidermal nevus**  *A brownish irregular plaque with a verrucous surface.*

## BENIGN DERMAL AND SUBCUTANEOUS NEOPLASMS AND HYPERPLASIAS

### LIPOMA

Lipomas are single or multiple, benign subcutaneous tumors that are easily recognized because they are soft, rounded, or lobulated and movable against the overlying skin (Figs. 9-49A and 9-49B). Many lipomas are small but may also enlarge to >6 cm. They occur especially on the neck, trunk, and on the extremities (Fig. 9-49B) but can occur anywhere on the body (Fig. 9-49A). Lipomas are composed of fat cells that have the same morphology as normal fat cells, and there is a connective tissue framework. Angiolipomas have a vascular component and may be tender in cold ambient temperature. These often require excision, whereas other lipomas should be excised only when considered disfiguring. Liposuction can also be performed when liposomas are soft and thus have only a minor connective tissue component. *Familial lipoma syndrome*, an autosomal dominant trait appearing in early adulthood, consists of hundreds of slowly growing nontender lesions. *Adipositas dolorosa*, or *Dercum's disease*, occurs in women in middle age; there are multiple tender, not circumscribed but rather diffuse fatty deposits. *Benign symmetric lipomatosis*, which affects middle-aged men, consists of many large nontender, coalescent poorly circumscribed lipomas, mostly on the trunk and upper extremities; they coalesce on the neck and may lead to a "horse-collar" appearance.

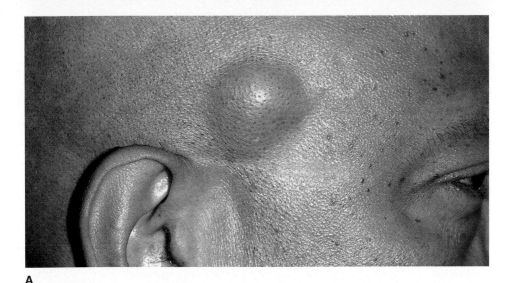

A

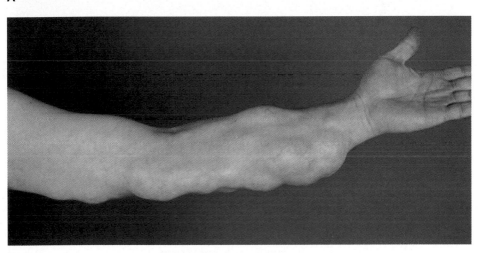

B

**FIGURE 9-49    Lipoma**    *A. Well-defined, soft, rounded tumor in the subcutis, movable both against the overlying skin and the underlying structures. B. Multiple lipomas on the lower arm in a 50-year-old male patient. In this patient lesions were symmetric and were also found on the trunk and lower extremities.*

## DERMATOFIBROMA        ■   ○

A dermatofibroma is a very common, button-like dermal nodule, usually occurring on the extremities, important only because of its cosmetic appearance or its being mistaken for other lesions, such as malignant melanoma when it is pigmented. The lesion may be tender.
*Synonyms*: Solitary histiocytoma, sclerosing hemangioma.

### EPIDEMIOLOGY AND ETIOLOGY

Very common, occurs mostly in adults. Females > males.
**Etiology**   Unknown. It is considered by many to represent a late histiocytic reaction to an arthropod bite.

### PHYSICAL EXAMINATION

#### Skin Lesions
Usually asymptomatic papule or nodule (Fig. 9-50), 3 to 10 mm in diameter. Surface variably domed but may be depressed below plane of surrounding skin. Texture of surface may be dull, shiny, or scaling. Top may be crusted or scarred secondary to excoriation or shaving. Borders ill defined, fading to normal skin. *Color*: variable—skin-colored, pink, brown, tan, dark chocolate brown (Fig. 9-51). Usually darker at center, fading to normal skin color at margin. Firm. *Dimple sign*: lateral compression with thumb and index finger produces a depression or "dimple" (Fig. 9-52).
***Distribution***   Legs > arms> trunk. Hardly ever occurs on head, palms, soles. Usually solitary; may be multiple, randomly scattered.

### LABORATORY EXAMINATION

**Dermatopathology**   Whorling fascicles of spindle cells with small amounts of pale blue cytoplasm and elongated nuclei. Some tumors extend to the panniculus. Pigmented dermatofibromas (Fig. 9-51) contain lipids or hemosiderin pigment in the histiocytes in addition to hyperpigmentation of the epidermis. Variable increase in vascular spaces. Overlying epidermis frequently hyperplastic.

### DIAGNOSIS AND DIFFERENTIAL DIAGNOSIS

Clinical findings— "dimple" sign (Fig. 9-52), but there are other lesions that can result in depression with lateral pressure, e.g., papulonodular lesions containing mucin, scar, blue nevus, pilar cyst, metastatic carcinoma, Kaposi's sarcoma, dermatofibrosarcoma protuberans.

### COURSE AND PROGNOSIS

Lesions appear gradually over several months, may persist without increase in size for years to decades, and may regress spontaneously.

### MANAGEMENT

Surgical removal is not usually indicated, as the resulting scar is often less cosmetically acceptable. Cryosurgery with a cotton-tip applicator is often effective and produces a cosmetically acceptable scar in most patients.

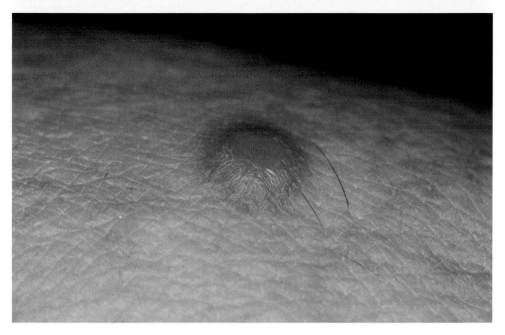

**FIGURE 9-50 Dermatofibroma** *A dome-shaped, slightly erythematous and tan nodule with a button-like, firm consistency.*

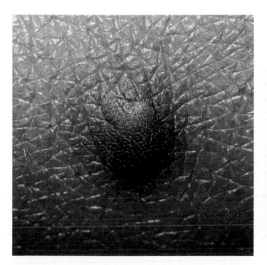

**FIGURE 9-51 Dermatofibroma** *This lesion is pigmented. Confused with blue nevus or even nodular melanoma. The pigment is melanin and hemosiderin.*

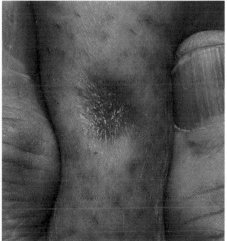

**FIGURE 9-52 Dermatofibroma: "dimple sign"** *Dimpling of the lesion is seen when pinched between two fingers.*

## HYPERTROPHIC SCARS AND KELOIDS    ■

Hypertrophic scars and keloids are exuberant fibrous repair tissues after a cutaneous injury. A *hypertrophic scar* remains confined to the site of original injury; a *keloid*, however, extends beyond this site, often with clawlike extensions. May be cosmetically very unsightly and pose a serious problem for the patient if the lesion is large and on the ear or face.

### EPIDEMIOLOGY AND ETIOLOGY

**Age of Onset**    Third decade, but all ages.
**Sex**    Equal incidence in males and females.
**Race**    Much more common in blacks and in persons with blood group A.
**Etiology**    Unknown. They usually follow injury to skin, i.e., surgical scar, laceration, abrasion, cryosurgery, and electrocoagulation as well as vaccination, acne, etc. Keloid may also arise spontaneously, without history of injury, usually in presternal site.

### HISTORY

**Skin Symptoms**    Usually asymptomatic. May be pruritic or painful if touched.

### PHYSICAL EXAMINATION

**Skin Lesions**
Papules to nodules (Figs. 9-53 and 9-54) to large tuberous lesions. Most often the color of the normal skin but also bright red (Fig. 9-53) or bluish. May be linear after traumatic or surgical injury (Fig. 9-53). Hypertrophic scars tend to be elevated and are confined to approximately the site of the original injury (Fig. 9-53). Keloids, however, may extend in a clawlike fashion far beyond any slight original injury (Fig. 9-55) or may be nodular; tumor-like (Fig. 9-56). Firm to hard; may be tender, surface smooth (Figs. 9-55 and 9-56).
**Distribution**    Earlobes, shoulders, upper back, chest.

### LABORATORY EXAMINATION

**Dermatopathology**    *Hypertrophic Scar* Whorls of young fibrous tissue and fibroblasts in haphazard arrangement.
*Keloid* Features of hypertrophic scar with added feature of thick, eosinophilic, acellular bands of collagen.

### DIAGNOSIS AND DIFFERENTIAL DIAGNOSIS

Clinical diagnosis; biopsy not warranted unless there is clinical doubt, because another biopsy may induce new hypertrophic scarring. Differential diagnosis includes dermatofibroma, dermatofibrosarcoma protuberans, desmoid tumor, scar with sarcoidosis, foreign-body granuloma.

### COURSE AND PROGNOSIS

Hypertrophic scars tend to regress, in time becoming flatter and softer. Keloids, however, may continue to expand in size for decades.

### MANAGEMENT

This is a real challenge, as no treatment is highly effective.
**Intralesional Glucocorticoids**    Intralesional injection of triamcinolone (10 to 40 mg/mL) every month may reduce pruritus or sensitivity of lesion, as well as reduce its volume and flatten it. This works quite well in small hypertrophic scars but less well in keloids. Can be

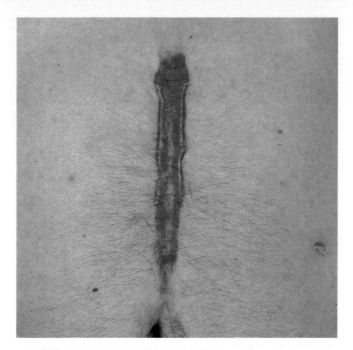

**FIGURE 9-53  Hypertrophic scar**  *A broad, raised scar developing at the site of surgical incision with telangiectatic blood vessels and a shiny atrophic epidermis.*

combined with cryotherapy whereby the lesion is initially frozen with liquid nitrogen, allowed to thaw, and then injected with triamcinolone (10 to 40 mg/mL). After freezing, the lesion becomes edematous and is much easier to inject.

**Surgical Excision**  Lesions that are excised surgically often recur larger than the original lesion. Excision with immediate postsurgical radiotherapy is beneficial.

**Silicone Cream and Silicone Gel Sheet**  Reported to be beneficial in keloids and is painless and noninvasive. Not very effective in authors' experience.

**Prevention**  Individuals prone to hypertrophic scars or keloids should be advised to avoid cosmetic procedures such as ear piercing. Scars from burns tend to become hypertrophic. Can be prevented by compression garments.

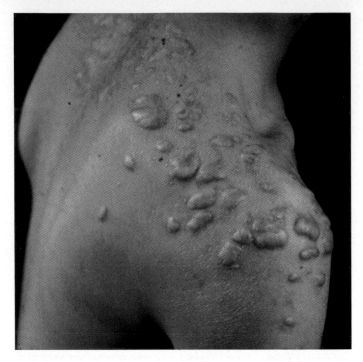

**FIGURE 9-54    Multiple hypertrophic scars**    *On the shoulders of a 20-year-old male with a history of severe acne conglobata.*

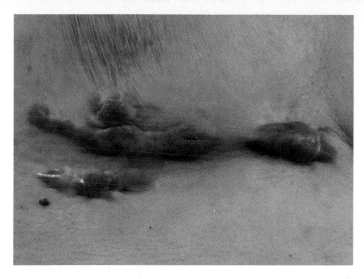

**FIGURE 9-55 Keloids** *Sausage-like red nodules, well-defined, with claw-like extensions, very hard on palpation in the presternal and mammary region in a 28-year-old man. These were "spontaneous" keloids arising without history of injury.*

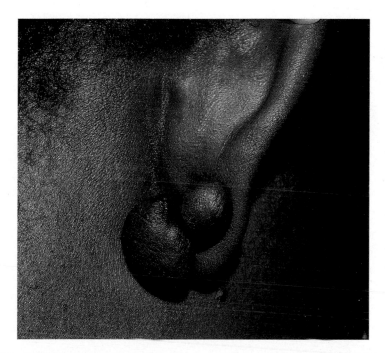

**FIGURE 9-56 Keloid, following ear piercing** *Firm, well-defined nodules on the earlobe of an African-American woman. Persons with susceptibility to developing keloids should not have their ears pierced.*

## SKIN TAG    ■    ○

*Synonyms*: Acrochordon, cutaneous papilloma, soft fibroma.

A skin tag is a very common, soft, skin-colored or tan or brown, round or oval, pedunculated papilloma (polyp) (Fig. 9-57); it is usually constricted at the base and may vary in size from >1 mm to as large as 10 mm. Histologic findings include a thinned epidermis and a loose fibrous tissue stroma. It occurs more often in the middle aged and in the elderly. A skin tag is usually asymptomatic but occasionally may become tender following trauma or torsion and may become crusted or hemorrhagic. More common in females and in obese patients and most often noted in intertriginous areas (axillae, inframammary, groin) and on the neck and eyelids; it occurs in acanthosis nigricans as an obligatory lesion. May be confused with a pedunculated seborrheic keratosis, dermal or compound melanocytic nevus, solitary neurofibroma, or molluscum contagiosum. Lesions tend to become larger and more numerous over time, especially during pregnancy. Following spontaneous torsion, autoamputation can occur. Management is accomplished with simple snipping with scissors, electrodesiccation, or cryosurgery.

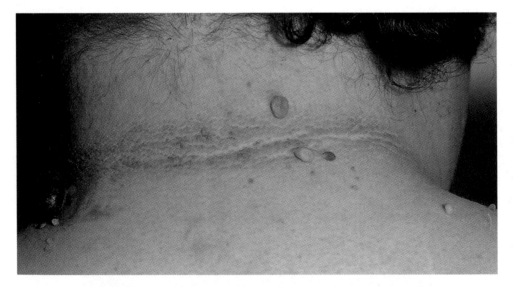

**FIGURE 9-57    Skin tags**  *Soft skin-colored and tan pedunculated papillomas. These are very common in the elderly obese and are an obligatory lesion in acanthosis nigricans, as in this patient.*

## CHONDRODERMATITIS NODULARIS HELICIS    ■   ◑

Usually occurs as a single elongated, exquisitely tender nodule of the free border of helix of the ear. Common, probably due to constant mechanical and environmental trauma. Appears spontaneously, enlarges quickly, measuring less than 1 cm (Fig. 9-58), firm, well-defined, round to oval with sloping margins. Either embedded in the skin or elevated several millimeters and with dome-shaped surface, white-waxy and translucent, and often covered with an adherent scale. More common in males than in females.

Spontaneous pain or tenderness is the initial presenting complaint. Can be intense and stabbing, paroxysmal or continuous. Lesion may ulcerate and spontaneous remission is rare. Differential diagnosis includes basal cell and squamous cells carcinoma, actinic keratosis and keratoacanthoma. One also has to think of tophus, rheumatoid and rheumatic nodules, and discoid lupus erythematosus.

**Management**   Includes intralesional injection of triamcinoloneacetonide, carbon dioxide laser, surgery. The definite treatment is excisional surgery including the underlying cartilage.

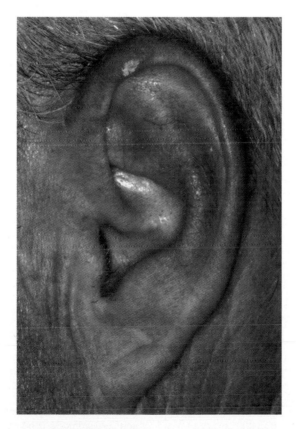

**FIGURE 9-58   Chondrodermatitis nodularis helicis**   *An exquisitely tender nodule on the helix of this 70-year-old male. The lesion is covered by a small, tightly adhering hyperkeratosis and can thus be mistaken for an actinic keratosis.*

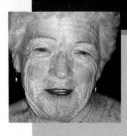

# PHOTOSENSITIVITY, PHOTO-INDUCED DISORDERS, AND DISORDERS BY IONIZING RADIATION

## SKIN REACTIONS TO SUNLIGHT

The term *photosensitivity* describes an abnormal response to light, usually sunlight, occurring within minutes, hours, or days of exposure and lasting up to weeks, months, and even longer. Cutaneous photosensitivity reactions require absorption of photon energy by appropriately shaped molecules leading to molecular deformity. Energy is either dispersed harmlessly or is directed to chemical reactions that lead to molecular, cellular, and tissue damage resulting in clinical disease. Absorbing molecules can be (1) exogenous agents applied topically or systemically, (2) endogenous molecules either usually present in skin or produced by an abnormal metabolism, or (3) a combination of exogenous and endogenous molecules that have acquired antigenic properties and thus elicit a photoradiation-driven immune reaction. *Photosensitivity disorders occur only in body regions exposed to solar radiation* (Image 10-1).

There are three broad types of *acute photosensitivity*:

1. A *sunburn*-type response with the development of morphologic skin changes simulating a normal sunburn with erythema, edema, and bullae, such as in phototoxic reactions to drugs or phytophotodermatitis.
2. A *rash* response to light exposure with development of varied morphologic expressions: macules, papules, or plaques, as in eczematous dermatitis. These are usually photoallergic in nature or belong to the so-called idiopathic photodermatoses such as polymorphous light eruption.
3. *Urticarial* responses that are typical for solar urticaria but may occur in erythropoietic porphyria.

*Chronic photosensitivity*: chronic repeated sun exposures over time result in polymorphic skin changes that have been termed *dermatoheliosis*, or photoaging. A classification of skin reactions to sunlight is shown in Table 10-1.

### BASICS OF CLINICAL PHOTOMEDICINE

The main culprit of solar radiation–induced skin pathology is the ultraviolet portion of the solar spectrum. Ultraviolet radiation (UVR) in photomedicine is divided into two principal types: UVB (290 to 320 nm), the "sunburn spectrum," and UVA (320 to 400 nm). UVA has been subdivided into UVA-1 (340 to 400 nm) and UVA-2 (320 to 340 nm). The unit of measurement of sunburn is the *minimum erythema dose* (MED), which is the minimum ultraviolet exposure that produces a clearly marginated erythema in the irradiated site 24 h after a single exposure. The MED is expressed as the amount of energy delivered per unit area: $mJ/cm^2$ (UVB) or $J/cm^2$ (UVA). The MED for UVB in Caucasians is 20 to 40 $mJ/cm^2$ (for a skin phototype I or II, about 20 min in northern latitudes at noon in June) and for UVA is 15 to 20 $J/cm^2$ (about 120 min in northern latitudes at noon in June). UVB erythema develops in 6 to 24 h and fades within 72 to 120 h. UVA erythema develops in 4 to 16 h and fades within 48 to 120 h.

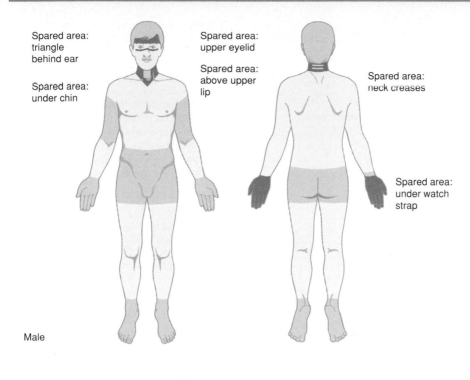

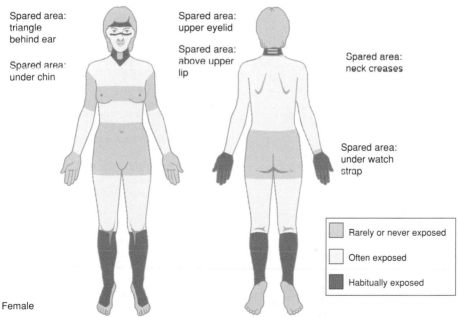

**IMAGE 10-1**   *Variations in solar exposure on different body areas.*

## TABLE 10-1  Simplified Classification of Skin Reactions to Sunlight

Phototoxicity
  Sunburn
  Drug-/chemical-induced
  Plant-induced (phytophotodermatitis)
Photoallergy
  Drug-/chemical-induced
  Chronic actinic dermatitis
  Solar urticaria[*]
Idiopathic
  Polymorphous light eruption
  Actinic prurigo[*]
  Hydroa vacciniforme[*]
Metabolic and nutritional
  Porphyria cutanea tarda
  Variegate porphyria
  Erythropoietic protoporphyria
  Pellagra[*]
DNA-deficient photodermatoses
  Xeroderma pigmentosum[*]
  Other rare syndromes[*]
Photoexacerbated dermatoses
Chronic photodamage
  Dermatoheliosis (photoaging)
  Solar lentigo
  Actinic keratoses
  Skin cancer[†]

[*]Conditions not dealt with here are marked with an asterisk and the reader is referred to IM Freedberg, AZ Eisen, K Wolff, KF Austen, LA Goldsmith, SI Katz (eds.): *Fitzpatrick's Dermatology in General Medicine*, 6th ed. New York, McGraw-Hill, 2003.
[†]For coverage of skin cancer, see Sections 11 and 12.

## Variations in Sun Reactivity in Normal Persons: Fitzpatrick's Skin Phototypes

(Table 10-2)

Sunburn is seen most frequently in individuals who have pale white or white skin and a limited capacity to develop *facultative*, or inducible, melanin pigmentation (tanning) after exposure to UVR. Basic skin color (*constitutive* melanin pigmentation) is divided into white, brown, and black. Not all persons with white skin have the same capacity to develop tanning, and this fact is the principal basis for the classification of "white" persons into four *skin phototypes* (SPT). The SPT is based on the basic skin color (Table 10-2) and on a *person's own estimate* of sunburning and tanning. One question permits the identification of the SPT: "Do you tan easily?" Persons with SPT I or II will say immediately, "No," and those with SPT III or IV will say, "Yes." Persons with SPT I or II are regarded as "melanocompromised," and those with SPT III or IV as "melanocompetent."

SPT I persons usually have pale white skin color, blond or red hair, and blue eyes; but, in fact, they may have dark brown hair and brown eyes, while their skin color is pale white. SPT I persons sunburn easily with short exposures and do not tan.

SPT II persons are a subgroup of SPT I and sunburn easily but *tan with difficulty*, whereas SPT III persons may have some sunburn with short exposures but can develop marked tanning. It is estimated that about 25% of white-skinned persons in the United States are SPT I and II. SPT IV persons tan with ease and do not sunburn with short exposures. SPT IV persons may have blond hair and blue eyes but more often have brown hair and brown eyes and light tan (beige) constitutive skin color. Persons with constitutive brown skin are termed SPT V and with black skin SPT VI. Note that sunburn depends on the amount of UVR energy absorbed. Thus, with excessive sun exposure, even SPT VI person can have a sunburn.

## TABLE 10-2  Classification of Fitzpatrick's Skin Phototypes (SPT)

| SPT | Basic Skin Color | Response to Sun Exposure |
| --- | --- | --- |
| I | Pale white | Do not tan, burn easily |
| II | White | Tan with difficulty, burn easily |
| III | White | Tan after initial sunburn |
| IV | Light brown/olive | Tan easily |
| V | Brown | Tan easily |
| VI | Black | Become darker |

## ACUTE SUN DAMAGE (SUNBURN)     ■    →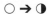

Sunburn is an acute, delayed, and transient inflammatory response of normal skin after exposure to UVR from sunlight or artificial sources. By nature it is a phototoxic reaction. Sunburn is characterized by erythema (Fig. 10-1) and, if severe, by vesicles and bullae, edema, tenderness, and pain.

### EPIDEMIOLOGY

Sunburn depends on the amount of UVR energy delivered and the susceptibility of the individual (SPT). It will therefore occur more often around midday, with decreasing latitude, increasing altitude, and decreasing SPT. Thus, the "ideal" setting for a sunburn to occur would be an SPT I individual (highest susceptibility) on Mt. Kenya (high altitude, close to the equator) at noon (UVR is highest). Of course, sunburn can occur at any latitude, but the probability for it to occur decreases with increasing distance from the equator. Sunburn is seen more often in those who frequent beaches or travel to sunny vacation areas. Sunburn also increases with respect to other ambient conditions, such as UVR reflectance from snow, water, or a glacier.

**Age**   Very young children and elderly persons are said to have a reduced capacity to sunburn, although this has not been thoroughly documented.

### PATHOGENESIS

The chromophores (molecules that absorb UVR) for UVB sunburn erythema are not known, but damage to DNA may be the initiating event. The damage to DNA results in excision of pyrimidine dimers, and that itself

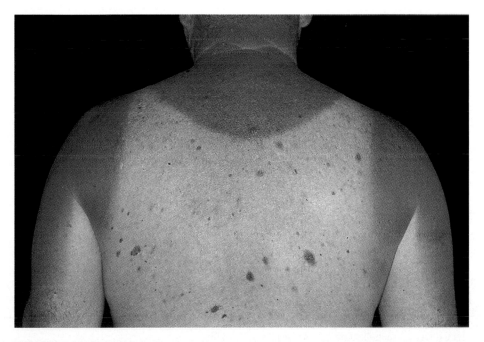

**FIGURE 10-1   Acute sunburn**   *Painful, tender, bright erythema with mild edema of the upper back with sharp demarcation between the sun-exposed and sun-protected white areas. Note large atypical melanocytic nevi. The patient is at risk for developing malignant melanoma.*

initiates a protective tanning response. The mediators that cause the erythema include histamine for both UVA and UVB. In UVB erythema, other mediators include serotonin, prostaglandins, lysosomal enzymes, and kinins. However, the cytokine interleukin 6 (IL-6), which peaks at 12 h, is probably the main mediator of the sunburn reaction in humans.

## HISTORY

Exposure to the sun or an artificial UV source. Onset of symptoms depends on intensity of exposure; erythema develops after 6 h and peaks after 24 h.

**Skin Symptoms**   Pruritus may be severe even in mild sunburn; pain and tenderness occur with severe sunburn.

**Constitutional Symptoms**   Headache, chills, feverishness, and weakness are not infrequent in severe sunburn; some SPT I and II persons develop headache and malaise even after short exposures.

## PHYSICAL EXAMINATION

**General Appearance**   In severe sunburn, the patient is "toxic"—with fever, weakness, lassitude, and a rapid pulse rate.

**Skin Lesions**
Confluent bright erythema always confined to sun-exposed areas and thus sharply marginated at the border between exposed and covered skin (Fig. 10-1). Edema, vesicles, and even bullae; always uniform erythema and no "rash," as occurs in most photoallergic reactions. Edematous areas are raised and tender.

*Distribution*   Strictly confined to areas of exposure; sunburn can occur in areas covered with clothing, depending on the degree of UV transmission through clothing, the level of exposure, and the SPT of the person.

**Mucous Membranes**   Sunburn of the tongue can occur rarely in mountain climbers who hold their mouth open "panting"; it is frequent on the vermilion border of the lips.

## LABORATORY EXAMINATIONS

**Dermatopathology**   "Sunburn" cells in the epidermis (apoptotic keratinocytes); also, exocytosis of lymphocytes, vacuolization of melanocytes and Langerhans cells. *Dermis*: endothelial cell swelling of superficial blood vessels. More prominent with UVA erythema, with a denser

mononuclear infiltrate and more severe vascular changes.

**Serology and Hematology**   To rule out systemic lupus erythematosus (SLE) obtain antinuclear antibody (ANA) level. Leukopenia may be present in SLE.

## DIAGNOSIS AND DIFFERENTIAL DIAGNOSIS

History of UVR exposure and sites of reaction on exposed areas. *Phototoxic erythema*: obtain history of medications that can induce phototoxic erythema. *SLE* can cause a sunburn-type erythema. *Erythropoietic protoporphyria* causes erythema, vesicles, edema, purpura, and, only rarely, urticarial wheals.

## COURSE AND PROGNOSIS

Sunburn, unlike thermal burns, cannot be classified on the basis of depth, i.e., first- second-, and third-degree. Third-degree burns after UVR do not occur, and none of the features of third-degree thermal burns are seen: scarring, loss of sensation, loss of sweating, hair loss. A permanent reaction from severe ultraviolet burns is mottled depigmentation, probably related to the destruction of melanocytes, and eruptive solar lentigines.

## MANAGEMENT

**Prevention**   Persons with SPT I or II should avoid sunbathing, especially between 11 A.M. and 2 P.M. Clothing: UV-screening cloth garments. There are now many highly effective topical chemical filters (sunscreens) in lotion, gel, and cream formulations. It is still not clear whether regular use of topical sunscreens can prevent melanoma of the skin, but there is reasonable proof that topical sunscreens reduce the induction of solar keratoses and, probably, squamous cell carcinoma.

**Moderate Sunburn**   *Topical*   Cool wet dressings, topical glucocorticoids.

*Systemic*   Acetylsalicylic acid, indomethacin.

**Severe Sunburn**   Bed rest. If very severe, a "toxic" patient may require hospitalization for fluid replacement, prophylaxis of infection, etc.

*Topical*   Cool wet dressings, topical glucocorticoids.

*Systemic*   Oral glucocorticoids are often given, but their efficacy has not been established by controlled studies. Indomethacin.

# DRUG-/CHEMICAL-INDUCED PHOTOSENSITIVITY

This describes the interaction of UVR with a chemical/drug within the skin. Two mechanisms are recognized: *phototoxic reactions*, which are photochemical reactions leading to skin pathology, and *photoallergic reactions*, where a photoallergen is formed that initiates an immunologic response and manifests in skin as a type IV immunologic reaction. The main clinical difference between phototoxic and photoallergic eruptions is that the former manifests like an irritant (toxic) contact dermatitis or sunburn and the latter like an allergic eczematous contact dermatitis (Table 10-3).

**TABLE 10-3   Characteristics of Phototoxicity and Photoallergy**

|  | Phototoxicity | Photoallergy |
|---|---|---|
| Clinical presentation | Sunburn reaction: erythema, edema, vesicles and bullae; frequently resolves with hyperpigmentation; burning, smarting | Eczematous lesions, papules, vesicles, scaling, crusting; usually pruritic |
| Histology | Necrotic keratinocytes, epidermal degeneration; sparse dermal infiltrate of lymphocytes, macrophages, and neutrophils | Spongiotic dermatitis, dense, dermal lymphohistio-cytic infiltrate |
| Pathophysiology | Direct tissue injury | Type IV delayed hypersensitivity reponse |
| Occurrence after first exposure | Yes | No |
| Onset of eruption after exposure | Minutes to hours | 24 to 48 h |
| Dosage of agent needed for eruption | Large | Small |
| Cross-reactivity with other agents | Rare | Common |
| Diagnosis | Clinical + phototests | Clinical + phototests + photopatch tests |

Adapted from H Lim, in IM Freedberg, AZ Eisen, K Wolff, KF Austen, LA Goldsmith, SI Katz (eds.): *Fitzpatrick's Dermatology in General Medicine*, 6th ed. New York, McGraw-Hill, 2003.

## PHOTOTOXIC DRUG-/CHEMICAL-INDUCED PHOTOSENSITIVITY

This describes an adverse reaction of the skin that results from simultaneous exposure to certain drugs (via ingestion, injection, or topical application) and to UVR or visible light. The chemicals may be therapeutic, cosmetic, industrial, or agricultural. There are two types of reaction: (1) systemic phototoxic dermatitis, occurring in individuals systemically exposed to a photosensitizing agent (drug) and subsequent UVR; and (2) local phototoxic dermatitis, occurring in individuals topically exposed to the photosensitizing agent and subsequent UVR. Both are *exaggerated sunburn responses* (erythema, edema, vesicles, and/or bullae). Systemic phototoxic dermatitis occurs in all *UVR-exposed sites*; local phototoxic dermatitis only in the *topical application sites*.

## SYSTEMIC PHOTOTOXIC DERMATITIS

### EPIDEMIOLOGY

Occurs in everyone after ingestion of a sufficient dose of a photosensitizing drug and subsequent UVR. Therefore all ages, both sexes, all races, and all types of skin color. Phototoxic drug reactions are more frequent than photoallergic drug sensitivity.

### ETIOLOGY AND PATHOGENESIS

Formation of toxic photoproducts such as free radicals or reactive oxygen species such as singlet oxygen. The principal sites of damage are nuclear DNA or cell membranes (plasma, lysosomal, mitochondrial). The action spectrum is UVA. Drugs eliciting systemic phototoxic dermatitis are listed in Table 10-4. Some drugs causing phototoxic reactions can also elicit photoallergic reactions (see below).

### HISTORY

An "exaggerated sunburn" after solar or UVR exposure that *normally would not elicit a sunburn in that particular individual*. Occurs usually within hours after exposure, with some agents such as psoralens after 24 h, and peaking at 48 h. Skin symptoms: burning, stinging, pruritus.

### PHYSICAL EXAMINATION

Skin Lesions
*Early*: The skin lesions are those of an "exaggerated sunburn." Erythema, edema (Fig. 10-2A), and vesicle and bulla formation (Fig. 10-2B) confined exclusively to areas exposed to light. An eczematous reaction is *not* seen in phototoxic reactions.

**Special Presentations: Pseudoporphyria**  With some drugs there is little erythema but pronounced blistering and skin fragility with erosions (see Fig. 20-11) and, upon repeated exposures, healing milia formation, particularly on the dorsa of hands and lower arms. Clinically indistinguishable from porphyria cutanea tarda (see Fig. 10-9)—hence the term *pseudoporphyria* (see Section 20).

**Nails**  Subungual hemorrhage and photoonycholysis can occur with certain drugs (psoralens, demethylchlortetracycline, benoxaprofen) (see Fig. 30-36).

**Pigmentation**  Marked brown epidermal melanin pigmentation may occur in the course of some eruptions. With certain drugs especially (chlorpromazine and amiodarone), a slate gray dermal melanin pigmentation develops (see Section 20).

### LABORATORY EXAMINATIONS

**Dermatopathology**  Inflammation, "sunburn cells" in the epidermis, epidermal necrobiosis, intraepidermal and subepidermal vesiculation. Absence of eczematous changes.

**Phototesting**  For verification of the incriminating agent, template test sites are exposed to increasing doses of UVA (phototoxic reactions are almost always due to UVA) while patient is on the drug. The UVA MED will be much lower than that for normal individuals of the same skin phototype. After drug is excreted and then eliminated from the skin, a repeat UVA phototest will reveal an *increase* in the UVA MED. This test may be important if patient is on multiple potentially phototoxic drugs.

**TABLE 10-4   Systemic Phototoxic Agents**[*]

| Property | Generic Name | Property | Generic Name |
|---|---|---|---|
| Antianxiety drugs | Alprazolam | | Hydrochlorothiazide |
| | Chlordiazepoxide | | **Dyazide** |
| Anticancer drugs | Adriamycin | Dyes | Fluorescein |
| | Dacarbazine | | Methylene blue |
| | Fluorouracil | Furocoumarins | Psoralens: |
| | Methotrexate | | **5-Methoxypsoralen** |
| | Vinblastine | | **8-Methoxypsoralen** |
| Antidepressants | Tricyclics: | | **4, 5′, 8-Trimethylpsoralen** |
| | Amitriptyline | Hypoglycemics | Sulfonylureas: |
| | Desipramine | | Acetohexamide |
| | Imipramine | | Chlorpropamide |
| Antifungals | Griseofulvin | | Glipizide |
| Antimalarials | Chloroquine | | Glyburide |
| | Quinine | | Tolazamide |
| Antimicrobials | Quinolones: | | **Tolbutamide** |
| | Ciprofloxacin | NSAIDs | Acetic acid derivative: |
| | Enoxacin | | Diclofenac |
| | Gemifloxacin | | Anthranilic acid derivative: |
| | **Lomefloxacin** | | Mefenamic acid |
| | Moxifloxacin | | Enolic acid derivative: |
| | **Nalidixic acid** | | **Piroxicam** |
| | Norfloxacin | | Propionic acid |
| | Ofloxacin | | derivatives: |
| | **Sparfloxacin** | | Ibuprofen |
| | Sulfonamides | | Ketoprofen |
| | Tetracyclines | | **Naproxen** |
| | **Demeclocycline** | | Oxaprozin |
| | **Doxycycline** | | Tiaprofenic |
| | Minocycline | | acid |
| | Tetracycline | | Salicylic acid |
| | Trimethoprim | | derivative: |
| Antipsychotic | Phenothiazines: | | Diflunisal |
| drugs | **Chlorpromazine** | | Others: |
| | Perphenazine | | Celecoxib |
| | **Prochlorperazine** | | **Nabumetone** |
| | Thioridazine | Photodynamic | **Porfimer** |
| | Trifluoperazine | therapy agents | **Verteporfin** |
| Cardiac | **Amiodarone** | | |
| medications | Quinidine | Retinoids | Acitretin |
| Diuretics | **Furosemide** | | Isotretinoin |
| | Thiazides: | | Etretinate |
| | Bendroflumethi- | Other | Flutamide |
| | azide | | Hypercin |
| | **Chlorothiazide** | | Pyridoxine (vitamin B6) |
| | | | Ranitidine |

[*]Commonly reported drugs are printed in bold

SOURCE: Adapted from H Lim, in IM Freedberg, AZ Eisen, K Wolff, KF Austen, LA Goldsmith, SI Katz, (eds): *Fitzpatrick's Dermatology in General Medicine*, 6th ed. New York, McGraw-Hill, 2003.

## DIAGNOSIS AND DIFFERENTIAL DIAGNOSIS

History of exposure to drugs is most important as are the types of morphologic changes in the skin characteristic of phototoxic drug eruptions: confluent erythema, edema, vesicles, bullae. Differential diagnosis includes regular sunburn, phototoxic reactions due to excess of endogenous porphyrins, and photosensitivity due to other diseases, e.g., SLE.

## COURSE AND PROGNOSIS

Phototoxic drug sensitivity is a major problem, since the abnormal reactions seriously limit or exclude the use of important drugs: diuretics, antihypertensive agents, drugs used in psychiatry. Whereas, as a rule, phototoxicity occurs in practically anyone who is on a phototoxic drug—in contrast to photoallergy, which occurs only in the sensitized—some individuals nonetheless show phototoxic reactions to a particular drug and others do not. It is not known why. Phototoxic drug reactions disappear after cessation of drug.

## MANAGEMENT

As for sunburn.

## TOPICAL PHOTOTOXIC DEMATITIS

Here there is inadvertent contact with or therapeutic application of a photosensitizer, followed by UVA irradiation (practically all topical photosensitizers have an action spectrum in the UVA range). The most common topical phototoxic agents are listed in Table 10-5, and the most common route of contact is either therapeutic or occupational exposure. Clinical presentation is like acute irritant contact dermatitis (see Section 2), with erythema, swelling, vesiculation, and blistering confined to the sites of contact with the phototoxic agent. Symptoms are smarting, stinging, and burning rather than itching. Healing usually results in pronounced pigmentation. The most common and thus important topical phototoxic dermatitis is phytophotodermatitis, described below.

**TABLE 10-5 Common Topical Phototoxic Agents**

| Agent | Exposure |
|---|---|
| Rose Bengal | Opthalmologic examination |
| Fluorescein | Dye |
| Furocoumarins | Occur naturally in plants (mostly *Compositae* spp.; *Umbiliferae* spp.; fruits and vegetables (lime, lemon, celery, fig, parsley, parsnip); used in perfumes and cosmetics (e.g., oil of bergamot); and used for topical photochemotherapy |
| Tar | Topical therapeutic agent, roofing materials, road tarring |

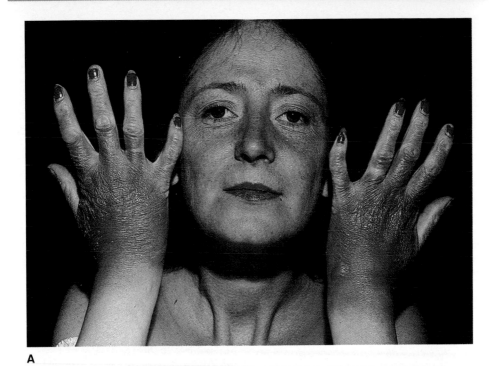

A

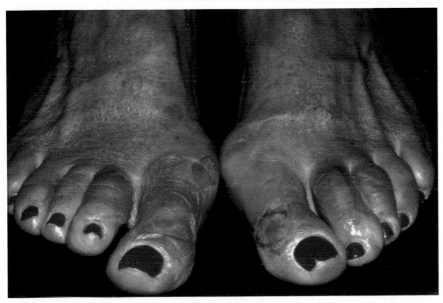

B

**FIGURE 10-2   Phototoxic drug-induced photosensitivity**   *A. Dusky erythema is seen on the dorsum of the hands of an individual who was treated with demethylchlortetracycline, which is used for acne. She had attended a sporting event and wore a hat that protected her head and neck; but she was holding onto a rail, thus increasing the exposure of her hands. There is, however, some erythema also on the bridge of the nose and on both cheeks. B. A bullous-erosive eruption on the toes of a cancer patient who had received adriamycin and later spent a considerable time outdoors wearing sandals that exposed her toes.*

# PHYTOPHOTODERMATITIS (PPD)

Phytophotodermatitis (plant + light = dermatitis) is an inflammation of the skin caused by contact with certain plants during recreational or occupational exposure to sunlight. The inflammatory response is a phototoxic reaction to photosensitizing chemicals in several plant families; a common type of PPD is due to exposure to limes.
*Synonyms*: Berloque dermatitis, lime dermatitis.

## EPIDEMIOLOGY AND ETIOLOGY

Common. Usually in spring and summer or all year in tropical climates. PPD can occur at any age.

**Race** All skin colors; brown- and black-skinned persons may develop only marked spotty dark pigmentation without erythema or bullous lesions.

**Occupation** Celery pickers, carrot processors, gardeners [exposed to carrot greens or to "gas plant" (*Dictamnus albus*)], and bartenders (lime juice) who are exposed to sun in outside bars.

**Etiology** Phototoxic reaction caused by photoactive furocoumarins (psoralens) contained in the plants (Table 10-5).

## HISTORY

The patient gives a history of exposure to certain plants (lime, lemon, wild parsley, celery, giant hogweed, parsnips, carrot greens, figs). Lime juice is a frequent cause: making lime drinks, hair rinses with lime juice. Women who use perfumes containing oil of bergamot (which contains bergapten, 5-methoxypsoralen) may develop streaks of pigmentation only in areas where the perfume was applied, especially the sides of the neck. This is called *berloque dermatitis* (French: *berloque*, "pendant"). Persons walking on beaches containing meadow grass and children playing in grassy meadows develop PPD on the legs; meadow grass contains agrimony.

**Skin Symptoms** Smarting, later pruritus.

## PHYSICAL EXAMINATION

**Skin Lesions**
Acute: erythema, edema, vesicles, and bullae (Fig. 10-3). Often bizarre streaks, artificial patterns that indicate an "outside job." Scattered areas on the sites of contact, especially the arms, legs, and face. Residual dark hyperpigmentation in bizarre streaks (Fig. 10-4).

## DIAGNOSIS AND DIFFERENTIAL DIAGNOSIS

Easily made if the pattern is recognized and a careful history is taken. Differential diagnosis is primarily acute irritant contact dermatitis, with streaky pattern poison ivy dermatitis (see p. 28), but this is eczematous with papules and vesicles whereas PPD is only vesicular.

## COURSE

May be an important occupational problem, as in celery pickers. The acute eruption has a short life and fades spontaneously, but the pigmentation may last for many weeks.

## MANAGEMENT

Wet dressings may be indicated in the acute vesicular stage. Topical glucocorticoids.

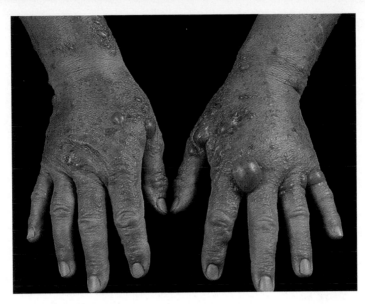

**FIGURE 10-3 Phytophotodermatitis (plant + light): acute with blisters** *These bullae were the result of exposure to both lime juice and the sun. This 50-year-old bartender was making drinks in an outside bar on a beach in the Bahamas. Lime contains bergapten (5-methoxypsoralen), which is a potent topical phototoxic chemical.*

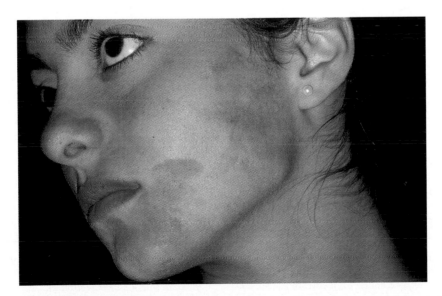

**FIGURE 10-4 Phytophotodermatitis: hyperpigmentation** *The patient had the oil from the rind of a lime on her fingers, which she then touched to her face while sunbathing ("lime" disease).*

# PHOTOALLERGIC DRUG-/CHEMICAL-INDUCED PHOTOSENSITIVITY   ▮   ◐

This results from interaction of a photoallergen and UVA radiation. In sensitized individuals exposure to a photoallergen and sunlight results in a pruritic eczematous eruption confined to exposed sites and clinically indistinguishable from allergic contact dermatitis. In most patients the eliciting drug/chemical has been applied topically, but systemic elicitation also occurs.

## EPIDEMIOLOGY

**Age of Onset**   More common in adults.
**Race**   All skin phototypes and colors.
**Incidence**   Photoallergic drug reactions occur much less frequently than do phototoxic drug reactions.

## ETIOLOGY AND PATHOGENESIS

Topically applied chemical/drug plus UVA radiation. The chemicals are disinfectants, antimicrobials, agents in sunscreens, perfumes in aftershaves, or whiteners (Table 10-6). The chemical agent present in the skin absorbs photons and forms a photoproduct; this then binds to a soluble or membrane-bound protein to form an antigen to which a type IV immune response is elicited. Since photoallergy depends on individual immunologic reactivity, it develops in only a small percentage of persons exposed to drugs and light and is elicited only in those who have been sensitized. Photoallergy can also be induced by systemic administration of a drug and elicited by topical administration of the same drug, and vice versa. UVA is always required.

## HISTORY

May be unclear in that the initial exposure induces sensitization to delayed-type hypersensitivity reactions, and the eruption occurs only on subsequent exposure. Topically applied photosensitizers are the most frequent cause of photoallergic eruptions, e.g., antibacterials or antifungals in soaps and other household products, fragrances or medications, sulfonamides (Table 10-6). Eruption is highly pruritic.

## PHYSICAL EXAMINATION

**Skin Lesions**
The morphology of the skin reaction is much different from that in phototoxic drug sensitivity. Acute photoallergic reaction patterns are clinically indistinguishable from allergic contact dermatitis (see Fig. 10-5): papular, vesicular, scaling, and crusted. Occasionally there can also be a lichenoid eruption similar to lichen planus. In chronic drug photoallergy, there is scaling, lichenification, and marked pruritus mimicking atopic dermatitis or, again, chronic allergic contact dermatitis (Fig. 10-5; see also "Eczema/Dermatitis," Section 2.)
***Distribution*** Confined primarily to areas exposed to light (distribution pattern of photosensitivity), but there may be spreading onto adjacent nonexposed skin; therefore, it not so well circumscribed as in phototoxic reactions.

## LABORATORY EXAMINATION

**Dermatopathology**   Acute and chronic delayed-type hypersensitivity reaction: epidermal spongiosis with lymphocytic infiltration.

## DIAGNOSIS

History of exposure to drug is most important, as well as the types of morphologic changes in the skin: this is essentially an allergic contact dermatitis pattern, while phototoxic drug eruptions mimic an exaggerated sunburn or an acute irritant contact dermatitis. In essence, the differential diagnosis between the two is identical to that described for toxic/irritant and allergic contact dermatitis (see Section 2).

Diagnosis requires the use of patch and photopatch tests. Photopatch tests are done in du-

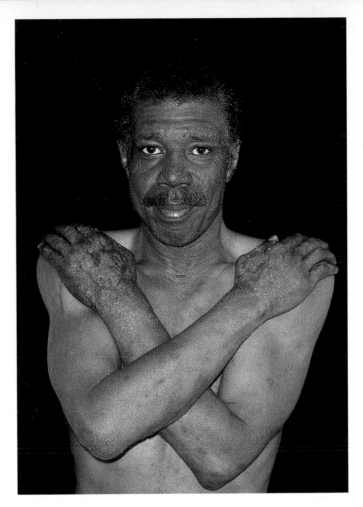

**FIGURE 10-5   Photoallergic drug-induced photosensitivity**   *This 51-year-old male with advanced HIV disease shows an eczematous dermatitis with hyperpigmentation in the sun-exposed sites (face, neck, dorsum of hands and wrist). He was taking trimethoprim-sulfamethoxazole as primary prophylaxis of* Pneumocystis carinii *pneumonia.*

plicate because photoallergens can also cause contact hypersensitivity. Photoallergens are applied to the skin and covered. After 24 h, one set of the duplicate test sites is exposed to UVA while the other set remains covered; test sites are read for reactions after 48 to 96 h. An eczematous reaction in the irradiated site but not in the nonirradiated site confirms photoallergy to the particular agent tested.

## COURSE AND PROGNOSIS

Photoallergic dermatitis can persist for months to years. This is known as *persistent light reaction,* or *chronic actinic dermatitis* (Fig. 10-6), and was first observed in soldiers in World War II in whom topical sulfonamides were used. It also occurs in patients with chronic chlorpromazine photoallergy. The classic generalized persistent light reactions were caused by exposure to soaps containing salicylanilides (Table 10-6). In *persistent light reaction*, the action spectrum usually broadens to involve UVB, and the condition persists despite discontinuation of the causative photoallergen, with each new UV exposure aggravating the condition. Chronic eczema-like lichenified and extremely itchy confluent plaques result (Fig. 10-6), which lead to gross disfigurement and a distressing situation for the patient. As the condition is now in-dependent of the original photoallergen and is aggravated by each new solar exposure, avoidance of photoallergen does not cure the disease. In contrast to earlier belief, chronic actinic dermatitis does not progress to lymphoma.

## MANAGEMENT

In severe cases, immunosuppression (azathioprine plus glucocorticoids or oral cyclosporine) is required.

### TABLE 10-6   Topical Photoallergens[*]

| Group | Chemical Name |
|---|---|
| Sunscreens | UVB absorbers:<br>**para-Aminobenzoic acids (PABA)**<br>Cinnamates<br>Salicylates<br>UVA absorbers:<br>Anthranilate<br>**Benzophenones** |
| Fragrances | **6-Methylcoumarin**<br>**Musk ambrette**<br>Sandalwood oil |
| Antibacterials | **Dibromosalicylanilide**<br>**Tetrachlorosalicylanilide**<br>Tribromosalicylanilide<br>Chlorhexidene<br>Dimethylol-dimethyl hydantoin<br>Hexachlorophene<br>**Bithionol**<br>Dichlorophene<br>Triclosan<br>**Sulfonamides** |
| Antifungals | Thiobischlorophenol<br>Buclosamide<br>Bromochlorosalicylanilide |
| Others | **Chlorpromazine**<br>Clioquinol<br>Ketoprofen<br>Olaquindox<br>Promethazine<br>Quinidine<br>Thiourea |

[*]Commonly reported drugs are printed in bold

SOURCE: Adapted from H Lim; in IM Freedberg, AZ Eisen, K Wolff, KF Austen, LA Coldsmith, SI Katz (eds); *Fitzpatrick's Dermatology in General Medicine*, 6th ed. New York, McGraw-Hill, 2003.

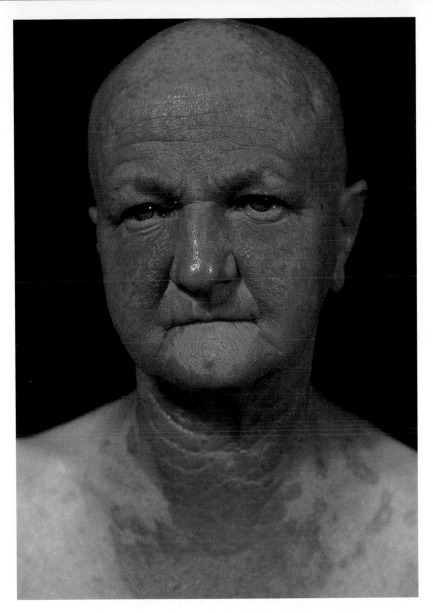

**FIGURE 10-6   Drug-induced photosensitivity: persistent light eruption**   *Thick erythematous plaques confined to the scalp, face, and exposed chest, sparing areas shaded by the nose. This female patient has excruciating prutius.*

# POLYMORPHOUS LIGHT ERUPTION     ■   ◑

Polymorphous light eruption (PMLE) is a term that describes a group of heterogeneous, idiopathic, acquired, acute recurrent eruptions characterized by delayed abnormal reactions to UVR and manifested by varied lesions, including erythematous macules, papules, plaques, and vesicles. However, in each patient the eruption is consistently monomorphous. By far the most frequent morphologic types are the papular and papulovesicular eruptions.

## EPIDEMIOLOGY

**Incidence.**   Most common photodermatosis. Prevalence from 10% in Boston, 14% in London, to 21% in Sweden. Average age is 23 years, much more common in females. All races, but most common in SPT I, II, III, and IV. In American Indians (North and South America) there is a *hereditary* type of PMLE that is called *actinic prurigo.*

**Geography**   PMLE is less frequently observed in areas that have high solar intensity throughout the year and in persons who have adapted to persistent sun exposures. In fact, PMLE often occurs for the first time in persons traveling for short vacations to tropical areas in winter from northern latitudes.

## PATHOGENESIS

Possibly a delayed-type hypersensitivity reaction to an (auto-) antigen induced by UVR; suggested by the morphology of the lesions and the histologic pattern, which shows an infiltration of T cells. More commonly, UVA is the action spectrum, but PMLE lesions have been evoked with UVB and with both UVA and UVB. Since UVA is transmitted through window glass, PMLE can be precipitated while riding in a car. Areas of the skin habitually exposed (face and neck) are often spared, despite severe involvement of the arms, trunk, and legs.

## HISTORY

**Onset and Duration of Lesions**   PMLE appears in spring or early summer, and not infrequently the eruption does not recur by the end of summer, suggesting a "hardening." PMLE most often appears within 18 to 24 h of exposure and, once established, persists for 7 to 10 days,

thereby limiting the vacationer's subsequent time in the sun. Symptoms are pruritus (may precede the onset of the rash) and paresthesia (tingling).

## PHYSICAL EXAMINATION

### Skin Lesions

The papular (Fig. 10-7) and papulovesicular types (Fig. 10-8) are the most frequent. Less common are plaques or urticarial plaques. The lesions are pink to red. In the individual patient, lesions are quite monomorphous, i.e., either papular or papulovesicular or urticarial plaques. Recurrences follow the original pattern.

*Distribution*   The eruption often spares the face and appears most frequently on the forearms, V area of the neck (Fig. 10-7), and arms (Fig. 10-8). The lesions may also occur on the trunk, if there has not been previous exposure.

## LABORATORY EXAMINATIONS

**Dermatopathology**   Edema of the epidermis, spongiosis, vesicle formation, and mild liquefaction degeneration of the basal layer. A dense lymphocytic infiltrate is present in the dermis, with occasional neutrophils. There is edema of the papillary dermis and endothelial swelling.

**Immunofluorescence (Direct)**   Negative. ANA negative. There is no leukopenia.

## DIAGNOSIS

The diagnosis is not difficult: delayed onset of eruption, characteristic morphology, histopathologic changes that rule out lupus erythematosus, and the history of disappearance of the eruption in days. In plaque-type PMLE, a biopsy and immunofluorescence studies are mandatory to rule out SLE. *Phototesting* is done with both UVB

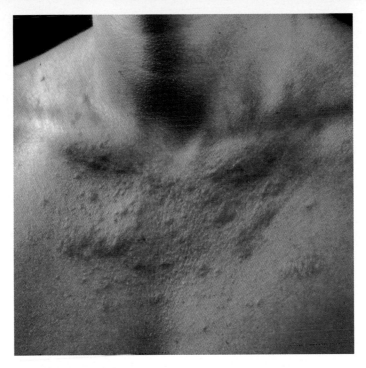

**FIGURE 10-7** **Polymorphic light eruption** *Clusters of confluent, extremely pruritic papules on the exposed chest, occurred the day following the first sun exposure of the season. The eruption also involved the dorsum of the arms, but spared the face and dorsal hands.*

and UVA. Test sites are exposed daily, starting with 2 MEDs of UVB and UVA, respectively, for 1 week to 10 days, using increments of the UV dose. In 50% of patients, a PMLE-like eruption will occur in the test sites, confirming the diagnosis. This also helps to determine whether the action spectrum is UVB, UVA, or both.

## COURSE AND PROGNOSIS

The course is chronic and recurrent and may, in fact, become worse each season. Although some patients may develop "tolerance" by the end of the summer, the eruption usually recurs the following spring and/or when the person travels to tropical areas in the winter. However, spontaneous improvement or even cessation of eruptions occurs after years.

## MANAGEMENT

**Prevention**  Sunblocks, even the potent UVA-UVB sunscreens, are not always effective but should be tried first in every patient.

**Systemic**  β-Carotene, 60 mg tid for 2 weeks before going in the sun and *antimalarials* (hydroxychloroquine, 200 mg bid 1 day before and daily while on vacation are rarely useful. Intramuscular triamcinolone acetonide, 40 mg, will suppress an eruption when administered a few days before a trip to a sunny region.

**PUVA Photochemotherapy**  This is very effective when given in early spring by inducing "tolerance" for the summer. PUVA treatments have to be given before the sunny season, have to be repeated each spring, but are usually not necessary for more than 3 or 4 years. *Narrowband UVB* (311 nm) has been used with equal success.

## PHOTOEXACERBATED DERMATOSES

Various wavelengths of UVR and/or visible light can elicit or aggravate a number of dermatoses. In these cases the eruption is invariably similar to that of the primary condition. An abbreviated list is given in alphabetical order in Table 10-7 below, but it should be emphasized that among these disorders SLE is by far the most important.

## TABLE 10-7    Diseases Exacerbated by Ultraviolet Irradiation

| | |
|---|---|
| Acne | Pellagra |
| Atopic eczema | Pemphigus foliaceus |
| Carcinoid syndrome | (erythematosus) |
| Cutaneous T-cell lymphoma | Pityriasis rubra pilaris |
| Darier's disease | Psoriasis |
| Dermatomyositis | Reticulate erythematous mucinosis |
| Disseminated superficial actinic | syndrome |
| porokeratosis | Rosacea |
| Erythema multiforme | Seborrheic dermatitis |
| Familial benign chronic pemphigus | Systemic lupus erythematosus |
| (Hailey-Hailey disease) | Transient acantholytic dermatosis |
| Keratosis follicularis (Darier's disease) | (Grover's disease) |
| Lichen planus | Viral infections |

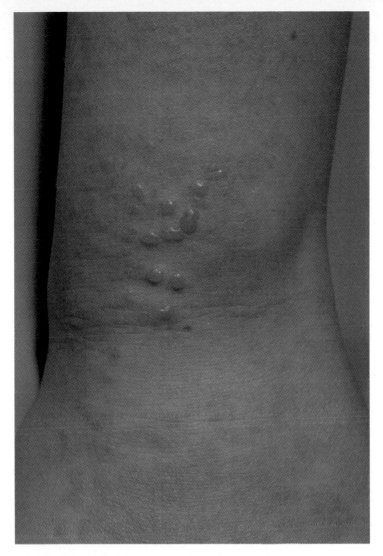

**FIGURE 10-8  Polymorphic light eruption**  *Clusters of pruritic papules and vesicles on the dorsal wrist and arm, and an erythematous plaque on the dorsum of the hand following first sun exposure of the season. The face is typically spared.*

# METABOLIC PHOTOSENSITIVITY

## PORPHYRIAS

### PORPHYRIA CUTANEA TARDA

Porphyria cutanea tarda (PCT) occurs mostly in adults. Patients do not present with characteristic photosensitivity but with complaints of "fragile skin," vesicles, and bullae, particularly on the dorsa of the hands, after minor trauma; the diagnosis is confirmed by the presence of a pinkish-red fluorescence in the urine when examined with a Wood's lamp. PCT is distinct from variegate porphyria (VP) and acute intermittent porphyria (AIP) in that patients with PCT do not have acute life-threatening attacks. Furthermore, the drugs that induce PCT are fewer than the drugs that induce VP and AIP. For classification of the porphyrias, see Table 10-8.

## EPIDEMIOLOGY

Onset 30 to 50 years, rarely in children; females on oral contraceptives; males on estrogen therapy for prostate cancer. Equal in males and in females.

**Heredity**   Most PCT patients have *type I (acquired)* induced by drugs or chemicals. *Type II (hereditary)*, autosomal dominant; possibly these patients actually have VP, but this is not yet resolved. There is also a "dual" type with VP and PCT in the same family.

## ETIOLOGY AND PATHOGENESIS

PCT is caused by either an inherited or acquired deficiency of UROGEN decarboxylase. In type I (sporadic, acquired PCT-symptomatic) the enzyme is deficient only in the liver; in type II (PCT-hereditary) it is also deficient in red blood cells (RBCs) and fibroblasts. *Chemicals and drugs that induce PCT:* Ethanol, estrogen, hexachlorobenzene (fungicide), chlorinated phenols, iron, tetrachlorodibenzo-*p*-dioxin. High doses of chloroquine lead to clinical manifestations in "latent" cases (low doses are used as treatment). *Other predisposing factors:* Diabetes mellitus (25%), hepatitis C virus.

## HISTORY

**Duration of Lesions**   No acute skin changes but gradual onset. Patients may present with fragility of skin and bullae on the hands and feet based on a photosensitivity reaction to sun and yet will have a suntan. Pain from erosions in easily traumatized skin ("fragile skin").

## PHYSICAL EXAMINATION

**Skin Lesions**
Tense bullae and erosions on normal-appearing skin (Fig. 10-9); slowly heal to form pink atrophic scars, milia (1 to 2 mm) on dorsa of hands and feet, nose, forehead, or (bald) scalp. Purple-red suffusion ("heliotrope") of central facial skin (Fig. 10-10), especially periorbital areas. Brown hypermelanosis, diffuse, on exposed areas (Figs. 10-10 and 10-11). Hypertrichosis of face (Fig. 10-11). Scleroderma-like changes, diffuse or circumscribed, waxy yellowish-white areas on exposed areas of face, neck, and trunk, sparing the doubly clothed area of the breast in females.

## LABORATORY EXAMINATIONS

**Dermatopathology**   Bullae, subepidermal with "festooned" (undulating) base. PAS staining

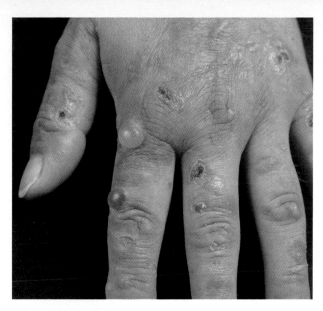

**FIGURE 10-9 Porphyria cutanea tarda** *Bullae and atrophic depigmented scars and milia on the knuckles and dorsum of the left hand and fingers. This is not an acute reaction to initial sun exposure but develops over time with repeated sun exposure and occurs after minor trauma. The patient presents with a history of "fragile" skin, and bullae. The hand changes developed in mid-summer while this patient was on a fishing trip during which he noticed that the skin on the back of his hands were easily damaged, with the skin slipping in spots. This condition is called the "fisherman's disease," in which there are three etiologic factors present: alcohol (beer drinking while fishing), sun exposure (while in a boat), and trauma to the back of the hands (reeling in the fish).*

reveals thickened vascular walls. Paucity of an inflammatory infiltrate.

**Immunofluorescence** IgG and other immunoglobulins at the dermal-epidermal junction and in and around blood vessels, in the sun-exposed areas of the skin.

**Chemictry** Plasma iron and liver enzymes may be increased. *Blood glucose* is increased in those patients with diabetes mellitus (25% of patients).

**Porphyrin Studies in Stool and Urine** (Table 10-8) Increased uroporphyrin (I isomer, 60%)

in urine and plasma. Increased isocoproporphyrin (type III) and 7-carboxylporphyrin in the feces. In contrast, VP has markedly elevated fecal protoporphyrin as the diagnostic hallmark. No increase in δ-aminolevulinic acid or porphobilinogen in the urine.

**Simple Test** Wood's lamp examination of the urine shows orange-red fluorescence (Fig. 10-12); to enhance, add a few drops of 10% hydrochloric acid.

**Liver Biopsy** Reveals porphyrin fluorescence and often fatty liver.

## DIAGNOSIS AND DIFFERENTIAL DIAGNOSIS

By clinical features, pink-red fluorescence of urine and elevated urinary porphyrins. Bullae on dorsa of hands and feet can occur in *pseudo-PCT* (see Section 20). Phototoxic reactions occur in chronic renal failure with hemodialysis. Tanning salon radiation (visible and UVA). May occasionally resemble dyshidrotic eczema but bullae are on the dorsa. *Epidermolysis bullosa acquisita* (see Section 6) has the same clinical picture (increased skin fragility, easy bruising, and light- and trauma-provoked bullae) and some of the histology (subepidermal bullae with little or no dermal inflammation).

### TABLE 10-8    Classification and Differential Diagnosis of Porphyrias

| | Erythropoietic Porphyrias | | Hepatic Porphyrias | | |
| --- | --- | --- | --- | --- | --- |
| | Congenital Erythropoietic Porphyria | Erythropoietic Protoporphyria | Porphyria Cutanea Tarda | Variegate Porphyria | Intermittent Acute Porphyria |
| Inheritance | Autosomal recessive | Autosomal dominant | Autosomal dominant (familial form) | Autosomal dominant | Autosomal dominant |
| Signs and symptoms | | | | | |
| Photosensitivity | Yes | Yes | Yes | Yes | No |
| Cutaneous lesions | Yes | Yes | Yes | Yes | No |
| Attacks of abdominal pain | No | No | No | Yes | Yes |
| Neuropsychiatric syndrome | No | No | No | Yes | Yes |
| Laboratory abnormalities | + | + | + | + | + |
| Red blood cells | | | | | |
| Fluorescence | + | + | − | − | − |
| Uroporphyrin | +++ | N | N | N | N |
| Coproporphyrin | ++ | + | N | N | N |
| Protoporphyrin | (+) | +++ | N | N | N |
| Plasma | | | | | |
| Fluorescence | + | + | − | + | − |
| Urine | | | | | |
| Fluorescence | − | − | + | ± | − |
| Porphobilinogen | N | N | N | (+++) | (+++) |
| Uroporphyrin | +++ | N | +++ | +++ | +++ |
| Feces | | | | | |
| Protoporphyrin | + | ++ | N | +++ | N |

NOTE: N, normal; +, above normal; ++, moderately increased; +++, markedly increased; (+++), frequently increased (depends on whether patient has an attack, or is in remission); (+), increased in some patients.

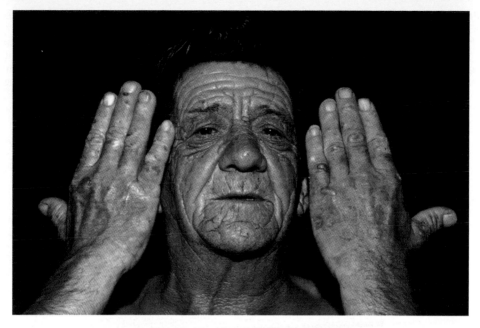

**FIGURE 10-10    Porphyria cutanea tarda**    *Periorbital and malar violaceous coloration, hyperpigmentation, and hypertrichosis on the face; bullae, crusts, and scars on the dorsa of the hands.*

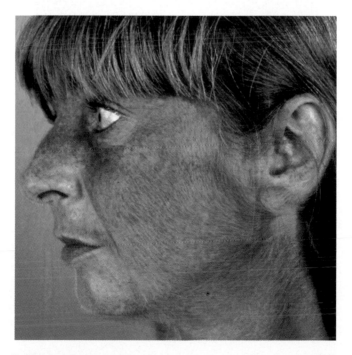

**FIGURE 10-11    Porphyria cutanea tarda** *Hyperpigmentation and hypertrichosis in a woman who had been on a prolonged regimen with estrogens. Under Wood's light her urine showed a bright coral-red fluorescence as shown in Fig. 10-12.*

## MANAGEMENT

1. Avoid ethanol, stop drugs that could be inducing PCT (such as estrogen), and eliminate exposure to chemicals (chlorinated phenols, tetrachlorodibenzo-*p*-dioxin). In some patients, complete avoidance of ethanol ingestion will result in a clinical and biochemical remission and in depletion of the high level of iron stores in the liver.
2. Phlebotomy is done by removing 500 mL of blood at weekly or biweekly intervals until the hemoglobin is decreased to 10 g. Clinical and biochemical remission occurs within 5 to 12 months after regular phlebotomy. Relapse within a year is uncommon (5 to 10%).
3. Low-dose chloroquine is used to induce re-

mission of PCT in patients in whom phlebotomy is contraindicated because of anemia. Since chloroquine can exacerbate the disease and, in higher doses, may even induce hepatic failure in these patients, this treatment requires considerable experience. However, long-lasting remissions and, in a portion of patients, clinical and biochemical "cure" can be achieved.

The best approach currently used by one of us (K.W.) is to start with a course of three consecutive phlebotomies every other day followed by 150 mg/d, of chloroquine PO. Close clinical and laboratory monitoring (transaminases, porphyrin excretion in urine), are required to adjust the chloroquine dose, which is eventually tapered to 150 mg twice a week and continued for several months.

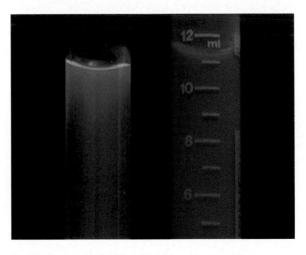

**FIGURE 10-12    Porphyria cutanea tarda: Wood's light**    *Coral-red fluorescence of the urine of a patient with PCT as compared to that of normal control.*

## VARIEGATE PORPHYRIA  □  (■*)  ◑ → ●

Variegate porphyria (VP) is a serious autosomal dominant disorder of heme biosynthesis characterized by skin lesions that are identical to those of PCT (vesicles and bullae, skin fragility, milia, and scarring of the dorsa of the hands and fingers), acute attacks of abdominal pain, neuropsychiatric manifestations, and increased excretion of porphyrins; especially characteristic are high levels of protoporphyrin in the feces.
*Synonym*: Porphyria variegata.

### EPIDEMIOLOGY

**Age of Onset**  At puberty; peak, second to fourth decades.
**Race**  All races; especially common in white South Africans (3:1000) (a large proportion of the present white population was descended from an early Dutch settler who emigrated to South Africa from Holland in 1680 to where VP can be traced).
**Incidence**  It is increasingly recognized in Europe (Finland) and the United States.
**Heredity**  Autosomal dominant.

### ETIOLOGY AND PATHOGENESIS

PROTOGEN oxidase defect resulting in an accumulation of protophyrinogen in the liver, which is excreted in the bile and is nonenzymatically converted to protoporphyrin; this accounts for the high fecal protoporphyrin.

The basic metabolic defect is accentuated by ingestion of certain drugs (sulfonamides, barbiturates, phenytoin, estrogens, alcohol, and others) (Table 10-9), with the resultant precipitation of acute attacks of abdominal pain and neuropsychiatric disorders (delirium, seizures, personality changes).

### HISTORY

**Change with Seasons**  Skin lesions occur during the summer season but may persist throughout the winter; lesions result from exposure to sunlight. Painful erosions, skin fragility.
**Systems Review**  Acute attacks of abdominal pain, constipation, nausea and vomiting, muscle weakness, seizures, confusional state, psychiatric symptoms (depression, coma); rarely, cranial nerve involvement, bulbar paralysis, sensory loss, and paresthesias.
**Drug Exposure**  See Table 10-9.

---

**TABLE 10-9  Drugs Hazardous to Patients with Variegate Porphyria**

| | |
|---|---|
| Anesthetics: barbiturates and halothane | Imipramine |
| Anticonvulsants: hydantoins, carbamazepine, ethosuximide, methsuximide, phensuximide, primidone | Methyldopa |
| | Minor tranquilizers: chlordiazepoxide, diazepam, oxazepam, flurazepam, meprobamate |
| Antimicrobial agents: chloramphenicol griseofulvin, novobiocin, pyrazinamide, sulfonamides | Pentazocine |
| Ergot preparations | Phenylbutazone |
| Ethyl alcohol | Sulfonylureas; chlorpropamide, tolbutamide |
| Hormones: estrogens, progestin, oral contraceptive preparations | Theophylline |

---

* In South Africa.

## PHYSICAL EXAMINATION

### Skin Lesions
PCT-like vesicles or, more commonly, bullae (Fig. 10-13); erosions, milia; sclerosis (scleroderma-like changes); scars (pink, atrophic). Periorbital heliotrope hue, diffuse melanoderma and hypertrichosis on exposed areas. Localization to dorsa of hands, fingers, and feet.

**Miscellaneous Findings**  Neurologic, especially peripheral neuropathy.

## LABORATORY EXAMINATIONS

**Dermatopathology**  As for PCT
**General Laboratory Examination**  *Porphyrins* (See Table 10-8).
*Plasma* Distinctive plasma fluorescence with emission maximum at 626 nm.
*Urine* Increased porphobilinogen during acute attacks.
*Stool* High protoporphyrin

## COURSE AND PROGNOSIS

Lifetime disease. Prognosis good, if exacerbating factors are avoided. Rarely, death can occur after ingestion or injection of drugs (e.g., barbiturates, general anesthesia) that induce increased amounts of cytochrome P450 and create a demand for increased synthesis of heme.

## DIFFERENTIAL DIAGNOSIS

Pseudoporphyria, scleroderma, acquired epidermolysis bullosa, hereditary coproporphyria, PCT.

## MANAGEMENT

None; oral β-carotene may or may not control the skin manifestations but has no effect on porphyrin metabolism or the important systemic manifestations.

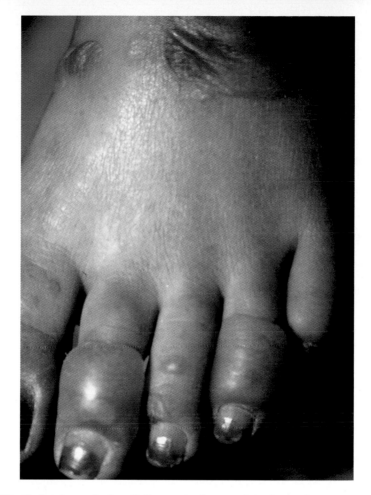

**FIGURE 10-13   Variegate porphyria**   *Bullae on the dorsum of the foot and toes, a common site of sun exposure in patients wearing open footwear. This 42-year-old female was diagnosed with porphyria cutanea tarda. The lesions in porphyria cutanea tarda are identical to the lesions in variegate porphyria. This patient, however, gave a history of recurrent attacks of abdominal pain, which was a clue to the diagnosis of variegate porphyria; this diagnosis was established by the detection of elevated stool protoporphyrins. Variegate porphyria (or South African porphyria) is akin to acute intermittent porphyria, in which there are no skin lesions but a fatal outcome may occur with ingestion of certain drugs (see Table 10-8). In South Africa every white patient who is scheduled for major surgery must have laboratory tests for porphyrins since variegate porphyria is common in that country.*

## ERYTHROPOIETIC PROTOPORPHYRIA

This hereditary metabolic disorder of porphyrin metabolism is unique among the porphyrias in that porphyrins or porphyrin precursors are not excreted in the urine. Also, erythropoietic protoporphyria (EPP) is characterized by an acute sunburn-like photosensitivity, in contrast to the other common porphyrias (PCT or VP), in which obvious acute photosensitivity is *not* a presenting complaint.

*Synonym*: Erythrohepatic protoporphyria.

## EPIDEMIOLOGY

**Incidence**   Not uncommon; series reported from Europe (in The Netherlands, 1:100, 000; Austria, United Kingdom), and the United States.

**Age of Onset**   Acute photosensitivity begins early in childhood; rarely, late onset in early adulthood.

**Sex**   Equal in males and females.

**Race**   All ethnic groups, including blacks.

**Heredity**   Autosomal dominant with variable penetrance.

## PATHOGENESIS

The defective enzyme is ferrochelatase. This defect occurs at the step in porphyrin metabolism in which protoporphyrin is converted to heme by ferrochelatase. This leads to an accumulation of protoporphyrin that is highly photosensitizing.

## HISTORY

Important sequence of symptoms: stinging, burning, and itching occur *within a few minutes* of sunlight exposure; erythema and edema appear only after 1 to 8 h. Children may choose not to go out in the direct sunlight after a few painful episodes, which may cause serious sociopsychologic problems. Symptoms occur when exposed to sunlight through window glass. Photosensitivity is less common in the winter months in temperate areas.

**Systems Review**   Biliary colic, even in children.

## PHYSICAL EXAMINATION

### SKIN CHANGES IN ACUTE REACTIONS TO SUNLIGHT EXPOSURE

Bright red erythema, later edema (swelling of hands especially), purpura [especially on the nose, cheeks (Fig. 10-14), backs of hands (Fig. 10-15), and tips of ears]. Urticaria uncommon; vesicles or bullae rarely occur. These changes appear within 1 to 8 h and after subjective symptoms and subside after several hours or days.

### SKIN CHANGES AFTER CHRONIC RECURRENT EXPOSURES

Shallow, often linear scars, on the nose and dorsa of the hands ("aged knuckles"). Diffuse wrinkling of the skin of the nose, around the lips, and the cheeks, with obvious thickening and a waxy color (Fig. 10-16). Crusted, erosive lesions may occur on the nose (Fig. 10-16) and lips. In contrast to PCT, absence of sclerodermoid changes, hypertrichosis, and hyperpigmentation.

### GENERAL MEDICAL FINDINGS

Hemolytic anemia with hypersplenism (rare). Cholelithiasis (12%), even in children; stones contain large amounts of protoporphyrin. Liver disease from massive deposition of protoporphyrin in hepatocytes occurs; fatal hepatic cirrhosis is rare, but occurs.

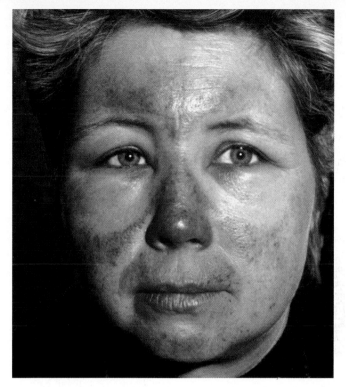

**FIGURE 10-14   Erythropoietic protoporphyria**   *Diffuse erythematous swelling of the nose, forehead, and cheeks with petechial hemorrhage and telangiectasia. There are no porphyrins in the urine. A clue to the diagnosis is the history of tingling and burning within 4 to 5 min of sun exposure.*

## LABORATORY EXAMINATIONS

**Porphyrin Studies**  (See Table 10-8) Increased protoporphyrin in red blood cells, plasma, and stools, but no excretion in the urine except in the rare cases with fatal hepatic cirrhosis. Decreased activity of the enzyme ferrochelatase in the bone marrow, liver, and skin fibroblasts.

**Liver Function**  Tests for liver function indicated. Liver biopsy: portal and periportal fibrosis and deposits of brown pigment and birefringent granules in hepatocytes and Kupffer cells. Cirrhosis and portal hypertension may develop.

**Radiography**  Gallstones may be present.

**Special Examination for Fluorescent Erythrocytes** RBCs in a blood smear exhibit a characteristic *transient* fluorescence when examined with a fluorescence microscope with a mercury or tungsten-iodide lamp that emits 400-nm radiation.

**Dermatopathology**  Marked eosinophilic homogenization and thickening of the blood vessels in the papillary dermis; there is an accumulation of an amorphous, hyaline-like eosinophilic substance in and around blood vessels.

## DIAGNOSIS

In EPP there is photosensitivity with an exaggerated sunburn response without blisters that appears much earlier than ordinary sunburn erythema. Also, the skin changes occur behind window glass. There is no other photosensitivity disorder in which the symptoms appear so rapidly (minutes after exposure to sunlight). Porphyrin examination establishes the diagnosis with elevated free protoporphyrin levels in the RBCs and in the stool. The fecal protoporphyrin is most consistently elevated, but urinary porphyrins are not. In chronic cases, the waxy thickening and wrinkling of facial skin is diagnostic.

**Differential Diagnosis**  Hyalinosis cutis et mucosae.

## COURSE AND PROGNOSIS

EPP persists throughout life, but the photosensitivity may become less apparent in late adulthood. Liver cirrhosis may become manifest in adults. Rarely, fatal outcome due to hepatic failure.

## MANAGEMENT

There is no treatment for the basic metabolic abnormality, but symptomatic relief of the photosensitivity can be achieved in most patients with oral β-carotene in divided doses of 180 mg/d. Therapeutic levels of carotenoids are achieved in 1 to 2 months. Patients on β-carotene can remain outdoors longer by a factor of 8 to 10 but will still burn if exposures are too long. Nevertheless, many patients can participate in outdoor activities for the first time. There is no toxicity with prolonged treatment with β-carotene. Protection by β-carotene can be considerably enhanced by PUVA-induced tanning.

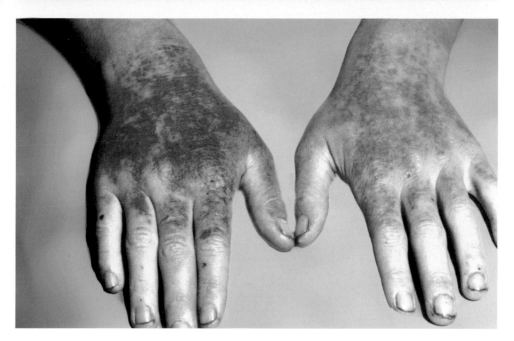

**FIGURE 10-15   Erythropoietic protoporphyria**   *Massive petechial, confluent hemorrhage on the dorsa of the hands of a 16-year-old 24 h after exposure to the sun.*

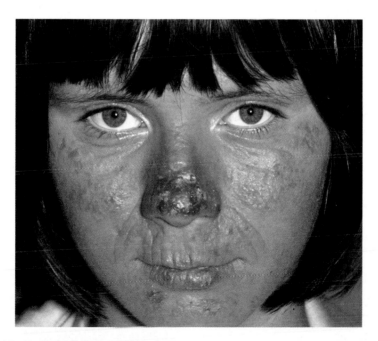

**FIGURE 10-16   Erythropoietic protoporphyria**   *Erythema, edema, erosion, crusting of the nose with less severe changes on the chin of a 15-year-old female. Deep wrinkling and a peculiar waxy thickening on the upper lip and cheeks make the patient look much older as they are similar to dermatoheliosis in photoaged skin.*

## CHRONIC PHOTODAMAGE

### DERMATOHELIOSIS ("PHOTOAGING")        ■    ○

Repeated solar injuries over many years ultimately can result in the development of a skin syndrome, *dermatoheliosis* (DHe). It occurs in persons with SPT I to III and in persons with SPT IV who have had heavy cumulative exposure to sunlight, such as lifeguards and outdoor workers, over a lifetime. DHe describes a polymorphic response of various components of the skin (especially cells in the epidermis, the vascular system, and the dermal connective tissue) to prolonged and/or excessive sun exposure. Its severity depends principally on the duration and intensity of sun exposure and on the indigenous (constitutive) skin color and the capacity to tan (facultative melanin pigmentation).

*Note*: If you want to demonstrate to an older patient the role of UVR in photoaging just have him/her undress and compare the quality of his/her facial skin to that of the suprapubic skin.

### EPIDEMIOLOGY

**Age of Onset**   Most often in persons >40 years; young white children (age 10) living in southern Borneo (cool climate with high UVR) have been observed to have DHe, including solar keratoses.

**Sex**   Higher incidence in males.

**Skin Phototype**   Persons with SPT I and II are most susceptible, but persons with SPT III and IV and even V (brown skin color) can develop DHe.

**Incidence**   Very common. The most susceptible persons with SPT I and II comprise about 25% of the white population in the United States.

**Occupation**   Farmers ("farmer's skin"), telephone linemen; sea workers ("sailor's skin"), construction workers, and lifeguards; tennis, swimming, and ski instructors; mountain guides, sportspersons, and "beach bums"; persons who spend considerable time in mountain or sea resorts.

**Geography**   DHe is more severe in white populations living in areas with high solar UVR (at high altitudes or in low latitudes).

### PATHOGENESIS

While UVB is the most obvious damaging UVR, UVA in high doses can produce connective tissue changes in mice. In addition, visible (400 to 700 nm) and infrared (1000 to 1,000,000 nm) radiations have been implicated. The action spectrum for DHe is not known for certain; there is some experimental evidence in mice that infrared radiation is implicated, in addition to UVB and UVA.

### HISTORY

**Personal History**   There is a history of intensive exposure to sun in youth (<20 years), even though sun exposure may have been quite limited in later adult life, and/or significant sun exposure in adulthood. Because skin phototypes are genetically determined, there is often a family history of DHe.

### PHYSICAL EXAMINATION

**Skin Lesions**
A combination of atrophy (of epidermis), hypertrophy (of papillary dermis due to elastosis), telangiectases, spotty depigmentation and hyperpigmentation, and spotty hperkeratosis in light-exposed areas. Skin appears wrinkled, wizened, leathery, "prematurely aged" (Fig. 10-17). Both fine, cigarette paper–like and deep furrow-like wrinkling (Fig. 10-17); skin is waxy, papular with a yellowish hue, and both glistening and rough. There may be telangiectasia and bruising due to fragility of small vessels. Macular

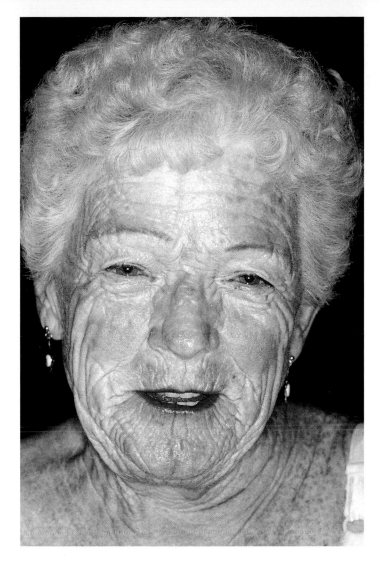

**FIGURE 10-17   Dermatoheliosis**   *Severe fine (periorbital) and deep wrinkling (cheeks, perioral, and neck). The skin appears waxy, papular with a yellowish hue (actinic elastosis). This 68-year-old Irish-American female with SPT I lived in New England near the sea and in her youth spent hours in the sun during an era in which it was believed that "sun was good for you."*

hyperpigmentations: *solar lentigines* (see below); macular hypopigmentations; *guttate hypomelanosis*, <3 mm in diameter, on the extremities. Comedones, particularly periorbital (termed *Favre-Racouchet disease*). Individuals with DHe invariably have actinic keratoses.

***Distribution*** Exposed areas, particularly face, periorbital and perioral areas, scalp (bald males). Nuchal area: cutis rhomboidalis ("red neck") with rhomboidal furrows; lower arms, dorsa of hands.

## LABORATORY EXAMINATION

**Dermatopathology**   Acanthosis of epidermis, increased horny layer. Flattening of the dermal-epidermal junction. Atypia of the keratinocytes. Loss of small vessels in the papillary dermis. *Elastosis:* Degraded elastic tissue with accumulation of coarse amorphous masses and increase in glycosaminoglycans in the upper dermis. Decrease in collagen.

## COURSE AND PROGNOSIS

The appearance of DHe marks a relatively young person as "old," a state that everyone tries to delay. DHe is inexorably progressive and irreversible, but some repair of connective tissue effects can occur if the skin is protected. Some processes leading to DHe continue to progress, however, even when sun exposures are severely restricted in later life; solar keratoses and lentigines develop in the sun-damaged skin that is now being protected by avoidance and sunblocks. Yet there are documented examples of spontaneous reversal of solar keratoses.

## MANAGEMENT

Current management is to prevent skin cancers and the development of DHe with the use of protective sunblocks, a change of behavior in the sun, and the use of topical chemotherapy (tretinoin) that reverses some of the changes of DHe.

**Topical Treatment**   *Tretinoin* in lotions, gels, and creams in varying concentrations reverses some aspects of DHe, especially in the connective tissue and vascular changes. Topical *tazarotene* has also been shown to reduce the effects of photoaging in short-term studies. Topical tretinoin can alter the progression of incipient epithelial skin cancers. *5-Fluorouracil* in lotions and creams is highly effective in causing a disappearance of solar keratoses.

**Prevention**   Persons of SPT I and II should be identified early in life and advised that they are susceptible to the development of DHe and skin cancers, including melanoma. These persons should never sunbathe and should, from an early age, adopt a daily program of self-protection using sun-filtering clothing and substantive and effective topical sun-protective solutions, gels, or lotions that can filter DNA-damaging UVB; effective UVA filters are now available. SPT I and II persons should avoid the peak hours of UVB intensity, which are the 2 h before and after solar noon (1200 GMT).

*Caution*: There is some experimental evidence that while sunscreens protect from sunburn, they do not protect from UV-induced local immunosuppression. Prevention of sunburn may lure individuals into exposing themselves to the sun for prolonged periods, which may abrogate immunosurveillance mechanisms in the skin. This has been linked to the rising incidence of melanoma but is not proven.

---

## SOLAR LENTIGO   ■   ○

---

Solar lentigo is a circumscribed 1- to 3-cm brown macule resulting from a localized proliferation of melanocytes due to acute or chronic exposure to sunlight.

## EPIDEMIOLOGY AND ETIOLOGY

**Age of Onset**   Usually >40 years but may be 30 years in sunny climates and in susceptible persons.

**Race**   Most common in Caucasians but seen also in Asians.

**Skin Phototype**   Generally correlated with skin phototypes I to III and duration and intensity of solar exposure.

**Etiology**   Solar lentigines may arise acutely after sunburns (Fig. 10-18) and after overdosage of PUVA (*PUVA lentigines*).

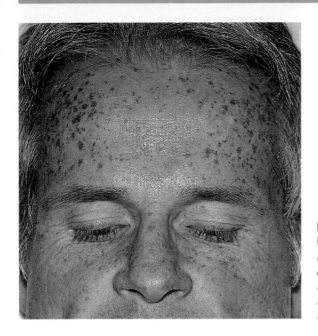

**FIGURE 10-18   Dermatoheliosis: solar lentigines**   *Multiple dark-brown macules on the forehead occurred after a sunburn. They are all of about the same size and sharply marginated that is characteristic of sunburn-induced solar lentigines.*

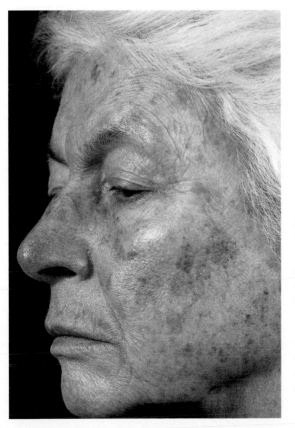

**FIGURE 10-19   Dermatoheliosis: solar lentigines**   *Multiple, variegated, tan-to-dark-brown macules on the malar and frontal areas in the face. Solar lentigines are not the same as ephelides (freckles)—they do not fade in the winter as freckles do. In contrast to the sharply marginated solar lentigines shown in Fig. 10-18, which are due to an acute sunburn, the solar lentigines shown here are of different sizes and partially ill defined and confluent, which is characteristic of chronic cumulative solar damage.*

## PHYSICAL EXAMINATION

**Skin Lesions**
Strictly macular (Fig. 10-18), 1 to 3 cm, and as large as 5 cm (Fig. 10-19). Light yellow, light brown, or dark brown; variegated mix of brown and not uniform color (Fig. 10-19), as in café au lait macules. Round, oval, with slightly irregular border, sharply (Fig. 10-18) but also ill defined (Fig. 10-19). Scattered, discrete lesions.
*Distribution* Exclusively exposed areas: forehead, cheeks, nose, dorsa of hands and forearms, upper back, chest, shins.

## LABORATORY EXAMINATION

**Dermatopathology** Club-shaped elongated rete ridges that show hypermelanosis and an in-creased number of melanocytes in the basal layer.

## DIFFERENTIAL DIAGNOSIS

**Brown Macules** "Flat," acquired, brown lesions on the exposed skin of the face, which may on cursory examination appear to be similar, have distinctive features: solar lentigo, freckles, seborrheic keratosis, spreading pigmented actinic keratosis (SPAK), lentigo maligna.

## MANAGEMENT

Cryosurgery or laser surgery are effective. No more than 10 s of liquid nitrogen should be administered; otherwise depigmentation of normal skin will occur.

---

## ACTINIC KERATOSIS    ■

These single or multiple, discrete, dry, rough, adherent scaly lesions occur on the habitually sun-exposed skin of adults, usually on a background of dermatoheliosis.
*Synonym*: Solar keratosis.

## EPIDEMIOLOGY

**Age of Onset** Middle age, although in Australia and southwestern United States solar keratoses may occur in persons <30 years.
**Sex** More common in males.
**Race** SPT I, II, and III; rare in SPT IV; almost never in blacks or South Indians.
**Occupation** Outdoor workers (especially farmers, ranchers, sailors) and outdoor sportspersons (tennis, golf, mountain climbing, deep-sea fishing).

## PATHOGENESIS

Prolonged and repeated solar exposure in susceptible persons (SPT I, II, and III) leads to cumulative damage to keratinocytes by the action of UVR, principally, if not exclusively, UVB (290 to 320 nm).

## HISTORY

**Duration of Lesions** Months to years.
**Skin Symptoms** Some lesions may be tender.

## PHYSICAL EXAMINATION

**Skin Lesions**
Adherent hyperkeratotic scale, which is removed with difficulty and pain (Fig. 10-20). May be papular. Skin-colored, yellow-brown, or brown (Fig. 10-20); often there is a reddish tinge. Rough, like coarse sandpaper, "better felt than seen" on palpation with a finger. Most commonly <1 cm, oval or round (Fig. 10-20).
*Special Presentation*: SPAK (spreading pigmented actinic keratosis). This lesion is best described as "looks like lentigo maligna but feels like actinic keratosis" (Fig. 10-21). It is a rather

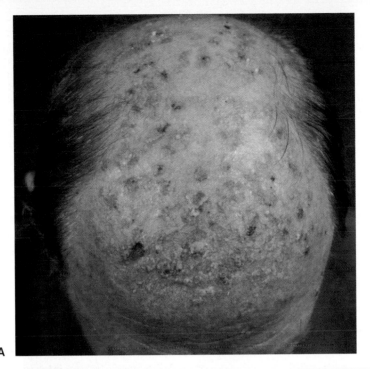

A

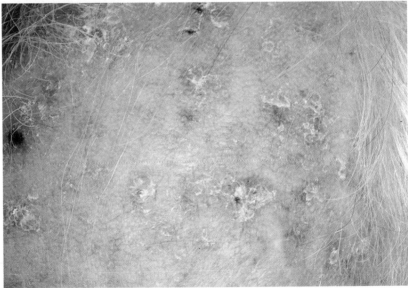

B

**FIGURE 10-20   Solar keratosis**   *A. Erythematous macules and papules with coarse, adherent scale become confluent on this bald scalp with dermatoheliosis. These hyperkeratoses are yellowish-greyish and have a tinge of hemorrhage; gently abrading lesions with a fingernail usually induces pain, even in early subtle lesions, a helpful diagnostic finding.* **B.** *Close up of solar keratosis revealing coarse scales on skin with dermatoheliosis.*

uncommon variant of actinic keratosis. The distinctive features of SPAK include size (>1.5 cm), pigmentation (brown to black and variegated), and history of lateral spreading, especially the verrucous surface. The lesion is important because it can mimic lentigo maligna (LM). It is, however, easily distinguished from LM because LM is completely flat without evidence of verrucous change. Biopsy is necessary to confirm the clinical diagnosis.

***Distribution*** Isolated single lesion or scattered discrete lesions. Face [forehead, nose, cheeks (Fig. 10-21), temples, vermilion border of lower lip], ears (in males), neck (sides), forearms, and hands (dorsa), shins, and the scalp in bald males (Fig. 10-20).

## LABORATORY EXAMINATION

**Dermatopathology**   Large bright-staining keratinocytes, with mild to moderate pleomorphism in the basal layer extending into follicles, atypical (dyskeratotic) keratinocytes, parakeratosis.

## DIAGNOSIS AND DIFFERENTIAL DIAGNOSIS

Usually made on clinical findings. Differential: Chronic cutaneous lupus erythematosus; irritated seborrheic keratosis, flat warts, Squamous cell carcinoma (SCC) in situ, superficial basal cell carcinoma. Highly hyperkeratotic lesions and SPAK may require biopsy to rule out SCC (in situ or invasive) or LM.

## COURSE AND PROGNOSIS

Solar keratoses may disappear spontaneously, but in general remain for years. The actual incidence of SCC arising in preexisting solar keratoses is unknown but has been estimated at one SCC developing annually in 1000 solar keratoses.

## MANAGEMENT

**Prevention**   Avoided by use of highly effective UVB/UVA sunscreens, which should be applied daily to the face, neck, and ears during the summer in northern latitudes for SPT I and SPT II persons and for those SPT III persons who sustain prolonged sunlight exposures.

**Topical Therapy**   *Cryosurgery*   Light spray or with cotton-tipped applicator is effective in most cases.

***5-Fluorouracil (5-FU) Cream 5%***   Effective, but difficult for many individuals. Treatment of facial lesions causes significant erythema and erosions, resulting in temporary cosmetic disfigurement. Apply bid for 2 to 4 weeks on face; may require longer period of therapy on dorsum of hands or lower legs. Efficacy can be increased and duration of treatment can be shortened if applied under occlusion and/or combined with topical tretinoin. This, however, leads to confluent erosions and may require hospitalization. Reepithelialization occurs after treatment is discontinued. Pretreatment with light cryosurgery to hyperkeratotic lesions may improve efficacy of 5-FU cream.

***Imiquimod (twice weekly for 16 weeks)***   Applied as 5-FU; also leads to irritation and erosions but is effective.

***Topical Retinoids***   Used chronically, may be effective for treatment of dermatoheliosis and superficial solar keratoses.

***Facial Peels***   Trichloroacetic acid (5 to 10%) effective for widespread lesions.

***Laser Surgery***   Erbium or carbon dioxide lasers. High cost. Usually effective for individual lesions. For extensive facial lesions, facial resurfacing is effective.

***Photodynamic Therapy***   Effective but painful and cumbersome.

**Systemic Therapy**   Acitretin or isotretinoin are effective in reducing the number of solar keratoses and SCC in situ in patients with advanced dermatoheliosis, many solar keratoses, especially in immunocompromised patients. Lesions recur once therapy is discontinued.

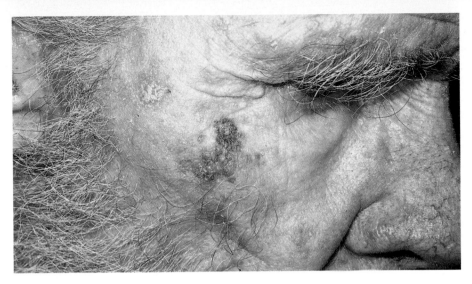

**FIGURE 10-21   Spreading pigmented actinic keratosis (SPAK)**   *"Looks like lentigo maligna" (see Fig. 12-9) but is rough and therefore "feels like actinic keratosis." A nonpigmented actinic keratosis is seen in the preauricular region.*

# SKIN REACTIONS TO IONIZING RADIATION

## RADIATION DERMATITIS

Radiation dermatitis is defined as skin changes resulting from exposure to ionizing radiation. There are *reversible effects*, i.e., erythema, epilation, suppression of sebaceous glands, and pigmentation that last for weeks to months to years, and *irreversible effects*, i.e., acute and chronic radiation dermatitis and radiation-induced cancers.

### Type of Exposure

Result of therapy (for cancer, formerly also used for acne and psoriasis), accidental, or occupational (e.g., formerly, in dentists who held the film in the mouth with their fingers). The radiation causing radiodermatitis includes superficial and deep x-ray radiation, electron-beam therapy, and grenz-ray therapy. It is a prevailing myth among some dermatologists that grenz rays are "soft" and not carcinogenic; it has been estimated that SCC can appear from >5000 cGy of grenz rays.

### Types of Reactions

**Acute**   Temporary erythema that lasts 3 days and then persistent erythema, which reaches a peak in 2 weeks (Fig. 10-22) and is painful; pigmentation appears about day 20; a late erythema can also occur beginning on day 35 to 40, and this lasts 2 to 3 weeks. Massive reactions lead to blistering and ulceration, also painful. Permanent scarring may result.

**Chronic**   After *fractional* but relatively intensive therapy with total doses of 3000 to 6000 rad, there develops an epidermolytic reaction in 3 weeks. This is repaired in 3 to 6 weeks, and scars and hypopigmentation develop; there is loss of all skin appendages and atrophy of the epidermis and dermis. During the next 2 to 5 years, the atrophy increases (Fig. 10-23); there is hyper- and hypopigmentation (poikiloderma), telangiectasia (Fig. 10-24), and superficial venules become ectatic. There are hyperkeratoses (x-ray keratoses) (Fig. 10-26). Necrosis and ulceration (Fig. 10-25A) are rare but occur in accidental exposure or error in dose: either one or a few accidentally high doses or multiple small doses at frequent intervals (monthly or weekly). When necrosis occurs, it is leathery, yellow, and adherent and the base and surrounding skin are extremely painful (Fig. 10-25A). Ulcerations have a very poor tendency to heal and usually require surgical intervention. Accidental exposure occurs mostly in occupational exposure and affects the hands, feet, and face. There is a destruction of the fingerprint pattern, xerosis, scanty hair (Fig. 10-23), atrophy of sebaceous and sweat glands, and development of keratoses (Fig. 10-26).

**Nails**   Longitudinal striations (Fig. 10-27) show thickening, dystrophy.

## COURSE, PROGNOSIS, AND MANAGEMENT

Chronic radiation dermatitis is permanent, progressive, and irreversible (Figs. 10-23 and 10-24). SCC may develop in 4 to 40 years (Figs. 10-25B, 10-26, and 10-27), with a median of 7 to 12 years, almost exclusively from the chronic repeated types of exposures. SCC always develops within the area of radiodermatitis, never in normal skin (Fig. 10-25B). Tumors metastasize in about 25%; despite extensive surgery (excision, grafts, etc.), the prognosis is poor, and recurrences are common. Basal cell carcinoma (BCC) may also occur in chronic radiation dermatitis and appears mostly in patients formerly treated with x-rays for acne vulgaris and acne cystica or epilation (tinea capitis) (Fig. 10-23). The tumors may appear 40 to 50 years after exposure. Excision and grafting are often possible before the cancer develops.

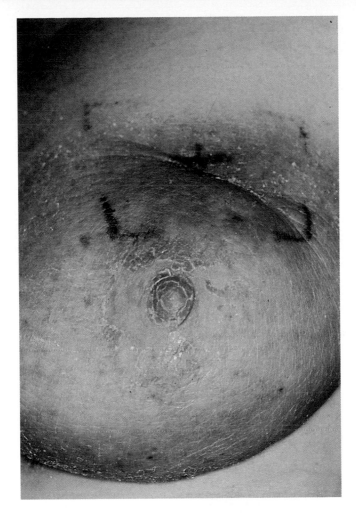

**FIGURE 10-22   Radiation dermatitis: acute**   *Localized area of erythema and edema in the radiation portal occurring at the end of radiotherapy treatment for breast cancer.*

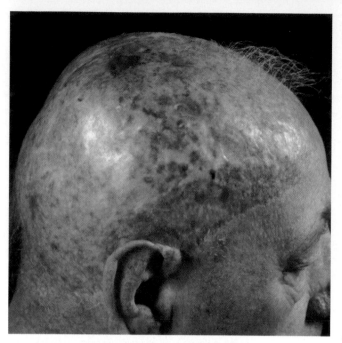

**FIGURE 10-23    Radiation dermatitis: chronic** *There is poikiloderma (brown: hyperpigmentation; white: hypopigmentation; and red: telangiectasia) combined with atrophy and sclerosis. Hairs are absent. These massive skin changes are the result of (overdosed) radiation therapy the patient received as a child for fungal infection of the scalp. He is a candidate for SCC in the future.*

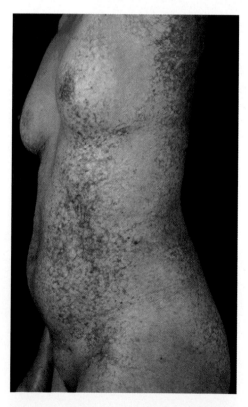

**FIGURE 10-24    Radiation dermatitis: chronic** *This poikilodermatous condition is the result of total body electron beam therapy for cutaneous T cell lymphoma. In this low power image, only the color changes are seen: hyper- and hypopigmentation and telangiectasias; not seen are the background of sclerosis and atrophy and hyperkeratoses.*

**FIGURE 10-27 (Across, Right)    Nail changes in site of radiation exposure** *Note the linear striations resulting from damage to the nail matrix. At the nailfold and extending proximally on the thumb, there is an irregular erythematous plaque that represents mostly SCCIS but, focally, also invasive SCC.*

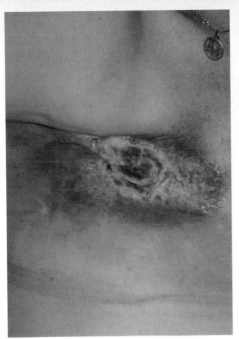
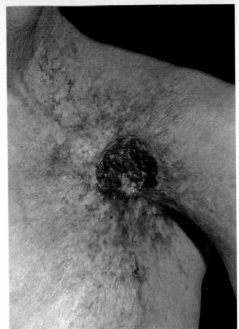

A                                                    B

**FIGURE 10-25    Radiation dermatitis: chronic**    *A. With a central necrosis that is leathery, yellow-ish-brown, and tightly adherent. Surgical removal will reveal a deep ulcer. The lesion is extremely painful. **B.** A large and deep ulcer in an area of atrophy, fibrosis, poikiloderma, and telangiectasia on the chest wall. This occurred 20 years after radical mastectomy, axillary lymph node dissection, and radiotherapy. The ulceration was primarily due to radionecrosis. Now the border of the ulcer is elevated and firm and so is the granulating base: this is SCC arising in this radiation dermatitis.*

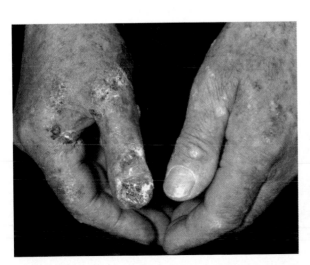
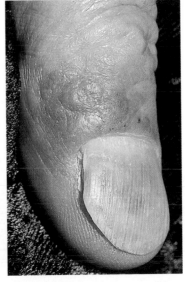

**FIGURE 10-26 (Left)    Chronic radiation dermatitis with SCC**    *These are the hands of an elderly radiologist who decades ago had disregarded precautionary measures and hardly wore gloves doing fluoroscopic work. There are multiple X-ray keratoses; the hyperkeratotic lesion on the right thumb has destroyed the nail and represents X-ray-induced SCC.*

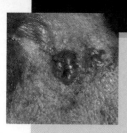

# PRECANCEROUS LESIONS AND CUTANEOUS CARCINOMAS

## EPIDERMAL PRECANCERS AND CANCERS

Cutaneous epithelial cancers [nonmelanoma skin cancer (NMSC)] are the easiest of all cancers to diagnose and treat. They originate most commonly in the epidermal germinative keratinocytes or adnexal structures (e.g., sweat apparatus, hair follicle). The two principal NMSCs are basal cell carcinoma (BCC) and squamous cell carcinoma (SCC). SCC often has its origin in an identifiable dysplastic in situ lesion that can be treated before frank invasion occurs. In contrast, in situ BCC is not known, but minimally invasive "superficial" BCCs are common.

The most common etiology of NMSC in fair-skinned individuals is sunlight, ultraviolet radiation (UVR), and human papillomavirus (HPV). Solar keratoses are the most common precursor lesions of SCC in situ (SCCIS) and invasive SCC occurring at sites of chronic sun exposure in individuals of northern European heritage (see Section 10). UVR and HPV cause the spectrum of changes ranging from epithelial dysplasia to SCCIS to invasive SCC. Much less commonly, NMSC can be caused by ionizing radiation (arising in sites of chronic radiation damage), chronic inflammation, hydrocarbons (tar), and chronic ingestion of inorganic arsenic; these tumors can be much more aggressive than those associated with UVR or HPV. In the increasing population of immunosuppressed individuals (those with HIV disease, organ transplant recipients, etc.), UVR- and HPV-induced SCCs are much more common and can be more aggressive.

## EPITHELIAL PRECANCEROUS LESIONS AND SCCIS

Dysplasia of epidermal keratinocytes in epidermis and squamous mucosa can involve the lower portion of the epidermis or the full thickness. Basal cells mature into dysplastic keratinocytes resulting in a hyperkeratotic papule, or plaque, clinically identified as "keratoses." A continuum exists from dysplasia to SCCIS to invasive SCC. These lesions have various associated eponyms such as Bowen's disease or erythroplasia of Queyrat, which as descriptive morphologic terms are helpful; terms such as UVR- or HPV-associated SCCIS, however, will be more meaningful but can be used only for those lesions with known etiology.

Epithelial precancerous lesions and SCCIS can be classified as follows:

- UVR-induced
  - Actinic solar keratoses
  - Spreading pigmented actinic keratoses (SPAK)
  - Lichenoid actinic keratoses
  - Bowenoid actinic keratoses
  - SCCIS (Bowen's disease)
- HPV-induced
  - Low-grade squamous intraepithelial lesion (LSIL)
  - High-grade squamous intraepithelial lesion (HSIL)
  - SCCIS (bowenoid papulosis)

- Arsenical keratoses
  Palmoplantar keratoses
  Bowenoid arsenical keratoses
- Hydrocarbon (tar) keratoses
  Bowenoid tar keratoses

- Thermal keratoses
  Bowenoid thermal keratoses
- Keratoses in chronic radiation dermatitis
- Bowenoid radiation keratoses
- Chronic cicatrix (scar) keratoses

## ACTINIC KERATOSIS

These single or multiple, discrete, dry, rough, adherent scaly lesions occur on the habitually sun-exposed skin of adults (Fig. 11-1).
*Synonym*: Solar keratosis.
For a full discussion of this condition, see Section 10, p. 262; Figs. 10-20 and 10-21.

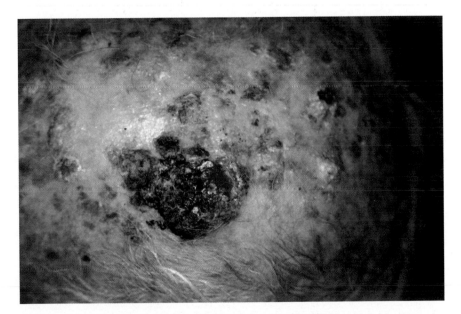

**FIGURE 11-1 Actinic keratoses and invasive squamous cell carcinoma** *Multiple, tightly adherent dirty-looking actinic keratoses. The large nodule is covered by hyperkeratoses and hemorrhagic crusts, it is partially eroded and firm. This nodule is invasive squamous cell carcinoma. The image is shown to demonstrate the transition from precancerous lesions to frank carcinoma.*

## CUTANEOUS HORN

A cutaneous horn (CH) is a *clinical* entity having the appearance of an animal horn with a papular or nodular base and a keratotic cap of various shapes and lengths. CHs most commonly represent hypertrophic solar keratoses. However, in situ or invasive SCC is often present at the base of a CH. CHs usually arise within areas of dermatoheliosis on the face, ear, dorsum of hands, or forearms. Non-precancerous CH formation can also occur in seborrheic keratoses, warts, and keratoacanthomas.

Clinically, CHs vary in size from a few millimeters to several centimeters (Fig. 11-2). The horn may be white, black, or yellowish in color and straight, curved, or spiral in shape. Histologically there is usually SCCIS or invasive SCC at the base. Because of the possibility of invasive SCC, a CH should always be excised.

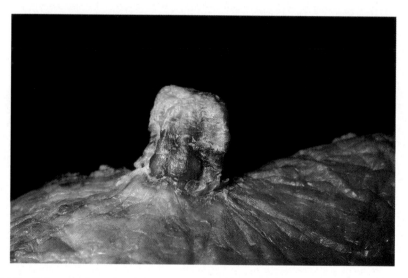

**FIGURE 11-2   Cutaneous horn, hand: hypertrophic actinic keratosis**   *A hornlike projection of keratin on a slightly raised base is the setting of advanced dermatoheliosis in an 83-year-old female. Excision showed actinic keratosis at the base in this case; however, in situ or invasive SCC is very often found at the base of CH.*

# SQUAMOUS CELL CARCINOMA IN SITU ■ ◑

SCCIS is most often caused by UVR or HPV infection, presenting as solitary or multiple macules, papules, or plaques, which may be scaling or hyperkeratotic. SCCIS commonly arises in epithelial dysplastic lesions such as solar keratoses or HPV-induced squamous intraepithelial lesions (SIL) (see Section 27 and Section 31) or arise de novo.

## ETIOLOGY

UVR, HPV, arsenic, tar, chronic heat exposure, chronic radiation dermatitis.

## HISTORY

Lesions are most often asymptomatic but may bleed. Nodule formation within SCCIS suggests progression to invasive SCC.

## PHYSICAL EXAMINATION

### Skin Findings

Appears as a sharply demarcated, scaling, or hyperkeratotic macule, papule, or plaque (Fig. 11-3). Solitary or multiple lesions are pink or red in color and have a slightly scaling surface, small erosions, and can be crusted. Such lesions are always well defined and are called *Bowen's disease* (Fig. 11-3).

Red, sharply demarcated, glistening macular or plaque-like SCCIS on the glans penis or labia minora are called *erythroplasia of Queyrat* (see Section 32). Anogenital HPV-induced SCCIS may be tan, brown, or black in color and are referred to as *bowenoid papulosis*. (see Section 32). Eroded lesions may have areas of crusting. SCCIS may be mistaken for a patch of eczema or psoriasis and go undiagnosed for years, resulting in large lesions with annular or polycyclic borders (Fig. 11-3). Once invasion occurs, nodular lesions appear within the plaque and the lesion is then commonly called *Bowen's carcinoma* (Fig. 11-4).

*Distribution* UVR-induced SCCIS commonly arises within a solar keratosis in the setting of photoaging (dermatoheliosis). HPV-induced SCCIS arises within an area of low-grade or high-grade SIL, mostly in the genital area but also periungually, most commonly on the thumb or in the nail bed.

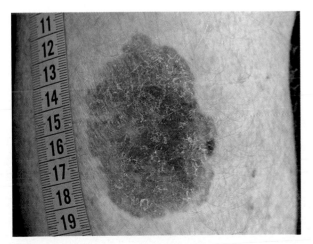

**FIGURE 11-3 Squamous cell carcinoma in situ: Bowen's disease** *A large, sharply demarcated, scaly, erythematous plaque simulating a psoriatic lesion on the calf.*

## LABORATORY EXAMINATION

**Dermatopathology**    Carcinoma in situ with loss of epidermal architecture and regular differentiation; keratinocyte polymorphism, single cell dyskeratosis, increased mitotic rate, multinuclear cells. Epidermis may be thickened but basement membrane intact.

## DIAGNOSIS AND DIFFERENTIAL DIAGNOSIS

Clinical diagnosis confirmed by dermatopathologic findings. Differential diagnosis includes all. Well-demarcated pink-red plaque(s): Nummular eczema, psoriasis, seborrheic keratosis, solar keratoses, verruca vulgaris, verruca plana, condyloma acuminatum, superficial BCC; amelanotic melanoma, Paget's disease.

## COURSE AND PROGNOSIS

Untreated SCCIS will progress to invasive SCC (Fig. 11-4). Lymph node metastasis can occur without demonstrable invasion.

## MANAGEMENT

**Topical Chemotherapy**    *5-Fluorouracil* cream applied qd or bid with or without tape occlusion is effective. So is *imiquimod,* but both require considerable time.

**Cryosurgery**    Highly effective. Lesions are usually treated more aggressively than solar keratoses and superficial scarring will result.

**Photodynamic Therapy**    Effective but cumbersome and painful.

**Surgical Excision**    Has the highest cure rate but the greatest chance of causing cosmetically disfiguring scars. It should be done in all lesions where invasion cannot be excluded by biopsy.

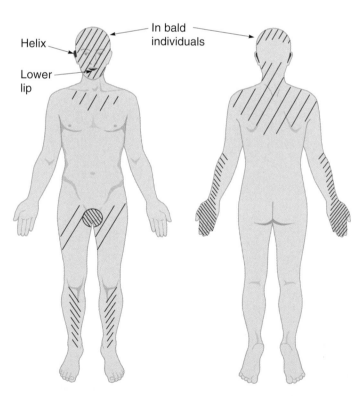

**IMAGE 11-1    Squamous cell carcinoma:** *predilection sites.*

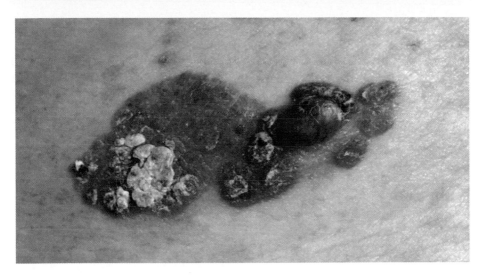

**FIGURE 11-4    Squamous cell carcinoma in situ: Bowen's disease and invasive SCC: Bowen's carcinoma**    *An orange plaque on the trunk, sharply defined, partially covered by yellowish, psoriasiform scale represents SCCIS or Bowen's disease. The red nodule on this plaque indicates that here the lesion is not any more an in situ lesion but that invasive carcinoma has developed.*

## INVASIVE SQUAMOUS CELL CARCINOMA   ■ ●

Invasive SCC is a malignant tumor of keratinocytes, arising in the epidermis, skin appendages, and other stratified squamous mucosa. SCC usually arises in epidermal precancerous lesions (see above) and, depending on etiology and level of differentiation, varies in its aggressiveness. The majority of UVR-induced lesions have a low rate of distant metastasis in otherwise healthy individuals. More aggressive SCC occur in immunosuppressed individuals with a greater incidence of metastasis.

### EPIDEMIOLOGY AND ETIOLOGY

#### Ultraviolet Radiation
**Age of Onset**   Older than 55 years of age in the United States; in Australia and New Zealand, persons in their twenties and thirties.
**Incidence**   Continental United States: 12 per 100,000 white males; 7 per 100,000 white females. Hawaii: 62 per 100,000 whites.
**Sex**   Males > females, but SCC can occur more frequently on the legs of females.
**Exposure**   Sunlight. Phototherapy, PUVA (oral psoralen + UVA). Excessive photochemotherapy can lead to promotion of SCC, particularly in patients with skin phototypes I and II or in patients with history of previous exposure to ionizing radiation or methotrexate treatment for psoriasis.
**Race**   Persons with white skin and poor tanning capacity (skin phototypes I and II) (see Section 10). Brown- or black-skinned persons can develop SCC from numerous etiologic agents other than UVR.
**Geography**   Most common in areas that have many days of sunshine annually, i.e., in Australia and southwestern United States.
**Occupation**   Persons working outdoors— farmers, sailors, lifeguards, telephone line installers, construction workers, dock workers.

#### Human Papillomavirus
Oncogenic HPV type-16, -18, -31, -33, -35, -39, -40, and -51 to -60 are associated with epithelial dysplasia, SCCIS, and invasive SCC. HPV-5, -8, -9 have also been isolated from SCCs.

#### Other Etiologic Factors
**Immunosuppression**   Solid organ transplant recipients, individuals with chronic immunosuppression of inflammatory disorders, and those with HIV disease are associated with an increased incidence of UVR- and HPV-induced SCCIS and invasive SCCs. SCCs in these individuals are more aggressive than in nonimmunosuppressed individuals.

**Chronic Inflammation**   Chronic cutaneous lupus erythematosus, chronic ulcers, burn scars, chronic radiation dermatitis, lichen planus of oral mucosa.
**Industrial Carcinogens**   Pitch, tar, crude paraffin oil, fuel oil, creosote, lubricating oil, nitrosoureas.
**Inorganic Arsenic**   Trivalent arsenic had been used in the past in medications such as Asiatic pills, Donovan's pills, Fowler's solution (used as a treatment for psoriasis). Arsenic is still present in drinking water in some geographic regions.

### HISTORY

Slowly evolving—any isolated keratotic or eroded papule or plaque in a suspect patient that persists for over a month is considered a carcinoma until proved otherwise. Also, a nodule evolving in a plaque that meets the clinical criteria of SCCIS (Bowen's disease), a chronically eroded lesion on the lower lip or on the penis, or nodular lesions evolving in or at the margin of a chronic venous ulcer or within chronic radiation dermatitis. Note that SCC is always asymptomatic. Potential carcinogens often can be detected only after detailed interrogation of the patient.

### PHYSICAL EXAMINATION

For didactic reasons, two types can be distinguished:

1. Highly differentiated SCCs, which practically always show signs of keratinization either within or on the surface (hyperkeratosis) of the tumor. These are firm or hard upon palpation.
2. Poorly differentiated SCCs, which do not show signs of keratinization and clinically appear fleshy, granulomatous, amd consequently are soft upon palpation.

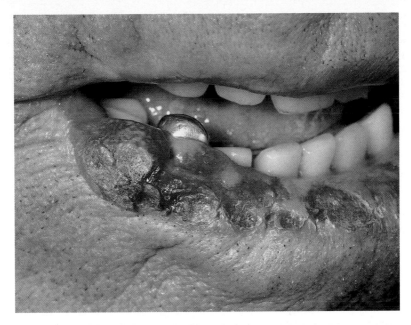

**FIGURE 11-5    Squamous cell carcinoma: invasive**    *A large but subtle nodule, which is better felt than seen, on the vermilion border of the lower lip with areas of hyperkeratosis and erosion, arising in the setting of dermatoheliosis of the lip (cheilitis actinica).*

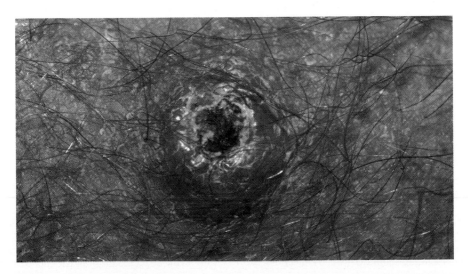

**FIGURE 11-6    Squamous cell carcinoma**    *A round nodule with central hyperkeratosis, firm and indolent. This lesion cannot be distinguished clinically from keratoacanthoma; it is easily distinguished from nodular BCC because BCC does not develop hyperkeratosis.*

### Differentiated SCC

**Lesions** Indurated papule, plaque, or nodule (Figs. 11-1, 11-5 to 11-8); adherent thick keratotic scale or hyperkeratosis (Fig. 11-1); when eroded or ulcerated, the lesion may have a crust in the center and a firm, hyperkeratotic, elevated margin (Figs. 11-5, 11-7, 11-8). Horny material may be expressed from the margin or the center of the lesion (Figs. 11-6 to 11-8). Erythematous, yellowish, skin color. Hard. Polygonal, oval, round (Fig. 11-6), or umbilicated and ulcerated.

*Distribution* Usually isolated but may be multiple. Usually exposed areas. Sun-induced keratotic and/or ulcerated lesions especially on the bald scalp (Fig. 11-1), cheeks, nose, lower lips (Fig. 11-5), tips of ears (Fig. 11-7), preauricular area, dorsa of the hands, forearms, trunk, and shins (females) (Fig. 11-8).

**Other Physical Findings** Regional lymphadenopathy due to metastases.

**Special Features** In UV-related SCC evidence of *dermatoheliosis* and *actinic keratoses*. SCCs of the lips develop from leukoplasia or actinic cheilitis; in 90% of cases they are found on the lower lip (Fig. 11-5). In chronic radiodermatitis they arise from radiation-induced keratoses (see Fig. 10-26); in individuals with a history of chronic intake of arsenic, from arsenical keratoses. Differentiated (i.e., hyperkeratotic) SCC due to HPV on genitalia (Fig. 11-9A); SCC due to excessive PUVA therapy on lower extremities (pretibial) or on genitalia (Fig. 11-9B). SCCs in scars from burns, in chronic stasis ulcers of long duration, and in sites of chronic inflammation are often difficult to identify. Suspicion is indicated when nodular lesions are hard and show signs of keratinization (Figs. 11-7 and 11-8). *Special form*: carcinoma cuniculatum, usually on the soles, highly differentiated, HPV-related.

**Histopathology** SCCs with various grades of anaplasia and keratinization.

### Undifferentiated SCC

**Lesions** Fleshy, granulating, easily vulnerable, erosive papules and nodules and papillomatous vegetations (Fig. 11-10). Ulceration with a necrotic base and soft, fleshy margin. Bleeds easily, crusting. Red. Soft. Polygonal, irregular, often cauliflower-like (Fig. 11-10).

*Distribution* Isolated but also multiple, particularly on the genitalia, where they arise from erythroplasia (see Fig. 32-17) and on the trunk (Fig. 11-4), lower extremities, or face (Fig. 11-10), where they arise from Bowen's disease.

**Miscellaneous Other Skin Changes** Lymphadenopathy as evidence of regional matastases is far more common than with differentiated, hyperkeratotic SCCs.

**Histopathology** Anaplastic SCC with multiple mitoses and little evidence of differentiation and keratinization.

## DIFFERENTIAL DIAGNOSIS

As stated previously, any persistent nodule, plaque, or ulcer, but especially when these occur in sun-damaged skin, on the lower lips, in areas of radiodermatitis, in old burn scars, or on the genitalia, must be examined for SCC. Keratoacanthoma may be clinically indistinguishable from differentiated SCC (Fig. 11-6).

## MANAGEMENT

**Surgery** Depending on localization and extent of lesion, excision with primary closure, skin flaps, or grafting. Microscopically controlled surgery in difficult sites. Radiotherapy should be performed only if surgery is not feasible.

## COURSE AND PROGNOSIS

**Recurrence and Metastases** SCC causes local tissue destruction but it has a significant potential for metastases. Metastases are directed to regional lymph nodes and appear 1 to 3 years after initial diagnosis. SCC in the skin has an overall metastatic rate of 3 to 4% and tends to occur with tumors that are large, recurrent, and involve deep structures of cutaneous nerves. High-risk SCCs are defined as having a diameter >2 cm, a depth >4 mm, and Clark levels IV or V[*]; tumor involvement of bone, muscle, and nerve; location on ear, lip, and genitalia; tumors arising in a scar or following ionizing radiation; and highly dedifferentiated tumors. Cancers arising in chronic osteomyelitis sinus tracts, in burn scars, and in sites of radiation dermatitis have a metastatic rate of 31, 20, and 18%, respectively. On the other hand, SCC arising in solar keratoses have the lowest potential for metastasis. A special group of high-risk SCCs are those in patients who are immunosuppressed.

---

[*]Clark level I, intraepidermal; level II, invades papillary dermis; level III, fills papillary dermis; level IV, invades reticular dermis; level V, invades subcutaneous fat.

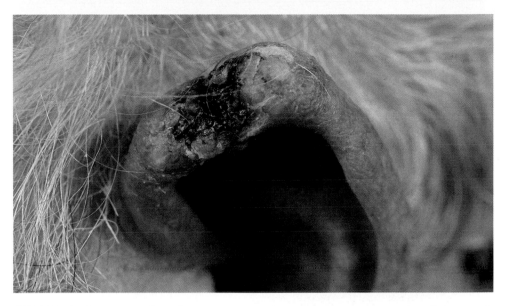

**FIGURE 11-7 Squamous cell carcinoma** *A large notch on the superior aspect of the helix, a nodule of SCC with hyperkeratosis and ulceration.*

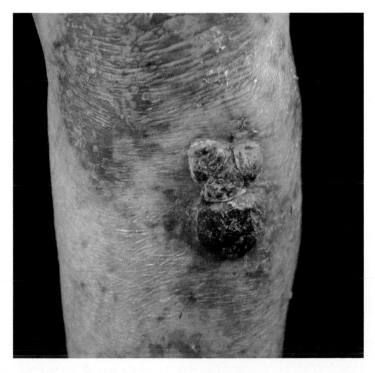

**FIGURE 11-8 Squamous cell carcinoma** *In a renal transplant recipient who also had psoriasis and had therefore spent considerable time in the sun. In addition to these fungating, firm, hyperkeratotic, and partially ulcerated nodules, the patient had seven smaller but similar nodules elsewhere on the legs and inguinal lymph node metastasis.*

**SCCs in Immunosuppression** Organ transplant recipients have a markedly increased incidence of NMSCs, primarily SCC, which is 40 to 50 times greater than in the general population. Risk factors include skin type, cumulative sun exposure, age at transplantation, male sex, HPV infections, and the degree and length of immunosuppression. Lesions are often multiple, usually in sun-exposed sites.

These tumors grow rapidly (see Fig. 11-8) and are aggressive; in one series of heart-transplant patients from Australia, 27% died of skin cancer.

Patients with AIDS have only a slight increased risk of NMSC. In one series a fourfold increase in their risk of developing lip SCC was noted. However, SCC of the anus is significantly increased in this population.

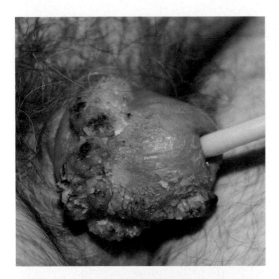

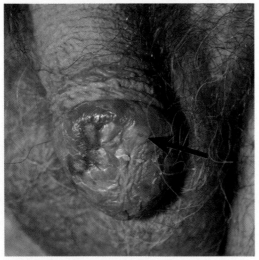

**FIGURE 11-9   Squamous cell carcinoma of the penis**   *A. Hyperkeratotic firm wartlike lesion that was associated with HPV.* *B. SCCIS (arrow) and invasive SCC (erosions) due to overexposure to ultraviolet radiation. Such lesions are a late and rare complication of excessive PUVA therapy in psoriatic patients in whom the genitalia were not covered during UVA-exposure.*

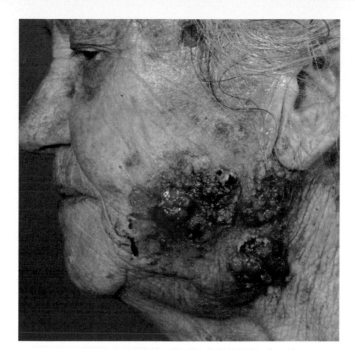

**FIGURE 11-10    Squamous cell carcinoma: invasive, poorly differentiated**    *Three large, ulcerated, fungating soft nodules that are friable and bleed easily. The submandibular swelling was due to lymph node metastasis.*

## BASAL CELL CARCINOMA    ■   ◑ → ●

BCC is the most common type of skin cancer. This malignant tumor is locally invasive, aggressive, and destructive, but there is a very limited capacity to metastasize. The reason for this is the tumor's growth dependency on its stroma, which on invasion of tumor cells into the vessels is not disseminated with the tumor cells. When tumor cells lodge at distant sites, they do not multiply and grow because of the absence of growth factors derived from their stroma. Exceptions occur when a BCC shows signs of dedifferentiation, for instance, after inadequate radiotherapy. BCC usually arises only from epidermis that has a capacity to develop (hair) follicles. Therefore, BCCs rarely occur on the vermilion border of the lips or on the genital mucous membranes.

### EPIDEMIOLOGY

**Age of Onset**   Older than 40 years.
**Sex**   Males > females.
**Incidence**   United States: 500 to 1000 per 100,000, higher in the sunbelt; >400,000 new patients annually.
**Race**   Rare in brown- and black-skinned persons.
**Predisposing Factors**   Skin phototypes I and II and albinos are highly susceptible to develop BCC with prolonged sun exposure. Also a history of heavy sun exposure in youth predisposes the skin to the development of BCC later in life. Previous therapy with x-rays for facial acne greatly increases the risk of BCC, even in those persons with a good ability to tan (skin phototypes III and IV). Superficial multicentric BCC occurs 30 to 40 years after ingestion of arsenic but also without apparent cause.

### PHYSICAL EXAMINATION

**Skin Lesions**
There are five clinical types: nodular, ulcerating, sclerosing (cicatricial), superficial, and pigmented.

- *Nodular BCC:* Papule or nodule, translucent or "pearly" (Fig. 11-11). Skin-colored or reddish, smooth surface with telangiectasia, well defined, firm (Figs. 11-11 and 11-12).
- *Ulcerating BCC:* Ulcer (often covered with a crust) with a rolled border (rodent ulcer), which again is translucent, pearly, smooth with telangiectasia, and firm (Figs. 11-12B and 11-13).
- *Sclerosing BCC:* Appears as a small patch of morphea or a superficial scar, often ill-defined, skin-colored, whitish but also with peppery pigmentation (Fig. 11-14). In this infiltrating

type of BCC there is an excessive amount of fibrous stroma. Histologically, finger-like strands of tumor extend far into the surrounding tissue, and excision therefore requires wide margins.
- *Superficial multicentric BCCs:* Appear as thin plaques (Figs. 11-15 and 11-16). Pink or red; characteristic fine threadlike border and telangiectasia can be seen with the aid of a hand lens. This is the only form of BCC that can exhibit a considerable amount of scaling.
- *Pigmented BCC:* May be brown to blue or black (Fig. 11-17). Smooth, glistening surface; hard, firm; may be indistinguishable from superficial spreading or nodular melanoma but is usually harder. *Cystic* lesions may occur: round, oval shape, depressed center ("umbilicated").

**Distribution**   Isolated single lesion; multiple lesions are not infrequent; >90% occur in the face (Image 11-2). Search carefully for "danger sites": medial and lateral canthi (Figs. 11-12C, 11-13A), nasolabial fold, behind the ears (Fig. 11-17). Superficial multicentric BCCs occur on the trunk (Fig. 11-16).

### LABORATORY EXAMINATION

**Dermatopathology**   Solid tumor consisting of proliferating atypical basal cells, large, oval, deep-blue staining on H&E, but with little anaplasia and infrequent mitoses; palisading arrangement at periphery; variable amounts of mucinous stroma.

### DIAGNOSIS AND DIFFERENTIAL DIAGNOSIS

Serious BCCs occurring in the danger sites [central part of the face (Fig. 11-13), behind the

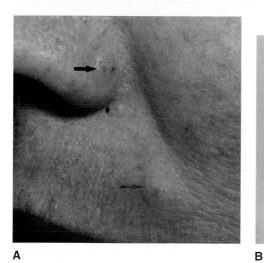

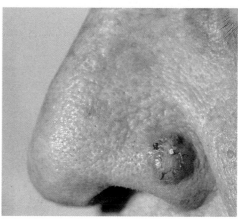

A                    B

**FIGURE 11-11   Basal cell carcinoma: nodular type**   *A. A small pearly papule (arrow) on the nostril and an even smaller one (small arrow) in the nasolabial fold. These are very early stages of BCC. The gray arrow denotes a dermal NMN. B. This is a farther advanced nodular BCC. A solitary, shiny, nodule with large telangiectatic vessels on the ala nasi, arising on skin with dermatoheliosis.*

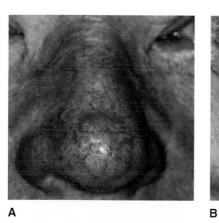

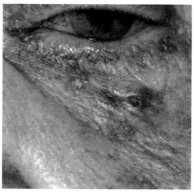

A                    B

C

**FIGURE 11-12   Basal cell carcinoma: nodular type**
*A. A glistening, smooth plaque on the tip of the nose with multiple telangiectasias. B. An oval, pearly nodule on the lower lid that starts to become erosive and will thus develop into a rodent ulcer. C. A smooth, pearly tumor with telangiectasia on the nose. Tumor feels hard, is well defined, and is asymptomatic.*

ears] are readily detectable by careful examination with good lighting, a hand lens, and careful palpation. Diagnosis is made clinically and confirmed microscopically. Differential diagnosis includes all smooth papules like dermal NMN, trichoepithelioma, dermatofibroma, and others; if pigmented, superficial spreading and nodular melanoma; if ulcerated, all nonpainful firm ulcers including SCC and a (extragenital) primary chancre of syphilis.

## MANAGEMENT

Excision with primary closure, skin flaps, or grafts. Cryosurgery and electrosurgery are options, but only for very small lesions and not in the danger sites or on the scalp.

For lesions in the danger sites (nasolabial area, around the eyes, in the ear canal, in the posterior auricular sulcus, in sclerosing BCC, and on the scalp), microscopically controlled surgery (Mohs surgery) is the best approach. Radiation therapy is an alternative only when disfigurement may be a problem with surgical excision (e.g., eyelids or large lesions in the nasolabial area) or in old age.

There are a variety of topical treatments that can be used for superficial BCCs but only for those tumors below the neck; *cryosurgery* is effective but leaves a white scar that remains for life. Electrocautery with curettage is also simple and effective, but it leaves scars. Topical 5-fluorouracil ointment and imiquimod cream (SBCC: 5 times a week for 6 weeks) are effective, do not cause scars, but require considerable time and may not radically remove all tumor tissue. Photodynamic therapy is effective but cumbersome, and radiation sessions (photodynamic dye + visible light) are painful.

## COURSE AND PROGNOSIS

BCC does not metastasize. Most lesions are readily controlled by various surgical techniques. Serious problems, however, may occur with BCC arising in the danger sites of the head. In these sites the tumor may invade deeply, cause extensive destruction of muscle and bone, and even invade to the dura mater. In such cases, death may result from hemorrhage of eroded large vessels or infection.

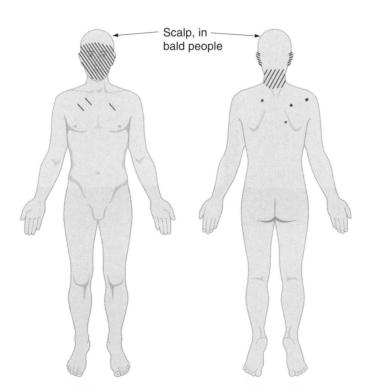

Scalp, in bald people

**IMAGE 11-2   Basal cell carcinoma:** *predilection sites. Dots indicate superficial multicentric BCCs.*

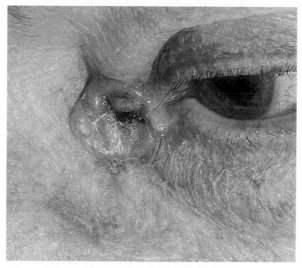

A

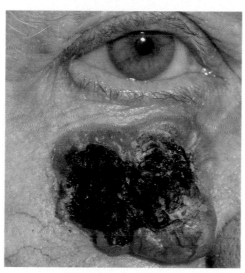

B

**FIGURE 11-13   Basal cell carcinoma in "danger" zone**   *A. Smooth, glistening, pearly tumor with telangiectasia. Basal cell carcinomas arising in the central area of the face, in the nasolabial folds, around the eye, and in the sulcus behind the ear ("danger zones") must be removed with Moh's surgery to prevent unmanageable recurrences, as these tumors move deeply along the fascial planes. B. Basal cell carcinoma: rodent-ulcer type. A large ulcer filled with black necrosis and hemorrhagic crusts is surrounded by a well-demarcated rolled border consisting of typical nodules of a BCC (translucency, teleangiectasia). It has destroyed almost the entire cheek.*

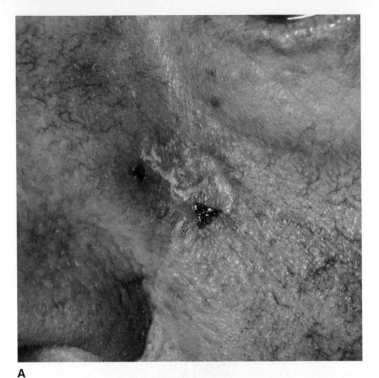

A

B

**FIGURE 11-14   Basal cell carcinoma: sclerosing type**   *A. A small inconspicuous area resembling a superficial scar, ill defined, with scaling and two tiny erosions covered by hemorrhagic crusts. Upon palpation, however, a platelike induration can be felt and this extends beyond the visible margins of the lesion. After verification of the diagnosis by biopsy will require excision with wide margins.* **B**. *A large depressed area resembling a scar or morphea; many small areas of pigmentation typical of BCC and telangiectasia are seen with the lesion, the lateral margin is slightly raised.*

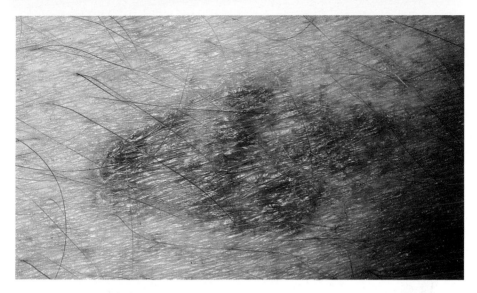

**FIGURE 11-15   Superficial basal cell carcinoma: solitary lesion**   *This bright red lesion has a slightly elevated rolled border that can be detected with "side lighting"; although this lesion is typical enough to be diagnosed clinically, a biopsy is necessary to verify the diagnosis.*

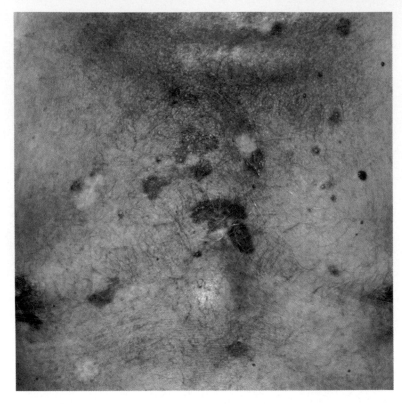

**FIGURE 11-16   Multiple superficial basal cell carcinomas**   *Many superficial basal cell carcinomas on the trunk. They appear as brightly erythematous, often scaling, flat lesions often without a rolled border. The hypopigmented areas represent superficial scars after cryotherapy of superficial BCCs.*

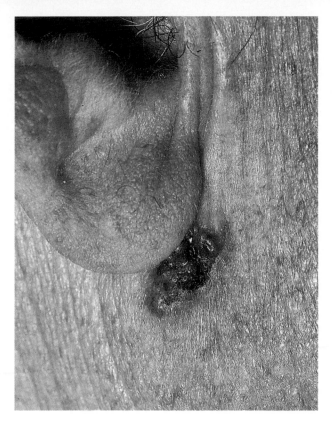

**FIGURE 11-17 Basal cell carcinoma, pigmented** *A nodule with irregular borders and variegation of melanin hues, easily confused with a malignant melanoma. Features indicating BCC are the areas of translucency and surface telangiectasia.*

## BASAL CELL NEVUS SYNDROME (BCNS)

*Synonyms*: Gorlin's syndrome, nevoid basal cell carcinoma syndrome.

This autosomal dominant disorder is caused by mutations in the patched gene that resides on chromosome 9q (9q22). It affects skin with multiple BCCs and so-called palmoplantar pits and has a variable expression of abnormalities in a number of systems, including skeletal malformations, soft tissue, eyes, CNS, and endocrine organs. The frequency is not known, but the condition is rare. BCCs may begin in late childhood, although several abnormalities are congenital. The syndrome occurs mostly in whites but also in African Americans and Asians, and there is an equal sex incidence. BCCs begin singly in childhood or early adolescence and continue throughout life. There are more BCCs on the sun-exposed areas of the skin, but they also occur in covered areas and there may be hundreds of lesions. Characteristic general features are frontal bossing, a broad nasal root, and hypertelorism. A systems review may reveal congenital anomalies including undescended testes and hydrocephalus. Other *extracutaneous lesions* are mandibular jaw odontogenic keratocysts, which may be multiple and may be unilateral or bilateral. There may be defective dentition, bifid or splayed ribs, pectus excavatum, short fourth metacarpals, scoliosis, and kyphosis. Eye lesions include strabismus, hypertelorism, dystopia canthorum, cataracts, glaucoma, and coloboma with blindness. There may be agenesis of the corpus callosum, medulloblastoma, and calcification of the falx. Mental retardation is rare, however. Fibrosarcoma of the jaw, ovarian fibromas, teratomas, and cystadenomas have been reported.

*Skin lesions* are small, pinpoint to larger nodular BCCs (Fig. 11-18), but "regular," nodular, ulcerating, and sclerosing BCCs also occur. Tumors on the eyelids, axillae, and neck tend to be pedunculated and are often symmetric on the face. There are characteristic palmoplantar lesions, which are present in 50% and are small pits that are pinpoint to several millimeters in size and 1 mm deep (Fig. 11-19).

The significance of the syndrome is that a large number of skin cancers create a lifetime problem of vigilance. The multiple excisions can cause a considerable amount of scarring. The tumors continue throughout life, and the patient must be followed carefully.

---

## MALIGNANT APPENDAGE TUMORS

---

Carcinomas of the eccrine sweat gland are rare and include eccrine porocarcinoma, syringoid eccrine carcinoma, mucinous carcinoma, and clear cell eccrine carcinoma. Carcinomas of the apocrine glands are rare, arising in axillae, nipples, vulva, and eyelids. Carcinomas of the sebaceous glands are equally rare, most commonly arising on the eyelids. These lesions are clinically indistinguishable from other carcinomas. They are usually more aggressive than other invasive cutaneous SCCs.

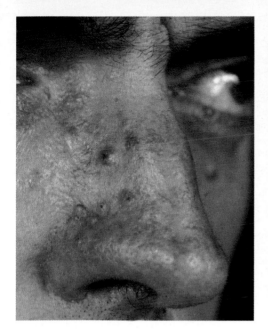

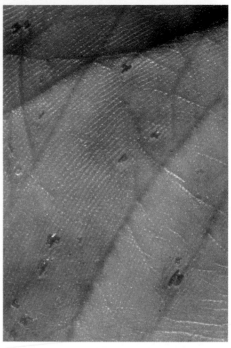

**FIGURE 11-18 Basal cell nevus syndrome: small basal cell carcinomas** *Multiple nodular BCCs on the right side of the nose; there were similar lesions on cheeks and forehead. This patient also had frontal bossing and odonto-genic cysts.*

**FIGURE 11-19 Basal cell nevus syndrome: palmar pits** *Palmar surface of hand showing 1- to 2-mm, sharply marginated, depressed lesions, i.e., palmar pits.*

## MERKEL CELL CARCINOMA     ☐  ●

Merkel cell carcinoma (MCC) (cutaneous neuroendocrine tumor) is a rare malignant solid tumor thought to be derived from a specialized epithelial cell, the Merkel cell. It is a nonkeratizing, "clear" cell present in the basal cell layer of the epidermis, free in the dermis, and around hair follicles as the hair disk of Pinkus. The etiology is unknown but may be related to chronic UVR damage. The tumor may be solitary or multiple and occurs on the head and on the extremities. There is a high rate of recurrence following excision, but, more important, it spreads to the regional lymph nodes in >50% of patients and is disseminated to the viscera and CNS.

MCC presents as a cutaneous to subcutaneous papule, nodule, or tumor (0.5 to 5 cm) (Figs. 11-20 and 11-21), which is pink, red to violet or reddish-brown, dome-shaped, and usually solitary. The overlying skin is intact, but larger lesions may ulcerate. They grow rapidly and usually occur in persons >50 years. Dermatopathology shows nodular or diffuse patterns of aggregated, deeply blue staining, small basaloid or lymphoma-like-looking cells that can also be arranged in sheets forming nests, cords, and trabeculae. Immunocytochemistry shows cytokeratin and neurofilament markers, chromogranin A, and neuron-specific enolase; electron microscopy reveals the characteristic organelles. Treatment is by excision or Moh's surgery, and sentinel node biopsy or prophylactic regional node dissection is advocated because of the high rate of regional metastases. Recurrence rates are high; in one series, even without a local recurrence, about 60% of patients developed regional node metastases, as did 86% of those patients with a local recurrence. Prognosis is guarded.

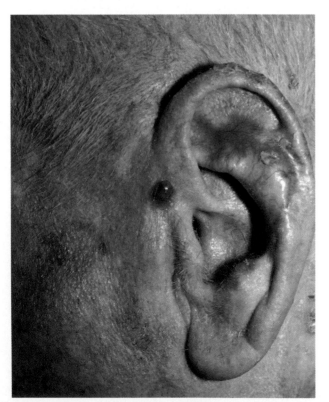

**FIGURE 11-20   Merkel cell carcinoma**   *A small violaceous nodule above the pinna that had been present for about 2 weeks. Sentinel lymph node biopsy revealed metastasis of neuroendocrine carcinoma. Also note actinic keratoses on the helix and concha.*

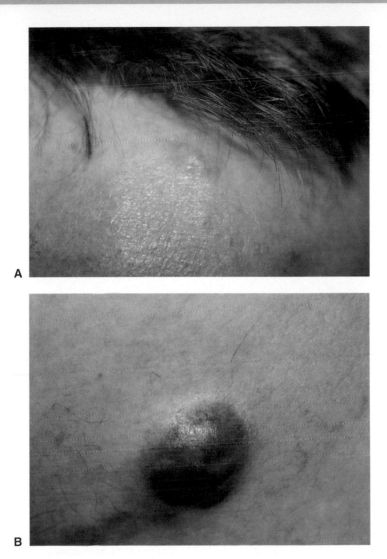

**FIGURE 11-21   Merkel cell carcinoma**   *A. A barely noticeable 6-mm slightly dermal nodule below the hairline that had been present for about 6 weeks. Preauricular lymph node metastasis was also present. **B.** A violaceous dermal nodule, 3 cm in diameter on the forearm of a 60-year-old man. There was metastasis to the axillary lymph nodes.*

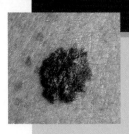

# MELANOMA PRECURSORS AND PRIMARY CUTANEOUS MELANOMA

## PRECURSORS OF CUTANEOUS MELANOMA

Precursors of melanoma are lesions that are benign per se but have the potential of turning malignant and thus giving rise to melanoma. Two such entities are recognized: (1) atypical nevomelanocytic nevi, and (2) congenital nevomelanocytic nevi.

## ATYPICAL MELANOCYTIC NEVUS (DYSPLASTIC NEVUS; CLARK'S NEVUS)   ■   ◑

Atypical melanocytic nevi (AMN) are a special type of acquired, circumscribed, pigmented lesions that represent disordered proliferations of variably atypical melanocytes. AMN arise de novo or as part of a compound melanocytic nevus. AMN are clinically distinctive from common acquired nevi: larger and more variegated in color, asymmetric in outline, irregular borders; they also have characteristic histologic features. AMN are regarded as potential precursors of superficial spreading melanoma and also as markers of persons at risk for developing primary malignant melanoma of the skin, either within the AMN or on "normal" skin. They occur either sporadically or in the context of the *familial AMN syndrome*: kindreds with familial multiple atypical melanocytic nevi and melanomas (formerly FAMMM, or B-K mole syndrome).

### EPIDEMIOLOGY

**Age of Onset**   Children and adults.
**Prevalence**   AMN are present in 5% of the general white population. They occur in almost every patient with familial cutaneous melanoma and in 30 to 50% of patients with sporadic nonfamilial primary melanomas of the skin.
**Sex**   Equal in males and females.
**Race**   White persons. Data on persons with brown or black skin are not available; AMN are rarely seen in the Japanese population.
**Transmission**   Autosomal dominant.

### PATHOGENESIS

Multiple loci, including 1p36 and 9p21, have been implicated in familial melanoma/AMN syndrome. The abnormal clone of melanocytes can be activated by exposure to sunlight. Immuno-suppressed patients (renal transplantation) with AMN have a higher incidence of melanoma. AMN favor the exposed areas of the skin, and this may be related to the degree of sun exposure.

### HISTORY

**Duration of Lesions**   AMN usually arise later in childhood than common acquired nevomelanocytic nevi (NMN), appearing first in late childhood, just before puberty. New lesions continue to develop over many years in affected persons; in contrast, common acquired NMN do not appear after middle age and disappear entirely in older persons. AMN are thought not to undergo spontaneous regression at all or at least much less than common acquired NMN.
**Precipitating Factors**   Exposure to sunlight is regarded by some as an inducing agent for AMN; nevertheless, AMN are not infrequently

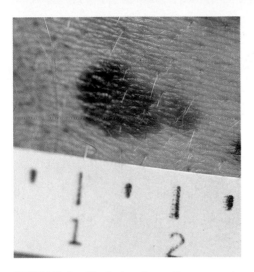

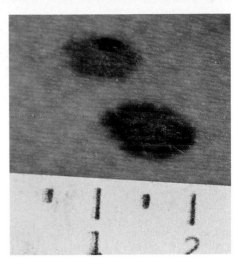

**FIGURE 12-1   Atypical melanocytic nevus**   *A large (1.2 cm), variegated, brown macule with a slightly raised area (10 o'clock), fuzzy margins, and oval but asymmetrical shape.*

**FIGURE 12-2   Atypical melanocytic nevi**   *Two large, variegated, brown very flat oval papules. Note notched border in the lower and eccentric dark brown color in the upper one.*

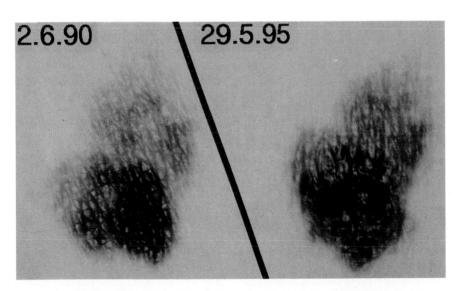

**FIGURE 12-3   Melanoma in situ: evolving in AMN**   *(Left) Image (2 June 1990) variegation of pigmentation and irregular borders. Five years later (29 May 1995), the lesion (right) shows darkening of melanin pigmentation, more irregularity in shape, and elevation in the most darkly pigmented region. Histologically, the lesion showed AMN evolving into melanoma in situ. Evolution of atypical nevi into in situ and/or invasive melanoma can occur within a period of months or many years.*

observed in completely covered areas such as the scalp and anogenital areas.

**Skin Symptoms**   Asymptomatic.

**Family History**   In the familial setting, family members can develop melanoma without the presence of AMN.

## PHYSICAL EXAMINATION

AMN show some of the features of common NMN and some of superficial spreading melanoma, so that they occupy an intermediary position between these two morphologies (Table 12-1). No single feature is diagnostic; rather, there is a constellation of findings. They are more irregular, lighter than common NMN, usually maculopapular, have distinct *and* indistinct borders (Figs. 12-1 and 12-2), and a greater complexity of color than common nevi (Figs. 12-1 and 12-2) but less than melanoma. "Fried-egg" and "targeted" types (see Table 12-1). Melanoma arising in an AMN appears initially as a small papule (often of a different color) or change in color pattern (Fig. 12-3) and massive color change within the precursor lesion (Fig. 12-4).

**Dermoscopy (Epiluminescence microscopy)** This noninvasive technique allows for clinical improvement of diagnostic accuracy in AMN by >50%. *Digital dermoscopy* permits computerized follow-up of lesions and immediate detection of any change over time, indicating developing malignancy.

## LABORATORY EXAMINATION

**Dermatopathology**   Hyperplasia and proliferation of melanocytes in a single-file, "lentiginous" pattern in the basal cell layer either as spindle cells or as epithelioid cells and as irregular and dyshesive nests. "Atypical" melanocytes, "bridging" between rete ridges by melanocytic nests; spindle-shaped melanocytes oriented parallel to skin surface. Lamellar fibroplasia and concentric eosinophilic fibrosis (not a constant feature). Histologic atypia do not always correlate with clinical atypia. AMN may arise in contiguity with a compound NMN (rarely, a junctional nevus) that is centrally located, i.e., AMN often have extension of intraepidermal melanocytic hyperplasia beyond the shoulder of the dermal nevus component; some AMN may not have a dermal nevus component.

## DIAGNOSIS AND DIFFERENTIAL DIAGNOSIS

The diagnosis of AMN is made by clinical recognition of typical distinctive lesions (see Table 12-1), and diagnostic accuracy is considerably improved by dermoscopy. The clinicopathologic correlations are now well documented. Siblings, children, and parents should also be examined for AMN once the diagnosis is established in a family member.

**Differential Diagnosis**   Congenital NMN, common acquired NMN, superficial spreading malignant melanoma, melanoma in situ, lentigo maligna, Spitz nevus, pigmented basal cell carcinoma.

**Association with Melanoma**   AMN are regarded as markers for persons at risk for melanoma and as precursors of superficial spreading melanoma. Anatomic association (in contiguity) of AMN has been observed in 36% of sporadic primary melanomas, in about 70% of familial primary melanomas, and in 94% of melanomas with familial melanoma and AMN.

**Lifetime Risks of Developing Primary Malignant Melanoma**

General population: 1.2%

Familial AMN syndrome with *two* blood relatives with melanoma: 100%

All other patients with AMN: 18%

The presence of *one* AMN doubles the risk for development of melanoma; with ≥10 AMN, the risk increases 12-fold.

## MANAGEMENT

Surgical excision of lesions with narrow margins. Laser or other types of physical destruction should *never* be used because they do not permit histopathologic verification of diagnosis. The following guidelines for selection of lesions to be excised are suggested:

- Lesions that are changing (increase in size, change in pigmentation pattern, changes in shape and/or border); decision is best and most reliably made by digital dermoscopy.
- Lesions that cannot be closely followed by the patient by self-examination (on the scalp, genitalia, upper back).

Patients with AMN in the familial melanoma setting need to be followed carefully: in familial AMN, every 3 months; in sporadic AMN, every 6 months to 1 year. Search for changes in existing AMN and development of new nevi. Photographic follow-up is important, with Polaroid prints of the trunk and extremities; also Polaroid prints (1:1) of larger lesions (>6 mm) and all lesions that have some variegation. Most reliable method is digitalized dermoscopy, which should be available in every pigmented lesion and melanoma center. Patients should be

**TABLE 12-1   Comparative Features of Common Nevomelanocytic Nevi (NMN), Atypical Melanocytic Nevi (AMN), and Superficial Spreading Melanoma (SSM)**

| Lesion | NMN (Figs. 9-1, 9-2) | AMN (Figs. 12-1, 12-2) | SSM (Figs. 12-12→12-18) |
|---|---|---|---|
| Number | Several or many | One or many | Single (1–2% have multiple) |
| Distribution | Mostly trunk, extremities | Mostly trunk, extremities | Anywhere but predominant upper back, legs |
| Onset | Childhood, adolescence | Early adolescence | Any age, most in adulthood |
| Type | Macules (junctional) Papules (compound, dermal) | Macules with raised portions (asymmetrically, maculopapular) | Plaque, irregular |
| A Asymmetry | Symmetry | Asymmetry | Greater asymmetry |
| B Border | Regular, well-defined | Irregular, ill- and well-defined | Irregular, well-defined |
| C Color | Tan, brown, dark brown, uniform, orderly pattern | Tan, brown, dark brown, pink, red, not uniform, variegated pattern, "fried egg," "targetoid" | Tan, brown, dark brown, black, pink, red, blue, white, usually a mix, highly variegated, spotted, speckled pattern |
| D Diameter | <5 mm, rarely <10 mm | Up to 15 mm | Most >5 mm (but, of course, starts smaller) |
| E Enlargement | Stops in adolescence | Continues in adulthood but limited | Growth in size at any age, unlimited |

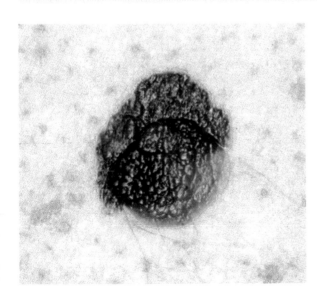

**FIGURE 12-4   Superficial spreading melanoma: arising within an atypical melanocytic nevus**   *The upper dark brown portion with a pinkish rim of this lesion is an atypical nevus; the variegated blue-black and pink plaque in the lower half of the lesion is the superficial spreading melanoma (0.9-mm thickness) arising within the atypical nevus.*

given color-illustrated pamphlets that depict the clinical appearance of AMN, malignant melanoma, and common acquired NMN. Patients with AMN (familial and nonfamilial) should not sunbathe and should use sunscreens when outdoors. They should not use tanning parlors. Family members of the patient should also be examined regularly.

## CONGENITAL NEVOMELANOCYTIC NEVUS   ■ → ▢*   ◐

Congenital nevomelanocytic nevi (CNMN) are pigmented lesions of the skin usually present at birth; rare varieties of CNMN can develop and become clinically apparent during infancy. CNMN may be any size from very small to very large. CNMN are benign nevomelanocytic neoplasms; but all CNMN, regardless of size, may be precursors of malignant melanoma.

## EPIDEMIOLOGY

**Prevalence**   Present in 1% of white newborns; the majority <3 cm in diameter. Larger CNMN are present in 1:2000 to 1:20,000 newborns. Lesions ≥9.9 cm in diameter have a prevalence of 1:20,000, and giant CNMN (occupying a major portion of a major anatomic site) occur in 1:500,000 newborns.

**Age of Onset**   Present at birth (congenital). Some CNMN become visible only after birth (*tardive*), "fading in" as a relatively large lesion over a period of weeks.

**Sex**   Equal prevalence in males and females.

**Race**   All races.

## PATHOGENESIS

Congenital and acquired nevomelanocytic nevi are presumed to occur as the result of a developmental defect in neural crest-derived melanoblasts. This defect probably occurs after 10 weeks in utero but before the sixth uterine month; the occurrence of the "split" nevus of the eyelid (Fig. 12-5) is an indication that nevomelanocytes migrating from the neural crest were in place in this site before the eyelids split (24 weeks).

## PHYSICAL EXAMINATION

### Small and Large CNMN

CNMN have a rather wide range of clinical features, but the following are typical (Figs. 12-5 to 12-7): CNMN usually distort the skin surface to some degree and are therefore a plaque with or without coarse terminal dark brown or black hairs (hair growth has a delayed onset). Sharply demarcated or merging imperceptibly with surrounding skin (Fig. 12-6); regular or irregular contours. Large lesions may be "wormy" or soft (Fig. 12-7), rarely firm (desmoplastic type). Skin surface smooth or "pebbly," mamillated, rugose, cerebriform, bulbous, tuberous, or lob-

ular (Fig. 12-7). These surface changes are observed more frequently in lesions that extend deep into the reticular dermis.

**Color**   Light or dark brown. With dermoscopy a fine speckling of a darker hue with a lighter surrounding brown hue is seen; often the pigmentation is follicular. "Halo" CNMN (see Fig. 9-5) are rare.

**Size**   Small (Fig. 12-5), large (>20 cm) (Fig. 12-6), or giant (Fig. 12-7). "Acquired" nevomelanocytic nevi >1.5 cm in diameter should be regarded as probably tardive CNMN or they represent AMN.

**Shape**   Oval or round.

**Distribution of Lesions**   Isolated, discrete lesion in any site (Figs. 12-5 and 12-6). Fewer than 5% of CNMN are multiple. Multiple lesions are more common in association with large CNMN. Numerous small CNMN occur in patients with giant CNMN, in whom there may be numerous small CNMN on the trunk and extremities away from the site of the giant CNMN (Fig. 12-7).

### Very Large ("Giant") CNMN (Fig. 12-7)

Giant CNMN of the head and neck may be associated with involvement of the leptomeninges with the same pathologic process; this presentation may be asymptomatic or manifested by seizures, focal neurologic defects, or obstructive hydrocephalus. Giant CNMN is usually a plaque with surface distortion, covering entire segments of the trunk, extremities, head, or neck.

### Melanoma in CNMN

A papule or nodule arises within CNMN (Fig. 12-8). Often melanoma arises in dermal or subcutaneous nevomelanocytes and can be far advanced when detected.

## DIFFERENTIAL DIAGNOSIS

Common acquired NMN, AMN, congenital blue nevus, nevus spilus, Becker's nevus, pigmented epidermal nevi, and café-au-lait macules should be considered in the differential diagnosis of CNMN. Small CNMN are virtually indistinguishable clinically from common

---

* Giant CNMC are rare.

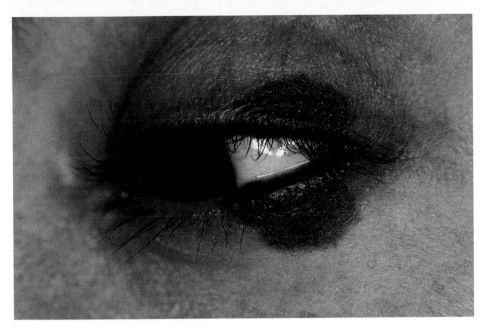

**FIGURE 12-5 Congenital nevomelanocytic nevus; "split" of the eyelid** *A sharply demarcated, brown plaque, involving the upper and lower eyelids in a 45-year-old Asian female. Nevomelanocytes migrate from the neural crest to the skin after the 10th week in utero but before 24 weeks when splitting of eyelids occurs.*

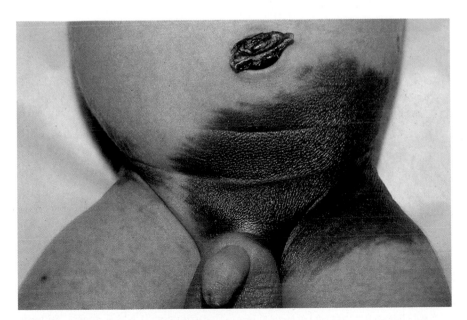

**FIGURE 12-6 Congenital nevomelanocytic nevus, large** *Sharply demarcated chocolate-brown hairless plaque with smudged borders in a newborn. With increasing age, lesions usually become elevated and hairy.*

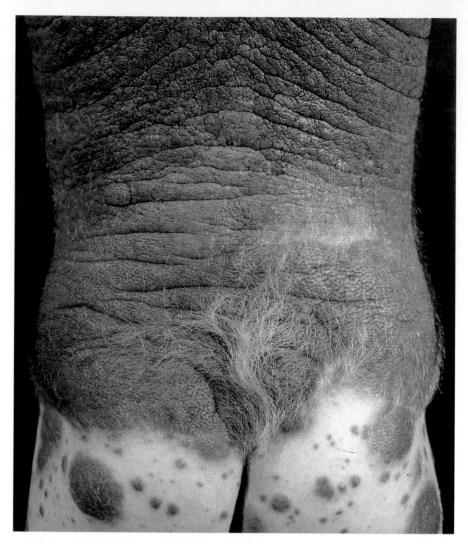

**FIGURE 12-7    Congenital nevomelanocytic nevus, giant**    *The lesion involves the majority of the skin, with complete replacement of normal skin on the back and multiple smaller CNMN on the buttocks and thighs. Note hypertrichosis of the sacral area. Melanoma developing in a giant CNMN is difficult to diagnose early in a setting of such highly abnormal tissue.*

acquired NMN except for size, and lesions >1.5 cm may be presumed to be either tardive CNMN or AMN.

## LABORATORY EXAMINATION

**Histopathology**    Nevomelanocytes occur as well-ordered clusters (*theques*) in the epidermis and in the dermis as sheets, nests, or cords. *A diffuse infiltration of strands of nevomelanocytes in the lower one-third of the reticular*

*dermis and subcutis is, when present, quite specific for CNMN.* In large and giant CNMN, the nevomelanocytes may extend into the muscle, bone, dura mater, and cranium.

## COURSE AND PROGNOSIS

By definition, CNMN appear at birth, but CNMN may arise during infancy (*tardive CNMN*). The life history of CNMN is not documented, but CNMN have been observed in

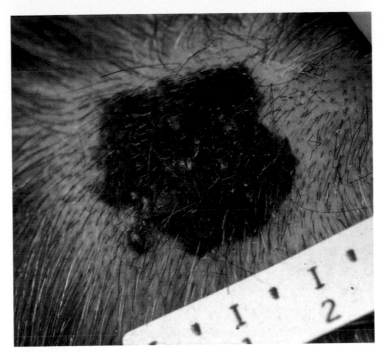

**FIGURE 12-8   Melanoma: arising in small CNMN**   *A black plaque on the scalp with irregular outlines. Note bulblike extension of the margin at 7 o'clock. This lesion had always been almost black since childhood and it was the increase in size and irregularity that alarmed this 36-year-old white female and prompted her to see a dermatologist.*

elderly persons, an age when the common acquired NMN have disappeared.

*Large or giant CNMN*: The lifetime risk for development of melanoma in large CNMN has been estimated to be at least 6.3%. In 50% of patients who develop melanoma in large CNMN, the diagnosis is made between the ages of 3 and 5 years. Melanoma that develops in a large CNMN has a poor prognosis because it is detected late.

*Small CNMN*: The lifetime risk of developing malignant melanoma is 1 to 5%. Based on the detection of congenital nevi in association with melanoma by means of histology and a careful history, a significantly increased risk is apparent for developing melanoma in persons with small CNMN. This risk is as high as 21-fold based on history and 3- to 10-fold based on histology. The expected association of small CNMN and melanoma is <1:171,000 based on chance alone. Nonetheless, small CNMN should be considered for prophylactic excision at puberty if there are no atypical features (variegated color and irregular borders); small CNMN with atypical features should be excised immediately.

## MANAGEMENT

**Surgical Excision**   The only acceptable method. *Small and large CNMN*: Excision, with full-thickness skin graft, if required; swing flaps, tissue expanders for large lesions. *Giant CNMN*: Risk of development of melanoma is significant even in the first 3 to 5 years of age, and thus giant CNMN should be removed as soon as possible. Individual considerations are necessary (size, location, degree of loss of function, or amount of mutilation). New surgical techniques utilizing the patient's own normal skin grown in tissue culture can now be used to facilitate removal of very large CNMN. Also, tissue expanders can be used.

## CUTANEOUS MELANOMA ■ ●

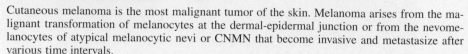

Cutaneous melanoma is the most malignant tumor of the skin. Melanoma arises from the malignant transformation of melanocytes at the dermal-epidermal junction or from the nevomelanocytes of atypical melanocytic nevi or CNMN that become invasive and metastasize after various time intervals.

### CLASSIFICATION OF MELANOMA

I. De novo melanoma
  A. Melanoma in situ (MIS)
  B. Lentigo maligna melanoma (LMM)
  C. Superficial spreading melanoma (SSM)
  D. Nodular melanoma (NM)
  E. Acral-lentiginous melanoma (ALM)
  F. Melanoma of the mucous membranes
  G. Desmoplastic melanoma

II. Melanoma arising from precursors
  A. Melanoma arising in atypical nevo-melanocytic nevi
  B. Melanoma arising in congenital nevo-melanocytic nevi

### FOUR IMPORTANT MESSAGES CONCERNING CUTANEOUS MELANOMA

#### 1. Melanoma of the Skin Is Approaching Epidemic Proportions

Melanoma is a common malignancy and its incidence is on the rise. In the United States the lifetime risk of invasive melanoma developing was only 1 in 1500 in 1935; in 1992 it was 1 in 105, in 2002 it was 1 in 75, and in 2010 it is estimated that it will be 1 in 50. In 2002 melanomas developed in about 88,000 Americans. Cutaneous melanoma currently represents 5% of newly diagnosed cancer in men. It is the leading fatal illness arising in the skin. In 2002 there were 7500 deaths due to melanoma in the United States, and U.S. cancer statistics show that melanoma had the second highest mortality rate increase among men ≥65 years old. On the other hand, deaths from melanoma occur at a younger age than deaths from most other cancers, and melanoma is among the most common types of cancer in young adults.

#### 2. Early Recognition and Excision of Primary Melanoma = Virtual Cure

Current cutaneous melanoma education stresses the detection of early melanoma, with high cure rates after surgical excision. Of all the cancers, melanoma of the skin is the most rewarding for detection of early curable primary tumors, thereby preventing metastatic disease and death. Early accessability to physicians is especially important because curability is directly related to size and depth of invasion of the tumor. At the present time, the most critical tool for conquering this disease is, therefore, the identification of early "thin" melanomas by clinical examination. Total skin examination for melanoma and its precursors should be done routinely.

About 30% of melanomas arise in a preexisting melanocytic lesion; 70% arise in normal skin. Almost all melanomas show an initial radial growth phase followed by a subsequent vertical growth phase. Since metastasis occurs only infrequently during the radial growth phase, detection of early melanomas (i.e., "thin" melanomas) during this phase is essential.

There is the paradox that even with a rising mortality rate, there has been an encouraging improvement in the overall prognosis of melanoma with very high 5-year survival rates (approaching 98%) for thin (<0.75 mm) primary melanoma and an 83% rate for all stages. The favorable prognosis is entirely attributable to early detection.

#### 3. All Physicians and Nurses Have the Responsibility of Detecting Early Melanoma

Early detection of primary melanoma assures increased survival; advanced primary melanoma has a poor prognosis and survival. The survival rate plummets when there is regional metastasis to lymph nodes. The seriousness of this disease thus places the responsibility on the health care provider in the pivotal role: not to overlook pigmented lesions. This is especially true for the primary care physician, the nurse, the physical therapist, or a health care provider who sees the total skin of the body. Therefore, it is recommended that in clinical practice, no matter what is the presenting complaint, total examination of the body

TABLE 12-2    Fitzpatrick's MMRISK

A mnemonic device for promoting melanoma risk awareness among physicians and patients. Each
letter represents one of the major risk factors for melanoma of the skin.

M    Moles: atypical (atypical nevus) (>5)
M    Moles: common moles (numerous, >50)
R    Red hair and freckling (often these persons have few or no moles)
I    Inability to tan: skin phototypes I and II
S    Sunburn: severe sunburn especially before age 14
K    Kindred: family history of melanoma

should be requested of all nonpigmented (i.e.,
white) patients at the time of the first encounter
and that all body regions, including the scalp,
toewebs, and orifices (mouth, anus, vulva), be
examined. It is helpful to question patients
according to a mnemonic list of melanoma risk
(Table 12-2).

### 4. Examination of All Acquired Pigmented Lesions According to the ABCDE Rule

This rule analyzes pigmented lesions according
to symmetry, border, color, diameter, growth
and elevation (see page 304). While it does not
apply to all types of melanoma it permits differential diagnostic separation of most
melanomas from common nevi and other pigmented lesions.

### ETIOLOGY AND PATHOGENESIS

The etiology and pathogenesis of cutaneous
melanoma are unknown. Epidemiologic studies
demonstrate a role for genetic predisposition
and sun exposure in melanoma development.
The major gene involved in melanoma development resides on chromosome 9p21. This gene,
known as CDKN2A, encodes two separate gene

products that are negative regulators of cell
cycle progression.

There is convincing evidence from epidemiologic studies that exposure to solar radiation is
the major cause of cutaneous melanoma. Cutaneous melanoma is a greater problem in light-
skinned whites (skin types I and II), and
sunburns during childhood and intermittent
burning exposure in unclimatized fair skin
seem to have a higher impact than cumulative
UV exposure over time. Other predisposing and
risk factors are the presence of precursor lesions (atypical melanocytic nevi and congenital
nevomelanocytic nevi) and a family history of
melanoma in parents, children or siblings. Risk
factors for melanoma are listed in Table 12-3.

### MELANOMA GROWTH PATTERNS

Almost all melanomas show an initial radial
growth phase followed by a subsequent vertical
growth phase. *Radial growth phase* refers to a
mostly intraepidermal, preinvasive, or minimally
invasive growth pattern; *vertical growth* refers to
growth into the dermis and thus into the vicinity
of vessels that serve as avenues for metastasis.
Since most melanomas produce melanin

TABLE 12-3    Risk Factors for the Development of Melanoma

• Genetic markers (CDKN2a mutation)
• Skin type I/II
• Family history of atypical nevi or melanoma
• Personal history of melanoma
• Ultraviolet irradiation, particularly sunburns during childhood and intermittent
  burning exposures
• Number (>50) and size (>5 mm) of melanocytic nevi
• Congenital nevi
• Number of atypical nevi (>5)
• Atypical melanocytic nevus syndrome

pigment, even preinvasive melanomas in their radial growth phase are clinically detectable by their color patterns. The prognostic difference among the clinical types of melanoma relates mainly to the duration of the radial growth phase, which may last from years to decades in lentigo maligna melanoma, from months to 2 years in superficial spreading melanoma, and 6 months or less in nodular melanoma.

## DATA AND FACTS[1]

- Melanoma represents 5% of all cancers by incidence in males and 4% in females.
- Number of new cases in the United States in 2004: invasive melanoma: 55,000
- U.S. lifetime risk of developing invasive melanoma: 2000:1/75; 2010:1/50.
- New melanoma deaths in United States, 2004: 7900.
- Most frequent sites (see Image 12-1)
  Whites
    Male: back, upper extremities.
    Female: back, lower legs.
  Blacks and Asians: soles, mucous membranes, palms, nail beds.

- Frequency of melanoma by type of tumor: superficial spreading melanoma: 70%; nodular melanoma: 15%; lentigo maligna melanoma: 5%; acral and unclassified melanoma: 10%.

## MELANOMA RECOGNITION

### Six Signs of Malignant Melanoma (ABCDE Rule)

A  *Asymmetry* in shape—one-half unlike the other half.

B  *Border* is irregular—edges irregularly scalloped, notched, sharply defined.

C  *Color* is not uniform; mottled—haphazard display of colors; all shades of brown, black, gray, red, and white.

D  *Diameter* is usually large—greater than the tip of a pencil eraser (6.0 mm).

E  *Elevation* is almost always present and is irregular—surface distortion is assessed by side-lighting. Melanoma in situ and acral lentiginous lesions initially flat.

*Enlargement*—a history of an increase in the size of lesion is one of the most important signs of malignant melanoma.

[1] Adapted from RGB Langley et al, in IM Freedberg, AZ Eisen, K Wolff, KF Austen, LA Goldsmith, SI Katz (eds): *Fitzpatrick's Dermatology in General Medicine*, 6th ed. New York, McGraw-Hill, 2003, p. 917.

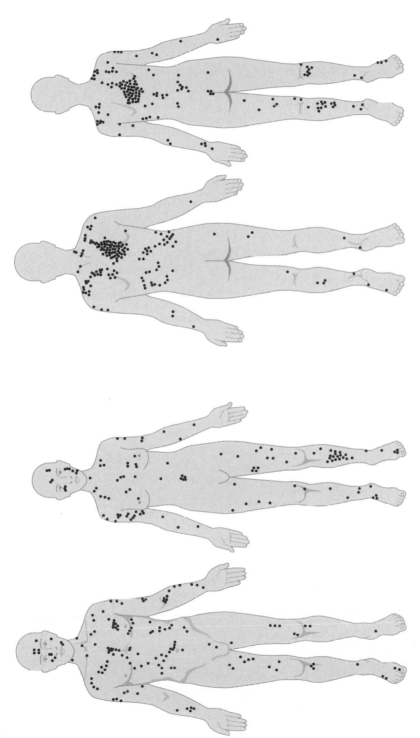

**IMAGE 12-1** *Localization of malignant melanoma in 731 males and females.*

## CLINICAL PRESENTATIONS OF MELANOMA

The clinical characteristics of the four major types of melanoma are summarized in Table 12-4. Also discussed in this section are melanoma in situ and desmoplastic melanoma.

### MELANOMA IN SITU (MIS)

The clinical features of MIS are not always clearly presented. MIS is primarily a histopathologic definition, and the term is used when melanoma cells are confined to the epidermis, above the basement membrane, and basilar melanocytic atypia, hyperplasia, and spread either occur in single-file alignment along the basal membrane or are distributed throughout the epidermis (pagetoid spread). Every melanoma starts as an in situ lesion, but MIS is clinically diagnosable only when the radial growth phase is long enough for it to become visually detectable. Such lesions are flat, within the level of the skin, and thus a *macule* (Fig. 12-9) or a macule with barely perceptible elevation (Fig. 12-11), with irregular borders and marked variegation of color: brown, dark brown, and black (Figs. 12-9 and 12-11A) or reddish tones (Fig. 12-11B) but without gray or blue, as this occurs only when melanin (within macrophages) or melanocytes are located in the dermis. The clinical distinction between melanoma in situ and severely atypical dysplastic nevi may be not be possible. Most life insurance companies at the present time do not regard this lesion as a malignancy, but it definitely is.

The clinical correlations of MIS are *lentigo maligna* (Fig. 12-9) and flat *superficial spreading melanoma* (Figs. 12-11A and B) and these are discussed in the respective sections below.

### LENTIGO MALIGNA MELANOMA (LMM)

Although LMM is the least common (<5%) of the three principal melanomas of white persons [superficial spreading melanoma (SSM), nodular melanoma (NM), and LMM], it is discussed first because it most clearly reveals the transition from the radial to the vertical growth phase and from a clinically recognizable MIS to invasive melanoma (Image 12-2). It occurs in older persons on the most sun-exposed areas—the face and forearms. Although there is still some debate about the role of sunlight in the pathogenesis of malignant melanoma, few question the role of sunlight in the pathogenesis of LMM; LMM always starts as *lentigo maligna* (LM), which represents a *flat* (macular) intraepidermal neoplasm and is an MIS (Fig. 12-9 and Image 12-2). LM is thus not a precursor but an evolving lesion of melanoma. Focal papular and nodular areas signal a switch from the radial to the vertical growth phase and thus invasion into the dermis; the lesion is now called LMM (Fig. 12-10 and Image 12-2). For the most important clinical characteristics, see Table 12-4.

**TABLE 12-4    Four Major Types of Melanoma**

| Type | Frequency, % | Site | Radial Growth | Vertical Growth |
|---|---|---|---|---|
| Superficial spreading | 70 | Any site, lower extremities, trunk | Months to 2 years | Delayed |
| Nodular | 15 | Any site, trunk, head, neck | No radial growth | Immediate |
| Lentigo maligna melanoma | 5 | Face, neck, dorsa of hands | Years | Much delayed |
| Acral lentiginous melanoma | 5–10 | Palms, soles, subungual | Months to years | Early but recognition delayed |

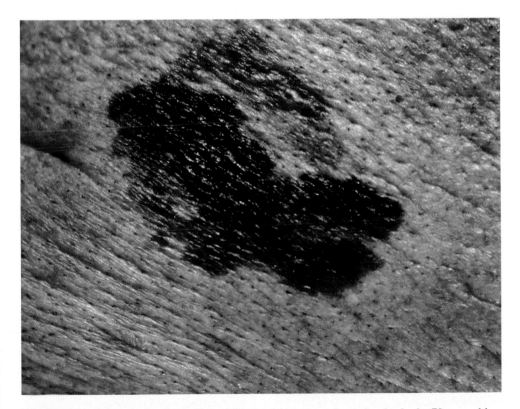

**FIGURE 12-9    Melanoma in situ: lentigo maligna**    *A large macule on the cheek of a 78-year-old male with highly irregular borders and striking variegation of pigmentation (white, tan, brown, dark brown, black).*

## EPIDEMIOLOGY

**Age of Onset** Median age is 65.

**Sex** Equal incidence in males and females.

**Race** Rare in brown- (e.g., Asians, East Indians) and extremely rare in black-skinned (African Americans and Africans) persons. Highest incidence in whites and skin phototypes I, II, and III.

**Incidence** 5% of primary cutaneous melanomas.

**Predisposing Factors** Same factors as in sun-induced nonmelanoma skin cancer: older population, outdoor occupations (farmers, sailors, construction workers).

## PATHOGENESIS

In contrast to SSM and NM, which appear to be related to intermittent high-intensity sun exposure and occur on the intermittently exposed areas (back and legs) of young or middle-aged adults, LM and LMM occur on the face, neck, and dorsa of the forearms or hands (Table 12-4); furthermore, LM and LMM occur almost always in older persons with evidence of heavily sundamaged skin (telangiectasia, marked freckling, atrophy, solar keratosis). The evolution of the lesion is shown in Image 12-2.

## HISTORY

LMM very slowly evolves from LM over a period of several years, sometimes up to 20 years.

## PHYSICAL EXAMINATION

**Skin Lesions**

*Lentigo Maligna* Uniformly *flat*, macule (Fig. 12-9); 3 cm or larger, up to 20 cm. Usually well defined, in some areas also blurred borders or highly irregular borders, often with a notch; "geographic" shape with inlets and peninsulas (Fig. 12-9). Striking variations in hues of brown and black (speckled), appears like a "stain"; haphazard network of black on a background of brown (Fig. 12-9). No hues of red and blue.

*Lentigo Maligna Melanoma* The clinical change that indicates the transition of LM to LMM is the appearance of variegated red, white and blue and of papules, plaques, or nodules (see Graph 12-2 and Fig. 12-11). Thus LMM is the same as LM *plus* (1) gray areas (indicates focal regression), and blue areas [indicating dermal pigment (melanocytes or melanin)], and (2) papules or nodules, which may be blue,

black, or pink (Fig. 12-11). Rarely, LMM may be nonpigmented. It is then skin-colored and patchy red and clinically not diagnosable.

***Distribution*** Single isolated lesion on the sun-exposed areas: forehead, nose, cheeks, neck, forearms, and dorsa of hands; rarely on lower legs.

**Other Skin Changes in Areas of Tumor** Sun-induced changes: solar keratosis, freckling, telangiectasia, thinning of the skin, i.e., dermatoheliosis.

**General Medical Examination**

Check for regional lymphadenopathy.

## LABORATORY EXAMINATION

**Dermatopathology** LM shows increased numbers of atypical melanocytes distributed in a single layer along the basal layer and above the basement membrane of an epidermis that shows elongation of rete ridges. Atypical melanocytes are usually singly dispersed but may also aggregate to small nests and extend into the hair follicles, reaching the mid-dermis, even in the preinvasive stage of LM. In LMM, they invade the dermis (vertical growth phase) and expand into the deeper tissues (see Image 12–2).

## DIFFERENTIAL DIAGNOSIS

**Variegate Tan-Brown Macule/Papule/Nodule** *Seborrheic keratoses* may be dark but are exclusively papules or plaques and have a characteristic stippled surface, often with a verrucous component, i.e., a "warty" but greasy surface that, when scratched, exhibits fine scales. *Solar lentigo*, although macular, does not exhibit the intensity or variegation of brown, dark brown, and black hues seen in LM. Dermoscopy is essential.

## PROGNOSIS

Summarized in Tables 12-6 and 12-7.

## MANAGEMENT

See also page 334.

1. Excise with 1-cm beyond the clinically visible lesion where possible and provided the flat component does not involve a major organ. Use of Wood's lamp helps in defining borders.

2. Sentinel node to be done in lesions >1.0 mm in terms of thickness.

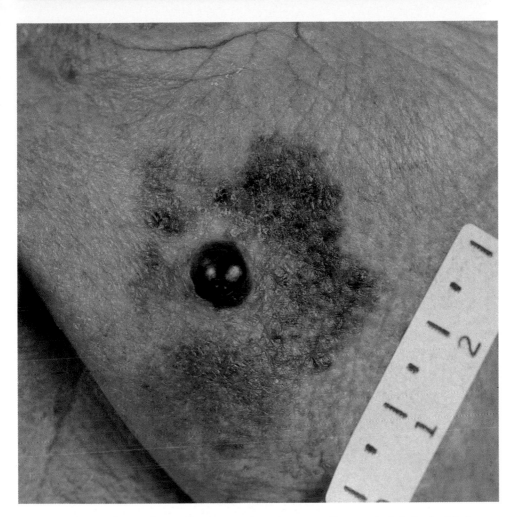

**FIGURE 12-10    Lentigo maligna melanoma**    *A large lentigo maligna on the left cheek with the typical variegation in color. The lesion is flat, macular, and represents in situ melanoma. In the center of the irregular lesion there is a pitch-black nodule indicating a switch from the radial to the vertical growth phase and thus invasiveness: the lesion is now called lentigo maligna melanoma.*

**TABLE 12-5　Melanoma TNM Classification**

| T Classification | Thickness, mm | Ulceration Status |
|---|---|---|
| T1 | ≤1.0 | a: Without ulceration and level II/III* |
| | | b: With ulceration or level IV/V/T2* |
| T2 | 1.01–2.0 | a: Without ulceration |
| | | b: With ulceration |
| T3 | 2.01–4.0 | a: Without ulceration |
| | | b: With ulceration |
| T4 | >4.0 | a: Without ulceration |
| | | b: With ulceration |

| N Classification | No. of Metastatic Nodes | Nodal Metastatic Mass |
|---|---|---|
| N1 | 1 | a: Micrometastasis |
| | | b: Macrometastasis |
| N2 | 2–3 | a: Micrometastasis |
| | | b: Macrometastasis |
| | | c: In-transit met(s)/satellite(s) without metastatic nodes |
| N3 | 4 or more metastatic nodes, or matted nodes, or in-transit met(s)/satellite(s) with metastatic node(s) | |

| M Classification | Site | Serum Lactate Dehydrogenase |
|---|---|---|
| M1a | Distant skin, subcutaneous, or nodal metastases | Normal |
| M1b | Lung metastases | Normal |
| M1c | All other visceral metastases | Normal |
| | Any distant metastasis | Elevated |

*Clark level I, Intraepidermal; level II, invades papillary dermis; level III, fills papillary dermis; level IV, invades reticular dermis; level V, invades subcutaneous fat.

SOURCE: Adapted from CM Balch et al: J Clin Oncol 19:3635, 2001.

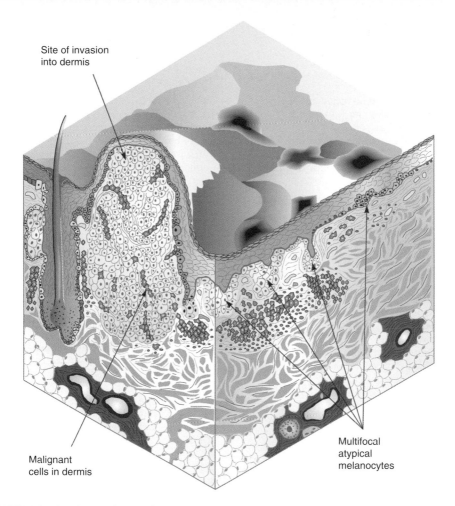

Site of invasion
into dermis

Malignant
cells in dermis

Multifocal
atypical
melanocytes

**IMAGE 12-2  Lentigo maligna melanoma** *Illustrated is a large, flat, variegated, freckle-like iacule (not elevated above the plane of the skin) with irregular borders. These areas show increased numbers of melanocytes, usually atypical and bizarre and distributed in a single layer along the basal layer (radial growth phase); at certain places in the dermis, malignant melanocytes have minimally invaded and formed nests. At the left is a large nodule that is composed of large epithelioid cells in this illustration; this nodule represents the vertical growth phase.*

## SUPERFICIAL SPREADING MELANOMA   ■  ●

Superficial spreading melanoma (SSM) is the most common melanoma (70%) in persons with white skin. It arises most frequently on the upper back and occurs as a moderately slow-growing lesion over a period up to 2 years. SSM has a distinctive morphology: an elevated, flat lesion (plaque). The pigment variegation of SSM is similar to, but more striking than, the variety of color present in most LMM. The color display is a mixture of brown, dark brown, black, blue, and red, with slate-gray or gray regions in areas of tumor regression. For most important clinical characteristics, see Table 12-4.

### EPIDEMIOLOGY

**Age of Onset**   30 to 50 (median, 37) years of age.
**Sex**   Slightly higher incidence in females.
**Race**   In world surveys, white-skinned persons overwhelmingly predominate. Only 2% brown- or black-skinned. Furthermore, brown and black persons have melanomas usually occurring on the extremities; half of brown and black persons have primary melanomas arising on the sole of the foot (see below).
**Incidence**   SSM constitutes 70% of all melanomas arising in white persons.
**Predisposing and Risk Factors**   (see Table 12-3) In order of importance these are *presence of precursor lesions* (AMN, CNMN; pages 294 and 298); *family history* of melanoma in parents, children, or siblings; *light skin color* (skin phototypes I and II); and *excessive sun exposure*, especially during preadolescence. Especially increased incidence in young urban professionals, with a frequent pattern of intermittent, intense sun exposure ("weekenders") or winter holidays near the equator.

### PATHOGENESIS

In the early stages of growth there is an intraepidermal, or radial growth phase, during which tumorigenic pigment cells are confined to the epidermis and thus cannot metastasize. At this stage SSM is an MIS (Fig. 12-11). This "grace period" of the radial growth phase, with potential for cure, is followed by the invasive vertical growth phase, in which malignant cells consist of a tumorigenic nodule that vertically invades the dermis with potential for metastasis (Image 12-3).

The pathophysiology of SSM is not yet understood. Certainly, in some considerable

number of SSMs, sunlight exposure is a factor, and SSM is related to occasional bursts of recreational sun exposure during a susceptible period (<14 years). About 10% of the roughly 6100 new SSMs each year in the United States occur in high-risk families. The rest of the cases may occur sporadically among persons without a specific genetic risk.

### HISTORY

The usual history of SSM is a change in a previously existing pigmented lesion (mostly an AMN). It should be noted, however, that 70% of melanomas arise in "normal" skin, but since initial growth is slow and melanomas often occur in persons with many nevi, an early SSM may be mistaken for a preexisting nevus by the patient. Often, a patient may offer a history of having had a mole at that particular site since childhood ("as long as I can remember"), but when a photograph of that particular age period and site is retrieved from a family album, no such "mole" can be detected.

The patient or a close relative may note a gradual darkening in one area of a "mole" (Fig. 12-4) or a change in shape (Fig. 12-3); and as the dark areas increase there will develop variegation of color with mixes of brown, dark brown, and black. Also, the borders of a previously regularly shaped lesion may become irregular with pseudopods and a notch.

With the switch from the radial to a vertical growth phase (Image 12-3), and thus invasion into the dermis, there is the clinical appearance of a papule and later nodule on top of the slightly elevated plaque of an SSM. Since many SSMs initially have the potential for a tumor-infiltrating lymphocyte (TIL)-mediated regression, albeit only partial, other areas of the SSM

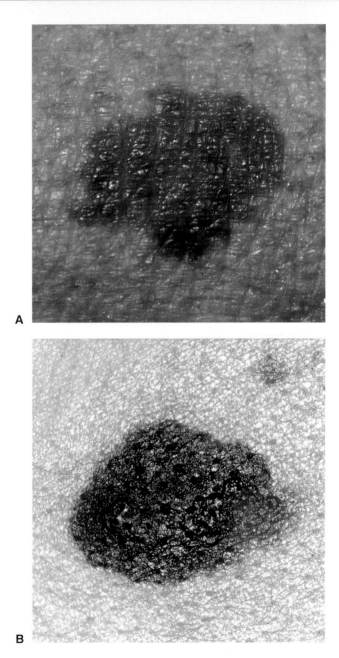

**FIGURE 12-11   Melanoma in situ, superficial spreading type**   *A. Barely elevated plaque on the arm of a 75-year-old white male was first noted 5 years previously, gradually increasing in size. The lesion is asymmetric and there is also asymmetry in the distribution of color that is variegated and shows dark-brown specks against a tan background. Dermatopathology of the lesion showed a superficial spreading melanoma in situ.* **B.** *An almost oval, barely elevated small plaque that has a relatively regular border but is striking with regard to the variegation in color: tan, dark brown, and even black with an orange portion on the right. Dermatopathology again showed MIS with a pagetoid growth pattern of intraepidermal melanoma cells.*

plaque may sink to the level of surrounding normal skin and the color mixes of brown to black are expanded by the addition of red, white, and the tell-tale blue and blue-gray.

## PHYSICAL EXAMINATION

Skin Lesions (Figs. 12-11 to 12-18)
SSM is the lesion to which the ABCDE rule (page 304) best applies. Initially a very flat plaque 5 to 12 mm or smaller; late lesions, 10 to 25 mm (Fig. 12-11). Asymmetric (one half unlike the other) (Figs. 12-13, 12-14, 12-16) or oval with irregular borders (Figs. 12-12 and 12-17) and often with one or more indentations (notches) (Figs. 12-12 to 12-17). Sharply defined. Dark brown, black, with admixture of pink, gray, and blue-gray hues—with marked variegation and a haphazard pattern. White areas indicate regressed portions (Figs. 12-17 and 12-18). An SSM is thus a flat plaque with all shades of brown to black plus the American flag or the tricolore (red, blue, white). *No benign pigmented lesion has these characteristics.* As the vertical growth phase progresses, additional papules (black, brown, red; Figs. 12-13 to 12-16) and nodules appear; eventually erosions and even superficial ulceration develop (Fig. 12-16).
*Distribution* Isolated, single lesions; multiple primaries are rare. Back (males and females); legs (females, between knees and ankles); anterior trunk and legs in males; relatively fewer lesions on covered areas, e.g., buttocks, lower abdomen, bra area (Graph 12-1).
**Dermoscopy** Increases diagnostic accuracy by 50%.
**General Examination** Always search for regional nodes.

## LABORATORY EXAMINATION

**Dermatopathology** Malignant melanocytes expand in a pagetoid pattern, i.e., in multiple layers within the epidermis (if confined to the epidermis, the lesion is an MIS) and superficial papillary body of the dermis—the radial growth phase. They occur singly and in nests (see Graph 12-3) and are S-100 and HMB-45 positive. In the vertical growth phase, presenting clinically as small nodules, they expand further into the reticular dermis and beyond (Graph 12-3). For microstaging see Table 12-5 and p. 333.

## COURSE AND PROGNOSIS

Left untreated, SSM develops deep invasion (vertical growth) over months to years. Prognosis is summarized in Tables 12-6 and 12-7, below.

## DIAGNOSIS

Clinically according to the ABCDE rule, verified by dermoscopy. In case of doubt, *biopsy*; total excisional biopsy with narrow margins is optimal biopsy procedure. Incisional or punch biopsy acceptable when total excisional biopsy cannot be performed or when lesion is large, requiring extensive surgery to remove the entire lesion.

## MANAGEMENT

**Surgical Treatment** See page 334.

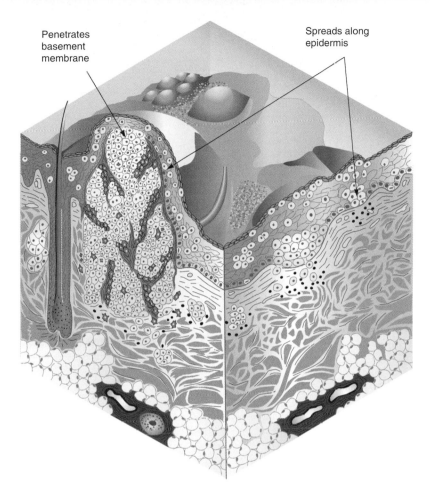

**IMAGE 12-3   Superficial spreading melanoma** *The border is irregular and elevated throughout its entirely; biopsy of the area surrounding the large nodule shows a pagetoid distribution of large melanocytes throughout the epidermis in multiple layers, occurring singly or in nests, and uniformly atypical. On the left is a large nodule, and scattered throughout the surrounding portion of the nodule are smaller papular and nodular areas. The nodules also may show epitheloid, spindle cells or small malignant melanocytes as in lentigo maligna melanoma and nodular melanoma.*

**Table 12-6    Cutaneous Melanoma: Stage Grouping and Prognosis**

| Stage | Clinical Staging | | | Pathologic Staging | | | Survival, % |
|---|---|---|---|---|---|---|---|
| | T | N | M | T | N | M | |
| 0 | Tis | N0 | M0 | Tis | N0 | M0 | |
| IA | T1a | N0 | M0 | T1a | N0 | M0 | 95 |
| IB | T1b | N0 | M0 | T1b | N0 | M0 | 90 |
| | T2a | N0 | M0 | T2a | N0 | M0 | |
| IIA | T2b | N0 | M0 | T2b | N0 | M0 | 78 |
| | T3a | N0 | M0 | T3a | N0 | M0 | |
| IIB | T3b | N0 | M0 | T3b | N0 | M0 | 65 |
| | T4a | N0 | M0 | T4a | N0 | M0 | |
| IIC | T4b | N0 | M0 | T4b | N0 | M0 | 45 |
| III | Any T | N1 | M0 | | | | |
| IIIA | | | | T1–4a | N1a | M0 | 60 |
| | | | | T1–4a | N2a | M0 | |
| IIIB | | | | T1–4b | N1a | M0 | |
| | | | | T1–4b | N2a | M0 | |
| | | | | T1–4a | N1b | M0 | 52 |
| | | | | T1–4a | N2b | M0 | |
| | | | | T1–4a/b | N2c | M0 | |
| IIIC | | | | T1–4b | N1b | M0 | |
| | | | | T1–4b | N2b | M0 | 26 |
| | | | | Any T | N3 | M0 | |
| IV | Any T | Any N | Any M1 | Any T | Any N | Any M1 | 7.5–11 |

SOURCE: Adapted from CM Balch et al: J Clin Oncol 19:3622-34, 2001.

**TABLE 12-7    8-Year Survival Rates for Patients with Clinical Stage I Melanoma (In the Vertical Growth Phase) Based on Tumor Thickness**

| Thickness, mm | 8-Year Survival Rate, % |
|---|---|
| <0.76 | 93.2 |
| 0.76–1.69 | 85.6 |
| 1.70–3.60 | 59.8 |
| >3.60 | 33.3 |

SOURCE: Adapted from WH Clark Jr et al: J Natl Cancer Inst 81:1893, 1989.

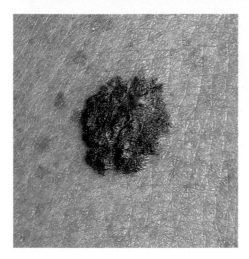

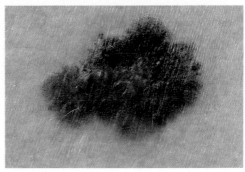

**FIGURE 12-13    Superficial spreading melanoma arising de novo**   *An asymmetrical, flat plaque with irregular and sharply defined margins. The melanin pigmentation ranges from light brown to pink, dark brown, black, and blue. A dark red-black nodule represents vertical growth and invasion of this SSM.*

**FIGURE 12-12    Superficial spreading melanoma arising de novo**   *A flat-topped, elevated, plaque on the trunk with sharply demarcated and irregular margins exhibiting variegation of melanin pigmentation, which ranges from light brown to dark brown and black as well as hues of red. The surface is irregular with a cobblestone pattern.*

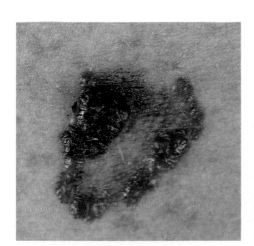

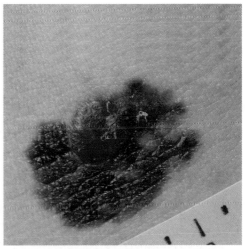

**FIGURE 12-14    Superficial spreading melanoma arising de novo**   *A lesion resembling a fried egg with a flat portion with color variegation (radial growth phase) with a black nodule arising within it (vertical invasive growth phase). The central, whitish-bluish area represents regression of the melanoma.*

**FIGURE 12-15    Superficial spreading melanoma arising within an atypical melanocytic nevus**
*A very flat plaque with a red-brown nodule arising within it: the flat portion (a preexisting atypical nevus) shows variegation of brown melanin pigmentation; the nodule shows slight erosion and crusting and represents the invasive vertical growth phase.*

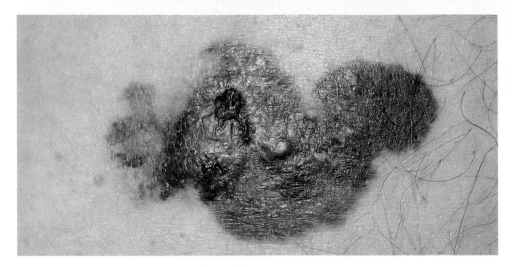

**FIGURE 12-16    Superficial spreading melanoma**   *A highly characteristic lesion with all features of SSM: asymmetry, borders that are highly irregular, colors that are widely variegated (black, brown, red, blue, white), diameter much greater than 1-cm, and elevation of the upper central portion. Note also small ulceration in the central portion of the lesion.*

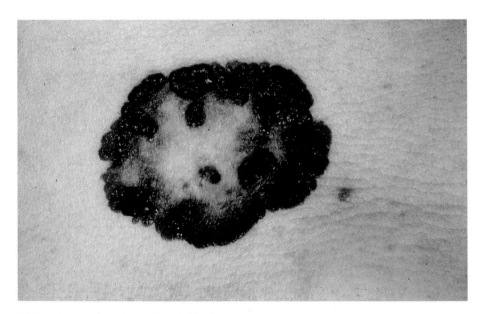

**FIGURE 12-17    Superficial spreading melanoma**   *An annular lesion with central resolution (regression) having a white scarlike appearance and peripheral extension with black, irregular scalloped borders. Note that there is brown, black, blue, white, and even red.*

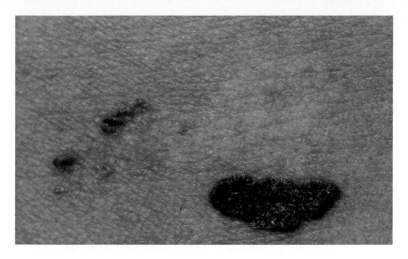

**FIGURE 12-18    Superficial spreading melanoma**    *This is one highly irregular lesion the greatest portion of which is a white, pinkish macule. At 6 o'clock there is a nearly oval but irregular black plaque with some brownish specks, at 9 o'clock there are some very small brownish and reddish papules. The whole lesion measured about 3 cm from left to right and represented an SSM that has 50% regressed (white area).*

## NODULAR MELANOMA   ■  ●

Nodular melanoma (NM) is second in frequency after SSM, occurring largely in middle life in persons with white skin and, as in SSM, on the less commonly exposed areas. The tumor from the beginning is in the vertical growth phase (Image 12-4). NM is uniformly elevated and presents as a thick plaque or an exophytic, polypoid or dome-shaped lesion. The color pattern is usually not variegated, and the lesion is uniformly blue or blue-black or, less commonly, can be very lightly pigmented or nonpigmented (amelanotic melanoma). NM is the one type of primary melanoma that arises quite rapidly (12 months to 2 years) from normal skin or from a melanocytic nevus as a nodular (vertical) growth without an adjacent epidermal component, as is always present in LMM and SSM (see Images 12-2 and 12-3).

For the most important clinical characteristics, see Table 12-4.

### EPIDEMIOLOGY

**Age of Onset**   Middle life.
**Sex**   Equal incidence in males and females.
**Race**   NM occurs in all races, but in the Japanese it occurs eight times more frequently (27%) than SSM (3%).
**Incidence**   NM constitutes 15% (up to 30%) of the melanomas in the United States.
**Predisposing and Risk Factors**   See page 303 and Table 12-3.

### PATHOGENESIS

Both SSM and NM occur in approximately the same sites (upper back in males, lower legs in females) (Graph 12-1), and presumably the same pathogenetic factors are operating in NM as were described in SSM. For the growth pattern of NM, see Graph 12-4. The reason for the high frequency of NM in the Japanese is not known.

### HISTORY

This type of melanoma may arise in a preexisting nevus, but more commonly arises de novo from normal skin. In contrast to SSM, NM evolves over a few months and is often noted by the patient as a new "mole" that was not present before.

### PHYSICAL EXAMINATION

#### Skin Lesions
Uniformly elevated "blueberry-like" nodule (Fig. 12-19) or ulcerated or "thick" plaque; may become polypoid. Uniformly dark blue, black, or "thundercloud" gray (Fig. 12-19); lesions may appear pink with a trace of brown or a black rim (amelanotic NM, Fig. 12-20). Early lesions are 1 to 3 cm in size but may grow much larger if undetected. Oval or round, usually with smooth, not irregular, borders, as in all other types of melanoma. Sharply defined.
**Distribution**   Same as SSM. In the Japanese, NM occurs on the extremities (arms and legs).
**General Medical Examination**   Always search for nodes.

### LABORATORY EXAMINATIONS

**Dermatopathology**   Malignant melanocytes, which appear as epithelioid, spindle, or small atypical cells, show little lateral (radial) growth within and below the epidermis and invade vertically into the dermis and underlying subcutaneous fat (see Graph 12-4). They are S-100 and usually HMB-45 positive. For microstaging, see page 333.
**Serology**   Serum levels of S-100 beta and melanoma-inhibiting activity (MIA), S-cysteinyldopa, and lactate dehydrogenase (LDH) levels are markers for *advanced* melanoma patients. LDH is the only statistically significant marker for *progressive* disease.

### DIAGNOSIS

Clinical and with the help of dermoscopy. However, dermoscopy may fail in uniformly black lesions. In case of doubt, *biopsy*. Total excisional biopsy with narrow margins is optimal

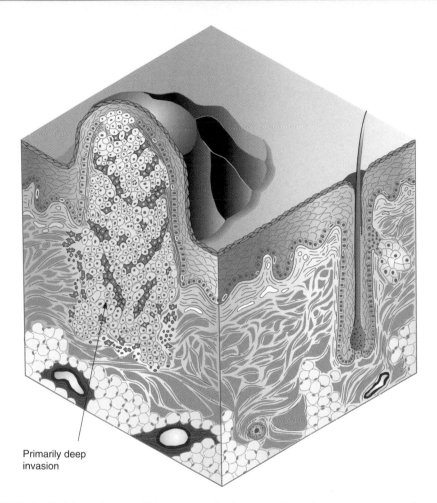

Primarily deep
invasion

**IMAGE 12-4   Nodular melanoma** *This arises at the dermal–epidermal junction and extends verti-cally in the dermis. The epidermis lateral to the areas of this invasion does not demonstrate atypi-cal melanocytes. As in lentigo maligna melanoma and superficial spreading melanoma, the tumor may show large epithelioid cells, spindle cells, small malignant melanocytes, or mixtures of all three.*

biopsy procedure, where possible. If biopsy is positive for melanoma, reexcision of site will be necessary (see Management, p. 334). Incisional or punch biopsy acceptable when total excisional biopsy cannot be performed or when lesion is large, requiring extensive surgery to remove the entire lesion.

## DIFFERENTIAL DIAGNOSIS

**Blue/Black Papule/Nodule**   NM can be confused with *hemangioma* (long history) and *pyogenic granuloma* (short history–weeks) and is sometimes almost indistinguishable from

*pigmented basal cell carcinoma*, although it is usually softer. However, any "blueberry-like" nodule of recent origin (6 months to 1 year) should be excised or, if large, an incisional biopsy is mandatory for histologic diagnosis.

## PROGNOSIS

Summarized in Tables 12-6 and 12-7.

## MANAGEMENT

**Surgical Treatment**   See page 334.

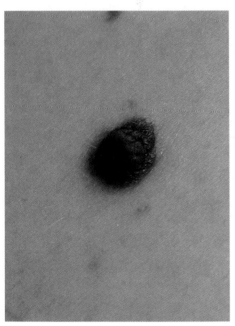

A

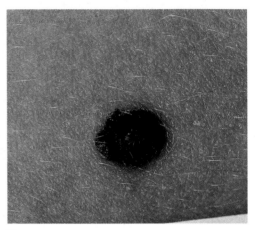

B

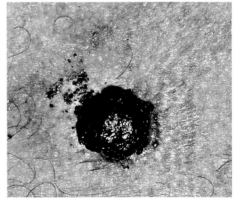

C

**FIGURE 12-19   Nodular melanoma arising de novo**   *A. A 5-mm domeshaped smooth nodule with a flatter portion at one o'clock arising on the back of a 38-year-old male. **B.** A 5-mm black papule on the posterior thigh of a 31-year-old female. The lesion had been present for less than 1 year. **C.** An eroded, bleeding, black nodule having a mushroom-like configuration with an eccentric, blue, noneroded, crescent-shaped portion between 3 and 6 o'clock. Such lesions can be mistaken for a vascular lesion such as a pyogenic granuloma, but the blue crescent at the base leaves no doubt that this is an NM.*

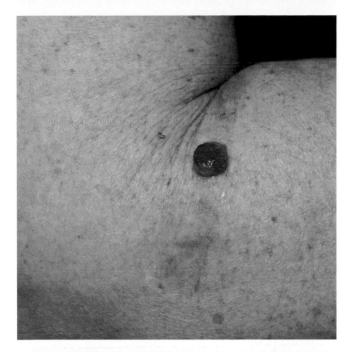

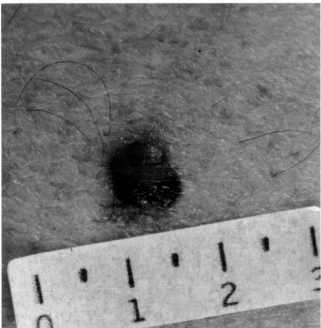

**FIGURE 12-20    Nodular melanoma: amelanotic**    *A. A cherry-red 6-mm nodule on the lower arm of a skin phototype I 59-year-old female. Due to the lack of pigment, a correct clinical diagnosis cannot be made except by suspicion. **B.** A similar, cherry-red nodule on the thigh of a 58-year-old male. In this case, the diagnosis is easy because of the dark brown crescent at the base between 3 and 9 o'clock.*

## DESMOPLASTIC MELANOMA    ☐  ●

The term *desmoplasia* refers to connective tissue proliferation and, when applied to malignant melanoma, describes (1) a dermal fibroblastic component of melanoma with only minimal melanocytic proliferation at the dermal-epidermal junction; (2) nerve-centered superficial malignant melanoma with or without an atypical intraepidermal melanocytic component; or (3) other lesions in which the tumor appears to arise in lentigo maligna or, rarely, in acral lentiginous melanoma or superficial spreading melanoma. Also, desmoplastic melanoma (DM) growth patterns have been noted in recurrent malignant melanoma. DM may be a variant of LMM in that most lesions occur on the head and neck in patients with dermatoheliosis. DM is more likely to recur locally and metastasize than LMM, however. DM is rare and occurs more frequently in women and persons >55 years of age.

At diagnosis DM lesions have been present from months to years. DM is asymptomatic, usually not pigmented and is therefore overlooked by the patient. Early lesions may appear as variegated lentiginous macules or plaques, at times with small blue-gray specks of color (Fig. 12-21). Later lesions may appear as dermal nodules, and although they commonly lack any melanin pigmentation and may have gray to blue papular elevations (Fig. 12-22). Borders, when discernible, are irregular as in LM.

The diagnosis requires an experienced dermatopathologist; S-100 immunoperoxidase-positive spindle cells need to be identified in the matrix collagen. HMB-45 staining may be negative. A typical junctional melanocytic proliferation, either individual or focal nests, occurs, resembling LM. S-100-positive spindle-shaped cells are embedded in matrix collagen that widely separates the spindle cell nuclei. Small aggregates of lymphocytes are commonly seen at the periphery of DM. Neurotropism is characteristic, i.e., fibroblast-like tumor cells around or within endoneurium of small nerves. Often, DM is seen with a background of severe solar damage to the dermis.

Diagnosis of DM is often delayed because of the bland clinical appearance and ill-defined margins. There are mixed views about the prognosis of DM. In one series, approximately 50% of patients experienced a local recurrence after primary excision of DM, usually within 3 years of excision; some patients experienced multiple recurrences. Lymph node metastasis occurs less often than local recurrence. In one series, 20% developed metastases, and DM was regarded as a more aggressive tumor than LMM. For management see page 334.

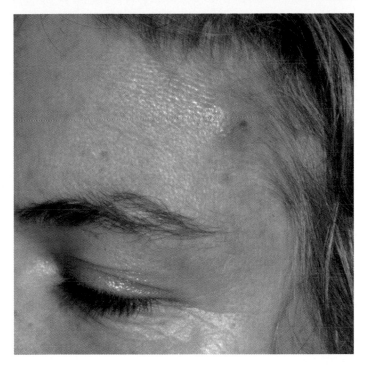

**FIGURE 12-21   Desmoplastic melanoma: amelanotic**   *A flat, skincolored nodule with a speck of brown in the center that appeared on the forehead of this 48-year-old female.*

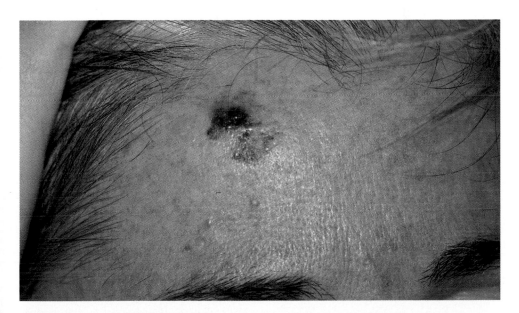

**FIGURE 12-22   Desmoplastic melanoma**   *A flat nodule with bluish-red and brown portion in an elderly male; lesions often are surrounded by a macular portion resembling lentigo maligna.*

## ACRAL LENTIGINOUS MELANOMA

Acral lentiginous melanoma (ALM) is a special presentation of cutaneous melanoma arising on the sole, palm, and fingernail or toenail bed. ALM occurs most often in Asians, sub-Saharan Africans, and African Americans, comprising 50 to 70% of the melanomas of the skin found in these populations. It occurs most often in older males (≥60 years) and often grows slowly over a period of years. The delay in development of the tumor is the reason these tumors are often discovered only when nodules appear or, in the case of nail involvement, the nail is shed; therefore, the prognosis is poor.

## EPIDEMIOLOGY

**Age of Onset**  Median age is 65.
**Incidence**  7 to 9% of all melanomas; in whites, 2 to 8%.
**Sex**  Male:female ratio, 3:1.
**Race**  The best data are on American blacks and Japanese brown-skinned persons, where the incidence of melanoma is about one-seventh that of white persons. ALM is the principal melanoma in the Japanese and in American and sub-Saharan African blacks. ALM accounts for 50 to 70% of melanomas in the Japanese.

## PATHOGENESIS

The pigmented macules that are frequently seen on the soles of African blacks could be comparable with AMN. ALM has a similar growth pattern as LMM (Graph 12-2).

## HISTORY

ALM is slow growing (about 2.5 years from appearance to diagnosis). The tumors occur on the volar surface (palm or sole) and in their radial growth phase may appear as a gradually enlarging "stain." ALM as subungual (thumb or great toe) melanoma appears first in the nail bed and involves, over a period of 1 to 2 years, the nail matrix, eponychium, and nail plate. In the vertical growth phase nodules appear; often there are areas of ulceration, and nail deformity and shedding of the nail may occur.

## PHYSICAL EXAMINATION

### Skin Lesions
**Acral and Palm/Sole**  Macular or slightly raised lesion in the radial growth phase (Fig. 12-23),

with focal papules and nodules developing during the vertical growth phase. Marked variegation of color including brown, black, blue, depigmented pale areas (Fig. 12-24A). Irregular borders as in LMM; usually well defined but not infrequently ill defined. This type of ALM occurs on soles, palms, dorsal and palmar/plantar aspects of fingers, and toes.
**Subungual**  Subungual macule beginning at the nail matrix and extending to involve the nail bed and nail plate. Papules, nodules, and destruction of the nail plate may occur in the vertical growth phase. Dark brown or black pigmentation that may involve the entire nail and surrounding skin looking like LM (Fig. 12-24A). As the lesion switches to the vertical growth phase, a papule or nodule appears and the nail is shed (Fig. 12-24A). Often the nodules or papules are unpigmented. Amelanotic ALM is often overlooked for weeks to months and, since there are no pigmentary changes, may first present as nail dystrophy (Fig. 12-24B).

## DIFFERENTIAL DIAGNOSIS

ALM (plantar type) is not infrequently regarded as a "plantar wart" and treated as such. Dermoscopy is of decisive help.
**Subungual Discoloration**  ALM (subungual) is usually considered to be traumatic bleeding under the nail, and subungual hematomas may persist for over 1 year; however, usually the whole pigmented area moves gradually forward. Distinction of ALM from subungual hemorrhage can easily be made by dermoscopy. With the destruction of the nail plate, the lesions are most often regarded as "fungal infection." When nonpigmented tumor nodules appear, they are misdiagnosed as pyogenic granuloma.

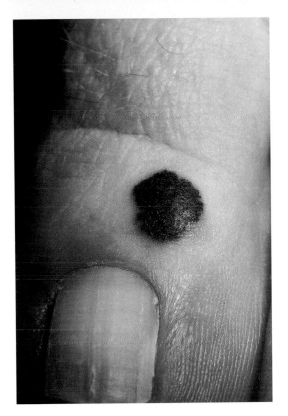

**FIGURE 12-23   Acral lentiginous melanoma arising on the toe**   *A black, only minimally raised papule with slightly irregular border of a 45-year-old white female of Celtic heritage. The lesion was treated with amputation of the toe at the metatarso-phalangeal joint.*

## LABORATORY EXAMINATION

**Dermatopathology**   The histologic diagnosis of the radial growth phase of the volar type of ALM may be difficult and may require large incisional biopsies to provide for multiple sections. There is usually an intense lymphocytic inflammation at the dermal-epidermal junction. Characteristic large melanocytes along the basal cell layer may extend as large nests into the dermis, along eccrine ducts. Invasive malignant melanocytes are often spindle shaped, so that ALM frequently has a desmoplastic appearance histologically.

## PROGNOSIS

The volar type of ALM can be deceptive in its clinical appearance, and "flat" lesions may be quite deeply invasive. Five-year survival rates are <50%. The subungual type of ALM has a better 5-year survival rate (80%) than does the volar type, but the data are probably not accurate. Poor prognosis for the volar type of ALM may be related to inordinate delay in the diagnosis.

## MANAGEMENT

In considering surgical excision, it is important that the extent of the lesion be ascertained by viewing the lesion with dermoscopy. Subungual ALM and volar-type ALM: amputation [toe(s), finger(s)]; volar and plantar ALM: wide excision with split skin grafting. Sentinel lymph node procedure necessary in most cases (see "Management of Melanoma," page 334).

A

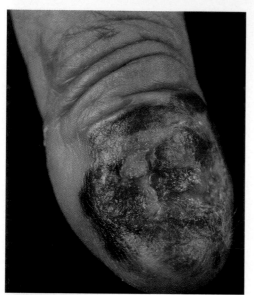

B

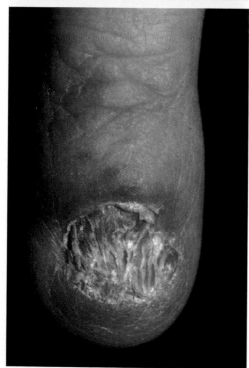

**FIGURE 12-24   Acral lentiginous melanoma**
*A. The tumor has replaced the entire nail bed and surrounding skin; the center is amelanotic and ulcerated and the peripheral parts are macular and of highly variegated color and resemble a lentigo maligna. This thumb was amputated and axillary lymphadenectomy revealed lymph node metastases. B. This is amelanotic ALM that has led to destruction of the nail matrix and was first diagnosed as nail dystrophy. Biopsy revealed the true nature of the lesion.*

## MALIGNANT MELANOMA OF THE MUCOSA    □  ●

Malignant melanomas arising in the mucosal epithelial lining of the respiratory tract and gastrointestinal and genitourinary tracts are very rare, with an annual incidence of 0.15% per 100,000 individuals. Major sites of the mucosal melanomas are the vulva and vagina (45%) and the nasal and oral cavity (43%). Mucosal melanomas are so rare that there are no large data bases compared to those for cutaneous melanoma; therefore, pathologic microstaging has not been possible, and the fine-tuning of the prognosis that has been useful in cutaneous melanoma (Breslow thickness) has so far not been possible in mucosal melanoma.

### Melanomas of the Oral Cavity

There is a delay in diagnosis of melanoma of the oral and nasal surfaces. Although melanosis of the mucosa is common in blacks and East Indians, it involves the buccal and gingival mucosa bilaterally (see "Disorders of Oropharynx," Section 31); when there is a single area of melanosis (see Fig. 31-10), a biopsy should be performed to rule out melanoma; this is also true of pigmented nevi in the oral cavity, which should be excised (see Disorders of Oropharynx, Section 31).

### Melanomas in the Genitalia

These melanomas mostly arise on the glans or prepuce (see Fig. 32-21) and the labia minora; there are fewer on the clitoris and the labia majora (see Fig. 32-22). Most tumors extend to the vagina at the mucocutaneous border. They look and evolve like LM and LMM (see Fig. 32-22). Vulva melanomas are often flat like LMM with large areas of melanoma in situ, and this is important to ascertain in planning excision of all the lesion to prevent recurrence. Dermoscopy should be used to outline the periphery of the lesion, as is done in LMM (see "Disorders of the Genitalia, Perineum, and Anus," Section 32).

### Anorectal Melanoma

Often presents with a localized, often polypoid or nodular primary tumor, but it may also present similarly to LMM.

## METASTATIC MELANOMA

Metastatic melanoma occurs in 15 to 26% of stage I and stage II melanoma (see below). The spread of disease from the primary site usually occurs in a stepwise sequence: primary melanoma → regional metastasis (Fig. 12-25) → distant metastasis. It should be noted that distant metastasis can occur, skipping the regional lymph nodes and indicating hematogenous spread. Distant metastases occur anywhere but usually in the following organs: lungs (18 to 36%), liver (14 to 29%), brain (12 to 20%), bone (11 to 17%), and intestines (1 to 7%). Most frequently, however, melanoma first spreads to distant lymph nodes, skin, and subcutaneous tissues (42 to 57%). Local recurrence occurs if excision has not been adequate (Fig. 12-26) or it can involve the skin of an entire region both with and without adequate surgical treatment (Fig. 12-27). *Metastatic melanoma without a primary tumor* is rare, 1 to 6%. It is the result of metastasis from a melanoma that underwent total spontaneous regression. *Melanoma may have a late recurrence* (≥10 years). The usual time is 14 years, but there have been "very late" recurrences (>15 years) in one series at the Massachusetts General Hospital, with 0.072% (20 of 2766 cases).

*Patients with a solitary metastasis* confined to the subcutaneous, nonregional lymph nodes or lung are most likely to benefit from surgical intervention.

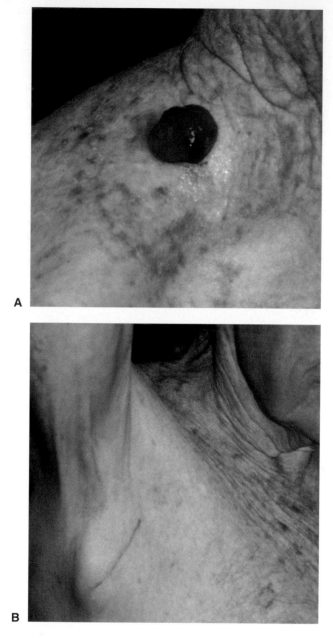

**FIGURE 12-25    Melanoma:    primary and regional metastasis** *A 75-year-old male presented with an axillary mass. Biopsy of the mass revealed lymph node metastasis of melanoma. The primary nodular melanoma on the right shoulder was detected after recurrence of axillary metastasis.* **A.** *Primary nodular melanoma on R-shoulder.* **B.** *R-axillary lymph node metastasis, recurrent.*

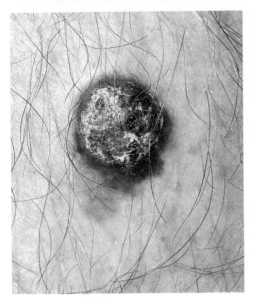 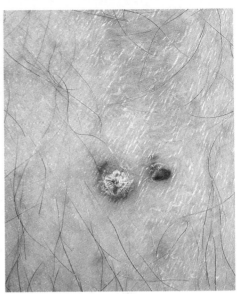

**FIGURE 12-26    Metastatic melanoma: recurring in excision scar**    *A. A pigmented lesion on the shin of a 35-year-old male, present for <2 years. Dermatopathology was initially interpreted as a spindle cell (Spitz) nevus. The primary lesion site was therefore not reexcised. **B.** Two papules are seen around the excision site scar, one of which has a blue-brown color. The histology from the excised lesion was reviewed and revised as a superficial spreading melanoma and the histopathology of the two papules seen here was metastatic melanoma.*

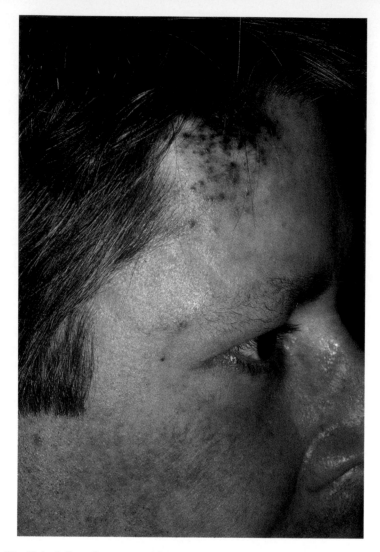

**FIGURE 12-27    Metastatic melanoma: multiple dermal metastases**    *Multiple blue and blue-gray dermal nodules on the forehead and throughout the scalp of a 45-year-old male. The patient bumped his scalp, resulting in a large ecchymosis 2½ months previously. As the ecchymosis resolved, the blue dermal nodules became apparent. Cervical lymph nodes were enlarged; needle aspiration demonstrated metastatic melanoma in the nodes as well. The primary melanoma presumably arose in the scalp but was not detected.*

# STAGING OF MELANOMA

Staging of melanoma depends on its TNM classification (primary *tumor*, regional *nodes*, *metastases*, Table 12-5). *Clinical staging* of melanoma differentiates between local, regional, and distant disease and is based on microstaging of the melanoma and clinical and imaging evaluation for metastases; *pathologic staging* consists of microstaging of the primary tumor and pathologic evaluation of regional lymph nodes (Tables 12-6 and 12-7). Staging of melanoma is strongly correlated with survival.

## Microstaging

*Microstaging* is done according to Breslow's method. The thickness of the primary melanoma is measured from the granular layer of the epidermis to the deepest part of the tumor. The thickness of melanoma (level of invasion) is the most important single prognostic variable and thus decisive for therapeutic decisions (Table 12-7).

Clark's microstaging* according to tissue level of invasion is no longer considered a significant prognostic variable.

## Sentinel Lymph Node Biopsy

Sentinel lymph node biopsy can predict the presence of clinically nondetectable metastatic melanoma within regional lymph nodes with the identification of malignant cells in H&E sections; staining for S-100 protein and HMB-45 and tyrosinase.

When the nodes are not palpable, it is not certain if there are micrometastases; these can be detected by the *sentinel node technique*. The hypothesis is that the *first* node draining a lymphatic basin, called the *sentinel node*, can predict the presence or absence of metastasis in other nodes in that basin. Either lymphatic mapping (LM) or sentinel lymphadenectomy (SL) is performed on the same day with a single injection of filtered $^{99m}$Tc subcutaneously into the site of the primary melanoma for probe-directed LM and SL. Alternatively, one day after lymphoscintigraphy, sentinel node biopsy is performed, guided by a gamma probe and blue dye also injected into the primary site; the sentinel node is subjected to histopathology and immunohistochemistry. LM is very useful in locating the drainage areas, especially in primary tumors on the trunk, which can drain on either side and to both the axillary and inguinal lymph nodes.

Lymph node dissection is performed only if metastasis is found in the sentinel node. The sentinel node technique is also essential in making a decision about the use of adjuvant therapy.

## WORKUP OF MELANOMA

I. Primary melanoma: Stage I or II (no nodes palpated)
   A. Chest roentgenogram, sonography of lymph nodes
   B. Liver function tests, LDH
   C. Lymphatic mapping and sentinel lymphadenectomy in stage 1 thickness >1.0 mm.

II. Primary melanoma with local-regional disease

   A. Stage III, satellites and local recurrence
     1. Complete blood count
     2. Liver function tests, LDH
     3. Chest roentgenogram
     4. Ultrasound and CT scans: abdomen, pelvis (with disease below the waist), neck (with disease in the head and neck); positron emission tomography (PET) scan
   B. Stage IV
     1. Same as for stage III
     2. CT scan of the chest
     3. MRI of the brain
     4. Bone scan
     5. GI series (on the basis of symptoms)

---

* Clark level I, intraepidermal; level II, invades papillary dermis; level III, fills papillary dermis; level IV, invades reticular dermis; level V, invades subcutaneous fat.

## PROGNOSIS OF MELANOMA

Prognosis of melanoma can be either excellent or grave, depending on whether the tumor is diagnosed early or late, when regional or distant metastases have occurred (Table 12-6). This emphasizes the importance of early diagnosis, of questioning patients for melanoma risks (Tables 12-2 and 12-3), of screening individuals belonging to risk groups, and of total-body examination of any patient seeing a physician for medical examination. Prognosis relating to stage grouping for cutaneous melanoma is shown in Table 12-6.

## MANAGEMENT OF MELANOMA

The only curative treatment of melanoma is early surgical excision.

### GUIDELINES FOR BIOPSY AND SURGICAL TREATMENT OF PATIENTS WITH MELANOMA

I. Biopsy
  A. Total excisional biopsy with narrow margins—optimal biopsy procedure, where possible.
  B. Incisional or punch biopsy acceptable when total excisional biopsy cannot be performed or when lesion is large, requiring extensive surgery to remove the entire lesion.
  C. When sampling the lesion: If raised, remove the most raised area; if flat, remove the darkest area.

II. Melanoma in situ
  A. Excise with 0.5-cm margin.

III. Lentigo maligna melanoma
  A. Excise with a 1-cm margin beyond the clinically visible lesion or biopsy scar—unless the flat component involves a major organ (e.g., the eyelid), in which case lesser margins are acceptable.
  B. Excise down to the fascia or to the underlying muscle where fascia is absent. Skin flaps or skin grafts may be used for closure.
  C. No node dissection is recommended unless nodes are clinically palpable and suspicious for tumor.
  D. See recommendation for sentinel node studies for thickness >1 mm (page 333).

IV. Superficial spreading melanoma, nodular melanoma, and acral melanoma
  A. Thickness <1 mm
    1. Excise with a 1-cm margin from the lesion edge.
    2. Excise down to the fascia or to the underlying muscle where fascia is absent. Direct closure without graft is often possible.
    3. Node dissection is not recommended unless nodes are clinically palpable and suspicious for tumor.
  B. Thickness 1 mm to 4 mm
    1. Excise 2 cm from the edge of the lesion, except on the face, where narrower margins may be necessary.
    2. Excise down to the fascia or to the underlying muscle where fascia is absent. Graft may be required.
    3. The sentinel node procedure for tumors with thickness >1 mm is recommended.
    4. Lymphadenectomy is selectively performed and only for those nodal basins with occult tumor cells (i.e., positive sentinel lymph node). If the sentinel node is negative, then the patient is spared a lymph node dissection.
    5. Therapeutic nodal dissection is recommended if nodes are clinically palpable and suspicious for tumor.
    6. If regional node is positive and completely resected with no evidence of distant disease, adjuvant therapy with interferon-α-2b (IFN-α-2b) is considered.

## ADJUVANT THERAPY

This is treatment of a patient after removal of all detectable tumor but the patient is considered at high risk for recurrence (i.e., stages IIb and III). As mentioned above, IFN-$\alpha$-2b (both high and low dose) is subject to intensive investigation; however, despite early promising results to date no clear benefit on overall survival has been convincingly demonstrated.

### Management of Distant Metastases (Stage IV)

Currently this can be considered palliative at best. Surgical removal of accessible metastases can provide excellent palliation. Chemotherapy encompasses a large list of drugs (dacarbazine/temozolomide, cisplatin, vindesine/vinblastine, fotemustine, taxol/taxotere) employed as single agents or in combination. Dacarbazine is still the most effective monotherapeutic agent, but all in all chemotherapeutic treatment of stage IV melanoma is disappointing, showing only a $\leq 20\%$ response rate and no effect on overall survival. There are a large number of melanoma vaccination trials presently being performed, and the field is rapidly expanding to include gene-therapeutic approaches such as anti-Bcl-2 oligonucleotide therapy. Increase of overall survival has, however, not been shown to date. Radiotherapy has only palliative effects also, but stereotactive radiosurgery with the gamma-knife has shown considerable palliation.

## FOLLOW-UP FOR PRIMARY MELANOMA

See Table 12-8.

### TABLE 12-8  Follow-up for Primary Melanoma

| Stage I (<1 mm) | Stages I (>1 mm) and II, Lymph Nodes Negative | Stage III, Lymph Nodes Positive |
|---|---|---|
| Every 3–6 months* for 3 years | Every 3–6 months* for 3 years | Every 3–6 months for 3 years; then 3–12 months for 2 years |
| Review of systems Physical examination | Review of systems Physical examination Liver function (LDH) Chest x-ray and CT scans every 6 months | Review of systems Physical examination CBC, liver function (LDH) Chest x-ray and CT scans every 6 months |
| Annual examination for life | Annual examination for life | Annual examination for life |

*Familial melanoma atypical nevus syndrome: every 3 months for 3 years, and then every 6 months for 5 years, and then annually for life.

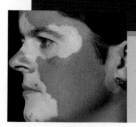
Normal skin color is composed of a mixture of four biochromes, namely, (1) *reduced hemoglobin* (blue), (2) *oxyhemoglobin* (red), (3) *carotenoids* (yellow; exogenous from diet), and (4) *melanin* (brown). The principal determinant of the skin color is melanin pigment, and variations in the amount and distribution of melanin in the skin are the basis of the three principal human skin colors: black, brown, and white. These three basic skin colors are genetically determined and are called *constitutive melanin pigmentation*; the normal basic skin color pigmentation can be increased deliberately by exposure to ultraviolet radiation (UVR) or pituitary hormones, and this is called *inducible melanin pigmentation*.

The combination of the constitutive and inducible melanin pigmentation determines what is called the *skin phototype* (SPT) (see Table 10-2). Ethnicity is not necessarily a part of the definition, e.g., African "black" ethnic persons can be SPT III and an East Indian Caucasian can be SPT IV or even V. *The skin phototype is a marker for skin cancer risk and should be recorded at the first patient visit.*

Increase of melanin in the epidermis results in a state known as *hypermelanosis*. This reflects one of two types of changes:

1. An increase in the number of melanocytes in the epidermis producing increased levels of melanin, which is called *melanocytotic hypermelanosis* (an example is *lentigo*).
2. *No* increase of melanocytes but an increase in the production of melanin only, which is called *melanotic hypermelanosis* (an example is *melasma*).

Hypermelanosis of both types can result from three factors: genetic; hormonal (as in Addison's disease), when it is caused by an increase in circulating pituitary melanotropic hormones; and UVR (as in tanning).

A decrease of melanin in the epidermis is called *hypomelanosis*. This reflects mainly two types of changes:

1. A decrease in the number or absence of melanocytes in the epidermis producing no or decreased levels of melanin. This is called *melanocytopenic hypomelanosis* (an example is vitiligo).
2. No decrease of melanocytes but a decrease of the production of melanin only that is called *melanopenic hypomelanosis* (an example is albinism).

Hypomelanosis also results from genetic (as in albinism), from autoimmune (as in vitiligo), or other inflammatory processes (as in postinflammatory leukoderma in psoriasis).

## VITILIGO  ■  ○ → ◑

Vitiligo is a major medical problem for brown and black persons that can result in severe difficulties in social adjustment. Vitiligo is characterized clinically by development of totally white macules, microscopically by complete absence of melanocytes, and medically by a not uncommon association with certain medical diseases, particularly thyroid disease.

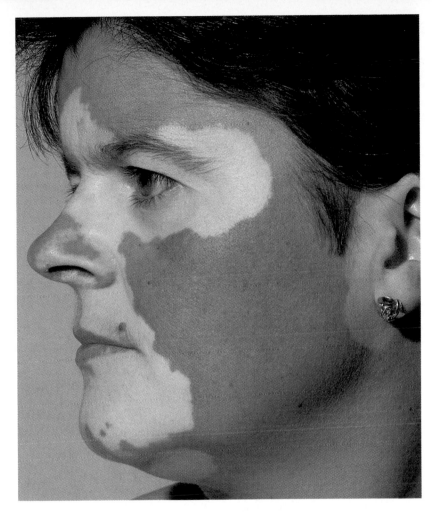

**FIGURE 13-1    Vitiligo: face**   *Extensive depigmentation of the central face. Involved vitiliginous skin has convex borders, extending into the normal pigmented skin. Note the chalkwhite color and sharp margination.*

## EPIDEMIOLOGY

**Sex**   Equal in both sexes. The predominance in women suggested by the literature likely reflects the greater concern of women about cosmetic appearance.

**Age of Onset**   May begin at any age, but in 50% of cases it begins between the ages of 10 and 30 years. A few cases have been reported to be present at birth; onset in old age also occurs but is unusual.

**Incidence**   Common. Affects up to 1% of the population.

**Race**   All races. The apparently increased prevalence reported in some countries and among darker-skinned persons results from a dramatic contrast between white vitiligo macules and dark skin and from marked social stigma in countries such as India, where even today the opportunities for advancement or marriage among affected individuals are limited.

**Inheritance**   Vitiligo has a genetic background; >30% of affected individuals have reported vitiligo in a parent, sibling, or child. Vitiligo in identical twins has been reported. Transmission is most likely polygenic with variable expression. The risk of vitiligo for children of affected individuals is unknown but may be <10%. Individuals from families with an increased prevalence of thyroid disease, diabetes mellitus, and vitiligo appear to be at increased risk for development of vitiligo.

## PATHOGENESIS

Three principal theories have been presented about the mechanism of destruction of melanocytes in vitiligo:

1. The *autoimmune theory* holds that selected melanocytes are destroyed by certain lymphocytes that have somehow been activated.
2. The *neurogenic hypothesis* is based on an interaction of the melanocytes and nerve cells.
3. The *self-destruct hypothesis* suggests that melanocytes are destroyed by toxic substances formed as part of normal melanin biosynthesis.

While the immediate mechanism for the evolving white macules involves progressive destruction of selected melanocytes by cytotoxic T cells, other genetically determined cytobiologic changes and cytokines must be involved. Because of differences in the extent and course of segmental and generalized vitiligo, the pathogenesis of these two types must be somewhat different.

## HISTORY

Many patients attribute the onset of their vitiligo to physical trauma (where vitiligo appears at the site of trauma—Koebner phenomenon), illness, or emotional stress. Onset after the death of a relative or after severe physical injury is often mentioned. A sunburn reaction may precipitate vitiligo.

## PHYSICAL EXAMINATION

### Skin Lesions

Macules, 5 mm to 5 cm *or more* in diameter (Figs. 13-1 and 13-2). "chalk" or pale white, sharply marginated. Newly developed macules may be "off-white" in color; this represents a transitional phase. The disease progresses by gradual enlargement of the old macules or by development of new ones. A variant is trichrome vitiligo (three colors: white, light brown, dark brown) but this represents different stages in the evolution of vitiligo. Pigmentation around a hair follicle in a white macule represents residual pigmentation or return of pigmentation (Fig. 13-3). Confetti-sized hypomelanotic macules may also be observed. *Inflammatory vitiligo* has an elevated erythematous margin and may be pruritic. Margins are *convex* (as if the pathologic process of depigmentation were flowing into normally pigmented skin).

***Distribution*** Depigmentation occurs in three general patterns. The *focal* type is characterized by one or several macules in a single site; this may be an early evolutionary stage of one of the other types in some cases. The *segmental* type is characterized by one or several macules in one band on one side of the body; this type is associated rarely with distant vitiligo macules or with further evolution of the disease to generalized vitiligo. The most common type is *generalized* vitiligo, characterized by widespread distribution of depigmented macules, often in a remarkable symmetry (Fig. 13-2). Typical macules occur around the eyes (Fig. 13-1) and mouth and on digits, elbows, and knees, as well as on the low back and in genital areas (Image 13-1). The *"lip-tip" pattern* involves the skin around the mouth as well as on distal fingers and toes; lips, nipples, genitalia (tip of the penis), and anus may be involved. Confluence of vitiligo results in large white areas, and extensive generalized vitiligo may leave only a few normally pigmented areas of skin—*vitiligo universalis* (Fig. 13-4).

**Segmental Vitiligo**   This is a special subset that usually develops in one unilateral region; usually does not extend beyond that initial one-sided region (though not always); and, once present, is very stable.

**Associated Cutaneous Findings**   White hair and prematurely gray hair. Circumscribed areas of white hair, analogous to vitiligo macules, are called *poliosis*. Alopecia areata and halo nevi. In older patients, photoaging as well as solar keratoses may occur in vitiligo macules in those with history of long exposures to sunlight. Squamous cell carcinoma, limited to the white macules, has rarely been reported.

**General Examination**   Not uncommonly associated with thyroid disease (up to 30% of all vitiligo cases: Hashimoto's thyroiditis, Graves' disease); also diabetes mellitus—probably <5%; pernicious anemia (uncommon, but increased risk); Addison's disease (uncommon); and multiple endocrinopathy syndrome (rare). Ophthalmologic examination may reveal evidence of healed chorioretinitis or iritis (probably <10% of all cases). Vision is unaffected.

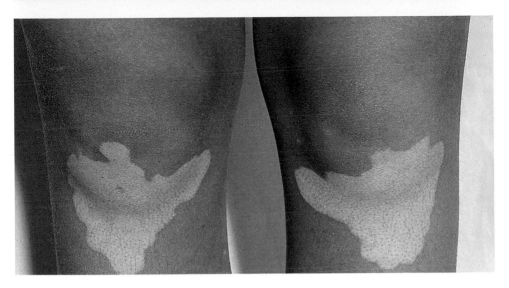

**FIGURE 13-2   Vitiligo: knees**   *Depigmented, sharply demarcated macules on the knees. Apart from the loss of pigment, vitiliginous skin appears normal. Note tiny follicular pigmented spots within the vitiligo areas that represent repigmentation.*

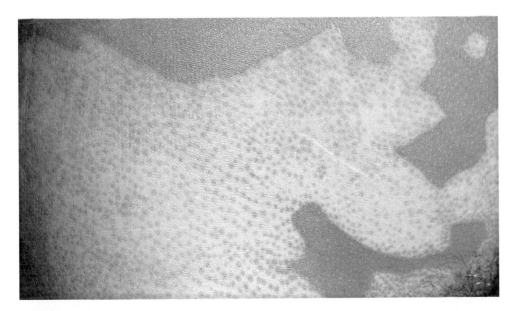

**FIGURE 13-3   Vitiligo repigmentation**   *A follicular pattern of repigmentation due to PUVA therapy occurring in a large vitiliginous macule. Melanocytes may persist in the hair follicle epithelium and serve to repopulate involved skin, spontaneously or with photochemotherapy.*

Hearing is normal. The *Vogt-Koyanagi-Harada syndrome* is vitiligo + poliosis + uveitis + dysacusia + alopecia.

## LABORATORY EXAMINATIONS

**Wood's Lamp Examination** Wood's lamp examination is required to evaluate macules, particularly in lighter skin types, and to identify macules, in sun-protected areas in all but the darkest skin types.

**Dermatopathology** In certain difficult cases, a skin biopsy may be required. Established vitiligo macules show normal skin except for an absence of melanocytes. Use special stains to identify melanocytes. There may be a mild lymphocytic response. These changes are not diagnostic for vitiligo, however, only consistent with it.

**Electron Microscopy** Absence of melanocytes and of melanosomes in keratinocytes; also changes in keratinocytes: spongiosis, exocytosis, basilar vacuopathy, and necrosis. Lymphocytes have been seen in the epidermis.

**Laboratory Studies** $T_4$, TSH (radioimmunoassay), fasting blood glucose, complete blood count with indices (pernicious anemia), ACTH stimulation test for Addison's disease, if suspected.

## DIAGNOSIS

Normally, diagnosis of vitiligo can be made readily on clinical examination of a patient with progressive, acquired, chalk-white, bilateral (usually symmetric), sharply defined macules in typical sites (periorbital, perioral, neck, penis, perineum, axillae, and points of pressure such as the elbow, malleoli, knees, lumbosacral area).

*Note*: Vitiligo is a sharply marginated, macular depigmentation of otherwise completely normal skin.

## DIFFERENTIAL DIAGNOSIS

*Pityriasis alba* (slight scaling, fuzzy margins, off-white color).

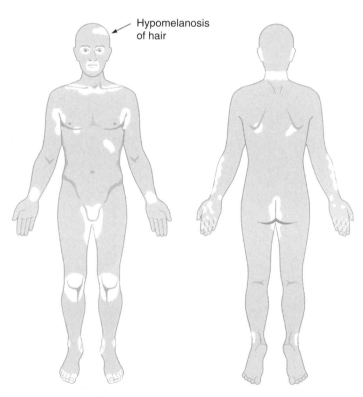

Hypomelanosis of hair

**IMAGE 13-1**    **Vitiligo:** *predilection sites.*

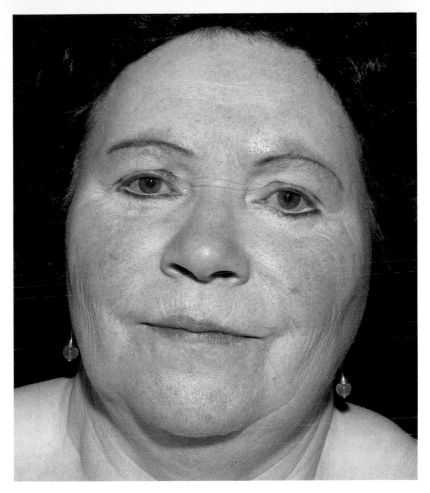

**FIGURE 13-4   Universal vitiligo**   *Vitiliginous macules have coalesced to involve all skin sites with complete depigmentation of skin and hair in a female. The patient is wearing a black wig and has darkened the brows with eyebrow pencil and eyelid margins with eye liner.*

*Pityriasis versicolor alba* (fine scales with greenish-yellow fluorescence under Wood's lamp, positive KOH.

*Chemical leukoderma* (history of exposure to certain phenolic germicides, confetti macules). This is a difficult differential diagnosis, as melanocytes are absent as in vitiligo.

*Leprosy* (endemic areas, off-white color, usually ill-defined *anesthetic* macules).

*Nevus depigmentosus* (stable, congenital, off-white macules, unilateral).

*Hypomelanosis of Ito* (bilateral, Blaschko's lines, marble cake pattern; 60 to 75% have systemic involvement–CNS, eyes, musculoskeletal system).

*Nevus anemicus* (does not enhance with Wood's lamp; does not show erythema after rubbing).

*Tuberous sclerosis* [stable, congenital off-white macules (polygonal, ash-leaf shape, occasional segmental macules, and confetti macules)].

*Piebaldism* (congenital, white forelock, stable, dorsal pigmented stripe on back, distinctive pattern with large hyperpigmented macules in the center of the hypomelanotic areas).

*Leukoderma associated with melanoma* (may not be true vitiligo inasmuch as melanocytes, although reduced, are usually present).

*Postinflammatory leukoderma* [off-white macules (usually a history of psoriasis or eczema in the same macular area), not so sharply, defined].

*Mycosis fungoides* (may be confusing as only depigmentation may be present and biopsy is necessary).

*Vogt-Koyanagi-Harada syndrome* (vision problems, photophobia, bilateral dysacousia).

*Waardenburg's syndrome* (commonest cause of congenital deafness, white macules and white forelock, iris heterochromia).

## COURSE AND PROGNOSIS

Vitiligo is a chronic disease. The course is highly variable, but rapid onset followed by a period of stability or slow progression is most characteristic. Up to 30% of patients may report some spontaneous repigmentation in a few areas—particularly areas that are exposed to the sun. Rarely is this sufficient to satisfy the cosmetic burden that the patient feels. Rapidly progressive or "galloping" vitiligo may quickly lead to extensive depigmentation with a total loss of pigment in skin and hair, but not eyes.

The treatment of vitiligo-associated disease (i.e., thyroid disease) has no impact on the course of vitiligo.

## MANAGEMENT

The approaches to the management of vitiligo are as follows:

### Sunscreens
The dual objectives of sunscreens are protection of involved skin from acute sunburn reaction and limitation of tanning of normally pigmented skin. Sunscreens with a sun protection factor >30 are reasonable choices to prevent sunburn for most patients. However, since their ability to limit the tanning reaction is inversely proportional to SPT, opaque sunscreens should be more effective in limiting the tanning reaction in fairer-skinned individuals. While all SPTs have a need for sun protection, sunscreens alone are often perfectly adequate management for those vitiligo patients with SPTs I, II, and sometimes III.

### Cosmetic Coverup
The objective of coverup with dyes or makeup is to hide the white macules so that the vitiligo is not apparent. Over-the-counter preparations come in many color shades, are easy to apply, and do not rub off but gradually wash or wear off. So-called self-tanning agents, which contain dihydroxyacetone, are available in a number of formulations.

### Repigmentation
The objective of repigmentation (Figs. 13-3 and 13-5) is the permanent return of normal melanin pigmentation. This may be achieved for local macules with topical glucocorticoids or topical psoralens and UVA (long-wave ultraviolet light) and for widespread macules with oral psoralens and UVA.

- *Topical glucocorticoids* Initial treatment with intermittent (4 weeks on, 2 weeks off) topical class I glucocorticoid ointments is practical, simple, and safe for single or a few macules. If there is no response in 2 months, it is unlikely to be effective. Monitor for signs of early steroid atrophy.

- *Topical photochemotherapy* Employs topical 8-methoxypsoralen (8-MOP) and UVA. This procedure should be undertaken for small macules only by experienced physicians and well-informed patients. As with oral psoralens, it may require ≥15 treatments to initiate response and ≥100 to finish.

- *Systemic photochemotherapy* For more widespread vitiligo, oral PUVA is more practical. Oral PUVA may be done using sunlight (in summer or in areas with year-round sunlight) and 5-methoxypsoralen (5-MOP) (available in Europe) or with artificial UVA and either 5-MOP or 8-MOP (Fig. 13-5). Outdoor and indoor PUVA therapy should be done only by experienced dermatologists who have had training in photochemotherapy and who are familiar with the short-and long-term side effects. A response to PUVA is signaled by the appearance of tiny, usually follicular macules of pigmentation (Fig. 13-3). When this occurs, it is a good prognostic sign for successful repigmentation. Oral PUVA photochemotherapy with either 8-MOP or 5-MOP is up to 85% effective in >70% of patients with vitiligo of the head, neck, upper arms and legs, and trunk. At least 1 year of treatment is required to achieve this result. Distal hands and feet and the "lip-tip" variant of vitiligo are poorly responsive and, when present alone, are not usually worth treating. Genital areas should be shielded and not treated. For risks of PUVA therapy see Section 3, "PUVA Therapy for Psoriasis".

- *Narrow-band UVB, 311 nm* This is just as effective as PUVA and does not require psoralens. It is the treatment of choice in children >6 years of age.

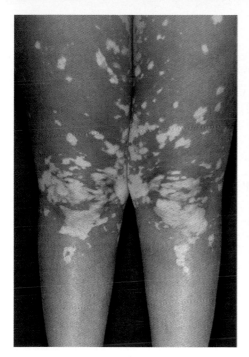 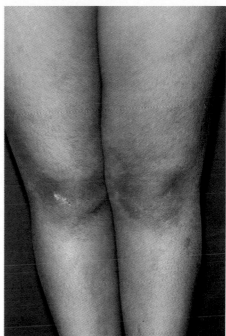

**FIGURE 13-5    Vitiligo: therapy-induced repigmentation**    *This 20-year-old Indian female is being treated with photochemotherapy (PUVA). There is slight erythema in the vitiliginous macules in the early phases (left) of therapy that will be followed by follicular pigmentation as in Fig. 13-3; after 1 year of treatment, vitiligo has completely repigmented but there is now hyperpigmentation of the knees (right). This, however, will fade with time and the color of the repigmented areas will blend with that of the surrounding skin.*

- Repigmentation has also been achieved with the topical calcineurin inhibitors tacrolimus and pimecrolimus, but large-scale trials have not yet been performed.

### Minigrafting
Minigrafting may be a useful technique for refractory and stable segmental vitiligo macules. PUVA may be required after the procedure to unify the color between the graft sites. The demonstrated occurrence of koebnerization in donor sites in generalized vitiligo restricts this procedure to those who have limited cutaneous areas at risk for vitiligo. "Pebbling" of the grafted site may occur.

### Depigmentation
The objective of depigmentation is "one" skin color in patients with extensive vitiligo or in those who have failed PUVA, who cannot use PUVA, or who reject the PUVA option.
***Bleaching*** Bleaching of *normally pigmented skin* with monobenzylether of hydroquinone 20% (MEH) cream is a permanent, irreversible process. Since application of MEH may be associated with satellite depigmentation, this treatment cannot be used selectively to bleach certain areas of normal pigmentation, since there is a real likelihood that new and distant white macules will develop over the months of use. The success rate is >90%. The end-stage color of depigmentation with MEH is chalk-white, as in vitiligo macules. The patient who may want bleaching with MEH is typically a skin phototype IV to VI with extensive repigmentation therapy–resistant vitiligo of the face and hands with residual areas of normal (dark) skin color who are happy with a uniform, albeit white skin color on the exposed regions. An occasional patient may wish to take 30 to 60 mg β-carotene per day to impart an off-white color to the vitiliginous skin.

All those who have bleached are at risk for sunburn from acute solar irradiation.

No long-term untoward effects have been reported from the use of MEH 20% cream, but note that the *depigmentation achieved is permanent.*

# ALBINISM

Albinism describes a group of genetic alterations of the melanin pigment system that affect skin, hair follicles, and eyes. It principally involves the synthesis of melanin in these sites, but a normal number of melanocytes are present; the CNS may also be affected in some forms. Albinism can affect the eyes: ocular albinism (OA); or the eyes and skin: oculocutaneous albinism (OCA); or the skin and other organ systems. The classification of albinism is shown in Table 13-1. OCA is by far the most common form of albinism and is the only form discussed here.

## OCULOCUTANEOUS ALBINISM (OCA)

### EPIDEMIOLOGY

**Classification**   See Table 13-1.
**Prevalence**   Estimated 1:20,000. OCA1 and OCA2 account for 40 to 50%.
**Inheritance**   Most autosomal recessive.

### PATHOGENESIS

The defect in melanin synthesis has been shown to result from absence of the activity of the enzyme tyrosinase. Tyrosinase is a copper-containing enzyme that catalyzes the oxidation of tyrosine to dopa and the subsequent conversion of dopa to dopa-quinone. Recent cloning of complementary DNAs encoding tyrosinase has made it possible to directly characterize the mutations in the tyrosinase gene responsible for deficient tyrosinase activity in several types of albinism (Table 13-1).

### HISTORY

**Duration**   Present at birth. Patients with albinism avoid the sun because of repeated sunburns and bright light because of problems with vision; otherwise, they live an essentially normal life.

### PHYSICAL EXAMINATION

**General Appearance**   "Poring" (eyes half closed, squinting) when in sunlight.
**Skin**   Varied, depending on the type: "Snow" white, creamy white, light tan (Table 13-1).
**Hair**   White (tyrosinase-negative); yellow, cream, or light brown (tyrosinase-positive); red; platinum.
**Eyes**   The eye changes are the essential physical finding that define the syndrome of OCA (Fig. 13-6).

Nystagmus, a feature always present, results from hypoplasia of the fovea with reduction of visual acuity and alteration in the formation of the optic nerves; this misrouting of the optic paths is also associated with an alternating strabismus and diminished stereoacuity. The diagnostic features in the eye that identify albinism are therefore nystagmus and iris translucency (Fig. 13-7), reduction of visual acuity, decreased retinal pigment, foveal hypoplasia, and strabismus.

### LABORATORY EXAMINATIONS

**Dermatopathology**   *Light Microscopy* Melanocytes are present in the skin and hair bulb in all types of albinism. The dopa reaction is markedly reduced or absent in the melanocytes of the skin and hair, depending on the type of albinism (tyrosinase-negative or tyrosinase-positive).
*Electron Microscopy* Melanosomes are present in melanocytes in all types of albinism, but depending on the type of albinism, there is a reduction of the melanization of melanosomes, with many melanosomes being completely unmelanized in tyrosinase-negative albinism. Melanosomes in the albino melanocytes are transferred in a normal manner to the keratinocytes.
**Molecular Testing**   Now available, and this makes it possible to classify the specific gene alteration in various types of albinism. However, it is not necessary for diagnosis or management of the problem.

### DIAGNOSIS

White persons with very fair skin (SPT I), blond hair, and blue eyes may mimic albinos,

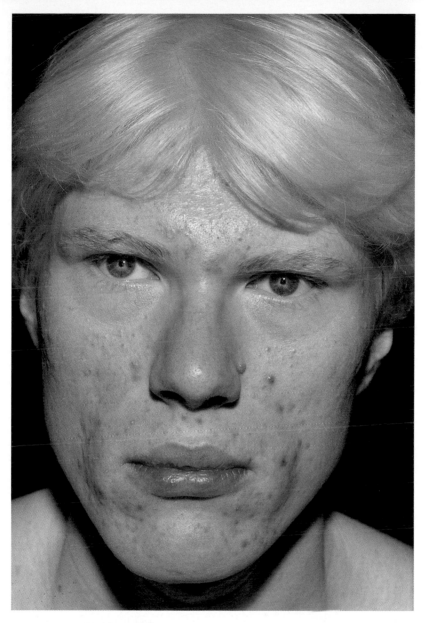

**FIGURE 13-6    Oculocutaneous albinism**    *White skin and white eyelashes; scalp hair and eyebrows have been darkened with dye. The irises appear translucent. Heme pigment gives the face a pinkish hue and carotene ingestion colors the central face a yellow-orange hue. The slight divergent strabism is due to nystagmus. Mild papulopustular acne is also present.*

but they do not have eye changes (iris translucency, nystagmus). Some persons with albinism who have constitutive black or brown skin color may have a dilution of their skin color from black to a light brown and have the capacity to tan; also, some types may have brown irides but still have iris translucency. Therefore, iris translucency and the presence of other eye findings in the fundus are the pathognomonic signs of albinism. The hair and skin color may vary from normal to absent melanin, and the various types are listed in Table 13-1. The special types of albinism are diagnosed on the basis of clinical presentation of the hair and skin pigmentation as well as hematologic studies (Hermansky-Pudlak syndrome).

## SIGNIFICANCE

Albinism is an important disease to recognize early in life in order to begin prophylactic measures to prevent dermatoheliosis and skin cancer, i.e., protective clothing, sunblocks, and sun avoidance in peak periods during the day (1 to 2 h either side of noon, depending on the latitude).

## COURSE AND PROGNOSIS

Albinos with tyrosinase-positive OCA form melanin pigment in the hair, skin, and eyes during early life, the hair becoming cream, yellow, or light brown, and the eye color changing from light gray to blue, hazel, or even brown.

### TABLE 13-1   Classification of Albinism

| Type | Subtypes | Gene Locus | Includes | Clinical Findings |
|------|----------|------------|----------|-------------------|
| OCA1 | OCA1A | *TYR* | Tyrosinase-negative OCA | White hair and skin, eyes (pink at birth → blue) |
|      | OCA1B | *TYR* | Minimal pigment OCA | White to near-normal skin and hair pigmentation |
|      |       |       | Platinum OCA | |
|      |       |       | Yellow OCA | Yellow (pheomelanin) hair, light red or brown hair |
|      |       |       | Temperature-sensitive OCA | May have near-normal pigment but not in axilla |
|      |       |       | Autosomal recessive OCA (some) | |
| OCA2 |       | *P* | Tyrosinase-positive OCA | Yellow hair, skin "creamy" white (Africa) |
|      |       |       | Brown OCA | Light brown/tan skin (Africa) |
| OCA3 |       | *TRP1* | Autosomal recessive OCA (some) | |
|      |       |       | Rufous OCA | Red and red-brown skin and brown eyes (Africa) |
| OCA4 |       | *MATP* | | |
| HPS  |       | *HPS* | Hermansky-Pudlak syndrome | Skin/hair as in OCA1A or OCA1B or OCA2, bleeding diathesis (Puerto Rico) |
| CHS  |       | *LYST* | Chédiak-Higashi syndrome | Silver hair/hypopigmentation/serious medical problems |
| OA1  |       | *OA1* | X-linked OA | Normal pigmentation of skin and hair |

NOTE: OCA, oculocutaneous albinism; TYR, tyrosinase; P, pink protein; TRP1, tyrosinase-related protein 1; OA, ocular albinism; MATP, membrane-associated transporter protein; LYST, lysosome trafficking.

source: Modified from P Bahadoran et al, Albinism in IM Freedberg, AZ Eisen, K Wolff, KF Austen, LA Goldsmith, SI Katz, (eds): *Fitzpatrick's Dermatology in General Medicine*, 6th ed. New York, McGraw-Hill, 2003.

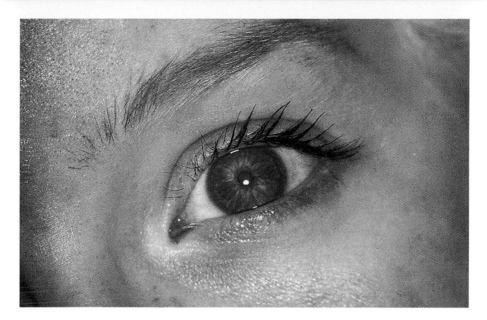

**FIGURE 13-7    Iris translucency with albinism**    *Iris translucency is a sine qua non in all types of oculocutaneous albinism, even in those patients in whom the iris is brown. The iris is rarely pink except in infants, and the diagnosis of albinism depends on the detection of iris translucency. This is best done in a dark room with a flashlight pointed at the sclera.*

Albinos living in central Africa who are unprotected from the sun develop squamous cell carcinomas early in life, and this significantly shortens their life span; few survive to the age of 40 years because of metastasizing squamous cell carcinoma. Dermatoheliosis and basal cell carcinomas are frequent in albinos living in temperate climates. Melanomas are, curiously, very rare in albinos living in Africa; when they occur, they are usually amelanotic. Melanocytic nevi occur in albinism and may also be amelanotic but may be pigmented, depending on the type of albinism.

## MANAGEMENT

Every albino should be under the care of an ophthalmologist for vision problems and a dermatologist to detect solar keratoses, skin cancers, and dermatoheliosis. Daily application of topical, potent, broad-spectrum SPF >30 sunblocks, including lip sunblocks. Avoidance of sun exposure in the high solar intensity season. Use of topical tretinoin for dermatoheliosis and for its possible prophylactic effect against sun-induced epithelial skin cancers. Treatment of solar keratoses to prevent the development of squamous cell carcinomas. Systemic β-carotene (30 to 60 mg tid) imparts a more normal color to the skin and may have some protective effect on the development of skin cancers, although this has been proved only in mice. It is helpful for albinos to belong to a national volunteer group of albinos, in the United States called the *N*ational *O*rganization for *A*lbinism and *H*ypomelanosis (NOAH). (Noah, the builder of the ark in the Old Testament, was alleged to be an albino.) This group assists albinos in various ways, especially in dealing with vision problems: obtaining driver's license, etc.

# MELASMA  ■ ○

Melasma (Greek: "a black spot") is an acquired light- or dark-brown hyperpigmentation that occurs in the exposed areas, most often on the face, and results from exposure to sunlight. It may be associated with pregnancy, with ingestion of contraceptive hormones, or possibly with certain medications such as diphenylhydantoin or it may be idiopathic.
*Synonyms*: Chloasma (Greek: "a green spot"), mask of pregnancy.

## EPIDEMIOLOGY

**Age of Onset**   Young adults.
**Sex**   Females > males; about 10% of patients with melasma are men.
**Race**   Melasma is more apparent or more frequent in persons with brown or black constitutive skin color (persons from Asia, the Middle East, India, South America).
**Incidence and Precipitating Factors**   Common, especially among persons with constitutive brown skin color who are taking contraceptive regimens and who live in sunny areas. Pregnancy causes melasma. Melasma has recently been appearing in menopausal women as a result of regimens for prevention of osteoporosis using a combination of estrogens *and* progesterone; melasma does not appear in those women who are given estrogen replacement treatment but without progesterone. Also in patients on diphenylhydantoin. Sun exposure required.

## PATHOGENESIS

Unknown.

## HISTORY

**Duration of Lesions**   The pigmentation usually evolves quite rapidly over weeks, particularly after exposure to sunlight.

## PHYSICAL EXAMINATION

**Skin Lesions**
Completely macular hyperpigmentation of the face, the hue and intensity depending largely on the skin phototype of the patient (Fig. 13-8). Light or dark brown or even black. Color is usually uniform but may be splotchy. Most often symmetric. Lesions have serrated, irregular, and geographic borders. Two-thirds on central part of the face: cheeks (Fig. 13-8), forehead, nose,

upper lip, and chin; a smaller percentage on the malar or mandibular areas of the face and occasionally the dorsa of the forearms.
**Wood's Lamp Examination** A marked accentuation of the hyperpigmented macules. *This contrast is not accentuated in patients with a normal brown or black skin.*

## DIFFERENTIAL DIAGNOSIS

Postinflammatory hypermelanotic macules.

## SIGNIFICANCE

While this is a strictly cosmetic problem, it is very disturbing to both males and females, especially persons with brown skin color and good tanning capacity.

## COURSE AND PROGNOSIS

Melasma may disappear spontaneously over a period of months after delivery or after cessation of contraceptive hormones. Melasma may or may not return with each subsequent pregnancy.

## MANAGEMENT

**Topical**   Commerically available preparations in the United States include: hydroquinone 3% solution and 4% cream; azelaic acid 20% cream; and a combination of flucinolone 0.01%, hydroquinone 4%, and tretinoin 0.05%. Hydroquinone 4% cream can be compounded with 0.05% tretinoin cream or glycolic acid by the pharmacist.
*Under no circumstances should monobenzylether of hydroquinone or the other ethers of hydroquinone (monomethyl- or monoethyl-) be used in the treatment of melasma because these drugs can lead to a permanent loss of melanocytes with the development of a disfiguring spotty leukoderma.*

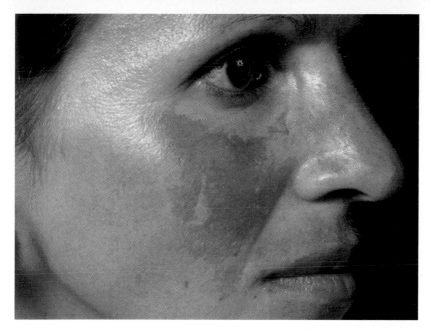

**FIGURE 13-8   Melasma**   *Well-demarcated, hyperpigmented macules are seen on the cheek, nose, and upper lip.*

**Prevention**   It is essential that the patient use, every morning, an *opaque* sunblock containing titanium dioxide and/or zinc oxide; the action spectrum of pigment darkening extends into the visible range, and even the potent transparent sunscreens (with high SPF) are completely ineffective in blocking visible radiation.

# HYPERPIGMENTATION AND HYPOPIGMENTATION FOLLOWING INFLAMMATION OF THE SKIN

## HYPERPIGMENTATION

*Postinflammatory epidermal melanin hyperpigmentation* (■ ◑) is a major problem for patients with skin phototypes IV, V, and VI (Figs. 13-9 and 13-10). This disfiguring pigmentation can develop with acne (Fig. 13-9), psoriasis, lichen planus (Fig. 13-10), atopic dermatitis, or contact dermatitis or after any type of trauma to the skin. It may persist for weeks to months but does respond to topical hydroquinone, which accelerates its disappearance.

The lesions are characteristically limited to the site of the preceding inflammation and have indistinct, feathered borders. Some drug eruptions may be associated with dermal melanin hyperpigmentation, which may also be associated with lichen planus and cutaneous lupus erythematosus. This dermal hyperpigmentation may be persistent, and there is no treatment.

*Riehl's melanosis* (melanodermitis toxica) (□ ◑) is a reticular, confluent black to brown-violet pigmentation of the face and neck (Fig. 13-11). It may be a result of contact sensitivity or photocontact sensitivity related to chemicals, particularly fragrance in cosmetics.

For *hypermelanosis due to phototoxic reactions* induced by psoralens (Berloque dermatitis), see Section 10, and for *non-melanin-based hyperpigmentation* due to drugs, see Section 20.

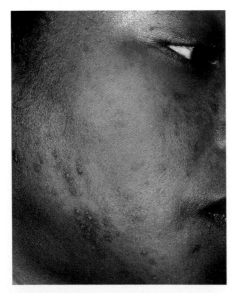

**Figure 13-9   Hypermelanosis with acne**   *This condition is a major complaint of this 18-year-old African American (skin phototype V). The acne is not the problem now; it is the disfiguring hypermelanosis. This hyperpigmentation can be markedly reduced with topical hydroquinone solution, 3%, applied daily. During the depigmentation, the patient must use an opaque sunblock daily to prevent the pigment darkening that occurs with daily sun exposure.*

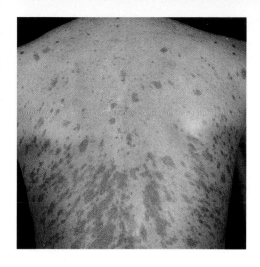

**FIGURE 13-10   Postinflammatory hyperpigmentation**   *May follow a drug eruption, psoriasis or lichen planus, especially in skin phototypes V and VI as was the case in this middle-age East Indian female. Postinflammatory hyperpigmentation is a major problem in young females with skin phototypes V and VI.*

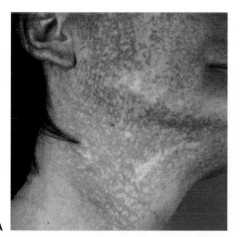

A

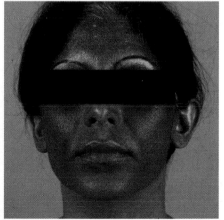

B

**FIGURE 13-11   Melanodermatitis toxica**   *A. A reticular confluent pigmentation on the face and neck of a 42-year-old female chemist who worked for a cosmetic industry and had applied, over years, most of the scented products she was involved in producing to her own skin. Since she lived in a sunny climate this increases the suspicion of a chronic photocontact sensitivity. B. In this Indian lady the mottled hyperpigmentation has coalesced to an almost uniform black color. For professional reasons this patient had also excessively used cosmetics.*

## HYPOPIGMENTATION

Postinflammatory hypomelanosis is always related to loss of melanin. It is a special feature of pityriasis versicolor (Fig. 13-12, see also Section 23), in which the hypopigmentation may also remain for weeks after the active infection has disappeared. Hypomelanosis is not uncommonly seen in atopic dermatitis, psoriasis (Fig. 13-13), guttate parapsoriasis, and pityriasis lichenoides chronica. It may also be present in cutaneous lupus erythematosus, alopecia mucinosa, mycosis fungoides, lichen striatus, and seborrheic dermatitis. Hypomelanosis may follow dermabrasion and chemical peels; in these conditions there is a "transfer block," in which melanosomes are present in melanocytes but are not transferred to keratinocytes, resulting in hypomelanosis. The lesions are usually not chalk white, as in vitiligo, but "off" white and have indiscrete margins. A common type of hypopigmentation is associated with *pityriasis alba* (Fig. 13-14). This is a macular hypopigmentation mostly on the face of children, off-white with a powdery scale. Relatively indistinct margins under Wood's light and scaling distinguish this eczematous dermatitis from vitiligo. It is self-limited. Hypomelanosis not uncommonly follows intralesional glucocorticoid injections; but when the injections are stopped, a normal pigmentation develops in the areas. Depending on the associated disorder, postinflammatory hypomelanosis may respond to oral PUVA photochemotherapy.

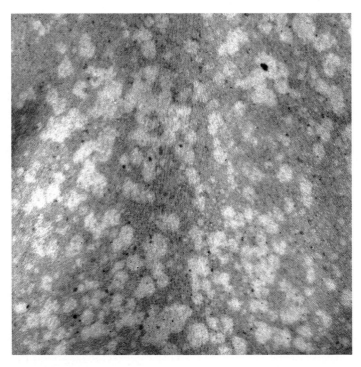

**FIGURE 13-12 Pityriasis versicolor** *Hypopigmented, sharply marginated, scaling macules on the back of an individual with brown skin. Gentle abrasion of the surface accentuates the scaling. This type of hypomelanosis can remain long after the eruption has been treated and the primary process is resolved.*

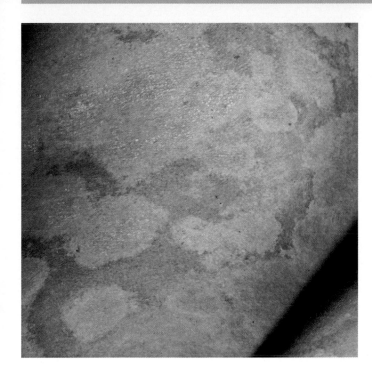

**FIGURE 13-13   Postinflammatory hypomelanosis (psoriasis)** *The hypomelanotic lesions correspond exactly to the antecedent eruption. There is some residual psoriasis within the lesions.*

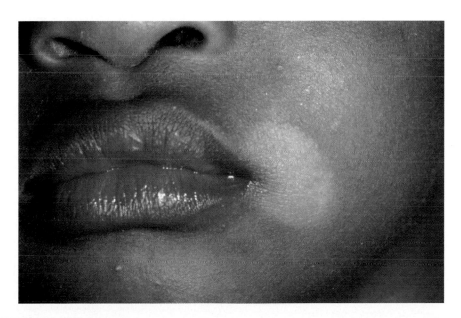

**FIGURE 13-14   Pityriasis alba** *A common disfiguring hypomelanosis, which, as the name indicates, is a white area (alba) with scaling (pityriasis). It is observed in a large number of children in the summer in temperate climates. It is mostly a cosmetic problem in persons with brown or black skin and commonly occurs on the face as in this child. Among 200 patients with pityriasis alba, 90% ranged from 6 to 12 years of age. In young adults, PA quite often occurs on the arms and trunk.*

# PART

## II

# DERMATOLOGY AND INTERNAL MEDICINE

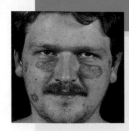

# SKIN SIGNS OF IMMUNE, AUTOIMMUNE, AND RHEUMATIC DISEASES

## SYSTEMIC AMYLOIDOSIS

Amyloidosis is an extracellular deposition in various tissues of amyloid fibril proteins and of a protein called *amyloid P component* (AP); the identical component of AP is present in the serum and is called *SAP*. These amyloid deposits can affect normal body function. *Acquired systemic amyloidosis* (AL), also known as *primary amyloidosis*, occurs in patients with B cell or plasma cell dyscrasias and multiple myeloma in whom fragments of monoclonal immunoglobulin light chains form amyloid fibrils. *Secondary amyloidosis* (AA) occurs in patients after chronic inflammatory disease, in whom the fibril protein is derived from the circulating acute-phase lipoprotein known as *serum amyloid A*. Clinical features of AL (primary amyloidosis) include a combination of macroglossia and cardiac, renal, hepatic, and GI involvement, as well as carpal tunnel syndrome and *skin lesions*. These occur in 30% of patients, and since they occur early in the disease, they are an important clue to the diagnosis. There are few or no characteristic skin lesions in AA (secondary amyloidosis), which usually affects the liver, spleen, kidneys, and adrenals; but there is a certain degree of overlap, and some skin lesions occur. In addition, skin manifestations may also be associated with a number of (rare) hederofamilial syndromes.

---

## ACQUIRED SYSTEMIC AMYLOIDOSIS, PRIMARY AMYLOIDOSIS (AL)  ▪

---

This occurs in many but not all patients with multiple myeloma and B cell and plasma cell dyscrasias.

### PHYSICAL EXAMINATION

#### Skin Lesions

Smooth, waxy papules (Fig. 14-1) but also nodules on the face, especially around the eyes (Fig. 14-2) but also elsewhere. Purpura following trauma, "pinch" purpura in waxy papules (Fig. 14-2) sometimes also involving large surface areas without nodular involvement. Predilection sites are around the eyes, central face, extremities, body folds, axillae, umbilicus, anogenital area. *Macroglossia*: diffusely enlarged and firm, "woody" (Fig. 14-3). This also occurs in AA.

**Systemic Symptoms** Include fatigue, weakness, anorexia, weight loss, malaise, dyspnea; symptoms related to hepatic, renal, and GI involvement; paresthesia related to carpal tunnel syndrome.

**General Examination** Kidney—nephrosis; nervous system—peripheral neuropathy, carpal tunnel syndrome; cardiovascular—partial heart block, congestive heart failure; hepatic—hepatomegaly; GI—diarrhea, sometimes hemorrhagic, malabsorption; lymphadenopathy.

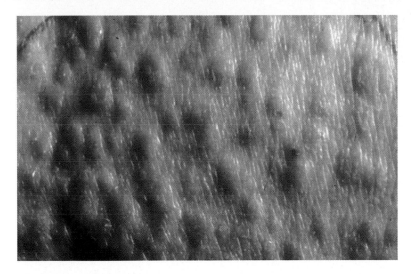

**FIGURE 14-1  Acquired systemic amyloidosis**  *Waxy papules on the trunk of a 58-year-old male patient with myeloma.*

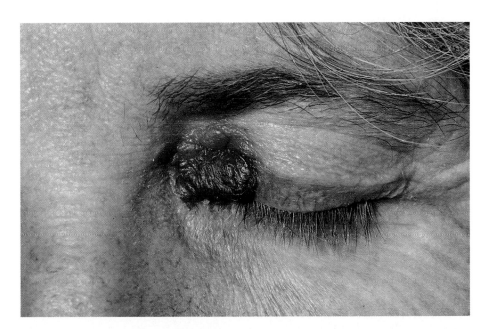

**FIGURE 14-2  Acquired systemic amyloidosis: "pinch purpura"**  *The topmost papule is yellowish and nonhemorrhagic; the lower portion is hemorrhagic. So-called "pinch purpura" of the upper eyelid can appear in amyloid nodules after pinching or rubbing the eyelid.*

## LABORATORY EXAMINATIONS

May reveal thrombocytosis >500,000/μL. Proteinuria and increased serum creatinine; hypercalcemia. Increased IgG. Monoclonal protein in two-thirds of patients with primary or myeloma-associated amyloidosis. Bone marrow: myeloma.

**Dermatopathology** Shows accumulation of faintly eosinophilic masses of amyloid in the papillary body near the epidermis, in the papillary and reticular dermis, in sweat glands, around and within blood vessel walls. Use thioflavin and examine the sections for an apple-green birefringence with a simple polarization microscope.

## DIAGNOSIS

Made by the combination of purpuric skin lesions (Fig. 14-2), waxy papules (Fig. 14-1), macroglossia (Fig. 14-3), carpal tunnel syndrome, and cardiac symptoms. A tissue diagnosis can be made from the skin biopsy. Scintigraphy after injection of [123]I-labeled SAP will reveal the extent of the involvement and can serve as a guide for treatment, which is that of the underlying disease.

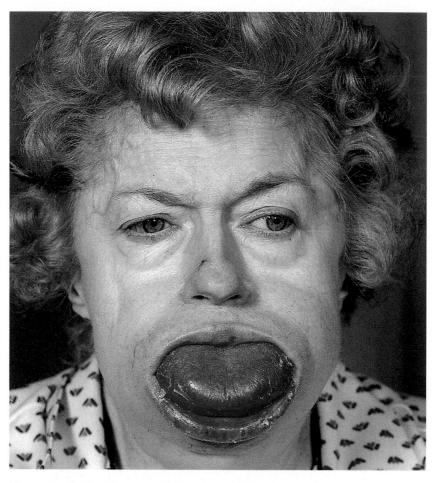

**FIGURE 14-3   Acquired systemic amyloidosis: macroglossia**   *Massive infiltration of the tongue with amyloid has caused immense enlargement; the tongue cannot be retracted completely into the mouth because of its size. (Courtesy of Evan Calkins, MD.)*

## SECONDARY AMYLOIDOSIS (AA)

There are no characteristic skin lesions in AA, except macroglossia and, occasionally, papules and hemorrhage; hyperpigmentation.

## LOCALIZED CUTANEOUS AMYLOIDOSIS   ▮  ◑

Three not uncommon varieties of localized amyloidosis that are unrelated to the systemic amyloidoses are *lichenoid amyloidosis* (discrete, very pruritic, brownish-red papules on the legs); *nodular amyloidosis* (single or multiple, smooth, nodular lesions with or without purpura on limbs, face, or trunk) (similar to that shown in Fig. 14-1); and *macular amyloidosis* [pruritic, gray-brown, reticulated macular lesions occurring principally on the upper back (Fig. 14-4); the lesions often have a distinctive "ripple" pattern]. In lichenoid and macular amyloidosis the amyloid fibrils in skin are keratin-derived. Although these three localized forms of amyloidosis are confined to the skin and unrelated to systemic disease, the skin lesions of nodular amyloidosis are identical to those that occur in AL, in which amyloid fibrils derive from immunoglobulin light chain fragments.

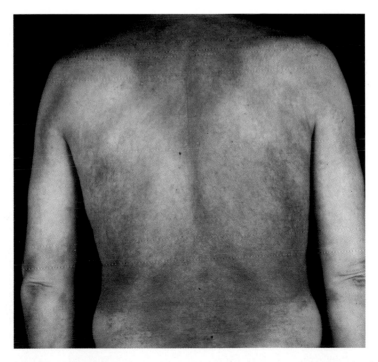

**FIGURE 14-4   Macular amyloidosis**  *Gray-brown, reticulated pigmentation on the back of a 52-year-old male of Arabian extraction.*

# URTICARIA AND ANGIOEDEMA ■ ◑ → ●

Urticaria is composed of wheals (transient edematous papules and plaques, usually pruritic and due to edema of the papillary body) (Fig. 14-5). The wheals are superficial, well defined. Angioedema is a larger edematous area that involves the dermis *and* subcutaneous tissue (Fig. 14-6) and is deep and ill defined. Urticaria and angioedema are thus the same edematous process but involving different levels of the cutaneous vascular plexus: papillary and deep. Urticaria and/or angioedema may be acute recurrent or chronic recurrent. There are some syndromes with angioedema in which urticarial wheals are rarely present (e.g., hereditary angioedema).

## EPIDEMIOLOGY AND ETIOLOGY

**Incidence**　15 to 23% of the population may have had this condition during their lifetime. Chronic urticaria is likely to be present at some time in about 25% of patients with urticaria.
**Etiology**　See Table 14-1.

## CLINICAL TYPES

**Acute Urticaria**　Acute onset and recurring over <30 days. Usually large wheals often associated with angioedema (Fig. 14-6); often IgE-dependent with atopic background; related to alimentary agents, parasites, and penicillin. Also, complement-mediated in serum sickness–like reactions (whole blood, immunoglobulins, penicillin). Often accompanied by angioedema. Common. (See also "Drug-Induced Acute Urticaria" Section 20.)
**Chronic Urticaria**　Recurring over >30 days. Small and large wheals (Figs. 14-5 and 14-7).

Rarely IgE-dependent but often due to anti-FcεR autoantibodies; etiology unknown in 80% and therefore considered idiopathic. Intolerance to salicylates, benzoates. Common. Chronic urticaria affects adults predominantly and is approximately twice as common in women as in men. Up to 40% of patients with chronic urticaria of >6 months' duration still have urticaria 10 years later.

## PHYSICAL EXAMINATION

### Skin Lesions
Sharply defined *wheals* (Fig. 14-5), small (<1 cm) to large (>8 cm), erythematous or white with an erythematous rim, round, oval, acriform, annular, serpiginous (Figs. 14-6 and 14-7), due to confluence and resolution in one area and progression in another (Figs. 14-7 and 20-4). Lesions are pruritic and transient.

### TABLE 14-1　Etiology and Classification of Urticaria/Angioedema

| | |
|---|---|
| Immunologic | Urticaria due to mast cell–releasing agents, |
| 　IgE-mediated urticaria | 　pseudoallergens, ACE inhibitors |
| 　Complement-mediated urticaria | Idiopathic urticaria |
| 　Autoimmune urticaria | Non-immune contact urticaria |
| 　Immune contact urticaria | Urticaria associated with vascular/connective |
| Physical | 　tissue autoimmune disease |
| 　Dermographism | Distinct angioedema (± urticaria) syndromes |
| 　Cold urticaria | 　Hereditary angioedema |
| 　Solar urticaria | 　Angioedema-urticaria-eosinophilia syndrome |
| 　Cholinergic urticaria | |
| 　Pressure angioedema | |
| 　Vibratory angioedema | |

NOTE: ACE, angiotensin-converting enzyme.

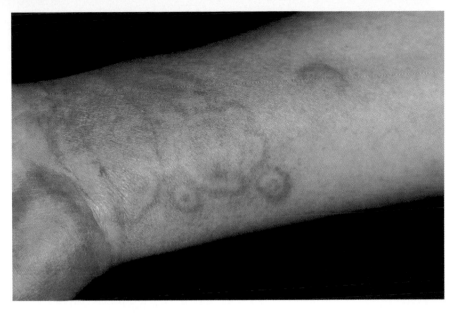

**FIGURE 14-5   Urticaria**   *Wheals with white-to-light-pink color centrally and peripheral erythema in a close-up view. These are the classic lesions of urticaria. It is characteristic that they are transient and highly pruritic.*

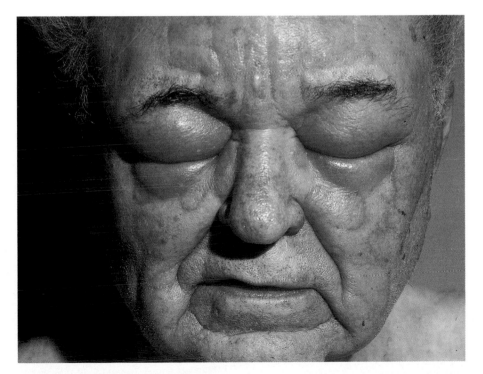

**FIGURE 14-6   Acute urticaria and angioedema**   *Note that there are both superficial wheals and deep, diffuse edema. Occurred after the patient had eaten shellfish. He had similar episodes previously but never considered seafood as the cause.*

*Angioedema*—skin-colored, transient enlargement of portion of face (eyelids, lips, tongue) (Figs. 14-6 and 20-4), extremity, or other sites due to subcutaneous edema.

**Distribution** Usually regional or generalized. Localized in solar, pressure, vibration, cold urticaria/angioedema and confined to the site of the trigger mechanism (see below).

## SPECIAL FEATURES/AS RELATED TO PATHOGENESIS

### Immunologic Urticaria

*IgE Mediated* Lesions in acute IgE-mediated urticaria result from antigen-induced release of biologically active molecules from mast cells or basophilic leukocytes sensitized with specific IgE antibodies (type I anaphylactic hypersensitivity). Released mediators increase venular permeability and modulate the release of biologically active molecules from other cell types. Often with atopic background. Antigens: food (milk, eggs, wheat, shellfish, nuts), therapeutic agents, drugs (penicillin) (see also "Drug-Induced Urticaria," Section 20), helminths. Most often acute (Figs. 14-6 and 20-4).

*Complement Mediated* By way of immune complexes activating complement and releasing anaphylatoxins that induce mast cell degranulation. Serum sickness, administration of whole blood, immunoglobulins. Acute.

*Autoimmune* Common, chronic. Autoantibodies against FcεRI and/or IgE. Positive autologous serum skin test. Clinically, patients with these autoantibodies (up to 40% of patients with chronic urticaria) are indistinguishable from those without them (Fig. 14-7). These autoantibodies may explain why plasmapheresis, intravenous immunoglobulins, and cyclosporine induce remission of disease activity in these patients.

*Immunologic Contact Urticaria* Usually in children with atopic dermatitis sensitized to environmental allergens (grass, animals) or individuals sensitized to wearing latex rubber gloves; can be accompanied by anaphylaxis.

### Physical Urticarias

*Dermographism (Factitious Urticaria)* Linear urticarial lesions occur after stroking or scratching the skin; they itch and fade in 30 min (Fig. 14-8). Although 4.2% of the normal population have it, symptomatic dermographism is a nuisance.

*Cold Urticaria* Usually in children or young adults; urticarial lesions confined to sites exposed to cold occurring within minutes after rewarming. "Ice cube" test (application of an ice cube for a few minutes to skin) establishes diagnosis.

*Solar Urticaria* Urticaria after solar exposure. Action spectrum from 290 to 500 nm; wheezing lasts for <1 h, may be accompanied by syncope; histamine is one of the mediators.

*Cholinergic Urticaria* Exercise to the point of sweating provokes typical small, papular, highly pruritic urticarial lesions (Fig. 14-9). May be accompanied by wheezing.

*Aquagenic Urticaria* Very rare. Contact with water of any temperature induces eruption similar to cholinergic urticaria.

*Pressure Angioedema* Erythematous swelling induced by sustained pressure (buttock swelling when seated, hand swelling after hammering, foot swelling after walking). Delayed (30 min to 12 h). Painful, may persist for several days, and interferes with quality of life. No laboratory abnormalities; fever may occur. Urticaria may occur in addition to angioedema.

*Vibratory Angioedema* May be familial (autosomal dominant) or sporadic. Rare. It is believed to result from histamine release from mast cells caused by a "vibrating" stimulus— rubbing a towel across the back produces lesions, but direct pressure (without movements) does not.

### Urticaria Due to Mast Cell–Releasing Agents and Pseudoallergens and Chronic Idiopathic Urticaria

Urticaria/angioedema and even anaphylaxis-like symptoms may occur with radiocontrast media and as a consequence of intolerance to salicylates, food preservatives and additives (e.g., benzoic acid and sodium benzoate), as well as several azo dyes, including tartrazine and sunset yellow (pseudoallergens) (Fig. 14-7); also to ACE inhibitors. May be acute and chronic. In chronic idiopathic urticaria, histamine derived from mast cells in the skin is considered the major mediator. Eicosanoids and neuropeptides may also play a part in producing the lesions, but direct measurement of these mediators has not been reported.

### Non-Immune Contact Urticaria

Due to direct effects of exogenous urticants penetrating into skin or blood vessels. Localized to site of contact. Sorbic acid, benzoic acid in eye solutions and foods, cinnamic aldehydes in cosmetics, histamine, acetylcholine, serotonin in nettle stings.

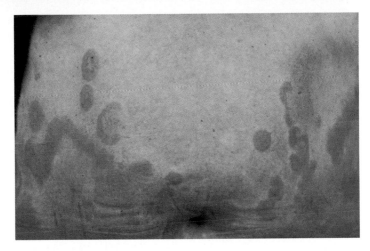

**FIGURE 14-7    Chronic urticaria**   *Chronic urticaria of 5-year duration in an otherwise healthy 50-year-old female. Eruptions occur on an almost daily basis and, as they are highly pruritic, greatly impair the patient's quality of life. Although suppressed by antihistamines, there is an immediate recurrence after treatment is stopped. Repeated laboratory and clinical examinations have not revealed an apparent cause.*

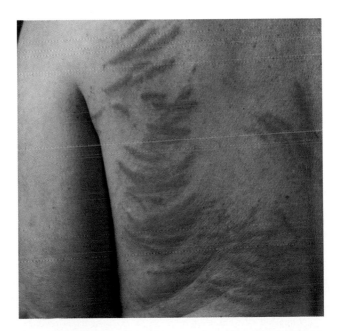

**FIGURE 14-8    Urticaria: dermographism**   *Urticaria as it appeared 5 min after the patient scratched himself because of itchiness of his otherwise normal skin. The patient had experienced generalized pruritus for several months with no spontaneously occurring urticaria.*

## Urticaria Associated with Vascular/Connective Tissue Autoimmune Disease

Urticarial lesions may be associated with systemic lupus erythematosus (SLE) and Sjögren's syndrome. However, in most instances they represent urticarial vasculitis (page 416). This is a form of cutaneous vasculitis associated with urticarial skin lesions that persist for >12 to 24 h. Slow changes in size and configuration, can be associated with purpura, and can show residual pigmentation due to hemosiderin after involution. Often associated with hypocomplementemia and renal disease.

### Distinct Angioedema (± Urticaria) Syndromes

*Hereditary Angioedema (HAE)* A serious autosomal dominant disorder; may follow trauma (physical and emotional). Angioedema of the face (Fig. 14-10) and extremities, episodes of laryngeal edema, and acute abdominal pain caused by angioedema of the bowel wall presenting as surgical emergency. Urticaria does not usually occur, but there may be an erythema marginatum–like eruption. Laboratory abnormalities involve the complement system: decreased levels of C1-esterase inhibitor (85%) or dysfunctional inhibitor (15%), low C4 value in the presence of normal C1 and C3 levels. Angioedema results from bradykinin formation, since C1-esterase inhibitor is also the major inhibitor of the Hageman factor and kallikrein, the two enzymes required for kinin formation. Episodes can be life threatening.

*Angioedema-Urticaria-Eosinophilia Syndrome* Severe angioedema, only occasionally with pruritic urticaria, involving the face, neck, extremities, and trunk that lasts for 7 to 10 days. There is fever and marked increase in normal weight (increased by 10 to 18%) owing to fluid retention. No other organs are involved. Laboratory abnormalities include striking leukocytosis (20,000 to 70,000/μL) and eosinophilia (60 to 80% eosinophils), which are related to the severity of attack. There is no family history. This condition is rare, prognosis is good.

## LABORATORY EXAMINATIONS

**Dermatopathology** Edema of the dermis or subcutaneous tissue, dilatation of venules but no evidence of vascular damage. Mast cell degranulation. The predominant perivascular inflammatory cell types are activated lymphocytes of the T helper phenotype.

**Serology** Search for hepatitis-associated antigen, assessment of the complement system, assessment of specific IgE antibodies by radioallergosorbent test (RAST), anti-FcεRI autoantibodies. Serology for lupus and Sjögren's syndrome.

**Hematology** The erythrocyte sedimentation rate (ESR) is often elevated in urticarial vasculitis, and there may be hypocomplementemia; transient eosinophilia in urticaria from reactions to foods, parasites, and drugs; high levels of eosinophilia in the angioedema-urticaria-eosinophilia syndrome.

**Complement Studies** Screening for functional C1 inhibitor in HAE.

**Ultrasonography** For early diagnosis of bowel involvement in HAE; if abdominal pain is present, this may indicate edema of the bowel.

**Parasitology** Stool specimen for presence of parasites.

## DIAGNOSIS

A detailed history (previous diseases, drugs, foods, parasites, physical exertion, solar exposure) is of utmost importance. History should differentiate between *type of lesions* — urticaria, angioedema or urticaria + angioedema; *duration of lesions* (<1 h or ≥1 h), *pruritus*; *pain* on walking (in foot involvement), *flushing*, *burning*, and *wheezing* (in cholinergic urticaria). *Fever* in serum sickness and in the angioedema-urticaria-eosinophilia syndrome; in angioedema, *hoarseness, stridor, dyspnea*. *Arthralgia* (serum sickness, urticarial vasculitis), *abdominal colicky pain* in HAE. A careful history of medications including penicillin, aspirin, nonsteroidal anti-inflammatory drugs, and ACE inhibitors should be obtained.

If *physical urticaria* is suspected, appropriate challenge testing should be performed. *Cholinergic urticaria* can best be diagnosed by exercise to sweating and intracutaneous injection of acetylcholine or mecholyl, which will produce micropapular whealing. *Solar urticaria* is verified by testing with UVB, UVA, and visible light. *Cold urticaria* is verified by a wheal response to the application to the skin of an ice cube or a test tube containing ice water. If urticarial wheals do not disappear in ≤24 h, urticarial vasculitis should be suspected and a biopsy done. The person with *angioedema-urticaria-eosinophilia syndrome* has high fever, high leukocytosis (mostly eosinophils), a striking increase in body

**FIGURE 14-9   Cholinergic urticaria**   *Small urticarial papules on pink skin (axon reflex erythema) occurring on the neck within 30 min of vigorous exercise.*

weight due to retention of water, and a cyclic pattern that may occur and recur over a period of years. *Hereditary angioedema* has a positive family history and is characterized by angioedema of the face and extremities as the result of trauma, abdominal pain, and decreased levels of C4 and C1-esterase inhibitor or a dysfunctional inhibitor.

Most difficult to evaluate is chronic urticaria. A practical approach to the diagnosis of chronic urticaria is shown in Table 14-2.

## COURSE AND PROGNOSIS

Half the patients with urticaria alone are free of lesions in 1 year, but 20% have lesions for >20 years. Prognosis is good in most syndromes except HAE, which may be fatal if untreated.

## MANAGEMENT

**Prevention**   Try to prevent attacks by elimination of etiologic chemicals or drugs: aspirin and food additives, especially in chronic recurrent urticaria—rarely successful; prevent trigger in physical urticarias.

**Antihistamines** $H_1$ blockers, e.g., hydroxyzine, terfenadine; or loratadine, cetirizine, fexofenadine. 180 mg/d of fexofenadine or 10 to 20 mg/d of loratadine usually controls most cases of chronic urticaria, but cessation of therapy usually results in a recurrence; if they fail, $H_1$ and $H_2$ blockers (cimetidine) and/or mast cell–stabilizing agents (ketotifen). Doxepin, a tricyclic antidepressant with marked $H_1$ antihistaminic activity, is valuable when severe urticaria is associated with anxiety and depression.

**Prednisone** In acute urticaria with angioedema; also for angioedema-urticaria-eosinophilia syndrome.

**Danazol** Long-term therapy for hereditary angioedema; whole fresh plasma or C1-esterase inhibitor in the acute attack.

TABLE 14-2　**Differential Diagnosis of Common Types of Chronic Urticaria**

| Type of Urticaria | Principal Clinical Features | Associated Angioedema | Diagnostic Test |
|---|---|---|---|
| Chronic idiopathic | Profuse or sparse generalized, pink or pale wheals, often annular with itching | Yes | In autoimmune urticaria: autologous serum skin test, anti-FcεRI autoantibodies |
| Symptomatic dermographism | Itchy, linear wheals with a surrounding bright-red flare at sites of scratching or rubbing | No | Light stroking of skin causes an immediate wheal with itching |
| Physical urticarias Cold | Itchy, pale or red wheal or swelling at sites of contact with cold surfaces or fluids | Yes | 10-min application of an ice pack causes a wheal within 5 min of the removal of ice |
| Pressure | Large, painful or itchy red swelling at sites of pressure (soles, palms, or waist) | No | Application of pressure perpendicular to skin produces persistent red swelling after a latent period of 1–4 h |
| Solar | Itchy, pale or red wheals or swelling at site of exposure to UV or visible light | Yes | Irradiation by a 2.5 kW solar simulator (290–690 nm) for 30–120 s causes wheals in 30 min |
| Cholinergic | Itchy, small (<5 mm) monomorphic pale or pink papular wheals on trunk, neck, and limbs | Yes | Exercise or a hot shower elicits an eruption, acute stressful situation |

SOURCE: Adapted from MW Greaves: N Engl J Med 332:1767, 1995.

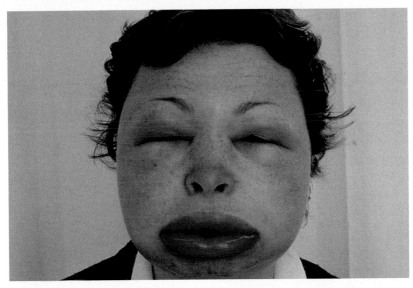

**A.**

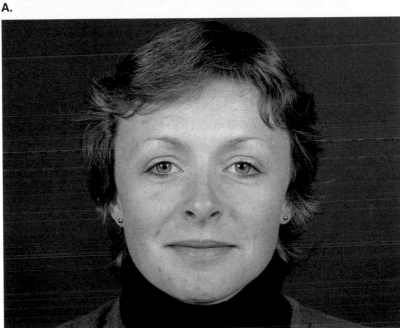

**B.**

**FIGURE 14-10   Hereditary angioedema**   *A. Severe edema of the face during an episode leading to grotesque disfigurement. **B.** Angioedema will subside within hours. The patient had a positive family history and had multiple similar episodes including colicky abdominal pain.*

# BEHÇET'S SYNDROME  

Behçet's syndrome (BS) is a perplexing multisystem vasculitic inflammation that has one basic major feature—recurrent oral aphthous ulcers (AUs)—and two of any of the following features: recurrent genital AU, eye lesions (anterior or posterior uveitis), skin lesions (erythema nodosum or pustules), and a positive pathergy test. Other manifestations include synovitis, neurologic disorders, and thrombophlebitis.
*Synonym*: Behçet's disease.

## EPIDEMIOLOGY

**Age of Onset**   Third and fourth decades.
**Prevalence**   Highest in Japan (1:10,000), Southeast Asia, the Middle East, southern Europe. Rare in northern Europe, United States.
**Sex**   Males > females, but dependent on ethnic background.

## PATHOGENESIS

Etiology unknown. In the eastern Mediterranean and East Asia, HLA-B5 and HLA-B51 association; in the United States and Europe, no consistent HLA association. The lesions are the result of leukocytoclastic (acute) and lymphocytic (late) vasculitis.

## HISTORY

Painful ulcers erupt in a cyclic fashion in the oral cavity and/or genital mucous membranes. Orodynophagia and oral ulcers may persist/recur weeks to months before other symptoms appear.

## PHYSICAL EXAMINATION

### Skin and Mucous Membranes
*Aphthous Ulcers* Punched-out ulcers (3 to >10 mm) with rolled or overhanging borders and necrotic base (Fig. 14-11); red rim; occur in crops (2 to 10) on oral mucous membrane (100%) (Fig. 14-11; see also Fig. 31-1), vulva, penis, and scrotum (Figs. 14-12 and 14-13); very painful.

*Erythema Nodosum–Like Lesions* Painful inflammatory nodules on the arms and legs (40%) (see Fig. 7-25).
*Other* Inflammatory pustules, superficial thrombophlebitis (see Fig. 16-5), *inflammatory plaques* resembling those in Sweet's syndrome (acute febrile neutrophilic dermatosis) (see Fig. 7-33), *pyoderma gangrenosum–like lesions* (see Fig. 7-27), *palpable purpuric lesions* of necrotizing vasculitis (see Fig. 14-34).

### Systemic Findings
*Eyes* Leading cause of morbidity. Posterior uveitis, anterior uveitis, retinal vasculitis, vitreitis, hypopyon, secondary cataracts, glaucoma, neovascular lesions.
*Musculoskeletal* Nonerosive, asymmetric oligoarthritis.
*Neurologic* Onset delayed, occurring in one-quarter of patients. Meningoencephalitis, benign intracranial hypertension, cranial nerve palsies, brainstem lesions, pyramidal/extrapyramidal lesions, psychosis.
*Vascular* Aneurysms, arterial occlusions, venous thrombosis, varices; hemoptysis. Coronary vasculitis: myocarditis, coronary arteritis, endocarditis, valvular disease.
*GI Tract* AUs throughout.

## LABORATORY EXAMINATIONS

**Dermatopathology** Leukocytoclastic vasculitis with fibrinoid necrosis of blood vessel walls in acute early lesions; lymphocytic vasculitis in late lesions.

**FIGURE 14-12 (Opposite page, bottom)   Behçet's syndrome: genital ulcers**   *Multiple large aphthous-type ulcers on the labial and perineal skin. In addition, this 25-year-old patient of Turkish extraction had aphthous ulcers in the mouth and previously experienced an episode of uveitis.*

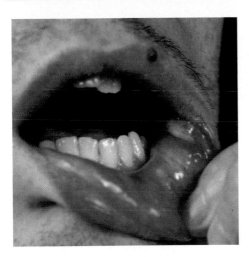
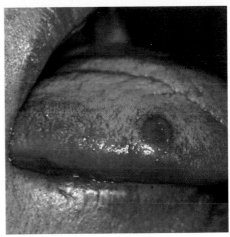

**FIGURE 14-11  Behçet's syndrome**  *Oral aphthous ulcers.* **A.** *These are highly painful, punched-out ulcers with a necrotic base on the buccal mucosa and lower and upper fornix in this 28-year-old Turkish male.* **B.** *A punched-out ulcer on the tongue of another patient.*

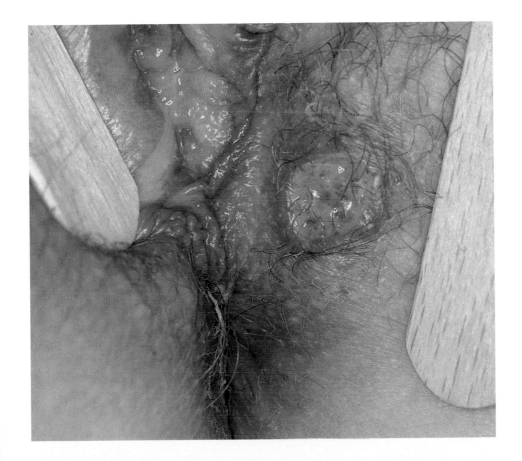

**Pathergy Test**   Positive pathergy test read by physician at 24 or 48 h, after skin puncture with a sterile needle. Leads to inflammatory pustule.

**HLA Typing**   Significant association with HLA-B5 and HLA-B51, in Japanese, Koreans, and Turks, and in the Middle East.

## DIAGNOSIS AND DIFFERENTIAL DIAGNOSIS

Proposed criteria for BS include the presence of oral AU plus two of the following: recurrent genital AU, eye lesions, skin lesions, or positive pathergy test.

**Differential Diagnosis**   *Ulcers*: Viral infection [herpes simplex virus (HSV), varicella-zoster virus (VZV)], hand-foot-and-mouth disease, herpangina, chancre, histoplasmosis, squamous cell carcinoma.

## COURSE AND PROGNOSIS

Highly variable course, with recurrences and remissions; the mouth lesions are always present; remissions may last for weeks, months, or years. In the eastern Mediterranean and East Asia, severe course, one of the leading causes of blindness. With CNS involvement, there is a higher mortality rate.

## MANAGEMENT

**Aphthous Ulcers**   Potent topical glucocorticoids. Intralesional triamcinolone, 3 to 10 mg/mL, injected into ulcer base. Thalidomide, 50 to 100 mg PO in the evening. Colchicine, 0.6 mg PO 2 to 3 times a day. Dapsone, 50–100 mg PO/day.

**Systemic Involvement**   Prednisone with or without azathioprine, cyclophosphamide, azathioprine alone, chlorambucil, cyclosporine.

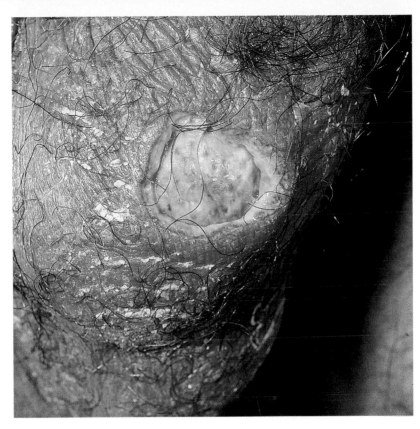

**FIGURE 14-13    Behçet's syndrome**    *A large, punched-out ulcer on the scrotum of a 40-year-old Korean. The patient also had aphthous ulcers in the mouth and pustules on the thighs and buttocks.*

# DERMATOMYOSITIS   □  ●

Dermatomyositis (DM) is a systemic disease belonging to the idiopathic inflammatory myopathies, a heterogenous group of genetically determined autoimmune diseases targeting the skin and/or skeletal muscles. DM is characterized by violaceous (heliotrope) inflammatory changes +/− edema of the eyelids and periorbital area; erythema of the face, neck, and upper trunk; and flat-topped violaceous papules over the knuckles. It is associated with polymyositis, interstitial pneumonitis, myocardial involvement, and vasculitis.

## EPIDEMIOLOGY AND ETIOLOGY

Rare. Incidence >6 cases per million, but this is based on hospitalized patients and does not include individuals without muscle involvement. Juvenile and adult (>40 years) onset.

**Etiology**   Unknown. In persons >55 years of age, often associated with malignancy.

**Clinical Spectrum**   Ranges from DM with only cutaneous inflammation (amyopathic DM) to polymyositis with only muscle inflammation. Cutaneous involvement occurs in 30 to 40% of adults and 95% of children with dermatomyositis/polymyositis. For classification, see Table 14-3.

## HISTORY

±Photosensitivity. Manifestations in skin disease may precede myositis or vice versa; often, both are detected at the same time. Muscle weakness, difficulty in rising from supine position, climbing stairs, raising arms over head, turning in bed. Dysphagia; burning and pruritus of the scalp.

## PHYSICAL EXAMINATION

### Skin Lesions

Periorbital heliotrope (reddish purple) flush, usually associated with some degree of edema (Fig. 14-14). May extend to involve scalp, entire face (Fig. 14-15A), upper chest, and arms.

In addition, papular dermatitis with varying degrees of violaceous erythema (Fig. 14-15A) in the same sites. Flat-topped, violaceous papules (Gottron's papule/sign) with various degrees of atrophy on the nape of the neck and shoulders and over the knuckles and interphalangeal joints (Fig. 14-15B). *Note*: In lupus, lesions usually occur in the interarticular region of the fingers (see Fig. 14-22). Periungual erythema with telangiectasia, thrombosis of capillary loops, infarctions. Lesions over elbows and knuckles may evolve into erosions and ulcers that heal with stellate scarring (particularly in juvenile DM with vasculitis). Long-lasting lesions may evolve into poikiloderma (mottled discoloration with red, white, and brown). Calcification in subcutaneous/fascial tissues common later in course of juvenile DM, particularly about elbows, trochanteric, and iliac region; may evolve into calcinosis universalis.

---

**TABLE 14-3   Classification of Dermatomyositis (DM)**

**Adult onset**
   Classic DM alone
   Classic DM with malignancy
   Classic DM of an overlap connective tissue disorder
   Amyopathic DM

**Juvenile onset**
   Classic DM
   Amyopathic DM
   Hypomyopathic DM

SOURCE: Adapted from RD Sontheimer, MI Costner, in IM Freedberg, AZ Eisen, K Wolff, KF Austen, LA Goldsmith, SI Katz (eds): *Fitzpatrick's Dermatology in General Medicine*, 6th ed. New York, McGraw-Hill, 2003.

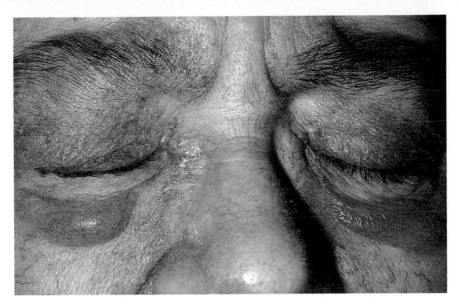

**FIGURE 14-14   Dermatomyositis**   *Heliotrope (reddish purple) erythema of upper eyelids and edema of the lower lids. This 55-year-old female had experienced severe muscle weakness of the shoulder girdle and presented with a lump in the breast that proved to be carcinoma.*

**Muscle**   ±Muscle tenderness, ±muscle atrophy. Progressive muscle weakness affecting proximal/limb girdle muscles. Difficulty or inability to rise from sitting or supine position without using arms. Difficulty in raising arms above head and difficulty in climbing stairs.

Occasional involvement of facial/bulbar, pharyngeal, and esophageal muscles. Deep tendon reflexes within normal limits.

**Disease Association**   Patients with DM have a higher than expected risk for malignancy, particularly ovarian cancer in females. Patients >50 years of age should be investigated for associated malignancy: carcinoma of the ovary, breast, bronchopulmonary, and GI tract. Most cancers detected within 2 years of diagnosis.

## LABORATORY EXAMINATIONS

**Chemistry**  During acute active phase: elevation of creatine phosphokinase (65%), which is most specific for muscle disease; also, of aldolase (40%), lactate dehydrogenase, glutamic oxaloacetic transaminase.

**Autoantibodies**  Autoantibodies to 155 kDa and/or Se in 80% and to Jo-1 in 20% (both have a high specificity for DM) and to (low specificity) antinuclear antibodies (ANA) in 40%.

**Urine**  Elevated 24-h creatine excretion (> 200 mg/24 h).

**Electromyography**  Increased irritability on insertion of electrodes, spontaneous fibrillations, pseudomyotonic discharges, positive sharp waves: excludes neuromyopathy. With evidence of denervation, suspect coexisting tumor.

**MRI**  MRI of muscles reveals focal lesions.

**ECG**  Evidence of myocarditis; atrial, ventricular irritability; atrioventricular block.

**X-Ray**  Chest: ±interstitial fibrosis. *Esophagus*: reduced peristalsis.

**Pathology**  *Skin* Flattening of epidermis, hydropic degeneration of basal cell layer, edema of upper dermis, scattered inflammatory infiltrate, PAS-positive fibrinoid deposits at dermal-epidermal junction and around upper dermal capillaries, accumulation of acid mucopolysaccharides in dermis (all these are compatible with DM but are not diagnostic).

*Muscle* Biopsy shoulder/pelvic girdle; one that is weak or tender, i.e., deltoid, supraspinatus, gluteus, quadriceps after marking by EMG or MRI. Histology—segmental necrosis within muscle fibers with loss of cross-striations; waxy/coagulative type of eosinophilic staining; with or without regenerating fibers; inflammatory cells, histiocytes, macrophages, lymphocytes, plasma cells. Vasculitis is seen in juvenile DM. MRI-guided needle biopsy of muscle may replace conventional muscle biopsy in the future.

## DIAGNOSIS AND DIFFERENTIAL DIAGNOSIS

Skin signs plus proximal muscle weakness with two of three laboratory criteria, i.e., elevated serum "muscle enzyme" levels, characteristic electromyographic changes, diagnostic muscle biopsy. Differential diagnosis is to seborrheic dermatitis, lupus erythematosus, mixed connective tissue disease, steroid myopathy, trichinosis, toxoplasmosis.

## COURSE AND PROGNOSIS

With treatment, prognosis is relatively good except in patients with malignancy and those with pulmonary involvement. With aggressive immunosuppressive treatment the 8-year survival rate is 70 to 80%. A better prognosis is seen in individuals who receive early systemic treatment. The early and aggressive use of glucocorticoids has reduced the mortality rates in children to <10%. The most common causes of death are malignancy, infection, cardiac and pulmonary disease. Successful treatment of an associated neoplasm is often followed by improvement/resolution of DM.

## MANAGEMENT

**Prednisone**  0.5 to 1 mg/kg body weight per day, increasing to 1.5 mg/kg if lower dose ineffective. Taper when "muscle enzyme" levels approach normal. Best if combined with azathioprine, 2 to 3 mg/kg per day.

**Alternatives**  Methotrexate, cyclophosphamide. High-dose IV immunoglobulin bolus therapy at monthly intervals spares glucocorticoid doses to achieve or maintain remissions.

*Note*: Steroid myopathy may occur after 4 to 6 weeks of therapy.

**FIGURE 14-15 (Opposite page)  Dermatomyositis**  *A. Violaceous erythema and papules on the face, neck, and upper chest. There is edematous swelling of the entire face. The patient could barely lift her arms and could not climb stairs. B. Violaceous erythema and Gottron's papules on the dorsa of the hands and fingers, especially over the metacarpophalangeal and interphalangeal joints; the light-protected areas of the forearms of this 28-year old male with severe muscle weakness were not involved. Periungual erythema and telangiectasis. This patient later developed severe calcinosis cutis.*

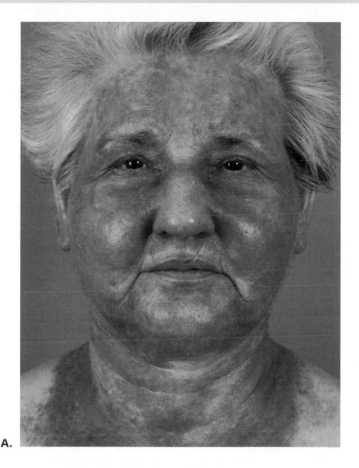

A.

B.

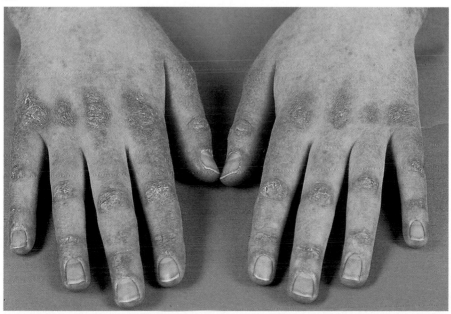

# GRAFT-VERSUS-HOST DISEASE

Graft-versus-host disease (GVHD) is an immune disorder caused by the reaction of histoin-compatible, immunocompetent donor cells against the tissues of an immunoincompetent host (graft-versus-host reaction, GVHR), characterized by acute cutaneous changes ranging from maculopapular eruption to toxic epidermal necrolysis, diarrhea, and liver dysfunction, as well as chronic changes comprising lichenoid eruptions and sclerodermatous changes.

## EPIDEMIOLOGY

**Incidence**    Allogeneic bone marrow transplantation (BMT): 60 to 80% of successful engraftments. Autologous BMT: mild cutaneous GVHD occurs in 8%. Low incidence after blood transfusion in immunosuppressed patients, maternal-fetal transfer in immunodeficiency disease.

---

## ACUTE GVHD

---

## PATHOGENESIS

With successful engraftment, there is replacement of host marrow by immunocompetent donor cells capable of mounting an inflammatory reaction against the foreign tissue antigens of the host. GVHR of specific host organs—skin, liver, or GI tract. Severity of GVHD related to histocompatibility match between donor and recipient and preparatory regimen used.

## HISTORY

During the first 3 months after BMT (usually between 14 and 21 days): mild pruritus, localized/generalized; pain on pressure, palms/soles. Nausea/vomiting, abdominal pain; watery diarrhea. Jaundice; dark yellow urine.

## PHYSICAL EXAMINATION

### Skin Lesions
Initially, subtle, discrete macules and/or papules on upper trunk, hands/feet (Fig. 14-16), especially palms/soles. Painful. Mild edema with violaceous hue, periungual and on pinna. If controlled/resolved, erythema diminishes with subsequent desquamation and postinflammatory hyperpigmentation. If progresses, macules/papules become generalized, confluent, and evolve into erythroderma. Subepidermal bullae, especially over pressure/trauma sites, palms/soles. Positive Nikolsky's sign. If bullae widespread with rupture/erosion, toxic epider-mal necrolysis–like (TEN-like, see Section 7) form of acute cutaneous GVHR (Fig. 14-17). For staging, see Table 14-4.

*Mucosa*    Lichen planus–like lesions in buccal mucosa; erosive stomatitis, oral and ocular sicca-like syndrome; esophagitis/esophageal strictures. Keratoconjunctivitis.

**General Findings**    Fever, jaundice, nausea, vomiting, right upper quadrant pain/tenderness, cramping, abdominal pain, diarrhea, serositis, pulmonary insufficiency, dark urine.

## LABORATORY EXAMINATIONS

**Chemistry**    Elevated SGOT, bilirubin, alkaline phosphatase.

**Dermatopathology**    Focal vacuolization of basal cell layer, apoptosis of individual keratinocytes; mild perivenular mononuclear cell infiltrate. Apposition of lymphocytes to necrotic keratinocytes (satellitosis); vacuoles coalesce to form subepidermal clefts → subepidermal blister formation. Endothelial cell swelling. Immunocytochemistry: HLA-DR expression of keratinocytes precedes morphologic changes and thus represents important, early diagnostic sign.

## DIAGNOSIS AND DIFFERENTIAL DIAGNOSIS

Clinical findings confirmed by skin biopsy.
**Differential Diagnosis**    Exanthematous drug reaction, viral exanthem, TEN, erythroderma.

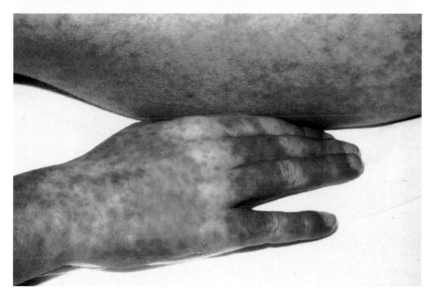

**FIGURE 14-16   Acute graft-versus-host disease**   *Discrete and confluent, erythematous, blanch-able macules and papules with relatively indistinct borders involving the hands and the trunk. Note the relative sparing over the metacarpophalangeal and proximal interphalangeal joints. These relatively mild cutaneous lesions were not associated with intestinal or hepatic involvement.*

### TABLE 14-4   Clinical Staging of Acute GVHD (SKIN)

1. Erythematous maculopapular eruption involving < 25% of body surface
2. Erythematous maculopapular eruption involving 25 to 50% of body surface
3. 50% of body surface, erythroderma
4. Bulla formation

## COURSE AND PROGNOSIS

Mild to moderate GVHD responds well to treatment. Prognosis of TEN–like GVHR is grave. Severe GVHD susceptible to infections—bacterial, fungal, viral (cytomegalovirus, HSV, VZV). Acute GVHD is primary or associated cause of death in 15 to 70% of BMT recipients.

## MANAGEMENT

**Topical Potent Glucocorticoids**   Symptomatic relief in mild to moderate cutaneous GVHD.
**Prednisone**   80 to 100 mg/d for mild to moderate cutaneous GVHD.
**Cyclosporine**   Added to prednisone for severe cutaneous GVHD, ±GI or liver GVHD.
**Extracorporeal Photopheresis**   Also effective.

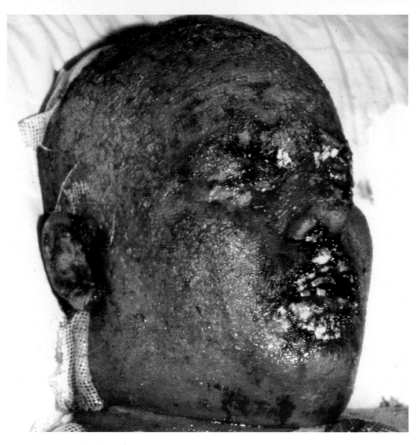

**FIGURE 14-17    Acute graft-versus-host disease**    *Confluent epidermal necrosis, sloughing, and bleeding resembling toxic epidermal necrolysis, on the face and entire trunk after allogeneic BMT. This is clearly a very severe condition.*

## CHRONIC GVHD

### HISTORY

>100 days after BMT. Evolving from acute GVHD or arising de novo. Acute GVHD not always followed by chronic GVHD. Clinical classification thus distinguishes between quiescent onset, progressive onset, and de novo chronic cutaneous GVHD. Chronic GVHD occurs in 25% of recipients of marrow from an HLA-identical sibling who survive >100 days.

### PHYSICAL EXAMINATION

#### Skin Lesions

Flat-topped (lichen planus–like) papules of violaceous color, initially on distal extremities but later generalized (Fig. 14-18) and/or confluent areas of dermal sclerosis (Fig. 14-19) with overlying scale resembling scleroderma mainly on trunk, buttocks, hips, and thighs. With more severe disease, severe generalized sclerodermoid

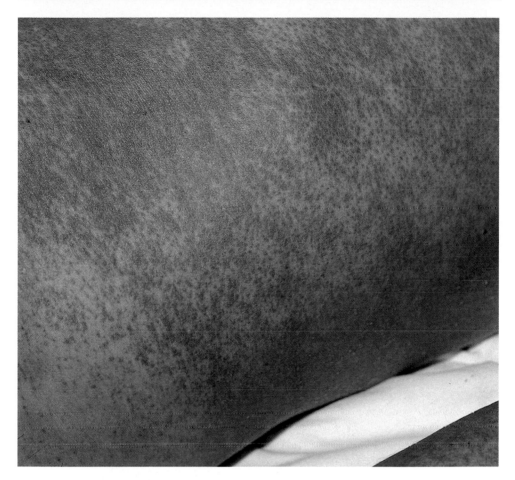

**FIGURE 14-18   Chronic graft-versus-host disease**   *Violaceous to brownish lichen planus-like, perifollicular papules becoming confluent on the trunk, occurring 3 months after allogeneic BMT.*

changes with necrosis and ulceration on acral and pressure sites. Hair loss; anhidrosis; nails: dystrophy, anonychia; vitiligo-like hypopigmentation.

**Mucosa**   Like erosive/ulcerative lichen planus.

**General Findings**   Chronic liver disease, general wasting.

### LABORATORY EXAMINATIONS

**Chemistry**   Elevated ALT, AST, γ-glutamyl-transferase.

**Dermatopathology**   Like *lichen planus*: hyperkeratosis, hypergranulosis, mild irregular acanthosis or atrophy, moderate basal vacuolization and epidermal apoptosis, mild perivascular mononuclear cell infiltrate, melanin incontinence; like *scleroderma*: dense dermal sclerosis. Loss of hair follicles, entrapment of sweat glands.

### COURSE AND PROGNOSIS

Sclerodermoid GVHD with tight skin/joint contracture may result in impaired mobility, ulcerations. Permanent hair loss; xerostomia, xerophthalmia, corneal ulcers, blindness. Malabsorption. Mild chronic cutaneous GVHD may resolve spontaneously. Chronic GVHD may be associated with recurrent and occasionally fatal bacterial infections.

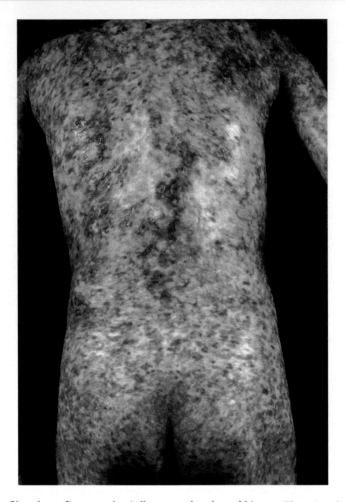

**FIGURE 14-19   Chronic graft-versus-host disease: sclerodermoid type**   *There is sclerosis and poikiloderma involving the entire skin. The porcelain white areas reflect sclerosis, the red is massive telangiectasias and erosions, and the brown is residual pigmentation after a lichenoid eruption with which the whole conditions started. Sclerosis of the tissue now supervenes, the skin feels bound down on palpation, similar to progressive systemic sclerosis (dSSc).*

## DIAGNOSIS AND DIFFERENTIAL DIAGNOSIS

Clinical, history, and histopathology. Differentiate from lichen planus, lichenoid drug reaction, scleroderma, all types of poikiloderma.

## MANAGEMENT

Topical glucocorticoids, PUVA, and extracorporeal photopheresis are very effective. Systemic immunosuppression with prednisone, cyclosporine, and azathioprine, in various combinations. Thalidomide.

## LIVEDO RETICULARIS □ → ◨ ○ → ●

Livedo reticularis (LR) is a mottled bluish (livid) discoloration of the skin that occurs in a net-like pattern. It is not a diagnosis in itself but a reaction pattern.

### CLASSIFICATION

*Idiopathic livedo reticularis (ILR)*: a purple/livid discoloration of the skin in a net-like pattern (diameter of mesh <3 cm) involving large areas of the lower, sometimes upper extremities and the trunk and disappearing after warming. A physiologic phenomenon. (*Synonym*: cutis marmorata.)

*Secondary (symptomatic) livedo reticularis (SLR)*: a purple discoloration occurring in a starburst or lightning-like pattern, netlike but with open (not annular) meshes; mostly, but not always, confined to the lower extremities and buttocks. A reaction pattern often indicative of serious systemic disease (Table 14-5). (*Synonym*: livedo racemosa.)

### ETIOLOGY

That of associated disorder.

### PATHOGENESIS

ILR pattern due to vasospasm or obstruction of perpendicular arterioles, perforating dermis

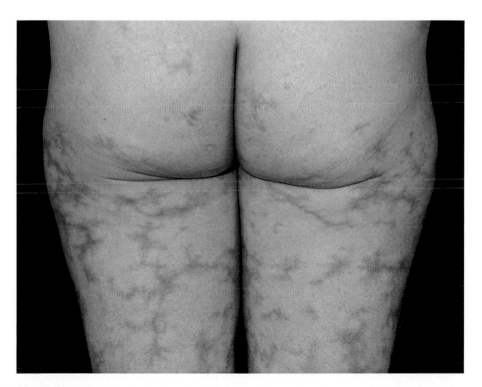

**FIGURE 14-20 Symptomatic livedo reticularis** *A netlike, arborizing pattern on the posterior thighs and buttocks defined by violaceous, erythematous streaks resembling lightning. The skin within the erythematous areas is normally pale. This occurred in a patient with labile hypertension and multiple cerebrovascular attacks and was thus pathognomonic for Sneddon's syndrome.*

**TABLE 14-5    Disorders Associated with Symptomatic Livedo Reticularis**

| Vascular Obstruction | Viscosity Changes | Drugs |
|---|---|---|
| Atheroemboli | Thrombocythemia | Amantadine |
| Arteriosclerosis | Polyglobulinemia | Quinine |
| Polyarteritis nodosa | Cryoglobulinemia | Quinidine |
| Cutaneous polyarteritis nodosa | Cold agglutinemia | |
| Rheumatoid vasculitis | Disseminated intravascular coagulation | |
| Livedoid vasculitis | Lupus erythematosus | |
| Sneddon's syndrome | Anticardiolipin syndrome | |
| | Leukemia/lymphoma | |

from below. Cyanotic periphery of each web of net caused by deoxygenated blood in surrounding horizontally arranged venous plexuses. When factors such as cold cause increased viscosity or flow rates in superficial venous plexus, further deoxygenation occurs and cyanotic reticular pattern becomes more pronounced. Elevation of limb decreases intensity of color due to increased venous drainage. SLR results from arteriolar disease causing obstruction to inflow and blood hyperviscosity or from obstruction to outflow of blood in venules.

## HISTORY

Appearance or worsening with cold exposure. ±Numbness, tingling associated. Worse during winter months.

## PHYSICAL EXAMINATION

**Skin Lesions, SLR**
Blotchy, arborizing, lightning-like, starburst, or mottled pattern of cyanosis (Fig. 14-20). Netlike webs are open (semicircular), and within webs, skin is normal to pallid and feels cool. Symmetric, arms/legs, buttocks; less commonly, body. On exposure to cold, livedo becomes more pronounced but never fades completely on warming. It never ulcerates. *Note*: When associated with *livedoid vasculitis* (see p. 484), ulceration about ankles and forefeet may occur.

**General Examination**    Symptoms of underlying disease (Table 14-5).

## LABORATORY EXAMINATIONS

**Laboratory**    Varies with associated disorders.
**Dermatopathology**    Vascular pathology of underlying disease.

## DIAGNOSIS AND DIFFERENTIAL DIAGNOSIS

Clinical diagnosis confirmed by laboratory data supporting diagnosis of associated disorder.
**Differential Diagnosis**    Cutis marmorata (idiopathic livedo reticularis), livedoid vasculitis (see page 484), erythema ab igne.

## COURSE AND PROGNOSIS

Course/prognosis of SLR depends on that of associated disorder.

## MANAGEMENT

- Keep from chilling. Pentoxifylline (400 mg PO tid), low-dose aspirin, and heparin may be helpful.
- Treat associated disorder.

# SNEDDON'S SYNDROME    □   ●

A potentially life-threatening disease of unknown etiology occurring more often in females than males and manifesting mainly in skin as livedo reticularis and in the central nervous system.

## EPIDEMIOLOGY

Rare but underdiagnosed.

## HISTORY

Skin lesions precede neurologic symptoms, often by years.

## PHYSICAL EXAMINATION

### Skin Lesions
These represent classical SLR on lower extremities, buttocks, sometimes arms (Fig. 14-20). ± Angiomatosis (mottled-purple discoloration of the face and other parts of the body).
*Note*: Sneddon's syndrome is not identical with antiphospholipid syndrome, although dermatologic manifestations (SLR) may be indistinguishable. May be associated with livedoid vasculitis—in this case, ulceration may occur around ankles or acrally (see page 484).

**Neurologic Symptoms**  Include headaches, labile hypertension, transient ischemic attacks, transient amnesia, transient aphasia, palsy, and cerebrovascular insult.

## LABORATORY EXAMINATION

**Dermatopathology**  Endothelitis → proliferation of subendothelial myofibroblasts → vascular occlusion and fibrosis. Cytotoxic anti-endothelial cell antibodies in a small percentage of patients. There may be antiphospholipid antibodies.

## MANAGEMENT

Longtime low-dose heparin, aspirin.

# LUPUS ERYTHEMATOSUS

Lupus erythematosus (LE) is the designation of a spectrum of diseases that are linked by distinct clinical findings and distinct patterns of cellular and humoral autoimmunity. It ranges from life-threatening manifestations of acute systemic lupus erythematosus (SLE) to the limited and exclusive skin involvement in chronic cutaneous lupus erythematosus (CCLE) (Graph 14-1). More than 85% of patients with LE have skin lesions, which can be classified into LE-specific and -nonspecific. An abbreviated version of Gilliam's classification of LE-specific skin lesions is given in Table 14-6.

## SYSTEMIC LUPUS ERYTHEMATOSUS    ◨   ●

This serious multisystem autoimmune disease is based on polyclonal B cell immunity, which involves connective tissue and blood vessels. The clinical manifestations include fever (90%); skin lesions (85%); arthritis; CNS, renal, cardiac, and pulmonary disease. SLE may uncommonly develop in patients with CCLE; on the other hand, lesions of CCLE are common in SLE (Graph 14-1).

## EPIDEMIOLOGY

**Age of Onset**   30 (females), 40 (males).
**Sex**   Male:female ratio 1:8.
**Race**   More common in blacks.
**Other Features**   Family history (<5%); an SLE syndrome can be induced by drugs (hydralazine, certain anticonvulsants, and procainamide), but rash is a relatively uncommon feature of drug-induced SLE.

## HISTORY

Lesions present for weeks (acute), months (chronic). Sunlight may cause an exacerbation of SLE (36%). Pruritus, burning of skin lesions. Fatigue (100%), fever (100%), weight loss, and malaise. Arthralgia or arthritis, abdominal pain, CNS symptoms.

## PHYSICAL EXAMINATION

**Skin Lesions**
Comprise acute cutaneous LE (ACLE) lesions (Table 14-6) in the acute phases of the disease and subacute (SCLE) and chronic cutaneous LE (CCLE) lesions. Whereas ACLE lesions occur only in acute or subacute SLE, SCLE and CCLE lesions are present in subacute and chronic SLE but may also occur in acute SLE. ACLE lesions are typically precipitated by sunlight.

**ACLE Lesions**   *Butterfly Rash*   Erythematous, confluent, macular butterfly eruption on the face (Fig. 14-21), sharply defined with fine scaling; erosions (acute flares) and crusts.
***Generalized ACLE***   Erythematous, discrete, papular or urticarial lesions on the face, on the dorsa of hands (Fig. 14-22), arms, and V of the neck.
***Others***   *Bullae*, often hemorrhagic (acute flares). *Papules* and *scaly plaques* as in SCLE (Fig. 14-23) and *discoid plaques* as in CCLE (Fig. 14-24), predominantly on the face and on the arms and scalp. Erythematous, sometimes violaceous, slightly scaling, densely set and *confluent papules* on the dorsa of the finger, usually with sparing of the articular regions (Fig. 14-22). Note difference to dermatomyositis (Fig. 14-15B). *Palmar erythema*, mostly on fingertips, *nailfold telangiectasias*. "Palpable" purpura (vasculitis), lower extremities (see Fig. 14-34). *Urticarial lesions* with purpura (urticarial vasculitis) (see Fig. 14-42).
**Hair**   Diffuse alopecia or discoid lesions associated with patchy alopecia.
**Mucous Membranes**   Ulcers arising in purpuric necrotic lesions on palate (80%), buccal mucosa, or gums (see Fig. 31-19).
***Sites of Predilection***   Localized or generalized, preferentially in light-exposed sites. Face (80%); scalp (discoid lesions); presternal, shoulders; dorsa of the forearms, hands, fingers, fingertips (see Image 14-2, p. 394).

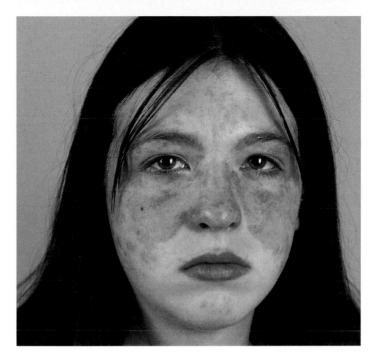

**FIGURE 14-21  Acute systemic lupus erythematosus**  *Bright red, sharply defined erythema with slight edema and minimal scaling in a "butterfly pattern" on the face. This is the typical "malar rash." Note also that the patient is female and young.*

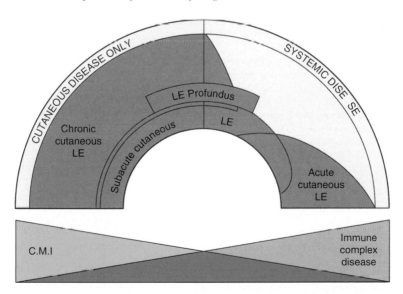

**IMAGE 14-1**  *The spectrum of lupus erythematosus, as envisaged by the late Dr. James N. Gilliam. The left comprises conditions that define cutaneous disease only and it can be seen that chronic cutaneous lupus extends into the systemic disease section. This is also true for lupus profundus and subacute cutaneous lupus, whereas acute cutaneous lupus is characteristic for systemic disease only. The bottom shows that immune complex disease dominate systemic disease and cell-mediated immunity (CMI) is predominant in the cutaneous disease manifestations.*

**Extracutaneous Multisystem Involvement** Arthralgia or arthritis (80%), renal disease (50%), pericarditis (20%), pneumonitis (20%), gastrointestinal (due to arteritis and sterile peritonitis), hepatomegaly (30%), myopathy (30%), splenomegaly (20%), lymphadenopathy (50%), peripheral neuropathy (14%), CNS disease (10%), seizures or organic brain disease (14%).

## LABORATORY EXAMINATIONS

**Pathology** *Skin* Atrophy of epidermis, liquefaction degeneration of the dermal-epidermal junction, edema of the dermis, dermal lymphocytic infiltrate, and fibrinoid degeneration of the connective tissue and walls of the blood vessels. *Immunofluorescence of Skin* The lupus band test (LBT, direct immunofluorescence demonstrating IgG, IgM, C3) shows granular or globular deposits of immune reactants in a bandlike pattern along the dermal-epidermal junction. Positive in lesional skin in 90% and in clinically normal skin (sun-exposed, 70 to 80%; non-sun-exposed, 50%).

**Serology** ANA positive (>95%); peripheral pattern of nuclear fluorescence. Anti-double-strand DNA antibodies, anti-Sm antibodies and rRNP antibodies specific for SLE; low levels of complement (especially with renal involvement). Anticardiolipin autoantibodies (lupus anticoagulant) in a specific subset (anticardiolipin syndrome); SS-A(Ro) autoantibodies have a low specificity for SLE but are specific in the subset of SCLE (see below).

**Hematology** Anemia [normocytic, normochromic, or rarely, hemolytic Coombs-positive, leukopenia (>4000/μL)], lymphopenia, thrombocytopenia, elevated ESR (a good guide to activity of the disease).

**Urinalysis** Persistent proteinuria, casts.

## DIAGNOSIS

Made on the basis of clinical findings, histopathology, lupus band test, and serology within the framework of the revised American Rheumatism Association (ARA) criteria for classification of SLE (Table 14-7).

---

**TABLE 14-6   Abbreviated Gilliam Classification of Skin Lesions of LE**

**I.** LE-specific skin disease [cutaneous LE* (CLE)]
  A. Acute cutaneous LE (ACLE)
    1. Localized ACLE (malar rash; butterfly rash)
    2. Generalized ACLE (maculopapular lupus rash, malar rash, photosensitive lupus dermatitis)
  B. Subacute cutaneous LE (SCLE)
    1. Annular SCLE
    2. Papulosquamous SCLE (disseminated DLE, subacute disseminated LE, maculopapular
       photosensitive LE)
  C. Chronic cutaneous LE (CCLE)
    1. Classic discoid LE (DLE)
      a. Localized DLE
      b. Generalized DLE
    2. Hypertrophic/verrucous DLE
    3. Lupus profundus
    4. Mucosal DLE
      a. Oral DLE
      b. Conjunctival DLE
    5. Lupus tumidus (urticarial plaque of LE)
    6. Chilblains LE (chilblains lupus)
    7. Lichenoid DLE (LE/lichen planus overlap)
**II.** LE-nonspecific skin disease
  These range from necrotizing and urticarial vasculitis to livedo reticularis, Raynaud's
  phenomenon, dermal mucinosis, and bullous lesions in LE.

*Alternative or synonymous terms are listed in parentheses; abbreviations are indicated in brackets.

SOURCE: Reprinted and modified from RD Sontheimer with permission from Stockton Journals, Macmillan Press, Ltd.

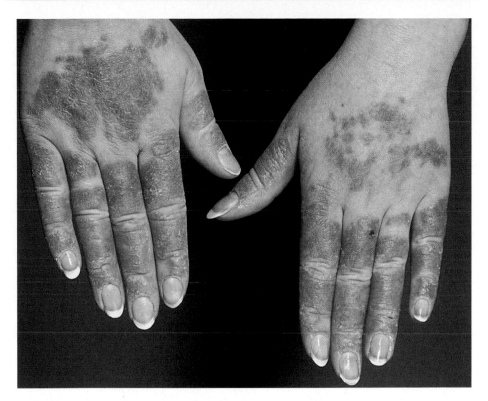

**FIGURE 14-22   Acute systemic lupus erythematosus**   *Red-to-violaceous, well-demarcated papules and plaques on the dorsa of the fingers and hands, characteristically sparing the skin overlying the joints. This is an important differential diagnostic sign when considering dermatomyositis, which characteristically involves the skin over the joints (compare with Fig. 14-15B).*

## PROGNOSIS

Five-year survival is 93%.

## MANAGEMENT

**General Measures**   Rest, avoidance of sun exposure.

**Indications for Prednisone**   (60 mg/d in divided doses): (1) CNS involvement, (2) renal involvement, (3) severely ill patients without CNS involvement, (4) hemolytic crisis, (5) thrombocytopenia.

**Concomitant Immunosuppressive Drugs**   Azathioprine or cyclophosphamide, depending on organ involvement and activity of disease. In renal disease, cyclophosphamide IV bolus therapy.

**Antimalarials**   Hydroxychloroquine is useful for treatment of the skin lesions in subacute and chronic SLE but does not reduce the need for prednisone. Observe precautions in the use of hydroxychloroquine.

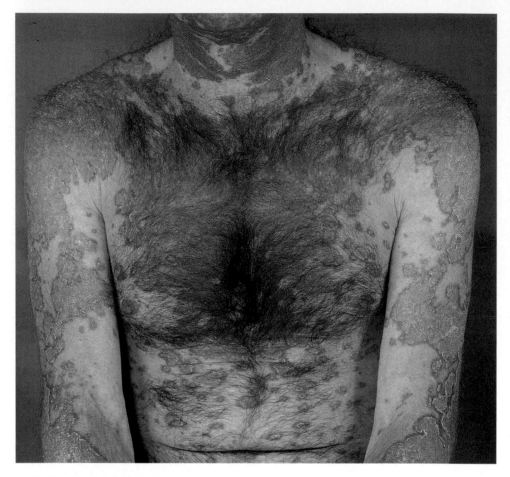

**FIGURE 14-23   Subacute cutaneous lupus erythematosus**   *Widely scattered, erythematous-to-violaceous, scaling, well-demarcated plaques on the trunk, neck, and arms, mimicking the clinical appearance of psoriasis vulgaris.*

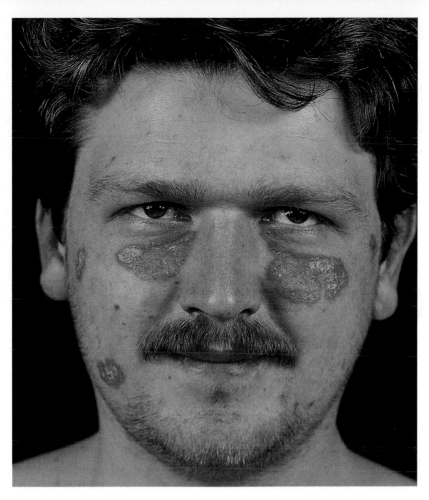

**FIGURE 14-24   Chronic cutaneous lupus erythematosus**   *Well-demarcated, erythematous, hyper-keratotic plaques with atrophy, follicular plugging, and adherent scale on both cheeks. This is the classic presentation of chronic discoid LE.*

**TABLE 14-7    1982 Revised ARA Criteria for Classification of Systemic Lupus Erythematosus**[*]

| Criterion | Definition |
|---|---|
| 1. Malar rash | Fixed erythema, flat or raised, over the malar eminences, tending to spare the nasolabial folds. |
| 2. Discoid rash | Erythematous raised patches with adherent keratotic scaling and follicular plugging; atrophic scarring may occur in older lesions. |
| 3. Photosensitivity | Skin rashes as a result of unusual reaction to sunlight, by patient history or physician observation. |
| 4. Oral ulcers | Oral or nasopharyngeal ulceration, usually painless, observed by a physician. |
| 5. Arthritis | Nonerosive arthritis involving two or more peripheral joints, characterized by tenderness, swelling, or effusion. |
| 6. Serositis | a. Pleuritis—convincing history of pleuritic pain or rub heard by a physician or evidence of pleural effusion *or* <br> b. Pericarditis—documented by ECG or rub or evidence of pericardial effusion. |
| 7. Renal disorder | a. Persistent proteinuria—0.5g/d or >3+ if quantitation not performed *or* <br> b. Cellular casts—may be red cell, hemoglobin, granular, tubular, or mixed. |
| 8. Neurologic disorder | a. Seizures—in the absence of offending drugs or known metabolic derangements, e.g., uremia, ketoacidosis, or electrolyte imbalance *or* <br> b. Psychosis—in the absence of offending drugs or known metabolic derangements, e.g., uremia, ketoacidosis, or electrolyte imbalance. |
| 9. Hematologic disorder | a. Hemolytic anemia—with reticulocytosis *or* <br> b. Leukopenia—<4000/$\mu$L total on two or more occasions *or* <br> c. Lymphopenia—<1500/$\mu$L on two or more occasions *or* <br> d. Thrombocytopenia—<100,000/$\mu$L in the absence of offending drugs. |
| 10. Immunologic disorder | a. Anti-DNA—antibody to native DNA in abnormal titer *or* <br> b. Anti-Sm—presence of antibody to Sm nuclear antigen *or* <br> c. Positive finding of antiphospholipid antibodies based on (1) an abnormal serum level of IgG or IgM anticardiolipin antibodies, (2) a positive test result for lupus anticoagulant using a standard method, or (3) a false-positive serologic test for syphilis known to be positive for at least 6 months and confirmed by negative *Treponema pallidum* immobilization or fluorescent treponemal antibody absorption test. |
| 11. Antinuclear antibody | An abnormal titer of antinuclear antibody by immunofluorescence of an equivalent assay at any point in time and in the absence of drugs known to be associated with "drug-induced lupus" syndrome. |

[*]The proposed classification is based on 11 criteria. For the purpose of identifying patients in clinical studies, a person shall be said to have SLE if any 4 or more of the 11 criteria are present, serially or simultaneously, during any interval of observation.

SOURCE: Reprinted from EM Tan et al: Arthritis Rheum 25:1271, 1982. Used by permission of the American College of Rheumatology.

# CUTANEOUS LUPUS ERYTHEMATOSUS

## SUBACUTE CUTANEOUS LUPUS ERYTHEMATOSUS (SCLE)

Skin lesions of SCLE are annular or psoriasiform (Fig. 14-23). Patients with SCLE may have a few of the criteria of SLE as defined by the ARA, including photosensitivity, arthralgias, serositis, renal disease, and serologic abnormalities, so that SCLE is not a purely cutaneous disease; practically all have anti-Ro (SS-A) and most have anti-La (SS-B) antibodies. The serious organ involvement of SLE is uncommon. The clinical skin lesions are the distinctive feature of SCLE (see Graph 14-1).

## EPIDEMIOLOGY

**Age of Onset**   Young and middle age.
**Race**   Uncommon in blacks or Hispanics.
**Sex**   Females > males.
**Incidence**   About 10% of the LE population.
**Precipitating Factors**   Sunlight exposure.

## HISTORY

Rather sudden onset with annular or psoriasiform plaques erupting on the upper trunk, arms, dorsa of the hands, usually after exposure to sunlight; mild fatigue, malaise; some arthralgia, fever of unknown origin.

## PHYSICAL EXAMINATION

### Skin Lesions
*Two types*: (1) *Psoriasiform papulosquamous*, sharply defined, with slight delicate scaling (Fig. 14-23), evolving into bright red confluent plaques that are oval, arciform, or polycyclic, just as in psoriasis; and (2) *annular*, bright red annular lesions with central regression and little scaling. In both there may be telangiectasia, but there is no follicular plugging and less induration than in CCLE. Lesions resolve with slight atrophy (no scarring) and hypopigmentation.
*Distribution*   Scattered, disseminated in light-exposed areas: shoulders, extensor surface of the arms, dorsal surface of the hands, upper back, V-neck area of the upper chest.
**Other Lesions**   Periungual telangiectasia, diffuse nonscarring alopecia.

## LABORATORY EXAMINATIONS

**Dermatopathology and Immunopathology**   As in ACLE, LBT positive in 60%.
**UV Testing**   Most patients have a lower than normal UVB minimum erythema dose (MED). Typical SCLE lesions may develop in UVB test sites.
**Serology**   ANA present in 60 to 80%. Antibodies to Ro(SS-A) positive in > 80%, to La (SS-B) in 30 to 50%; high levels of circulating immune complexes
**Other Laboratory Tests**   Patients with SCLE, particularly those with manifest systemic involvement, may have a number of laboratory abnormalities, including anemia, leukopenia, lymphopenia, hematuria, proteinuria, and depressed complement levels.

## DIAGNOSIS AND DIFFERENTIAL DIAGNOSIS

Clinical findings confirmed by histology and immunopathology. The extensive involvement is far more than is ever seen in CCLE, and the distinctive eruption is a marker for SCLE.
**Differential Diagnosis**   Red plaques of dermatomyositis, secondary syphilis, psoriasis, seborrheic dermatitis, tinea corporis.

## COURSE AND PROGNOSIS

A better prognosis than for SLE in general. Some patients with renal (and CNS) involvement have a guarded prognosis. The skin lesions can disappear completely, but occasionally, a vitiligo-like leukoderma remains for some months. Women with Ro(SS-A)-positive SCLE may give birth to babies with neonatal lupus and congenital heart block.

## MANAGEMENT

**Topical**  Anti-inflammatory glucocorticoids are only partially helpful.

**Topical Pimecrolimus and Tacrolimus**  Partially effective.

**Systemic**  Systemic treatment usually required. *Thalidomide* (100 to 300 mg/d) is very effective for skin lesions but not for systemic involvement. *Hydroxychloroquine*, 400 mg/d; if this does not control the skin lesions, quinacrine hydrochloride, 100 mg/d, can be added. The bizarre yellow skin color caused by quinacrine can be somewhat modified by β-carotene, 60 mg tid.

## CHRONIC CUTANEOUS LUPUS ERYTHEMATOSUS (CCLE)

This chronic, indolent skin disease is characterized by sharply marginated, scaly, infiltrated, and later atrophic red ("discoid") plaques, usually occurring on habitually exposed areas (Fig. 14-24). This disorder, in most cases, is purely cutaneous without systemic involvement (Graph 14-1). However, CCLE lesions may occur in SLE. CCLE may manifest as chronic discoid LE (CDLE) or LE panniculitis (Table 14-6).

## CLASSIC CHRONIC DISCOID LE (CDLE)

### EPIDEMIOLOGY

**Age of Onset**  20 to 45 years.
**Sex**  Females > males.
**Race**  Possibly more severe in blacks.

### HISTORY

Can be precipitated by sunlight but to a lesser extent than ACLE or SCLE. Lesions last for months to years. Usually no symptoms, sometimes slightly pruritic or smarting. No general symptoms.

### PHYSICAL EXAMINATION

#### Skin Lesions
Bright red papules evolving into plaques, sharply marginated, with adherent scaling (Fig. 14-24). Scales are difficult to remove and show spines on the undersurface (magnifying lens) resembling carpet tacks. Plaques are round or oval, annular or polycyclic, with irregular borders and expand in the periphery and regress in the center, resulting in depression of lesions, atrophy, and eventually scarring (Fig. 14-25). Follicular plugging and dilated follicles may persist in atrophic lesions but eventually disappear so that smooth, whitish scars result that are partially surrounded by a still active inflammatory and raised border (Fig. 14-25). "Burned out" lesions may be pink or white (hypomelanosis) macules and scars, but scarred lesions may also show hyperpigmentation, especially in persons with brown or black skin (Fig. 14-26).
***Distribution and Sites of Predilection*** CDLE may be localized or generalized, occurring predominantly on the face and scalp; dorsa of forearms, hands, fingers, toes, and less frequently, the trunk (Image 14-2).
**Scalp**  Scarring alopecia with residual inflammation and follicular plugging (Fig. 14-26).
**Mucous Membranes**  < 5% of patients have lip involvement (hyperkeratosis, hypermelanotic scarring, erythema) and atrophic erythematous or whitish areas with or without ulceration on the buccal mucosa, tongue, and palate.

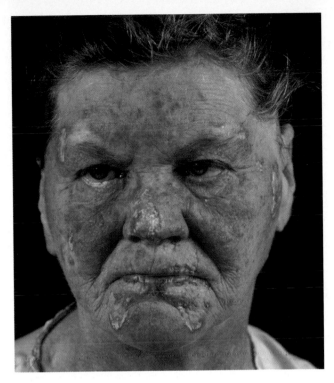

**FIGURE 14-25   Chronic cutaneous lupus erythematosus: scarring**   *There are multiple scarred plaques that have a depressed center and an active, still erythematous and scaly margin in the face of this 60-year-old female farmer. Scarring has led to considerable disfigurement.*

## LABORATORY EXAMINATIONS

**Dermatopathology** Hyperkeratosis, atrophy of the epidermis, follicular plugging, liquefaction degeneration of the basal cell layer. Edema, dilatation of small blood vessels, and perifollicular and periappendageal lymphocytic inflammatory infiltrate. Strong PAS reaction of the subepidermal, thickened basement zone.

**Immunofluorescence** LBT positive in 90% of active lesions at least 6 weeks old and not recently treated with topical glucocorticoids. LBT negative in burned-out (scarred) lesions and in the normal skin, both sun-exposed and nonexposed.

**Serology** Low incidence of ANA in a titer >1:16.

**Hematology** Occasionally leukopenia (<4500/μL).

## DIAGNOSIS AND DIFFERENTIAL DIAGNOSIS

Clinical findings confirmed by histopathology and immunopathology. The discoid lesions of CDLE may closely mimic *actinic keratosis*. *Plaque psoriasis* and scaling discoid LE without atrophy and scarring may be difficult to distinguish, especially on the dorsa of the hands; histopathology permits distinction. *Polymor-phous light eruption* LE (PMLE) may pose a problem. PMLE does not develop atrophy or follicular plugging, and does not occur in unexposed areas—mouth, hairy scalp. *Lichen planus* can be confusing, but the biopsy is distinctive. *Lupus vulgaris* and *tinea facialis.*

## COURSE AND PROGNOSIS

Only 1 to 5% may develop SLE; with localized lesions, complete remission occurs in 50%; with generalized lesions, remissions are less frequent (<10%). *Note again*: CCLE lesions may be the presenting cutaneous sign of SLE.

## MANAGEMENT

**Prevention** Topical sunscreens (SPF > 30) routinely.

**Local Glucocorticoids** Topical fluorinated glucocorticoids (with caution). Intralesional triamcinolone acetonide, 3 to 5 mg/mL, for small lesions.

**Antimalarials** Hydroxychloroquine, ≤6.5 mg/kg body weight per day. If hydroxychloroquine is ineffective, add quinacrine, 100 mg tid. Monitor for side effects.

**Retinoids** Hyperkeratotic CDLE lesions respond well to systemic acitretin (1 mg/kg body weight).

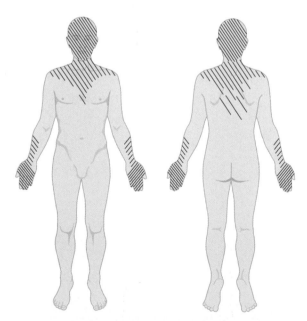

**IMAGE 14-2** *Predilection sites of cutaneus lupus erythematosus.*

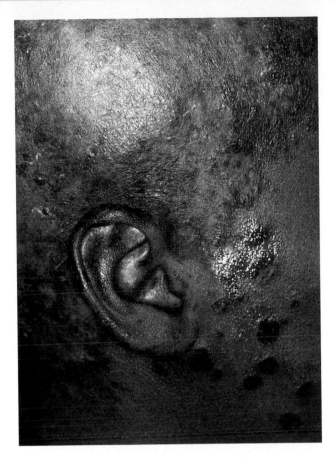

**FIGURE 14-26    Chronic cutaneous lupus erythematosus**    *Widespread involvement of the scalp has led to complete hair loss with residual erythema, atrophy, and scarring. Sharp demarcation of the confluent lesions in the periphery and the raised border indicate that these lesions originally were CDLE plaques, as can still be seen on the cheek. Note the intense lesional hyperpigmentation that can occur in Africans.*

## CHRONIC LUPUS PANNICULITIS

Chronic lupus panniculitis is a form of CCLE in which there are firm, circumscribed subcutaneous nodules occurring in addition to typical lesions of DLE but also in their absence. Usually a form of cutaneous lupus, but 35% of patients have mild SLE (see Image 14-1).
*Synonym*: Lupus erythematosus profundus.

### HISTORY

May precede or follow the onset of discoid lesions by several years. Nodules are asymptomatic, tender, or sometimes painful.

### PHYSICAL EXAMINATION

#### Skin Lesions

Deep-seated nodules or platelike infiltrations with or without grossly visible epidermal changes or change of color; indolent and firm, sometimes tender or painful, and are better felt than seen. The overlying skin may be normal, erythematous, or brownish or exhibit typical lesions of CDLE. Lesions evolve into deep depressions (Fig. 14-27) but may also ulcerate; in this case there is scarring.

*Distribution* Scalp, face, upper arms (Fig. 14-27), trunk (especially the breasts), thighs, and buttocks.

**Systems Review**   Mild SLE may be present (35%).

### LABORATORY EXAMINATIONS

**Dermatopathology**   Subcutaneous layer. Necrobiosis with fibrinoid deposits, dense lymphocytic infiltrates, and vasculitis; later, hyalinization of the fat lobules; fibrosis; there may be considerable mucinous deposits.

**Other**   In patients with SLE there are typical hematologic and serologic abnormalities.

### DIFFERENTIAL DIAGNOSIS

Morphea, erythema nodosum, sarcoid, miscellaneous types of panniculitis.

### MANAGEMENT

- Antimalarials
- Systemic glucocorticoids (short course)

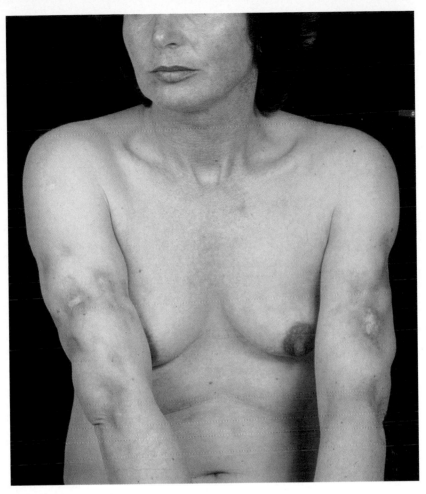

**FIGURE 14-27   Lupus panniculitis**   *Chronic panniculitis with atrophy of the subcutaneous tissue, resulting in large sunken areas of overlying skin, representing resolving lesions. Where erythema is still visible, palpation reveals firm subcutaneous nodules and plaques. Also, some lesions reveal scarring in the center.*

# SCLERODERMA  

Scleroderma is a multisystem disorder characterized by inflammatory, vascular, and sclerotic changes of the skin and various internal organs, especially the lungs, heart, and GI tract. *Synonyms*: Progressive systemic sclerosis, systemic sclerosis, systemic scleroderma.

## EPIDEMIOLOGY

**Age of Onset**   30 to 50 years.
**Sex**   Female:male ratio, 4:1.

## CLASSIFICATION

Systemic scleroderma can be divided into two subsets: *limited systemic scleroderma* (lSSc) and *diffuse systemic scleroderma* (dSSc). lSSc patients comprise 60%; patients are usually female; older than those with dSSc; and have a long history of Raynaud's phenomenon with skin involvement limited to hands, feet, face, and forearms (acrosclerosis) and a high incidence of anticentromeric antibodies. lSSc includes the CREST syndrome, and systemic involvement may not appear for years; patients usually die of other causes. dSSc patients have a relatively rapid onset and diffuse involvement, not only of hands and feet but also of the trunk and face, synovitis, tendosynovitis, and early onset of internal involvement Anticentromere antibodies are uncommon, but Scl-70 (antitopoisomerase I) antibodies are present in 33%.

## ETIOLOGY AND PATHOGENESIS

Unknown. Primary event might be endothelial cell injury in blood vessels, the cause of which is unknown. Early in course, target organ edema occurs, followed by fibrosis; cutaneous capillaries are reduced in number; remainder dilate and proliferate, becoming visible telangiectasia. Fibrosis due to overproduction of collagen by fibroblasts.

## HISTORY

Raynaud's phenomenon (see p. 402) with digital pain, coldness. Pain/stiffness of fingers, knees. Migratory polyarthritis. Heartburn, dysphagia, especially with solid foods. Constipation, diarrhea, abdominal bloating, malabsorption, weight loss. Exertional dyspnea, dry cough.

## PHYSICAL EXAMINATION

### Skin
*Hands/Feet Early*: Raynaud's phenomenon with triphasic color changes, i.e., pallor, cyanosis, rubor (Fig. 14-28). Precedes sclerosis by months and years. Nonpitting edema of hands/feet. Painful ulcerations at fingertips ("rat bite necrosis") (Fig. 14-29), knuckles; heal with pitted scars. *Late*: sclerodactyly with tapering of fingers (madonna fingers) with waxy, shiny, hardened skin, which is tightly bound down and does not permit folding or wrinkling (Fig. 14-28); leathery crepitation over joints, flexion contractures; periungual telangiectasia, nails grow clawlike over shortened distal phalanges. Bony resorption and ulceration results in loss of distal phalanges (Fig. 14-28).

    As sclerosis proceeds proximally, there are loss of sweat glands with anhidrosis and thinning and complete loss of hair on distal extremities.

*Face Early*: periorbital edema. *Late*: edema and fibrosis result in loss of normal facial lines, masklike (patients look younger than they are) (Fig. 14-30), thinning of lips, microstomia, radial perioral furrowing, beak-like sharp nose. Telangiectasia (Fig. 14-31) and diffuse hyperpigmentation.

*Trunk* In dSSc the chest and proximal upper and lower extremities are involved early. Tense, stiff, and waxy appearing skin that cannot be folded (Fig. 14-30). Impairment of respiratory movement of chest wall and of joint mobility.

### Other Changes
*Cutaneous Calcification* Occurs on fingertips or over bony prominences or any sclerodermatous site; may ulcerate and exude white paste.
*Color Changes* Hyperpigmentation that may be generalized and on the extremities may be accompanied by perifollicular hypopigmentation.
*Mucous Membranes* Sclerosis of sublingual ligament; uncommonly, painful induration of gums, tongue.
*Distribution of Lesions* Early: in lSSc early involvement is seen on fingers, hands, and face, and in many patients scleroderma remains confined to

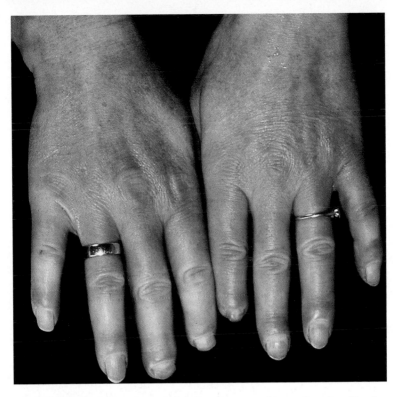

**FIGURE 14-28   Scleroderma (lSSc): Raynaud's phenomenon and acrosclerosis**   *Hands and fingers are edematous (nonpitting) with both erythema and vasoconstriction (blue and white); skin is shiny, bound down. Distal fingers are tapered and the phalanges on some fingers shortened (index fingers), which is associated with bony resorption. Nail dystrophy.*

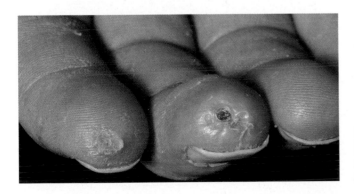

**FIGURE 14-29   Scleroderma (lSSc): acrosclerosis**   *Typical "rat bite" necroses and ulcerations of fingertips.*

these regions. *Late*: the distal upper and lower extremities may be involved and occasionally the trunk. In dSSc sclerosis of the extremities and the trunk may start soon or soon after or concomitant with acral involvement.

**Clinical Variant**   CREST syndrome, i.e., *c*alcinosis cutis + *R*aynaud's phenomenon + *e*sophageal dysfunction + *s*clerodactyly + *t*elangiectasia. Matlike telangiectasia, especially the face (Fig. 14-31), upper trunk, and hands; also in the entire GI tract. Calcinosis over bony prominences, fingertips, elbows, and trochanteric regions.

## GENERAL EXAMINATION

**Esophagus**   Dysphagia, diminished peristalsis, reflux esophagitis.

**Gastrointestinal System**   Small intestine involvement may produce constipation, diarrhea, bloating, and malabsorption.

**Lung**   Pulmonary fibrosis and alveolitis. Reduction of pulmonary function due to restricted movement of chest wall.

**Heart**   Cardiac conduction defects, heart failure, pericarditis.

**Kidney**   Renal involvement occurs in 45%. Slowly progressive uremia, malignant hypertension.

**Musculoskeletal System**   Carpal tunnel syndrome. Muscle weakness.

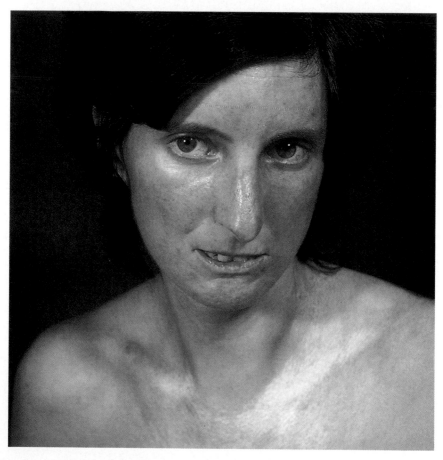

**FIGURE 14-30   Scleroderma (dSSc)**   *Masklike facies with stretched, shiny skin and loss of normal facial lines giving a younger appearance than actual age; the hair and eyebrows are dyed black. Thinning of the lips and perioral sclerosis result in a small mouth, which is asymmetric, creating a snarling appearance. Sclerosis (whitish, glistening areas) and multiple telangiectases (not visible at this magnification) are also present on the shoulders and chest.*

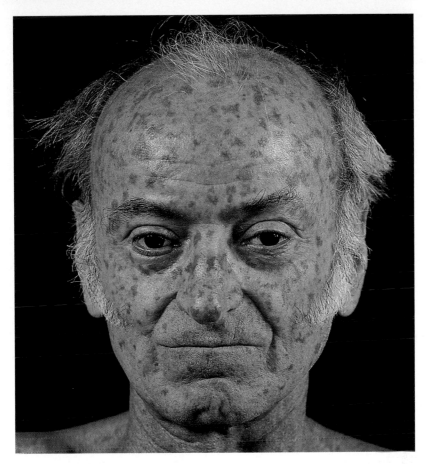

**FIGURE 14-31 Scleroderma: CREST syndrome** *Numerous macular or matlike telangiectases without other findings of scleroderma on the face. Complete features include calcinosis cutis, Raynaud's phenomenon, esophageal dysmotility, sclerosis, and telangiectasia.*

## LABORATORY EXAMINATIONS

**Dermatopathology** *Early*: mild cellular infiltrate around dermal blood vessels, eccrine coils, and at the dermal subcutaneous interphase. *Late*: broadening and homogenization of collagen bundles, obliteration and decrease of interbundle spaces, thickening of dermis with replacement of upper or total subcutaneous fat by hyalinized collagen. Paucity of blood vessels, thickening/hyalinization of vessel walls.

**Autoantibodies** Patients with dSSc have circulating autoantibodies by ANA testing. Autoantibodies react with centromere proteins or DNA topoisomerase I; fewer patients have antinucleolar antibodies. Anticentromeric autoantibodies occur in 21% of dSSc and 71% of CREST patients, DNA topoisomerase I (Scl-70) antibodies in 33% of dSSc and 18% of CREST patients.

## DIAGNOSIS AND DIFFERENTIAL DIAGNOSIS

Clinical findings confirmed by dermatopathology.

**Differential Diagnosis** *Diffuse sclerosis*: mixed connective tissue disease, eosinophilic fasciitis, scleromyxedema, morphea, porphyria cutanea tarda, chronic GVHD, lichen sclerosus et atrophicus, polyvinyl chloride exposure, adverse drug reaction (pentazocine, bleomycin).

## COURSE AND PROGNOSIS

Course characterized by slow, relentless progression of skin and/or visceral sclerosis; the 10-year survival rate is > 50%. Renal disease is the leading cause of death, followed by cardiac and pulmonary involvement. Spontaneous remissions do occur. lSSc, which includes the CREST syndrome, progresses more slowly and has a more favorable prognosis; some cases do not develop visceral involvement.

## MANAGEMENT

Systemic glucocorticoids may be of benefit for limited periods early in the disease. All other systemic treatments (EDTA, aminocaproic acid, D-penicillamine, *para*-aminobenzoate, colchicine, immunosuppressive drugs) have not been shown to be of lasting benefit. Currently, interferon-γ is being tested clinically, as is photopheresis.

## SCLERODERMA-LIKE CONDITIONS

A dSSc-like condition occurs in persons exposed to polyvinyl chloride. Bleomycin also produces pulmonary fibrosis and Raynaud's phenomenon. Cutaneous changes indistinguishable from dSSc-like sclerosis of skin, accompanied by myalgia, pneumonitis, myocarditis, neuropathy, and encephalopathy, are related to the ingestion of certain lots of L-tryptophan (*arthralgia-myalgia syndrome*); the *toxic oil syndrome* that occurred in an epidemic in Spain in 1981 affecting 25,000 people was due to the consumption of denatured grape seed oil. After an acute phase, with rash, fever, pneumonitis, and myalgia, the syndrome progresses to a condition with neuromuscular abnormalities and scleroderma-like skin lesions.

# RAYNAUD'S DISEASE/RAYNAUD'S PHENOMENON   ■

Raynaud's phenomenon (RP) is digital ischemia that occurs on exposure to cold and/or as a result of emotional stress. The various causes of RP are listed in Table 14-8. *Rheumatic disorders* [systemic scleroderma (85%), SLE (35%), dermatomyositis (30%), Sjögren's syndrome, rheumatoid arthritis, polyarteritis nodosa], *diseases with abnormal blood proteins* (cryoproteins, cold agglutinins, macroglobulins), *drugs* (β-adrenergic blockers, nicotine), and *arterial diseases* (arteriosclerosis obliterans, thromboangiitis obliterans) are the most common. When no etiology is found for RP, the term *Raynaud's disease* (RD) is used. It is primarily RD that is summarized below.

## EPIDEMIOLOGY

**Age of Onset**   Young adults or at menopause.
**Sex**   Female > male.
**Incidence**   As high as 20% in young women.
**Occupation**   May occur in persons using vibratory tools (chain saw users), meat cutters, typists, and pianists.
**Precipitating Factors**   Cold, mental stress, certain occupations (see above), smoking.

## PATHOGENESIS

The vasomotor tone is regulated by the sympathetic nervous system. The centers for vasomotor tone are located in the brain, the spinal cord, and the peripheral nerves. Vasodilatation occurs only on withdrawal of the sympathetic activity. It is conjectured that there may be a "local fault" in which blood vessels are abnormally sensitive to cold.

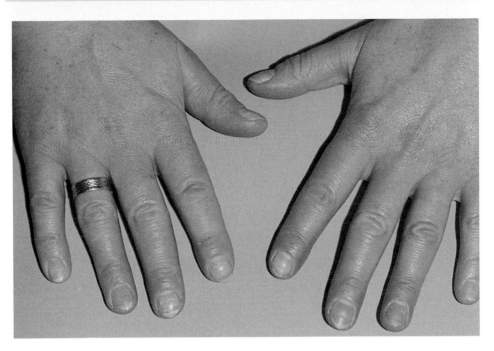

**FIGURE 14-32 Raynaud's disease** *The left hand exhibits a distal cyanosis compared to the right hand; it is seen especially well in the nailbeds. Unilateral episodes such as this one may occur after contact with a cold object.*

## HISTORY

Numbness and/or pain worse in winter in temperate climates, in the cold (meat cutters); previous treatment (drugs), occupation (using vibratory tools) have to be explored. Careful review is important to detect diseases in which RP is associated: arthralgia, fatigue, dysphagia, muscle weakness, etc.

## PHYSICAL EXAMINATION

### Types of Skin Changes

*The Episodic Attack* There is blanching or cyanosis of the fingers or toes, extending from the tip to various levels of the digits. The finger distal to the line of ischemia is white or blue and cold (Fig. 14-32); the proximal skin is pink and warm. When the digits are rewarmed, the blanching may be replaced by cyanosis because of slow blood flow; at the end of the attack, the normal color or a red color reflects the reactive hyperemic phase. To recapitulate, the sequence of color changes is white → blue → red. Rarely, the tip of the nose, earlobes, or the tongue may be involved. Blanching may occur in one or two digits or in all the digits; often the thumb is spared. The feet are involved in only 40%.

*Repeated or Persistent Vascular Vasospasm* Patients with RP often have a persistent vasospasm rather than episodic attacks. Skin changes include trophic changes with development of taut, atrophic skin, pterygium, clubbing and shortening of the terminal phalanges, sclerodactyly-like in lSSc. Acrogangrene is rare in RD (< 1%), but in RP associated with scleroderma, painful ulcers. Sequestration of the terminal phalanges or the development of gangrene (Fig. 14-33) may lead to autoamputation of the fingertips.

### TABLE 14-8   Causes of Raynaud's Phenomenon

| | |
|---|---|
| Connective tissue disease | Drugs (*continued*) |
|    Scleroderma |    Methysergide |
|    Systemic lupus erythematosus |    Bleomycin and vinblastine |
|    Dermatomyositis and polymyositis |    Clonidine |
|    Mixed connective tissue disease |    Bromocriptine |
|    Rheumatoid arthritis |    Cyclosporine |
|    Polyarteritis and vasculitis | Trauma |
|    Sjögren syndrome |    Vibratory tools |
| Obstructive arterial disease |    Hypothenar hammer syndrome |
|    Arteriosclerosis obliterans |    Pianists, typists |
|    Thromboangiitis obliterans |    Meat cutters |
|    Arterial embolism | Hematologic causes |
|    Thoracic outlet syndrome |    Cryoproteins |
| Neurogenic disorders |    Cold agglutinins |
|    Carpal tunnel syndrome |    Macroglobulins |
|    Reflex sympathetic dystrophy |    Polycythemia |
|    Hemiplegia | Miscellaneous |
|    Poliomyelitis |    Hypothyroidism |
|    Multiple sclerosis |    Vinyl chloride disease |
|    Syringomyelia |    Neoplasms |
| Drugs |    Vasculitis and hepatitis B antigenemia |
|    β-Adrenergic blockers |    Arteriovenous fistula |
|    Ergot preparations |    Intraarterial injections |

SOURCE: TD Coffman: Cutaneous changes in peripheral vascular disease, in Fitzpatrick et al. (eds): *Dermatology in General Medicine*, 4th ed. New York, McGraw-Hill, 1993, Chapter 167.

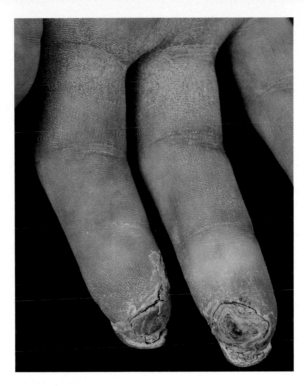

**FIGURE 14-33   Raynaud's phenomenon: acrogangrene**   *Persistent vasospasm of medium-sized arterioles can sometimes lead to gangrene of the terminal digits as illustrated in this patient with scleroderma.*

## LABORATORY EXAMINATION

**Serology**   Should be performed.

## DIAGNOSIS

Diagnosis is based on the vascular changes that are characteristic; ANA and other tests to rule out scleroderma and other conditions (Table 14-8). When no other disease is discovered, the diagnosis is RD.

## PROGNOSIS

RP/RD may disappear spontaneously; it progresses in about a third of patients.

## MANAGEMENT

**Prevention**   Education regarding the use of loose-fitting clothing and avoiding cold and pressure on the fingers. Giving up smoking is mandatory.
**Therapy**   Drug therapy (e.g., reserpine and nifedipine) should be used only in patients who have severe RD.

# VASCULITIS

## HYPERSENSITIVITY VASCULITIS

Hypersensitivity vasculitis (HV) encompasses a heterogeneous group of vasculitides associated with hypersensitivity to antigens from infectious agents, drugs, or other exogenous or endogenous sources (Table 14-9). It is characterized pathologically by involvement of postcapillary venules and inflammation and fibrinoid necrosis. Clinically, skin involvement is characteristic, manifested by "palpable purpura." Systemic vascular involvement occurs, chiefly in the kidney, muscles, joints, GI tract, and peripheral nerves. Schönlein-Henoch purpura is a type of HV associated with IgA.

*Synonyms*: Allergic cutaneous vasculitis, necrotizing vasculitis.

### EPIDEMIOLOGY AND ETIOLOGY

**Age of Onset**   All ages.
**Sex**   Equal incidence in males and females.
**Etiology**   See Table 14-9; idiopathic 50%.

### PATHOGENESIS

A postulated mechanism for necrotizing vasculitis is the deposition in postcapillary venules of circulating immune complexes. Initial alterations in venular permeability, due to the release of vasoactive amines from platelets, basophils, and/or mast cells, facilitate the deposition of immune complexes and these may activate the complement system or may interact directly with Fc receptors on endothelial cell membranes. When the complement system is activated, the generation of anaphylatoxins C3a and C5a can degranulate mast cells. Also, C5a can attract neutrophils that release lysosomal enzymes during phagocytosis of complexes and subsequently damage vascular tissue.

### HISTORY

A new drug taken during the few weeks before the onset of HV is a likely etiologic agent, as may be an infection, a known vascular/connective tissue disease, or paraproteinemia (see Table 14-9). Onset and course: acute (days, as in drug-induced or idiopathic), subacute (weeks, especially urticarial types), chronic (recurrent over years). Symptoms are pruritus, burning pain; there may be no symptoms or there may be fever, malaise; symptoms of peripheral neuritis, abdominal pain (bowel ischemia), arthralgia, myalgia, kidney involvement (microhematuria), CNS involvement.

### PHYSICAL EXAMINATION

#### Skin Lesions
The hallmark is *palpable purpura*. This term describes palpable petechiae that present as bright red, well-demarcated macules and papules with a central, dotlike hemorrhage (Fig. 14-34) (petechiae due to coagulation defects or thrombocytopenia are strictly macular and, therefore, not palpable). Lesions are scattered, discrete or confluent, and are primarily localized to the lower legs and the ankles (Figs. 14-34 and 14-35) but may spread to the buttocks and arms (Graph 14-2). Stasis aggravates or precipitates lesions. Purpuric lesions do not blanch (with a glass slide). Red initially, they turn purple and even black in the center (Fig. 14-35). In the case of massive inflammation, purpuric papules convert to hemorrhagic blisters, become necrotic (Fig. 14-35), and even ulcerate.

### LABORATORY EXAMINATIONS

**Hematology**   Rule out thrombocytopenic purpura.
**ESR**   Elevated.

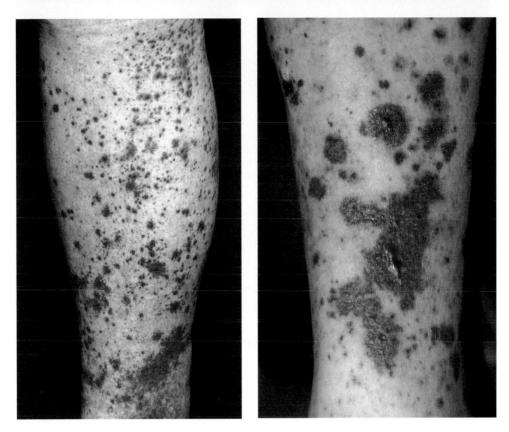

**FIGURE 14-34  (Left)   Hypersensitivity vasculitis**   *Cutaneous vasculitis presents clinically as "palpable purpura" on the lower extremities. Although appearing to the eye as macules, the lesions can be palpated, and this contrasts with petechiae, for instance, in thrombocytopenic purpura. The lesions shown here have central punctum that is a darker red and do not blanch with a glass slide, indicating hemorrhage.*


**FIGURE 14-35 (Right)   Hypersensitivity vasculitis**   *This is a more advanced stage. Lesions have progressed to hemorrhagic bullae and some have become necrotic. The lesions may progress to ulceration.*

**Serology** Serum complement is reduced or normal in some patients, depending on associated disorders.

**Urinalysis** RBC casts, albuminuria.

**Others** Depending on underlying disease.

**Dermatopathology** *Necrotizing vasculitis*. Deposition of eosinophilic material (fibrinoid) in the walls of postcapillary venules in the upper dermis, and perivenular and intramural inflammatory infiltrate consisting predominantly of neutrophils. Extravasated RBC and fragmented neutrophils ("nuclear dust"). Frank necrosis of vessel walls. Intramural C3 and immunoglobulin deposition is seen with immunofluorescent techniques.

## DIAGNOSIS AND DIFFERENTIAL DIAGNOSIS

Based on clinical appearance and histopathology.

**Differential Diagnosis** Thrombocytopenic purpura, rash such as exanthematous drug eruption in setting of thrombocytopenia, disseminated intravascular coagulation (DIC) with purpura fulminans, septic vasculitis (rickettsial spotted fevers), septic emboli (infective endocarditis), bacteremia [disseminated gonococcal infection, meningococcemia (acute/chronic)], other noninfectious vasculitides.

## COURSE AND PROGNOSIS

Depends on underlying disease. In the idiopathic variant, multiple episodes can occur over the course of years. Usually self-limited, but irreversible damage to kidneys can occur.

## MANAGEMENT

**Antibiotics** Antibiotics for patients in whom vasculitis follows bacterial infection.

**Prednisone** For patients with moderate to severe disease.

**Cytotoxic Immunosuppressives** Cyclophosphamide, azathioprine are used, usually in combination with prednisone.

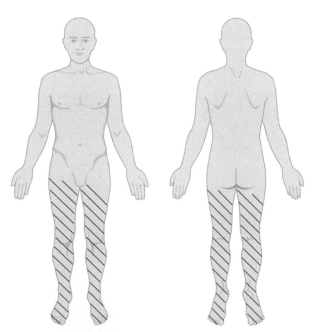

**IMAGE 14-3** *Predilection sites of hypersensitivity vasculitis.*

**TABLE 14-9 Classification of Hypersensitivity Vasculitis**

Associated with infections
   Hepatitis B virus
   Hepatitis C virus
   Group A hemolytic streptococcus
   *Staphylococcus aureus*
   *Mycobacterium leprae*
   Others
Associated with drugs
   Sulfonamides
   Penicillin
   Serum
   Others

Associated with neoplasms
   Lymphoproliferative disease
   Carcinoma of kidney
Associated with autoimmune connective tissue disease
   SLE
   Rheumatoid arthritis
   Sjögren's syndrome
Associated with dysproteinemias
   Cryoglobulinemia
   Paraproteinemia
   Hypergammaglobulinemia
   Congenital deficiencies of
      complement
Idiopathic

## SCHÖNLEIN-HENOCH PURPURA ☐ ●

This is a specific subtype of hypersensitivity vasculitis that occurs mainly in children but also affects adults. There is a history of upper respiratory tract infection (75%), involving group A streptococci. The disorder consists of palpable purpura accompanied by bowel angina (diffuse abdominal pain that is worse after meals) or bowel ischemia, usually including bloody diarrhea, kidney involvement (hematuria and red cell casts), and arthritis. Histopathologically, there is necrotizing vasculitis and the immunoreactants deposited in skin are IgA. Long-term morbidity may result from progressive renal disease (5%).

## POLYARTERITIS NODOSA ☐ ●

Polyarteritis nodosa (PAN) is a multisystem, necrotizing vasculitis of small- and medium-sized muscular arteries with involvement of the renal and visceral arteries.
*Synonyms*: Periarteritis nodosa, panarteritis nodosa.

## EPIDEMIOLOGY AND ETIOLOGY

**Age of Onset**   Mean age 45 years.
**Sex**   Male:female ratio 2.5:1.
**Etiology**   Unknown.
**Clinical Variants**   *Cutaneous PAN* is a rare variant with symptomatic vasculitis limited to skin and at times peripheral nerves.

## PATHOGENESIS

Necrotizing inflammation of small- and medium-sized muscular arteries; may spread circumferentially to involve adjacent veins. Lesions segmental, tend to involve bifurcations of arteries. About 30% of cases associated with hepatitis B antigenemia, i.e., immune complex formation.

## HISTORY

**Chronic Disease Syndrome**   With internal organ involvement and associated symptoms (see below).
**Cutaneous PAN**   Pain in nodules, ulcers; aching during flares and physical activity. Myalgia. Neuralgia, numbness, mild paresthesia.

## PHYSICAL EXAMINATION

**Skin Lesions**
Occur in 15% of cases. Subcutaneous inflammatory, bright red to bluish nodules (0.5 to 2 cm) that follow the course of involved arteries. Violaceous, become confluent to form painful subcutaneous plaques (Fig. 14-36), and accompanied by livedo reticularis; "starburst" livedo is pathognomonic and marks a cluster of nodular lesions. Ulcers follow ischemia of nodules (Fig. 14-36). Usually bilaterally on lower legs, thighs. Other areas: arms, trunk, head, neck, buttocks. Livedo reticularis may extend to trunk. Duration—days to months. Resolves with residual violaceous or postinflammatory hyperpigmentation. Skin lesions in systemic and cutaneous PAN are identical.

## GENERAL EXAMINATION

**Cardiovascular**   Elevated blood pressure; congestive heart failure, pericarditis, conduction system defects, myocardial infarction.

**Neurologic**   Cerebrovascular accident. Peripheral nerves: mixed motor/sensory involvement with mononeuritis multiplex pattern.
**Muscles**   Diffuse myalgias (excluding shoulder and hip girdle), lower extremities.
**GI System**   Nausea, vomiting, abdominal pain, hemorrhage, infarction.
**Eyes**   Hypertensive changes, ocular vasculitis, retinal artery aneurysm, optic disc edema/atrophy.
**Kidney**   BUN $\uparrow$, keratinin clearance $\downarrow$.
**Testes**   Pain and tenderness.

## LABORATORY EXAMINATIONS

**Dermatopathology**   *Best yield: biopsy of nodular skin lesion* (deep wedge biopsy). Polymorphonuclear neutrophils infiltrate all layers of muscular vessel wall and perivascular areas; later, mononuclear cells. Fibrinoid necrosis of vessel wall with compromise of lumen, thrombosis, infarction of tissues supplied by involved vessel, with or without hemorrhage. Skin pathology is identical in systemic and cutaneous PAN.
**CBC**   Commonly neutrophilic leukocytosis; rarely, cosinophilia; anemia of chronic disease. $\pm$ Elevated ESR.
**Serology**   Antineutrophil cytoplasmic autoantibodies (p-ANCA) in some cases. Hepatitis B surface antigenemia in 30% of cases.
**Chemistry**   Elevated creatinine, BUN.
**Arteriography**   Aneurysms in small- and medium-sized muscular arteries of kidney/hepatic/visceral vasculature.

## DIFFERENTIAL DIAGNOSIS

Other vasculitides and panniculitides.

## COURSE AND PROGNOSIS

Untreated, very high morbidity and mortality rates characterized by fulminant deterioration or by relentless progression associated with intermittent acute exacerbations. Death from renal failure, bowel infarction and perforation, cardiovascular complications, intractable hypertension. *Cutaneous PAN*: chronic relapsing benign course.

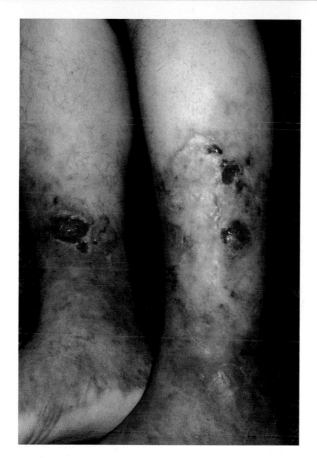

**FIGURE 14-36   Polyarteritis nodosa**   *Multiple, confluent, dermal and subcutaneous nodules with ulceration occurring on the medial and lateral aspects of the lower legs; a starburst pattern can still be seen in the pretibial region of the left leg. These lesions represent cutaneous infarction.*

## MANAGEMENT

**Systemic PAN**   *Combined therapy:* prednisone, 1 mg/kg body weight per day, and cyclophosphamide, 2 mg/kg per day.

**Cutaneous PAN**   Nonsteroidal anti-inflammatory agents, prednisone. In severe cases, as for systemic PAN.

# WEGENER'S GRANULOMATOSIS          □  ●

Wegener's granulomatosis (WG) is a systemic vasculitis, defined by a clinical triad of manifestations comprising involvement of the upper airways, lungs, and kidneys and by a pathologic triad consisting of necrotizing granulomas in the upper respiratory tract and lungs, vasculitis involving both arteries and veins, and glomerulitis.

## EPIDEMIOLOGY AND ETIOLOGY

**Age of Onset**  Mean age 40 years, but occurs at any age.
**Sex**  Male:Female ratio 1.3:1.
**Race**  Rare in blacks.
**Etiology**  Unknown.
**Clinical Variants**  One variant is limited to kidneys, i.e., glomerulitis occurs in 15% of cases; another is limited to respiratory tract.

## PATHOGENESIS

Immunopathogenesis unclear. Possibly an aberrant hypersensitivity response to an exogenous or endogenous antigen that enters through or resides in upper airways. Clinical symptomatology caused by necrotizing vasculitis of small arteries and veins. Pulmonary involvement: multiple, bilateral, nodular infiltrates. Similar infiltrates in paranasal sinuses, nasopharynx.

## HISTORY

Chronic disease syndrome. Fever. Paranasal sinus pain, purulent or bloody nasal discharge. Cough, hemoptysis, dyspnea, chest discomfort.

## PHYSICAL EXAMINATION

### Skin Lesions
Overall in 50% of patients but in only 13% of patients at initial presentation. *Ulcers with jagged, undermined borders* most typical; resemble pyoderma gangrenosum (Fig. 14-37). *Papules, vesicles, palpable purpura* as in hypersensitivity (necrotizing) vasculitis (Fig. 14-38), subcutaneous nodules, plaques, noduloulcerative lesions as in PAN. Most common on lower extremities. Also, face, trunk, upper limbs.
*Mucous Membranes* Oral ulcerations (Fig. 14-39). Often first symptom. ±Nasal mucosal

ulceration, crusting, blood clots; nasal septal perforation; saddle-nose deformity. Eustachian tube occlusion with serous otitis media; ±pain. External auditory canal: pain, erythema, swelling. Marked gingival hyperplasia.
*Eyes* 65%. Mild conjunctivitis, episcleritis, scleritis, granulomatous sclerouveitis, ciliary vessel vasculitis, retroorbital mass lesion with proptosis.
*Nervous System* Cranial neuritis, mononeuritis multiplex, cerebral vasculitis.
*Renal Disease* 85%. Signs of renal failure in advanced WG.

## DIFFERENTIAL DIAGNOSIS

**Cutaneous Necrosis + Respiratory Tract Disease**
Other vasculitides, Goodpasture's syndrome, tumors of the upper airway/lung, infectious/noninfectious granulomatous diseases (especially blastomycosis), midline granuloma, angiocentric lymphoma, allergic granulomatosis.

## LABORATORY EXAMINATIONS

**Hematology**  Mild anemia. Leukocytosis. ± Thrombocytosis.
**ESR**  Markedly elevated.
**Chemistry**  Impaired renal function.
**Urinalysis**  Proteinuria, hematuria, RBC casts.
**Serology**  Antineutrophil cytoplasmic autoantibodies (ANCA) are seromarkers for WG. Two ANCA patterns occur in ethanol-fixed neutrophils: cytoplasmic pattern (c-ANCA) and perinuclear pattern (p-ANCA). A 29-kDa protease (PR-3) is the major antigen for c-ANCA; myeloperoxidase, for p-ANCA. c-ANCA has been associated predominantly with WG and is considered specific for this condition; p-ANCA with microscopic polyarteritis, PAN, other vasculitides, idiopathic necrotizing and crescentic glomerulonephritis. Titers correlate

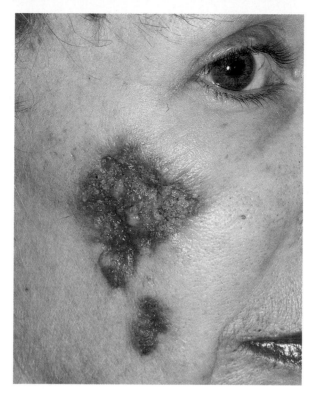

**FIGURE 14-37    Wegener's granulomatosis**    *A pyoderma gangrenosum-like irregular ulceration with jagged and undermined borders is often the first manifestation of Wegener's granulomatosis.*

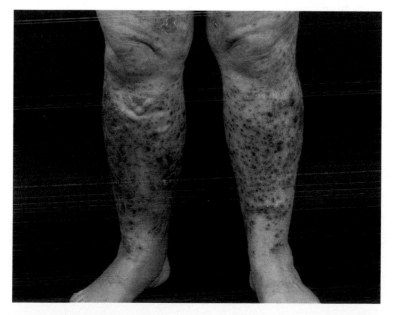

**FIGURE 14-38    Wegener's granulomatosis**    *Palpable purpura with necrotic lesions on the legs as in hypersensitivity vasculitis (compare with Fig. 14-35).*

with disease activity. Hypergammaglobuline-mia, particularly IgA class.

**Pathology**    All involved tissues including skin: necrotizing vasculitis of small arteries/veins with intra- or extravascular granuloma formation. Kidneys: focal/segmental glomerulonephritis.

**Imaging**    *Paranasal sinuses*: opacification, with or without sclerosis. *Chest*: pulmonary infiltrates, nodules; consolidation, cavitation; upper lobes.

## COURSE AND PROGNOSIS

Untreated, usually fatal because of rapidly progressive renal failure. With combination cyclophosphamide plus prednisone therapy, long-term remission is achieved in 90% of cases.

## MANAGEMENT

**Treatment of Choice**    Cyclophosphamide plus prednisone.

*Cyclophosphamide* 2 mg/kg body weight per day. Dose should be adjusted to keep leukocyte count >5000/$\mu$L (neutrophil count >1500/$\mu$L) to avoid infections associated with neutropenia. Therapy should be continued for 1 year after complete remission, then tapered and discontinued. *Alternative drug*: azathioprine in similar doses if cyclophosphamide is not tolerated.

*Prednisone* 1 mg/kg body weight per day for 1 month, and then changed to alternate-day doses which are tapered and then discontinued after 6 months of therapy.

*Trimethoprim-sulfamethoxazole* As adjunctive therapy and/or prevention of upper airway bacterial infections that promote disease flare.

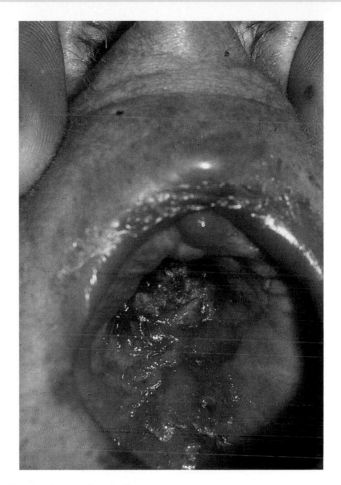

**FIGURE 14-39    Wegener's granulomatosis**    *A large ulcer on the palate covered by a dense, adherent, necrotic mass; note accompanying edema of the upper lip. Similar lesions occur in the sinuses and tracheobronchial tree.*

## GIANT CELL ARTERITIS    □    ●

Giant cell arteritis is a systemic granulomatous vasculitis of medium- and large-sized arteries, most notably the temporal artery and other branches of the carotid artery, characterized by headaches, fatigue, fever, anemia, and high ESR, in elderly patients.
*Synonyms*: Temporal arteritis, cranial arteritis.

### EPIDEMIOLOGY AND ETIOLOGY

**Age of Onset**   Elderly, usually >55 years.
**Sex**   Females > males.
**Etiology**   Unknown. Probably via cell-mediated immunity.

### HISTORY

Fatigue. Fever. Chronic disease syndrome. Headache usually bilateral. Scalp pain. Claudication of jaw/tongue while talking/chewing. Eye involvement: transient impairment of vision, ischemic optic neuritis, retrobulbar neuritis, persistent blindness. Systemic vasculitis: claudication of extremities, stroke, myocardial infarction, aortic aneurysms/dissections, visceral organ infarction. *Polymyalgia rheumatica syndrome:* stiffness, aching, pain in the muscles of the neck, shoulders, lower back, hips, thighs.

### PATHOGENESIS

Systemic vasculitis of multiple medium- and large-sized arteries. Symptoms secondary to ischemia.

### PHYSICAL EXAMINATION

**Skin Lesions**
Superficial temporal arteries are swollen, prominent, tortuous, ±nodular thickenings (Fig. 14-40). Tender. Initially, involved artery pulsates; later, occluded with loss of pulsation. ±Erythema of overlying skin. Gangrene, i.e., skin infarction of the area supplied by affected artery in the temporal/parietal scalp with sharp, irregular borders; ulceration with exposure of bone (Fig. 14-41). Scars at sites of old ulcerations. Postinflammatory hyperpigmentation over involved artery.
**General Examination**   Findings in other organ systems related to tissue ischemia/infarction (see "History," above).

### LABORATORY EXAMINATIONS

**CBC**   Normochromic/slightly hypochromic anemia.
**ESR**   Markedly elevated.
**Temporal Artery Biopsy**   Biopsy tender nodule of involved artery with or without overlying affected skin after Doppler flow examination. Lesions focal. Panarteritis with inflammatory mononuclear cell infiltrates within the vessel wall with frequent giant cell granuloma formation. Intimal proliferation with vascular occlusion, fragmentation of internal elastic lamina, extensive necrosis of intima and media.

### COURSE AND PROGNOSIS

Untreated, can result in blindness secondary to ischemic optic neuritis. Excellent response to glucocorticoid therapy. Remission after several years.

### MANAGEMENT

**Prednisone**   Initially, 40 to 60 mg/d; taper when symptoms abate; continue 7.5 to 10 mg/d for 1 to 2 years.
**Methotrexate**   Observations indicate that low-dose (15 to 20 mg) methotrexate, once a week, may have a considerable glucocorticoid-sparing effect in giant cell arteritis.

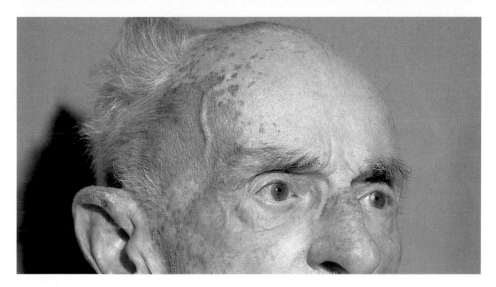

**FIGURE 14-40   Giant cell arteritis**   *The superficial temporal artery is prominent and on palpation is tender and pulseless in an elderly male who has excruciating headaches and progressive impairment of vision.*

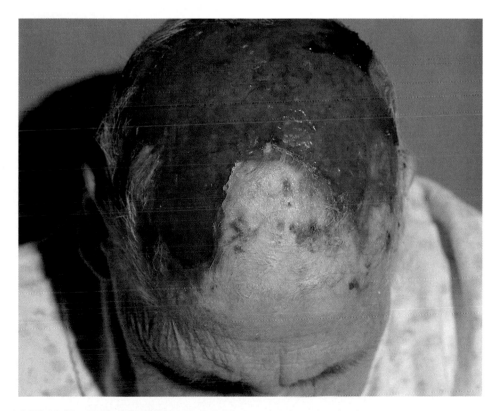

**FIGURE 14-41   Giant cell arteritis**   *Extensive bilateral infarction and ulceration of the scalp of an elderly female secondary to occlusion of temporal arteries.*

## URTICARIAL VASCULITIS          □   ◑

Urticarial vasculitis is a multisystem disease characterized by cutaneous lesions resembling urticaria, except that wheals persist for >24 h. Fever, arthralgia, elevated ESR, and histologic findings of a leukocytoclastic vasculitis are also present. The syndrome is often accompanied by various degrees of extracutaneous involvement. May be cutaneous manifestations of SLE. *Synonym*: Urticaria perstans.

### EPIDEMIOLOGY AND ETIOLOGY

**Age of Onset**   Majority 30 to 50 years.
**Sex**   Female:male ratio 3:1.
**Etiology**   In patients with serum sickness; in collagen vascular diseases, in particular, lupus erythematosus; with certain infections (e.g., hepatitis B); and idiopathic.
**Incidence**   <5% of patients with urticaria.

### PATHOGENESIS

Thought to be an immune complex disease, similar to hypersensitivity vasculitis (see page 406).

### HISTORY

Lesions may be associated with itching, burning, stinging sensation, pain, tenderness. Fever (10 to 15%). Arthralgias with or without arthritis in one or more joints (ankles, knees, elbows, wrists, small joints of fingers). Nausea, abdominal pain. Cough, dyspnea, chest pain, hemoptysis. Pseudotumor cerebri. Cold sensitivity. Renal involvement: diffuse glomerulonephritis.

### PHYSICAL EXAMINATION

**Skin Lesions**
Urticaria-like (i.e., edematous plaques and wheals), occasionally indurated, erythematous, circumscribed (Fig. 14-42); occasionally with angioedema. Eruption occurs in transient crops, usually lasting >24 h and up to 3 to 4 days. They change shape slowly, often reveal purpura on blanching (glass slide), and resolve with a yellowish-green color and hyperpigmentation.
**General Examination**   Extracutaneous manifestations: joints (70%), GI tract (20 to 30%), CNS (>10%), ocular system (>10%), kidneys (10 to 20%), lymphadenopathy (5%).

### LABORATORY EXAMINATIONS

**Dermatopathology**   Inflammation of dermal venules primarily with neutrophils *without* necrotizing vasculitis. Later, frank leukocytoclastic vasculitis.
**Urinalysis**   10% of patients—microhematuria, proteinuria.
**ESR**   Elevated.
**Serologic Findings**   Hypocomplementemia (70%); circulating immune complexes.

### DIAGNOSIS AND DIFFERENTIAL DIAGNOSIS

Clinical suspicion confirmed by skin biopsy. Urticaria, serum sickness, other vasculitides, SLE, urticaria in acute hepatitis B infection.
**Disease Associations**   SLE and other collagen vascular autoimmune disease.

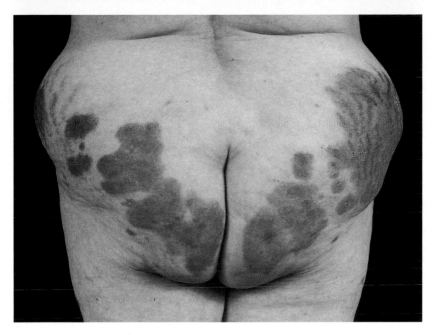

**FIGURE 14-42 Urticarial vasculitis** *Erythematous plaques and wheals on the buttocks that, in part, do not blanch on diascopy (compression of the lesional skin with glass that indicate hemorrhage. This contrasts urticaria. Also, in contrast to lesions of urticaria, which usually resolve within 24 h, those of urticarial vasculitis persist for up to 3 days before resolving with residual hyperpigmentation (hemosiderin deposition). Lesions of urticaria change shape in a short time, while those of urticarial vasculitis change slowly.*

## COURSE AND PROGNOSIS

Most often this syndrome has a chronic (months to years) but benign course. Episodes recur over periods ranging from months to years. Renal disease occurs only in hypocomplementemic patients.

## MANAGEMENT

Rule out vascular/connective tissue disease.

**First Line** $H_1$ and $H_2$ blockers [doxepin (10 mg bid to 25 mg tid) *plus* cimetidine (300 mg tid)/ranitidine (150 mg bid)] *plus* a nonsteroidal anti-inflammatory agent [indomethacin (75 to 200 mg/d)/ibuprofen (1600 to 2400 mg/d)/ naprosyn (500 to 1000 mg/d)].

**Second Line** Colchicine, 0.6 mg bid or tid *or* dapsone, 50 to 150 mg/d.

**Third Line** Prednisone.

**Fourth Line** Cytotoxic immunosuppressive agents (azathioprine, cyclophosphamide).

# NODULAR VASCULITIS          □   ◑

Nodular vasculitis is a form of lobular panniculitis associated with subcutaneous blood vessel vasculitis with subsequent ischemic changes that produce lipocyte injury, necrosis, inflammation, and granulation. Synonyms are *erythema induratum* and *Bazin's disease*, but these terms are now reserved for those cases of nodular vasculitis that are associated with *Mycobacterium tuberculosis*.

## EPIDEMIOLOGY AND ETIOLOGY

**Age of Onset**   Middle-aged to older persons.
**Sex**   Usually females.
**Etiology**   Immune complex–mediated vascular injury due to bacterial antigens has been implicated. Immunoglobulins, complement, and bacterial antigens have been found by immunofluorescence and in some cases mycobacterial DNA sequences by PCR. Bacterial cultures are invariably negative.

## HISTORY

Chronic, recurrent, often bilateral, subcutaneous nodules and plaques with ulceration of the legs. Usually asymptomatic but may be tender. Often in middle-aged females with stubby column-like legs who work in the cold.

## PHYSICAL EXAMINATION

Skin Lesions
Initially erythematous, tender, or asymptomatic subcutaneous nodules or plaques (Fig. 14-43) on the calves, rarely on shins and thighs (Image 14-4). Lesions become bluish red in color, are firm, and fluctuate before ulcerating. Ulcers drain serous/oily fluid, are ragged, punched-out, and have violaceous or brown margins (Fig. 14-43). They persist for prolonged periods before healing with atrophic scars.
*Associated Findings*  Follicular perniosis, livedo, varicose veins, and a cool, edematous skin.
**General Examination**   Patients are usually healthy.

## LABORATORY EXAMINATIONS

**Dermatopathology**   Tuberculoid granulomas, foreign-body giant cell reaction, and necrosis of fat lobules. Medium-sized vessel vasculitis, predominantly venular but sometimes arterial, in the septal areas. Fibrinoid necrosis or a granulomatous chronic inflammatory infiltrate invades between the fat cells, gradually replacing adipose tissue and leading to fibrosis.
**Skin Testing**   Patients with an association with mycobacterial infection are highly sensitive to tuberculin and purified protein derivative (PPD); therefore, skin testing to mycobacterial antigens should be performed. In such patients, mycobacterial DNA sequences can be found by PCR.

## DIAGNOSIS AND DIFFERENTIAL DIAGNOSIS

By clinical findings and biopsy.
**Differential Diagnosis**   *Red nodules on legs*: Erythema nodosum, other forms of panniculitis, cutaneous panarteritis nodosa. *Note*: Erythema nodosum is hot, very tender, and never ulcerates.

## COURSE AND PROGNOSIS

Chronic recurrent, scarring.

## MANAGEMENT

Antituberculous therapy in those cases where a mycobacterial etiology is proved. In other cases, bed rest, tetracyclines, and potassium iodide have proved effective. Systemic glucocorticoids are sometimes necessary for remission. In some cases dapsone is effective.

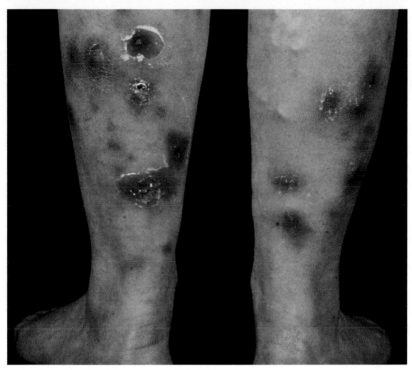

**FIGURE 14-43    Nodular vasculitis**    *Multiple, deep-seated, brown to bluish nodules, particularly on the posterior aspects of both lower legs. The lesions, which are relatively asymptomatic, may undergo necrosis forming slowly healing ulcers. Varicose veins are also seen on the right calf.*

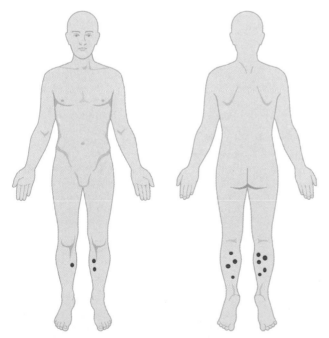

**IMAGE 14-4**    *Predilection sites of nodular vasculitis.*

# KAWASAKI'S DISEASE □ (→ ■*) ●

Kawasaki's disease (KD) is an acute febrile illness of infants and children, characterized by cutaneous and mucosal erythema and edema with subsequent desquamation, cervical lymphadenitis, and complicated by coronary artery aneurysms (20%).
*Synonym*: Mucocutaneous lymph node syndrome.

## EPIDEMIOLOGY AND ETIOLOGY

**Age of Onset** Peak incidence at 1 year, mean 2.6 years, uncommon after 8 years. Most cases of KD in adults probably represent toxic shock syndrome.
**Sex** Male predominance, 1.5:1.
**Race** In United States: Japanese > African Americans > whites.
**Etiology** Idiopathic.
**Season** Winter and spring.
**Geography** First reported in Japan, 1961; United States, 1971. Epidemics.

## PATHOGENESIS

Generalized vasculitis. Endarteritis of vasa vasorum involves adventitia/intima of proximal coronary arteries with ectasia, aneurysm formation, vessel obstruction, and distal embolization with subsequent myocardial infarction. Other vessels: brachiocephalic, celiac, renal, iliofemoral arteries. Increased activated helper T cells and monocytes, elevated serum soluble interleukin (IL) 2 receptor levels, elevated levels of spontaneous IL-1 production by peripheral blood mononuclear cells, anti-endothelial antibodies, and increased cytokine-inducible activation antigens on the vascular endothelium occur in KD. T cell response is driven by a superantigen.

## HISTORY AND CLINICAL PHASES

**Phase I: Acute Febrile Period** Abrupt onset of fever, lasting approximately 12 days, followed (usually within 1 to 3 days) by most of the other principal features. Constitutional symptoms of diarrhea, arthritis, photophobia.
**Phase II: Subacute Phase** Lasts approximately until day 30 of illness; fever, thrombocytosis, desquamation, arthritis, arthralgia, carditis; highest risk for sudden death.
**Phase III: Convalescent Period** Begins within 8 to 10 weeks after onset of illness when all signs

of illness have disappeared and ends when ESR returns to normal; very low mortality rate during this period.

## PHYSICAL EXAMINATION

### Skin Lesions
**Phase I** Lesions appear 1 to 3 days after onset of fever. Duration 12 days average. Nearly all mucocutaneous abnormalities occur during this phase.
***Exanthem*** Erythema usually first noted on palms/soles, spreading to involve trunk and extremities within 2 days. First lesions: erythematous macules; lesions enlarge and become more numerous (Fig. 14-44). Type: urticaria-like lesions most common; morbilliform pattern second most common; scarlatiniform and erythema multiforme–like in <5% of cases. Confluent macules to plaque-type erythema on perineum, which persist after other findings have resolved. Edema of hands/feet: deeply erythematous to violaceous; brawny swelling with fusiform fingers. Palpation: lesions may be tender.
***Mucous Membranes*** Bulbar conjunctivae: bilateral vascular dilatation (conjunctival injection); noted 2 days after onset of fever; duration, 1 to 3 weeks (throughout the febrile course) (Fig. 14-45). Lips: red, dry, fissured (Fig. 14-45), hemorrhagic crusts; duration, 1 to 3 weeks. Oropharynx: diffuse erythema. Tongue: "strawberry" tongue (erythema and protuberance of papillae of tongue).
**Phase II** Desquamation highly characteristic; follows resolution of exanthem (Fig. 14-46). Begins on tips of fingers and toes at junction of nails and skin; desquamating sheets of palmar/plantar epidermis are progressively shed.
**Phase III** Beau's lines (transverse furrows on nail surface) may be seen. Possible telogen effluvium.
**General Findings** Meningeal irritation. Pneumonia. Lymphadenopathy, usually cervical nodes: ≥1.5 cm, slightly tender, firm. Arthritis/arthralgias, knees, hips, elbows. Pericardial

---

* This indicates that KD is not uncommon when there are epidemics.

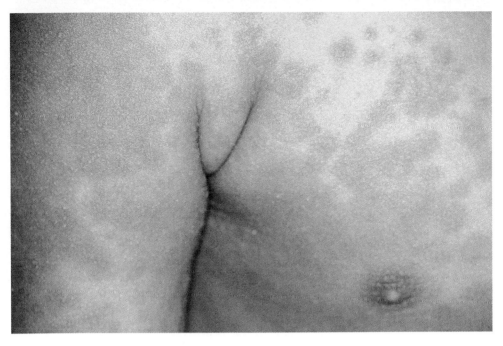

**FIGURE 14-44   Kawasaki's disease**   *Blotchy erythema on the trunk of a child; bulbar conjunctivitis, lymphadenopathy, and "strawberry" tongue were also present.*

tamponade, dysrhythmias, rubs, congestive heart failure, left ventricular dysfunction.

## LABORATORY EXAMINATIONS

**Chemistry**   Abnormal liver function tests.
**Hematology**   Leukocytosis   ($>18,000/\mu L$). Thrombocytosis after the tenth day of illness. Elevated ESR in phase II. ESR returns to normal in phase III.
**Urinalysis**   Pyuria.
**Dermatopathology**   Arteritis involving small and medium-sized vessels with swelling of endothelial cells in postcapillary venules, dilatation of small blood vessels, lymphocytic/monocytic perivascular infiltrate in arteries/arterioles of dermis.
**Electrocardiography**   Prolongation of PR and QT intervals; ST-segment and T-wave changes.
**Echocardiography and Angiography**   Coronary aneurysms in 25% of cases.

## DIAGNOSIS AND DIFFERENTIAL DIAGNOSIS

Diagnostic criteria: fever spiking to $>39.4°$ C, lasting $\geq 5$ days without other cause, associated with four of five criteria: (1) bilateral conjunctival injection; (2) at least one of following mucous membrane changes: injected/fissured lips, injected pharynx, "strawberry" tongue; (3) at least one of the following extremity changes: erythema of palms/soles, edema of hands/feet, generalized/periungual desquamation; (4) diffuse scarlatiniform or deeply erythematous maculopapular rash, iris lesions; and (5) cervical lymphadenopathy (at least one lymph node $\geq 1.5$ cm in diameter).

**Differential Diagnosis**   Juvenile rheumatoid arthritis, infectious mononucleosis, viral exanthems, leptospirosis, Rocky Mountain spotted fever, toxic shock syndrome, staphylococcal scalded-skin syndrome, erythema multiforme, serum sickness, SLE, Reiter's syndrome.

## COURSE AND PROGNOSIS

Clinical course triphasic. Uneventful recovery occurs in majority. Cardiovascular system complications in 20%. Coronary artery aneurysms occur within 2 to 8 weeks, associated with myocarditis, myocardial ischemia/infarction, pericarditis, peripheral vascular occlusion, small bowel obstruction, stroke. Case fatality rate, 0.5 to 2.8% of cases, and is associated with coronary artery aneurysms.

## MANAGEMENT

Diagnosis should be made early and attention directed at prevention of the cardiovascular complications.
**Hospitalization**   Recommended during the phase I illness, monitoring for cardiac and vascular complications.
**Systemic Therapy**   *Intravenous Immunoglobulin* 2 g/kg as a single infusion over 10 h together with aspirin.
*Aspirin* 100 mg/kg per day until fever resolves or until day 14 of illness, followed by 5 to 10 mg/kg per day until ESR and platelet count have returned to normal.
*Glucocorticoids Contraindicated* Associated with a higher rate of coronary aneurysms.

**FIGURE 14-45 (Opposite page, top)   Kawasaki's disease**   *Cherry-red lips with hemorrhagic fissures, in a little boy with prolonged high fever. This child also had a generalized morbilliform eruption, infected conjunctivae and "strawberry" tongue (not shown). Note erythema and edema of fingertips.*

**FIGURE 14-46 (Opposite page, bottom)   Kawasaki's disease**   *Shedding of the epidermis on the palm of this child 10 days after the acute illness.*

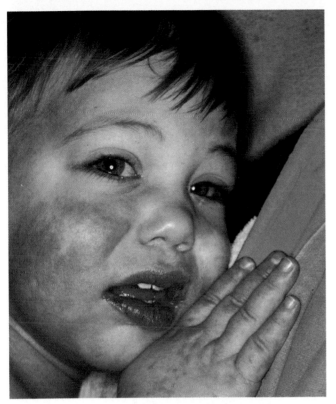

**FIGURE 14-45**

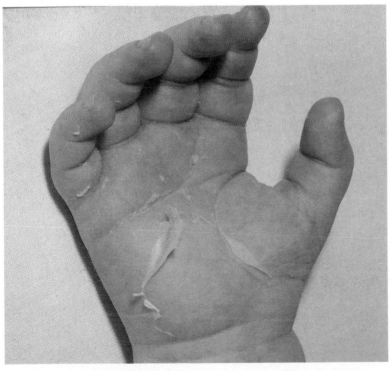

**FIGURE 14-46**

# REITER'S SYNDROME   □ ◐

Reiter's syndrome (RS) is defined by an episode of peripheral arthritis of >1 month's duration occurring in association with urethritis and/or cervicitis and frequently accompanied by keratoderma blennorrhagicum, circinate balanitis, conjunctivitis, and stomatitis. The classic triad is arthritis, urethritis, and conjunctivitis.

## EPIDEMIOLOGY AND ETIOLOGY

**Age of Onset**   22 years (median) in postvenereal type.
**Sex**   90% of patients are males (postvenereal type).
**Race**   Most common in Caucasians from northern Europe; rare in Asians and African blacks.
**Genetic Diathesis**   HLA-B27 occurs in up to 75% of Caucasians with RS but in only 8% of healthy Caucasians. Patients who are HLA-B27-negative have a milder course, with significantly less sacroiliitis, uveitis, and carditis.
**Associated Disorders**   Incidence of RS may be increased in HIV-infected individuals.
**Etiology**   Unknown.

## PATHOGENESIS

RS appears linked to two factors: (1) *genetic factors*, i.e., HLA-B27 and (2) *enteric pathogens* such as *Salmonella enteritidis, S. typhimurium, S. heidelberg*; *Yersinia enterolitica, Y. pseudotuberculosis*; *Campylobacter fetus*; *Shigella flexneri*; or genitourinary pathogens (such as *Chlamydia* or *Ureaplasma urealyticum*). Two patterns are observed: the *epidemic form*, which follows venereal exposure, the most common type in the United States and the United Kingdom; and the *postdysenteric form* following GI infection, the most common type in continental Europe and North Africa.

## HISTORY

Onset 1 to 4 weeks after infection: enterocolitis; nongonococcal urethritis. Urethritis and/or conjunctivitis usually first to appear, followed by arthritis.

Symptoms consist of malaise, fever, dysuria, urethral discharge. Eyes: red, slightly sensitive.

Arthritis: tendon/fascia inflammation results in pain over ischial tuberosities, iliac crest, long bones, ribs; heel pain at site of attachment of plantar aponeurosis and/or Achilles tendon; back pain; joint pains.

## PHYSICAL EXAMINATION

**Skin Lesions**
Resemble those of psoriasis, especially on palms/soles, glans penis.
   *Keratoderma blennorrhagicum*: brownish-red papules or macules, sometimes topped by vesicles that enlarge; centers of lesions become pustular and/or hyperkeratotic, crusted (Fig. 14-47), i.e., resembling mollusk shells, mainly on palms and soles. Scaling erythematous, psoriasiform plaques on scalp, elbows, and buttocks. Erosive patches resembling pustular psoriasis may occur, especially on shaft of penis, scrotum. *Circinate balanitis* (Fig. 14-48): shallow erosions with serpiginous, micropustular borders if uncircumcised; crusted and/or hyperkeratotic plaques if circumcised, i.e., psoriasiform.
**Nails**   Small subungual pustules; →onycholysis and subungual hyperkeratosis.
**Mucous Membranes**   *Urethra* Sterile serous or mucopurulent discharge.
*Mouth*   Erosive lesions on tongue or hard palate, resembling migratory glossitis.
*Eyes*   Conjunctivitis, mild, evanescent, bilateral; anterior uveitis.
**Systemic Findings**   Arthritis: oligoarticular, asymmetric; most commonly knees, ankles, small joints of feet; diffuse swelling of fingers and toes.

## LABORATORY EXAMINATIONS

**Hematology**   Nonspecific findings: anemia, leukocytosis, thrombocytosis, elevated ESR.

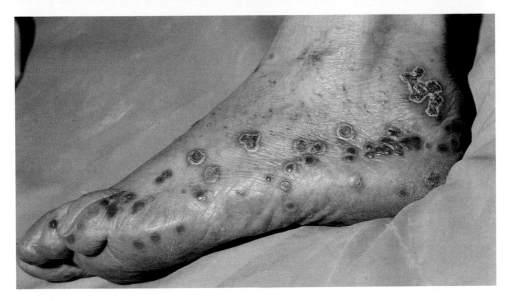

**FIGURE 14-47    Reiter's syndrome: keratoderma blennorrhagicum**    *Red-to-brown papules, vesicles, and pustules with central erosion and characteristic crusting and peripheral scaling on the dorso-lateral and plantar foot.*

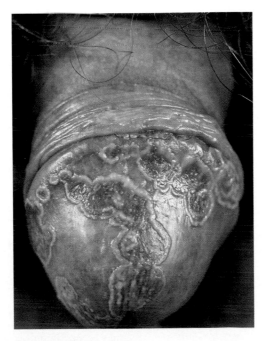

**FIGURE 14-48    Reiter's syndrome: balanitis circinata**    *Moist, well-demarcated erosions with a slightly raised micropustular circinate border on the glans penis.*

**Culture**  Urethral culture negative for gonococcus, may be positive for *Chlamydia* or *Ureaplasma*. Stool culture: may be positive for *Shigella, Yersinia,* and others.

**Serology**  ANA, rheumatoid factor negative. Rule out HIV infection.

**Dermatopathology**  Spongiosis, vesiculation; later, psoriasiform epidermal hyperplasia, spongiform pustules, parakeratosis. Perivascular neutrophilic infiltrate in superficial dermis; edema.

### DIAGNOSIS AND DIFFERENTIAL DIAGNOSIS

Clinical findings: arthritis and skin lesions ruling out other spondylo- and reactive arthropathies: psoriasis vulgaris with psoriatic arthritis, disseminating gonococcal infection, SLE, ankylosing spondylitis, rheumatoid arthritis, gout, Behcet's disease.

### COURSE AND PROGNOSIS

Only 30% develop complete triad of arthritis, urethritis, conjunctivitis; 40% have only one manifestation, i.e., incomplete RS. Majority have self-limited course, with resolution in 3 to 12 months. RS may relapse over many years in 30%. Chronic deforming arthritis in 10 to 20%.

### MANAGEMENT

**Prior Infection**  Role of antibiotic therapy unproven in altering course of postvenereal RS.

**Cutaneous Manifestations**  Similar to management of psoriasis (see Section 3). Balanitis: low-potency glucocorticoids. Palmar/plantar: potent glucocorticoid preparations, which are more effective under plastic occlusion. Extensive or refractory disease: systemic retinoids (acitretin, 0.5 to 1 mg/kg body weight), phototherapy, and PUVA.

**Prevention of Articular Inflammation/Joint Deformity**  Rest, nonsteroidal anti-inflammatory agents. Occasionally, phenylbutazone is indicated, methotrexate, acitretin. In HIV-infected individuals, highly active antiviral therapy may ameliorate RS.

## SARCOIDOSIS

Sarcoidosis is a chronic granulomatous inflammation affecting diverse organs, but it presents primarily as skin lesions, eye lesions, bilateral hilar lymphadenopathy, and pulmonary infiltration.

### EPIDEMIOLOGY

**Age of Onset**  Under 40 years (range 12 to 70 years).

**Sex**  Equal incidence in males and females.

**Race**  All races. In the United States and South Africa, much more frequent in blacks. The disease occurs worldwide; frequent in Scandinavia.

**Other Factors**  Etiology unknown. The disease can occur in families.

### HISTORY

Onset of lesions: days (presenting as acute erythema nodosum) or months (presenting as asymptomatic sarcoidal papules or plaques on skin or pulmonary infiltrate discovered on routine chest radiography). Constitutional symptoms such as fever, fatigue, weight loss, arrhythmia.

### PHYSICAL EXAMINATION

Skin Lesions

Brownish, purple infiltrated plaques that may be annular, polycyclic, serpiginous, and occur mainly on extremities, buttocks, and trunk (Fig. 14-49). Central clearing with slight atrophy may occur. Multiple scattered maculopapular or papular lesions, 0.5 to 1 cm, yellowish brown, or purple occur mainly on the face (Fig. 14-50)

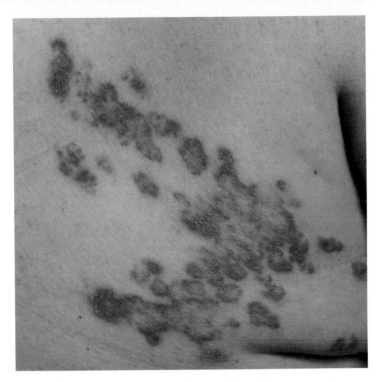

**FIGURE 14-49  Sarcoidosis: granulomatous lesions**  *Multiple, circinate, confluent, firm, brownish-red, infiltrated plaques that show a tendency to resolve in the center. Thus, the annular appearance. The lesions are diascopy positive, i.e., an "apple-jelly" tan-pink color remains in lesions after compression with glass.*

and extremities. Occasionally, nodules, firm, purple or brown, may arise on the face, trunk, or extremities, particularly hands (Fig. 14-52); and diffuse, violaceous, soft doughy infiltrations may occur on the nose, cheeks, or earlobes (*lupus pernio*) (Fig. 14-51). Swelling of individual digits (Fig. 14-52). Sarcoidosis tends to infiltrate old scars, which then exhibit translucent purple-red or yellowish papules or nodules. *Note*: On blanching with glass slide, all cutaneous lesions of sarcoidosis reveal "apple jelly" yellowish brown color. On the scalp sarcoidosis may cause scarring alopecia.

**Systems Review**  Enlarged parotids, pulmonary infiltrates, cardiac dyspnea, neuropathy, uveitis, kidney stones. In acute bilateral hilar sarcoidosis, particularly in young women, the first clinical manifestations of sarcoidosis may be erythema nodosum and arthritis. This combination is called *Löfgren syndrome*. The *Heerfordt syndrome* describes patients with fever, parotid enlargement, uveitis, and facial nerve palsy.

### LABORATORY EXAMINATIONS

**Dermatopathology**  Large islands of epithelioid cells with a few giant cells and lymphocytes (so-called naked tubercles). Asteroid bodies in large histiocytes; occasionally fibrinoid necrosis.

**Skin Tests**   Intracutaneous tests for recall antigens usually but not always negative.

**Imaging**   Systemic involvement is verified radiologically by gallium scan and transbronchial, liver, or lymph node biopsy. In 90% of patients: hilar lymphadenopathy, pulmonary infiltrate. Cystic lesions in phalangeal bones (osteitis cystica).

**Blood Chemistry**   Increased level of serum angiotensin-converting enzyme, hypergammaglobulinemia, hypercalcemia.

## DIAGNOSIS

Tissue biopsy of skin or lymph nodes is the best criterion for diagnosis of sarcoidosis.

## MANAGEMENT

**Systemic Sarcoidosis**   Systemic glucocorticoids for active ocular disease, active pulmonary disease, cardiac arrhythmia, CNS involvement, or hypercalcemia.

**Cutaneous Sarcoidosis**   *Glucocorticoids Local*: intralesional triamcinolone, 3 mg/mL, effective for small lesions. *Systemic*: glucocorticoids for widespread or disfiguring involvement.

***Hydroxychloroquine*** 100 mg bid for widespread or disfiguring lesions refractory to intralesional triamcinolone. Only sometimes effective.

***Methotrexate*** Low-dose for widespread skin and systemic involvement. Not always effective.

***Anti-TNF-α Monoclonal Antibodies*** Anecdotally effective.

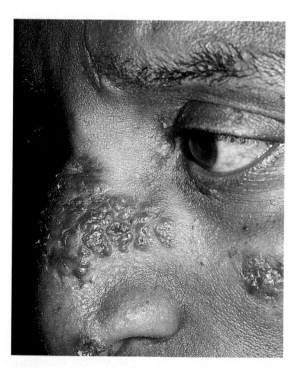

**FIGURE 14-50   Sarcoidosis**   *Brownish-to-purple papules coalescing to irregular plaques, occurring on the face of this man who also had massive pulmonary involvement. Blanching with a glass slide reveals "apple-jelly" color in the lesions.*

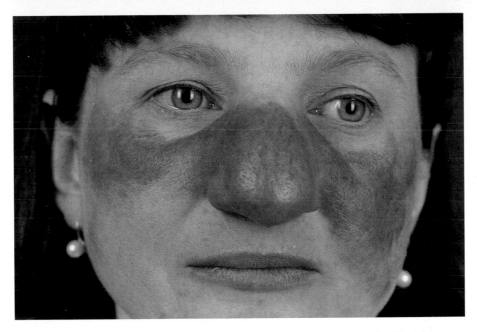

**FIGURE 14-51   Sarcoidosis**   *This is the classic appearance of "lupus pernio" with violaceous, soft, doughy infiltrations on cheeks and nose, which is grossly enlarged.*

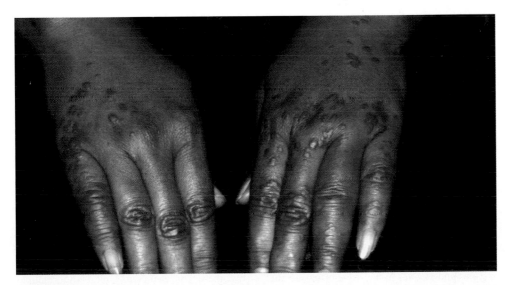

**FIGURE 14-52   Sarcoidosis**   *Papular brownish to violaceous lesions on the dorsa of a 40-year-old woman who also had pulmonary involvement. Note swelling of the fourth digit of the left hand and of the fifth digit of the right hand.*

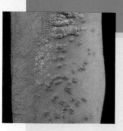

# ENDOCRINE, METABOLIC, NUTRITIONAL, AND GENETIC DISEASES

## DISEASES IN PREGNANCY

### PRURITIC URTICARIAL PAPULES AND PLAQUES OF PREGNANCY   ■  ◑

Pruritic urticarial papules and plaques of pregnancy (PUPPP) is a distinct pruritic eruption of pregnancy that usually begins in the third trimester, most often in primigravidae (76%). There is no increased risk of fetal morbidity or mortality. The disease is common, estimated to be 1 in 120 to 240 pregnancies. The etiology and pathogenesis are not understood.

*Synonyms*: Polymorphic eruption of pregnancy, toxemic rash of pregnancy, late-onset prurigo of pregnancy.

### HISTORY AND PHYSICAL EXAMINATION

Average time of onset is 36 weeks of gestation, usually 1 to 2 weeks before delivery. However, *symptoms and signs can start in the postpartum period*. Pruritus develops on the abdomen, often in the striae distensae, and is severe enough to disrupt sleep. The skin lesions evolve over 1 to 2 weeks and taper off over 7 to 10 days.

*Skin lesions* consist of erythematous papules, 1 to 3 mm, quickly coalescing into urticarial plaques (Fig. 15-1) with polycyclic shape and arrangement; blanched halos around the periphery of lesions. Tiny vesicles, 2 mm, may occur in the plaques, but bullae are absent. Target lesions are observed in 19%. Although pruritus is the chief symptom, excoriations are infrequent. 50% of the women affected have papules and plaques in the striae distensae; the abdomen, buttocks, thighs (Fig. 15-1), upper inner arms, and lower back may also be affected. The face, breasts, palms, and soles are rarely involved. The periumbilical area is usually spared. There are no mucous membrane lesions. Differential diagnosis includes all pruritic abdominal rashes in pregnancy: pemphigoid gestationis, adverse cutaneous drug reaction, allergic contact dermatitis, metabolic pruritus, atopic dermatitis.

*Laboratory findings* are noncontributory, as are histopathology and immunohistopathology.

The majority of women studied do not have a recurrence in the postpartum period or with subsequent pregnancies or with the use of oral contraceptives. If a recurrence occurs, is usually much milder than the original episode. The symptoms usually resolve within 10 days of delivery and there are no premature or postmature infants or spontaneous abortions; neither are these consistent congenital abnormalities with this condition.

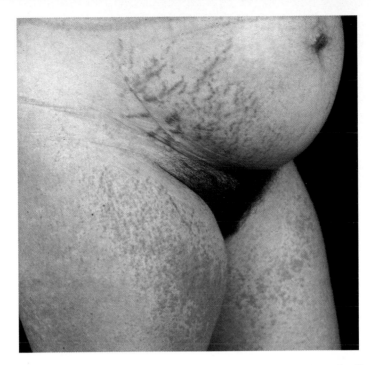

**FIGURE 15-1   Pruritic urticarial papules and plaques of pregnancy**   *Small papules distributed and confluent within striae distensae on the abdomen in a pregnant woman (35 weeks of gestation). Similar urticarial papules are present on both thighs where they coalesce to urticarial plaques. Lesions were extremely pruritic, causing sleepless nights and great stress, yet there are no excoriations.*

## MANAGEMENT

Consists of high-potency topical steroids that often can be tapered off after 1 week of therapy. Oral prednisone in doses of 10 to 40 mg/d has been used for severe cases; often the symptoms are relieved in 24 h. Oral antihistamines are generally ineffective. The symptoms can be so severe and exhausting for the pregnant woman that early delivery may be a consideration; often, however, the patient is better within several days of therapy.

## PEMPHIGOID GESTATIONIS

Pemphigoid gestationis (PG) is a pruritic polymorphic inflammatory dermatosis of pregnancy and the postpartum period. It is an autoimmune process with circulating complement-fixing IgG antibodies in the serum. The condition is described in Section 6 and illustrated in Fig. 6-13.

# DIABETES MELLITUS

## SKIN DISEASES ASSOCIATED WITH DIABETES MELLITUS[1]

### *ACANTHOSIS NIGRICANS* (page 86) AND *LIPODYSTROPHY*

Associated with insulin resistance in diabetes mellitus (DM). Insulin–like epidermal growth factors may cause epidermal hyperplasia.

### *ADVERSE CUTANEOUS DRUG REACTIONS IN DIABETES* (see Section 20)

*Insulin*: local reactions—lipodystrophy with decreased adipose tissue at sites of subcutaneous injection; Arthus-like reaction with urticarial lesion at site of injection.

*Systemic insulin allergy*: Urticaria, serum sickness-like reactions.

*Oral hypoglycemic agents*: Exanthematous eruptions, urticaria, erythema multiforme, photosensitivity.

### *CALCIPHYLAXIS* (page 440)

### CUTANEOUS PERFORATING DISORDERS

Rare conditions in which horny plugs perforate into the dermis or dermal debris is eliminated through the epidermis.

### *DIABETIC BULLAE* (*Bullosis diabeticorum*) (page 435)

### *DIABETIC DERMOPATHY* (page 437)

### *ERUPTIVE XANTHOMAS* (page 450)

### *GRANULOMA ANNULARE* (page 128)

### *INFECTIONS* (see Sections 22 and 23)

Poorly controlled DM associated with increased incidence of primary (furuncles, carbuncles) and secondary *Staphylococcus aureus* infections (paronychia, wound/ulcer infection), cellulitis (*S. aureus*, group A streptococcus), erythrasma, dermatophytoses (tinea pedis, onychomycosis), candidiasis (mucosal and cutaneous), mucormycosis with necrotizing nasopharyngeal infections.

### *NECROBIOSIS LIPOIDICA* (page 438)

### *PERIPHERAL NEUROPATHY* (Diabetic foot) (page 436)

### *PERIPHERAL VASCULAR DISEASE* (see Section 16)

*Small-vessel vasculopathy (microangiopathy):* Involves arterioles, venules, and capillaries. Characterized by basement membrane thickening and endothelial cell proliferation. Presents clinically as acral erysipelas-like erythema, ±ulceration.

Large-vessel vasculopathy: Incidence greatly increased in DM. Ischemia is most often symptomatic on lower legs and feet with gangrene and ulceration. Predisposes to infections.

### *SCLEREDEMA*

*Synonym*: Scleredema adultorum of Buschke. Need not be associated with DM. Onset correlates with duration of DM and with presence of microangiopathy. Skin findings: poorly demarcated scleroderma-like induration of the skin and subcutaneous tissue of the upper back, neck, proximal extremities. Rapid onset and progression.

---

[1] Figures in parentheses indicate page numbers where these conditions are dealt with.

## DIABETIC BULLAE

Large, intact bullae arise spontaneously on the lower legs, feet, dorsa of the hands and fingers on noninflamed bases (Fig. 15-2). When ruptured, oozing bright red erosions result but heal after several weeks. Localization on dorsa of hand and fingers suggests porphyria cutanea tarda, but abnormalities of porphyrin metabolism are not found. Neither trauma nor an immunologic mechanism has been implicated. Histologically, bullae show intra- or subepidermal clefting without acantholysis. The 46-year-old diabetic male shown in Fig. 15-2 had the toes of the right foot amputated because of gangrene. One year after surgery he started to develop bullae in the pretibial areas and dorsum of the feet and on the amputation stump of the left great toe, as shown in the illustration.

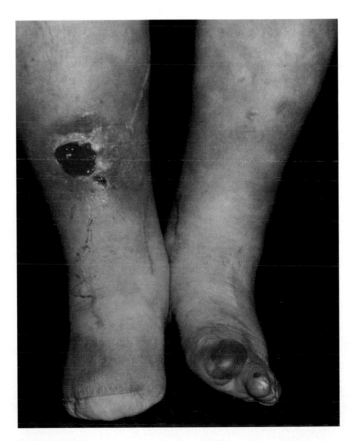

FIGURE 15-2   Diabetic bulla   *A large, intact bulla is seen on the stump of the left amputated great toe and a large erosion on the pretibial skin on the right lower leg. The patient has many of the vascular complications of diabetes mellitus, i.e., renal failure, retinopathy, and atherosclerosis obliterans resulting in amputation of the right forefoot and the left big toe.*

## "DIABETIC FOOT" AND DIABETIC NEUROPATHY    ■    ◑

Peripheral neuropathy is responsible for the "diabetic foot." Other factors are angiopathy, atherosclerosis, and infection and most often they are combined. Diabetic neuropathy is combined motor and sensory. Motor neuropathy leads to weakness and muscle wasting distally. Autonomic neuropathy accompanies sensory neuropathy and leads to anhidrosis, which may not be confined to the distal extremities. Sensory neuropathy predisposes to neurotropic ulcers over bony prominences of feet, usually on the great toe and sole as shown here (Fig. 15-3). Ulcers are surrounded by a ring of callus and may extend to interlying joint and bone, leading to osteomyelitis.

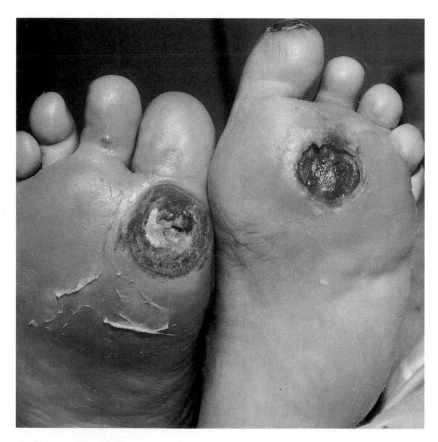

**FIGURE 15-3    Diabetic, neuropathic ulcers on the soles**    *Two large ulcers overlying the first right and second left metacarpophalangeal joints. The patient, a 56-year-old male with diabetes mellitus of 20 years' duration, has significant sensory neuropathy of the feet and lower legs as well as peripheral vascular disease.*

## DIABETIC DERMOPATHY    ◨    ◐

Circumscribed, atrophic, slightly depressed lesions on the anterior lower legs that are asympto-matic (Fig. 15-4). They arise in crops and gradually resolve, but new lesions appear and occa-sionally may ulcerate. The pathogenic significance of diabetic angiopathy remains to be established, but it is often accompanied by microangiopathy.

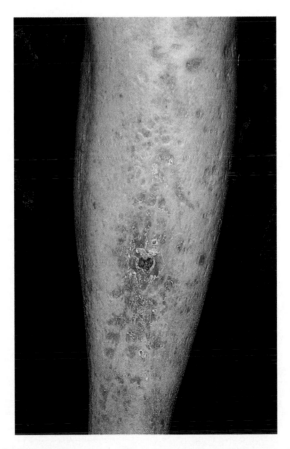

**Figure 15-4    Diabetic dermopathy**    *A crusted erosion at the site of traumatic injury and many old pink depressed areas and scars are seen on the anterior leg of a 56-year-old male with diabetes mellitus. The other leg had identical findings.*

# NECROBIOSIS LIPOIDICA   

Necrobiosis lipoidica (NL) is a cutaneous disorder often, but not always, associated with diabetes mellitus. The lesions are distinctive, sharply circumscribed, multicolored plaques occurring on the anterior and lateral surfaces of the lower legs.

## EPIDEMIOLOGY AND ETIOLOGY

**Age of Onset**   Young adults, early middle age, but not uncommon in juvenile diabetics.

**Sex**   Female:male ratio 3:1 in both diabetic and nondiabetic forms.

**Incidence**   From 0.3 to 3% of diabetic individuals. NL may occur in individuals without manifest diabetes. *Relationship to DM*: One-third of patients have clinical DM, one-third have abnormal glucose tolerance only, one-third have normal glucose tolerance.

**Etiology**   Unknown.

**Precipitating Factors**   A history of preceding trauma to the site can be a factor in the initial development of the lesions.

## PATHOGENESIS

The arteriolar changes in the areas of necrobiosis of the collagen have been thought by some to be precipitated by aggregation of platelets. The granulomatous inflammatory reaction is believed to be due to alterations in the collagen. The severity of NL is not related to the severity of DM. Furthermore, control of the diabetes has no effect on the course of NL.

## HISTORY

Slowly evolving and enlarging over months, persisting for years. Cosmetic disfigurement; pain in lesions that develop ulcers.

## PHYSICAL EXAMINATION

**Skin Lesions**

Lesion starts as brownish-red or skin-colored papule that slowly evolves into a well-demarcated waxy plaque of variable size (Fig. 15-5). The sharply defined and slightly elevated border retains a brownish-red color, whereas the center becomes depressed and acquires a yellow-orange hue. Through the shiny and atrophic epidermis, multiple telangiectasias of variable size are seen. Larger lesions formed by centrifugal enlargement or merging of smaller lesions acquire a serpiginous or polycyclic configuration. Ulceration commonly occurs within the plaques (Fig. 15-6), and healed ulcers result in depressed scars. Burned-out lesions appear as tan areas with telangiectasia.

**Distribution**   Usually 1 to 3 lesions; >80% occur on the shin; at times symmetric. Less commonly, on feet, arms, trunk, or face and scalp; rarely may be generalized.

## LABORATORY EXAMINATIONS

**Dermatopathology**   Sclerosis, obliteration of the bundle pattern of collagen → necrobiosis, surrounded by concomitant granulomatous infiltration in lower dermis. Fat-containing foam cells are often present, imparting the yellow color to the clinical lesion. Dermal blood vessels show microangiopathy with endothelial thickening and focal deposits of PAS-positive material. Presence of immunoglobulins and complement (C3) in the walls of the small blood vessels.

**Chemistry**   Abnormal glucose tolerance test in two-thirds of patients.

## DIAGNOSIS AND DIFFERENTIAL DIAGNOSIS

The lesions are so distinctive that biopsy confirmation is not necessary; however, biopsy may be required in early stages to rule out granuloma annulare (which frequently coexists with NL), sarcoidosis, or xanthoma.

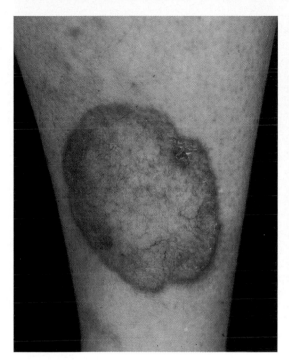 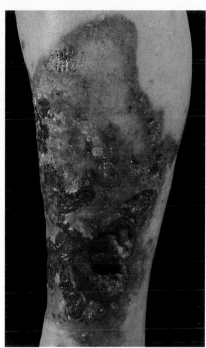

**Figure 15-5 (Left)   Necrobiosis lipoidica diabeticorum: early**   *A large, symmetric plaque with active tan-pink, well-demarcated, raised, firm borders and a yellow center in the pretibial regions of a 28-year-old diabetic female. The central parts of the lesions are depressed with atrophic changes of epidermal thinning and telangiectasis against yellow background.*

**Figure 15-6 (Right)   Necrobiosis lipoidica: late with ulceration**   *A very extensive plaque of necrobiosis lipoidica on the lower leg of a diabetic female. The lower portion has undergone necrosis with extensive, deep ulceration. These lesions can become very painful.*

## COURSE AND PROGNOSIS

The lesions are indolent and can enlarge to involve large areas of the skin surface unless treated. The lesions are unsightly, and patients are often upset about the cosmetic appearance. Ulcerated areas within NL are painful.

## MANAGEMENT

**Glucocorticoids**   *Topical* The application of potent glucocorticoids under occlusion is helpful in some cases; however, ulcerations may occur when NL is occluded.
*Intralesional* Intralesional triamcinolone, 5 mg/mL, into active lesions or lesion margins usually arrests extension of plaques of NL. This is the best treatment, with 3 to 5 mg/mL triamcinolone suspension.
**Ulceration**   Most ulcerations within NL lesions heal with local wound care; if not, excision of entire lesion with grafting may be required.

## CALCIPHYLAXIS   

Calciphylaxis is characterized by progressive cutaneous necrosis associated with small- and medium-sized vessel calcification occurring in the setting of end-stage renal disease, DM, and hyperparathyroidism.

## EPIDEMIOLOGY

**Age of Onset**   Middle to old age.
**Sex**   Equal.

## PATHOGENESIS

The pathogenesis is poorly understood. In animal models, calciphylaxis is described as a condition of induced systemic hypersensitivity in which tissues respond to appropriate challenging agents with calcium deposition. Calciphylaxis is associated with chronic renal failure, secondary hyperparathyroidism, and an elevated calcium phosphate end product. Implicated "challenging agents" include glucocorticoids, albumin infusions, intramuscular tobramycin, iron dextran complex, calcium heparinate, immunosuppressive agents, and vitamin D.

## HISTORY

Even early infarctive lesions are exquisitely tender and painful.
**Disease Associations**   Occurs in end-stage renal disease. Most patients are diabetic. Onset often closely follows initiation of hemo- or peritoneal dialysis. Hyperparathyroidism.

## PHYSICAL EXAMINATION

**Skin Lesions**
Initially preinfarctive ischemic plaques occur, appearing as mottling or having a livedo reticularis pattern, dusky red to violaceous. Bullae may form over ischemic tissue, which eventually becomes necrotic. Central infarcted sites have a tightly adherent black or yellowish, leathery slough (Fig. 15-7). Lesions gradually enlarge over weeks to months; when debrided, deep ulcers reaching down to the fascia result. Ischemic skin frequently becomes secondarily infected; infection can remain localized or become invasive, causing cellulitis and bacteremia. In addition, large areas of induration can be defined on palpation as platelike subcutaneous masses that extend beyond infarcted or ulcerated areas (Fig. 15-7).
***Distribution***   Distal extremities, most commonly on the lateral and posterior calves; abdomen, buttocks; fingers; glans penis.

## LABORATORY EXAMINATIONS

**Chemistry**   Azotemia. Calcium $\times$ phosphate ion product usually elevated.
**Parathormone (PTH)**   Levels usually elevated.
**Cultures**   Rule out secondary infection.
**Dermatopathology**   Incisional, deep biopsy shows calcification of the media of small- and medium-sized blood vessels in the dermis and subcutaneous tissue. Intraluminal fibrin thrombi are present. Ischemia results in intralobular or septal fat necrosis, accompanied by a sparse lymphohistiocytic infiltrate.
**Imaging**   Radiographs of affected extremities show calcium deposition outlining small and large vessels. Microcalcification of calciphylaxis is difficult to visualize.

## DIAGNOSIS AND DIFFERENTIAL DIAGNOSIS

Made on history of renal failure, clinical findings, elevated PTH level, elevated calcium $\times$ phosphate ion product, and histologic features.
**Differential Diagnosis**   Panniculitis, vasculitides, necrobiosis lipoidica with ulceration, dystrophic calcinosis cutis, scleroderma, atheroembolization, atherosclerosis obliterans, disseminated intravascular coagulation (purpura fulminans), pyoderma gangrenosum, warfarin necrosis, heparin necrosis. *Vibrio vulnificus* cellulitis, other necrotizing cellulitides.

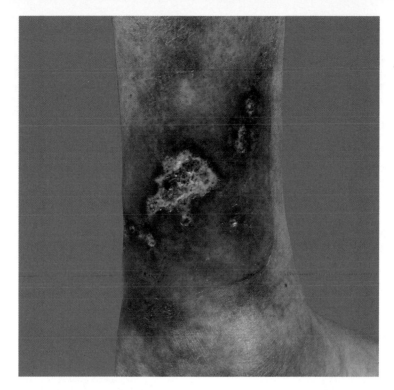

**Figure 15-7  Calciphylaxis**  *A jagged ulceration of the right lower leg, surrounded by a mottled violaceous zone of ischemia and several smaller ulcers in a diabetic male with renal failure. The ulcer is sharply demarcated with an eschar and extends into the subcutaneous fat; the lesion is extremely painful and, secondarily infected. The reticulated and mottled surrounding skin is indurated and represents a platelike subcutaneous mass that is appreciated only on palpation. It may also become necrotic.*

## COURSE AND PROGNOSIS

Slowly progressive despite all therapeutic interventions. Pain is a constant feature. In advanced disease, gangrenc of fingers, toes, and penis may result in autoamputation. Local infection and sepsis are common comlications. Overall, the prognosis is poor, and the mortality rate is very high.

## MANAGEMENT

Calciphylaxis is best managed by early diagnosis, treatment of renal failure, partial parathyroidectomy when indicated, aggressive debridement of necrotic tissue, and avoidance of precipitating factors such as systemic glucocorticoids.

## CUSHING'S SYNDROME AND HYPERCORTICISM

Cushing's syndrome (CS) is characterized by truncal obesity, moon face, acne, abdominal striae, hypertension, decreased carbohydrate tolerance, protein catabolism, psychiatric disturbances, and amenorrhea and hirsutism in females; it is associated with excess adrenocorticosteroids of endogenous or exogenous source. *Cushing's disease* refers to CS associated with pituitary adrenocorticotropic hormone (ACTH)-producing adenoma. *CS medicamentosum* refers to CS caused by exogenous administration of glucocorticoids.

A plethoric obese person with a "classic" habitus that results from the redistribution of fat: moon facies (Fig. 15-8), "buffalo" hump, truncal obesity, and thin arms. Purple striae, mostly on the abdomen and trunk; atrophic skin with easy bruising and telangiectasia; facial hypertrichosis with pigmented hairs and often increased lanugo hairs on the face and arms; androgenetic alopecia in females. Acne of recent onset (without comedones) or flaring of existing acne. General symptoms consist of fatigue and muscle weakness, hypertension, personality changes, amenorrhea in females, polyuria, and polydipsia. Work-up includes determination of blood glucose, serum potassium, and free cortisol in 24-h urine. Abnormal dexamethasone suppression test with failure to suppress endogenous cortisol secretion when dexamethasone is administered. Elevated ACTH. CT scan of the abdomen and the pituitary. Assessment of osteoporosis. Management consists of elimination of exogenous glucocorticoids or the detection and correction of underlying endogenous cause.

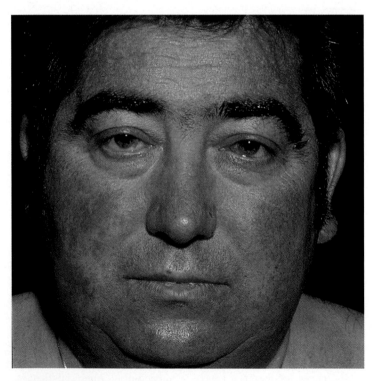

**Figure 15-8   Cushing's syndrome**   *Plethoric moon facies with erythema and telangiectases of cheek and forehead; the face and neck and supraclavicular areas (not depicted here) show increased deposition of fat.*

# GRAVES' DISEASE AND HYPERTHYROIDISM   ◧  ◐

Graves' disease (GD) is a disorder with three major manifestations: hyperthyroidism with diffuse goiter, ophthalmopathy, and dermopathy. The manifestations often do not occur together,
may not occur at all, and run courses that are independent of each other.

**Dermopathy (Pretibial Myxedema)**   Early lesions: bilateral, asymmetric, firm, non-pitting
nodules and plaques that are pink, skin-colored,
or purple (Fig. 15-9, *right*). Late lesions: confluence of early lesions, which symmetrically
involve the pretibial regions and may, in extreme cases, result in grotesque involvement of
entire lower legs and dorsa of feet; smooth surface with orange peel– like appearance, later
becomes verrucous (Fig. 15-9, *right*). *Note*:
pretibial myxedema may also occur *after* treatment of hyperthyroidism.

**Fingers**   Fingers show acropachy, which represents diaphyseal proliferation of the periosteum
and clubbing (Fig. 15-9, *left*).

**Ophthalmopathy**   GD ophthalmopathy has two
components, spastic (stare, lid lag, lid retraction) and mechanical [proptosis (Fig. 15-9, *top*),
ophthalmoplegia,   congestive   oculopathy,
chemosis, conjuctivitis, periorbital swelling, and
potential complications of corneal ulceration,
optic neuritis, optic atrophy]. Exophthalmic
ophthalmoplegia: ocular muscle weakness with
inward gaze, convergence, strabismus, diplopia.

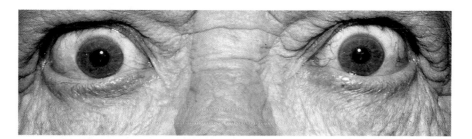

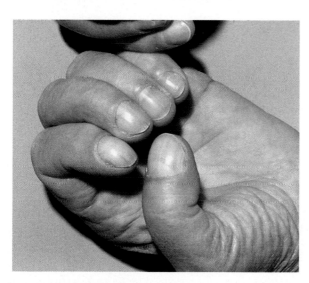

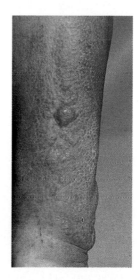

**Figure 15-9   Graves' disease**   *A composite image illustrates: proptosis, lid retraction; thyroid
acropachy (osteoarthropathy) with clubbing; and the pink- and skin-colored papules, nodules and
plaques in the pretibial region.*

**Thryoid**   Diffuse toxic goiter, asymmetric, lobular. Asymmetric and lobular thyroid enlargement, often with the presence of a bruit.

## MANAGEMENT

**Thyrotoxicosis**   Antithyroid agents block thyroid hormone synthesis. Ablation of thyroid tissue, surgically or by radioactive iodine.

**Ophthalmopathy**   Symptomatic treatment in mild cases. Severe cases: prednisone 100 to 120 mg/d initially, tapering to 5 mg/d. Orbital radiation. Orbital decompression.

**Dermopathy**   Topical glucocorticoid preparations under plastic occlusion for several months are usually effective. Low-dose oral glucocorticoids (prednisone, 5 mg/d). Intralesional triamcinolone 3 to 5 mg/mL for smaller lesions.

# HYPOTHYROIDISM AND MYXEDEMA

Myxedema results from insufficient production of thyroid hormones and can be caused by multiple disturbances. Hypothyroidism may be *thyroprivic* (e.g., congenital, primary idiopathic, postablative); *goitrous* (e.g., heritable biosynthetic defects, maternally transmitted, iodine deficiency, drug-induced or chronic thyroiditis); *trophoprivic* (e.g., pituitary); or *hypothalamic* [e.g., infection (encephalitis), neoplasm].

Early symptoms of *myxedema* are often overlooked: fatigue, lethargy, cold intolerance, constipation, stiffness and cramping of muscles, carpal tunnel syndrome, menorrhagia; slowing of intellectual and motor activity, decline in appetite, increase in weight, and deepening of voice. There is a dull, expressionless facies (Fig. 15-10), with puffiness of eyelids. Skin appears swollen, cool, waxy, dry, coarse, and pale with increased skin creases (Fig. 15-10). Palms and soles are yellow-orange due to carotenemia. The hair is dry, coarse, and brittle. Thinning of the scalp, beard (Fig. 15-10), and sexual areas. Eyebrows: alopecia of the lateral one-third. Nails brittle and slow growing. Large, smooth, red, and clumsy tongue. Work-up includes thyroid function tests, thyroid-stimulating hormone (TSH), scintigraphic imaging, and serum cholesterol ($\uparrow$).

Management is by replacement therapy.

# ADDISON'S DISEASE

Addison's disease is a syndrome resulting from adrenocortical insufficiency. It is insidious and is characterized by progressive generalized brown hyperpigmentation, slowly progressive weakness, fatigue, anorexia, nausea, and, frequently, GI symptoms (vomiting and diarrhea).

Suggestive laboratory changes include low serum sodium, high serum potassium, and elevation of the blood urea nitrogen. The diagnosis is confirmed by specific tests of adrenal insufficiency.

The patient may appear completely normal except for a generalized brown hyperpigmentation: (1) in areas where pigmentation normally occurs either habitually or UV-induced: around the eyes, face, dorsa of hands (Fig. 15-11), nipples, in the linea nigra (abdomen), axillae, and anogenital areas in males and females (the intensity of the pigmentation is related to skin phototype); and (2) in new areas: gingival or buccal mucosa, creases of palms, bony prominences. Also in new scars following surgery.

The differential diagnosis includes hemochromatosis; porphyria cutanea tarda; chronic renal failure; hepatic cirrhosis; benign endocrine tumors, such as chromophobe adenomas that produce ACTH and associated peptides [i.e., Nelson's syndrome, metastatic cancers (especially lung), carcinoid]; vitamin $B_{12}$ deficiency; chemotherapy (doxorubicin, busulfan, bleomycin, 5-fluorouracil); and systemic scleroderma. A screening test used for diagnosis is plasma cortisol 30 to 60 min after 250 $\mu$g cosyntropin intramuscularly or intravenously. This disease should be managed by an endocrinologist.

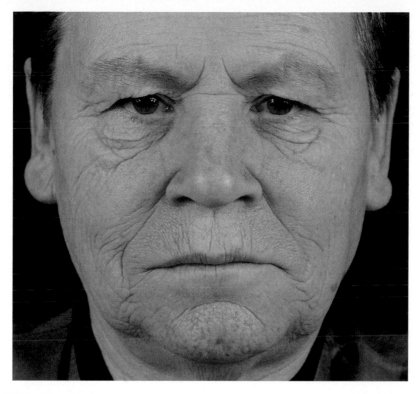

**Figure 15-10    Myxedema**    *Dry, pale skin; thinning of the lateral eyebrows; puffiness of the face and eyelids; increased number of skin creases; dull, expressionless, beardless facies.*

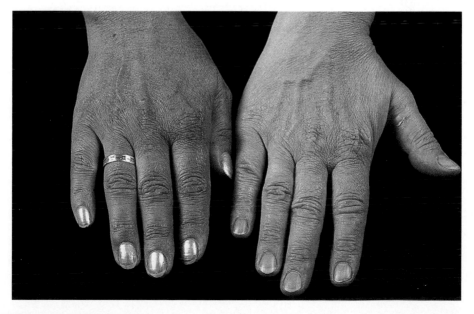

**FIGURE 15-11    Addison's disease**    *Hyperpigmentation representing an accentuation of normal pigmentation of the hand of a patient with Addison's disease (left). For comparison, the hand of a normal individual, matched for ethnic pigmentation, is shown on the right.*

# XANTHOMAS

Cutaneous xanthomas are yellow-brown, pinkish, or orange macules, papules, plaques, nodules, or infiltrations in tendons. They are characterized histologically by accumulations of xanthoma cells—macrophages containing droplets of lipids. Xanthomas may be symptoms of a general metabolic disease, a generalized histiocytosis, or a local fat phagocytosing storage process. The classification of metabolic xanthomas is based on this principle: (1) xanthomas due to hyperlipidemia and (2) normolipidemic xanthomas. The cause of xanthomas in the first group may be a primary hyperlipidemia, mostly genetically determined (Table 15-1), or secondary hyperlipidemia, associated with certain internal diseases such as biliary cirrhosis, diabetes mellitus, chronic renal failure, alcoholism, hyperthyroidism, and monoclonal gammopathy, or with intake of certain drugs such as beta-blockers and estrogens.

Some of the xanthomas are associated with high plasma low-density lipoprotein (LDL)-cholesterol levels, and therefore with a serious risk of atheromatosis and myocardial infarction. For that reason laboratory investigation of plasma lipid levels is always necessary. In some cases an apoprotein deficiency is present. Table 15-2 shows correlations of clinical xanthoma type and lipoprotein disturbances.

**TABLE 15-1   Classification of Genetic Hyperlipidemias**

| Frederickson Type | Classification | Lipid Profile |
|---|---|---|
| I | Familial lipoprotein lipase deficiency (hyperchylomicronemia, hypertriglyceridemia) (FLD) | TG++, C normal, CM++, HDL −/normal |
| IIa | Familial hypercholesterolemia (FH) | TG normal, C+, LDL+ |
| IIb | Familial combined hyperlipidemia (FCHL) | TG+, C+, LDL+, VLDL+ |
| III | Familial dysbetalipidemia (remnant particle disease) (FD) | TG+, C+, IDL+, CM remnants+ |
| IV | Familial hypertriglyceridemia (FHTG) | TG+, C normal/+, LDL++, VLDL++ |
| V | Familial combined hypertriglyceridemia (FHT) | TG+, C+, VLDL++, CM++ |

NOTE: TG, triglycerides; C, cholesterol; CM, chylomicrons; HDL, high-density lipoproteins; LDL, low-density lipoproteins; VLDL, very low density lipoproteins; IDL, intermediate-density lipoproteins; +, raised; −, lowered.

# XANTHELASMA   ■   ○

Most common of all xanthomas. In most cases an isolated finding unrelated to hyperlipidemia. Occurs in individuals >50 years; however, when in children or young adults, it is associated with familial hypercholesterolemia (FH) or familial dysbetalipidemia (FD).
*Synonyms*: Xanthelasma palpebrarum, periocular xanthoma.

Skin lesions are asymptomatic. Soft, polygonal yellow-orange papules and plaques localized to upper and lower eyelids (Fig. 15-12) and around inner canthus. Slow enlargement from tiny spots over months to years.

Cholesterol should be estimated in plasma; if enhanced, screening for type of hyperlipidemia (FH or FD). If due to hyperlipidemia, complication with atherosclerotic cardiovascular disease may be expected. However, in >50% of these patients, no metabolic disturbances are found.

## MANAGEMENT

Laser, excision, electrodesiccation, or topical application of trichloroacetic acid. Recurrences are not uncommon.

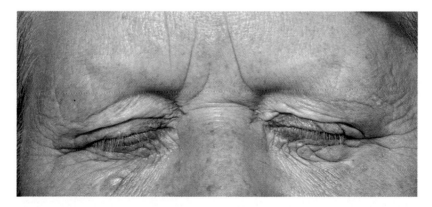

**FIGURE 15-12   Xanthelasma**   *Multiple, longitudinal, creamy-orange, slightly elevated dermal papules on the eyelids of a normolipemic individual.*

## XANTHOMA TENDINEUM     □  ◑

These subcutaneous tumors are yellow or skin-colored and move with the extensor tendons (Fig. 15-13). They are a symptom of familial hypercholesterolemia (FH) that presents as type IIa hyperlipidemia. This condition is autosomal recessive with a different phenotype in the heterozygote and homozygote. In the homozygote, the xanthomata appear in early childhood and the cardiovascular complications in early adolescence; the elevation of the LDL content of the plasma is extreme. These patients rarely attain ages above 20 years.
*Synonym*: Tendinous xanthoma.
*Management*: A diet low in cholesterol and saturated fats, supplemented by cholestyramine or statins. In extreme cases, measures such as portacaval shunt or liver transplantation have to be considered.

## XANTHOMA TUBEROSUM      ◑

This condition comprises yellowish nodules (Fig. 15-14) located especially on the elbows and knees by confluence of concomitant eruptive xanthomas. They are to be found in patients with FD, FHT, and FH (Table 15-2). In homozygous patients with FH, the tuberous xanthomas are flatter and skin colored. They are not accompanied by eruptive xanthomas.
*Synonym*: Tuberous xanthoma.
*Management*: Treatment of the underlying condition.

**TABLE 15-2   Relation of Xanthoma Type to Lipoprotein Disturbances**

| | |
|---|---|
| Xanthelasma palpebrarum | Normolipemic (~50%) or FH, FD |
| Xanthoma tendineum | FH (type IIa) |
| Xanthoma tuberosum | FD, FHT, FH (if homozygous) (type III, V, IIa) |
| Xanthoma eruptivum (or tuberoeruptivum) | FD, FHT, FLD (rare) |
| Xanthoma striatum palmare | FD (type III) |
| Xanthoma planum (generalized) | Patients often develop a monoclonal gammopathy associated with myeloma (type III), macroglobulinema, or lymphoma, and with normal plasma lipid levels. Less commonly, FHT may be present. |

NOTE: FH, familial hypercholesterolemia; FD, familial dysbetalipidemia; FHT, familial combined hypertriglyceridemia; FLD, familial lipoprotein lipase deficiency.

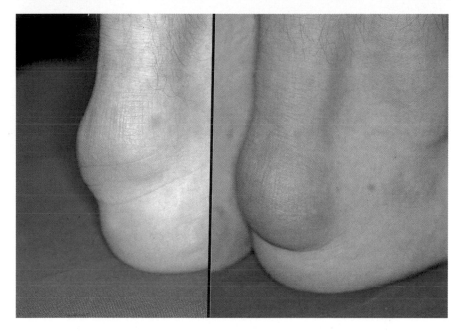

**FIGURE 15-13   Tendinous xanthomas**   *Large subcutaneous tumors adherent to the Achilles tendons.*

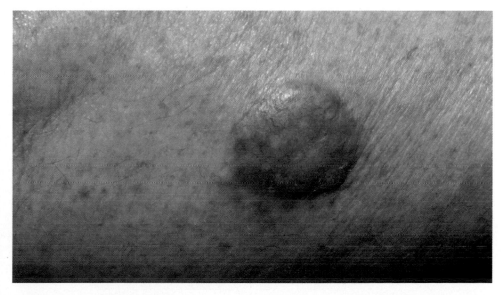

**FIGURE 15-14   Tuberous xanthoma**   *Flat-topped, yellow, firm tumor with an erythematous margin.*

## ERUPTIVE XANTHOMA

These discrete inflammatory-type papules "erupt" suddenly and in showers, appearing typically on the buttocks, elbows, lower arms (Fig. 15-15) and knees. A sign of FHT, FD, the very rare FLD (Tables 15-1 and 15-2), and diabetes out of control.

Papules are dome-shaped, discrete, initially red, then yellow center with red halo. Lesions may be scattered, discrete, in a localized region [e.g., elbows (Fig. 15-15), buttocks] or appear as "tight" clusters that become confluent to form nodular "tuberoeruptive" xanthomas. *Management*: React very favorably to a low-calorie and low-fat diet.

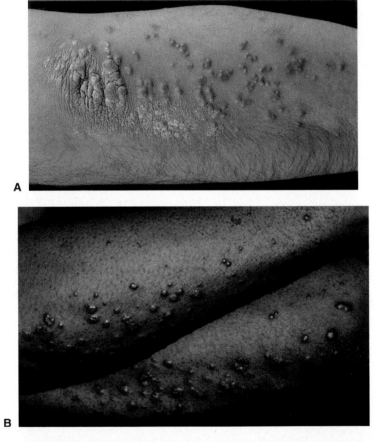

**FIGURE 15-15    Papular eruptive xanthomas**    *A. Multiple, discrete, red-to-yellow papules becoming confluent on the elbow of an individual with uncontrolled diabetes mellitus; lesions were present on both elbows and buttocks. **B.** Papular eruptive xanthomas on the elbows and lower arms in an African American. This image is shown to demonstrate the color of xanthomas in black skin.*

**FIGURE 15-16 (Opposite page, left)    Xanthoma striatum palmare**    *The palmar creases are yellow, often a subtle lesion noticeable only upon close examination.*

## XANTHOMA STRIATUM PALMARE   □ ◑

This condition is characterized by yellow-orange, flat or elevated infiltrations of the volar creases of palms and fingers (Fig. 15-16). Pathognomonic for FD (type III) (Table 15-2). Next to xanthoma striatum palmare, FD also presents with tuberous xanthoma (Fig. 15-14) and xanthelasma palpebrarum (Fig. 15-12).

Patients with FD are prone to atherosclerotic cardiovascular disease, especially ischemia of the legs and coronary vessels.

*Management*: Patients with FD react very favorably to a diet low in fats and carbohydrates. If necessary, this may be supplemented with statins, fibrates, or nicotinic acid.

## NORMOLIPEMIC PLANE XANTHOMA

Xanthoma planum is a normolipemic xanthoma that consists of diffuse orange-yellow pigmentation and slight elevations of the skin (Fig. 15-17). There is a recognizable border. These lesions can be idiopathic or secondary to leukemia, but the most common association is with multiple myeloma. The lesions may precede the onset of multiple myeloma by many years.

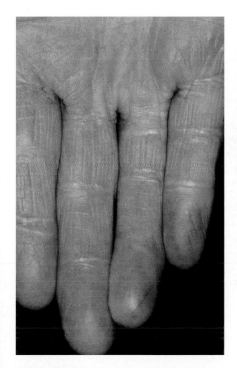

**FIGURE 15-16**

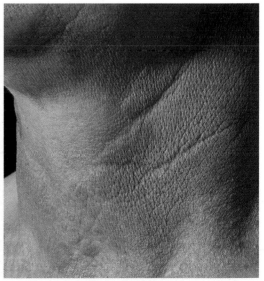

**FIGURE 15-17   Plane xanthoma**   *Yellowish-red, slightly elevated plaques on the neck, noticeable mainly because of the accentuation of the skin texture in a normolipemic patient with lymphoma. Plane xanthomas occur most commonly on the upper trunk and neck and also occur in individuals with myeloma.*

# SCURVY  □  ●

Scurvy is an acute or chronic disease of infancy and of middle and old age caused by dietary deficiency of ascorbic acid (vitamin C). The disorder is characterized principally by anemia, hemorrhagic manifestations in the skin (ecchymoses and perifollicular hemorrhage) and in the musculoskeletal system (hemorrhage into periosteum and muscles), and changes in the gums (loosening of teeth, bleeding gums).
*Synonym*: Vitamin C deficiency.

Humans are unable to synthesize ascorbic acid and require it as an essential dietary vitamin. Total-body pool of vitamin C varies from 1.5 to 3 g. First symptoms of depletion occur when pool size is <0.5 g. Deficiency of vitamin C leads to impairment of peptidyl hydroxylation of procollagen, reduction in collagen formation with associated capillary fragility.

Scurvy occurs in infants or children on a diet consisting of only processed milk with no added citrus fruit or vegetables as a result of parental neglect; or in edentulous adult persons who live alone, and do not eat salads and uncooked vegetables. *Precipitating factors* are pregnancy, lactation, and thyrotoxicosis when there are increased requirements of ascorbic acid; most common in alcoholism. With no vitamin C intake, symptoms of scurvy occur after 1 to 3 months. Lassitude, weakness, arthralgia, and myalgia.

*Skin lesions* consist of petechiae, follicular hyperkeratosis with perifollicular hemorrhage, especially on the lower legs (Fig. 15-18). Hair becomes fragmented and buried in these perifolliculár hyperkeratotic papules (corkscrew hairs); also, extensive ecchymoses (Fig. 15-19), which can be generalized. Nails: splinter hemorrhages. Gingiva: swollen, purple, spongy, and bleeds easily; findings occur in more advanced scurvy. Loosening and loss of teeth.

Hemorrhage occurring into periosteum of long bones and into joints causes painful swellings and, in children, epiphyseal separation. Sternum may sink inward: scorbutic rosary (elevation at rib margins). Retrobulbar, subarachnoid, intracerebral hemorrhage can cause death.

*Differential diagnosis* includes thrombocytopenia, senile purpura, coagulopathy, anticoagulant drug therapy (warfarin, heparin), cryoglobulinemia, vasculitis and gingival hypertrophy due to poor dental hygiene, drug-induced gingival hyperplasia, leukemia, pregnancy.

*Laboratory examinations* show normocytic, normochromic anemia resulting from bleeding into tissues. Folate deficiency is also common, resulting in macrocytic anemia. Positive capillary fragility test. Platelet ascorbic acid level usually <25% of normal value; serum ascorbic acid level zero. X-ray findings are diagnostic. Unless treated, scurvy is fatal. On treatment, spontaneous bleeding ceases within 24 h, muscle and bone pain fade quickly, bleeding from gums stops in 2 to 3 days.

## MANAGEMENT

In suspected cases, blood should be obtained for ascorbic acid level and therapy begun immediately.
**Ascorbic Acid**  100 mg 3 to 5 times daily until 4 g is given; then 100 mg/d is curative in days to weeks.

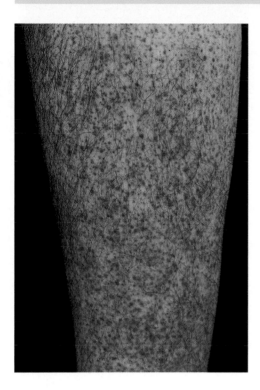

**FIGURE 15-18   Scurvy**   *Perifollicular hemorrhage on the leg. The follicles are often plugged by keratin (perifollicular hyperkeratosis). This eruption occurred in a 46-year-old alcoholic, homeless male, who also had bleeding gums and loose teeth.*

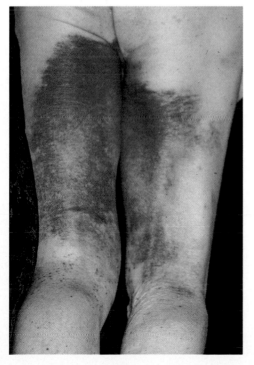

**FIGURE 15-19   Scurvy**   *These extensive ecchymoses occurred in an edentulous 65-year-old male who lived alone and whose food intake consisted mainly of biscuits soaked in water.*

## ZINC DEFICIENCY AND ACRODERMATITIS ENTEROPATHICA     □ ●

Acrodermatitis enteropathica (AE) is a genetic disorder of zinc absorption, presenting in infancy, characterized by a triad of acral dermatitis (face, hands, feet, anogenital area), alopecia, and diarrhea; nearly identical clinical findings occur in older individuals with acquired zinc deficiency (AZD) due either to dietary deficiency or failure of intestinal absorption.

### EPIDEMIOLOGY AND ETIOLOGY

**Age of Onset**   *AE*: in infants bottle-fed with bovine milk, days to few weeks. In breast-fed infants, soon after weaning. *AZD*: older individuals.

**Etiology**   *AE*: autosomal recessive trait resulting in failure to absorb zinc. *AZD*: secondary to reduced dietary intake of zinc, malabsorption (regional enteritis, after intestinal bypass surgery for obesity), chronic alcoholism, increased urinary loss (nephrotic syndrome), hypoalbuminemic states, penicillamine therapy, high catabolic states (trauma, burns, surgery), hemolytic anemias; adolescents who eat dirt, prolonged parenteral nutrition without supplemental zinc.

### PATHOGENESIS

In AE, patients do not absorb enough zinc from the diet. The specific ligand involved in basic transport mechanisms for zinc that might be abnormal in AE is not known. The defect appears to be somewhere in the early stages of zinc nutriture, where zinc is presented to the intestinal brush border. This defect can be overcome by increased zinc supply in the diet. It is not known how zinc deficiency leads to skin and other lesions.

### HISTORY

*AE* usually starts when infant is weaned and placed on cow's milk. *AZD* concomitant with dietary change or underlying illness.

### PHYSICAL EXAMINATION

**Skin Findings**
Patches and plaques of dry, scaly, sharply marginated and brightly red, eczematous dermatitis evolving into vesiculobullous, pustular, erosive, and crusted lesions (Figs. 15-20 and 15-21A). Initially occur in the perioral and anogenital areas. Later, scalp, hands and feet, flexural regions, trunk. Fingertips glistening, erythematous, with fissures and secondary paronychia. Perlèche. Lesions become secondarily infected with *Candida albicans*, *S. aureus*. Impaired wound healing.

**Hair and Nails**   Diffuse alopecia, graying of hair. Paronychia, nail ridging, loss of nails.

**Mucous Membranes**   Red, glossy tongue; superficial aphthous-like erosions; secondary oral candidiasis.

**General Examination**   Photophobia; irritable, depressed mood. Children with AE whine and cry constantly. Failure of growth.

### LABORATORY EXAMINATIONS

**CBC**   Anemia.

**Chemistry**   Low serum/plasma zinc levels.

**Urine**   Reduced urinary zinc excretion.

**Dermatopathology**   Psoriasiform dermatitis with large, pale keratinocytes in the upper epidermis; prominent parakeratosis. There may be intraepidermal clefts with acantholysis and blisters. Sparse, superficial, perivascular lymphohistiocytic infiltrate and tortuous capillaries in the papillary dermis.

### DIAGNOSIS AND DIFFERENTIAL DIAGNOSIS

Clinical diagnosis confirmed by zinc blood levels and histopathology.

**Differential Diagnosis**   Atopic dermatitis, seborrheic dermatitis, psoriasis, mucocutaneous candidiasis, glucagonoma syndrome.

### COURSE AND PROGNOSIS

Before it was known that AE is due to deficient zinc uptake from the diet, it was usually fatal in infancy or early childhood. Patients failed to thrive and suffered from severe

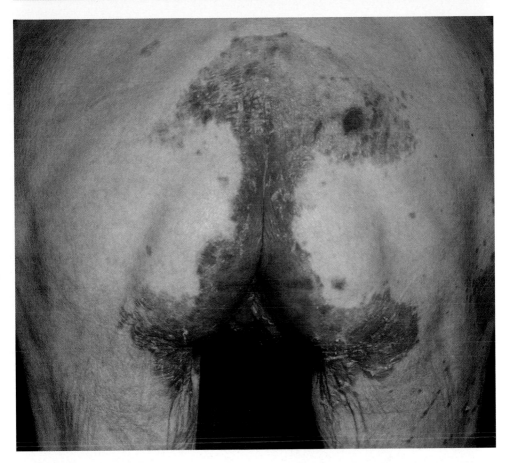

**FIGURE 15-20   Zinc deficiency**   *Well-demarcated, psoriasiform and eczematous–like plaques with scaling and erosions overlying the sacrum, intergluteal cleft, buttocks, and hip in a 60-year-old alcoholic female whose diet had consisted of pickles and cheap wine. She also had a similar eruption around the mouth, perlèche, atrophic glossitis, and had glistening, shiny, oozing fingertips.*

candidal and bacterial infections. After zinc replacement, severely infected and erosive skin lesions heal within 1 to 2 weeks (Fig. 15-21B), diarrhea ceases, and irritability and depression of mood improve within 24 h.

## MANAGEMENT

Dietary or IV supplementation with zinc salts in 2 to 3 times the required daily amount restores normal zinc status in days to weeks.

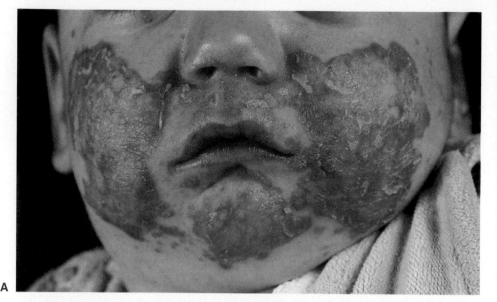

A

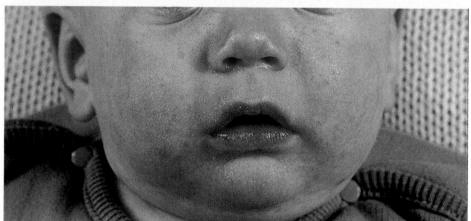

B

**FIGURE 15-21   Acrodermatitis enteropathica**   *A. Sharply demarcated, symmetric, partially erosive, scaly, and crusted plaques on the face of an infant after weaning. Similar lesions were also found in the perigenital and perianal regions and on the fingertips. The child was highly irritable, whining, and crying and had diarrhea. B. Within 24 h after zinc replacement, the irritability and diarrhea ceased and the infant's mood improved; and after 10 days (shown here) the perioral and perigenital lesions had healed.*

# PELLAGRA   □  ◑

Pellagra is related to niacin deficiency. Niacinamide is an important constituent of coenzyme I (NAD) and coenzyme II (NADP), which function in oxidation-reduction reactions as a hydrogen ion donor and acceptor, respectively. The essential amino acid tryptophan is converted in the body to niacin. Pellagra may arise from a diet deficient in niacin or tryptophan, or both. A predominantly maize-based diet is usually implicated, but only when the maize is steamed or cooked. Pellagra is characterized by the 3 Ds: *d*ermatitis, *d*iarrhea, and *d*ementia. Skin changes are determined by exposure to sunlight and pressure. The disorder begins with a symmetric itching and smarting erythema on the dorsa of the hands, neck, and face. Vesicles and bullae may erupt and break, so that crusting occurs and lesions become scaly (Fig. 15-22). Later, skin becomes indurated, lichenified, rough, covered by dark scales and crusts; there are cracks and fissures and a sharp demarcation from normal skin (Fig. 15-22). The distribution is striking: dorsa of hands and fingers ("gauntlet" of pellagra), bandlike around the neck ("Casal's necklace"), dorsa of feet up to malleoli with sparing of the heel, and butterfly region of the face.

*Management*: Diagnosis is verified by detection of decreased levels of urinary metabolites. Oral administration of 100 to 300 mg niacinamide plus other vitamins of the B complex lead to complete resolution.

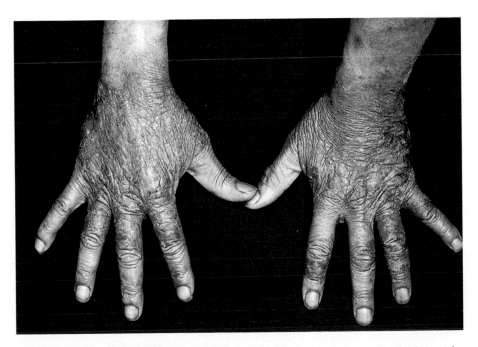

**FIGURE 15-22   "Gauntlet" of pellagra**   *Indurated, lichenified, pigmented, and scaly skin on the dorsa of the hands in a patient with niacin deficiency.*

# PSEUDOXANTHOMA ELASTICUM

Pseudoxanthoma elasticum (PXE) is a serious hereditary disorder of connective tissue that involves the elastic tissue in the skin, blood vessels, and eyes. The principal skin manifestations are a distinctive *peau d'orange* surface pattern resulting from closely grouped clusters of yellow (chamois-colored) papules in a reticular pattern on the neck, axillae, and other body folds. The effects on the vascular system include GI hemorrhage, hypertension occurring in young persons and resulting from involvement of renal arteries, and claudication. Ocular manifestations ("angioid" streaks and retinal hemorrhages) can lead to blindness.

## EPIDEMIOLOGY

**Age of Onset** 20 to 30 years.
**Incidence** 1:40,000 to 1:100,000.
**Inheritance** Autosomal recessive (most common) and autosomal dominant.

## ETIOLOGY AND PATHOGENESIS

Pathogenic mutation in the *ABCC6* gene, which encodes MRP6, a member of the ATPase-dependent transmembrane transporter family of proteins. MRP6 can serve as an efflux pump transporting small-molecular-weight glutathione conjugates, which may facilitate calcification of elastic fibers. This may result in fragmented elastic fibers in skin, eyes, arteries.

## HISTORY

Asymptomatic skin lesions, usually present by age 30 but may go undetected until old age. There may be symptoms relating to multisystem involvement. Decreased visual acuity in a young person. Coronary artery disease: angina pectoris, myocardial infarction. Peripheral vascular disease: claudication. Others such as symptoms associated with hypertension, hematemesis, and melena. History of miscarriages.

## PHYSICAL EXAMINATION

### Skin Lesions
Yellow, chamois-colored papules, coalescing to form larger plaques on the sides of neck (Fig. 15-23), axillae, groin, abdomen, and thighs. Papules are arranged in a reticulated or linear pattern with furrows between individual plaques (Fig. 15-23). Skin of involved sites becomes redundant, lax, soft, and may hang in folds.

**Mucous Membranes** Yellow papules on the soft palate, labial mucosa, rectum, and vagina.
**Eyes** Angioid streaks (Fig. 15-24): slate-gray or yellowish, wider than blood vessels, and extend across the fundus, radiating from the optic disc (represent rupture of Bruch's membrane). Macular degeneration. Retinal hemorrhages. Diminished visual acuity; blindness. Alteration of retinal pigmentation.
**General Examination** Decreased or absent peripheral pulses. Hypertension. Mitral valve prolapse.

## LABORATORY EXAMINATIONS

**Dermatopathology** Biopsy of a scar can detect characteristic changes of PXE *before typical skin changes are apparent.* Swelling and irregular clumping and basophilic staining of elastic fibers in reticular dermis; with von Kossa stain, elastic fibers appear curled and "chopped up" with calcium deposition.
**Imaging** X-ray: extensive calcification of the peripheral arteries of the lower extremities. Arteriography of symptomatic vessels.

## DIAGNOSIS AND DIFFERENTIAL DIAGNOSIS

By the skin lesions, which are distinctive, confirmed by biopsy. Angioid streaks are also characteristic.
**Differential Diagnosis** Cutis laxa, Ehlers-Danlos syndrome; diffuse normolipemic plane xanthoma.

## COURSE AND PROGNOSIS

The course is inexorably progressive. Gastric artery hemorrhage occurs commonly, resulting

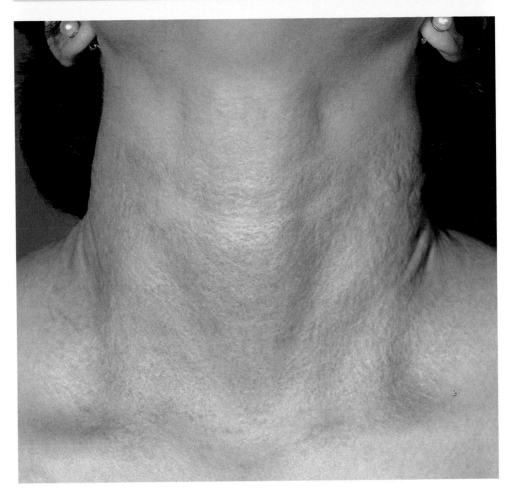

**FIGURE 15-23   Pseudoxanthoma elasticum**   *Multiple, confluent, chamois-colored or yellow papules (pseudoxanthomatous) created a large, circumferential, pebbled plaque on the neck of a 32-year-old woman. Changes in the connective tissue in this condition led to excessive folds on the lateral neck.*

in hematemesis. Peripheral vascular disease presents as premature cerebrovascular accidents, atherosclerosis obliterans, or bowel angina. Pregnancies are complicated by miscarriage, cardiovascular complications. Blindness. Life span is often shortened due to myocardial infarction or massive GI hemorrhage.

## MANAGEMENT

Genetic counseling. Evaluate family members for PXE. Obstetrician should be aware of PXE diagnosis and follow patient carefully. Regular reevaluation by primary care physician and ophthalmologist is mandatory.
*Support organization:* PXE International, *www.pxe.org*

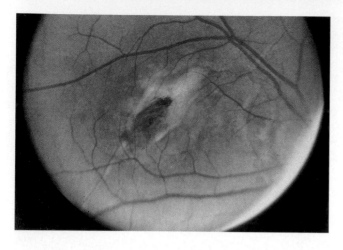

**FIGURE 15-24   Pseudoxanthoma elasticum: angioid streaks in retina**  *Yellowish streaks wider than blood vessels extend across the fundus in a distribution more or less radial from the optic disk.*

# TUBEROUS SCLEROSIS

Tuberous sclerosis is an autosomal dominant disease arising from a genetically programmed hyperplasia of ectodermal and mesodermal cells and manifested by a variety of lesions in the skin, CNS (hamartomas), heart, kidney, and other organs. The principal early manifestations are the triad of seizures, mental retardation, and congenital white spots. Facial angiofibromata are pathognomonic but do not appear until the third or fourth year.

## EPIDEMIOLOGY

**Incidence**   In institutions, 1:100 to 1:300; in general population, 1:20,000 to 1:100,000.
**Age of Onset**   Infancy.
**Sex**   Equal incidence.
**Race**   All races.
**Heredity**   Autosomal dominant. The genes for tuberous sclerosis have been mapped to chromosomes 16p13 and 9q34.

## PATHOGENESIS

Genetic alterations of ectodermal and mesodermal cells with hyperplasia, with a disturbance in embryonic cellular differentiation.

## HISTORY

White macules are present at birth or appear in infancy (>80% occur by 1 year of age, 100% appear by 2 years); >20% of angiofibromata are present at 1 year of age, 50% occur by 3 years. Seizures (infantile spasms) occur in 86%; the earlier the onset of seizures, the worse the mental retardation. Mental retardation (49%).

## PHYSICAL EXAMINATION

**Skin Lesions**   96% incidence.
*Hypomelanotic Macules*  "Off-white"; one or many, usually more than three. Polygonal or "thumbprint," 0.5 to 2 cm; lance ovate or "ash-leaf" spots (Fig. 15-25), 3 to 4 cm (up to 12 cm); tiny white "confetti" macules, 1 to 2 mm (Fig. 15-26). White macules occur on trunk (56%), lower extremities (32%), upper extremities (7%), head and neck (5%). White macules shine up with Wood's light.
*Papules/Nodules*  0.1 to 0.5 cm, dome-shaped and smooth, exhibiting red or skin color (Fig. 15-27). Occur in the center of the face. They are firm and disseminated but may coalesce; termed *adenoma sebaceum* but represent angiofibromas (present in 70%).
*Plaques*  Represent connective tissue nevi ("shagreen" patch), present in 40%; skin colored; occur on the back and buttocks.

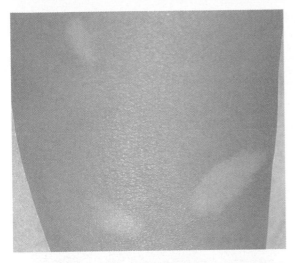

**Figure 15-25    Tuberous sclerosis: ash-leaflet hypopigmented macules**   *Three well-demarcated, elongated (ash-leaflet shaped), hypomelanotic macules on the lower leg of a child with tan skin.*

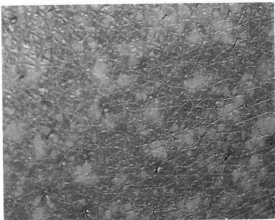

**FIGURE 15-26    Tuberous sclerosis: "confetti" macules**   *Multiple, discrete, small, confetti–like, hypopigmented macules of variable size on the leg. These lesions are pathognomonic.*

*Periungual Papules or Nodules* Ungual fibromas (Koenen's tumors) present in 22%, arise late in childhood and have the same pathology (angiofibroma) as the facial papules. (See Fig. 30-28).

## ASSOCIATED SYSTEMS

CNS (tumors producing seizures), eye (gray or yellow retinal plaques, 50%), heart (benign rhabdomyomas), hamartomas of mixed cell type (kidney, liver, thyroid, testes, and GI system).

## LABORATORY EXAMINATIONS

**Dermatopathology**   *White Macules* Decreased number of melanocytes, decreased melanosome size, decreased melanin in melanocytes and keratinocytes.

*Angiofibromata* Proliferation of fibroblasts, increased collagen, angioneogenesis, capillary dilatation, absence of elastic tissue.

**Brain Pathology**   "Tubers" are gliomas.

**Imaging**

*Skull X-Ray* Multiple calcific densities.

*CT Scan* Ventricular deformity and tumor deposits along the striothalamic borders.

*MRI* Subependymal nodules.

*Electroencephalography* Abnormal.

*Renal Ultrasound* Reveals renal hamartoma.

## DIAGNOSIS

The diagnosis may be difficult or impossible in an infant or child if one or two white macules

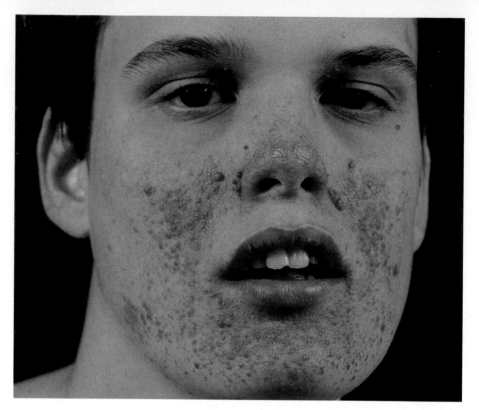

**FIGURE 15-27    Tuberous sclerosis: angiofibromas**  *Confluent, small, angiomatous (erythematous, glistening) papules on the lower half of the face. These lesions were not present during the first few years of life; appeared only after the age of 4 years.*

are the only cutaneous finding. More than five is highly suggestive. Even when typical white "ash-leaf" or "thumbprint" macules (Fig. 15-25) are present, it is necessary to confirm the diagnosis. Confetti spots (Fig. 15-26) are virtually pathognomonic. A pediatric neurologist can then evaluate the patient with a study of the family members and by obtaining various types of imaging as well as electroencephalography. Mental retardation and seizures may be absent.

### DIFFERENTIAL DIAGNOSIS

**White Spots**   Focal vitiligo, nevus anemicus, tinea versicolor, nevus depigmentosus, postinflammatory hypomelanosis.
**Angiofibromas**   Tricholemmoma, syringoma, skin-colored papules on the face, dermal nevi. *Note*: angiofibromata of the face (Fig. 15-27) have been mistaken for and treated as acne vulgaris.

**Periungual Fibromas**   Verruca vulgaris.

### COURSE AND PROGNOSIS

A serious autosomal disorder that causes major problems in behavior, because of mental retardation, and in therapy, to control the serious seizure problem present in many patients.

In severe cases, 30% die before the fifth year of life, and 50 to 75% die before reaching adult age. Malignant gliomas are not uncommon. Genetic counseling is imperative.

### MANAGEMENT

**Prevention**   Counseling.
**Treatment**   Laser surgery for angiofibromas.
**Support   organization:**   *http://www.support-group.com*

# NEUROFIBROMATOSIS

Neurofibromatosis (NF) is an autosomal dominant trait manifested by changes in the skin, nervous system, bones, and endocrine glands. These changes include a variety of congenital abnormalities, tumors, and hamartomas. Two major forms of NF are recognized: (1) classic von Recklinghausen's NF, termed *NF1*; and (2) central, or acoustic NF, termed *NF2*. Both types have café-au-lait macules and neurofibromas, but only NF2 has *bilateral* acoustic neuromas (unilateral acoustic neuromas are a variable feature of NF1). An important diagnostic sign present only in NF1 is pigmented hamartomas of the iris (Lisch nodules).
*Synonym*: von Recklinghausen's disease.

## EPIDEMIOLOGY

**Incidence**   *NF1*: 1:4000; *NF2*: 1:50,000.
**Race**   All races.
**Sex**   Males slightly more than females.
**Heredity**   Autosomal dominant; the gene for NF1 is on chromosome 17 (q 1.2) and the gene codes for a protein named neurofibromin. The gene for NF2 is on chromosome 22 and codes for a protein called merlin.

## PATHOGENESIS

Action of an abnormal gene on cellular elements derived from the neural crest: melanocytes, Schwann cells, endoneurial fibroblasts.

## HISTORY

Café-au-lait (CAL) macules are not usually present at birth but appear during the first

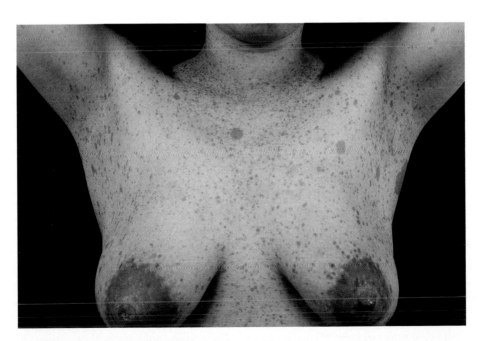

**FIGURE 15-28    Neurofibromatosis (NF1)**    *Several larger (>1 cm) café-au-lait macules on the upper chest and multiple small macules on the axillae (axillary "freckling") in a brown-skinned female. Myriads of early, small, pink-tan neurofibromas on the chest, breasts, and neck.*

3 years; neurofibromata appear during late adolescence. Clinical manifestations in various organs are related to pathology: hypertensive headaches (pheochromocytomas), pathologic fractures (bone cysts), mental retardation, brain tumor (astrocytoma), short stature, precocious puberty (early menses, clitoral hypertrophy).

## PHYSICAL EXAMINATION

### Skin Lesions

*CAL Macules* Light or dark brown *uniform* melanin pigmentation with sharp margination. Lesions vary in size from multiple "freckle-like" tiny macules <2 mm (Fig. 15-28), to very large brown macules >20 cm (Fig. 15-29). The common size, however, is 2 to 5 cm. CAL macules also vary in number, from a few to hundreds. Tiny freckle–like lesions in the axillae are highly characteristic ("axillary freckling") (Fig. 15-28).

*Papules/Nodules (Neurofibromas)* Skin-colored, pink, or brown (Fig. 15-29); flat, dome-shaped or pedunculated; soft or firm, sometimes tender; "buttonhole sign"—invagination with the tip of the index finger is pathognomonic.

*Plexiform Neuromas* Drooping, soft, doughy (Fig. 15-30); may be massive, involving entire extremity, the head, or a portion of the trunk.

*Distribution* Randomly distributed (Fig. 15-29) but may be localized to one region (segmental NF1). The segmental type may be heritable or a localized hamartoma.

**Other Physical Findings** *Eyes* Pigmented hamartomas of the iris (Lisch nodules) begin to appear at age 5 and are present in 20% of children with NF before age 6 but can be found in 95% of patients with NF1 in adolescence. They are not present in NF2. Lisch nodules are visible only with slit-lamp examination and appear as "glassy," transparent, dome-shaped, yellow-to-brown papules up to 2 mm. They do not correlate with the severity of the disease.

*Musculoskeletal* Cervicothoracic kyphoscoliosis, segmental hypertrophy.

*Adrenal Pheochromocytoma* Elevated blood pressure and episodic flushing.

*Peripheral Nervous System* Elephantiasis neuromatosa (gross disfigurement from neurofibromatosis of the nerve trunks).

*Central Nervous System* Optic glioma, acoustic neuroma (rare in NF1 and unilateral, but bilateral in NF2), astrocytoma, meningioma, neurofibroma.

## LABORATORY EXAMINATIONS

**Dermatopathology** More than 10 *melanin macroglobules* per 5 high-power fields in "split" dopa preparations.

**Wood's Lamp Examination** In white persons with pale skin, the CAL macules are more easily visualized with Wood's lamp examination.

## DIAGNOSIS AND DIFFERENTIAL DIAGNOSIS

Two of the following criteria:

1. Multiple CAL macules—more than six lesions with a diameter of 1.5 cm in adults and more than five lesions with a diameter of 0.5 cm or more in children younger than 5 years.
2. Multiple freckles in the axillary and inguinal regions.
3. Based on clinical and histologic grounds, two or more neurofibromas of any type, or one plexiform neurofibroma.
4. Sphenoid wing dysplasia or congenital bowing or thinning of long bone cortex, with or without pseudoarthrosis
5. Bilateral optic nerve gliomas
6. Two or more Lisch nodules on slit-lamp examination
7. First-degree relative (parent, sibling, or child) with NF1 by the preceding criteria

**Differential Diagnosis** Brown CAL-type macules: Albright's syndrome (polyostotic fibroma, dysplasia, and precocious puberty); a few CAL macules (three or less) may be present in 10 to 20% of normal population.

## COURSE AND PROGNOSIS

It is important to establish the diagnosis in order to do genetic counseling and to follow patients for development of malignancy. Also, neurofibromatosis support groups help with social adjustment in severely affected persons.

There is variable involvement of the organs affected over time, from only a few pigmented macules to marked disfigurement with thousands of nodules, segmental hypertrophy, and plexiform neuromas. The mortality rate is higher than in the normal population, principally because of the development of neurofibrosarcoma during adult life. Other serious complications are relatively infrequent.

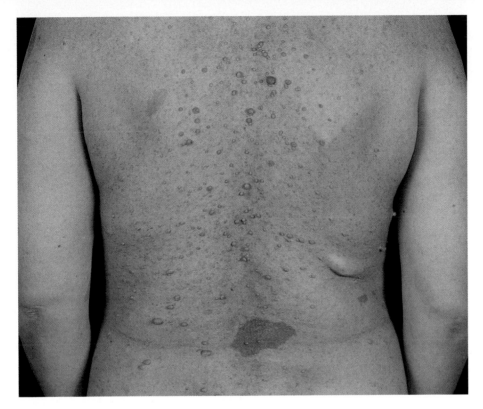

**FIGURE 15-29 Neurofibromatosis (NF1)** *Skin-colored and pink-tan, soft papules and nodules on the back are neurofibromas. The lesions first appeared during late childhood. Two large café au lait macules on the back. The large, soft, ill-defined, subcutaneous nodule on the right lower back and on the right posterior axillary line are plexiform neuromas.*

## MANAGEMENT

An orthopedic physician should manage the two major bone problems: kyphoscoliosis and tibial bowing. A plastic surgeon can do reconstructive surgery on the facial asymmetry. The language disorders and learning disabilities should be evaluated by a psychologist. Close follow-up annually should be mandatory to detect sarcomas that may arise within plexiform neuromas. Surgical removal of pheochromocytoma.

Support group: *http://www.support-group.com*

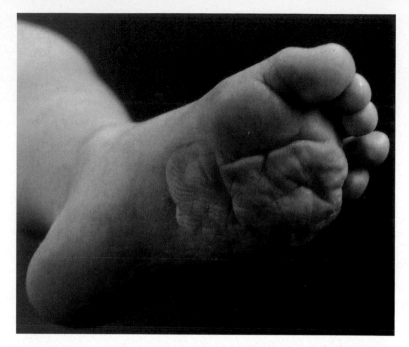

**FIGURE 15-30   Neurofibromatosis (NF1)**   *Plexiform neuroma on the sole of the foot of a child. This ill-defined subcutaneous mass is soft and asymptomatic. The patient has café au lait macules and multiple neurofibromas.*

## HEREDITARY HEMORRHAGIC TELANGIECTASIA

Hereditary hemorrhagic telangiectasia is an autosomal dominant condition affecting blood vessels, especially in the mucous membranes of the mouth and the GI tract. The disease is frequently heralded by recurrent epistaxis that appears often in childhood. The diagnostic lesions are small, pulsating, macular and papular, usually punctate, telangiectases (Fig. 15-31) on the lips, tongue, face, palms/soles, fingers/toes, nail beds, tongue, conjunctivae, nasopharynx, and throughout the GI and genitourinary tracts. In the 18-year-old male, shown in Fig. 15-31A, there had been repeated epistaxis, but the telangiectasias had gone unnoticed until the patient was evaluated for anemia. Careful history then revealed that the patient's father had a minor form of the same condition. Pulmonary arteriovenous fistulas may occur. Chronic blood loss results in anemia. Electrocautery and pulse dye laser are used to destroy cutaneous and accessible mucosal lesions. Estrogens have been used to treat recalcitrant bleeding.
*Synonym*: Osler-Weber-Rendu syndrome.

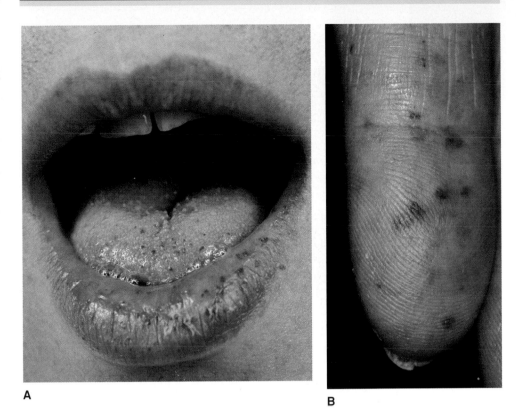

A

B

**FIGURE 15-31   Hereditary hemorrhagic telangiectasia**   *A. Multiple 1- to 2 mm, discrete, red macular and papular telangiectases on the lower lip and tongue. B. Multiple pinpoint telangiectases on the index finger of another patient. Using dermatoscopy or a glass slide the lesions can be shown to pulsate.*

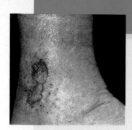

# SKIN SIGNS OF VASCULAR INSUFFICIENCY

## ATHEROSCLEROSIS, ATHEROEMBOLIZATION, AND ARTERIAL INSUFFICIENCY

Atherosclerosis obliterans (ASO), especially of the lower extremities, is associated with a spectrum of cutaneous findings, ranging from slowly progressive ischemic changes to the sudden appearance of ischemic lesions following atheroembolization. Atheroembolism is the phenomenon of dislodgment of atheromatous debris from an affected artery or aneurysm with centrifugal microembolization and resultant ischemic and infarctive cutaneous lesions.

### EPIDEMIOLOGY

**Age of Onset**  Middle age to elderly.

**Sex**  Males > females.

**Incidence**  Atherosclerosis is the cause of 90% of arterial disease in developed countries, affecting 5% of men >50 years; 10% (20% of diabetics) of all men with atherosclerosis develop critical limb ischemia.

**Risk Factors for Atherosclerosis**  Cigarette smoking, hyperlipidemia, low high-density lipoprotein (HDL), high cholesterol, high low-density lipoprotein (LDL), hypertension, diabetes mellitus, hyperinsulinemia, abdominal obesity, family history of premature ischemic heart disease, personal history of cerebrovascular disease or occlusive peripheral vascular disease.

**Diabetes Mellitus and Lower Leg Ischemia**  Gangrene of lower extremities is estimated to be up to 8 to 150 times more frequent in diabetic than in nondiabetic individuals, most often occurring in those who smoke.

### PATHOGENESIS

Atherosclerosis is the most common cause of arterial insufficiency and may be generalized or localized to the coronary arteries, aortic arch vessels to the head and neck, or those supplying the lower extremities, i.e., femoral, popliteal, anterior and posterior tibial arteries. Atheromatous narrowing of arteries supplying the upper extremities is much less common. Atheromatous deposits and thromboses occur commonly in the femoral artery in Hunter's canal and in the popliteal artery just above the knee joint. The posterior tibial artery is most often occluded where it rounds the internal malleolus, the anterior tibial artery where it is superficial and becomes the dorsalis pedis artery. Atheromatous material in the abdominal or iliac arteries can also diminish blood flow to the lower extremities as well as break off and embolize downstream to the lower extremities (atheroembolization). Detection of atherosclerosis is often delayed until an ischemic event occurs, related to critical decrease in blood flow.

In addition to large-vessel arterial obstruction, individuals with diabetes mellitus often have microvasculopathy associated with endothelial cell proliferation and basement membrane thickening of arterioles, venules, and capillaries.

**Atheroembolism**  Multiple small deposits of fibrin, platelet, and cholesterol debris embolize from proximal atherosclerotic lesions or aneurysmal sites. Occurs spontaneously or after intravascular surgery or procedures such as arteriography, fibrinolysis, or anticoagulation. Emboli tend to lodge in small vessels of skin and muscle and usually do not occlude large vessels.

### HISTORY

**Symptoms**  *Atherosclerosis of Lower Extremity Arteries*  Pain on exercise, i.e., *intermittent claudication*. With progressive arterial insuffi-

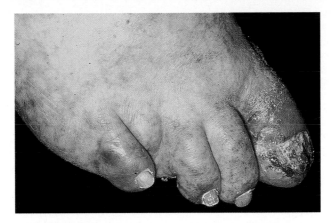

**FIGURE 16-1   Atherosclerosis obliterans with ischemic skin changes**   *The great toe shows ischemic and preinfarctive changes and early ulceration. The forefoot is white; there is mottled, livedoid erythema distally and livid erythema on the tips of the toes. The fourth digit had been amputated previously because of gangrene. In this 68-year-old diabetic woman, the iliac artery was occluded.*

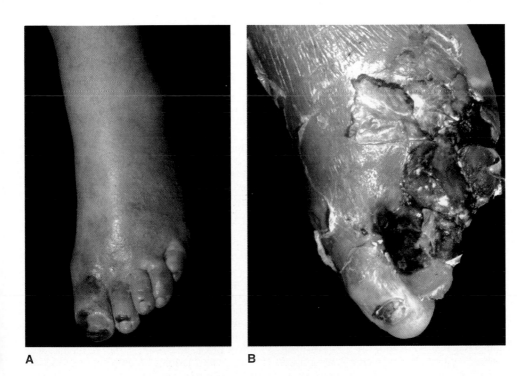

A                                                                                     B

**FIGURE 16-2   Atherosclerosis obliterans**   *A. There is pallor of the forefoot and mottled erythema distally with incipient gangrene on the great toe and the second digit. This is a female diabetic with partial occlusion of the femoral artery. The patient was a smoker. B. More advanced gangrene of the second to the fifth toe, the great toe is ebony white and will also turn black.*

ciency, pain and/or paresthesias at rest occur in leg and/or foot, especially at night. Individuals with arterial insufficiency of the lower extremities often have symptoms of ischemic heart disease (coronary artery disease or arteriosclerotic heart disease), diabetes mellitus.

*Atheroembolism* Acute pain and tenderness at site of embolization. "Blue toe," "purple toe" syndrome: peripheral ischemia, livedo reticularis of sudden onset may be accompanied by embolization to kidney, pancreas, muscle, etc.

## PHYSICAL EXAMINATION

### Atherosclerosis/Arterial Insufficiency

**Skin Lesions**   General findings associated with ischemia include pallor, cyanosis, livedoid vascular pattern (Fig. 16-1), loss of hair on affected limb. Earliest infarctive changes include well-demarcated maplike areas of epidermal necrosis. Later, dry black gangrene may occur over the infarcted skin (purple cyanosis → white pallor → black gangrene) (Fig. 16-2). With shedding of slough, well-demarcated ulcers with underlying structures such as tendons can be seen.

**General Examination**   *Pulses* Pulse of large vessels usually diminished or absent. In diabetics with mainly microangiopathy, gangrene may occur in the setting of adequate pulses. Temperature of foot: cool to cold.

*Buerger's Sign* With significant reduction in arterial blood flow, limb elevation causes pallor (best noted on plantar foot); dependency causes delayed and exaggerated hyperemia. Auscultation over stenotic arteries reveals bruits.

*Pain* Ischemic ulcers are painful; in diabetics with neuropathy and ischemic ulcers, pain may be minimal or absent.

*Distribution* Ischemic ulcers may first appear between toes at sites of pressure and beginning on fissures on plantar heel. Dry gangrene of feet, starting at the toes or at pressure sites (Fig. 16-2).

### Atheroembolization

**Skin Lesions**   Violaceous livedo reticularis on legs, feet, but also as high up as buttocks. Ischemic changes with poor return of color after compression of skin. "Blue toe" (Fig. 16-3): indurated, painful plaques often following livedo reticularis on calves and thighs that may undergo necrosis (Fig. 16-4), become black and crusted, and ulcerate. Cyanosis and gangrene of digits.

**General Examination**   *Pulses* Distal pulses may remain intact.

## LABORATORY EXAMINATIONS

**Hematology**   Rule out anemia, polycythemia.

**Lipid Studies**   Hypercholesterolemia (>240 mg/dL), often associated with rise in LDL. Hypertriglyceridemia (250 mg/dL), often associated with rise in very low-density lipoproteins (VLDLs) and remnants of their catabolism (mainly intermediate-density lipoprotein, IDL).

**Dermatopathology of Atheroembolism**   Deep skin and muscle biopsy specimen shows arterioles occluded by fibrosis with multinucleated giant cells surrounding biconvex, needle-shaped clefts corresponding to cholesterol crystal microemboli.

**Doppler Studies**   Show reduced or interrupted blood flow.

**Digital Plethysmography**   With exercise can unmask significant atherosclerotic involvement of lower extremity arteries.

**X-Ray**   Calcification can be demonstrated intramurally.

**Arteriography**   Atherosclerosis is best visualized by angiography. Ulceration of atheromatous plaques seen in abdominal aorta or more distally.

## DIAGNOSIS AND DIFFERENTIAL DIAGNOSIS

Clinical suspicion confirmed by arteriography and deep skin biopsy (atheroembolism).

**Differential Diagnosis**   *Intermittent Claudication* Pseudoxanthoma elasticum, Buerger's disease (thromboangiitis obliterans), arthritis, gout.

*Painful Foot* Gout, interdigital neuroma, flat feet, calcanean bursitis, plantar fasciitis, rupture of plantar muscle.

*Ischemic and Infarctive Lesions of Leg/Foot* Vasculitis, Raynaud's phenomenon (vasospasm), disseminated intravascular coagulation, cryoglobulinemia, hyperviscosity syndrome (macroglobulinemia), septic embolization (infective endocarditis), nonseptic embolization (ventricular mural thrombus with myocardial infarction, atrial thrombus with atrial fibrillation), aneurysms (dissecting, thrombosed), drug-induced necrosis (warfarin, heparin), ergot poisoning, intraarterial injection, livedo reticularis syndromes, external compression (popliteal entrapment).

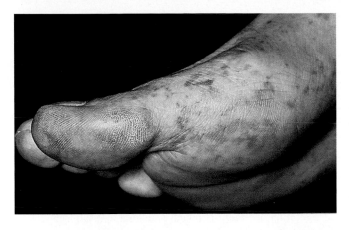

**FIGURE 16-3   Atheroembolism after angiography**   *A mottled ("blue toe"), violaceous, vascular pattern on the forefoot and great toe. The findings were noted after intravascular catheterization and angiography in an individual with ASO.*

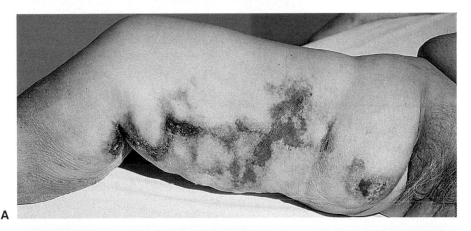

A

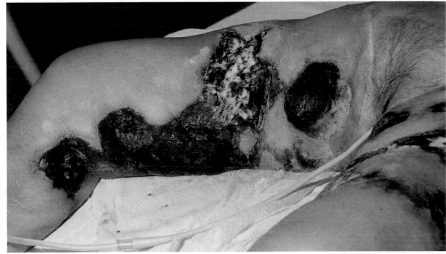

B

**FIGURE 16-4   Atheroembolism with cutaneous infarction**   *A. Violaceous discoloration and cutaneous infarctions with a linear arrangement on the medial thigh of a 73-year-old woman with atherosclerosis, heart failure, and diabetes. B. Within 48 h the initial changes progressed to become far more extensive with large areas of infarction and necrosis.*

## COURSE AND PROGNOSIS

*Arterial insufficiency* is a slowly progressive disease, punctuated by episodes of complete occlusion or embolism. Approximately 5% per year of individuals with intermittent claudication progress to pain at rest or gangrene. A much higher percentage die from other complications of atherosclerosis such as ischemic heart disease.

Infection from interdigital tinea pedis, leg/foot ulcers, or small breaks and fissures in the skin. Chronic lymphedema, prior saphenous venous harvesting, and prior episodes of cellulitis increase the likelihood of cellulitis.

Atherosclerosis of coronary and carotid arteries usually determines survival of patient, but involvement of lower extremity arteries causes significant morbidity. Balloon angioplasty, endarterectomy, and bypass procedure have improved prognosis of patients with atherosclerosis. Amputation rates have been lowered from 80% to <40% by aggressive vascular surgery. *Atheroembolism* may be a single episode if atheroembolization follows intraarterial procedure. May be recurrent if spontaneous and associated with significant tissue necrosis.

## MANAGEMENT

**Prevention**   Goal of management is prevention of atherosclerosis.

*Diet* First step in management of primary hyperlipidemia: Reduce intake of saturated fats and cholesterol as well as calories.

*Exercise* Useful adjunct to diet. Walking increases new collateral vessels in ischemic muscle.

*Hypertension* Reduce elevated blood pressure.

*Cigarette Smoking* Discontinue.

*Blood* Correct anemia or polycythemia.

*Drug Therapy* Recommended for adults with LDL cholesterol >190 mg/dL or >160 mg/dL in the presence of two or more risk factors after an adequate trial of at least 3 months of diet therapy alone.

**Intermittent Claudication**   *Medical Management* Encourage walking to create new collateral vessels.

*Surgical Management* Endarterectomy or bypass for aortic iliac occlusions and for extensive femoral popliteal disease.

**Ischemia/Infarction of Foot/Leg**   *Positioning of Ischemic Foot* As low as possible without edema.

*Medical Management* Heparin and warfarin. IV prostacyclins. Analgesics.

*Surgical Management* Distal bypass surgery of crural arteries. Response to surgical revascularization or thrombolytic therapy often poor in atheroembolization. Debridement of necrotic tissue locally. Remove or bypass atherosclerotic vessel or aneurysm. Amputation of leg/foot: indicated when medical and surgical management has failed.

**FIGURE 16-5 (Opposite page, left)   Superficial phlebitis**   *A linear painful erythematous cord extending from the popliteal fossa to the mid-calf in a 35-year-old man who had moderate varicosities. Phlebitis occurred after a 15-h flight.*

**FIGURE 16-6 (Opposite page, right)   Deep venous thrombosis**   *The leg is swollen, pale, with a blotchy cyanotic discoloration, and is painful. The episode occurred after abdominal surgery (the circular marks are from a compression bandage).*

# THROMBOPHLEBITIS AND DEEP VENOUS THROMBOSIS

Superficial phlebitis is an inflammatory thrombosis of a superficial *normal* vein, usually due to infection or trauma from needles and catheters, or of a *varicose* vein usually in the context of the chronic venous insufficiency (CVI) syndrome. Deep venous thrombosis (DVT) is due to thrombotic obstruction of a vein with or without an inflammatory response and occurs due to slow blood flow, hypercoagulability, or changes in the venous walls. The most common causes are shown in Table 16-1

## ETIOLOGY AND PATHOGENESIS

The thrombus originates in an area of low venous flow. An occlusion of a vein by thrombus imposes a block to venous return, which leads to increased venous pressure and edema in the distal limb. An inflammatory response to the thrombus causes pain and tenderness. If the venous pressure is too high, arterial limb flow may rarely be compromised and ischemia of the distal limb may occur. The thrombus in the vein often has a free-floating tail, which may break off to produce a pulmonary embolus. Organization of the thrombus in the vein destroys the venous walls, and this leads to postthrombotic syndrome.

## HISTORY

Patients complain of pain or aching in the involved limb or notice limb swelling. Some patients may have no symptoms. Pulmonary embolus may be the first indication of DVT.

## CLINICAL MANIFESTATIONS

Superficial thrombophlebitis is diagnosed by the characteristic induration of a superficial vein with

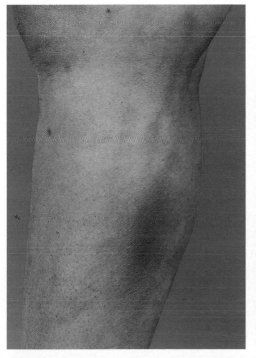

**FIGURE 16-5**

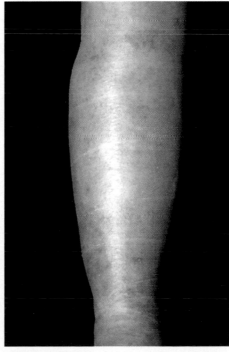

**FIGURE 16-6**

redness, tenderness, and increased heat (Fig. 16-5). DVT presents with a swollen, warm, tender limb (Fig. 16-6) with prominent distended collateral veins. Pitting edema may occur but is not always present, and a tender cord may be felt where the vein is thrombosed. With iliofemoral thrombophlebitis the limb is swollen from the foot to the inguinal region and tenderness is not present in the limb, but collateral veins may form from the thigh to the abdominal wall. Two types are recognized: the limb may be very pale and painful (*phlegmasia alba dolens*) or may be cyanotic and painful with cold digits if the arterial inflow is compromised (*phlegmasia coerulea dolens*). In thrombosis of calf veins the calf and foot are swollen and warm, and there is deep tenderness of the calf, often without a palpable cord (Fig. 16-6).

*Migratory phlebitis* describes an inflammatory induration of superficial veins that migrates within a defined region of the body; may be associated with thromboangiitis obliterans and malignancies. *Mondor's disease* is an indurated, subcutaneous vein from the breast to the axillary region that during healing leads to a shortening of the venous cord, which puckers the skin.

## LABORATORY EXAMINATIONS

Venous imaging by color-coded duplex ultrasound and Doppler examination reveals an absence of flow or of the normal respiratory venous flow variations in proximal venous occlusions. For thrombophlebitis of the calf veins, intravenous [$^{125}$I] fibrinogen or a venogram gives a definite diagnosis.

## DIFFERENTIAL DIAGNOSIS

Lymphedema, cellulitis, erysipelas, superficial phlebitis, lymphangitis. An uncommon differential diagnosis is rupture of the plantar muscle, which produces pain, swelling, and ecchymotic areas in the dependent ankle area.

## MANAGEMENT

The treatment of DVT is anticoagulation. IV heparin at a loading dose of 5000 U and approximately 1000 U/h thereafter. The partial thromboplastin time (PTT) should be 1.5 to 2 times normal. Low-molecular-weight heparin is also effective. Warfarin can be started orally at the same time and should overlap heparin for 5 days until the necessary factors for blood clotting are depressed. Patients should be treated for at least 3 months with anticoagulation. Elastic stockings and compression are mandatory and should be worn for at least 3 months; ambulation should be started as soon as symptoms subside.

---

### TABLE 16-1   Predisposing Factors in Deep Venous Thrombosis

**Common Factors**

| | |
|---|---|
| Major surgery | Oral contraceptives |
| Fractures | Malignancies |
| Congestive heart failure | Venous varicosities |
| Acute myocardial infarction | Previous history of venous thrombosis |
| Stroke | Leiden factor 5 mutation |
| Pregnancy and postpartum | Severe pulmonary insufficiency |
| Spinal cord injuries | Prolonged immobilization |
| Shock | |

**Less Common Factors**

| | |
|---|---|
| Sickle cell anemia | Antithrombin III deficiency |
| Homocystinuria | Antiphospholipid antibodies |
| Protein C or S deficiency | Ulcerative colitis |

SOURCE: TD Coffman, RT Eberhardt, in IM Freedberg, AZ Eisen, K Wolff, KF Austen, LA Goldsmith, SI Katz (eds): *Fitzpatrick's Dermatology in General Medicine*, 6th ed. New York, McGraw-Hill, 2003.

# CHRONIC VENOUS INSUFFICIENCY ■ ◑

Chronic venous insufficiency (CVI) results from failure of return of venous blood and increased capillary pressure; the resultant changes include edema, stasis dermatitis, hyperpigmentation, fibrosis of the skin and subcutaneous tissue (lipodermatosclerosis) of the leg, and ulceration.

## EPIDEMIOLOGY AND ETIOLOGY

Varicose veins: peak incidence of onset 30 to 40 years. Varicose veins are three times more common in women than in men.

**Etiology** CVI is most commonly associated with varicose veins and the postphlebitic syndrome. Varicose veins are an inherited characteristic.

**Aggravating Factors** Pregnancy, increased blood volume, increased cardiac output, increased venocaval pressure, progesterone.

## PATHOGENESIS

The damaged valves of the deep veins of the calf are incompetent at restricting backflow of blood. Damaged communicating veins connecting deep and superficial calf veins also cause CVI in that blood flows from deep veins to superficial venous plexus. Fibrin is deposited in the extravascular space and undergoes organization, resulting in sclerosis and obliteration of lymphatics and microvasculature. Perivascular fibrosis results in diminished nutrition of the epidermis, which breaks down with ulcer formation.

This cycle repeats itself: initial event → aggravation of venous stasis and varicose vein dilatation → lipodermatosclerosis → thrombosis → stasis dermatitis → ulceration.

## HISTORY

Prior episode(s) of superficial phlebitis and DVT. Risk factors are listed in Table 16-1.

CVI commonly associated with heaviness or aching of leg, which is aggravated by standing (dependency) and relieved by walking. Lipodermatosclerosis may limit movement of ankle and cause pain and limitation of movement, which in turn increases stasis. Leg edema aggravated by dependency (end of the day, standing), summer season. Shoes feel tight in the evening. Night cramps.

## PHYSICAL EXAMINATION

A simple staging system for CVI is shown in Table 16-2. Superficial leg veins are enlarged, tortuous, with incompetent valves; best evaluated with the patient standing (Fig. 16-7).

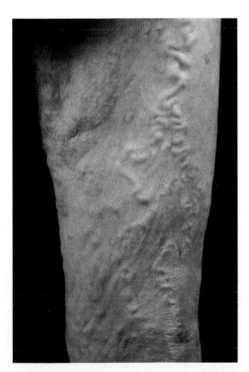

**FIGURE 16-7   Varicose veins**   *There are meandering irregular varicose veins on the thigh of a 70-year-old man who also had varicosities, lipodermatosclerosis, and venous ulcers in the lower legs.*

"Blow-out" at sites of incompetent communicating veins. Tourniquet test: A tourniquet is applied to the leg that has been elevated to empty the veins; when the patient stands up and the tourniquet is released, there is instant filling of a varicose vein due to absent or ill-functioning valves.

### Skin Lesions

**Edema**   Dependent; improved or resolved in the morning after a night in the horizontal position. Dorsa of feet, ankles, lower legs.

**Eczematous (Stasis) Dermatitis**   Occurs in setting of CVI about the lower legs and ankles (Fig. 16-8). It is a classic eczematous dermatitis with inflammatory papules, scaly and crusted erosions; in addition, there is pigmentation, stippled with recent and old hemorrhages (Fig. 16-9); dermal sclerosis; and excoriations due to scratching. It must be distinguished from contact dermatitis secondary to topical agents, with which it is often combined. In addition, there may be concomitant irritant dermatitis due to secretion from stasis ulcer (see below) and bacterial colonization. If extensive, may be associated with generalized eczematous dermatitis, i.e., "id" reaction or autosensitization (see Section 2).

**Atrophie Blanche**   Small ivory-white depressed plaques (Fig. 16-9) on the ankle and/or foot; stellate and irregular, coalescing; stippled pigmentation; hemosiderin-pigmented border, usually within stasis dermatitis. Often following trauma.

**Lipodermatosclerosis**   Inflammation, induration, pigmentation of lower third of leg creating "champagne bottle" or "piano leg" appearance with edema above and below the sclerotic region (Fig. 16-10). "Groove sign" created by varicose veins meandering through sclerotic tissue. A verrucous epidermal change can occur overlying the sclerosis; if it is combined with chronic lymphedema, it is referred to as *elephantiasis nostras verrucosa*. In long-standing sclerosis, calcification can occur.

**Ulceration**   Occurs in 30% of cases; very painful "hyperalgesic micro-ulcer" in area of atrophie blanche (Fig. 16-9); larger superficial or deep ulcers, sharply defined with deep margin, necrotic base surrounded by atrophie blanche, stasis dermatitis, and lipodermatosclerosis (Fig. 16-11). Venous ulcers usually occur medially and above ankles (Fig. 16-11). Venous ulcers and their differential diagnosis are discussed in more detail below (p. 480).

## LABORATORY EXAMINATIONS

**Doppler and Color-Coded Duplex Sonography**   These detect incompetent veins, venous occlusion due to thrombus.

**Phlebography**   Contrast medium is injected into veins to detect incompetent veins and venous occlusion.

**Imaging**   X-ray may show subcutaneous calcification (10% of chronic cases), i.e., postphlebitic subcutaneous calcinosis. Bony changes include periostitis underlying ulceration, osteoporosis as a result of disuse, fibrous ankylosis of ankle. Osteomyelitis.

**Dermatopathology**   *Early*: small venules and lymphatic spaces appear dilated; edema of extracellular space with swelling and separation of collagen bundles. *Subsequently*: capillaries dilated, congested with tuft formation and tortuousity of venules; deposition of fibrin. *Endothelial cell hypertrophy*: may be associated with venous thrombosis; angioendotheliomatous proliferation mimicking Kaposi's sarcoma. In all stages, extravasation of red blood cells that break down forming hemosiderin, which is taken up by macrophages. Lymphatic vessels become encased in a fibrotic stroma, i.e., lipodermatosclerosis. Calcification of fat and fibrous tissue may occur.

## DIAGNOSIS

Usually made on history, clinical findings, Doppler and color-coded Duplex sonography, phlebography.

---

#### TABLE 16-2   Staging of CVI (According to Widmer)

| | |
|---|---|
| I | Edema, subfascial congestion, ankle flare (phlebectasia around ankle) |
| II | Lipodermatosclerosis, pigmentation, stasis dermatitis, atrophie blanche |
| III | All of the above plus ulcers, scars |

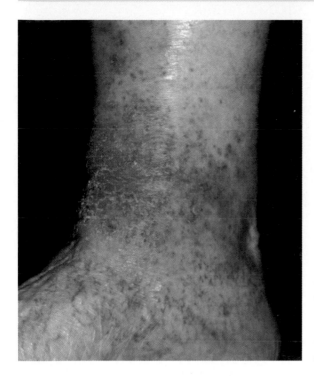

**FIGURE 16-8   Stasis dermatitis in CVI**   *A patch of eczematous dermatitis overlying venous varicosities on the medial ankle in a 59-year-old woman. The lesion is papular, scaly, and itching.*

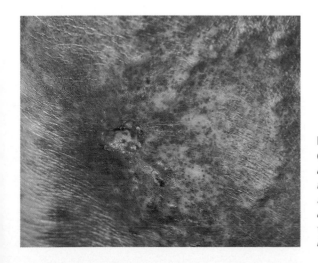

**FIGURE 16-9   Chronic venous insufficiency**   *Small varicose veins meandering through an area of diffuse and mottled pigmentation due to hemosiderin and ivory-white patches of atrophie blanche and a small ulcer with a necrotic base. Such lesions are both itchy and painful.*

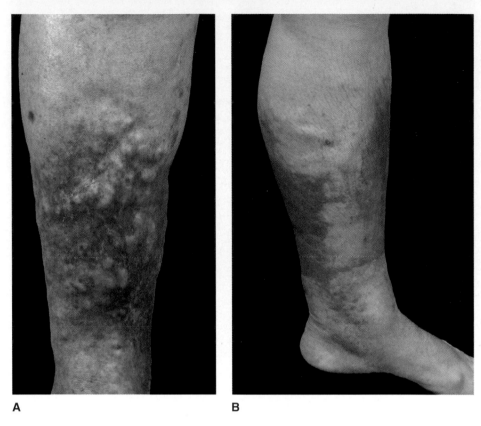

A                                    B

**FIGURE 16-10   Chronic venous insufficiency and lipodermatosclerosis**   *The ankle is relatively thin and the upper calf edematous, creating a "champagne bottle" or "piano leg" appearance.*
***A.*** *Varicose veins are embedded in pigmented, sclerotic tissue. There are also areas of atrophie blanche.* ***B.*** *Varicose veins are less visible here but can be easily palpated in the sclerotic plaque encasing the entire calf ("groove" sign). There is also pigmentation and minor papular stasis dermatitis.*

## MANAGEMENT

**Prerequisite**   Compression dressings or stockings.
**Atrophie Blanche**   Avoid trauma to area involved. Intralesional triamcinolone into painful lesions. Compression.
**Varicose Veins** *Injection Sclerotherapy* A sclerosing agent such as tetradecyl sulfate is injected into varicosities, followed by prolonged compression. Used mainly to treat minor branch varicosities not associated with saphenous incompetence and new branch vein varicosities developing after surgery. Recurrence is common within 5 years.

*Vascular Surgery* Incompetent perforating veins are identified, ligated, and cut, followed by stripping long and/or short saphenous veins out of the main trunk. Residual perforating veins are the main cause of recurrences after surgery. In patients with combined arterial and CVI, bypass or angioplasty may prove beneficial.
**Endovascular Techniques**   These new technologies encompass endoscopic subfascial dissection of perforating veins (employed primarily in the elimination of insufficient perforating veins in CVI); and endoscopic endovenous diode laser or radiofrequency thermal heating, which leads to occlusion of varicose vein.

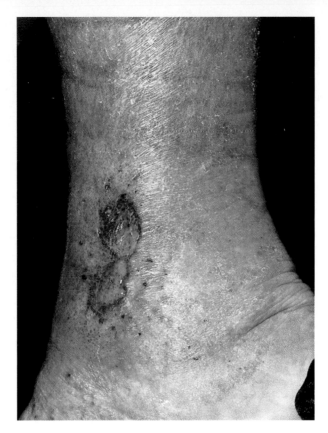

**FIGURE 16-11 Venous insufficiency** *Two coalescing ulcers with a necrotic base in an area of atrophie blanche, lipodermatosclerosis, and stasis dermatitis. Scratch marks indicate itchiness of surrounding skin, while the ulcers are painful.*

## MOST COMMON LEG/FOOT ULCERS ■ ◑

Leg ulcers occur relatively commonly in late middle and old age, arising in association with CVI, chronic arterial insufficiency, or peripheral sensory neuropathy; in some patients, a combination of these factors. Leg ulcers are common. An estimated 2½ million persons in the United States have leg ulcers, with an estimated loss of 2 million workdays per year. Leg ulcers are associated with significant long-term morbidity and often do not heal unless the underlying problem(s) is corrected.

**Venous Ulcers**  The prevalence of venous ulcers is estimated to be approximately 1%. It rises with patient age, obesity, previous leg injury (fractures), DVT, and phlebitis. Patients complain of limb heaviness, swelling associated with standing and worsening in the evening, and pain. Venous ulcers are associated with at least one or all of the symptoms of CVI (Fig. 16-11 and Table 16-2) and may be single or multiple; they are commonly found on the medial lower aspect of the calf, especially over the malleolus (medial > lateral), in the area supplied by incompetent perforating veins (Fig. 16-11). They can be large, involving the circumference of the entire lower leg. They are sharply defined, irregularly shaped, relatively shallow with a sloping border, and usually painful. The base is usually covered by fibrin and necrotic material (Fig. 16-11), and there is always secondary bacterial colonization. Stasis ulcers can also develop in the most dependent parts of a pendulous abdominal panniculus in a massively obese individual. Squamous cell carcinoma (SCC) can arise in a longstanding venous ulcer (Fig. 16-12) of the leg.

**Arterial Ulcers**  Arterial ulcers are associated with peripheral arterial disease (atherosclerosis obliterans, see p. 468), which has an age-adjusted prevalence of 12%. Associated with intermittent claudication and pain, even at rest, as disease progresses. Characteristically painful at night and often quite severe; may be worse when legs are elevated, improving on dependency. They occur on the lower leg, usually over sites of pressure and trauma: pretibial, supramalleolar (usually lateral), and at distant points, such as toes. These ulcers are painful. Punched out, with sharply demarcated borders (Fig. 16-13). A tissue slough is often present at the base, under which tendons can be seen. Exudation minimal. Associated findings of ischemia: loss of hair on feet and lower legs, shiny atrophic skin. Stasis pigmentation and lipodermatosclerosis are absent. Pulses diminished or absent.

A special type of arterial ulcer is *Martorell's ulcer*, which is associated with labile hypertension and lacks signs of atherosclerosis obliterans. Ulcer(s) start with a black eschar surrounded by erythema and after sloughing of necrotic tissue are punched out with sharply demarcated borders, with surrounding erythema; very painful on the anterior lateral lower leg

**Combined Arterial and Venous Ulcers**  These ulcers arise in patients who have both CVI and atherosclerosis obliterans and thus show a combination of signs and symptoms of both venous and arterial insufficiency and ulceration (Fig. 16-14). Symptoms include intermittent claudication, pain both at elevated and dependent position of the leg, both pallor and cyanosis of the foot, stasis dermatitis, and lipodermatosclerosis associated with both sloped and punched out ulcers reaching down to tendons (Fig. 16-14).

**Neuropathic Ulcers**  Soles, toes, heel. Most commonly associated with diabetes of many years' duration. Early symptoms of neuropathy include paresthesia, pain, anesthesia of leg and foot. Patients are often unaware of prior trauma that commonly precedes ulcerations of heel, plantar metatarsal area, or great toe. Neuropathic ulcers are discussed in Section 15 (see Fig. 15-3).

### DIFFERENTIAL DIAGNOSIS

A differential diagnosis of the three main types of leg/foot ulcers is shown in Table 16-3. Other differential diagnostic considerations include ulcerated SCC (note that SCC can arise in a longstanding venous ulcer) (Fig. 16-12), basal cell carcinoma, injection drug use (skin popping), pressure ulcer (ski boot). Ulcerations also occur in vasculitis (particularly polyarteritis nodosa), erythema induratum, calciphylaxis, and various infections [ecthyma, Buruli ulcer, *Mycobacterium marinum* infection, gumma, leprosy, invasive fungal infection, chronic herpes simplex virus (HSV) ulcer] and in sickle cell anemia, polycythemia vera, pyoderma

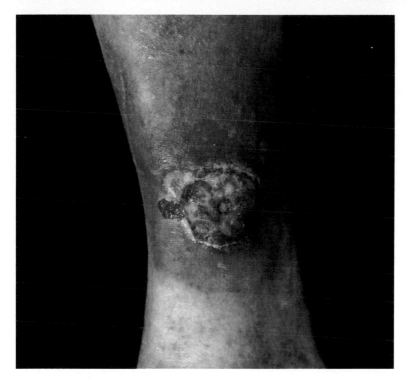

**FIGURE 16-12  Squamous cell carcinoma in chronic venous ulcer**  *A venous ulcer had been present >10 years in an area of lipodermatosclerosis and stasis dermatitis. Eventually the base of the ulcer became elevated, hard, less painful. Deep biopsy (circular mark in the center) revealed necrosis and at the base invasive squamous cell carcinoma.*

**TABLE 16-3    Differential Diagnosis of Three Major Types of Leg Ulcers**

|  | Lesion | Site | Surrounding Skin | General Examination |
|---|---|---|---|---|
| Venous | Irregular<br>Sloped borders<br>Necrotic base<br>Fibrin | Malleolar and<br>supramalleolar<br>(medial) | Lipodermatosclerosis<br>Stasis dermatitis<br>Atrophie blanche<br>Pigmentation<br>Lymphedema | Varicose veins<br>Pain, worse in<br>  dependent state |
| Arterial | Punched out<br>Necrotic base | Pressure sites:<br>distal (toes),<br>pretibial,<br>supramalleolar<br>(lateral) | Atrophic, shiny<br>Hair loss<br>Pallor or reactive<br>  hyperemia | Weak/absent pulses<br>Pallor on elevation<br>  of leg<br>Pain worse on<br>  elevation of leg |
| Neuropathic | Punched out | Pressure sites<br>Plantar | Callus before<br>  ulceration and<br>  surrounding ulcer | Peripheral neuropathy<br>Decreased sensation<br>No pain |

gangrenosum, necrobiosis lipoidica with ulceration, factitia.

## COURSE AND PROGNOSIS

Course and prognosis are dependent on underlying disease. With correction of underlying causes, ulcers heal with initial formation of pink granulation tissue at the base, which is re-epithelialized by epithelium from either residual skin appendages or surrounding epidermis. Venous ulcers can heal with a pseudoepitheliomatous epidermal hyperplasia within the scar, which can mimic SSC.

## MANAGEMENT

**General Management**   In general, factors such as anemia and malnutrition should be corrected to facilitate healing. Control hypertension, weight reduction in the obese, exercise; mobilize patient; correct edema caused by cardiac, renal, or hepatic dysfunction. Of utmost importance is treatment of underlying disease. Arterial ulcers do not heal unless arterial blood flow is corrected by endarterectomy to remove localized atheromatous plaques or bypass of occluded areas (see "Management" of atherosclerosis

obliterans, p. 472). Arterial ulcers at acral sites that do not heal despite arterial reconstruction or where arterial reconstruction cannot be performed may require amputation. Venous ulcers tend to be recurrent unless underlying risk factors are corrected, i.e., corrective surgery and/or elastic stockings worn on a daily basis (see "Management" of chronic venous insufficiency, p. 478). Beware of excess compression in patients with additional underlying arterial occlusion; leg elevation; intermittent pneumatic compression. In neuropathic ulcers, underlying diabetes has to be corrected. Rule out or treat underlying osteomyelitis. Distribute weight of pressure points with special shoes in neuropathic ulcers. *Note:* diabetic patients are particularly predisposed to ulcers and frequently have several etiologic factors in play, i.e., peripheral vascular disease, neuropathy, infection, and impaired healing.

Secondary infection should be treated with antibiotics both topically and systemically in all ulcers. Ulcers provide an easy portal of entry for systemic infection, which should be suspected if pain appears or increases in intensity. Infection can occur relatively superficially in ulcer base or more invasively with cellulitis and possible lymphangitis and bacteremia.

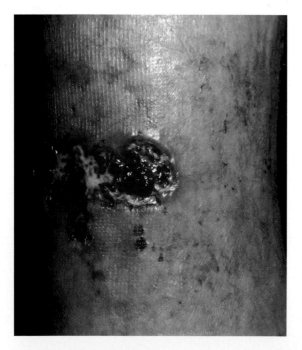

**FIGURE 16-13   Chronic arterial insufficiency with a sharply defined, "punched out" ulcer with irregular outlines**.   *The extremity was pulseless, and there was massive ischemia on the toes.*

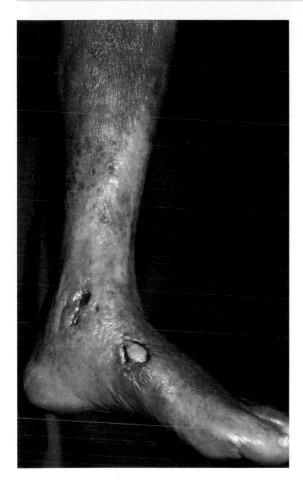

**FIGURE 16-14   Chronic arterial and venous insufficiency, "combined" arterial and venous ulcers** *Note pronounced lipodermatosclerosis and ulceration on the supramalleolar lower leg (venous component) and purple discoloration of forefoot and toes with punched-out ulcer revealing tendon over metatarsal site (arterial component).*

### Local Treatment of Ulcer and Surrounding Skin

Treat stasis dermatitis (or irritant, or allergic contact dermatitis) in CVI with wet dressings in the acute exudative phase and subsequently with moderate to potent glucocorticoid ointment. In all ulcers debride necrotic material mechanically (surgically) or by enzymatic debriding agents, including collagenase and papain; use antiseptics and antibiotics to counteract infection. Granulating but only slowly epithelializing ulcers are treated by surgical procedures either by pinch grafts, split-thickness skin grafts, epidermal grafts, cultured keratinocyte allografts, or composite grafts.

## LIVEDOID VASCULITIS

Livedoid vasculitis is a thrombotic vasculopathy of dermal vessels confined to the lower extremities and starting mostly in the ankle region. It is characterized by a triad of livedo reticularis, atrophie blanche, and very painful, small punched-out ulcers that have a very poor tendency for healing (Fig. 16-15). Atrophie blanche in livedoid vasculitis is clinically indistinguishable from that seen in CVI, except for varicose veins (compare Figs. 16-15 and 16-9). It is a reaction pattern of the skin that often recurs in winter or summer ("livedo reticularis with winter and summer ulcerations"). Histologically, it is characterized by fibrin thrombi in small- and medium-sized dermal veins and arteries with wedge-shaped necrosis and hyalinization of the vessel walls (segmental hyalinizing vasculitis). Livedoid vasculitis may be idiopathic or may be associated with Sneddon's syndrome (see p. 383), antiphospholipid antibody syndrome, or conditions of hypercoagulability or hyperviscosity. Treatment consists of bed rest, analgesics, low-dose heparin, and platelet aggregation inhibitors. Pain can be relieved and healing accelerated by systemic glucocorticoids. Anabolic agents such as danazol and stanazolol have been anecdotally reported to be effective. Larger ulcers will have to be excised and grafted.

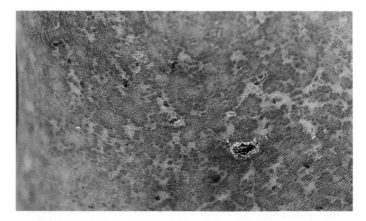

**FIGURE 16-15    Livedoid vasculitis**   *This is characterized by the triad of livedo reticularis, atrophie blanche and small, painful, crusted ulcers. This is clinically indistinguishable from atrophie blanche seen in CVI except for the absence of varicose veins.*

# PRESSURE ULCERS    ■  ◐ → ●

Pressure ulcers develop at body-support interfaces over bony prominences as a result of external compression of the skin, shear forces, and friction, which produce ischemic tissue necrosis. Pressure ulcers occur in patients who are obtunded mentally or have diminished sensation (as in spinal cord disease) in the affected region. Secondary infection results in localized cellulitis, which can extend locally into bone or muscle or into the bloodstream.
*Synonyms*: Pressure sore, bed sore, decubitus ulcer.

## EPIDEMIOLOGY

**Age of Onset**  Any age, but the greatest prevalence of pressure ulcers is in elderly, chronically bedridden patients.
**Sex**  Equally prevalent in both sexes.
**Prevalence**  Acute care hospital setting, 3 to 14%; long-term care settings, 15 to 25%; home-care settings, 7 to 12%; spinal cord units, 20 to 30%.

## PATHOGENESIS

Risk factors for developing pressure ulcers: inadequate nursing care, diminished sensation/immobility (obtunded mental status, spinal cord disease), hypotension, fecal or urinary incontinence, presence of fracture, hypoalbuminemia, and poor nutritional status. The mean skin capillary pressure is approximately 25 mmHg. External compression with pressures >30 mmHg occludes the blood vessels so that the surrounding tissues become anoxic and eventually necrotic. Amount of damage is proportional to extent and duration of pressure. Repositioning the patient every 1 or 2 h prevents the interface skin over a bony prominence from becoming ischemic, with subsequent ulcer formation. Secondary bacterial infection can enlarge the ulcer rapidly, extend to underlying structures (osteomyelitis), and invade the bloodstream, with bacteremia and septicemia. Infection also impairs or prevents healing.

## HISTORY

Ulcers often develop within the first 2 weeks of acute hospitalization and more rapidly if the patient experiences significant immobilization. Painful unless there is altered sensorium.

## PHYSICAL EXAMINATION

### Skin Lesions
***Clinical Categories of Pressure Ulcers*** Early change: localized erythema that blanches on pressure.

   Stage I: Nonblanching erythema of intact skin.
   Stage II: Necrosis, superficial or partial-thickness involving the epidermis and/or dermis. Bullae → necrosis of dermis (black) → shallow ulcer.
   Stage III: Deep necrosis, crateriform ulceration with full-thickness skin loss (Fig. 16-16); damage or necrosis can extend down to, but not through, fascia.
   Stage IV: Full-thickness necrosis (→ ulceration) with involvement of supporting structures such as muscle and bone (Fig. 16-17). May enlarge to many centimeters. May or may not be tender. Borders of ulcers may be undetermined.

Well-established pressure ulcers are widest at the base and taper to a cone shape at the level of skin. Ulcers with devitalized tissue at the base (eschar) have a higher chance of secondary infection. Purulent exudate and erythema surrounding the ulcer suggest infection. Foul odor suggests anaerobic infection.
***Distribution*** Occur over bony prominences: sacrum (60%) (Fig. 16-17) > ischial tuberosities, greater trochanter (Fig. 16-16), heel > elbow, knee, ankle, occiput.
**General Examination**  Fever, chills, or increased pain of ulcer suggests possible cellulitis or osteomyelitis.

## LABORATORY EXAMINATIONS

**Hematologic Studies** Elevated white blood cell count and erythrocyte sedimentation rate suggest infection (osteomyelitis or bacteremia).

**Wound Culture** Infection must be differentiated from colonization. Culture of the ulcer base detects only surface bacteria. Optimal culture technique: Deep portion of punch biopsy specimen obtained from the ulcer base is minced and cultured for aerobic and anaerobic bacteria. Most infections are polymicrobial and anaerobes may be present. Viral culture to rule out chronic herpes simplex virus ulcer.

**Blood Culture** Bacteremia often follows manipulation of ulcer (within 1 to 20 min of beginning the debridement); resolves within 30 to 60 min.

**Pathology** *Skin Biopsy* Epidermal necrosis with eccrine duct and gland necrosis. Deep ulcers show wedge-shaped infarcts of the subcutaneous tissue, obstruction of the capillaries with microthrombi, and endothelial cell swelling followed by endothelial cell necrosis and secondary inflammation.

***Bone Biopsy*** Essential for diagnosing continuous osteomyelitis; specimen is examined histologically and microbiologically.

**Imaging** It is difficult to distinguish osteomyelitis from chronic pressure-related changes by radiogram or scan.

## DIAGNOSIS AND DIFFERENTIAL DIAGNOSIS

Usually made clinically. Complications are assessed with data on cultures, biopsies, and imaging. Differential diagnosis includes infectious ulcer (actinomycotic infection, deep fungal infection, chronic herpetic ulcer), thermal burn, malignant ulcer (cutaneous lymphoma, basal cell carcinoma or SCC), pyoderma gangrenosum, rectocutaneous fistula.

## COURSE AND PROGNOSIS

If pressure is relieved, some changes are reversible; intermittent periods of pressure relief increase resistance to compression. Osteomyelitis occurs in nonhealing pressure ulcers (32 to 81%). Septicemia is associated with a high mortality rate. Overall, patients with pressure ulcers have a fourfold risk of prolonged hospitalization and of dying when compared with patients without ulcers. With proper treatment, stages I and II ulcers heal in 1 to 4 weeks and stages III and IV ulcers heal in 6 to >12 weeks.

## MANAGEMENT

**Prophylaxis in At-Risk Patients** Reposition patient every 2 h (more often if possible); massage areas prone to pressure ulcers while changing position of patient; inspect for areas of skin breakdown over pressure points.

- Use interface air mattress to reduce compression.
- Minimize friction and shear forces by using proper positioning, transferring, and turning techniques.
- Clean with mild cleansing agents, keeping skin free of urine and feces.
- Minimize skin exposure to excessive moisture from incontinence, perspiration, or wound drainage.
- Maintain head of the bed at a relatively low angle of elevation ($<30°$).
- Evaluate and correct nutritional status; consider supplements of vitamin C and zinc.
- Mobilize patients as soon as possible.

**Stages I and II Ulcers** Topical antibiotics (not neomycin) under moist sterile gauze may be sufficient for early erosions. Normal saline wet-to-dry dressings may be needed for debridement. Hydrogels or hydrocolloid dressings.

**Stages III and IV Ulcers** Surgical management: debridement of necrotic tissue, bony prominence removal, flaps and skin grafts.

**Infectious Complications** Prolonged course of antimicrobial agent depending on sensitivities, with surgical debridement of necrotic bone in osteomyelitis.

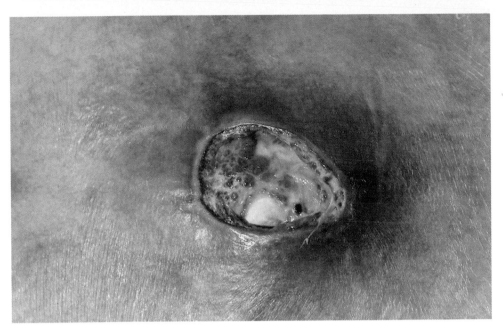

**FIGURE 16-16    Pressure ulcer, stage III**    *Well-demarcated crateriform ulcer with full thickness skin loss extending down to fascia over greater trochanteric region.*

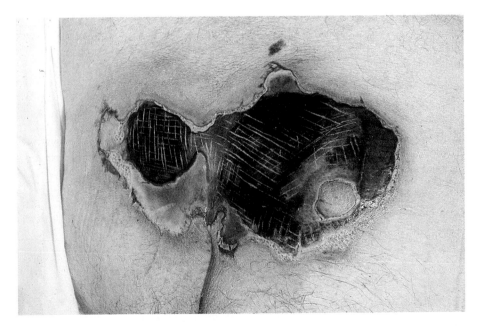

**FIGURE 16-17    Pressure ulcer, stage IV**    *Huge black necrosis over sacral area in a patient who had been bedridden after a stroke. The criss-cross marks in the necrotic area are from attempts to mechanically debride necrotic tissue. Surgical debridement of necrotic tissue under anesthesia revealed involvement of fascia and bone.*

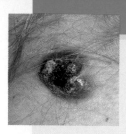

# SKIN SIGNS OF SYSTEMIC CANCERS

## MUCOCUTANEOUS SIGNS OF SYSTEMIC CANCERS

Mucocutaneous findings may suggest systemic cancers in several ways: associations of heritable mucocutaneous disorders with systemic cancers; by action at a distance, i.e., paraneoplastic syndromes; or spread of cancer to skin or mucosal sites by direct, lymphatic, or hematogenous extension (cutaneous metastasis).

---

## CLASSIFICATION OF SKIN SIGNS OF SYSTEMIC CANCER[1]

### METASTATIC CANCERS

**Persistent tumor. Lymphatic extension, hematogenous spread**
**Direct extension. Paget's disease, extramammary Paget's disease**
*Lymphomas with secondary skin involvement* (p. 534)

### HERITABLE DISORDERS

**Cowden's syndrome**
**Peutz-Jeghers syndrome**
*Neurofibromatosis* (p. 463)
*Tuberous sclerosis* (p. 460)
Multiple endocrine neoplasia (MEN) (types 1 and 2b)

### PARANEOPLASTIC SYNDROMES

**Malignant acanthosis nigricans, tripe palms**
Bazex's syndrome
Muir-Torre syndrome
Gardner's syndrome
Carcinoid syndrome
Erythema gyratum repens
Hypertrichosis lanuginosa
Ectopic ACTH syndrome
**Glucagonoma syndrome**

*Sweet's syndrome* (p. 156)
*Pyoderma gangrenosum* (p. 152)
**Paraneoplastic pemphigus**
*Dermatomyositis* (p. 372)
*Pruritus* (p. 1052)
Palmar keratoses
Acquired ichthyosis
*Vasculitis* (p. 406)

---

[1] Conditions covered in this section are printed in *bold*, conditions dealt with in other sections are in *bold italics*. Numbers in parentheses indicate page numbers. Conditions not discussed in this book are described in IM Freedberg, AZ Eisen, K Wolff, K Frank Austen, LA Goldsmith, SP Katz (eds): *Fitzpatrick's Dermatology in General Medicine*, 6th ed. New York, McGraw-Hill, 2003.

# METASTATIC CANCER TO THE SKIN

Metastatic cancer to the skin is characterized by solitary or multiple dermal or subcutaneous nodules, occurring as metastatic cells from a distant noncontiguous primary malignant neoplasm, that are transported to and deposited in the skin or subcutaneous tissue by hematogenous or lymphatic routes, or by contiguous spread across the peritoneal cavity or other tissues.

## EPIDEMIOLOGY

**Age of Onset**   Any age, but usually older.
**Sex**   Frequency of primary tumors varies with sex.
**Incidence**   In principle almost any cancer can metastasize to skin. Skin metastases occur in up to 10% of all patients with cancer. The frequency of metastases according to type of tumor and gender are shown in Tables 17-1 and 17-2.

## PATHOGENESIS

Includes detachment of cancer cells from primary tumor, invasion, intravasation into blood or lymphatic vessel, $\rightarrow$ circulation, stasis within vessel, migration across vessel wall, invasion into tissue, proliferation at metastatic site. The growth of metastases depends on proliferation of metastatic cells, cytokine and growth factor release from cancer and stromal cells, angiogenesis, and immune reactions. Three patterns of metastases are observed: mechanical tumor stasis (anatomic proximity and lymphatic draining), site-specific (selective attachment of tumor cells to specific organ), nonselective (independent of mechanical or organ-specific factors).

## HISTORY

Prior history of primary internal cancer or cancer chemotherapy or may be first sign of visceral cancer.

## PHYSICAL EXAMINATION

### Skin Lesions
Nodule (Figs. 17-1 and 17-2), raised plaque, thickened fibrotic area. First detected when <5 mm. Fibrotic area may resemble morphea; occurring on scalp, may produce alopecia. Initially, epidermis is intact (Fig. 17-1), stretched over nodule; in time, surface may become ulcerated or hyperkeratotic (Fig. 17-2). May appear inflammatory, i.e., pink to red (Figs. 17-1 and 17-2) or hemorrhagic (Fig. 17-3). Metastatic melanoma to dermis: blue to gray to black nodules (see Fig. 12-26). Firm to indurated. May be solitary, few, or multiple.
*Distribution* Anywhere. Lung cancer preferentially to trunk, scalp. Hypernephroma to scalp, operative scar.
### Special Patterns of Cutaneous Involvement
*Breast*

> *Inflammatory metastatic carcinoma* (carcinoma erysipelatoides): erythematous patch or plaque with an active spreading border (Fig. 17-4). Most often with breast cancer that may spread within lymphatics to skin of involved breast, resulting in inflammatory plaques resembling erysipelas (hence the designation carcinoma erysipelatoides). Breast most common primary (Fig. 17-4), but occurs with others as well [pancreas, parotid, tonsils, colon, stomach, rectum, melanoma, pelvic organs, ovary (Fig. 17-5), uterus, prostate, lung].
>
> *Telangiectatic metastatic carcinoma* (carcinoma telangiectaticum): breast cancer appearing as pinpoint telangiectases with dilated capillaries within carcinoma erysipelatoides. Violaceous papules or papulovesicles resembling lymphangioma circumscriptum (Fig. 17-5).
>
> *En cuirasse metastatic carcinoma*: diffuse morphea–like induration of skin. Usually local extension of breast cancer occurring in breast and presternal region. Sclerodermoid plaque may encase chest and resembles a metal breastplate of a cuirassier. Also occurs with primary of lung, GI tract, kidney.
>
> *Breast carcinoma of inframammary crease*: cutaneous exophytic nodule resembling primary squamous cell carcinoma (SCC) or basal cell carcinoma of skin.
>
> *Paget's disease*: sharply demarcated plaque or patch of erythema and scaling occurring

on nipple or areola associated with underlying breast cancer (see below).

*Alopecia neoplastica*: occurs via *hematogenous spread*. On scalp, areas of hair loss resembling alopecia areata; well-demarcated, red-pink, smooth surface.

**Large Intestine** Often presents on skin of abdomen or perineal regions; also, scalp or face. Most originate in rectum. May present with metastatic inflammatory carcinoma (like carcinoma erysipelatoides) of inguinal region, supraclavicular area, or face and neck. Less commonly, sessile or pedunculated nodules on buttocks, grouped vascular nodules of groin or scrotum, or facial tumor. Rarely, cutaneous fistula after appendectomy or resembling hidradenitis suppurativa.

**Lung Carcinoma** May produce a large number of metastatic nodules in a short period. Most commonly, reddish nodule(s) (Fig. 17-1) on scalp. Trunk: symmetric; along direction of intercostal vessels, may be zosteriform; in scar (thoracotomy site or needle aspiration tract).

**Hypernephroma** Can produce solitary lesion; also widespread. Usually appear vascular, ±pulsatile, ±pedunculated (Fig. 17-3); can resemble pyogenic granuloma. Most common on head (scalp) and neck; also trunk and extremities.

**Malignant Melanoma** May spread from primary cutaneous site to distant cutaneous site by lymphatic vessels. Primary sites also can be noncutaneous: eye, cervix, oral cavity. Cutaneous metastases of unknown primary melanoma also occur. Nodules, single or multiple. Usually deeply pigmented; black, blue, slate gray (see Fig. 12-26), amelanotic variants pink or red.

**Carcinoma of Bladder, Ovary** Can spread contiguously to abdominal and inguinal skin similarly to breast cancer, as described above, and look like erysipelas (Fig. 17-5).

**Miscellaneous Patterns** With dilation of lymphatics and superficial hemorrhage, may resemble lymphangioma. With lymph stasis and dermal edema, resembles pigskin or orange peel. May metastasize hematogenously to scalp, forming many subcutaneous nodules with "bag of marbles" feel to scalp.

*Sister Mary Joseph nodule* is metastatic carcinoma to umbilicus from intraabdominal carcinoma, most commonly stomach, colon, ovary, pancreas (Fig. 17-6); however, primary may be in breast. Easier to detect by palpation than by visual detection. Can be firm to indurated nodule, ±fissuring, ±ulceration, ±vascular appearance (Fig. 17-6), ±discharge. In 15% may be initial presentation of primary malignancy.

**TABLE 17-1**   **Percent of Patients with Cutaneous Metastases**

| Type of Primary Malignancy | Patients with Cutaneous Metastases, % |
|---|---|
| Melanoma | 44.8 |
| Breast | 30.0 |
| Nasal sinuses | 20.0 |
| Larynx | 16.3 |
| Endocrine glands | 12.5 |
| Oral cavity | 11.5 |
| Esophagus | 8.6 |
| Kidney | 4.6 |
| Stomach | 2.0 |

SOURCE: Adapted from DP Lookingbill et al: J Am Acad Dermatol 29:228, 1993.

**TABLE 17-2**   **Ranking of Underlying Primary Malignancies in Patients with Cutaneous Metastasis According to Gender**

| Primary Malignancy | Patients with Cutaneous Metastases, % | |
|---|---|---|
| | Male | Female |
| Breast | 2.4 | 70.7 |
| Melanoma | 32.3 | 12.0 |
| Lung | 11.8 | 2.0 |
| Colon/rectum | 11.0 | 1.3 |
| Ovary | – | 3.3 |
| Unknown | 8.7 | 3.0 |

SOURCE: Adapted from DP Lookingbill et al: J Am Acad Dermatol 29:228, 1993.

[Important differential diagnosis: endometriosis of skin (Fig. 17-7).]

## DIFFERENTIAL DIAGNOSIS

**"Blueberry Muffin Baby"** Neuroblastoma, congenital leukemia.

**Multiple Smooth Nodules on Scalp** (Prostate adenocarcinoma, lung cancer, breast cancer): Cylindromas (rare adnexal tumors of the scalp mimicking marbles tucked under the skin), trichilemmal (pilar) cysts.

**Kaposi's Sarcoma-Like Lesions** Cancer of kidney.

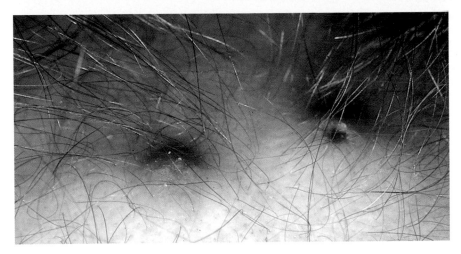

**FIGURE 17-1   Metastatic cancer to the skin: bronchogenic cancer**   *Dermal nodules on the scalp of a patient undergoing chemotherapy for metastatic lung cancer; the nodules were only apparent following loss of hair during chemotherapy. The nodule on the left is asymptomatic, erythematous, but noninflamed. The nodule on the right has a central depression marking a biopsy site.*

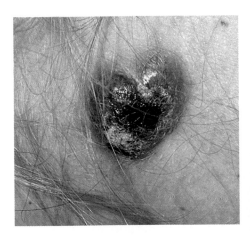

**FIGURE 17-2   Metastatic cancer to the skin: breast cancer**   *Large, hyperkeratotic nodule on the posterior neck in a 40-year-old woman with metastatic breast cancer, present for 6 months; became ulcerated; similar but smaller lesions were present on the scalp and back.*

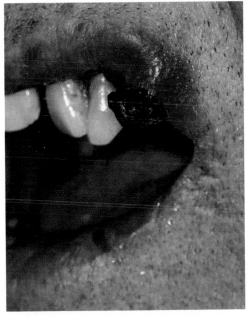

**FIGURE 17-3   Metastatic cancer to the skin, hypernephroma**   *Hypernephroma metastases often localize to the head and have an angiomatous appearance mimicking pyogenic granuloma as in this lesion on the upper lip of a 66-year-old man. This was the first indication that the patient had cancer of the kidney.*

**Pyogenic Granuloma-Like Lesions**   Amelanotic melanoma, renal cancer.

**Alopecia Areata-Like Lesions**   Breast cancer.

**Lymphangioma-Like Lesions**   Cancer of breast, lung, cervix, ovary.

**Morphea-Like Lesions**   Cancer of breast, stomach, lung, mixed tumors, lacrimal gland.

## LABORATORY EXAMINATION

**Dermatopathology** At times, cell differentiation and architectural structure sufficient to predict primary site; however, many times cells anaplastic. Employ monoclonal antibodies to differentiate solid carcinoma metastases from lymphoma, neuroendocrine carcinoma, melanoma, anaplastic angiosarcoma, and sarcomas.

## COURSE AND PROGNOSIS

In individuals with known cancer, cutaneous metastases are indicative of a poor prognosis.

Average survival after detection of cutaneous metastasis only 3 months except for contiguous spread of breast cancer, which may last for years. In individuals with unknown cancer, skin metastases may help to detect primary tumor.

## MANAGEMENT

With solitary or few lesions and if patient not terminal, excision may be indicated.

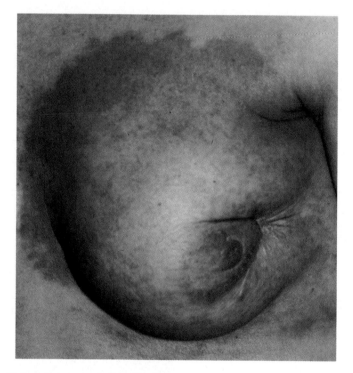

**FIGURE 17-4 Metastatic cancer to the skin: inflammatory breast cancer (carcinoma erysipelatoides)** *The breast has a depression and scar in the left lower quadrant from limited breast surgery and a well-defined, irregularly margined erythema resembling cellulitis or erysipelas on most of the surface; the cancer has spread via the cutaneous lymphatics.*

**FIGURE 17-6 (Opposite page, left) Sister Mary Joseph nodule** *Is a metastasis to the umbilicus usually, but not always, from abdominal carcinoma. Usually an indurated nodule, often vascular as in this 72-year-old woman with carcinoma of the colon.*

**FIGURE 17-7 (Opposite page, right) Endometriosis of the umbilicus** *A bluish-brown nodule that at times bleeds. This image of the umbilicus of a 36-year-old woman is shown for differential diagnostic reasons because the most important lesion from which it has to be distinguished is the Sister Mary nodule (Fig. 17-6).*

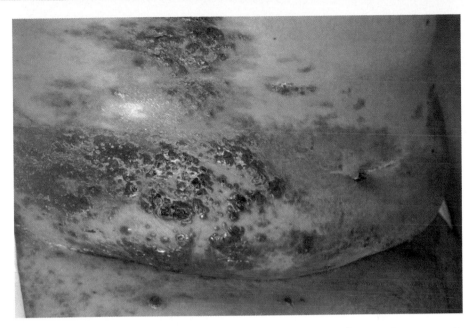

**FIGURE 17-5   Metastatic cancer to the skin: carcinoma erysipelatoides from ovarian cancer**   *In addition to the erysipelas-like inflammatory erythema there are multiple, grouped papules, and nodules resembling lymphangioma circumscriptum on the abdomen of a 65-year-old woman. The patient had lost weight but was otherwise asymptomatic. Biopsy revealed metastatic cancer and general workup disclosed ovarian cancer with peritoneal carcinomatosis.*

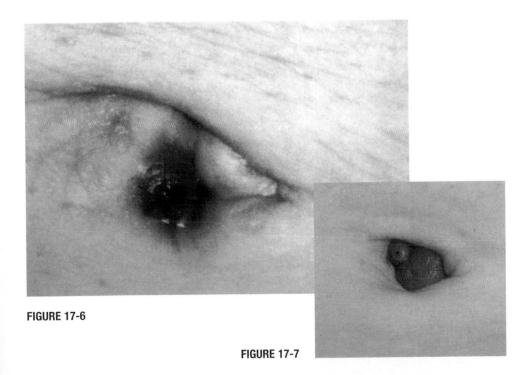

**FIGURE 17-6**

**FIGURE 17-7**

# PAGET'S DISEASE

## MAMMARY PAGET'S DISEASE ◼ ●

Mammary Paget's disease (MPD) is a malignant neoplasm that unilaterally involves the nipple or areola and simulates a chronic eczematous dermatitis; it represents contiguous spread of underlying intraductal carcinoma of the breast (1 to 4% of breast cancers). Usually occurring in females (>50 years), there are rare examples in males.

Onset is insidious over several months or years. May be asymptomatic or there may be pruritus, pain, burning, discharge, bleeding, ulceration, nipple invagination. Skin lesion represents as red, scaling plaque, rather sharply marginated, oval with irregular borders. When scale is removed, the surface is moist and oozing (Fig. 17-8). Lesions range in size from 0.3 to 15 cm. In early stages there is no induration of the plaque; later, induration and infiltration develop and nodules may be palpated in breast. At initial presentation an underlying breast mass is palpable in fewer than one-half of patients. May be bilateral. Lymph node metastases occur more often when MPD is associated with an underlying palpable mass.

Differential diagnosis includes eczematous dermatitis, psoriasis, benign ductal papilloma, nipple-areola retention hyperkeratosis, impetigo, SCC in situ, familial pemphigus.

*Eczematous dermatitis of the nipples* is usually bilateral; it is without any induration and responds rapidly to topical glucocorticoids. Nevertheless, be suspicious of Paget's disease if "eczema" persists for >3 weeks. Diagnosis verified by biopsy showing neoplastic cells in epidermis following a pathognomonic pattern of spread. Define underlying intraductal carcinoma by mammography.

Management consists of surgery, radiotherapy, and/or chemotherapy as in any other breast carcinomas. Lymph node dissection if regional nodes are palpable. Prognosis varies. When breast mass is not palpable, 92% of patients survive 5 years after excision; 82%, 10 years. When breast mass is palpable, 38% survive 5 years; 22%, 10 years. Prognosis worse when there is lymphadenopathy.

## EXTRAMAMMARY PAGET'S DISEASE ☐ ●

Extramammary Paget's disease (EPD) is a neoplasm of the anogenital and axillary skin, histologically identical and clinically similar to Paget's disease of the breast, often representing an intraepidermal extension of a primary adenocarcinoma of underlying apocrine glands or of the lower gastrointestinal, urinary, or female genital tracts. Often, however, it is unassociated with underlying cancer.

The histogenesis of EPD is not uniform. Paget cells in the epidermis may occur as an in situ upward extension of an in situ adenocarcinoma in deeper glands (25%). Alternatively, EPD may have a multifocal primary origin in the epidermis and its related appendages. Primary

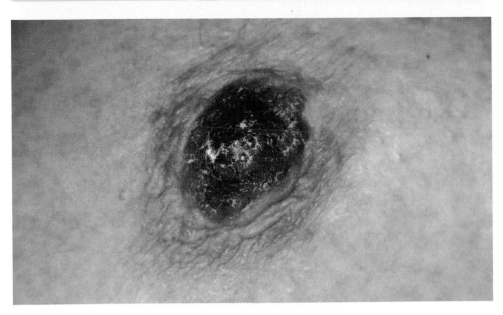

**FIGURE 17-8    Mammary Paget's disease**    *A sharply demarcated red plaque mimicking eczema or psoriasis on the nipple. The plaque is slightly indurated and there is slight scaling; any red, eczema-like lesion on the nipple and areola that does not respond to topical corticosteroids should be biopsied.*

tumors in the anorectum can arise within the rectal mucosa or intramural glands.

There is an insidious onset, slow spread, +itching. The lesion presents as erythematous plaque, +scaling, +erosion (Fig. 17-9), +crusting, +exudation; eczematous-appearing lesions but borders are sharply defined (Fig. 17-9), geographic configuration. Lesions should always be biopsied. Histopathologically, characteristic Paget cells are dispersed between keratinocytes, occur in clusters, extend down into adnexal structures (hair follicles, eccrine ducts). Adnexal adenocarcinoma is often found when carefully searched for. In perineal/perianal EPD, underlying carcinoma should be searched for by *rectal examination, proctoscopy, sigmoidoscopy, barium enema*. In genital EPD, search for underlying carcinoma by *cystoscopy, intravenous pyelogram*; in vulvar EPD, by *pelvic examination*.

Differential diagnosis includes all red plaques: eczematous dermatitis, lichen simplex chronicus, lichen sclerosus et atrophicus, lichen planus, inverse pattern psoriasis, *Candida* intertrigo, SCC in situ (erythroplasia of Queyrat), human papilloma virus–induced SCC in situ, (amelanotic) superficial spreading melanoma.

EPD is usually much larger than is apparent clinically. Surgical excision must be controlled histologically (Mohs' microscopic surgery). If Paget cells are in dermis and regional lymph nodes are palpable, lymph node dissection may improve prognosis, which is related to underlying adenocarcinoma. EPD remains in situ in the epidermis and adnexal epithelium in >65% of cases. When no underlying neoplasm is present, there is nonetheless a high recurrence rate, even after apparently adequate excision; this is due to the multifocal origin in the epidermis and adnexal structures.

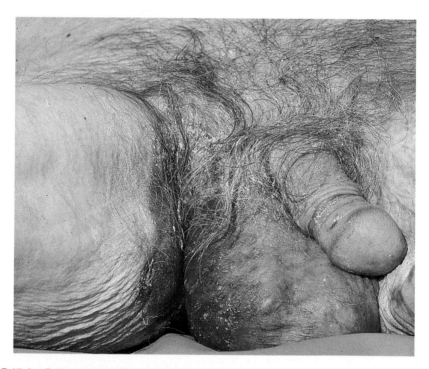

**FIGURE 17-9   Extramammary Paget's disease**   *Moist, well-demarcated, eroded, oozing, erythematous plaque on the scrotum and inguinal fold in an older male. The lesion is commonly mistaken for* Candida intertrigo *and unsuccessfully treated as such.*

# COWDEN'S SYNDROME (MULTIPLE HAMARTOMA SYNDROME)  □  ◑

Cowden's syndrome (named after the propositus) is a rare, autosomal dominant heritable cancer syndrome with variable expressivity in a number of systems in the form of multiple hamartomatous neoplasms of ectodermal, mesodermal, and endodermal origin. Germ line mutations in the tumor-suppressor gene *PTEN* are located on chromosome 10q22–23 in most cases. There is a special susceptibility for breast and thyroid cancers, and the skin lesions are important markers because they portend the onset of breast and thyroid cancers.

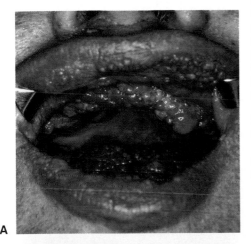

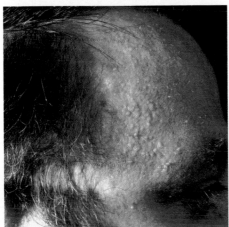

Skin lesions may appear first in childhood but develop over time. They consist of *tricholemmomas*, skin-colored, pink (Fig. 17-10), or brown papules having the appearance of flat warts on the central area of the face, perioral areas, lips near the angles of the mouth, and the ears; *translucent punctate keratoses* of the palms and soles; and *hyperkeratotic, flat-topped papules* on the dorsa of the hands and forearms. Mucous membrane lesions are characteristic: *papules* of the gingival, labial (Fig. 17-10), and palatal surfaces that coalesce, giving a "cobblestone" appearance. *Papillomas* of the buccal mucosa and the tongue.

In addition to breast cancer (20%), which is often bilateral, and thyroid cancer (8%), there are various internal hamartomas:

*Breast*—fibrocystic disease, fibroadenomas, adenocarcinoma, gynecomastia in males

*Thyroid*—goiter, adenomas, thyroglossal duct cysts, follicular adenocarcinoma

*GI tract*—hamartomatous polyps throughout tract but increased in large bowel, adenocarcinoma arising in polyp

*Female genital tract*—ovarian cysts, menstrual abnormalities

*Musculoskeletal*—craniomegaly, kyphoscoliosis, "adenoid" facies, high-arched palate

*CNS*—mental retardation, seizures, neuromas, ganglioneuromas, and meningiomas of the ear canal.

It is important to establish the diagnosis of Cowden's syndrome so that these patients can be followed carefully to detect breast and thyroid cancers.

**FIGURE 17-10  Cowden's syndrome**  *A. Multiple reddish, confluent papules on the oral mucosa giving a cobblestone appearance. B. Multiple skin-colored warty papules on the face, which represent tricholemmonas.*

## PEUTZ-JEGHERS SYNDROME

Peutz-Jeghers syndrome (PJS) is a familial (autosomal dominant, spontaneous mutation in 40%) polyposis characterized by many small, pigmented brown macules (lentigines) on the lips, oral mucous membranes (brown to bluish black), and on the bridge of the nose, palms, and soles.

Macules on the lips may disappear over time, but not the pigmentation of the mouth; therefore the mouth pigmentation is the sine qua non for the diagnosis (Fig. 17-11). The gene has been mapped to 19p13.3. There are usually, but not always, multiple hamartomatous polyps in the small bowel, as well as in the large bowel and stomach, that cause abdominal symptoms such as pain, GI bleeding, anemia. Whereas pigmented macules are congenital or develop in infancy and early childhood, polyps come on in late childhood or before age 30. Adenocarcinoma may develop in polyps, and there is an increased incidence of breast, ovarian, and pancreatic cancer.

There is a normal life expectancy unless carcinoma develops in the GI tract. Malignant neoplasms may be more frequent in Japanese patients with this syndrome, and prophylactic colectomy has been recommended for these patients.

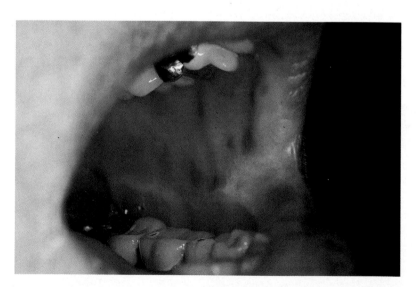

**FIGURE 17-11    Peutz-Jeghers syndrome**  *Multiple, dark-brown lentigines on the vermilion border of the lip and the buccal mucosa. This patient had GI bleeding due to hamartomatous polyps in the small bowel.*

## GLUCAGONOMA SYNDROME

Glucagonoma syndrome is a rare but well-described clinical entity caused by excessive production of glucagon in an α cell tumor of the pancreas, characterized by superficial migratory necrolytic erythema (MNE) with erosions that crust and heal with hyperpigmentation, a beefy-red tongue, and angular cheilitis. Most cases are associated with glucagonoma, but the pathogenesis of MNE is not known. There exists MNE without glucagonoma.

### Skin Lesions

Consist of inflammatory red plaques (Fig. 17-12) of gyrate, circinate, arcuate, or annular shape that enlarge with central clearing, resulting in geographic areas that become confluent (Fig. 17-13). Borders show vesiculation to bulla formation, crusting, and scaling (Figs. 17-12 and 17-13). Lesions involve perioral and perigenital regions and flexures and intertriginal areas. Fingertips red, shining, erosive. There is glossitis, angular cheili-tis (Fig. 17-12), blepharitis, and general examination reveals wasting, malnutrition.

### DIFFERENTIAL DIAGNOSIS

Includes all moist red plaque(s): acrodermatitis enteropathica, zinc deficiency, pustular psoriasis, mucocutaneous candidiasis, Hailey-Hailey disease (familial pemphigus).

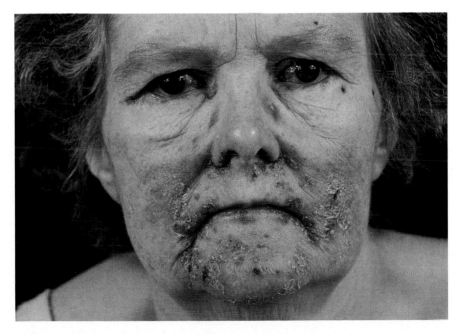

**FIGURE 17-12   Glucagonoma syndrome: migratory necrolytic erythema**   *Inflammatory dermatosis with angular cheilitis, inflammatory, scaly, erosive and crusted plaques and fissures around the nose, mouth, and medial aspects of the eyes. Marginal blepharitis.*

Fasting plasma glucagon level increased to >1000 ng/L (normal 50 to 250 ng/L) and makes the diagnosis. There is also hyperglycemia, reduced glucose tolerance. Associated findings include severe malabsorption, gross hypoaminoacidemia, low serum zinc. CT scan angiography will locate tumor within pancreas and metastases in the liver.

Dermatopathology of early skin lesions shows bandlike upper epidermal necrosis with retention of pyknotic nuclei and pale keratinocyte cytoplasm.

Prognosis depends on the aggressiveness of the glucagonoma. Hepatic metastases have occurred in 75% of patients at the time of diagnosis. If these are slow-growing, patients may have prolonged survival, even with metastatic disease.

MNE responds poorly to all types of therapy. Some cases have responded partially to zinc replacement. MNE resolves after tumor excision. However, surgical excision of glucagonoma achieves cure in only 30% of cases because of persistent metastases (usually liver). Surgery also reduces tumor masses and associated symptoms. There is poor response to chemotherapy.

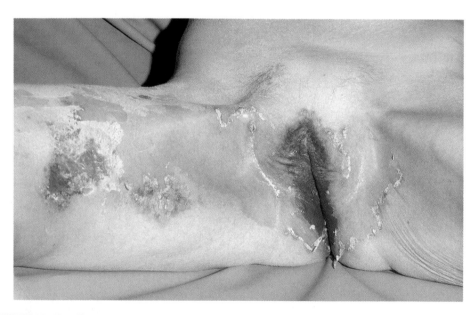

**FIGURE 17-13   Glucagonoma syndrome: migratory necrolytic erythema**   *Polycyclic erosions in the anogenital gluteal and sacral regions. Sharply defined with necrotic flaccid epidermis still covering part of these erosions.*

## MALIGNANT ACANTHOSIS NIGRICANS   □

Like other forms of acanthosis nigricans (AN) (see Section 5), malignant AN starts as a diffuse, velvety thickening and hyperpigmentation chiefly on the neck, axillae and other body folds, as well as on the perioral and periorbital, umbilical, mamillary, and genital areas, giving the skin a dirty appearance (Fig. 17-14; see also Fig. 5-1). Hyperpigmentation and hyperkeratosis soon lead to a rugose, mamillated, and papillomatous surface (Fig. 17-14); verrucous growths also involve the vermilion border of the lips (Fig. 17-15); and the knuckles and the palms show maximal accentuation of the palmar ridges (tripe hands) (Fig. 17-16). On the oral mucous membranes there is a velvety texture with delicate furrows, and there are warty papillomatous thickenings periorally.

Malignant AN differs from other forms of AN primarily because of (1) the more pronounced velvety hyperkeratosis and hyperpigmentation, (2) the pronounced mucosal involvement and involvement of the mucocutaneous junction, (3) tripe hands, and (4) weight loss and wasting due to the underlying malignancy.

AN may precede by 5 years other symptoms of a malignancy, usually adenocarcinoma of the GI or GU tract, bronchocarcinoma, or, less commonly, lymphoma. Malignant AN is a truly paraneoplastic disease, and a search for underlying malignancies is imperative. Removal of malignancy is followed by regression of AN.

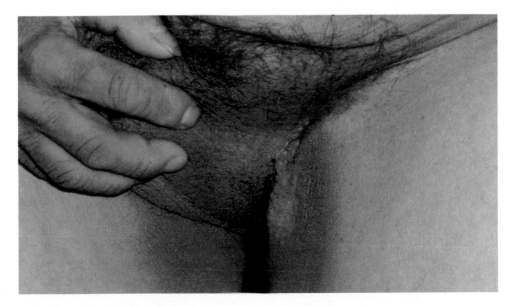

**FIGURE 17-14   Acanthosis nigricans: malignant**   *Poorly defined, velvety, verrucous and papillomatous, dark chocolate-brown plaques on the medial thighs and scrotum. Similar changes were also present in the axillae and neck and the vermilion border of the lips was covered with velvety, raspberry-like growths.*

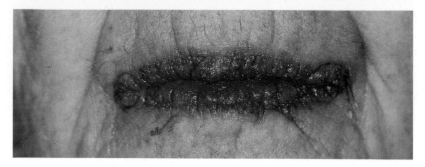

**FIGURE 17-15    Acanthosis nigricans: malignant** *Verrucous and mamillated growths on the vermilion border of the lips in a patient with carcinoma of the stomach. The gastric cancer was suspected because of these raspberry-like growths, acanthosis nigricans of the major skin folds, and weight loss. There is still a suture at the site of a biopsy.*

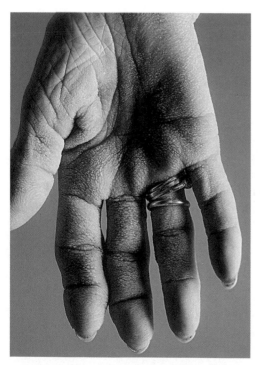

**FIGURE 17-16    Acanthosis nigricans: tripe palm** *The palmar ridges of the palm show maximal accentuation, thus resembling the mucosa of the stomach of a ruminant (tripe palm).*

# PARANEOPLASTIC PEMPHIGUS (PNP)    □   ●

Mucous membranes primarily and most severely involved. Lesions combine features of pemphigus vulgaris (page 100) and erythema multiforme (page 140), clinically, histologically, and immunopathologically. Most prominent clinical findings consist of severe oral (Fig. 17-17) and conjunctival erosions in a patient with an underlying neoplasm, usually a lymphoma. Patients with PNP may also have clinical and serologic evidence of myasthenia gravis and autoimmune cytopenias. PNP sera contain autoantibodies to plakin antigens (in the intercellular plaque of desmosomes), envoplakin and periplakin, and to desmoplakin I and II. Less commonly patient sera may also recognize bullous pemphigoid antigen (BPAG1e) (230 kDa), plectin and plakoglobin, and an unidentified 170-kDa antigen. Autoantibodies of PNP cause blistering in neonatal mice and are detected by indirect immunofluorescence on rodent urinary bladder epithelium. Treatment is directed toward elimination or suppression of malignancy but may also require systemic glucocorticoids.

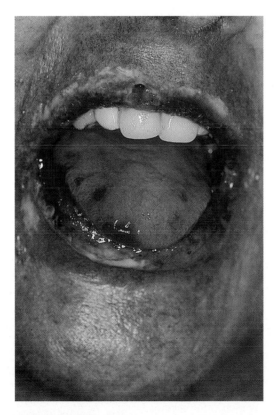

**FIGURE 17-17   Paraneoplastic pemphigus**   *Severe erosions covering practically the entire mucosa of the oral cavity with partial sparing of the dorsum of the tongue. Lesions are extremely painful interfering with adequate food intake. This patient had non-Hodgkin's lymphoma as underlying malignancy.*

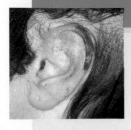

# SKIN SIGNS OF HEMATOLOGIC DISEASES

## THROMBOCYTOPENIC PURPURA

Thrombocytopenic purpura (TP) is characterized by cutaneous hemorrhages occurring in association with a reduced platelet count; clinically, hemorrhages are usually small (petechiae) but at times larger (ecchymoses) and occur at sites of minor trauma/pressure (platelet count < 40,000/μL) or spontaneously (platelet count < 10,000/μL).

### EPIDEMIOLOGY

**Age of Onset** Acute idiopathic thrombocytopenic purpura (ITP) mostly in children; drug-induced and autoimmune TP in adults.
**Sex** Both sexes; HIV-associated TP—homosexual men > heterosexual females.

### ETIOLOGY AND PATHOGENESIS

Due to either decreased platelet production, splenic sequestration, or increased platelet destruction.

1. *Decreased platelet production.* Direct injury to bone marrow, drugs (cytosine arabinoside, daunorubicin, cyclophosphamide, busulfan, methotrexate, 6-mercaptopurine, vinca alkaloids, thiazide diuretics, ethanol, estrogens), replacement of bone marrow, aplastic anemia, vitamin deficiencies, Wiskott-Aldrich syndrome.
2. *Splenic sequestration.* Splenomegaly, hypothermia.
3. *Increased platelet destruction. Immunologic:* autoimmune TP, drug hypersensitivity (sulfonamides, quinine, quinidine, carbamazepine, digitoxin, methyldopa), after transfusion. *Nonimmunologic:* infection, prosthetic heart valves, disseminated intravascular coagulation, thrombotic thrombocytopenic purpura.

Platelet plugs by themselves effectively stop bleeding from capillaries and small blood vessels but are incapable of stopping hemorrhage from larger vessels. Platelet defects therefore produce problems with small-vessel hemostasis, small hemorrhages in the skin or in the CNS.

### HISTORY

Usually sudden appearance of asymptomatic hemorrhagic skin and/or mucosal lesions.

### PHYSICAL EXAMINATION

**Skin Lesions**
*Petechiae*—small (pinpoint to pinhead), red, nonblanching macules that are not palpable and turn brown as they get older (Fig. 18-1); later acquiring a yellowish-green tinge. *Ecchymoses*—black-and-blue spots; larger area of hemorrhage. *Vibices*—linear hemorrhages (Fig. 18-1), due to trauma or pressure. Most common on legs and upper trunk, but may be anywhere.
**Mucous Membranes** *Petechiae*—most often on palate (Fig. 18-2), gingival bleeding.
**General Examination** Possible CNS hemorrhage, anemia.

### LABORATORY EXAMINATIONS

**Hematology** Thrombocytopenia.
**Bone Marrow Aspiration** Defines state of platelet production.
**Serology** Rule out HIV disease.
**Lesional Skin Biopsy** May be contraindicated due to postoperative hemorrhage; however,

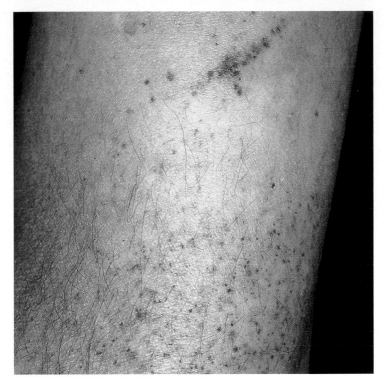

**FIGURE 18-1    Thrombocytopenic purpura**    *Myriads of petechiae on the upper arm of an HIV-infected 25-year-old male were the presenting manifestation of his disease. The linear arrangement of petechiae at the site of minor trauma are called vibices.*

usually can be controlled by suturing biopsied site and applying pressure.

## DIAGNOSIS

Clinical suspicion confirmed by platelet count.

## DIFFERENTIAL DIAGNOSIS

**Nonhemorrhagic Blanching Vascular Lesions** Telangiectasia/erythema, spider nevi, Osler's disease.
**True Hemorrhagic Lesions** Actinic or senile purpura, purpura of scurvy, progressive pigmentary purpura (Schamberg's disease), purpura following severe Valsalva maneuver (coughing, vomiting/retching), traumatic purpura, factitial or iatrogenic purpura, Gardner-Diamond syn-drome (autoerythrocyte sensitization syndrome), *palpable nonblanching purpura = vasculitis.*

## COURSE AND PROGNOSIS

Depends on and varies with the etiology.

## MANAGEMENT

Identify underlying cause and correct, if possible. If platelet count is very low ($<$10,000/$\mu$L), bed rest to reduce risk of hemorrhage.
**Oral Glucocorticoids, High-Dose IV Immunoglobulins**
**Platelet Transfusions** If the platelet count $<$10,000/$\mu$L, platelet transfusion may be indicated.
**Chronic ITP** Splenectomy may be indicated.

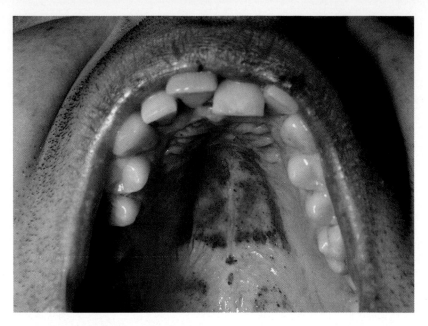

**FIGURE 18-2  Thrombocytopenic purpura**  *Can first manifest on the oral mucosa or conjunctiva. Here multiple petechial hemorrhages are seen on the palate.*

# DISSEMINATED INTRAVASCULAR COAGULATION   ☐   ●

Disseminated intravascular coagulation (DIC) is a widespread blood clotting disorder occurring within blood vessels, associated with a wide range of clinical circumstances (bacterial sepsis, obstetric complications, disseminated malignancy, massive trauma), and manifested by purpura fulminans (cutaneous infarctions and/or acral gangrene) or bleeding from multiple sites. The spectrum of clinical symptoms associated with DIC ranges from relatively mild and subclinical to explosive and life-threatening.

*Synonyms*: Purpura fulminans, consumption coagulopathy, defibrination syndrome, coagulation-fibrinolytic syndrome.

## EPIDEMIOLOGY

**Age of Onset**   All ages; occurs in children. Antecedent or concomitant infections due to bacteria (scarlet fever, group A streptococcal, staphylococcal, pneumococcal, vibrio, and meningococcal bacteremia; less commonly varicella).

## ETIOLOGY AND PATHOGENESIS

- *Events that initiate DIC* Tumor products, crushing trauma, extensive surgery, severe intracranial damage; retained contraception products, placental abruption, amniotic fluid embolism; certain snake bites; hemolytic transfusion reaction; acute promyelocytic leukemia; burn injuries.
- *Extensive destruction of endothelial surfaces, exposure to foreign surfaces* Vasculitis in Rocky Mountain spotted fever, meningococcemia, or occasionally gram-negative septicemia; group A streptococcal infection, heat stroke, malignant hyperthermia; extensive pump oxygenation (repair of aortic aneurysm); eclampsia, preeclampsia; giant hemangioma (Kasabach-Merritt syndrome); immune complexes; postvaricella purpura gangrenosa.
- *Events that complicate and propagate DIC* Shock, complement pathway activation.

Uncontrolled activation of coagulation results in thrombosis and consumption of platelets/clotting factors II, V, VIII. Secondary fibrinolysis. If the activation occurs slowly, excess activated products are produced, predisposing to vascular infarctions/venous thrombosis. If the onset is acute, hemorrhage surrounding wound sites and IV lines/catheters or bleeding into deep tissues is usually seen.

## HISTORY

Hours to days; rapid evolution. Fever, chills associated with onset of hemorrhagic lesions.

## PHYSICAL EXAMINATION

### Skin Lesions

*Infarction (purpura fulminans)* (Fig. 18-3): massive ecchymoses with sharp, irregular ("geographic") borders with deep purple color and erythematous halo, ± evolution to hemorrhagic bullae and blue to black gangrene (Fig. 18-4); multiple lesions are often symmetric; distal extremities, areas of pressure; lips, ears, nose, trunk; peripheral acrocyanosis followed by gangrene on hands, feet, tip of nose, with subsequent autoamputation if patient survives.

*Hemorrhage* from multiple cutaneous sites, i.e., surgical incisions, venipuncture or catheter sites.

**Mucous Membranes**   Hemorrhage from gingiva.

**General Examination**   High fever, tachycardia, ± shock. Multitude of findings depending on the associated medical/surgical problem.

## LABORATORY EXAMINATIONS

**Dermatopathology**   Occlusion of arterioles with fibrin thrombi. Dense PMN infiltrate around infarct and massive hemorrhage.

**Hematologic Studies   *CBC***   Schistocytes (fragmented RBCs), arising from RBC entrapment and damage within fibrin thrombi, seen on blood smear; platelet count low. Leukocytosis.

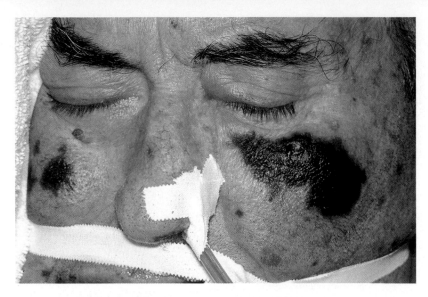

**FIGURE 18-3   Disseminated intravascular coagulation: purpura fulminans**   *Geographic cutaneous infarctions on the cheeks with smaller lesions on the forehead; lesions were also present on the hands, elbows, thighs, and feet. The patient was a diabetic with* Staphylococcus aureus *sepsis and died within 24 h after onset of the purpuric lesions.*

*Coagulation Studies* Reduced plasma fibrinogen; elevated fibrin degradation products; prolonged prothrombin time, partial thromboplastin time, and thrombin time.
**Blood Culture**   For bacterial sepsis.

## DIAGNOSIS AND DIFFERENTIAL DIAGNOSIS

Clinical suspicion confirmed by coagulation studies. Differential diagnosis of *large cutaneous infarctions*: necrosis after initiation of warfarin therapy, heparin necrosis, calciphylaxis, atheroembolization.

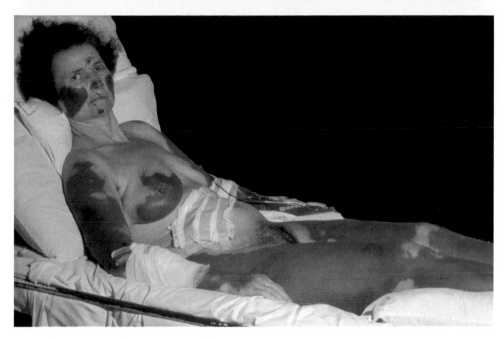

**FIGURE 18-4   Disseminated intravascular coagulation: purpura fulminans**   *Extensive geographic areas of cutaneous infarction with hemorrhage involving the face, breast, and extremities; although the patient looked alert, she died within several days. This catastrophic event followed sepsis after abdominal surgery.*

## COURSE AND PROGNOSIS

Mortality rate is high. Surviving patients require skin grafts or amputation for gangrenous tissue. Common complications: severe bleeding, thrombosis, tissue ischemia/necrosis, hemolysis, organ failure.

## MANAGEMENT

Correct reversible cause. Vigorous antibiotic therapy for infections. Control bleeding or thrombosis: heparin, pentoxifylline, protein C concentrate. Prevent recurrence in chronic DIC.

# CRYOGLOBULINEMIA

Cryoglobulinemia (CG) is the presence of serum immunoglobulin (precipitates at low temperature and redissolves at 37°C) complexed with other immunoglobulins or proteins. Associated clinical findings include purpura in cold-exposed sites, Raynaud's phenomenon, cold urticaria, acral hemorrhagic necrosis, bleeding disorders, vasculitis, arthralgia, neurologic manifestations, hepatosplenomegaly, and glomerulonephritis. Precipitation of cryoglobulins (when present in large amounts) causes vessel occlusion, also associated with hyperviscosity; immune complex deposition followed by complement activation and inflammation; platelet aggregation/consumption of clotting factors by cryoglobulins, causing coagulation disorder; small vessel thromboses and vasculitis produced by immune complexes.

Cryoglobulinemia can be due to three types of cryoglobulins:

*Type I Cryoglobulins*: Monoclonal immunoglobulins (IgM, IgG, IgA, light chains). *Associated with*: plasma cell dyscrasias such as multiple myeloma, Waldenström's macroglobulinemia, lymphoproliferative disorders such as chronic lymphocytic leukemia.

*Type II Cryoglobulins*: Mixed cryoglobulins: two immunoglobulin components, one of which is monoclonal (usually IgG, less often IgM) and one polyclonal; components interact and cryoprecipitate. *Associated with*: multiple myeloma, Waldenström's macroglobulinemia, chronic lymphocytic leukemia; rheumatoid arthritis, systemic lupus erythematosus, Sjögren's syndrome.

*Type III Cryoglobulins*: Polyclonal immunoglobulins that form cryoprecipitate with polyclonal IgG or a nonimmunoglobulin serum component occasionally mixed with complement and lipoproteins. Probably represents immune complex disease. *Associated with*: autoimmune diseases; connective tissue diseases; wide variety of infectious diseases, i.e., hepatitis B, hepatitis C, Epstein-Barr virus infection, cytomegalovirus infection, subacute bacterial endocarditis, leprosy, syphilis, β-hemolytic streptococcal infections.

There is cold sensitivity in <50% of cases. Chills, fever, dyspnea, diarrhea may occur following cold exposure. Purpura also may follow long periods of standing or sitting. Due to other organ system involvement, arthralgia, renal symptoms, neurologic symptoms, abdominal pain, arterial thrombosis.

Skin lesions consist of the following:

*Noninflammatory purpura* (usually type I), occurring at cold-exposed sites, e.g., helix (Fig. 18-5), tip of nose.
*Acrocyanosis* and *Raynaud's phenomenon*, with or without severe resultant gangrene of fingertips and toes (usually types I or II) (Fig. 18-6).
*Palpable purpura* (usually types II and III) as in hypersensitivity vasculitis, occurring in crops on lower extremities with extension to thighs, abdomen; precipitated by

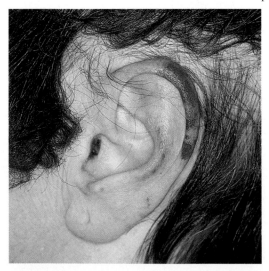

**FIGURE 18-5   Cryoglobulinemia: monoclonal (type I)**   *This noninflamed, purpuric lesion on the helix appeared on the first cold day in the fall.*

standing up (Fig. 18-7), less commonly by cold.

*Livedo reticularis* mostly on lower and upper extremities.

*Urticaria* induced by cold, associated with purpura.

Between 30 and 60% of individuals with essential mixed CG (type II) develop renal disease with hypertension, edema, or renal failure. Neurologic involvement manifests as peripheral sensorimotor polyneuropathy, presenting as paresthesias or foot drop. Arthritis. Hepatosplenomegaly.

Diagnosis is confirmed by determination of cryoglobulins (blood drawn into warmed syringe, RBC removed via warmed centrifuge; plasma refrigerated in a Wintrobe tube at 4°C for 24 to 72 h, then centrifuged and cryocrit determined) and diagnosis of underlying disease. The course is characterized by cyclic eruptions induced by cold or fluctuations of the activity of the underlying disease. Treatment is that of the underlying disease.

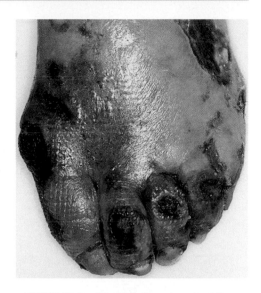

**FIGURE 18-6   Cryoglobulinemia: mixed (type II)**   *Associated Raynaud's phenomenon and arterial occlusion have resulted in extensive necroses, hemorrhage, and ulcerations on the skin of the foot.*

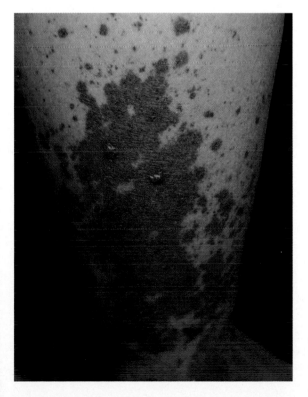

**FIGURE 18-7   Cryoglobulinemia: polyclonal (type III)**   *Palpable purpura with widespread hemorrhage and hemorrhagic blister formation as in any other type of hypersensitivity vasculitis (compare with Fig. 14-35).*

## LEUKEMIA CUTIS

Leukemia cutis (LC) is a localized or disseminated skin infiltration by leukemic cells. It is usually a sign of dissemination of systemic disease or relapse of existing leukemia. Reported incidence varies from <5 to 50%, depending on the type of leukemia, both acute and chronic, including the leukemic phase of non-Hodgkin's lymphoma and hairy cell leukemias. Most commonly occurs with acute monocytic leukemia M5 and acute myelomonocytic leukemia M4.

Pattern of presentation of skin lesions in LC is variable and may have features that overlap with other (inflammatory) eruptions. Most common lesions are small (2 to 5 mm) papules (Figs. 18-8 and 18-9), nodules (Figs. 18-10 and 18-11), or plaques. LC lesions are usually somewhat more pink, violaceous, or darker than normal skin, always palpable, indurated,

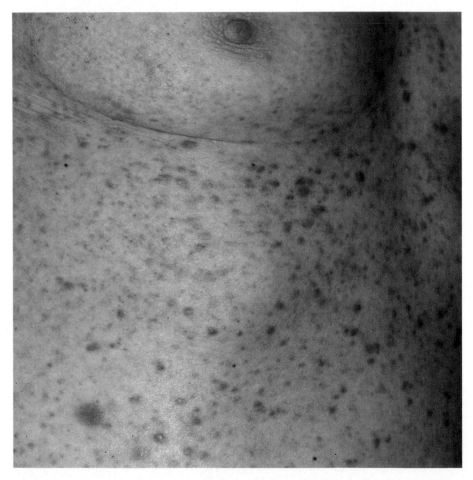

**FIGURE 18-8   Leukemia cutis**   *Hundreds of tan-pink papules and a nodule on the trunk of a female with acute myelogenous leukemia arose during a 1-week interval. Per se, these lesions are "nonspecific" and do not present a diagnosis; but when such an eruption is seen, one should perform a peripheral blood count and a biopsy.*

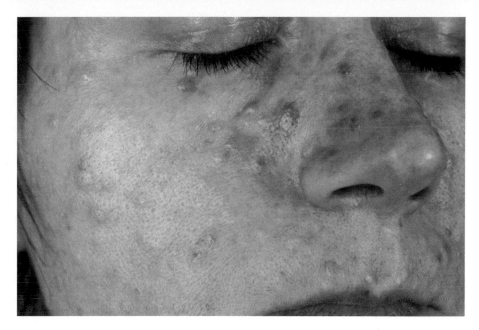

**FIGURE 18-9   Leukemia cutis**   *Multiple skin-colored and erythematous papules in a 38-year-old febrile woman that had erupted about 1 week before this picture was taken. The patient had acute myelogenous leukemia.*

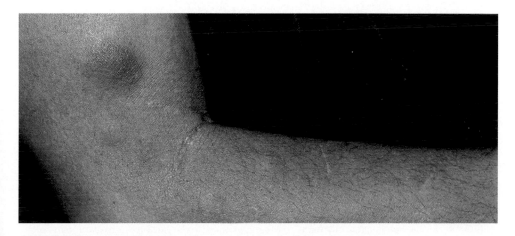

**FIGURE 18-10   Leukemia cutis**   *A large, dark brown nodule on the upper arm of a male with acute myelogenous leukemia; six similar nodules were also present on the trunk.*

firm, or guttate psoriasiform or lymphomatoid papulosis–like lesions, but usually not tender. Localized or disseminated; usually on trunk (Fig. 18-8), extremities (Fig. 18-10), and face (Fig. 18-9) but may occur at any site. May be hemorrhagic when associated with thrombocytopenia or may ulcerate (Fig. 18-11). Erythroderma may (rarely) occur. Leukemic gingival infiltration (hypertrophy) occurs with acute monocytic leukemia. Similar lesional morphologies occur with different types of leukemia or a specific type of leukemia may present with a variety of morphologies.

*Inflammatory disorders* occurring in patients with leukemia are modified by the participation of leukemic cells in the infiltrate, resulting in unusual presentations of such disorders, e.g., psoriasis with hemorrhage or erosions/ulcerations. Also there are a number of cutancous inflammatory diseases that may be associated with leukemia: Sweet's syndrome, bullous pyoderma gangrenosum, urticaria, and necrotizing vasculitis.

Systemic symptoms are those associated with hematologic malignancy. Not infrequently, cutaneous manifestation may be the initial presenting symptom and may contribute importantly to the diagnosis.

The *diagnosis* is made by suspicion and verified by skin biopsy, immunophenotyping, and B or T cell receptor rearrangement studies. Hematologic studies with complete analysis of bone marrow aspirate and peripheral blood smear are then needed to make the diagnosis. If cutaneous findings precede any systemic disease, careful assessment of peripheral blood smears and bone marrow biopsies must be made.

The prognosis for LC is directly related to the prognosis for the systemic disease. Therapy is usually directed at the leukemia itself. However, systemic chemotherapy sufficient for bone marrow remission may not treat the cutaneous lesions effectively. Thus, a combination of systemic chemotherapy and local electron beam therapy or PUVA may be necessary for chemotherapy-resistant LC lesions.

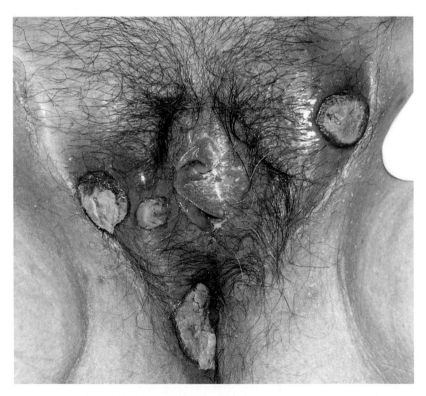

**FIGURE 18-11   Leukemia cutis: chloroma**   *Large, ulcerated, green-hued tumors (chloromas) in the inguinal and perineal regions of a female with acute myelogenous leukemia; similar lesions were also present in the axillae and on the tongue.*

# LANGERHANS CELL HISTIOCYTOSIS

Langerhans cell histiocytosis (LCH) is an idiopathic group of disorders characterized histolog-ically by proliferation and infiltration of tissue by Langerhans cell-type histiocytes that fuse into multinucleated giant cells and form granulomas with eosinophils. LCH is characterized clini-cally by cutaneous findings that range from soft tissue swelling to seborrheic dermatitis–like changes to ulceration and by lytic bony lesions.

## CLASSIFICATION

The disorders of xanthohistiocytic proliferation involving histiocytes, foam cells, and mixed in-flammatory cells are divided into Langerhans cell histiocytosis (LCH; formerly, histiocytosis X) and non-Langerhans cell histiocytosis (non-histiocytosis X). A simplified classification of LCH is presented in Table 18-1.

## EPIDEMIOLOGY AND ETIOLOGY

**Age of Onset**   *Unifocal LCH* Most commonly, childhood and early adulthood.
*Multifocal LCH* Most commonly, childhood.
*Letterer-Siwe Syndrome* More commonly, in-fancy and childhood. Also, adult form.
**Sex**   Males > females.
**Etiology**   Unknown.
**Incidence**   Rare, 0.5 per 100,000 children in the United States (estimate).

## PATHOGENESIS

The stimulus for the proliferation of Langer-hans cells is unknown.

## HISTORY

**Unifocal LCH**   Systemic symptoms uncommon. Pain and/or swelling over underlying bony le-sion. Disruption of teeth with mandibular dis-ease, fracture, otitis media due to mastoid involvement.
**Multifocal LCH**   Erosive skin lesions are ex-udative, pruritic, or painful and may have of-fensive odor. Otitis media caused by destruction of temporal and mastoid bones, proptosis due to orbital masses, loose teeth with infiltration of maxilla or mandible, pitu-itary dysfunction with involvement of sella turcica associated with growth retardation, diabetes insipidus. Triad of lytic skull lesions, proptosis, and diabetes insipidus: *Hand-Schüller-Christian disease.* Lung involvement associated with chronic cough, pneumotho-rax.
**LSS**   Child (or very rarely an adult) is system-ically ill with a course that resembles a sys-temic infection or malignancy. Hepatomegaly, petechiae, and purpura, generalized skin eruption.

## TABLE 18-1   Classification of LCH

| | |
|---|---|
| **Unifocal LCH** | Most commonly manifested by a single osteolytic bony lesion. Skin and soft tissue lesions not so uncommon (known as *eosinophilic granuloma*). |
| **Multifocal LCH** | Similar to unifocal LCH; however, bony lesions are multiple and interfere with function of neighb-oring structures. Multifocal LCH involves bones, skin (second most frequently involved organ), soft tissue, lymph nodes, lungs, and pituitary glands. |
| **Letterer-Siwe Syndrome** (LSS) | The most aggressive of multifocal LCH forms, with skin and internal organ involvement. |
| **Hashimoto-Pritzger Syndrome** | A benign, self-healing variant of LCH. |

## PHYSICAL EXAMINATION

### Skin Lesions

***Unifocal LCH*** (formerly called *eosinophilic granuloma*)

- Swelling over bony lesion (e.g., humerus, rib, mastoid), tender.
- Cutaneous/subcutaneous nodule, yellowish, may be tender and break down, occurring anywhere.
- Sharply marginated ulcer, usually in genital and perigenital regions or oral mucous membrane (gingiva, hard palate). Necrotic base, draining, tender (Fig. 18-12).

***Multifocal LCH*** As in unifocal LCH; in addition, regionally localized (head) or generalized (trunk) eruptions. Papulosquamous, seborrheic dermatitis–like (scaly, oily), eczematous dermatitis–like lesions (Fig. 18-13); sometimes vesicular or purpuric (Fig. 18-14). Turn necrotic and may become heavily crusted. Removal of crusts leaves small, shallow punched-out ulcers (Fig. 18-14). Intertriginous lesions coalesce, may be erosive and exudative, become secondarily infected and ulcerate. Mandibular and maxillary bone involvement may result in loss of teeth (Fig. 18-12). Ulceration of vulva and/or anus (Fig. 18-15).

**LSS** Skin lesions as in multifocal LCH but more widespread, disseminated (Fig. 18-14), and ulcerating in intertriginous regions (Fig. 18-15).

**General Findings** *Multifocal LCH* Bony lesions occur in calvarium, sphenoid bone, sella turcica, mandible, long bones of upper extremities, and vertebrae. Associated findings of pituitary involvement.

*LSS* Hepatosplenomegaly, lymphadenopathy, involvement of lungs and other organs, bone marrow; thrombocytopenia.

## LABORATORY EXAMINATIONS

**Histopathology** Constant histologic feature of LCH is proliferation of Langerhans cells with abundant pale eosinophilic cytoplasm and indistinct cell borders; a folded, indented, kidney-shaped nucleus with finely dispersed chromatin; Langerhans cells in LCH have to be recognized by morphologic, ultrastructural (Birbeck granules), histochemical, and immunohistochemical markers (ATPase, S-100 protein, $\alpha$-D-mannosidase, peanut agglutinin, CD1a).

## DIAGNOSIS

Confirmation of diagnosis by biopsy (skin, bone, or soft tissue/internal organs). Since skin is the organ most frequently involved after bone, skin biopsies have great diagnostic significance.

## COURSE AND PROGNOSIS

**Unifocal LCH** Benign course with excellent prognosis for spontaneous resolution.

**Multifocal LCH** Spontaneous remissions possible. Prognosis poorer at extremes of age and with extrapulmonary involvement.

**LSS** Commonly fulminant and fatal. Spontaneous remissions uncommon but there is a rare benign, self-healing variant of LCH in infants, termed *Hashimoto-Pritzger syndrome.* Current scoring systems for evaluation of prognosis are based on number of organs involved, presence or absence of organ dysfunction, and age. The worst prognosis is in the very young with multifocal LCH and organ dysfunction and in LSS.

## MANAGEMENT

**Unifocal LCH** Curettage with or without bony chip packing. Low-dose (300 to 600 rad) radiotherapy. Extraosseous soft tissue lesions: surgical excision or low-dose radiotherapy.

**Multifocal LCH** Diabetes insipidus and growth retardation treated with vasopressin and human growth hormone. Low-dose radiotherapy to bony lesions. Systemic treatment with glucocorticoids and/or vinblastine, mercaptopurine, and methotrexate, given as single agents or in combination, also with epipodophyllotoxin (etoposide). Topical glucocorticoids for discrete cutaneous lesions. Cutaneous lesions respond best to PUVA or topical nitrogen mustard but also to oral thalidomide.

**LSS** Only a few controlled studies of chemotherapy exist. The use of vinblastine results in complete or partial remission in 55%; combination chemotherapy in 70%. PUVA is effective in cutaneous lesions.

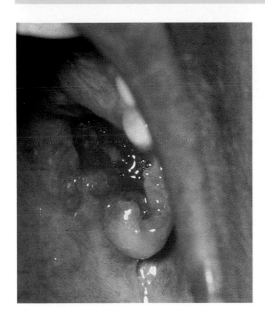

**FIGURE 18-12   Langerhans cell histiocytosis: eosinophilic granuloma**   *Solitary, ulcerated nodule with loss of teeth on the gingival ridge near the palate, associated with involvement of the maxillary bone. Lesion was asymptomatic and only when the molars were lost did the patient consult a physician.*

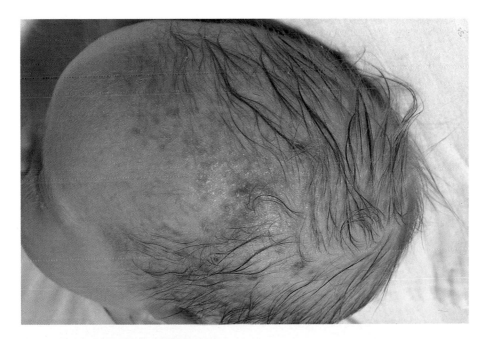

**FIGURE 18-13   Langerhans cell histiocytosis**   *Small, yellow-pink papules with a greasy scale on the scalp in this infant. These were the only lesions at first presentation and were mistaken for infantile seborrheic dermatitis. After lesions proved refractory to topical treatment and additional purpuric and crusted lesions appeared on the trunk, a biopsy was performed and the correct diagnosis was established.*

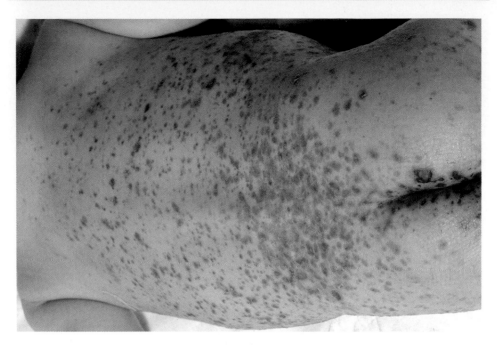

**FIGURE 18-14    Langerhans cell histiocytosis: Letterer-Siwe syndrome**    *Erythematous papules with purpura, crusting, and ulceration becoming confluent on the trunk and the intergluteal fold of a young child.*

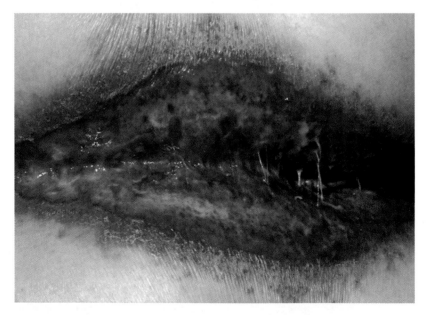

**FIGURE 18-15    Langerhans cell histiocytosis: Letterer-Siwe syndrome**    *Confluent erythematous papules with hemorrhage, necrosis, scaling, and ulceration in the anogenital and perineal region in a 65-year-old female.*

## MASTOCYTOSIS SYNDROMES  ▯ ◑

Mastocytosis is an abnormal accumulation of mast cells in the skin and at various systemic sites, which, because of pharmacologically active substances, is manifested clinically by local cutaneous (urticarial swelling) and systemic symptoms (flushing, vomiting, diarrhea, headache, syncope). The WHO classification that divides mastocytosis into a number of categories is given in Table 18-2. A classification of *cutaneous mastocytosis* (CM) is shown in Table 18-3.

Most patients with mastocytosis have only skin involvement, and most of these have no systemic symptoms. However, up to half of patients with systemic mastocytosis may not have any skin findings.

**TABLE 18-2  Abbreviated WHO Classification of Mastocytosis**

Cutaneous mastocytosis (CM)
Indolent systemic mastocytosis (ISM)
Systemic mastocytosis with an associated clonal hematologic
   non-mast cell lineage disease
Aggressive systemic mastocytosis (ASM)
Mast cell sarcoma (MCS)
Mast cell leukemia (MCL)
Extracutaneous mastocytoma

**TABLE 18-3  Classification of Cutaneous Mastocytosis (CM)**

| | |
|---|---|
| Localized | Nodular CM (mastocytoma, NCM) |
| Generalized | Maculopapular CM |
| |     Papular plaque CM (PPCM) |
| |     Urticaria pigmentosa (UP) |
| |     Telangiectasia macularis eruptiva perstans (TMEP) |
| |     Diffuse CM (DCM) |

## EPIDEMIOLOGY

**Age of Onset**   Between birth and 2 years of age (55%) (NCM, PPCM, UP), but mastocytosis can occur at any age; infancy-onset mastocytosis rarely associated with systemic mastocytosis.
**Sex**   Slight male:female predominance.
**Prevalence**   Unknown.

## PATHOGENESIS

Human mast cell proliferation depends on Kit ligand and Kit is the receptor for stem cell factor. c-*kit* mutations have been identified in blood and tissues of patients with mastocytosis. Mast cells contain several pharmacologically active substances that are associated with the clinical findings in mastocytosis: histamine (urticaria, GI symptoms), prostaglandin $D_2$ (flush, cardiovascular symptoms, bronchoconstriction, GI symptoms), heparin (bleeding into tissue, osteoporosis), neutral protease/acid hydrolases (patchy hepatic fibrosis, bone lesions).

## HISTORY

Stroking lesion causes it to itch and to wheal (*Darier's sign*). Various drugs are capable of causing mast cell degranulation and release of pharmacologically active substances that exacerbate skin lesions (whealing, itching) and cause flushing: alcohol, dextran, polymyxin B, morphine, codeine, scopolamine, D-tubocuratin, NSAIDs. Flushing episode can also be elicited by heat or cold and may be accompanied by headache, nausea, vomiting, diarrhea, dyspnea/wheezing, syncope. Systemic involvement may lead to symptoms of malabsorption; portal hypertension. Bone pain. Neuropsychiatric symptoms (malaise, irritability).

## PHYSICAL EXAMINATION

### Skin Lesions (CM)

**Localized**   *NCM* Macular to papular to nodular lesions (mastocytoma) (Fig. 18-16), often solitary; may be multiple, but few. Yellow to tan-pink, which become erythematous and raised (urticate) when stroked due to degranulation of mast cells (Darier's sign); in some patients, lesions become bullous.
**Generalized**   *PPCM* Tan, occasionally yellowish plaques, up to 2 to 5 cm, sharply defined with irregular outlines. Darier's sign positive (Fig. 18-17). No scaling, occasionally with bulla formation after rubbing. Occurs mostly in infants and children.
*UP* Tan macules to slightly raised tan to brown papules (Fig. 18-18). Disseminated, few or >100 with widespread symmetric distribution. Darier's sign (whealing) after rubbing; in infants may become bullous. Occurs in infancy and/or de novo in adults. Bright red diffuse flushing occurring spontaneously, after rubbing of skin, or after ingestion of alcohol or mast cell–degranulating agents.
*TMEP* Freckle-like, brownish to reddish macules (Fig. 18-19) with fine telangiectasia in long-standing lesions. Hundreds of lesions, trunk > extremities; lesions may be confluent. Urticate with gentle stroking. Dermatographism. Occur only in adults.
*DCM* Yellowish, thickened appearance of large areas of skin; "doughy." Smooth with scattered elevation, resembling leather, "pseudoxanthomatous mastocytosis," skin folds exaggerated, especially in axilla/groin. Large bullae may occur after trauma or spontaneously. DCM may present as erythroderma (Fig. 18-20). Very rare, occurs at all ages.
**Systemic Symptoms**   Flushing, accompanied by wheezing, headache, asthmatic attacks, nausea,

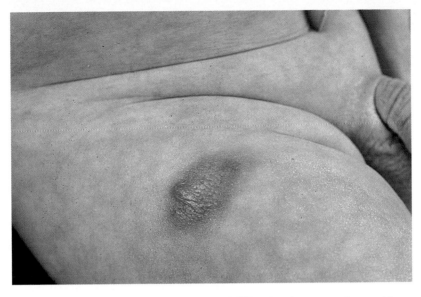

**FIGURE 18-16   Mastocytosis: solitary mastocytoma (NCM)**   *A solitary, tan plaque with poorly demarcated borders on the thigh of a young child. When stroked very vigorously, the lesion became red, more elevated and a blister developed.*

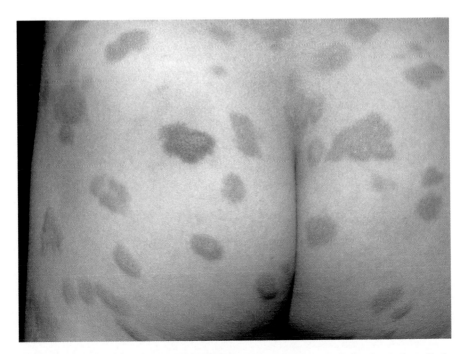

**FIGURE 18-17   Mastocytosis: generalized (PPCM)**   *Multiple, flattopped papules and small plaques of brownish color on the buttocks of a child. Lesions are asymptomatic. Rubbing one of the lesions has resulted in urtication and an axon flare, a positive Darier's sign.*

vomiting, diarrhea, syncope. Bone pain/spontaneous fractures with osteolytic lesions. Neuropsychiatric symptoms, malaise, irritability. Malabsorption, weight loss.

## LABORATORY EXAMINATIONS

**Dermatopathology**   Accumulation of normal-looking mast cells in dermis. Mast cell infiltrates may be sparse (spindle-shaped mast cells) or densely aggregated (cuboidal shape) and have a perivascular or nodular distribution. Pigmentation due to increased melanin in basal layer.
**CBC**   Systemic mastocytosis: anemia, leukocytosis, eosinophilia.
**Blood**   Tryptase levels↑, coagulation parameters.
**Urine**   Patients with extensive cutaneous involvement may have increased 24-h urinary histamine excretion.

**Bone Scan and Imaging**   Define bone involvement (lytic bone lesions, osteoporosis, or osteosclerosis), and endoscopy for small bowel involvement.
**Bone Marrow**   Smear and/or biopsy for morphology and mast cell markers.

## DIAGNOSIS

Clinical suspicion, positive Darier's sign, confirmed by skin biopsy.

## DIFFERENTIAL DIAGNOSIS

**NCM**   Juvenile xanthogranuloma, Spitz nevus.
**Flushing**   Carcinoid syndrome.
**UP, PPCM, TMEP**   Langerhans cell histiocytosis, secondary syphilis, papular sarcoid, generalized eruptive histiocytoma, non-Langerhans cell histiocytosis of childhood.

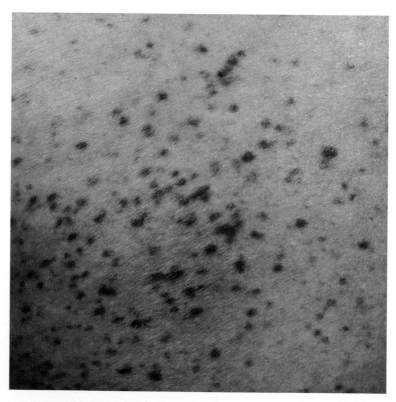

**FIGURE 18-18   Mastocytosis: urticaria pigmentosa (UP)**   *Multiple, generalized tan to brown papules in a 38-year-old male. The patient had occasional syncopes, diarrhea, and wheezing; work-up revealed systemic mastocytosis.*

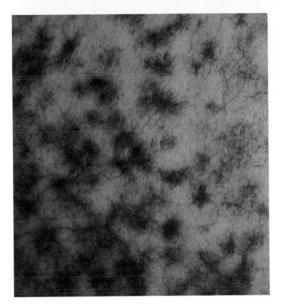

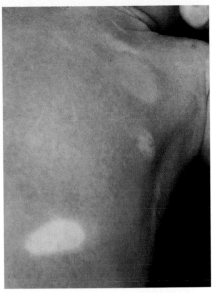

**FIGURE 18-19   Mastocytosis: telangiectasia macularis eruptiva perstans** *Small, stellate erythematous macules and telangiectases on the back of a 45-year-old woman who had systemic (indolent) mastocytosis.*

**FIGURE 18-20   Mastocytosis: diffuse cutaneous mastocytosis** *The skin of this infant is uniformly erythematous (erythroderma) secondary to infiltrating mast cells with several spared, white areas of normal skin. In this child there were systemic symptoms associated with the flare of this erythroderma: syncope, wheezing, and diarrhea.*

**DCM** Cutaneous T cell lymphoma, pseudoxanthoma elasticum, forms of erythroderma.

### COURSE AND PROGNOSIS

Most cases of solitary mastocytosis and generalized UP and PPCM in children resolve spontaneously. They rarely have systemic involvement. Adults with onset of UP or TMEP with extensive cutaneous involvement have a higher risk for development of systemic mastocytosis. In young children, acute and extensive degranulation may be life-threatening (shock).

### MANAGEMENT

Avoidance of drugs that may cause mast cell degranulation and histamine release (see above).

Antihistamines, both $H_1$ and $H_2$, either alone or with ketotifen. Disodium cromoglycate, 200 mg qid, may ameliorate pruritus, flushing, diarrhea, abdominal pain, and disorders of cognitive function but not skin lesions. PUVA treatment is effective for disseminated skin lesions, but recurrence is common. Vascular collapse is treated with epinephrine. NCM responds to potent glucocorticoid ointments under occlusion or to intralesional triamcinolone acetonide but may eventually recur.

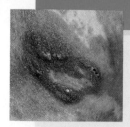

# CUTANEOUS LYMPHOMAS AND SARCOMA

## LYMPHOMATOID PAPULOSIS    □   ◑

Lymphomatoid papulosis is an asymptomatic, chronic, self-healing, polymorphous eruption of unknown etiology characterized by recurrent crops of lesions that regress spontaneously, with histologic features of lymphocytic atypia. It is a low-grade, self-limited T cell lymphoma with a low but real risk of progression to more malignant forms of lymphoma.

### EPIDEMIOLOGY

**Incidence**   1.2 to 1.9 cases per million, occurring sporadically in both sexes from childhood to old age; average age 40 years.

### PATHOGENESIS

Unknown; considered to be a low-grade lymphoma perhaps induced by chronic antigenic stimulation and controlled by host mechanisms. It may thus begin as a chronic, reactive, polyclonal lymphoproliferative phenomenon that sporadically overwhelms host immune defenses and evolves into a clonal, antigen-independent, true lymphoid malignancy. It belongs in the spectrum of primary cutaneous Ki-1+ lymphoproliferative disorders, including pseudo-Hodgkin's disease of the skin, regressing atypical histiocytosis, Hodgkin's lymphoma, and Ki-1+ large cell lymphoma.

### HISTORY

Usually asymptomatic; occasionally, lesions are pruritic, tender, or painful. If weight loss, anorexia, fever, sweating are present, pursue workup for systemic lymphoma.

### PHYSICAL EXAMINATION

**Skin Findings**
Close clinical resemblance to pityriasis lichenoides et varioliformis acuta (see Fig. 7-18).

Erythematous to red-brown papules (Fig. 19-1) and nodules, 2 to 5 mm in diameter, which are initially smooth and hemorrhagic, later hyperkeratotic, with central, black necrosis, crusting (Fig. 19-1), and ulceration. Few to hundreds of lesions, arranged at random and often grouped, appear in crops of recurrent eruptions primarily on trunk and extremities; rarely, oral and genital mucosa. Individual lesions evolve over a 2- to 8-week period and resolve spontaneously at any point in their evolution. Atrophic hyper- or hypopigmented scarring following ulcerated lesions.
**Other Organ Systems**   Uninvolved.

### LABORATORY EXAMINATIONS

**Dermatopathology**   Superficial or deep, perivascular or interstitial mixed cell infiltrate, wedge-shaped. Cytologically, atypical cells may comprise 50% of infiltrate. *Type A*: large, atypical histiocytic-looking lymphocytes with abundant cytoplasm, convoluted nucleus with occasional binucleation, multipolar mitosis, and Reed-Sternberg cell apppearance. *Type B*: smaller, atypical lymphocytes with cerebriform nuclei, epidermotropism, and occasional mitosis.
**Immunohistochemistry**   Predominantly activated, interleukin(IL) 2 receptor–positive, HLA-DR-positive, Ki-1 (CD30)-positive T helper cells (CD4). Also, there is often a loss of T cell antigens as in T cell lymphomas. Large atypical CD30+ cells are polyclonal, whereas smaller CD30− T cells are monoclonal.

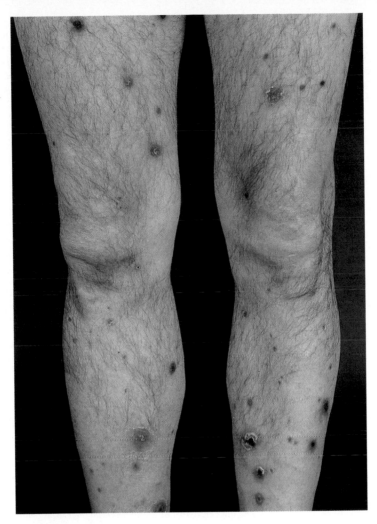

**FIGURE 19-1   Lymphomatoid papulosis**   *Crops of reddish-brown papules appear in waves involving the entire body. Lesions are asymptomatic, become hyperkeratotic, crusted, and necrotic in the center. Since lesions arise asynchronously, all stages in this evolution are present simultaneously.*

**Other**   Negative workup for systemic involvement.

## DIAGNOSIS AND DIFFERENTIAL DIAGNOSIS

Based on typical histology and immunohistochemistry, lack of systemic involvement by history and physical examination. May necessitate periodic biopsy to rule out blastic transformation, especially with tumor formation. No reliable histologic, immunohistochemical, or genotypic test available for prediction of risk of progression to lymphoma.

**Multiple Papules/Nodules in Various Stages of Development**   *Pityriasis lichenoides et varioliformis acuta. Various lymphomas, large cell anaplastic T cell lymphoma, regressing atypical histiocytosis;* papular mycosis fungoides; also Langerhans cell histiocytosis, papular drug eruption, papular urticaria, rickettsiosis, arthropod bites, and scabies.

## COURSE AND PROGNOSIS

May remit in 3 weeks or continue for decades. Patients may experience periods without lesions or have continuous, repetitive outbreaks. In 10 to 20% of patients, lymphomatoid papulosis is preceded by, associated with, or followed by another type of lymphoma: mycosis fungoides, Hodgkin's disease, or CD30+ large cell lymphoma. May persist despite systemic chemotherapy for concurrent lymphoma.

## MANAGEMENT

No treatments have proved consistently effective, as is evidenced by the multiple reported therapies. Topical agents include glucocorticoids and carmustine (BCNU). Electron-beam irradiation has been employed as well. PUVA may control the disease but does not affect the long-term prognosis. Tetracyclines, sulfones, systemic glucocorticoids, and even acyclovir have been anecdotally reported as effective. Also, a wide spectrum of other systemic agents has been used, including retinoids, methotrexate, chlorambucil, cyclophosphamide, cyclosporine, and interferon-α2b, none with lasting effect.

# ADULT T CELL LEUKEMIA/LYMPHOMA    □   ●

Adult T cell leukemia/lymphoma (ATLL) is a neoplasm of CD4+ T cells, caused by human T cell lymphotrophic virus I (HTLV-I), manifested by skin infiltrates, hypercalcemia, visceral involvement, lytic bone lesions, and abnormal lymphocytes on peripheral smears.

HTLV-I is a human retrovirus. Malignant cells are activated CD4+ T cells with an increased expression of the α chain of the IL-2 receptor. Infection by the virus does not usually cause disease, which suggests that other environmental factors are involved. Immortalization of some infected CD4+ T cells, increased mitotic activity, genetic instability, and impairment of cellular immunity can all occur after infection with HTLV-I. These events may increase the probability of additional genetic changes, which, by chance, may lead to the development of leukemia 20 to 40 years after infection in some people (≤5%). Most of these effects have been attributed to the HTLV-I-encoded protein tax.

ATLL occurs in southwestern Japan (Kyushu), Africa, the Caribbean Islands, southeastern United States. Transmission is by sexual intercourse, perinatally, or by exposure to blood or blood products (same as HIV).

There are four main categories. In the relatively indolent *smoldering* and *chronic* forms, the median survival is ≥2 years. In the *acute* and *lymphomatous* forms, it ranges from only 4 to 6 months.

Symptoms include fever, weight loss, abdominal pain, diarrhea, pleural effusion, ascites, cough, sputum. Skin lesions occur in 50% of patients with ATLL. Single to multiple small, confluent erythematous, violaceous papules (Fig. 19-2), ±purpura; firm violaceous to brownish nodules (Fig. 19-3); papulosquamous lesions, large plaques, ±ulceration; trunk > face > extremities; generalized erythroderma; poikiloderma; diffuse alopecia. Lymphadenopathy (75%) sparing mediastinal lymph nodes. There is hepatomegaly (50%) and splenomegaly (25%).

Patients are seropositive (ELISA, Western blot) to HTLV-I; in IV drug users, up to 30% have dual retroviral infection with both HTLV-I and HIV. WBC ranges from normal to 500,000/μL. Peripheral blood smears show polylobulated lymphocytic nuclei ("flower cells"). *Dermatopathology* reveals lymphomatous infiltrates composed of many large abnormal lymphocytes, ±giant cells, ±Pautrier's microabscesses. There is hypercalcemia—in 25% at time of diagnosis of ATLL and in >50% during clinical course; this is thought to be due to osteoclastic bone resorption.

*Diagnosis* is based on characteristic clinical findings, seropositivity to HTLV-I, confirmation of integration of HTLV-I proviral DNA in the cellular DNA of the ATLL cells. Course may be smoldering or chronic for prolonged period or progressive lymphoma. Mean survival with acute crisis in hypercalcemic patients 12.5 weeks (range 2 weeks to 1 year); if normocalcemic, 50 weeks. Cause of death: opportunistic infections, disseminated intravascular coagulation.

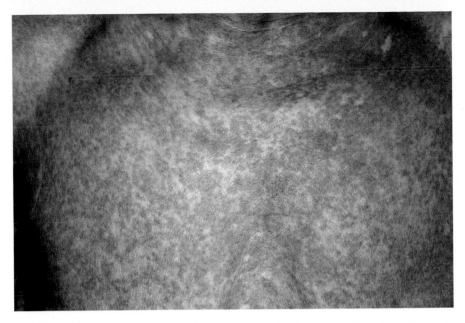

**FIGURE 19-2   Adult T cell leukemia/lymphoma**   *A generalized eruption of small, confluent violaceous papules with a predilection for the trunk. The patient had fever, weight loss, abdominal pain, massive leukocytosis with "flower cells" in smear, lymphadenopathy, hepatosplenomegaly and hypercalcemia.*

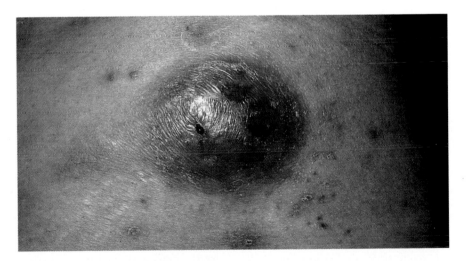

**FIGURE 19-3   Adult T cell leukemia/lymphoma**   *Firm, violaceous to brownish nodules as shown here are another cutaneous manifestation of ATLL. These nodules may ulcerate.*

Management consists of various regimens of cytotoxic chemotherapy; the rates of complete response are <30% and responses lack durability, but excellent results have been obtained with the combination of oral zidovudine and subcutaneous interferon-α in acute and lymphoma-type ATLL patients.

# CUTANEOUS T CELL LYMPHOMA   ▯ ●

Cutaneous T cell lymphoma (CTCL) is a term that applies to T cell lymphoma first manifested in the skin, but since the neoplastic process involves the entire lymphoreticular system, the lymph nodes and internal organs become involved in the course of the disease. CTCL is a malignancy of helper T cells (CD4+). In the classic form of CTCL, called *mycosis fungoides* (MF), the malignant cells are cutaneous CD4+ cells, but the old clinical entity of MF has now been expanded to the spectrum of CTCL including non-MF cutaneous T cell lymphomas. Whereas all MF is CTCL not all CTCLs are MF. Only the classic MF form is discussed here. *Synonym*: Mycosis fungoides.

## EPIDEMIOLOGY AND ETIOLOGY

**Age of Onset**   50 years (range 5 to 70 years).
**Sex**   Male:female ratio 2:1.
**Incidence**   Uncommon but not rare.
**Etiology**   Unknown, but HTLV in some patients. CTCL is a malignancy of skin-homing T cells.

## HISTORY

For months to years, often preceded by various diagnoses such as psoriasis, nummular dermatitis, and "large plaque" parapsoriasis. Symptoms: pruritus, often intractable, but may be none.

## PHYSICAL EXAMINATION

### Skin Findings
Randomly distributed, scaling or nonscaling patches or plaques in different shades of red (Fig. 19-4). Well- or ill-defined; at first superficial, much like eczema or psoriasis or mimicking dermatophytosis ("mycosis") (Fig. 19-5), and later becoming thicker (Fig. 19-6). Round, oval, but often also arciform, annular, and of bizarre configuration (Figs. 19-5 and 19-6). Lesions are randomly distributed but in early stages often spare exposed areas.

Later lesions consist of nodules (Fig. 19-6) and tumors, with or without ulceration (Fig. 19-7). Extensive infiltration can cause leonine facies (Fig. 19-8). Confluence may lead to erythroderma (see Section 8). There is palmoplantar keratoderma and there may be hair loss. Poikiloderma may be present from the onset or develop later (Fig. 19-9).

**General Examination**   Lymphadenopathy, usually after thick plaques and nodules have appeared.

**Sézary's Syndrome**   This is a leukemic form of CTCL described on page 534.

**Pageoid Reticulosis (Woringer-Kolopp Disease)**   This is a special variant of CTCL consisting of localized patches and plaques (Fig. 19-10), with a proliferation of neoplastic T cells, that expand intraepidermally following a pattern similar to Paget's disease. Extracutaneous dissemination has not been observed, and there is an excellent prognosis.

## LABORATORY EXAMINATIONS

**Dermatopathology**   In early stages repeated and multiple biopsies are often necessary to finally establish the diagnosis. Bandlike and patchy infiltrate in upper dermis of atypical lymphocytes (mycosis cells) extending to epidermis and skin appendages. The classic finding is the epidermotropism of this T cell infiltrate, which will form microabscesses in the epidermis (Pautrier's microabscesses). In the plaque and tumor stage the infiltrate extends deep into the dermis and beyond. Mycosis cells are T cells with hyperchromatic, irregularly shaped (cerebriform) nuclei. Mitoses vary from rare to frequent.

Mycosis cells are activated monoclonal CD4+ T cells. However, lesions of CTCL often have a CD8+ T cell component, and these cells are considered to reflect an antitumor response; improved long-term prognosis has been correlated with the presence of such CD8+ tumor-infiltrating lymphocytes. Immunophenotypically, there are also other forms of CTCL syndromes: CD8+ T cell lymphomas, gamma-delta T cell lymphomas, and cutaneous natural killer cell lymphomas.

**Hematology**   Eosinophilia, 6 to 12%, can increase to 50%. Buffy coat: abnormal circulating T cells (Sézary type) and increased WBC

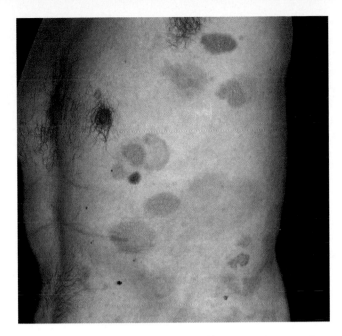

**FIGURE 19-4   Cutaneous T cell lymphoma/mycosis fungoides**   *In early stages lesions consist of randomly distributed, well- and/or ill-defined plaques as shown here in a 37-year-old male. They may be scaly and appear in various shades of red. They mimic eczema, psoriasis, or dermatophytosis.*

(20,000/µL). Bone marrow examination is not helpful in early stages.

**Chemistry**   Lactic dehydrogenase isoenzymes 1, 2, and 3 increased in erythrodermic stage.

**Chest X-Ray**   Search for hilar lymphadenopathy.

**Imaging**   In stage I and stage II disease, diagnostic imaging (CT, gallium scintigraphy, liver-spleen scan, and lymphangiography) does not provide more information than biopsies of lymph nodes.

*CT Scan*   With more advanced disease, to search for retroperitoneal nodes in patients with extensive skin involvement, lymphadenopathy.

## DIAGNOSIS AND DIFFERENTIAL DIAGNOSIS

In the early stages, the diagnosis of CTCL is a problem. Clinical lesions may be typical, but histologic confirmation may not be possible for years despite repeated biopsies. Tissue should be sent for immunophenotyping of infiltrating T cells by use of monoclonal antibodies and T cell receptor rearrangement studies. Lymphadenopathy and the detection of abnormal circulating T cells in the blood appear to correlate well with *internal* organ involvement.

**Differential Diagnosis**   Mainly *scaling plaques* (see Figs. 19-4 and 19-5). High index of suspicion is needed in patients with atypical or refractory "psoriasis," "eczema," and poikiloderma. CTCL often mimics psoriasis in being a scaly plaque and disappearing with exposure to sunlight.

**Patient Evaluation in CTCL and Staging**   This has to focus on an evaluation of tumor burden, the degree of atypia of malignant cells, and the state of immunocompetence of the patient. Table 19-1 shows a flow sheet of patient evaluation,

## TABLE 19-1    Patient Evaluation

Skin
    Body surface area assessment
    Routine histology
    Immunophenotyping
    Polymerase chain reaction for T cell
        receptor rearrangement
Blood
    Complete blood count with smear
        examination
    Immunophenotyping
Lymph node
    Palpate all nodes
    Measure enlarged nodes by CT scan
    Biopsy enlarged nodes

SOURCE: JA Latkowski, P Heald, in IM Freedberg, AZ
    Eisen, K Wolff, KF Austen, LA Goldsmith, SI Katz
    (eds): *Fitzpatrick's Dermatology in General Medicine*,
    6th ed. New York, McGraw-Hill, 2003.

Table 19-2 the TNM classification of CTCL and
Table 19-3 the staging of CTCL.

## COURSE AND PROGNOSIS

Unpredictable; CTCL (pre-CTCL) may be
present for years. Course varies with the source
of the patients studied. At the NIH there was a
median survival time of 5 years from the time
of the histologic diagnosis, while in Europe a
less malignant course is seen (survival time, up
to 10 to 15 years). This, however, may be due to
patient selection. Prognosis is much worse
when (1) tumors are present (mean survival, 2.5
years), (2) there is lymphadenopathy (mean
survival, 3 years), (3) >10% of the skin surface
is involved with pretumor-stage CTCL, and (4)
there is a generalized erythroderma. Patients
<50 years have twice the survival rate of pa-
tients >60 years.

## MANAGEMENT

In the pre-CTCL stage, in which the histologic
diagnosis is only compatible, but not confirmed, PUVA photochemotherapy is the most
effective treatment, but narrowband UVB treatment is also effective. For histologically proven
plaque-stage disease with no lymphadenopathy
and no abnormal circulating T cells, PUVA
photochemotherapy is also the method of
choice, either alone or combined with oral
isotretinoin or subcutaneous interferon-$\alpha$. Also
used at this stage are topical chemotherapy
with nitrogen mustard in an ointment base
(10 mg/dL) and total-body electron-beam therapy, singly or in combination. Isolated tumors
that may develop should be treated with local

## TABLE 19-2    TNM Classification of CTCL [Mycosis Fungoides (MF)]

| T: Skin | $T_0$ | Clinically and/or histologically suspicious lesions |
|---|---|---|
| | $T_1$ | Limited plaques, papules, or eczematous patches covering <10% of the skin surface |
| | $T_2$ | Generalized plaques, papules, or erythematous patches covering >10% of the skin surface |
| | $T_3$ | Tumors (1 or more) |
| | $T_4$ | Generalized erythroderma |
| N: Lymph nodes | $N_0$ | No clinically abnormal peripheral nodes, pathology negative for MF |
| | $N_1$ | Clinically abnormal peripheral lymph nodes, pathology negative for MF |
| | $N_2$ | No clinically abnormal peripheral lymph nodes, pathology positive for MF |
| | $N_3$ | Clinically abnormal peripheral lymph nodes, pathology positive for MF |
| B: Blood | $B_0$ | <5% atypical circulating lymphocytes |
| | $B_1$ | >5% atypical circulating lymphocytes (Sézary's) |
| M: Visceral organs | $M_0$ | No visceral organ involvement |
| | $M_1$ | Histologically proven visceral involvement |

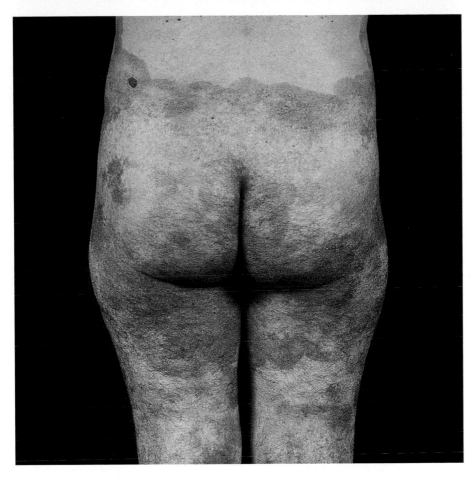

**FIGURE 19-5   Cutaneous T cell lymphoma/mycosis fungoides**   *More advanced stages show confluence of plaques with bizarre configuration and areas of poikiloderma. This patient had been treated unsuccessfully for psoriasis for 2 years. Morphologically, he could also have extensive, confluent dermatophytosis (compare with Fig. 23-10) but the ill-defined plaques and poikiloderma in the popliteal fossae (not shown here) and a negative KOH preparation ruled out this diagnosis. Only after a biopsy had been done was the correct diagnosis of CTCL made.*

**TABLE 19-3   Staging System for CTCL**

| Stage | T | N | M |
|-------|-----|-------|-------|
| IA  | $T_1$     | $N_0$     | $M_0$ |
| IB  | $T_2$     | $N_0$     | $M_0$ |
| IIA | $T_{1-2}$ | $N_1$     | $M_0$ |
| IIB | $T_3$     | $N_{0-1}$ | $M_0$ |
| III | $T_4$     | $N_{0-1}$ | $M_0$ |
| IVA | $T_{1-4}$ | $N_{2-3}$ | $M_0$ |
| IVB | $T_{1-4}$ | $N_{0-3}$ | $M_1$ |

x-ray or electron-beam therapy. For extensive plaque stage with multiple tumors or in patients with lymphadenopathy or abnormal circulating T cells, electron-beam plus chemotherapy is probably the best combination for now; randomized, controlled studies of various combinations are in progress. Also, extracorporeal PUVA photochemotherapy is being evaluated in patients with Sézary's syndrome.

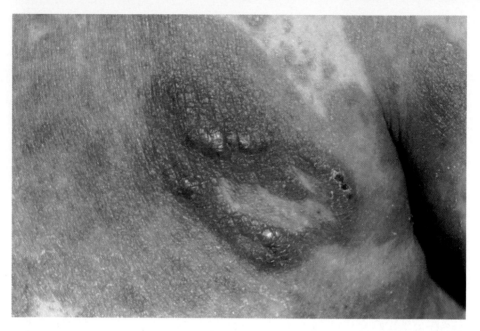

**FIGURE 19-6   Cutaneous T cell lymphoma/mycosis fungoides**   *Early nodular stage with reddish-brownish smooth, or scaly, and crusted nodules within a psoriasis-like plaque.*

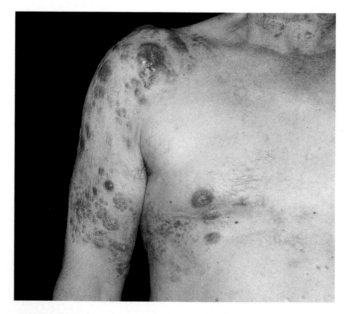

**FIGURE 19-7   Cutaneous T cell lymphoma/mycosis fungoides: tumor stage**   *Scaly and crusted eczema-like plaques seen on the arm and chest have turned nodular on the shoulder. This patient had similar lesions elsewhere and was staged IIB ($T_3 N_1 M_0$).*

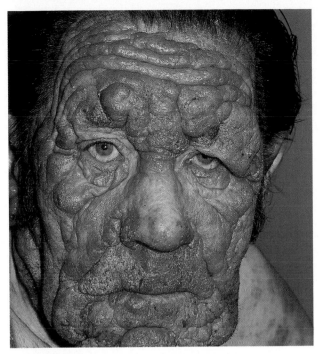

**FIGURE 19-8   Cutaneous T cell lymphoma/mycosis fungoides: leonine facies**   *In this 50-year-old patient the disease had started with extremely pruritic, generalized eczema-like plaques on the trunk that had been treated as eczema over a course of 4 years. Massive nodular infiltration of the face occurred only recently leading to a leonine facies.*

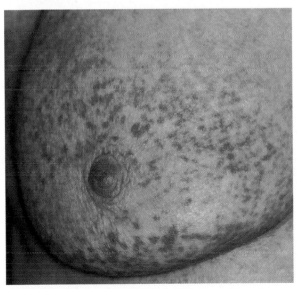

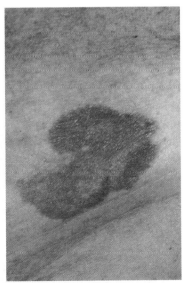

**FIGURE 19-9   (Left)   Cutaneous T cell lymphoma/mycosis fungoides: poikilodermatous lesions**
*Small reticulated, confluent papules mixed with superficial atrophy give the impression of poikiloderma. This patient had plaques elsewhere on the body similar to those shown in Fig. 19-4.*

**FIGURE 19-10   (Right)   Cutaneous T cell lymphoma: pagetoid reticulosis**   *This singular plaque on the abdomen of a 62-year-old male looks like psoriasis but is irregular with notched margins. It was asymptomatic and had been present for 8 months. Histopathology revealed intraepidermal T cells in a pagetoid pattern.*

# SÉZARY'S SYNDROME □ ●

Sézary's syndrome is a rare special variant of cutaneous T cell lymphoma (CTCL, mycosis fungoides) characterized by universal erythroderma, peripheral lymphadenopathy, and cellular infiltrates of atypical lymphocytes (Sézary cells) in the skin and in the blood. The disease may arise de novo or, less commonly, result from extension of a preexisting circumscribed CTCL. It usually occurs in patients >60 years and more commonly in males than in females.

Patients appear sick, shivering, and scared and there is generalized scaling erythroderma with considerable thickening of the skin. Because of the bright red color, the syndrome has been called the "red man syndrome" (see Section 8 and Fig. 8-3). There is diffuse hyperkeratosis of palms and soles, diffuse hair loss that can lead to baldness, and generalized lymphadenopathy.

*Dermatopathology*: the same as CTCL. The lymph nodes may contain nonspecific inflammatory cells (dermatopathic lymphadenopathy) or there can be a complete replacement of the nodal pattern by Sézary cells. The cell infiltrates in the viscera in CTCL are the same as are present in the skin. *Immunophenotyping*: CD4+ T cells; T cell receptor rearrangement: monoclonal process. There may be a moderate leukocytosis or a normal WBC. The buffy coat contains from 15 to 30% atypical lymphocytes (Sézary cells). Diagnosis rests on three features: erythroderma, generalized lymphadenopathy, and presence of increased numbers of atypical lymphocytes in the buffy coat. But note that any exfoliative dermatitis can mimic Sézary's syndrome (see Section 8).

Without treatment, the course is progressive and patients die from opportunistic infections. Management is as in CTCL, plus appropriate supportive measures required for erythroderma (see Section 8).

# CUTANEOUS B CELL LYMPHOMA □ ●

A clonal proliferation of B lymphocytes can be confined to the skin or more often is associated with systemic B cell lymphoma. Rare. Occurs in individuals >50 years and consists of crops of asymptomatic nodules and plaques, red to plum color (Fig. 19-11) with a smooth surface, firm, nontender, cutaneous or subcutaneous. Dermatopathology shows dense nodular or diffuse monomorphous infiltrates of lymphocytes usually separated from the epidermis by a zone of normal collagen ("grenz zone"). B cell–specific monoclonal antibody studies facilitate differentiation of cutaneous B cell lymphoma from pseudolymphoma and cutaneous T cell lymphoma and permit more accurate classification of the cell type. Most cases react with CD19, 20, 22, and 28. Gene-typing studies confirm diagnosis with immunoglobulin gene rearrangement.

Patients should be investigated thoroughly for nodal and extracutaneous disease; if found, bone marrow, lymph node, and peripheral blood studies will show morphologic, cytochemical, and immunologic features similar to those of the cutaneous infiltrates. Management consists of x-ray therapy to localized lesions and chemotherapy for systemic disease.

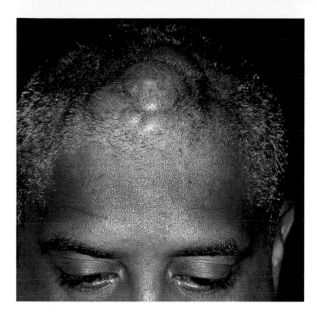

**FIGURE 19-11   Cutaneous B cell lymphoma**  *Smooth, cutaneous and subcutaneous nodules on the scalp. They were asymptomatic and firm and were the first signs of B cell lymphoma (leukemia).*

## CUTANEOUS Ki-1+ LYMPHOMA  □

Ki-1+ lymphomas are cutaneous lymphomas consisting of large tumor cells that express CD30 antigen and have no evidence or history of lymphomatoid papulosis, mycosis fungoides, or other types of CTCL. They occur in adults and present as solitary, reddish to brownish nodules and tumors, which frequently tend to ulcerate (Fig. 19-12). The nodular infiltrates are nonepidermotropic, and neoplastic cells show an anaplastic morphology. At least 75% of the neoplastic cells are CD30+ and additionally express the CD4+ phenotype. CD30+ cutaneous large cell lymphomas have a favorable prognosis with a disease-related 5-year survival rate of 90%. Treatment is radiotherapy, but successful treatment with PUVA in combination with interferon-α has been reported.

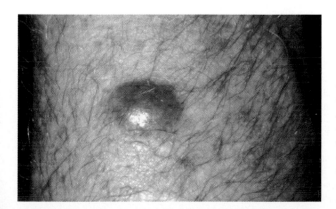

**FIGURE 19-12   Ki-1+ lymphoma**  *A solitary violaceous, reddish nodule on the forearm of a 46-year-old male patient. Histopathology revealed nonepidermotropic anaplastic mononuclear cells, most of which were of the CD4+, CD30+ phenotype. The lesion was excised and there was no recurrence.*

# KAPOSI'S SARCOMA     ▣  ◑ → ●

Kaposi's sarcoma (KS) is a multisystem vascular neoplasia characterized by mucocutaneous violaceous lesions and edema as well as involvement of nearly any organ. Many individuals with KS are in some degree immunocompromised, especially those with HIV disease. *Synonym*: Multiple idiopathic hemorrhagic sarcoma.

## ETIOPATHOGENESIS

DNA of human herpesvirus type 8 (HHV-8) has been identified in tissue samples of all variants of KS. There is seroepidemiologic evidence that this virus is involved in the pathogenesis.

## CLASSIFICATION AND CLINICAL VARIANTS

**Classic or European KS**   Occurs in elderly males of eastern European heritage (Mediterranean and Ashkenazi Jewish). Not so uncommon in eastern and southern Europe; rare in the United States. Peak incidence after sixth decade. Males > females. Predominantly arises on the legs but also occurs in lymph nodes and abdominal viscera; slowly progressive.

**African-Endemic KS**   Between 9 and 12.8% of all malignancies in Zaire. Two distinct age groups: young adults, mean age 35; and young children, mean age 3 years. Males > females. No evidence of underlying immunodeficiency. Four clinical patterns (see below).

**HIV-Associated KS**   In HIV-infected individuals, the risk for KS is 20,000 times that of the general population, 300 times that of other immunosuppressed individuals. Early in the HIV epidemic in the United States and Europe, 50% of homosexual men at the time of initial diagnosis of AIDS had KS; currently, the incidence is 18% in this risk group. Young adults. HIV-associated KS occurs almost exclusively in homosexual males; rarely women may have HIV-associated KS when they acquire HIV infection via heterosexual exposure from a bisexual male. Associated with HIV infection, rapid progression, extensive systemic involvement. At the time of initial presentation, one in six HIV-infected individuals with KS have CD4+ T cell counts of ≤500/μL.

**Iatrogenic Immunosuppression-Associated KS**   Rare. Most commonly in solid-organ transplant recipients as well as individuals treated chronically with immunosuppressive drugs. Arises on average 16.5 months after transplantation. Resolves on cessation of immunosuppression.

## PATHOGENESIS

KS cells likely are derived from the endothelium of the blood/lymphatic microvasculature. Not a true malignancy but rather a widespread reactive cellular proliferation in response to angiogenic substances. KS lesions produce factors that promote their own growth as well as the growth of other cells, but it is not known how HHV-8 induces/promotes proliferation of endothelial cells.

## HISTORY

Mucocutaneous lesions are usually asymptomatic but are associated with significant cosmetic stigma. At times lesions may ulcerate and bleed easily. Large lesions on palms or soles may impede function. Lesions on the lower extremities that are tumorous, ulcerated, or associated with significant edema often give rise to moderate to severe pain. Urethral or anal canal lesions can be associated with obstruction. GI involvement rarely causes symptoms. Pulmonary KS can cause bronchospasm, intractable coughing, progressive respiratory failure, shortness of breath.

## PHYSICAL EXAMINATION

### Skin Lesions
KS most often begins as an ecchymotic-like macule (Fig. 19-13). Macules evolve into papules, plaques (Fig. 19-14), nodules, and tumors that are violaceous, red, pink, or tan and become purple-brownish (Figs. 19-13 and 19-15) with a greenish hemosiderin halo as they age. Almost all KS lesions are palpable, feeling firm to hard even when they are in a macular stage. Often oval initially, and on the trunk often arranged parallel to skin tension lines (Fig. 19-16). Lesions may initially occur at sites of trauma,

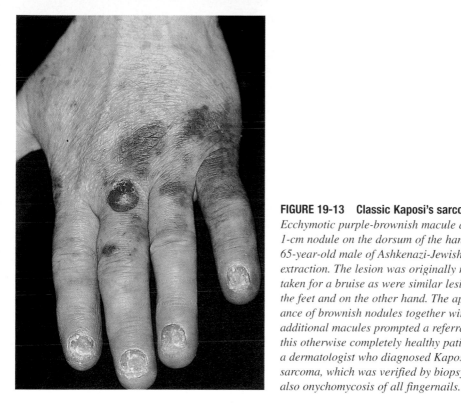

**FIGURE 19-13   Classic Kaposi's sarcoma**
*Ecchymotic purple-brownish macule and a 1-cm nodule on the dorsum of the hand of a 65-year-old male of Ashkenazi-Jewish extraction. The lesion was originally mistaken for a bruise as were similar lesions on the feet and on the other hand. The appearance of brownish nodules together with additional macules prompted a referral of this otherwise completely healthy patient to a dermatologist who diagnosed Kaposi's sarcoma, which was verified by biopsy. Note also onychomycosis of all fingernails.*

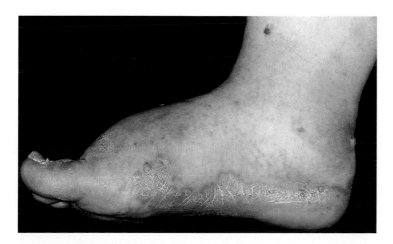

**FIGURE 19-14   Classic Kaposi's sarcoma**   *Brownish confluent plaques on the sole have become hyperkeratotic and pea-sized purplish nodules have arisen on the lower leg. Involvement of lymphatics has led to pronounced edema of the forefoot, which indicates that the disease process is further advanced than in the patient shown in Figure 19-13.*

usually in the acral regions. In time, individual lesions may enlarge and become confluent, forming tumor masses. Secondary changes to larger nodules and tumors include erosion, ulceration, crusting, and hyperkeratosis.

*Lymphedema* usually occurs on the lower extremities (Fig. 19-14) and results from confluent masses of lesions due to deeper involvement of lymphatics and lymph nodes. Distal edema may initially be unilateral but later becomes symmetric and involves not only the lower legs but also the genitalia and/or face.

*Distribution* Widespread or localized. In classic KS, lesions almost always occur on the feet and legs or the hands and slowly spread centripetally (Figs. 19-13 and 19-14). Tip of nose, periorbital areas, ears, and scalp as well as penis and legs may also be involved, but involvement of the trunk is rare. In HIV-associated KS there is early involvement of the face (Fig. 19-15) and widespread distribution on the trunk (Fig. 19-16)

**Mucous Membranes**   Oral lesions are the first manifestation of KS in 22% of cases; in HIV-associated KS often a marker for CD4+ T cell counts of <200/μL. Very common (50% of individuals) on hard palate, appearing first as a violaceous stain, which evolves into papules and nodules with a cobblestone appearance. Lesions also arise on soft palate, uvula, pharynx, gingiva, and tongue. Conjunctival lesions uncommon.

**Special Features of African-Endemic KS**   (Non-HIV-Associated) Four clinical patterns are recognized:

*Nodular type*: Runs a rather benign course with a mean duration of 5 to 8 years and resembles classic KS.

*Florid or vegetating type*: Characterized by more aggressive biologic behavior; is also nodular but may extend deeply into the subcutis, muscle, and bone.

*Infiltrative type*: Shows an even more aggressive course with florid mucocutaneous and visceral involvement.

*Lymphadenopathic type*: Predominantly affects children and young adults. Frequently confined to lymph nodes and viscera, but occasionally also involves the skin and mucous membrane.

**General Examination**   *Viscera* KS lesions of the viscera, though common, are often asymptomatic. This is particularly true for classic KS. At autopsy of HIV-infected individuals with mucocutaneous KS, 75% have visceral involvement (bowel, liver, spleen, lungs).

*Lymph Nodes* Lymph nodes are involved in half of cases of HIV-associated KS and in all cases of African lymphadenopathic type KS.

*Urogenital Tract* Prostate, seminal vesicles, testes, bladder, penis, scrotum.

*Lung* Pulmonary infiltrates, particularly in HIV-associated KS.

*GI Tract* GI hemorrhage, rectal obstruction, protein-losing enteropathy can occur.

*Other* Heart, brain, kidney, adrenal glands.

## LABORATORY EXAMINATIONS

**Skin Biopsy**   Vascular channels lined by atypical endothelial cells among a network of reticulin fibers and extravasated erythrocytes with hemosiderin deposition. Three histologic stages are described:

*Patch stage*: Proliferation of small, irregular, and jagged endothelial-lined spaces surrounding normal dermal vessels and adnexal structures; variable, inflammatory lymphocytic infiltrate (±plasma cells).

*Plaque stage*: Spindle cells expand throughout dermal collagen bundles forming irregular, cleftlike, angulated vascular channels that contain variable numbers of RBCs. Hemosiderin deposits; eosinophilic hyaline globules. Peripheral perivascular inflammatory infiltrate.

*Nodular stage*: Spindle cells in sheets and fascicles with mild to moderate cytologic atypia, single cell necrosis, trapped RBCs within an extensive network of slitlike vascular spaces.

**Imaging**   For internal organ involvement.

## DIAGNOSIS AND DIFFERENTIAL DIAGNOSIS

Confirmed on lesional skin biopsy.
**Differential Diagnosis**   Includes single pigmented lesions: dermatofibroma, pyogenic granuloma, hemangioma, bacillary (epithelioid) angiomatosis, melanocytic nevus, ecchymosis, granuloma annulare, insect bite reactions, stasis dermatitis.

## COURSE AND PROGNOSIS

**Classic KS**   Average survival, 10 to 15 years; death usually from unrelated causes. Secondary malignancies arise in >35% of cases.

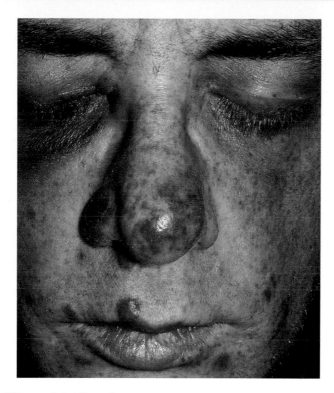

**FIGURE 19-15   HIV-associated Kaposi's sarcoma** *Multiple bruise-like purplish and brownish macules, papules and nodules are present not only on the face but also on the trunk and the extremities of this 29-year-old male homosexual with AIDS. Note also swelling of the nose. Early involvement of the face is typical for HIV-associated KS.*

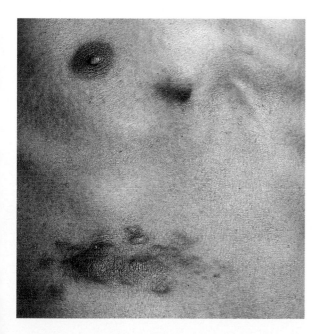

**FIGURE 19-16   HIV-associated Kaposi's sarcoma** *Multiple purplish plaques and nodules on the trunk of a homosexual AIDS patient. The patient had CD4+ T cell counts <200/μL and marked mucous membrane involvement,* Pneumocystis carinii *pneumonia, and* Candida.

**African-Endemic KS**   Mean survival in young adults, 5 to 8 years; young children, 2 to 3 years.

**Iatrogenic Immunosuppression-Associated KS**
Course may be chronic or rapidly progressive; KS usually resolves after immunosuppressive drugs are discontinued.

**HIV-Associated KS**   HIV-infected individuals with high CD4+ T cell counts can have stable or slowly progressive disease for many years. Rapid progression of KS can occur after decline of CD4+ T cell counts to low values, prolonged systemic glucocorticoid therapy, or illness such as *pneumocystis carinii* pneumonia. KS of the bowel and/or lungs is the cause of death in 10 to 20% of patients. Patients with only a few lesions, present for several months, without history of opportunistic infections, and CD4+ T cell counts $>200/\mu L$ tend to respond better to therapy and have a better overall prognosis. At time of initial diagnosis, 40% of KS patients have GI involvement; 80% at autopsy. Reduced survival rate in patients with GI involvement. Pulmonary KS has high short-term mortality rate, i.e., median survival <6 months.

## MANAGEMENT

The goal of therapy for KS is to control symptoms of the disease, not cure. A number of local and systemic therapeutic modalities are effective in controlling symptoms. Classic KS responds well to radiotherapy of involved sites. African-endemic KS, when symptomatic, responds best to systemic chemotherapy. Immunosuppressive drug–associated KS regresses or resolves when drug dosages are reduced or discontinued. HIV-associated KS usually responds to a variety of local therapies; for extensive mucocutaneous involvement or visceral involvement, chemotherapy is indicated.

Local therapy is usually directed at individual lesions that are cosmetically disturbing (e.g., on the face), bulky, bleeding, cause functional disturbance on the palms or soles, or cause lymphatic obstruction and lymphedema.

### Limited Intervention

**Radiotherapy**   Indicated for tumorous lesions, confluent lesions with a large surface area, large lesions on distal extremity, large oropha-ryngeal lesions. Dosing: 8 Gy in a single fraction for small lesions, 800 to 3000 rad in single or divided dose.

**Cryosurgery**   Indicated for deeply pigmented, protruding nodules. Best results with two freeze-thaw cycles. Pain is moderate during freeze cycle. Treated lesions heal with crust formation. KS often persists in deeper portions of lesion. Violaceous lesion is replaced with a white scar. Secondary infection is uncommon.

**Laser Surgery**   Pulsed-dye laser effective for small superficial lesion.

**Electrosurgery**   Effective for ulcerated, bleeding nodular lesion; must use a smoke evacuator in conjunction.

**Excisional Surgery**   Effective for selected small lesions. Not a realistic approach to the patient with many lesions.

**Intralesional Cytotoxic Chemotherapy**   *Vinblastine* 0.1 mg (0.5 mL of a 0.2-mg/mL solution) injected per square centimeter of lesion; for refractory lesions, incremental doses of up to 0.2 mg/cm$^2$ can be given. Most effective for small, early, papular lesions. Larger nodular lesions respond more slowly. The maximal total vinblastine dose injected should not exceed 2 mg per clinic visit. Some lesions heal with blister formation, crusting, and scarring. Inadvertent injection near a cutaneous sensory nerve can result in a neutric pain that can last up to a month. *Vincristine and Bleomycin* Have also been used for intralesional therapy.

### Aggressive Intervention

#### Single-Agent Chemotherapy

Adriamycin, 20 mg/m$^2$.
Vinblastine, IV bolus 0.1 mg/kg weekly.
Lipid formulations of daunorubicin and doxorubicin.
Etoposide (VP16), given orally.
Paclitaxel (Taxol), given intravenously every 3 weeks.

#### Combination Chemotherapy

Vincristine (2 mg) + bleomycin (15 U/m$^2$) + adriamycin (20 mg/m$^2$) is given every other week in patients with relatively advanced KS.
Interferon-$\alpha$ (15 million U/d) + zidovudine (600 mg/d).

## DERMATOFIBROSARCOMA PROTUBERANS   □ ◑

A rare, recurring, and locally aggressive tumor that usually presents as indurated plaque with firm smooth protuberant nodules, varying from flesh color to reddish-brown (Fig. 19-17), and often measuring several centimeters in diameter. Initially often presenting as an atrophic, depressed, scarlike lesion, it develops into nodular masses, firm and irregular. Most commonly occurs on the trunk. The tumor histologically shows cartwheel–like arrangements of fibroblasts, seen as short fascicles running at right angles to one another. The tumor may be monomorphous—often mimicking scarred tissue—but mitosis may be present. Immunohistochemistry nearly always shows CD34 positivity.

*Management*: By wide and deep (to the fascia) surgical excision and split skin grafting. Recurrences occur and require a second surgical procedure.

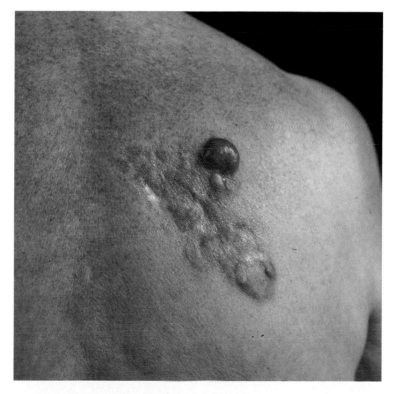

**FIGURE 19-17   Dermatofibrosarcoma protuberans**   *This firm, flesh- to reddish-brown colored irregular nodular plaque started as a firm papule and was completely asymptomatic. The patient consulted a physician for cosmetic reasons only. Excision with 3-cm margins and split-skin grafting resulted in a cure.*

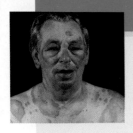

# ADVERSE CUTANEOUS DRUG REACTIONS

Adverse cutaneous drug reactions (ACDRs) are common in hospitalized patients (2 to 3% experience ACDRs) as well as in ambulatory patients. Complications of drug therapy, overall, are the most common adverse event for hospitalized individuals, accounting for 19% of such events. ACDRs in an ambulatory practice occur frequently, many commonly used drugs having reaction rates of > 1%. Most reactions are mild, accompanied by pruritus, and resolve promptly after the offending drug is discontinued. However, severe, life-threatening ACDRs do occur and are unpredictable. *Drug eruptions can mimic virtually all the morphologic expressions in dermatology and must be the first consideration in the differential diagnosis of a suddenly appearing symmetric eruption.* Drug eruptions are caused by immunologic or nonimmunologic mechanisms and are provoked by systemic or topical administration of a drug. The majority are based on a hypersensitivity mechanism and are thus immunologic and may be of types I, II, III, or IV.

## CLASSIFICATION

**Immunologically Mediated ACDR** See Table 20-1. It should be noted, however, that classification of immunologically mediated ACDR according to the Gell and Coombs classification is an oversimplification because in most reactions both cellular and humoral immune reactions are involved.

### Nonimmunologic Drug Eruptions

*Idiosyncrasy* Reactions due to hereditary enzyme deficiencies.

*Cumulation* Reactions are dose dependent, based on the total amount of drug ingested: pigmentation due to gold, amiodarone, or minocycline.

*Reactions due to combination of a drug with ultraviolet irradiation (photosensitivity)* Reactions may have a toxic or immunologic (allergic) pathogenesis (see Section 10).

*Irritancy/toxicity of a topically applied drug* 5-Fluorouracil, imiquimod.

*Individual idiosyncrasy to a topical or systemic drug.* Mechanisms not yet known.

## GUIDELINES FOR ASSESSMENT OF POSSIBLE ACDRs[1]

- Exclude alternative causes, especially infections, in that many infections (especially viral) are difficult to distinguish clinically from the adverse effects of drugs used to treat infections.
- Examine interval between introduction of a drug and onset of the reaction.
- Note any improvement after drug withdrawal.
- Determine whether similar reactions have been associated with the same compound.
- Note any reaction on readministration of the drug.

## FINDINGS INDICATING POSSIBLE LIFE-THREATENING ACDR[1]

### Cutaneous

Confluent erythema
Facial edema or central facial involvement
Skin pain
Palpable purpura
Skin necrosis

[1]Source: From JC Roujeau, RS Stern: N Engl J Med 331:1272, 1994.

**TABLE 20-1    Immunologically Mediated Adverse Cutaneous Drug Reactions***

| Type of Reaction | Pathogenesis | Examples of Causative Drug | Clinical Patterns |
|---|---|---|---|
| Type I | IgE-mediated; immediate-type immunologic reactions | Penicillin | Urticaria/angioedema of skin/mucosa, edema of other organs, and anaphylactic shock |
| Type II | Drug + cytotoxic antibodies cause lysis of cells such as platelets or leukocytes | Penicillin, sulfonamides, quinidine, isoniazid | Petechiae due to thrombocytopenic purpura, drug-induced pemphigus |
| Type III | IgG or IgM antibodies formed to drug; immune complexes deposited in small vessels activate complement and recruitment of granulocytes | Immunoglobulins, antibiotics | Vasculitis, urticaria, serum sickness |
| Type IV | Cell-mediated immune reaction; sensitized lymphocytes react with drug, liberating cytokines, which trigger cutaneous inflammatory response | Sulfamethoxazole, anticonvulsants, allopurinol | Morbilliform exanthematous reactions, fixed drug eruption, lichenoid eruptions, Stevens-Johnson syndrome, toxic epidermal necrolysis |

* After the Gell and Coombs classification of immune reactions.

Blisters of epidermal detachment
Positive Nikolsky's sign (epidermis separates readily from dermis with lateral pressure)
Mucous membrane erosions
Urticaria
Swelling of the tongue

### General

High fever (temperature $>40°C$)
Enlarged lymph nodes
Arthralgias or arthritis
Shortness of breath, wheezing, hypotension

### CLINICAL TYPES OF ADVERSE DRUG REACTIONS

ACDR can be exanthematous and can manifest as urticaria/angioedema, anaphylaxis and ana-

phylactoid reactions, or serum sickness; they can mimic or cause dermatoses that can also have other causes; they can present as cutaneous necrosis, pigmentation, alopecia, hypertrichosis; and they can induce nail changes. An overview is presented in Table 20-2.

### LABORATORY EXAMINATIONS

**Hematology**    Eosinophil count $> 1000/\mu L$. Lymphocytosis with atypical lymphocytes.
**Chemistry**    Abnormal results of liver function tests.

### DIAGNOSIS

Usually made on clinical findings. Lesional skin biopsy is helpful in defining the type of reaction

**TABLE 20-2  Types of Clinical ACDRs**

| Type | Drugs | Comment |
|---|---|---|
| **BASIC REACTIONS** | | |
| Exanthematous reactions | Any | Most common; initial reaction usually <14 days after drug intake; recurs after rechallenge; drug hypersensitivity syndrome, initially indistinguishable (see page 548) |
| Fixed drug eruptions | See Table 20-4 | See p. 556 |
| Urticaria/angioedema | Aspirin, NSAIDs, codeine, penicillin, opiates, amphetamine, polymyxine B, atropine, hydralazine, pentamidine, quinine, radiocontrast media, ACE inhibitors (see Table 20-3) | Second most common; usually within 36 h after initial exposure; within minutes after rechallenge (see page 553) |
| Anaphylaxis and anaphylactoid reactions | Antibiotics, extracts of allergens, radiocontrast media, monoclonal antibodies (see Table 20-3) | Most serious type of ACDR, within minutes and hours; more common with oral than parenteral drug administration. Intermittent administration of drug may predispose to anaphylaxis |
| Serum sickness | IV Ig, antibiotics, bovine serum albumin (used for oocyte retrieval in in vitro fertilization), cefaclor, cefprozil, bupropion, minocycline | 5 to 21 days after initial exposure *Minor form*: fever, urticaria, arthralgia *Major (complete) form*: fever, urticaria, angioedema, arthralgia, arthritis, lymphadenopathy, eosinophilia, ±nephritis, ±endocarditis. |
| **ACDR MIMICRY OF OTHER DERMATOSES** | | |
| Acneiform eruption | Glucocorticoids, anabolic steroids, contraceptives, halogens, isoniazid, lithium, azathioprine, danazol | See Section 1 |
| Bullous eruptions | Naproxene, nalidixic acid, furosemide, oxaprozin, penicillamine, piroxicam, tetracyclines | Fixed drug eruption, drug-induced vasculitis, SJS, TEN, porphyria, pseudoporphyria, drug-induced pemphigus, drug-induced pemphigoid, drug-induced linear IgA disease, bullae over pressure areas in sedated patients |

*(continued)*

**TABLE 20-2   Types of Clinical ACDRs (*Continued*)**

| Type | Drugs | Comment |
|------|-------|---------|
| Dermatomyositis-like reactions | Penicillamine, NSAIDs, carbamazepine | See Section 14 |
| Drug hypersensitivity syndrome | Antiepileptic drugs, sulfonamides, and others | Mimics exanthematous reactions; systemic involvement (see page 560) |
| Eczematous eruptions | Ethylenediamine, antihistamines, aminophylline/ aminophylline suppositories; procaine/benzocaine; iodides, iodinated organic compounds, radiographic contrast media/iodine; streptomycin, kanamycin, paramomycin, gentamicin/neomycin sulfate; nitroglycerin tablets/ nitroglycerin ointment; disulfuram/thiuram | Systemic administration of a drug to an individual who has been previously sensitized to the drug by topical application can provoke a widespread eczematous dermatitis (systemic contact-type dermatitis, see Section 2) or urticaria |
| Erythema multiforme, Stevens-Johnson syndrome (SJS), toxic epidermal necrolysis (TEN) | Anticonvulsants, sulfonamides, allopurinol, NSAIDs (piroxicam) | See Section 7, pages 140 and 144 |
| Erythema nodosum | Sulfonamides, other antimicrobial agents, analgesics, oral contraceptives, G-CSF | See Section 7, page 148 |
| Exfoliative dermatitis and erythroderma | Sulfonamides, antimalarials, phenytoin, penicillin | See Section 8 |
| Lichenoid eruptions | Gold, beta blockers, ACE inhibitors, especially captopril; see also Table 7-1 | See Section 7. May be extensive, occurring weeks to months after initiation of drug therapy; may progress to exfoliative dermatitis. Adnexal involvement may result in alopecia, anhidrosis. Resolution after discontinuation slow, 1 to 4 months; up to 24 months after gold. May be photodistributed or bullous. Oral involvement occurs with some drugs |
| Lupus erythematosus (LE) | Procainamide, hydralazine, isoniazid, minocycline, acebutolol, $Ca^{2+}$ channel blockers, ACE inhibitors | See Section 14. 5% of cases of systemic LE are drug-induced Cutaneous manifestations, including photosensitivity; however, urticaria, erythema |

(*continued*)

**TABLE 20-2**    Types of Clinical ACDRs (*Continued*)

| Type | Drugs | Comment |
|------|-------|---------|
| | | multiforme-like lesions, Raynaud's phenomenon are not common |
| Photosensitivity | See Tables 10-4 to 10-6 | See Section 10. Phototoxic, photoallergic, or photocontact |
| Pityriasis rosea–like eruptions | Gold, captopril, and others | For clinical appearance, see Section 7 |
| Pseudolymphoma | Phenytoin, carbamazepine, allopurinol, antidepressants, phenothiazines, benzodiazepam, antihistamines, beta blockers, lipid-lowering agents, cyclosporine, D-penicillamine | Papular eruptions with a histology mimicking lymphoma |
| Pseudoporphyria | Tetracycline, furosemide, naproxene | See Section 10 and page 565 |
| Psoriasiform eruption | Antimalarials, beta blockers, lithium salts, NSAIDs, interferon, penicillamine, methyldopa | See Section 3 |
| Purpura | Penicillin, sulfonamides, quinine, isoniazid | See Section 18. Hemorrhage into morbilliform ACDR occurs not uncommonly on the legs. Progressive pigmented purpura also reported associated with drugs (see Section 7) |
| Pustular eruptions | Ampicillin, amoxicillin, macrolides, tetracyclines, beta blockers, $Ca^{2+}$ channel blokers | Toxic pustuloderma, acute generalized exanthematous pustulosis (AGEP). Must be differentiated from pustular psoriasis; eosinophil in the infiltrate suggests AGEP |
| Scleroderma-like reactions | Penicillamine, bleomycin, bromocryptine, Na-valproate, 5-hydroxytryptophan, acetanilide – containing rapeseed cooking oil | See Section 14 |
| **ACDR-RELATED PIGMENTATION** | | |
| ACDR-pigmentation | Amiodarone, minocycline, clofazimine zidovudine, hydantoins, cytotoxic agents, heavy metals, hormones, chlorpromazine | See page 562. Associated with postinflammatory hyperpigmentation, increased melanin synthesis, increased lipofuscin |

(*continued*)

**TABLE 20-2   Types of Clinical Acdrs (*Continued*)**

| Type | Drugs | Comment |
|---|---|---|
| | | synthesis, or cutaneous deposition of drug-related material |
| | **ACDR-RELATED NECROSIS** | |
| ACDR necrosis | Warfarin, heparin, interferon-$\alpha$, cytotoxic agents | See page 566. Associated with post inflammatory hyperpigmentation, increased melanin synthesis, increased lipofuscin synthesis, or cutaneous deposition of drug-related materials |
| | **Others** | |
| ACDR related to chemotherapy | | See page 568 |
|   Alopecia | | See Section 29 |
|   Hypertrichosis | | See Section 29 |
|   Nail changes | | See Section 30 |

NOTE: NSAIDs, nonsteroidal anti-inflammatory drugs; ACE, angiotensin-converting enzyme; G-CSF, granulocyte colony-stimulating factor.

pattern occurring but not in identifying the offending drug. Skin tests and radioallergosorbent tests are helpful in diagnosing IgE-mediated type I hypersensitivity reactions, more specifically to penicillins.

## MANAGEMENT

In most cases, the implicated or suspected drug should be discontinued. In some, such as with morbilliform eruptions, the offending drug can be continued and the eruption may resolve. In cases of urticaria/angioedema or early Stevens–Johnson syndrome (SJS)/toxic epidermal necrolysis (TEN), the ACDR can be life-threatening, and the drug must be discontinued.

# EXANTHEMATOUS DRUG REACTIONS ■

An exanthematous drug reaction (eruption) is an adverse hypersensitivity reaction to an in-gested or parenterally administered drug characterized by a cutaneous eruption that mimics a measles-like viral exanthem (Fig. 20-1); systemic involvement is low. (See Table 20-2.)
*Synonyms*: Morbilliform drug reaction, maculopapular drug reaction.

## EPIDEMIOLOGY AND ETIOLOGY

**Age of Onset** Less common in the very young.
**Incidence** Most common type of cutaneous drug reaction.
**Etiology** *Drugs with a high probability of reaction* (3 to 5%): penicillin and related antibiotics, carbamazepine, allopurinol, gold salts (10 to 20%). *Medium probability*: sulfonamides (bacteriostatic, antidiabetic, diuretic), nonsteroidal anti-inflammatory drugs (NSAIDs), hydantoin derivatives, isoniazid, chloramphenicol, erythromycin, streptomycin. *Low probability* (≤1%): barbiturates, benzodiazepines, phenothiazines, tetracyclines.

## PATHOGENESIS

Exact mechanism unknown. Probably delayed hypersensitivity. In Epstein-Barr virus (EBV) and cytomegalovirus (CMV) mononucleosis, exanthematous drug reactions occur very frequently but are probably not allergic.

## HISTORY

**Mononucleosis** Up to 100% of patients with primary EBV or CMV infection (infectious mononucleosis syndrome) given ampicillin or amoxicillin develop an exanthematous drug eruption.
**HIV Infection** 50 to 60% of HIV-infected patients who receive sulfa drugs (i.e., trimethoprim-sulfamethoxazole) develop an eruption. With immune restitution with highly-active antiretroviral therapy (HAART), previously tolerant individuals may develop ACDR as CD4+ cell count rises.
**Drug History** Increased incidence of reactions in patients on allopurinol given ampicillin/amoxicillin.
**Prior Drug Sensitization** Patients with prior history of exanthematous drug eruption will most likely develop a similar reaction if rechallenged with same drug. About 10% of patients sensitive to penicillins who are given cephalosporins will exhibit cross-drug sensitivity and develop eruption. Patients sensitized to one sulfa-based drug may cross-react with another category of the drug in 20% of cases.
**Onset** *Early Reaction* In previously sensitized patient, eruption starts within 2 or 3 days after readministration of drug.
*Late Reaction* Sensitization occurs during administration or after completing course of drug; peak incidence at ninth day after administration. However, ACDR may occur at any time between the first day and 3 weeks after the beginning of treatment. Reaction to penicillin can begin ≥ 2 weeks after drug is discontinued.
**Skin Symptoms** Usually quite pruritic, disturbs sleep. Painful skin lesions suggest development of a more serious ACDR, such as TEN.
**Systems Review** ± Fever, chills.

## PHYSICAL EXAMINATION

### Skin Lesions
Macules and/or papules, a few millimeters to 1 cm in size (Fig. 20-1). Bright or "drug" red. Resolving lesions have hues of tan and purple. In time, lesions become confluent forming large macules, polycyclic/gyrate erythema, reticular eruptions, sheetlike erythema, erythroderma; also erythema multiforme–like. Purpura may be seen in lesions of lower legs. In individuals with thrombocytopenia, exanthematous eruptions can mimic vasculitis because of intralesional hemorrhage. Scaling and/or desquamation may occur with healing.
*Distribution* Symmetric (Fig. 20-1). Almost always on trunk and extremities. Confluent lesions in intertriginous areas, i.e., axilla, groin, inframammary area. Palms and soles variably involved. In children, may be limited to face and extremities. May spare face, nipple, periareolar area, surgical scar. Reactions to ampicillin usually appear initially on the elbows, knees, and trunk, extending symmetrically to most areas of the body.

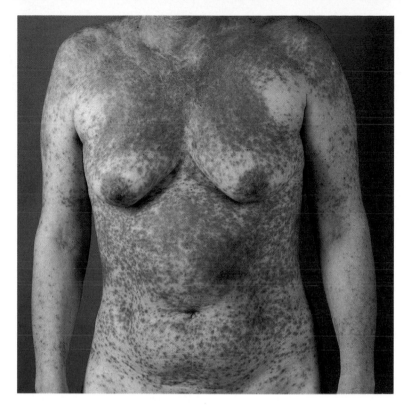

**FIGURE 20-1   Exanthematous drug eruption: ampicillin**  *Symmetrically arranged, brightly erythematous macules and papules, discrete in some areas and confluent in others on the trunk and discretely on the extremities.*

**Mucous Membranes** Enanthem on buccal mucosa.

**Reactions to Specific Drugs** *Ampicillin, Amoxicillin* Up to 100% of patients with EBV or CMV mononucleosis syndrome given ampicillin, amoxicillin developed drug eruptions.

*NSAIDS* Incidence: 1 to 3%. Site: trunk, pressure areas. Onset: 1 to 2 weeks after beginning therapy.

*Barbiturates* Site: face, trunk. Onset: few days after initiation of therapy. Cross-reactivity with other barbiturates: not universal.

*Nitrofurantoin* Associated findings: fever, peripheral eosinophilia, pulmonary edema, chest pain, dyspnea. Onset: 2 weeks after initiation of therapy; within hours if previously sensitized.

*Hydantoin Derivatives* Macular or confluent erythema. Begins on face, spreads to trunk and extremities. Onset: 2 weeks after initiation of therapy. Associated findings: fever, peripheral eosinophilia; facial edema; lymphadenopathy (can mimic lymphoma histologically).

*Isoniazid* Morbilliform; may evolve to exfoliative dermatitis. Associated findings: fever; hepatitis.

*Benzodiazepines* Incidence: very low. Onset: few days after initiation of therapy. Rechallenge: frequently rash does not occur.

*Phenothiazines* Begins on face, spreads to trunk (mainly back) and extremities. Onset: between second and third weeks after initiation of therapy. Associated findings: periorbital edema. Rechallenge: rash may not occur. Cross-reactivity: common.

*Carbamazepine* Morphology: diffuse erythema; severe erythroderma may follow. Site:

begins on face, spreads rapidly to all areas; may occur in photodistribution. Onset: 2 weeks after initiation of therapy. Associated findings: facial edema.

*Sulfonamides* Incidence: common in up to 50 to 60% of HIV-infected patients. Morphology: morbilliform, erythema multiforme–like.

*Allopurinol* Incidence: 5%. Morphology: morbilliform. Begins on face, spreads rapidly to all areas; may occur in photodistribution. Onset: 2 to 3 weeks after initiation of therapy. Associated findings: facial edema; systemic vasculitis, especially involving kidneys. Rash may fade in spite of continued administration.

*Gold Salts* Incidence: 10 to 20% of patients; dose-related. Morphology: diffuse erythema; exfoliative dermatitis, lichenoid, hemorrhagic, bullous, or pityriasis rosea–like eruptions may follow.

**General Examination**   Drug fever. Findings associated with the indication for drug administration.

## LABORATORY EXAMINATIONS

**Hemogram**   Peripheral eosinophilia.
**Dermatopathology**   Perivascular lymphocytes and eosinophils.

## DIAGNOSIS AND DIFFERENTIAL DIAGNOSIS

Clinical diagnosis, at times confirmed by histologic findings, correlated with history of drug administration.

**Differential Diagnosis**   Includes all exanthematous eruptions: Viral exanthem (often begins on face, progresses to trunk; may be accompanied by conjunctivitis, lymphadenopathy, fever), secondary syphilis, atypical pityriasis rosea, early widespread allergic contact dermatitis.

## COURSE

After discontinuation of drug, rash usually fades; however, it may worsen for a few days. The eruption may also begin after the drug has been discontinued. Occasionally fades even though drug is continued. Eruption usually recurs with rechallenge, although not always. In some cases of exanthematous ampicillin reactions, readministration of the drug does not cause the eruption. Duration of ampicillin eruption after discontinuation of drug: 3 to 5 days. If drug is continued, exfoliative dermatitis may develop. Of more concern, a morbilliform eruption may be the initial presentation of a more serious eruption, i.e., SJS, TEN, drug hypersensitivity syndrome, or serum sickness.

## MANAGEMENT

The definitive step in management is to identify the offending drug and discontinue it.

**Indications for Discontinuation of Drug**   Urticaria (concern for anaphylaxis), facial edema, pain, blisters, mucosal involvement, ulcers, palpable or extensive purpura, fever, lymphadenopathy.

**Symptomatic Treatment**   Oral antihistamine to alleviate pruritus.

**Glucocorticoids**   *Potent Topical Preparation* May help speed resolution of eruption, especially if secondary changes of eczematous dermatitis have occurred due to scratching.

*Oral or IV* Provides symptomatic relief. If offending drug cannot be substituted or omitted, systemic glucocorticoids can be administered to treat the ACDR; also, to induce more rapid remission.

**Prevention**   Patients must be aware of their specific drug hypersensitivity and that other drugs of the same class can cross-react. Although an exanthematous drug eruption may not recur if the drug is given again, readministration is best avoided by using a different agent. Wearing a medical alert bracelet is advised.

**FIGURE 20-2 (Opposite page)   Pustular drug eruption: acute generalized exanthematous pustulosis (AGEP)**   *A close-up of the lesions of AGEP reveals multiple tiny nonfollicular pustules against the background of diffuse erythema that first appeared in the large folds and then covered the entire trunk and the face. This 58-year-old female had fever and leukocytosis and had taken ampicillin for an upper respiratory tract infection.*

## PUSTULAR ERUPTIONS    □ ◑

*Acneiform eruptions* are associated with iodides, bromides, adrenocorticotropic hormone (ACTH), glucocorticoids, isoniazid, androgens, lithium, actinomycin D, and phenytoin (see Section 1). Drug-induced acne may appear in atypical areas, such as on the arms and legs, and is most often monomorphous. Comedones are usually absent. *Acute generalized exanthematous pustulosis* (AGEP) is an acute febrile eruption that is often associated with leukocytosis (Fig. 20-2). After drug administration, it may take 1 to 3 weeks before skin lesions appear; however, in previously sensitized patients, the skin symptoms may occur within 2 to 3 days. AGEP typically presents with nonfollicular sterile pustules occurring on a diffuse, edematous erythema (Fig. 20-2) predominantly in the folds and/or on the face. Fever and elevated blood neutrophils are common. Histopathology typically shows spongiform subcorneal and/or intraepidermal pustules; a marked edema of the papillary dermis; and eventually vasculitis, eosinophils, and/or focal necrosis of keratinocytes. Onset is acute, most often following drug intake, but viral infections can also trigger the disease. Pustules resolve spontaneously in <15 days and generalized desquamation occurs approximately 2 weeks later. The estimated incidence rate of AGEP is approximately 1 to 5 cases per million per year. Differential diagnosis includes pustular psoriasis, the hypersensitivity syndrome reaction with pustulation, subcorneal pustular dermatosis (Sneddon-Wilkinson disease), pustular vasculitis, or TEN, especially in severe cases of AGEP. Pustular eruptions also occur with monoclonal antibodies used in cancer treatment (Fig. 20-3).

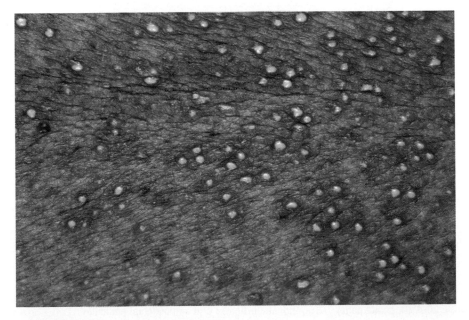

**FIGURE 20-2**

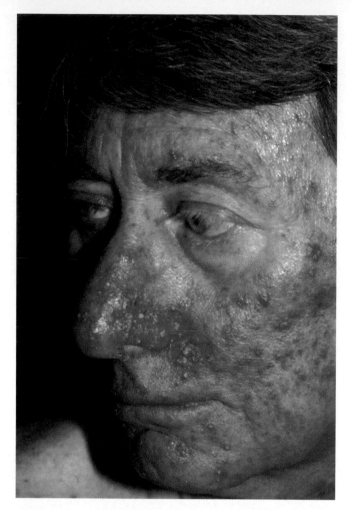

**FIGURE 20-3    Pustular drug eruption: cetuximab**   *This pustular eruption occurred in a patient who had received an anti-EGF monoclonal antibody for cancer of the colon. Although occurring also on other sites of the body it could be classified among the acneiform drug eruptions seen after the ingestion of bromides, iodides, isoniazid, and others.*

**FIGURE 20-4  (Opposite page)    Drug-induced urticaria and angioedema: penicillin**   *Large, urticarial wheals on the face, neck, and trunk with angioedema in the periorbital region.*

# DRUG-INDUCED ACUTE URTICARIA, ANGIOEDEMA, EDEMA, AND ANAPHYLAXIS (See also Section 14)    ■   ◗ → ●

Drug-induced urticaria and angioedema occur due to a variety of mechanisms (see Table 20-2) and are characterized clinically by transient wheals and larger edematous areas that involve the dermis and subcutaneous tissue (angioedema). In some cases, cutaneous urticaria/angioedema is associated with systemic anaphylaxis, which is manifested by respiratory distress, vascular collapse, and/or shock. Drugs causing urticaria/angioedema and anaphylaxis are listed in Table 20-3.

## CLASSIFICATION OF URTICARIAL/ ANGIOEDEMA ACDRs

1. Immune-Mediated
   a. IgE mediated: penicillin
   b. Complement- and immune complex– mediated: penicillin, immunoglobulins, whole blood

2. Nonallergic urticarial ACDR
   a. Analgesics/NSAIDs inhibit/block cyclooxygenase in prostaglandin synthesis
   b. Radio contrast media
   c. ACE inhibitors: inhibition of kinin metabolism
   d. Calcium channel blockers
   e. Drugs releasing histamine

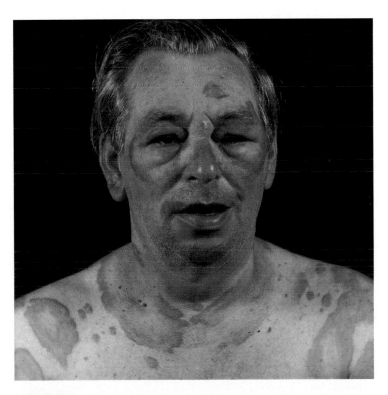

**FIGURE 20-4**

## HISTORY

### Time from Initial Drug Exposure to Appearance of Urticaria
*IgE-Mediated* Initial sensitization, usually 7 to 14 days; urticaria may occur while the drug is still being administered or after it is discontinued. In previously sensitized individuals, usually within minutes or hours.
*Immune Complex-Mediated* Initial sensitization, usually 7 to 10 days, but as long as 28 days; in previously sensitized individuals, symptoms appear 12 to 36 h after drug is readministered.
*Analgesics/Anti-Inflammatory Drugs* Occurs after administration of drug by 20 to 30 min (up to 4 h).

### Prior Drug Exposure
*Radiographic Contrast Media* 25 to 35% probability of repeat reaction in individuals with history of prior reaction to contrast media.

### Duration of Lesions   Hours.

### Skin Symptoms
Pruritus, burning of palms/soles, auditory canal. With airway edema, difficulty breathing.

### Constitutional Symptoms
IgE-mediated: flushing, sudden, fatigue, yawning, headache, weakness, dizziness; numbness of tongue, sneezing, bronchospasm, substernal pressure, palpitations; nausea, vomiting, crampy abdominal pain, diarrhea.

### Systems Review   Arthralgia.

## PHYSICAL EXAMINATION

### Skin Lesions
Urticaria and angioedema are described in Section 14. Large wheals (Fig. 20-4) that appear and resolve within a few hours, spontaneously or with therapy. Extensive tissue swelling with involvement of deep dermal and subcutaneous tissues. Often pronounced on face with skin-colored enlargement of portion of face (eyelids, lips, tongue) (Fig. 20-4).

### General Findings
*IgE-Mediated Reactions* Hypotension. Bronchospasm, laryngeal edema.

## LABORATORY EXAMINATIONS

**Dermatopathology**   As in urticaria.
**Complement Levels**   Decreased in serum sickness.
**Ultrasonography**   For early diagnosis of bowel involvement; presence of abdominal pain may indicate edema of the bowel.

## DIAGNOSIS

Clinical diagnosis. *Differential diagnosis* is of acute edematous red pruritic plaque (s): Allergic contact dermatitis (poison ivy, poison oak dermatitis), cellulitis, insect bite(s).

## COURSE AND PROGNOSIS

Drug-induced urticaria/angioedema usually resolves within hours to days to weeks after the causative drug is withdrawn.

## MANAGEMENT

The offending drug should be identified and withdrawn as soon as possible.
**Prevention**   *Previously Sensitized Individuals* The patient should carry information listing drug sensitivities (wallet card, bracelet).
*Radiographic Contrast Media* Avoid use of contrast media known to have caused prior reaction. If not possible, pretreat patient with antihistamine and prednisone (1 mg/kg) 30 to 60 min before contrast media exposure.

### Treatment of Acute Severe Urticaria/Anaphylaxis
*Epinephrine* 0.3 to 0.5 mL of a 1:1000 dilution subcutaneously, repeated in 15 to 20 min. Maintain airway. Intravenous access.

**Antihistamines**   $H_1$ blockers or $H_2$ blockers or combination.

**Systemic Glucocorticoids**   *Intravenous* Hydrocortisone or methylprednisolone for severe symptoms.
*Oral* Prednisone, 70 mg, tapering by 10 or 5 mg daily over 1 to 2 weeks, is usually adequate.

**TABLE 20-3    Drugs Causing Urticaria/Angioedema/Anaphylaxis**

| Drug Type | Specific Drugs |
|---|---|
| Antibiotics and chemotherapeutic agents | Penicillins: ampicillin, amoxicillin, dicloxacillin, mezlocillin, penicillin G, penicillin V, tricarcillin. Cephalosporins, including third-generation sulfonamides and derivatives |
| Cardiovascular drugs | Amiodarone, procainamide |
| Immunotherapeutics, vaccines | Antilymphocyte serum, levamisole, horse serum, monoclonal antibodies |
| Cytostatic agents | L-Asparaginase, bleomycin, cisplatin, daunorubicin, 5-fluorouracil, procarbazine,thiotepa |
| Angiotensin-converting enzyme inhibitors | Captopril, enalopril, lininopril |
| Calcium-channel blockers | Nifedipine, diltiazem, verapamil |
| Drugs releasing histamine | Centrally acting drugs: morphine, meperidine, atropine, codeine, papaverine, propanidid, alfaxalone<br>Muscle relaxants: D-tubocurarine, succinylcholine<br>Sympathomimetics: amphetamine, tyramine<br>Hypotensive agents: hydralazine, tolazoline, trimethaphan camsylate<br>Antimicrobial agents: pentamidine, propamidine, stilbamidine, quinine, vancomycin<br>Radiographic contrast media and others |

# FIXED DRUG ERUPTION  ▯ ◑

A fixed drug eruption (FDE) is an adverse cutaneous reaction to an ingested drug, characterized by the formation of a solitary (but at times multiple) erythematous patch, plaque, bulla, or erosion; if the patient is rechallenged with the offending drug, the FDE occurs repeatedly at the identical skin site (i.e., fixed) within hours of ingestion. Most commonly implicated agents are listed in Table 20-4.

## PATHOGENESIS

Unknown.

## HISTORY

**Drug History**  Patients frequently give a history of identical lesion(s) occurring at the identical location. FDEs may be associated with the following: (1) a headache for which the patient takes a barbiturate containing analgesic, (2) constipation for which the patient takes a phenolphthalein-containing laxative, or (3) a cold for which the patient takes an over-the-counter medication containing a yellow dye. The offending "drug" in food dye–induced FDE may be difficult to identify, e.g., yellow dye in Galliano liqueur or phenolphthalein in maraschino cherries; quinine in tonic water.
**Skin Symptoms**  Usually asymptomatic. May be pruritic, painful, or burning. Painful when eroded.
**Time to Onset of Lesion(s)**  Occur from 30 min to 8 h after ingestion of drug in previously sensitized individual.
**Duration of Lesion(s)**  Lesions persist if drug is continued. Resolve days to few weeks after drug is discontinued.

## PHYSICAL EXAMINATION

### Skin Lesions
The characteristic early lesion is a sharply demarcated macule (Fig. 20-5A), round or oval in shape, occurring within hours after ingestion of the offending drug. Initially erythema, then dusky red to violaceous (Fig. 20-5B). Most commonly, lesions are solitary (Fig. 20-5A) and can spread to become quite large (Fig. 20-6), but they may be multiple (Fig. 20-7) with random distribution; numerous lesions may simulate TEN (Fig. 20-7). Lesions become edematous, thus forming a plaque, which may evolve to become a bulla (Fig. 20-5A) and then an erosion. Eroded lesions, especially on genitals or oral mucosa, are quite painful. After healing, dark brown with violet hue postinflammatory hyperpigmentation. Genital skin is most commonly involved site, but any site may be involved; perioral, periorbital. Occur in conjunctivae, oropharynx.

## LABORATORY EXAMINATIONS

**Dermatopathology**  Similar to findings in erythema multiforme and/or TEN.
**Patch Test**  Suspected drug can be placed as a patch test at a previously involved site; an inflammatory response occurs in only 30% of cases.

---

**TABLE 20-4   Most Commonly Implicated Agents in Fixed Drug Eruptions**

---

Antimicrobial agents
  Tetracyclines (tetracycline, minocycline)
  Sulfonamides, including
    "nonabsorbable" drugs;
    cross-reactions with antidiabetic and
    diuretic sulfa drug may occur
  Metronidazole
  Nystatin
Anti-inflammatory agents
  Salicylates
  NSAIDs
  Phenylbutazone
  Phenacetin
Psychoactive agents
  Barbiturates, including Fiorinal
    Quaalude, Doriden
Oral contraceptives
Quinine (including quinine in tonic water),
  quinidine
Phenolphthalein
Food coloring: in food or medications

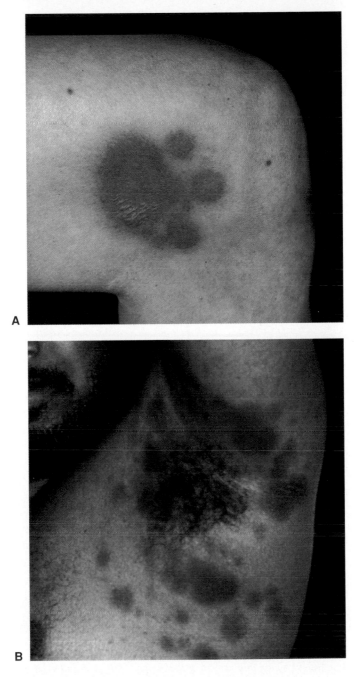

**FIGURE 20-5   Fixed drug eruption:**   *A.* **Tetracycline** *A well-defined plaque on the knee, merging with three "satellite" lesions. The large plaque exhibits epidermal wrinkling, a sign of incipient blister formation. This was the second such episode following ingestion of a tetracycline. No other lesions were present.* ***B.*** **Tylenol** *Multiple violaceous lesions in both axillae following the ingestion of Tylenol. Erosive mouth lesions were also present.*

## DIAGNOSIS

Made on clinical grounds. Readministration of the drug confirms diagnosis but should be avoided.

Solitary genital erosion to be differentiated from recurrent herpetic lesion; multiple erosions from SJS, TEN; oral erosion(s) from aphthous stomatitis, primary herpetic gingivostomatitis, erythema multiforme.

## COURSE AND PROGNOSIS

FDE resolves within a few weeks of withdrawing the drug. Recurs within hours after ingestion of a single dose of the drug.

## MANAGEMENT

Identify and withhold the offending drug. Noneroded lesions can be treated with a potent topical glucocorticoid ointment. Eroded cutaneous lesions can be treated with bacitracin or other antimicrobial ointment and a dressing until the site is reepithelialized. For widespread, generalized, and highly painful mucosal lesions, oral prednisone 1 mg/kg body weight tapered over a course of 2 weeks.

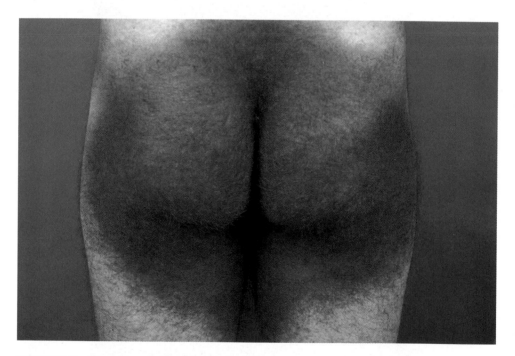

**FIGURE 20-6   Fixed drug eruption: phenolphthalein** *A large area of dusky, violaceous erythema covering the entire gluteal region and extending to the upper thighs. It followed the ingestion of a phenolphthalein-containing laxative.*

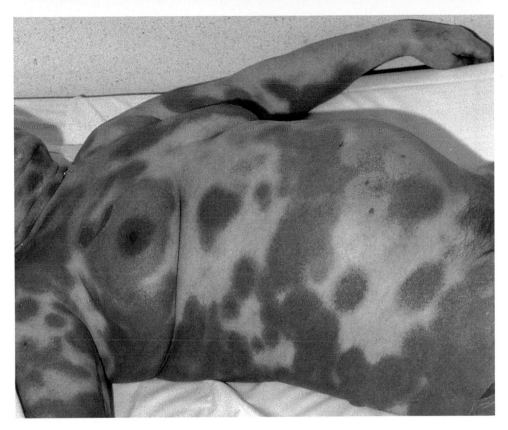

**FIGURE 20-7    Generalized fixed drug eruption: tetracycline**    *Multiple, confluent, violaceous-red, oval erythematous areas, some of which later became bullous. The eruption may be difficult to distinguish from toxic epidermal necrolysis.*

# DRUG HYPERSENSITIVITY SYNDROME

Hypersensitivity syndrome is an idiosyncratic adverse drug reaction that begins acutely in the first 2 months after initiation of drug and is characterized by fever, severe disease with characteristic infiltrated papules and facial edema or an exfoliative dermatitis, lymphadenopathy, hematologic abnormalities (eosinophilia, atypical lymphocytes), and organ involvement (hepatitis, carditis, interstitial nephritis, or interstitial pneumonitis). The mortality rate is 10% if unrecognized and untreated. Lesional biopsy specimens show a lymphocytic infiltrate, at times mimicking a cutaneous lymphoma.
*Synonym*: Drug rash with eosinophilia and systemic symptoms (DRESS).

## EPIDEMIOLOGY AND ETIOLOGY

**Race**   Reactions to antiepileptic drugs may be higher in black individuals.
**Etiology**   Most commonly: antiepileptic drugs (phenytoin, carbamazepine, phenobarbital; cross-sensitivity among the three drugs is common) and sulfonamides (antimicrobial agents, dapsone, sulfasalazine). Less commonly: allopurinol, gold salts, sorbinil, minocycline, zalcitabine, calcium-channel blockers, ranitidine, thalidomide, mexiletine.

## PATHOGENESIS

Some patients have a genetically determined inability to detoxify the toxic arene oxide metabolic products of anticonvulsant agents. Slow N-acetylation of sulfonamide and increased susceptibility of leukocytes to toxic hydroxylamine metabolites are associated with higher risk of hypersensitivity syndrome.

## HISTORY

**Onset**   2 to 6 weeks after drug is initially used, and later than most other serious skin reactions.
**Prodrome**   Fever. rash.
**Systems Review**   Fever.

## PHYSICAL EXAMINATION

### Skin Lesions
*Early*: morbilliform eruption (Fig. 20-8) on face, upper trunk, upper extremities; cannot be distinguished from exanthematous drug eruption. May progress to generalized exfoliative dermatitis/erythroderma, especially if drug is not discontinued. Eruption becomes infiltrated with edematous follicular accentuation. Facial edema (especially periorbitally) is characteristic.

Dermal edema may result in blister formation. Sterile folliculocentric as well as nonfollicular pustules may occur. Eruption may become purpuric on legs. Scaling and/or desquamation may occur with healing.
*Distribution*   Symmetric. Almost always on trunk and extremities. Lesions may become confluent and generalized.
**Mucous Membranes**   Cheilitis, erosions, erythematous pharynx, enlarged tonsils.
**General Examination**   Elevated temperature (drug fever).
*Lymph Nodes* Lymphadenopathy frequent ± tender; usually due to benign lymphoid hyperplasia.
*Other* Involvement of liver, heart, lungs, joints, muscles, thyroid, brain also occurs.

## LABORATORY EXAMINATIONS

**Hemogram and Chemistries**   Eosinophilia (30% of cases). Leukocytosis. Mononucleosis-like atypical lymphocytes. Signs of hepatitis and nephritis.
**Histology**   *Skin* Lymphocytic infiltrate, dense and diffuse or superficial and perivascular. ±Eosinophils or dermal edema. In some cases, bandlike infiltrate of atypical lymphocytes with epidermotropism, simulating cutaneous T cell lymphoma.
*Lymph Nodes* Benign lymphoid hyperplasia. Uncommonly atypical lymphoid hyperplasia, pseudolymphoma.
*Liver* Eosinophilic infiltrate or granulomas.
*Kidney* Interstitial nephritis.

## DIAGNOSIS

**Proposed Diagnostic Criteria** (1) Cutaneous drug eruption; (2) hematologic abnormalities (eosinophilia $\geq$1500/$\mu$L or presence of atypical lymphocytes); (3) systemic involvement

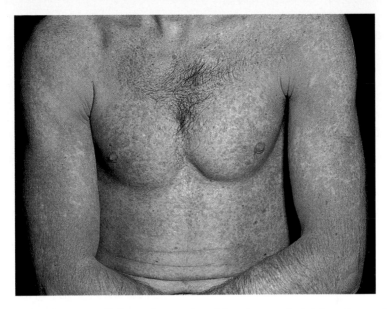

**FIGURE 20-8 Drug hypersensitivity syndrome: phenytoin** *Symmetric, bright red, exanthematous eruption, confluent in some sites; the patient had associated lymphadenopathy.*

[adenopathies ≥2 cm in diameter or hepatitis (SGOT ≥ 2 $N$) or interstitial nephritis or interstitial pneumonitis or carditis]. Diagnosis is confirmed if three criteria are present.

## DIFFERENTIAL DIAGNOSIS

**Early** That of morbilliform eruptions. Can mimic early measles or rubella.
**Later** Serum sickness, drug-induced vasculitis, Henoch-Schönlein purpura, cryoglobulin-associated vasculitis, vasculitis associated with infection, and collagen vascular diseases.
**Rash Plus Lymphadenopathy** Rubella, primary EBV or CMV mononucleosis syndrome.

## COURSE AND PROGNOSIS

Rash and hepatitis may persist for weeks after drug is discontinued. In patients treated with systemic glucocorticoids, rash and hepatitis may recur as glucocorticoids are tapered. Lymphadenopathy usually resolves when drug is withdrawn; however, rare progression to lymphoma has been reported. Rarely, patients die from systemic hypersensitivity such as with eosinophilic myocarditis. Clinical findings recur if drug is given again.

## MANAGEMENT

Identify and discontinue the offending drug.
**Symptomatic Treatment** Oral antihistamine to alleviate pruritus.
**Glucocorticoids** *Topical* High-potency topical glucocorticoids applied bid are usually helpful in relieving cutaneous symptoms of pruritus but do not alter systemic hypersensitivity.
*Systemic* Prednisone (0.5 mg/kg per day) usually results in rapid improvement of symptoms and laboratory parameters.
**Future Drug Therapy** Cross-sensitivity between various aromatic antiepileptic drugs occurs, making it difficult to select alternative anticonvulsant therapy.
**Prevention** The individual must be aware of his or her specific drug hypersensitivity and that other drugs of the same class can cross-react. These drugs must never be readministered. Patient should wear a medical alert bracelet.

# DRUG-INDUCED PIGMENTATION

Drug-induced alterations in pigmentation are relatively common, resulting from a variety of endogenous and exogenous pigments, and can be of significant cosmetic concern to the patient.

## CAUSATIVE DRUGS

The following drugs are capable of inducing hyperpigmentation of skin and/or mucosa:

Antiarrhythmic: amiodarone
Antimalarial: chloroquine, hydroxychloroquine, quinacrine, quinine
Antimicrobial: minocycline, clofazimine, zidovudine
Antiseizure: hydantoins
Cytostatic: bleomycin, cyclophosphamide, doxorubicin, daunorubicin, busulfan, 5-fluorouracil, dactinomycin
Heavy metals: silver, gold, mercury
Hormones: adrenocorticotropic hormone (ACTH), estrogen/progesterone
Psychiatric: chlorpromazine

## PHYSICAL EXAMINATION

### Skin Findings

**Amiodarone**   >75% of patients after 40-g cumulative dose after >4 months of therapy. More common in skin phototypes I and II. Low-grade or minimal photosensitivity; phototoxic erythema limited to the light-exposed areas in a small proportion (8%) of patients. Dusky-red erythema and, later, blue-gray dermal melanosis (ceruloderma) (Fig. 20-9) in exposed areas (face and hands). Lipofuscin-type pigment deposited in macrophages and endothelial cells.
*Other Adverse Effects of Amiodarone* Pulmonary fibrosis, pneumonitis, hepatotoxicity, thyroid disturbances, neuropathy, and myopathy.
*Course* The low-grade photosensitivity disappears 12 to 24 months after drug is discontinued; the long period results from the gradual elimination of the photoactive drug from the lysosomal membranes. The pigmentation also disappears after 1 to 3 years if drug is discontinued and sun is avoided.
**Minocycline**   Onset delayed, usually after total dose of >50 g, but may occur after a small dose. Not melanin but an iron-containing brown pigment, located in the dermal macrophages; stippled or diffuse. Blue-gray or slate-gray pigmentation (Fig. 20-10). Distributed on extensor legs, ankles, dorsa of feet, face, especially around eyes; sites of trauma or inflammation such as acne scars, contusions, abrasions; hard palate, teeth; nails.
*Internal Sites* Bones, cartilage, thyroid ("black thyroid").
*Course* Discoloration gradually disappears over a period of months after drug is discontinued.
**Clofazimine**   Orange, reddish brown (range, pink to black) discoloration, ill-defined on light-exposed areas; conjunctivae; accompanied by red sweat, urine, feces. Subcutaneous fat is orange.
**Zidovudine**   Brown macules on lips or oral mucosa; longitudinal brown bands in nails.
**Antimalarials (Chloroquine, Hydroxychloroquine, Quinacrine)**   Occurs in 25% of individuals who take the drug for >4 months. Brownish, gray-brown, and/or blue-black discoloration due to melanin, hemosiderin. With quinacrine: yellow, yellow-green due to quinacrine-containing complexes. Over shins; face, nape of neck; hard palate (sharp line of demarcation at soft palate); under finger- and toenails (see Fig. 30-35); may also occur in cornea and retina; quinacrine: skin and sclerae (resembling icterus); yellow-green fluorescence of nail bed with Wood's lamp. Discoloration disappears within a few months after drug is discontinued; quinacrine dyschromia can fade after 2 to 6 months even though drug is continued.
**Phenytoin**   *Dose* High dose over a long period of time (>1 year). *Discoloration* is spotty, resembling melasma, in light-exposed areas and is due to melanin.
**Bleomycin**   Mechanism unknown. Tan to brown to black and due to increase in epidermal melanin at sites of minor inflammation, i.e., parallel linear streaks at sites of dermatographism induced by excoriation ("flagellate" pigmentation), most commonly on the back, elbows, small joints, nails.

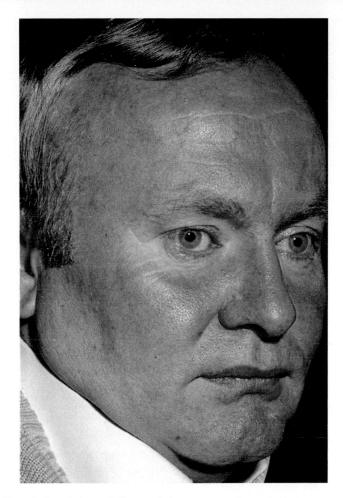

**FIGURE 20-9    Drug-induced pigmentation: amiodarone**   *A striking slate-gray pigmentation in a photodistribution of the face. The blue color (ceruloderma) is due to the deposition of melanin and lipofuscin contained in macrophages and endothelial cells in the dermis. The pigmentation is reversible, but it may take up to a year or more to complete resolution. In this patient it took 33 months for the ceruloderma to disappear.*

**Cyclophosphamide (Cytoxan)**   Brown. Diffuse or discrete macules on elbows; palms with Addisonian–like pigmentation (see Fig. 15-11) and macules.

**Busulfan (Myleran)**   Occurs in 5% of treated patients. Addisonian–like pigmentation.

*Distribution*   Face, axillae, chest, abdomen, oral mucous membranes.

**ACTH**   Addisonian pigmentation of skin and oral mucosa. First 13 amino acids of ACTH are identical to α-melanocyte-stimulating hormone (MSH) (see Fig. 15-11).

**Estrogens/Progesterone**   Caused by endogenous and exogenous estrogen combined with progesterone, i.e., during pregnancy or with oral contraceptive therapy. Sunlight causes marked darkening of pigmentation. Tan/brown (melasma or chloasma) (see page 348 and Fig. 13-8).

**Chlorpromazine and Other Phenothiazines**   Occurs after long-term (>6 months), high-dose (>500 mg/d) therapy. Phototoxic reaction. Slate-gray, blue-gray, or brownish in areas exposed to light, i.e., chin and cheeks. After

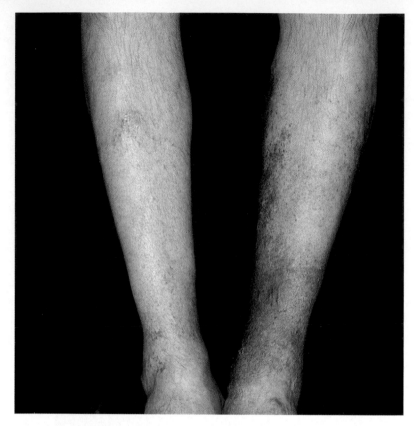

**FIGURE 20-10   Drug-induced pigmentation: minocycline**   *Stippled, blue-gray macular pigmentation on the lower legs. The patient had taken minocycline for years for rosacea. The pigmentation was much more pronounced on the left leg, associated with varicose veins, chronic venous insufficiency, and chronic edema. A melon-sized inguinal hernia was also present with striking pigmentation of the enlarged scrotum.*

discontinuation of drug, discoloration usually fades slowly.

**Silver (Argyria or Argyrosis)**   *Source*: Silver nitrate nose drops; silver sulfadiazine applied as an ointment. Silver sulfide (silver nitrate converted into silver sulfide by light, as in photographic film). Blue-gray discoloration. Primarily areas exposed to light, i.e., face, dorsa of hands, nails, conjunctiva; also diffuse.

**Gold (Chrysiasis)**   *Source*: Organic colloidal gold preparations used in therapy of rheumatoid arthritis. 5 to 25% of all treated patients. Dose-dependent. In high-dose therapy, appears in a short time; with lower dose, occurs after months. Blue-gray to purple discoloration. In light-exposed areas; sclerae. Persists long after drug is discontinued.

**Iron**   *Source*: IM iron injections; multiple blood transfusions. Brown or blue-gray discoloration. Generalized; also, local deposits at site of injection.

**Carotene**   Ingestion of large quantities of β-carotene-containing vegetables; β-carotene tablets. Yellow-orange discoloration. Most apparent on palms and soles.

# PSEUDOPORPHYRIA    □ ◑

Pseudoporphyria is a condition that clinically presents with cutaneous manifestations of porphyria cutanea tarda (PCT) (see Section 10) without the characteristic abnormal porphyrin
excretion. It is a bullous drug-induced photosensitivity reaction. This disorder develops on
the dorsa of hands and feet with characteristic tense bullae that rupture and leave erosions
(Fig. 20-11) and heal with scars and milia formation. Pseudo-PCT is associated with ingestion of drugs such as furosemide and nalidixic acid (Table 20-5). It is characterized by
subepidermal blistering with little or no dermal inflammation and, in contrast to true PCT, little or no deposition of immunoreactants around upper dermal blood vessels and capillary
walls.

A bullous dermatosis that is morphologically and histologically indistinguishable from PCT
also occurs in patients with chronic renal failure receiving maintenance hemodialysis.

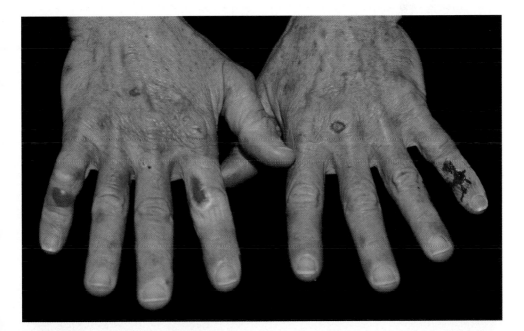

**FIGURE 20-11    Pseudoporphyria: non-
steroidal anti-inflammatory agents**    *In this
20-year-old male blisters appeared on the
dorsa of both hands that led to erosions,
crusting, and were clinically indistinguishable
from porphyria cutanea tarda. However, there
was no urinary fluorescence, and porphyrin
studies were negative. The patient had taken
an NSAID for arthritis and had impaired kidney function.*

**TABLE 20-5    Drugs Causing Pseudoporphyria**

| | |
|---|---|
| Naproxen | Diflunisal |
| Nabumetone | Celecoxib |
| Oxaprozin | Tetracyclines |
| Ketoprofen | Nalidixic acid |
| Mefenamic acid | Amiodarone |
| Tiaprofenic acid | Furosemide |

## ACDR-RELATED NECROSIS

Drugs can cause cutaneous necrosis when given orally or at sites of injection. Warfarin-induced cutaneous necrosis is a rare reaction with onset between the third and fifth days of anticoagulation therapy with the warfarin derivatives and indandione compounds, manifested by sharply demarcated, purpuric cutaneous infarction. *Risk factors*: higher initial dosing, obesity, female sex; individuals with hereditary deficiency of protein C, protein S or antithrombin III deficiency. Idiosyncratic reaction. In individuals with hereditary deficiency of protein C, a natural anticoagulant protein, warfarin greatly depresses protein C levels before decreasing other vitamin K–dependent coagulation factors, inducing a transient hypercoagulable state and thrombus formation. Lesions vary with severity of reaction: petechiae to ecchymoses to tender hemorrhagic infarcts to extensive necrosis. *Early*: large indurated dermal plaque(s). *Later*: quickly evolve to well-demarcated, deep purple to black, geographic areas of necrosis (Fig. 20-12). Hemorrhagic bullae, large erosions may complicate infarcts. Later, deep tissue sloughing and ulceration if lesions are not debrided and grafted. Often single; may present as two lesions. *Distribution*: areas of abundant subcutaneous fat: breasts (Fig. 20-12), buttocks, abdomen, thighs, calves; acral areas are spared. *Histology*: epidermal necrosis, thrombosis, and occlusion of most blood vessels, scanty inflammatory response. *Coagulation studies*: usually within normal limits. *Differential diagnosis*: Purpura fulminans (disseminated intravascular coagulation), hematoma/ecchymosis in overly anticoagulated patient, necrotizing soft tissue infection, vasculitis, rare necrosis after vasopressin treatment, brown recluse spider bite. Depending on severity of reaction, lesions may subside, heal by granulation, or require surgical intervention. If area of necrosis is large in an elderly, debilitated patient, may be life-threatening. If warfarin is inadvertently readministered, reaction recurs.

Cutaneous necrosis can occur at sites of injection of several drugs. Heparin can cause cutaneous necrosis, usually at the site of subcutaneous injection (Fig. 20-13). Interferon-α can cause necrosis and ulceration at injection sites, often in the lower abdominal panniculus (Fig. 20-14). Necrosis also occurs in ergotism where ergotamine-containing medications lead to acral gangrene, ergotamine-containing suppositories after prolonged use cause extremely painful anal and perianal black eschars (Fig. 20-15).

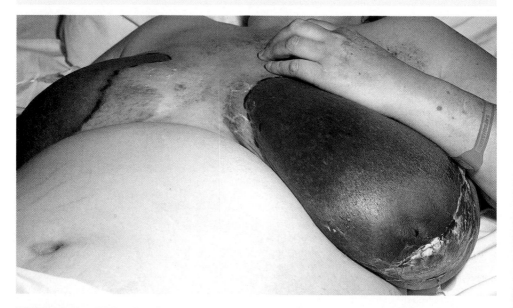

**FIGURE 20-12    ADCR-related cutaneous necrosis: coumarin**  *Bilateral areas of cutaneous infarction with purple-to-black coloration of the breast surrounded by an area of erythema occurred on the fifth day of coumarin therapy.*

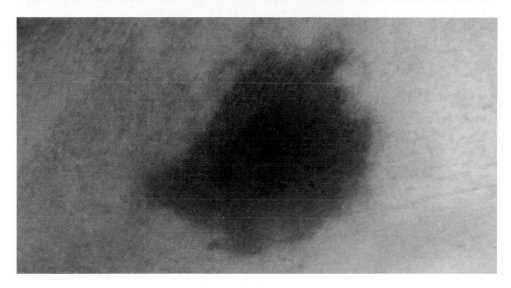

**FIGURE 20-13    ADCR-related cutaneous necrosis: heparin**   *An area of irregular dark-red ery-thema with central hemorrhagic necrosis on the abdomen occurring postoperatively in a female treated with heparin.*

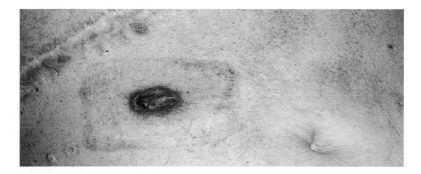

**FIGURE 20-14    ADCR-related cutaneous necrosis: interferon α**   *An ulcer on the abdomen at the site of interferon injection. The patient had liver transplantation and acquired hepatitis C virus infection during the procedure.*

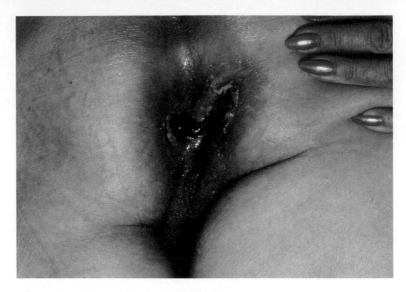

**FIGURE 20-15   ADCR-related cutaneous necrosis: ergotamine**   *This 53-year-old female had used ergot-containing suppositories for pain relief over many months. Painful black necrosis and ulceration developed on the anus and paraanally and extended into the rectum.*

## ACDR RELATED TO CHEMOTHERAPY

Chemotherapy may induce local and systemic skin toxicity with a wide range of cutaneous manifestations from benign to life threatening. A diversity of drugs are used to treat neoplastic and inflammatory disease, and the ACDR can be related to overdose, pharmacologic side effects, cumulative toxicity, delayed toxicity, or drug–drug interactions. Clinical manifestations range from alopecia (see Section 29) and nail changes (see Section 30) to mucositis and acral erythema, known as erythrodysesthesia. Chemotherapeutic agents are also responsible for inflammation and ulceration at sites of extravasation of intravenous medications, such as doxorubicin or taxol, which can be followed by skin necrosis with ulceration (Fig. 20-16). Other reactions are radiation recall or enhancement (as with methotrexate), erosion or ulceration of psoriasis due to an overdose of methotrexate, inflammation and sloughing of actinic keratosis due to 5-fluorouracil, or erosions due to cisplatin plus 5-fluorouracil (Fig. 20-17).

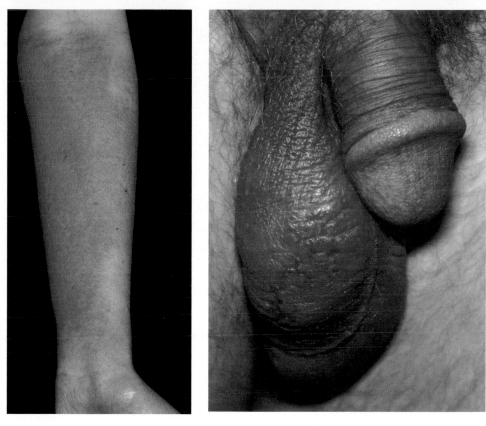

**FIGURE 20-16 (Left)   ADCR-related cellulitis: taxol**   *This extremely painful cellulitis appeared after a paravenous taxol infusion.*

**FIGURE 20-17 (Right)   ADCR-related erosions: cisplatin and 5FU**   *This patient had received chemotherapy with cisplatin and 5FU. Painful erosive lesions appeared on the scrotum and there was also erosive mucositis.*

## CUTANEOUS SIGNS OF INJECTING DRUG USE    ◫ ◐

Injecting drug users often develop cutaneous stigmata as a result of their habit, whether injecting subcutaneously or intravascularly. Cutaneous lesions range from foreign body response to
injected material, infections, and scars.

### Cutaneous Injection Reactions

*Cutaneous Injury* Multiple punctures at sites of
cutaneous injection, often linear over veins
(Fig. 20-18).

*Foreign Body Granuloma* Subcutaneous injection of adulterants (talc, sugar, starch, baking
soda, flour, cotton fibers, glass, etc.) can elicit a
foreign body response ± granuloma ± ulceration (Fig. 20-19).

### Intravascular Injection Reactions

*Venous Injury* Intravenous injection can result
in thrombosis, thrombophlebitis, septic
phlebitis. Chronic edema of the upper extremity
is common.

*Arterial Injury* Chronic intraarterial injection
can result in injection site pain, cyanosis, erythema, sensory and motor deficits, and vascular compromise (vascular insufficiency/-
gangrene).

### Infections

*Transmission of Infectious Agents* Injecting
drug use can result in transmission of HIV, hepatitis B virus (HBV), and hepatitis C virus
(HCV) with subsequent life-threatening systemic infections.

*Injection Site Infections* Local infections include cellulitis (Fig. 20-19), abscess formation,
lymphangitis, septic phlebitis/thrombophlebitis.
The most common organisms are those from the
drug users, e.g., *Staphylococcus aureus* and
group A streptococcus. Less common microbes:
enteric organisms, anaerobes, *Clostridium botulinum*, oral flora, fungi (*Candida albicans*), and
polymicrobial infections.

*Systemic Infections* Intravenous injection of
microbes can result in infection of vascular endothelium, most commonly heart valve with infectious endocarditis.

### Scars

*Linear Scars* Multiple cutaneous punctures result in linear scarring along the course of veins,
i.e., "needle tracks" (Fig. 20-18). These are
found on the forearms, dorsum of the hands,
wrists, antecubital/popliteal fossae, penis.

*Atrophic Punched-Out Scars* Result from subcutaneous injections (i.e., "skin popping") after
an inflammatory (sterile or infected) response
to injected material.

*Tattoos* Carbon on needles (after flame sterilization) can result in inadvertent tattooing and
pigmented linear scars.

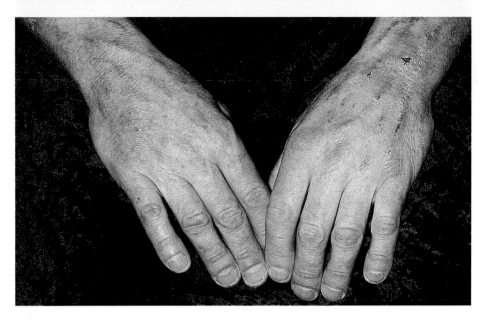

**FIGURE 20-18    Injecting drug use: injection tracks over veins on the dorsum of the hand**    *Linear tracks with punctures, fibrosis, and crusts were created by daily injections into the superficial veins.*

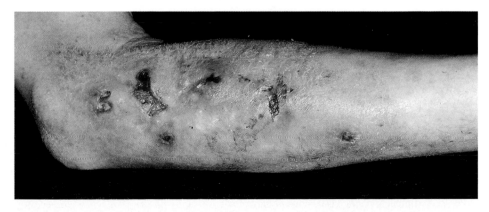

**FIGURE 20-19    Injecting drug use: cellulitis and foreign body response at injection site**    *The patient injected into the subcutaneous tissue as well as veins of the forearm, resulting in foreign body response and* S. aureus *cellulitis with associated bacteremia and infectious endocarditis.*

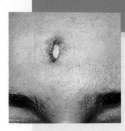

# DISORDERS OF PSYCHIATRIC ETIOLOGY

## CLASSIFICATION OF DISORDERS OF PSYCHIATRIC ETIOLOGY

Delusions
  Dysmorphic syndrome
  Delusions of parasitosis

Compulsive habits
  Neurotic excoriations
Factitious syndromes

## DYSMORPHIC SYNDROME (DS)  □  ◑

Patients with dysmorphic syndrome regard their image as distorted in the eyes of the public; this becomes almost an obsession. The patient with DS does not consult a psychiatrist but a dermatologist or plastic surgeon. The typical patient with DS is a single, female, young adult who is an anxious and unhappy person. Common dermatologic complaints are facial (wrinkles, acne, scars, hypertrichosis, dry lips), scalp (incipient baldness, increased hair growth), genital [normal sebaceous glands on the penis, red scrotum (males), red vulva, vaginal odor (females)], hyperhidrosis, and bromhidrosis. Management is a problem. One strategy is for the dermatologist to agree with the patient that there is a problem and thus establish rapport; in a few visits the complaint can be explored and further discussed. If the patient and physician do not agree that the complaint is a vastly exaggerated skin or hair change, then the patient should be referred to a psychiatrist; this latter plan is usually not accepted, in which case the problem may persist indefinitely.

**FIGURE 21-1  (Opposite page)    Delusions of parasitosis**  *Usually patients collect small pieces of debris from their skin by scratching with their nails or an instrument and submit them to the doctor for examination for parasites. Occasionally this can progress to an aggressive behavior such as depicted in this case where the patient posed to demonstrate how she removes the "parasites" from her skin with a mirror and tweezers. "Objects" are then meticulously collected on a piece of paper that is submitted for examination. In the majority of cases, patients are not dissuaded from their monosymptomatic delusion.*

## DELUSIONS OF PARASITOSIS   □  ◑

This rare disorder, which occurs in adults and is present for months or years, is associated with pain or paresthesia and is characterized by the presence of numerous skin lesions, mostly excoriations, which the patient truly believes are the result of a parasitic infestation (Fig. 21-1). The onset of the initial pruritus or paresthesia may be related to xerosis or, in fact, to a previously treated infestation. Patients pick with their fingernails or dig into their skin with needles or tweezers to remove the "parasites." It is important to rule out other causes of pruritus. This problem is serious; patients truly suffer and are opposed to seeking psychiatric help (Fig. 21-2). Patients may sell their houses to move away from the offending parasite.

The patient should see a psychiatrist for at least one visit and for recommendations of drug therapy: pimozide plus an antidepressant. Treatment is difficult and usually unsuccessful.

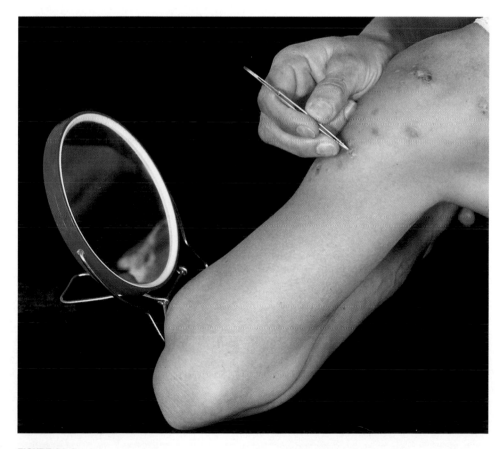

**FIGURE 21-1**

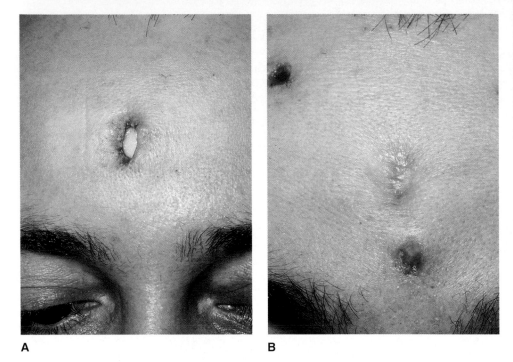

A                                              B

**FIGURE 21-2    Delusions of parasitosis**    *A. A sharply marginated ulcer on the forehead extending to the skull in a 32-year-old male. The patient saw fat lobules, considered them as parasites and picked them out with a needle. Similar lesions were also present on the neck. The ulcer had recently been excised by a plastic surgeon; however, the patient resumed picking at the site shortly after the procedure. **B**. The ulcer was occluded for 3 weeks preventing manipulation; the ulcer healed completely but new excoriations are seen. The patient was a successful businessman; he refused psychiatric consultation.*

## NEUROTIC EXCORIATIONS

Neurotic excoriations are not an uncommon problem, occurring in females more than in males and in the third to fifth decades. They may relate the onset to a specific event or to chronic stress; patients deny picking and scratching. The clinical lesions are an admixture of several types of lesions, principally excoriations, all produced by habitual picking of the skin with the fingernails (Figs. 21-3 through 21-5); most common on the face (Fig. 21-3), back (Fig. 21-4), and extremities but also at other sites (Fig. 21-5). There may be depigmented (Fig. 21-4) atrophic or hyperpigmented macules → scars. *The lesions are located only on sites that the hands can reach, thus sparing the center of the back.* The diagnosis can be deceptive, and what prima facie appears to be neurotic excoriations could be a serious cause of pruritus. Psychiatric guidance may be necessary if the problem is not solved, as it can be very disfiguring on the face and disruptive to the patient and the family. The course is prolonged, unless life adjustments are made. Pimozide has been helpful but must be used with caution and with the advice and guidance of a psychopharmacologist. Also, antidepressant drugs may be used.

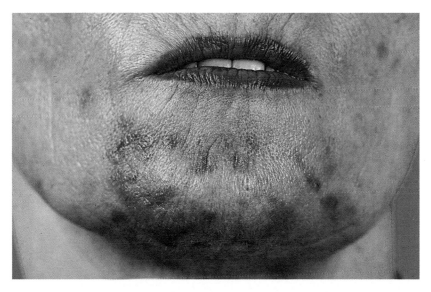

**FIGURE 21-3   "Neurotic" excoriations: chin**   *Multiple erythematous and pigmented macules and a few crusted erosions on the chin of a 45-year-old female with mild facial acne. No primary lesions are seen. The patient, who is moderately depressed, has mild acneiform lesions, which she compulsively picks with her fingernail.*

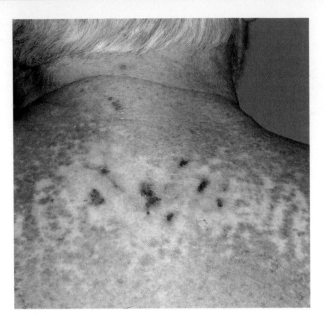

**Figure 21-4   "Neurotic" excoriations: upper back**   *Excoriations of the upper mid-back and linear areas of postinflammatory depigmentation and scarring in a 66-year-old diabetic female. Lesions have been present for at least 10 years but resolved for one month with intralesional triamcinolone and cloth tape occlusion. Once the protection was removed, the patient resumed excoriating the site.*

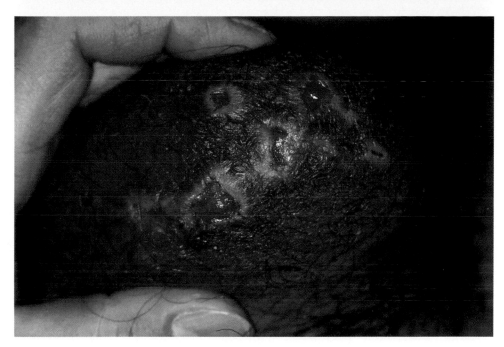

**FIGURE 21-5   "Neurotic" excoriations: scrotum**   *Large circular ulcerations on the scrotum of a severely depressed 55-year-old male. The lesions had been present for several years, worsening after the death of his wife. The lesions resolved with occlusion of the site but recurred whenever he had access to the skin. He was unable to control his compulsive behavior of picking at the site with his fingernails.*

# FACTITIOUS SYNDROMES (MUNCHAUSEN'S SYNDROME)

The term *factitial* means "artificial," and in this condition there is a self-induced dermatologic lesion(s); either the patient claims no responsibility or it is determined that the patient is deliberately mutilating the skin. It occurs in young adults, females > males. The history is vague ("hollow" history) of the evolution of the lesions. The lesions may be present for weeks to months to years (Fig. 21-6).

Patient may be normal looking and act normally in every respect, although frequently there is a strange affect and bizarre personality. The skin lesions consist of scars, ulcers, sphacelus (dense adherent necrotic membrane) (Fig. 21-6). The shape of the lesions may be linear, bizarre shapes, geometric patterns, single or multiple, and rarely occurring on the face. It is important to rule out chronic infections, granulomas, and vasculitis. The diagnosis can be difficult, but the nature of the lesions (bizarre shapes) may immediately suggest an artificial etiology. It is important to rule out every possible cause and perform a biopsy before assigning the diagnosis of *dermatosis artefacta*, both for the benefit of the patient and because the physician may be at risk for malpractice if he or she fails to diagnose a true pathologic process. This makes the task difficult. There is often serious personality and/or psychosocial stress.

The condition demands the utmost tact on the part of the physician, who can avert a serious outcome (i.e., suicide) by attempting to gain enough empathy with the patient to ascertain the cause. This varies with the nature of the psychiatric problem. The condition may persist for years in a patient who has selected his or her skin as the target organ of his or her conflicts. Consultation and management with a psychiatrist are mandatory in most patients.

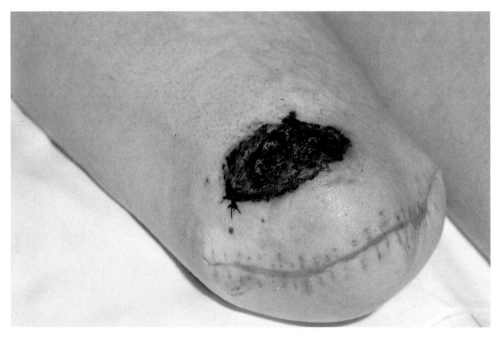

**FIGURE 21-6  Factitious syndrome**  *This sharply demarcated necrosis was self-inflicted by the covert application of potassium hydroxide incorporated into soap and applied to the skin with a tightly fitting bandage. Similar ulcers had previously been present first on the toes and later on the lower extremities and had led to successive steps of amputation.*

# DISEASES DUE TO MICROBIAL AGENTS

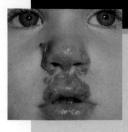
# BACTERIAL INFECTIONS INVOLVING THE SKIN

## SUPERFICIAL CUTANEOUS INFECTIONS

Three superficial bacterial "infections" occur in the stratum corneum and hair follicles, associated with overgrowth of normal flora at sites of occlusion and high surface humidity: erythrasma, pitted keratolysis, and trichomycosis. Trichomycosis, a misnomer in that the causative agents are corynebacteria and not fungi, presents as adherent granular nodules of hairs in the axillae (trichomycosis axillaris) or pubic area; the underlying skin is normal. Intertrigo is a nonspecific inflammation of naturally opposed skin, the diagnosis being made after specific infectious causes such as erythrasma or candidiasis are ruled out.

## ERYTHRASMA

Erythrasma (Greek, "red spot") is a chronic bacterial infection caused by *Corynebacterium minutissimum* affecting the intertriginous areas of the webspace of the feet, groins, axillae, and submammary areas, which mimics epidermal dermatophyte infections. The organism rarely causes invasive infections.

### EPIDEMIOLOGY AND ETIOLOGY

**Age of Onset**   Adults
**Etiology**   *C. minutissimum*, gram-positive (diphtheroid), non-spore-forming, aerobic or facultatively anaerobic bacillus; part of normal skin flora, which causes superficial infection under certain conditions.
**Predisposing Factors**   Humid cutaneous microclimate: warm and/or humid climate or season; occlusive clothing/shoes; obesity, hyperhidrosis.

### HISTORY

**Symptoms**   Usually asymptomatic. Duration: weeks to months to years.

### PHYSICAL EXAMINATION

**Skin Lesions**
Macule, sharply marginated (Fig. 22-1). Scaling at sites not continuously occluded. In web-spaces of feet, may be macerated (Fig. 22-2), eroded, or fissured. Often symmetric or in multiple webspaces. Red or brownish red; postinflammatory hyperpigmentation in more heavily melanized individuals. If pruritic, secondary changes of excoriation, lichenification. Dermatophytosis and/or candidiasis may also be present.
***Sites of Predilection***   Toe webspaces (Fig. 22-2) >> groin folds (Fig. 22-1) > axillae; also, intertriginous skin under panniculus, intergluteal, inframammary.

### DIFFERENTIAL DIAGNOSIS

**Well-Demarcated Intertriginous Plaque**   Dermatophytosis, intertriginous candidiasis, pityriasis versicolor, pitted keratolysis, inverse-pattern psoriasis, seborrheic dermatitis, acanthosis nigricans.

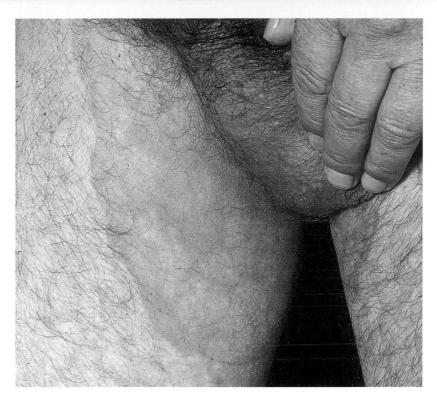

**FIGURE 22-1   Erythrasma: groins**   *Sharply marginated, brownish-red, slightly scaling macular patch on the medial thigh (infectious intertrigo) appears bright coral-red when examined with a Wood's lamp. KOH preparation was negative for hyphae.*

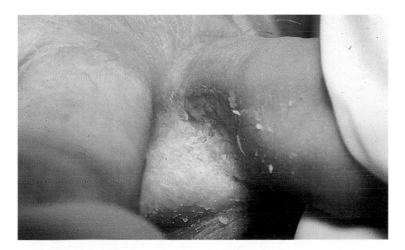

**FIGURE 22-2   Erythrasma: webspace**   *This macerated interdigital webspace (infectious intertrigo) appeared bright coral-red when examined with a wood's lamp; KOH preparation was negative for hyphae. The webspace is the most common site for erythrasma in temperate climates. In some cases, interdigital tinea pedis and/or pseudomonal intertrigo may coexist.*

## LABORATORY EXAMINATIONS

**Wood's Lamp**   The diagnosis is made by demonstration of the characteristic coral-red fluorescence (attributed to coproporphyrin III). May not be present if patient has bathed recently.
**Direct Microscopy**   Negative for fungal forms on KOH preparation of skin scraping. In the webspaces of the feet, concomitant interdigital tinea pedis may also be present. Gram or Giemsa stains may show fine bacterial filaments.
**Bacterial Culture**   Heavy growth of *Corynebacterium*. Rules out *Staphylococcus aureus*, group A streptococcus, and *Candida* infection. In some cases, concomitant *Pseudomonas aeruginosa* webspace infection (feet) is also present.

## DIAGNOSIS

Clinical findings, absence of fungi on direct microscopy, positive Wood's lamp examination.

## COURSE

Relapse occurs if predisposing causes are not corrected. Secondary prophylaxis usually indicated.

## MANAGEMENT

**Prevention/Prophylaxis**   Wash with benzoyl peroxide (bar or wash). Medicated powders (do not use cornstarch powder). Topical antiseptic alcohol gels: isopropyl, ethanol.
**Topical Therapy**   Preferable. Benzoyl peroxide (2.5%) gel daily after showering for 7 days. Topical erythromycin or clindamycin solution bid for 7 days. Sodium fusidate ointment, mupirocin ointment or cream. Topical antifungal agents: clotrimazole, miconazole, or econazole.
**Systemic Antibiotic Therapy**   Erythromycin or tetracycline, 250 mg qid for 14 days. Clarithromycin.

---

## PITTED KERATOLYSIS (KERATOLYSIS SULCATA)    ▮  ○

Pitted keratolysis (PK) presents as defects in the thickly keratinized skin of the plantar foot with eroded pits of variable depth, depending on the thickness of the stratum corneum, usually associated with pedal hyperhidrosis, caused by *Kytococcus sedentarius*.

## EPIDEMIOLOGY AND ETIOLOGY

**Etiology**   *K. sedentarius*
**Age of Onset**   Young adults
**Sex**   Males > females
**Predisposing Factors**   Hyperhidrosis of the feet; occlusive footwear. *K. sedentarius* produces two extracellular proteases that can digest keratin.

## HISTORY

**Skin Symptoms**   Usually asymptomatic. Foot odor, sliminess of feet. Uncommonly, itching, burning, tenderness. Often mistaken for tinea pedis.

## PHYSICAL EXAMINATION

**Skin Lesions**
Crater-like pits in stratum corneum, 1 to 8 mm in diameter (Fig. 22-3). Pits can remain discrete or, more often, become confluent, forming large areas of eroded stratum corneum. Involved areas are white when stratum corneum is fully hydrated (Fig. 22-4). Symmetric or asymmetric involvement of both feet.
***Distribution***   Pressure-bearing areas, ventral aspect of toe, ball of foot, heel. Friction areas: interface of toes.

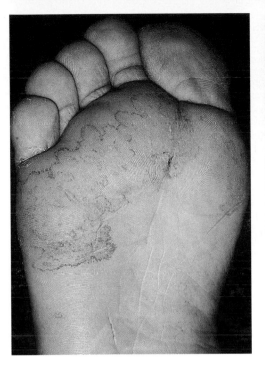

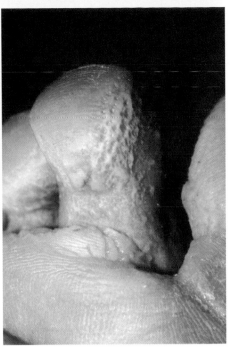

**FIGURE 22-3   Pitted keratolysis: plantar**
*The stratum corneum of the anterior plantar foot shows loss of keratinization with well-dermarcated scalloped margins, formed by the confluence of multiple, confluent "pits" (defects in the stratum corneum).*

**FIGURE 22-4   Pitted keratolysis: toe**   *Pitted epidermis of an intertriginous toe, associated with hyperhidrosis.*

## DIFFERENTIAL DIAGNOSIS

**Erosion in Multiple Webspaces of Feet**   Interdigital tinea pedis, *Candida* intertrigo, erythrasma, *Pseudomonas* webspace infection.

## LABORATORY EXAMINATIONS

**Direct Microscopy**   KOH preparation negative for hyphae.
**Wood's Lamp Examination**   Negative for bright coral-red fluorescence (erythrasma).
**Culture**   In some cases, rules out *S. aureus*, group A streptococcus, or *P. aeruginosa* infection.

## DIAGNOSIS

Clinical diagnosis ruling out other causes.

## COURSE AND PROGNOSIS

Persists and recurs until the underlying predisposing factors are corrected. Secondary prophylaxis usually indicated.

## MANAGEMENT

See "Erythrasma."

## INTERTRIGINOUS INFECTIONS AND INTERTRIGO

Intertrigo (Latin *inter*, "between," *trigo*, "rubbing") is a nonspecific inflammation of opposed skin, occurring in the inframammary regions, axillae, groins, and gluteal folds (Figs. 22-5 to 22-8) and between redundant skin. With increased moisture and maceration, the stratum corneum becomes eroded. The problem is common in obese individuals with overlapping abdominal panniculus. Intertriginous infections caused by bacteria (groups A and B streptococcus, *C. minutissimum*, *P. aeruginosa*) and fungi (dermatophytes, *Candida*, and *Malassezia furfur*) must be ruled out. Dermatoses such as psoriasis vulgaris (inverse pattern), seborrheic dermatitis, and atopic dermatitis also occur in body folds, presenting as erythema or erythematous plaques.

Intertrigo is diagnosed in the presence of erythema ± symptoms of pruritus, tenderness, or increased sensitivity, excluding infectious causes. For acutely symptomatic intertrigo, moist dressings and/or Castellani's paint give immediate symptomatic relief. Powders with antibacterial/antifungal activity are helpful for preventing recurrence. In some cases, zinc oxide ointment reduces friction at involved sites. Topical glucocorticoid preparations should be avoided because of the risk of cutaneous atrophy at these naturally occluded sites. Topical pimecrolimus and tacrolimus may be effective, without risk of atrophy. Weight reduction is ideal but often not possible.

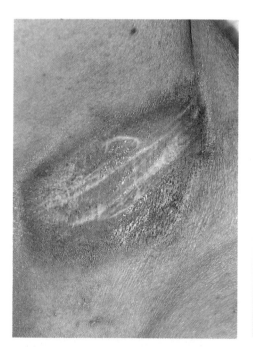

**FIGURE 22-5   Axillary intertrigo: group A streptococcus**   *A painful erythematous plaque with purulent exudate in the axilla of an HIV-infected woman.*

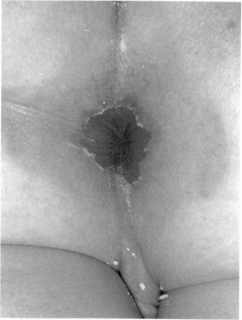

**FIGURE 22-6   Perineal intertrigo: group A streptococcus**   *Well-dermarcated erythema and erosion in the perineum of an 8-year-old boy associated with pruritus and tenderness (perianal streptococcal "cellulitis").*

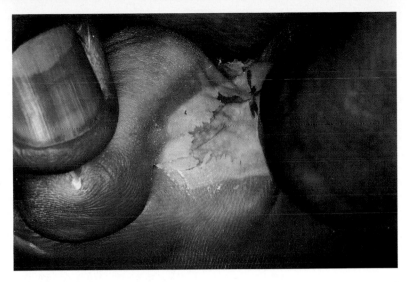

**FIGURE 22-7    Webspace intertrigo: _C. albicans_**  _Maceration of a webspace of the foot of a female with diabetes. KOH preparation showed yeast with pseudomycelial forms;_ C. albicans _was isolated on culture._

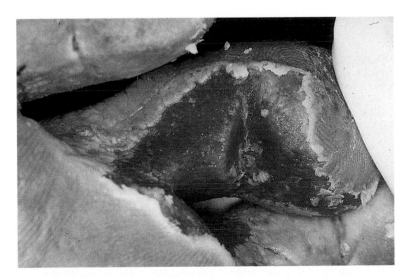

**FIGURE 22-8    Webspace intertrigo: _P. aeruginosa_**  _Erosion of a webspace of the foot with a bright red base and surrounding erythema. Tinea pedis (interdigital and moccasin-patterns) and hyperhidrosis were also present, which facilitated growth of_ Pseudomonas.

# PYODERMAS

## ETIOPATHOGENESIS

Normal skin is heavily colonized by bacterial flora such as coagulase-negative staphylococci (CoNS), more numerous in occluded than exposed sites. Colonization of the skin by *S. aureus* and group A β-hemolytic streptococcus (GAS) (*Streptococcus pyogenes*) is promoted by warm weather/climate, high humidity, presence of skin disease (especially atopic dermatitis), age of patient, prior antibiotic therapy, poor hygiene, crowded living conditions, and neglected minor trauma. *S. aureus* and GAS cause a variety of syndromes, including superficial and deep pyogenic infections, and systemic intoxications.

- CoNS, which colonize the skin shortly after birth have been subdivided into 32 species, 15 of which are indigenous to humans. The most common CoNS are *S. epidermidis* (65 to 90% of individuals), *S. hominis*, *S. haemolyticus*, *S.warneri*, and *S. lugdunensis*. CoNS have lower pathogenicity in the skin and mucosa but increasingly cause infection of artificial devices such as percutaneous intervenous catheter (PIC) lines and heart valves.
- *S. aureus* does not normally reside on the skin, but may be present transiently, inoculated from colonized sites such as the nares (Fig. 22-9). Colonization occurs on the mucous membranes of the anterior nasopharynx of 30% of otherwise healthy persons. Other commonly colonized sites include axillae, vagina (5 to 15%, and up to 30% during menses), damaged skin, perineum. Colonization is usually intermittent; 10 to 20% of individuals have persistent colonization; 10 to 20% are never colonized. Colonization rates are higher among health care workers, dialysis patients, patients with type 1 diabetes, injection drug users, persons with HIV disease, those with atopic dermatitis (90% in dermatitis, 70% of nonlesional skin). Colonization rate is higher (30 to 50%) after 2 weeks in hospital, and organisms are more likely methicillin-resistant *S. aureus* (MRSA).
- MRSA has been emerging as a nosocomial as well as a community-acquired pathogen and has a higher associated morbidity and mortality than methicillin-sensitive *S. aureus* (MSSA). In some report of community-acquired infection, MRSA was isolated in more than half of isolates. Infection usually presents as abscess or cellulitis.
- GAS usually colonizes the skin first and then the nasopharynx. An intact stratum corneum is the most important defense against invasion of pathogenic bacteria. Group B and group G β-hemolytic streptococci (GBS, GGS) colonize the perineum of some individuals and may cause superficial and invasive infections.

Carriers of *S. aureus* and/or GAS are at increased risk for pyodermas, (impetigo/ecthyma; furuncles, carbuncles, abscesses; folliculitis) and soft tissue infections (erysipelas, cellulitis, gangrenous cellulitis). Frequent hand washing reduces the risk of person-to-person transmission of cutaneous pathogens.

## COMPLICATIONS OF PYODERMAS

Vascular invasion may result in bacteremia and subsequent infectious endocarditis, abscesses of abdominal viscera, brain abscess, meningitis, septic arthritis, osteomyelitis, epidural abscess, mycotic aneurysm.

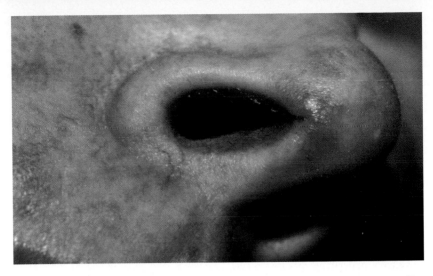

**FIGURE 22-9    Impetigo: *S. aureus* nasal colonization**    *Colonization of the nares in usually asymptomatic. This patient had tenderness and erythema of the skin adjacent to the nares, indicative of superficial infection rather than colonization.*

## IMPETIGO AND ECTHYMA    ■

*S. aureus* and GAS (*S. pyogenes*) cause superficial infections of the epidermis (*impetigo*), which may extend into the dermis (*ecthyma*), characterized by crusted erosions or ulcers. They may arise as primary infections in minor superficial breaks in the skin or as secondary infections of preexisting dermatoses (impetiginization, or secondary infection).

### EPIDEMIOLOGY AND ETIOLOGY

**Age of Onset**    Primary infections more common in children. Secondary infections, any age. Bullous impetigo: children, young adults.

**Etiology**    *S. aureus* most commonly; also, GAS or mixed *S. aureus* and GAS. Bullous impetigo: 80% caused by *S. aureus* phage group 2 (types 71 and 55), which produce exfoliative toxins and also cause staphylococcal scalded-skin syndrome.

**Predisposing Factors**    Topical glucocorticoids have little effect on the microflora of the skin, except in those with atopic dermatitis; topical glucocorticoids applied to atopic dermatitis usually reduce the density of *S. aureus*. Ecthyma: lesion of neglect—develops in excoriations; insect bites; minor trauma in diabetics, elderly patients, soldiers, and alcoholics.

**Portals of Entry of Infection**    *Primary Impetigo*   Arises at minor breaks in the skin.

*Secondary Impetigo (Impetiginization)* Arises in a variety of underlying dermatoses and traumatic breaks in the integrity of the epidermis.

### Inflammatory Dermatoses

Atopic dermatitis, stasis dermatitis, psoriasis vulgaris, chronic cutaneous lupus erythematosus, pyoderma gangrenosum.

### Bullous Disease

Pemphigus vulgaris, bullous pemphigoid, sunburn, porphyria cutanea tarda.

### Ulcers

Pressure, stasis.

### Chronic Lymphedema

### Cutaneous Infections

Herpes simplex, varicella, herpes zoster; dermatophytosis (tinea pedis, tinea capitis).

### Trauma/Wounds

Surgical wounds; abrasion; laceration; puncture; bites: human, animal, insect; burns; ulcers; umbilical stump.

## HISTORY

**Duration of Lesions**   Impetigo: days to weeks. Ecthyma: weeks to months.
**Symptoms**   Impetigo: variable pruritus, especially associated with atopic dermatitis. Ecthyma: pain, tenderness.

## PHYSICAL EXAMINATION

### Skin Lesions

*Nonbullous Impetigo* Transient superficial small vesicles or pustules rupture, resulting in erosions, which in turn become surmounted by a crust (Fig. 22-10). Golden-yellow crusts are often seen in impetigo but are not pathognomonic (Fig. 22-11). 1- to 3-cm lesions; central healing often apparent if lesions present for several weeks. *Arrangement*: scattered, discrete lesions; without therapy, lesions may become confluent; satellite lesions occur by autoinoculation.
*Bullous Impetigo* Vesicles (Fig. 22-12) and bullae (Fig. 22-13) containing clear yellow or slightly turbid fluid without surrounding erythema, arising on normal-appearing skin. With rupture, bullous lesions decompress. If roof of bulla is removed, shallow moist *erosion* forms. *Distribution*: more common in intertriginous sites.

*Ecthyma* Ulceration with a thick adherent crust (Fig. 22-14). Lesions may be tender, indurated. *Distribution*: more common on distal extremities.

### Miscellaneous Physical Findings

At times, lymphangitis and/or regional lymphadenopathy.

## DIFFERENTIAL DIAGNOSIS

**Erosion ± Crust/Scale-Crust**   Excoriation, perioral dermatitis, seborrheic dermatitis, allergic contact dermatitis, herpes simplex, epidermal dermatophytosis, scabies. *The majority of lesions with "honey-colored crusts" are not impetigo.*
**Intact Bulla(e)**   Allergic contact dermatitis, insect bites, thermal burns, herpes simplex, herpes zoster, bullous pemphigoid, porphyria cutanea tarda (PCT) (dorsa of hands), pseudo-porphyria.
**Ulcer ± Crust/Scale-Crust**   Chronic herpetic ulcers, excoriated insect bites, neurotic excoriations, cutaneous diphtheria, PCT, venous (stasis) and atherosclerotic ulcers (legs).

## LABORATORY EXAMINATIONS

**Gram Stain**   Gram-positive cocci, in chains or clusters, within neutrophils.
**Culture**   *S. aureus*, commonly; GAS (especially from older lesions). Failure of oral antibiotic may be indication of infection by MRSA.
**Dermatopathology**   Impetigo: gram-positive cocci in blister fluid, erosion, or ulceration.

## DIAGNOSIS

Clinical findings confirmed by Gram's stain or culture.

## COURSE AND PRSOGNOSIS

Untreated, lesions of impetigo progress for several weeks. Untreated or neglected impetigo can progress to ecthyma. With adequate treatment, prompt resolution. Lesions can progress to invasive infection with lymphangitis, suppurative lymphadenitis, cellulitis or erysipelas, bacteremia, septicemia. Nonsuppurative complications of GAS infection include guttate psoriasis, scarlet fever, and glomerulonephritis. Recurrence may occur because of failure to eradicate organism or reinfection from a family member. Ecthyma often heals with scar. Recurrent *S. aureus* or GAS infections can occur by

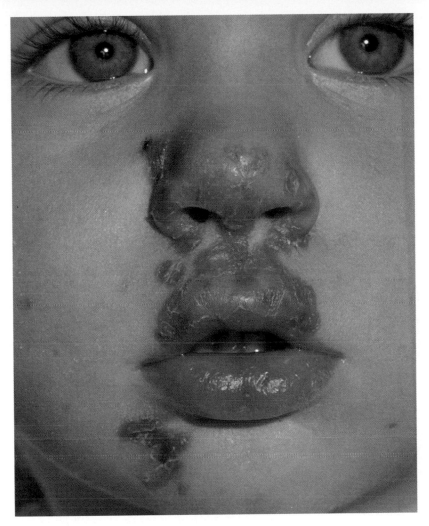

**FIGURE 22-10    Impetigo: *S. aureus***   *Crusted erythematous erosions becoming confluent on the nose, cheek, lips, and chin in a child with nasal carriage of* S. aureus *and mild facial eczema.*

recolonization from a family member or a family dog. MRSA infection has higher morbidity and mortality.

### MANAGEMENT

**Prevention**   Daily bath. Benzoyl peroxide wash (bar). Check family members for signs of impetigo. Ethanol or isopropyl gel for hands and/or involved sites.

**Topical Treatment**   Mupirocin (pseudomonic acid) ointment is highly effective in eliminating both GAS and *S. aureus*, including MRSA, from the nares and cutaneous lesions. Apply three times daily to involved skin and to nares for 7 to 10 days.

**Systemic Antimicrobial Treatment**   See Table 22-1. For MRSA, sensitivities of the isolated organism and personal history of antibiotic allergies determine drug of choice and alternatives.

## TABLE 22-1 Organisms, Antimicrobial Agents of Choice, and Alternatives

| Infecting Organism | Antimicrobial Agent(s) of First Choice | Alternative Antimicrobial Agents |
|---|---|---|
| *Staphylococcus aureus* or *epidermidis* Non-penicillinase producing | Penicillin G or V | A cephalosporin; clindamycin; vancomycin; imipenem; a fluoroquinolone |
| Penicillinase-producing | A penicillinase-resistant penicillin. PO: dicloxacillin, cloxacillin. IV for severe infections; nafcillin, oxacillin | A cephalosporin; vancomycin; amoxicillin/clavulanic acid; ticarcillin/clavulanic acid; piperacillin/ tazobactam; ampic-illin/sulbactam; imipenem; clindamycin; a fluoroquinolone |
| Methicillin-resistant | Vancomycin ± gentamicin ± rifampin | Trimethoprim-sulfamethox-azole; a fluoroqui-nolone; minocycline; linezolid; quinupristin/dalfopristin |
| *Streptococcus pyogenes* (group A) and groups C and G | Penicillin G or V | An erythromycin, clarithromycin, azithromycin; a cephalosporin; vancomycin; clindamycin |
| *Streptococcus, group B* | Penicillin G or ampicillin | A cephalosporin, vancomycin, an erythromycin |
| *Streptococcus pneumoniae (pneumococcus)* | Penicillin G or V | A cephalosporin erythro mycin; azithromycin; clarithromycin; a fluoroquinolone; meropenem; imipenem; trimethoprim-sulfameth-oxazole; clindamycin; a tetracycline |
| Penicillin-susceptible (MIC <0.1 µg/mL) Penicillin-intermediate resistance | Penicillin G IV (12 million U/d for adults) *or* ceftriaxone *or* cefotaxime | Levofloxacin; vancomycin; clindamycin |
| Penicillin-high level resistance (MIC ≥ 2 µg/mL) | Meningitis: vancomycin + ceftriaxone *or* cefotaxime ± rifampin Other infections: varicomycin ± ceftri-axone *or* cefotaxime; *or* levofloxacin | Meropenem; imipenem; clindamycin Quinupristin/dalfopristin; linezolid |

*(continued)*

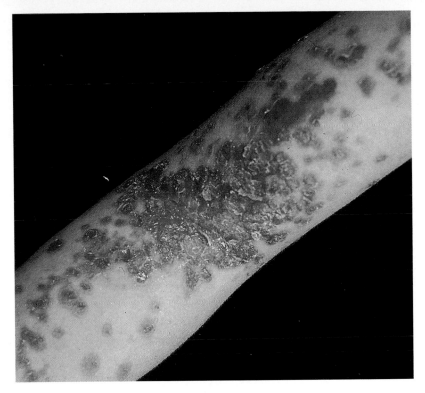

**FIGURE 22-11    Impetiginization of atopic dermatitis: *S. aureus***    *Atopic dermatitis on the antecubital fossae with secondary* S. aureus *infection (impetiginization).*

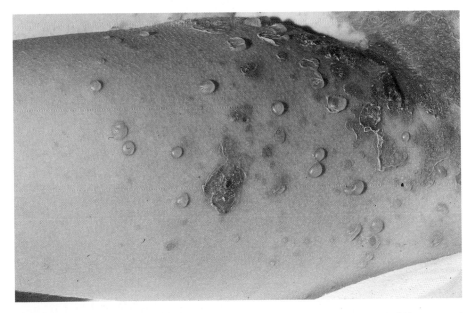

**FIGURE 22-12    Bullous impetigo: *S. aureus***    *Scattered, discrete, intact thin-walled blisters on the thigh of a child; lesions in the groin have ruptured, resulting in superficial erosions.*

**TABLE 22-1  Organisms, Antimicrobial Agents of Choice, and Alternatives (*Continued*)**

| Infecting Organism | Antimicrobial Agent(s) of First Choice | Alternative Antimicrobial Agents |
|---|---|---|
| *Erysipelothrix rhusiopathiae* | Penicillin G | Erythromycin, a cephalosporin, a fluoroquinolone |
| *Haemophilus influenzae* | | |
| Meningitis, epiglottitis, arthritis, and other serious infections | Cefotaxime *or* ceftriaxone | Cefuroxime (not for meningitis); chloramphenicol; meropenem |
| Upper respiratory infections and bronchitis | Trimethoprim-sulfamethoxazole | Cefuroxime; amoxicillin/clavulanic acid; cefuroxime axetil; cefpodoxime; cefaclor; cefotaxime, ceftizoxime; ceftriaxone; cefixime; a tetracycline; clarithromycin; azithromycin; a fluoroquinolone; ampicillin or amoxicillin |
| *Pasteurella multocida* | Penicillin G | A tetracycline; a cephalosporin; amoxicillin /clavulanic acid; ampicillin/sulbactam |
| *Pseudomonas aeruginosa* | Ciprofloxacin; ticarcillin, mezlocillin *or* piperacillin + tobramycin, gentamicin *or* amikacin | Carbenicillin, ticarcillin, piperacillin *or* mezlocillin; ceftazidime; cefepime; imipenem *or* meropenem; aztreonam; tobramycin; gentamicin; amikacin |
| *Vibrio vulnificus* | A tetracycline | Cefotaxime |
| *Neisseria gonorrhoeae* (**gonococcus**) | Ceftriaxone *or* cefixime *or* ciprofloxacin *or* ofloxacin | Cefotaxime; spectinomycin; penicillin G; cefotaxime; ceftizoxime; ceftriaxone |
| *Neissera meningitis* (**meningococcus**) | Penicillin G | Chloramphenicol; a sulfonamide; a fluoroquinolone |
| *Mycobacterium tuberculosis* | Isoniazid + rifampin + pyrazinamide + ethambutol *or* streptomycin | Levofloxacin, ofloxacin *or* ciprofloxacin; cycloserine; capreomycin *or* kanamycin *or* amikacin; ethionamide; clofazimine; aminosalicylic acid |
| *Mycobacterium fortuitum/chelonae* complex | Amikacin + clarithromycin | Cefoxitin; rifampin; a sulfonamide; doxycycline; ethambutol |
| *Mycobacterium marinum (balnie)* | Minocycline | Trimethoprim-sulfamethoxazole; rifampin; clarithromycin; doxycycline |

(*continued*)

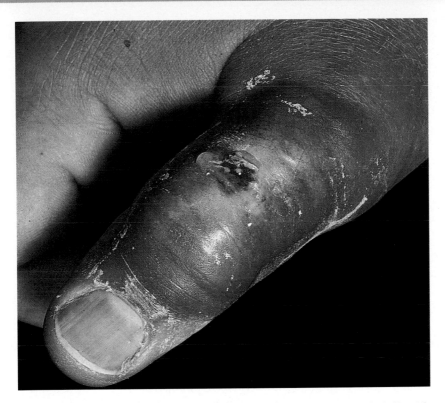

**FIGURE 22-13   Bullous Impetigo (blistering dactylitis): *S. aureus***   *A large, single bulla with surrounding erythema and edema on the thumb of a child; the bulla has ruptured only in the center and clear serum exudes from it.*

**TABLE 22-1   Organisms, Antimicrobial Agents of Choice, and Alternatives (*Continued*)**

| Infecting Organism | Antimicrobial Agent(s) of First Choice | Alternative Antimicrobial Agents |
|---|---|---|
| *Mycobacterium leprae* (leprosy) | Dapsone + rifampin + clofazimine | Minocycline ofloxacin; sparfloxacin; clarithromycin |
| *Actinomyces israelii* (actinomycosis) | Penicillin G | A tetracycline; erythromycin; clindamycin |
| *Nocardia* | Trimethoprim-sulfamethoxazole | Sulfasoxazole; amikacin; a tetracycline; imipenem *or* meropenem; cycloserine |

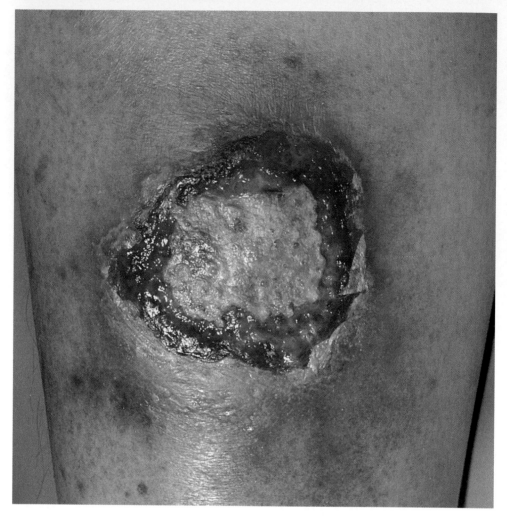

**FIGURE 22-14    Ecthyma: *S. aureus*** *A large, circumscribed chronic ulcer with surrounding erythema in the pretibial region.*

# ABSCESS, FURUNCLE, AND CARBUNCLE    ■  ◑

An *abscess* is an acute or chronic localized inflammation, associated with a collection of pus and tissue destruction. A *furuncle* is an acute, deep-seated, red, hot, tender nodule or abscess that evolves from a staphylococcal folliculitis. A *carbuncle* is a deeper infection composed of interconnecting abscesses usually arising in several contiguous hair follicles.
*Synonym*: Boil.

## EPIDEMIOLOGY AND ETIOLOGY

**Age of Onset**  Children, adolescents, and young adults.
**Sex**  More common in boys.
**Etiology**  Most commonly MSSA. MRSA infections becoming more common. Much less commonly, other organisms. Sterile abscess can occur as a foreign body response (splinter, ruptured inclusion cyst, injection sites). Cutaneous odontogenic sinus can appear anywhere on the lower face, even at sites distant from the origin.
**Predisposing Factors**

• Chronic *S. aureus* carrier state (nares, axillae, perineum, vagina)
• Diabetes mellitus
• Obesity
• Poor hygiene
• Bactericidal defects (e.g., chronic granulomatous disease)
• Chemotactic defects
• Hyper-IgE syndrome (Job's syndrome)
• HIV disease, especially MRSA infection

## PATHOGENESIS

Folliculitis, furuncles, and carbuncles represent a continuum of severity of *S. aureus* infection. Portal of entry: hair follicle, break in the integrity of skin. MRSA infections often have high morbidity due to delay in administration of effective antibiotic. Control/eradication of carrier state treats/prevents folliculitis, furuncle, and carbuncle formation.

## HISTORY

**Duration of Lesions**  Days to weeks to months.
**Skin Symptoms**  Throbbing pain and invariably exquisite tenderness.

**Constitutional Symptoms**  Carbuncles may be accompanied by low-grade fever and malaise.

## PHYSICAL EXAMINATION

### Skin Lesions
Lesions are red, hot, and painful/tender.
*Abscess*  May arise in any organ or structure. Abscesses that present on the skin arise in the dermis, subcutaneous fat, muscle, or a variety of deeper structures. Initially, a tender red nodule forms. In time (days to weeks), pus collects within a central space (Fig. 22-15). A well-formed abscess is characterized by fluctuance of the central portion of the lesion and can occur at any cutaneous site. At sites of trauma. Upper trunk for abscesses in ruptured inclusion cysts. Single or multiple.
*Furuncle*  Initially, a firm tender nodule, up to 1 to 2 cm in diameter (Fig. 22-16) with a central necrotic plug. In many individuals, furuncles occur in setting of staphylococcal folliculitis in beard area or neck. Nodule becomes fluctuant, with abscess formation below necrotic plug often topped by a central pustule. After rupture or drainage of pustule and discharge of necrotic plug, a nodule with cavitation remains. A variable zone of cellulitis may surround the furuncle. May arise in any hair-bearing region: beard area (Fig. 22-17), posterior neck and occipital scalp, axillae, buttocks. Single or multiple (Fig. 22-18).
*Carbuncle*  Evolution is similar to that of furuncle. Composed of several to multiple, adjacent, coalescing furuncles (Fig. 22-19). Characterized by multiple loculated dermal and subcutaneous abscesses, superficial pustules, necrotic plugs, and sieve-like openings draining pus.

## DIFFERENTIAL DIAGNOSIS

**Painful Dermal/Subcutaneous Nodule**   Ruptured epidermoid or pilar cyst, hidradenitis suppurativa (axillae, groin, vulva), necrotizing lymphangitis.

## LABORATORY EXAMINATIONS

**Gram's Stain**   Gram-positive cocci within PMN leukocytes.

**Bacterial Culture**   Culture of pus isolates *S. aureus*. Sensitivities to antimicrobial agents may determine management.

*Antibiotic Sensitivities*   Identifies MRSA and need for changing usual antibiotic therapy.

**Dermatopathology**   Pyogenic infection arising in hair follicle and extending into deep dermis and subcutaneous tissue (furuncle) and with loculated abscesses (carbuncle).

## DIAGNOSIS

Clinical findings confirmed by findings on Gram's stain and culture.

## COURSE AND PROGNOSIS

Most cases resolve with incision and drainage and systemic antibiotic treatment. At times, however, furunculosis is complicated by bacteremia and possible hematogenous seeding of heart valves, joints, spine, long bones, and viscera (especially kidneys). *S. aureus* can disseminate hematogenously via venous drainage to cavernous sinus with resultant cavernous venous thromboses and meningitis. Some individuals are subject to recurrent furunculosis, particularly diabetics.

## MANAGEMENT

The treatment of an abscess, furuncle, or carbuncle is incision and drainage plus systemic antimicrobial therapy.

**Prevention**   Mupirocin ointment is effective for eliminating nasal carriage.

**Surgery**   Incision and drainage are often adequate for treatment of abscesses, furuncles, or carbuncles. Scissors or scalpel blade can be used to drain loculated pus in carbuncles; if this is not done, resolution of pain and infection can be delayed despite systemic antibiotic therapy. Dental abscesses are often associated with devitalized tooth pulp, which must be removed or the tooth extracted. All foreign matter must be removed: comedone, keratinaceous debris, foreign body.

**Adjunctive Therapy**   Application of heat to the lesion promotes localization/consolidation and aids early spontaneous drainage.

**Systemic Antimicrobial Treatment**   In healthy individuals, incision and drainage are often adequate therapy. Systemic antibiotics speed resolution in healthy individuals and are mandatory in any individual at risk for bacteremia (e.g., immunosuppressed patients). See Table 22-2.

**Recurrent Furunculosis**   Usually related to persistent *S. aureus* in the nares, perineum, and body folds.

*Topical Therapy* Shower with providone iodine soap or benzoyl peroxide (bar or wash). Apply mupirocin ointment daily to the inside of nares and other sites of *S. aureus* carriage.

*Systemic Therapy* Appropriate antibiotic treatment is continued until all lesions have resolved. Secondary prophylaxis may be given once a day for many months.

*Carrier State* Rifampin: 600 mg PO for 7 to 10 days for eradication of carrier state.

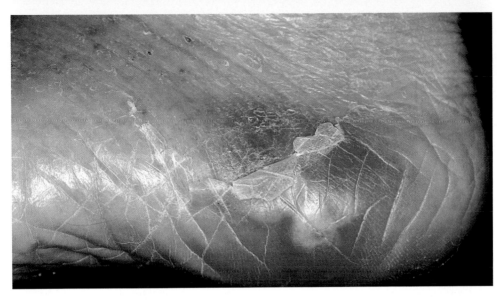

**FIGURE 22-15   Abscess: _S. aureus_**  *A very tender abscess with surrounding erythema on the heel. The patient was a diabetic with sensory neuropathy; a sewing needle in the heel had provided a portal of entry.*

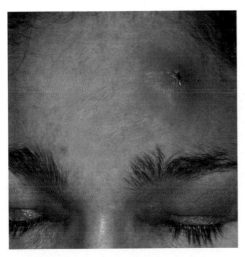 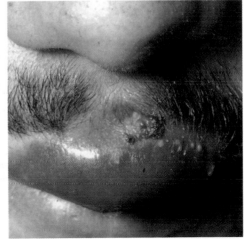

**FIGURE 22-16 (Left)   Furuncle: _S. aureus_**  *Soft-tissue swelling of the forehead with central abscess formation, nearing rupture.*

**FIGURE 22-17 (Right)   Furuncles: _S. aureus_**  *Multiple areas of folliculitis in the moustache area, extending to become furuncles.*

TABLE 22-2 Oral Antimicrobial Agents for Bacterial Infections

| Antimicrobial Agent | Dosing (PO Unless Indicated), Usually For 7 to 14 Days |
|---|---|
| **Natural penicillins** | |
| Penicillin V | 250–500 mg tid/qid for 10 days |
| Penicillin G | 600,000–1.2 million U IM qd for 7 days |
| Benzathine penicillin G | 600,000 U IM in children ≤6 years, 1.2 million units if ≥7 years, if compliance is a problem |
| **Penicillinase-resistant penicillins** | |
| Cloxacillin | 250–500 mg (adults) qid for 10 days |
| Dicloxacillin | 250–500 mg (adults) qid for 10 days |
| Nafcillin | 1.0–2.0 g IV q4h |
| Oxacillin | 1.0–2.0 g IV q4h |
| **Aminopenicillins** | |
| Amoxicillin | 500 mg tid or 875 mg q12h |
| Amoxicillin plus clavulanic acid (β-lactamase inhibitor) | 875/125 mg bid; 20 mg/kg per day tid for 10 days |
| Ampicillin | 250–500 mg qid for 7–10 days |
| **Cephalosporins** | |
| Cephalexin | 250-500 mg (adults) qid for 10 days; 40–50 mg/kg per day (children) for 10 days |
| Cephradine | 250–500 mg (adults) qid for 10 days; 40–50 mg/kg per day (children) for 10 days |
| Cefaclor | 250–500 mg q8h |
| Cefprozil | 250–500 mg q12h |
| Cefuroxime axetil | 125–500 mg q12h |
| Cefixime | 200–400 mg q12–24h |
| **Erythromycin group** | |
| Erythromycin ethylsuccinate | 250–500 mg (adults) qid for 10 days; 40 mg/kg per day (children) qid for 10 days |
| Clarithromycin | 500 mg bid for 10 days |
| Azithromycin | Azithromycin: 500 mg on day 1, then 250 mg qd days 2–5 |
| **Clindamycin** | 150-300 mg (adults) qid for 10 days; 15 mg/kg per day (children) qid for 10 days |
| **Tetracylines** | |
| Minocycline | 100 mg bid for 10 days |
| Doxycycline | 100 mg bid |
| Tetracycline | 250–500 mg qid |
| **Miscellaneous agents** | |
| Trimethoprim-sulfamethoxazole | 160 mg TMP + 800 mg SMX bid |
| Metronidazole | 500 mg qid |
| Ciprofloxacin | 500 mg bid for 7 days |

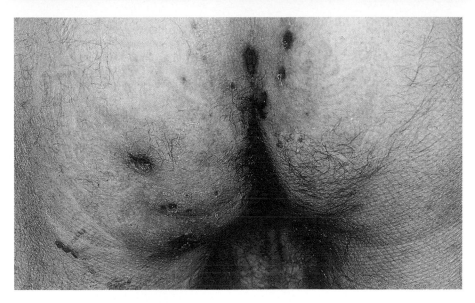

**FIGURE 22-18  Multiple furuncles: MRSA**  *Multiple, painful ulcerated nodules on the buttocks of a 20-year-old male, occurring during hospitalization for ulcerative colitis.*

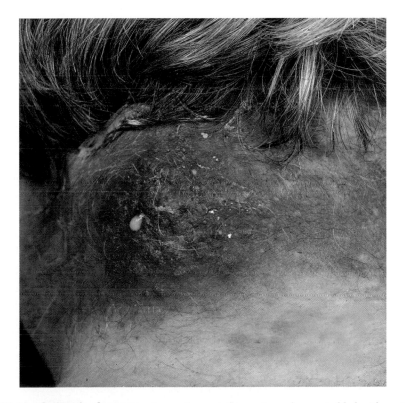

**FIGURE 22-19  Carbuncle: S. aureus**  *A very large, inflammatory plaque studded with pustules, draining pus, on the nape of the neck. Infection extends down to the fascia and has formed from a confluence of many furuncles.*

## SOFT TISSUE INFECTIONS: CLASSIFICATION/DEFINITIONS

Soft tissue infections (STIs), or cellulitides, are characterized by an acute, diffuse, spreading, edematous, suppurative inflammation of the dermis and subcutaneous tissues, often associated with systemic symptoms of malaise, fever, and chills. Non-necrotizing STIs are treated with antibiotics, drainage of abscesses, and supportive measures. Necrotizing STIs are often life-threatening and require, in addition, extensive surgical debridement. See Table 22-3.

**Erysipelas** A distinct type of superficial cutaneous cellulitis with marked dermal lymphatic vessel involvement presenting as a painful, bright red, raised, edematous, indurated plaque with advancing raised borders, sharply marginated from the surrounding normal skin (see Figs. 22-20, 22-22). Usually caused by group A β-hemolytic streptococcus (GAS) (very uncommonly group C or G streptococcus) and rarely due to *S. aureus*. Group B streptococci can cause erysipelas in the newborn. Most common cause of virulent STI in a healthy host, sometimes without evident portal of entry. *Sites of predilection*: face, lower legs, areas of preexisting lymphedema, umbilical stump.

**Cellulitis** Has many of the features of erysipelas but extends into the subcutaneous tissues. Cellulitis is differentiated from erysipelas by two physical findings: cellulitis lesions are primarily not raised, and demarcation from uninvolved skin is indistinct. The tissue feels hard on palpation and is extremely painful. In some cases, even with antibiotic therapy, the overlying epidermis undergoes bulla formation (see Fig. 22-23) or necrosis, resulting in extensive areas of epidermal sloughing and superficial erosion. In other cases, with or without therapy, infection may localize in the soft tissue, with dermal and subcutaneous abscess formation (see Fig. 22-23) or necrotizing fasciitis. *S. aureus* and GAS are by far the most common etiologic agents, but occasionally other bacteria are implicated [e.g., GBS in the newborn, pneumococcus (*Streptococcus pneumoniae*), a variety of gram-negative bacilli, and *Cryptococcus*].

**Lymphangitis** Inflammation of the lymphatic vessels, usually beginning on acral sites such as hands or feet; presents as erythematous streaking on the volar or dorsal aspect of the arm proximal to a finger or hand infection (see Figs. 22-29 and 22-30).

**Gangrenous Cellulitis** Characterized by necrosis of the dermis, subcutaneous fat (hypodermis), fascia, or muscle. Classified as *necrotizing fasciitis, clostridial soft tissue infections*, and *progressive bacterial synergistic gangrene*.

**Necrotizing Soft Tissue Infection (NSTI)** Differs from other variants because of significant tissue necrosis, lack of response to antimicrobial treatment alone, and need for surgical debridement of devitalized tissues. Starts with erythema and painful induration of underlying soft tissues; rapid development of black eschar, which transforms into liquefied black and malodorous necrotic mass (see Figs. 22-27, 22-28). Divided into three categories: *necrotizing cellulitis, necrotizing fasciitis, myonecrosis*. In that the presence of fascial necrosis can be determined only by surgical exploration and histopathologic examination of involved tissue, necrotizing cellulitis cannot be differentiated from necrotizing fasciitis on clinical grounds alone. NSTI in the genital area is called *Fournier's gangrene*.

**Ecthyma Gangrenosum** An NSTI, most commonly caused by *Pseudomonas aeruginosa*, characterized by a cutaneous infarction progressing to large ulcerated gangrenous lesions (see Fig. 22-25). Occurs most commonly in the setting of profound prolonged neutropenia and is often followed by *P. aeruginosa* bacteremia. Patients are often immunocompromised.

**TABLE 22-3   Etiology of Soft Tissue Infections (STIs)**

| Type of Infection | Most Common Cause(s) | Uncommon Causes |
|---|---|---|
| **Erysipelas** | Group A streptococcus (GAS) | Group B, C, and G streptococci (GBS, GCS, GGS) *S. aureus* |
| **Cellulitis** | *S. aureus*, GAS | GBS, GCS, GGS<br>*Erysipelothrix rhusiopathiae*<br>Pneumococcus<br>*Haemophilus influenzae* (children)<br>*E. coli*<br>*Campylobacter jejuni*<br>*Moraxella*<br>*Serratia*, *Proteus*,other Enterobacteriaceae<br>*Cryptococcus neoformans*<br>*Legionella pneumophila*, *L. micdadei*<br>*Bacillus anthracis* (anthrax)<br>*Aeromonas hydrophila*<br>*Vibrio vilnificus*, *V. alginolyticus* |
| **Cellulitis in children**<br>  Facial/periorbital cellulitis<br>  Perianal cellulitis | *S. aureus*, GAS<br>*H. influenzae* (young children)<br>GAS | GBS (neonates)<br>*Neisseria meningitidis*<br>*S. aureus* |
| **Cellulitis secondary to bacteremia** | *P. aeruginosa* | *V. vulnificus*<br>*Streptococcus pneumoniae* GAS, GBS |
| **Crepitant cellulitis** | *Clostridia* spp. (*C. perfringens*, *C. septicum*) | *Bacteroides* spp.<br>Peptostreptococci<br>*E. coli*, *Klebsiella* |
| **Cellulitis associated with water exposure** | *E. rhusiopathiae* (erysipeloid)<br>*V. vulnificus*<br>*Aeromonas hydrophila*<br>*Mycobacterium marinum* (nodular lymphangitis)<br>*M. fortuitum* complex | Seal finger (etiology unknown) |
| **Gangrenous cellulitis**<br>  (infectious gangrene)<br>    Necrotizing fasciitis (NF)<br>      Streptococcal gangrene<br>      Nonstreptococcal NF | <br><br><br>GAS<br>Mixed infection with one or more anaerobes (*Peptostreptococcus* or *Bacteroides*) plus at least one facultative species (non-group A streptococci; members of the Enterobacteriaceae such as *Enterobacter or Proteus*) | <br><br><br>GBS, GCS, GGS<br>*Bacillus cereus* (agranulocytic patients) |

*(continued)*

**TABLE 22-3    Etiology of Soft Tissue Infections (STIs) (*Continued*)**

| Type of Infection | Most Common Cause(s) | Uncommon Causes |
|---|---|---|
| Synergistic necrotizing cellulitis* (necrotizing cutaneous myositis, synergistic nonclostridial anaerobic myonecrosis) | Polymicrobial with aerobic and anaerobic organisms that originate in the intestine<br>One-third of patients have positive blood cultures, usually a coliform, *Bacteroides*, or *Peptostreptococcus* | |
| Aerobes | Coliforms: *E. coli*, *Proteus*, *Klebsiella* | |
| Anaerobes | *Bacteroides*, *Peptostreptococcus*, *Clostridium*, *Fusobacterium* | |
| Fournier's gangrene | Similar to nonstreptococcal NF | |
| Clostridial STI | *C. perfringens*<br>Other histotoxic clostridial spp. | |
| Anaerobic cellulitis<br>Anaerobic myonecrosis (GAS gangrene) | | |
| Spontaneous, nontraumatic anaerobic myonecrosis | *C. septicum* (bacteremic) | |
| Nonclostridial anaerobic cellulitis | Various *Bacteroides* spp.<br>Peptostreptococci<br>Peptococci | |
| Progressive bacterial synergistic gangrene (Meleney's gangrene) | Mixed bacterial infection | |
| Ulcer base | *S. aureus* | *Proteus* spp.<br>Other gram-negative bacilli |
| Advancing margin | Microaerophilic or anaerobic streptococci | |
| Gangrenous cellulitis in the immunosuppressed individual | *P. aeruginosa* (ecthyma gangrenosum) | Mucoraceae (*Mucor*, *Rhizopus*, *Absidia*) Bacillus spp. |

*Essentially the same as nonstreptococcal NF but with same involvement of adjacent skeletal muscle.

## ERYSIPELAS AND CELLULITIS ■ ◑ → ●

Erysipelas and cellulitis are acute, spreading infections of dermal and subcutaneous tissues, characterized by a red, hot, tender area of skin, often originating at the site of bacterial entry, caused most frequently by GAS (erysipelas) or *S. aureus*.*

### EPIDEMIOLOGY AND ETIOLOGY

**Age of Onset** Any age. Children <3 years; older individuals.
**Etiology** Adults: *S. aureus*, GAS. Children: *H. influenzae* type b (Hib), GAS, *S. aureus*.

*Less Commonly* Group B streptococci (GBS), pneumococci, *E. rhusiopathiae* (erysipeloid). In patients with diabetes or impaired immunity: *E. coli, Proteus mirabilis, Acinetobacter, Enterobacter, P. aeruginosa, Pasteurella multocida, Vibrio vulnificus; Mycobacterium fortuitum* complex, *C. neoformans*. In children: pneumococci, *N. meningitidis* group B (periorbital).

*Opportunistic Pathogens Helicobacter cinaedi* (HIV disease); *C. neoformans; Fusarium, Proteus, Pseudomonas* spp.
*Dog and Cat Bites P. multocida* and other *Pasteurella* spp.; *S. aureus*.

**Portals/Source of Infection** (See Table 22-4). Mucocutaneous, subjacent, bacteremic.
*Mucocutaneous*

* *Underlying dermatoses*: Bullous disease (pemphigus vulgaris, bullous pemphigoid, sunburn); chronic lymphedema; dermatophytosis (epidermal dermatophytosis/ tinea pedis, tinea capitis, tinea barbae); viral infections (herpes simplex, varicella, herpes zoster); inflammatory dermatoses (atopic dermatitis, contact

### TABLE 22-4 Anatomic Variants of Cellulitis/Causes of Predisposition

|  | Location | Likely Bacterial Cause |
|---|---|---|
| Periorbital cellulitis | Periorbital | *S. aureus*, pneumococci, GAS |
| Buccal cellulitis | Cheek | *H. influenzae* |
| Cellulitis complicating ear piercing | Ear, nose, umbilicus | *S. aureus*, GAS |
| Mastectomy (with axillary node dissection) for breast cancer; lumpectomy | Ipsilateral arm | *S. aureus*. Non-group A hemolytic streptococci |
| Harvest of saphenous vein for coronary artery bypass | Ipsilateral leg | GAS or non-group A hemolytic streptococci |
| Liposuction | Thigh, abdominal wall | GAS, peptostreptococci, *M. fortuitum* complex |
| Postoperative (very early) wound infection | Abdomen, chest, hip | GAS |
| Injection-drug use (IDU) ("skin popping") | Extremities, neck, penis | *S. aureus*; streptococci (groups A. F. G) |
| Perianal "cellulitis" (intertrigo) | Perineum, inguinal | GAS |
| Crepitant cellulitis | Trunk, extremities | See text |
| Gangrenous cellulitis | Trunk, extremities | See text |
| Erythema migrans (Lyme disease) | Extremities, trunk | *Borrelia burgdorferi* |

*See Swartz M: N Engl J Med 350:904, 2004.

dermatitis, stasis dermatitis, pyoderma gangrenosum); superficial pyoderma (impetigo, folliculitis, furunculosis, carbuncle, ecthyma); ulcers (pressure, chronic venous insufficiency, ischemic, neuropathic); umbilical stump

- *Trauma*: Abrasion; bites (human, animal); insect bites; burns; laceration; puncture
- *Surgical wound*: Surgical incisions; PIC lines
- *Mucosal infection*: Oropharynx, nasal mucosa; middle ear
- *Injecting drug use (IDU)*: "Skin popping" sites
- *Water exposure*: *V. vulnificus*, *V. cholerae* non-01 and non-0139. *Aeromonas hydrophilia*.

**Subjacent** Osteomyelitis, cutaneous odontogenic sinus, abdominal infection
**Bacteremic** Sepsis, infectious endocarditis. *S. pneumoniae*, *V. vulnificus*, and *C. neoformans*.
**Risk Factors** Drug and alcohol abuse, cancer and cancer chemotherapy, chronic lymphedema (postmastectomy, postcoronary artery grafting, previous episode of cellulitis/erysipelas), cirrhosis, diabetes mellitus, nephritic syndrome, iatrogenic immunosuppression, neutropenia, immunodeficiency syndromes, malnutrition, renal failure, systemic atherosclerosis.
**Human Bites** Most common in young males. Most bites occur on the hands: clenched-first or occlusional injuries. Multiple organisms often isolated from wound site, including *Streptococcus anginosus*, *S. aureus*, *E. corrodens*, *Fusobacterium nucleatum*, and *Prevotella melaninogenica*. *Fusobacterium*, *Peptostreptococcus*, and *Candida* spp. more frequently from occlusional bites than from clenched-fist injuries.

## PATHOGENESIS

After entry, infection spreads to tissue spaces and cleavage planes as hyaluronidases break down polysaccharide ground substances, fibrinolysins digest fibrin barriers, lecithinases destroy cell membranes. Local tissue devitalization, e.g., trauma, is usually required to allow for significant anaerobic bacterial infection. The number of infecting organisms is usually small, suggesting that cellulitis may be more of a reaction to cytokines and bacterial superantigens than to overwhelming tissue infection.

## HISTORY

**Incubation Period** Few days.
**Prodrome** Malaise, anorexia; fever, chills can develop rapidly, before cellulitis is apparent clinically. Higher fever (38.5°C) and chills usually associated with GAS.
**Immune Status** Immunocompromised patients susceptible to infection with pathogens of low pathogenicity.
**History** Local pain and tenderness. Necrotizing infections associated with more local pain and systemic symptoms.

## PHYSICAL EXAMINATION

### Skin Lesions
**Portals of Entry** Red, hot, edematous and shiny plaque, and very tender area of skin of varying size (Figs. 22-20, 22-22); borders usually sharply defined, irregular, and slightly elevated; bluish purple color with *H. influenzae* (Fig. 22-21). Vesicles, bullae, erosions, abscesses, hemorrhage, and necrosis may form in plaque. Lymphangitis. *Lymph nodes*: Can be enlarged and tender, regionally.
**Distribution** *Adults* Lower leg (Fig. 22-22); most common site, following interdigital tinea (Fig. 22-22). Arm: in young male, consider IV drug use; in female; postmastectomy. Trunk: operative wound site. Face: following rhinitis, conjunctivitis (Fig. 22-20).
*Children* Cheek, periorbital area, head, neck most common: usually *H. influenzae* (Fig. 22-21). Extremities: *S. aureus*, group A streptococci.

### Variants in Infecting Organism
**S. aureus** Often a portal of entry is apparent; usually a focal infection (Figs. 22-22 and 22-23). Most common pathogen in injection drug user. Toxin syndromes (scalded-skin syndrome, TSS) may occur. Endocarditis may follow bacteremia.
**Group A Streptococcus** Incidence of invasive GAS infections is increasing. The morbidity and mortality rates are significant: 37% of patients have necrotizing fasciitis and 25% meet the criteria for streptococcal TSS; mortality rate reported to be 21%.
**Group B Streptococcus (S. agalactiae)** Colonizes anogenital region. Causes anogenital cellulitis, which may extend into pelvic tissues. Following childbirth, known as *puerperal sepsis*. Cellulitis occurs in neonates; high morbidity and mortality.
**S. pneumoniae (Pneumococcus)** Occurs more commonly in individuals with systemic lupus erythematosus, complement deficiency, HIV disease, glucocorticoid therapy, drug or alcohol abuse. Infected sites show bulla formation, brawny erythema, violaceous hue.
**E. rhusiopathiae: Erysipeloid** Painful, swollen plaque with sharply defined irregular raised

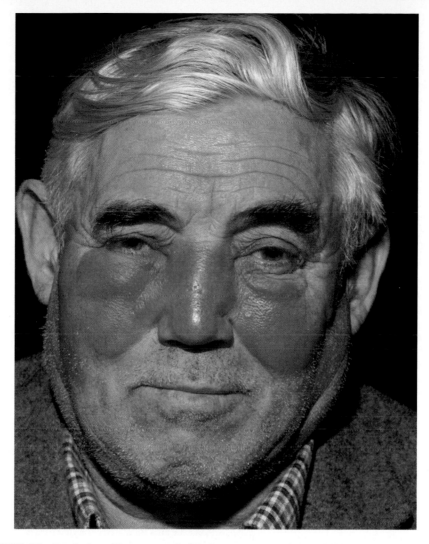

**FIGURE 22-20  Erysipelas of face: group A streptococcus**  *Painful, well-defined, shiny, erythematous, edematous plaques involving eyelids, cheeks, and the nose of an elderly febrile male. On palpation the skin is hot and tender. Portal of entry was conjunctivitis.*

border occuring at the site of inoculation, i.e., finger or hand (Fig. 22-24), spreading to wrist and forearm. Color: purplish red acutely; brownish with resolution. Enlarges peripherally with central fading. Usually no systemic symptoms. Uncommonly, associated with bacteremia and aortic valvulitis. Occurs in individuals who handle game, poultry, fish.

***P. aeruginosa*** (See "Cutaneous *P. aeruginosa* infections") Ecthyma gangrenosum begins as erythematous macule (cutaneous ischemic lesion) that quickly evolves to a bluish or gunmetal gray plaque with an erythematous halo (infarction) (Fig. 22-25A and 25B). The epidermis overlying the ischemic area forms a bulla. Epidermis eventually sloughs, forming an ulcer. *Distribution:* most commonly in the axilla, groin, perineum. Usually occurs as solitary lesion but may occur as a few lesions. Lesions associated with *Pseudomonas* septicemia: rose spotlike lesions (erythematous macules and/or papules on trunk as in typhoid fever, occur with *Pseudomonas* infection of GI tract, i.e., diarrhea, headache, high fever); painful clustered vesicular to bullous lesions; multiple painful nodules representing small embolic lesions.

***H. influenzae***    Occurs mainly in children <2 years. Cheek, periorbital area, head, neck most common sites (Fig. 22-21). Clinically, swelling, characteristic violaceous erythema hue. Use of Hib vaccine has dramatically reduced incidence.

***V. vulnificus, V. cholerae* non-01 and non-0139**    Underlying disorders: cirrhosis, diabetes, immunosuppression, hemochromatosis, thalassemia. Follows ingestion of raw/undercooked seafood, gastroenteritis, bacteremia with seeding of skin; also exposure of skin to sea water. Characterized by bulla formation, necrotizing vasculitis (Fig. 22-26). Usually on the extremities; often bilateral.

***A. hydrophila***    Water-associated trauma; preexisting wound. Immunocompromised host. Lower leg. Necrotizing STIs.

***C. canimorsus***    Immunosuppression or asplenia; exposure to a dog.

***P. multocida***    Follows cat bite.

***Clostridium* Spp.**    Associated with trauma, contamination by soil or feces, malignant intestinal tumor. Infection may be characterized by gas, marked systemic toxicity.

***M. chelonei–M. fortuitum* Complex**    History of recent surgery, injection, penetrating wound. Low-grade cellulitis. Systemic findings lacking.

***C. neoformans***    Patient always immunocompromised. Red, hot, tender, edematous plaque on extremity. Rarely multiple noncontiguous sites.

**Mucormycosis**    Usually occurring in individual with uncontrolled diabetes.

General Findings
Fever, signs of sepsis.

## DIFFERENTIAL DIAGNOSIS

**Erysipelas/Cellulitis**    Deep vein thrombophlebitis, stasis dermatitis, early contact dermatitis, giant urticaria, insect bite (hypersensitivity response), fixed drug eruption, erythema nodosum, acute gout, erythema migrans (Lyme borreliosis), prevesicular herpes zoster, Well's syndrome (eosinophilic cellulitis), familial Mediterranean fever–associated cellulitis-like erythema, cutaneous anthrax, pyoderma gangrenosum, Sweet's syndrome (acute febrile neutrophilic dermatosis), Kawasaki disease, carcinoma erysipeloides.

**Necrotizing STIs**    Vasculitis, embolism with infarction of skin, peripheral vascular disease, purpura fulminans, calciphylaxis, warfarin necrosis, traumatic injury, cryoglobulinemia, fixed drug eruption, pyoderma gangrenosum, brown recluse spider bite.

## LABORATORY EXAMINATIONS

**Direct Microscopy**    *Smears* Gram's stain of exudate, pus, bulla fluid, aspirate, or touch preparation may show bacteria. GAS: chains of gram-positive cocci. *S. aureus*: clusters of gram-positive cocci. Clostridia: gram-negative rods, few neutrophils.

*"Touch" Preparation*    Lesional skin biopsy specimen touched to microscope slide. Potassium hydroxide applied; examined for yeast and mycelial forms of fungus; detects *Candida, Cryptococcus, Mucor*. Gram's stain: detects bacteria.

**Cultures**    *Cellulitis*: aspirate or biopsy of leading edge of inflammation, identifies pathogen in up to 20% of cases. Fungal and mycobacterial cultures indicated in atypical case. *Portal of entry* (ulcers, etc., adjacent to cellulitis: similar result to culture of cellulitis. *Blood cultures*: yield very low, ≤2 to 4%, highest in GAS infections. Yields higher in the setting of chronic

**FIGURE 22-21 (Opposite page, top)    Cellulitis of cheek: *H. influenzae***    *Erythema and edema of the cheek of a young child, associated with fever and malaise.* H. influenzae *was isolated on culture of the nasopharynx. (Courtesy of Sandy Tsao, MD.)*

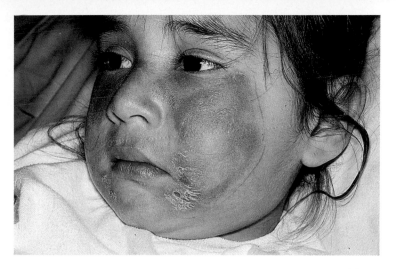

**FIGURE 22-21**

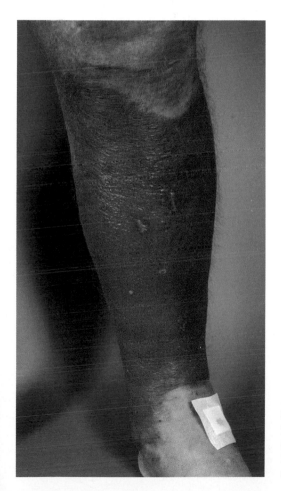

**FIGURE 22-22   Erysipelas of leg: *S. aureus***
*The lower leg is red, hot, tender, and edematous. Erythematous plaque is well defined. The infection is recurrent with interdigital tinea pedis as the portal of entry.*

lymphedema and in patients with buccal or periorbital cellulitis.

**Hematology** White blood count (WBC) and erythrocyte sedimentation rate (ESR) may be elevated.

**Dermatopathology** Frozen sections of lesional biopsies may be helpful in ruling out noninfectious inflammatory dermatoses. Open surgical inspection with debridement defines the extent and severity of NF; tissue is obtained for histologic examination, Gram staining, and culture. In necrotizing STI: vasculitis without thrombosis, paucity of neutrophils at site of infection; bacilli found in media and adventitia, but usually not in intima, of vessel. Helpful with cryptococcal cellulitis.

**Imaging** MRI may be helpful in diagnosis of severe acute infectious cellulitis, identifying pyomyositis, necrotizing fasciitis, and infectious cellulitis with or without subcutaneous abscess formation. Soft tissue radiography, CT, MRI, and ultrasonographic imaging can detect localized abscess, gas in tissue, and subjacent osteomyelitis but do not define NF or myonecrosis.

## DIAGNOSIS

Clinical diagnosis based on morphologic features of lesion and the clinical setting [travel history, animal exposure, history of bite, age, underlying disease(s)]. Confirmed by culture in only 29% of cases in immunocompetent patients. Suspicion of NF requires immediate deep biopsy and frozen-section histopathology.

## COURSE AND PROGNOSIS

When occurring as a local infection in the absence of bacteremia, prognosis is much more favorable. Dissemination of infection (lymphatics, hematogenously) with metastatic sites of infection occurs if treatment is delayed. Abnormal or prosthetic heart valve may be colonized and infected. In the preantibiotic era, the mortality rate was very high. In immuncompromised patients, prognosis depends on prompt restoration of altered immunity, usually on correction of neutropenia. Without surgical debridement, NF is fatal. If neutropenia exists, prognosis depends on recovery of neutrophil count.

## MANAGEMENT

See guidelines for the treatment of skin and soft tissue infections by the Infectious Diseases Society of America at http://www.journals.uchicago.edu./IDSA/guidelines/

**Prophylaxis** *Primary* Status postsaphenous vein harvest (especially with tinea pedis): Wash with benzoyl peroxide bar daily or apply topical antifungal cream or alcohol gel. *Pneumococcus*: Immunize those at risk. *Hib*: Chemoprophylaxis for household contacts <4 years of age if unimmunized. *Vibrio* spp.: Diabetics, alcoholics, cirrhotics should avoid eating undercooked seafood.

*Secondary Individuals with prior episodes of cellulitis* (especially in sites of chronic lymphedema): Support stockings or sleeve, antiseptics to skin (Purell), chronic secondary antimicrobial prophylaxis (penicillin G, dicloxacillin, or erythromycin, 500 mg/d). *Interdigital tinea pedis*: Treat and institute prophylaxis against recurrent tinea pedis.

**Supportive** Rest, immobilization, elevation, moist heat, analgesia.

**Dressings** Cool sterile saline dressings for removal of purulent exudate and necrotic tissue.

**Surgical Intervention** Drain abscesses. Debride necrotic tissue. Early/aggressive surgical exploration/debridement is lifesaving in suspected necrotizing STIs. Deep structures are visualized, necrotic tissue removed, compartment decompressed, tissues obtained for Gram stain and aerobic and anaerobic cultures.

**Antimicrobial Therapy** In that most cases of cellulitis are caused by *S. aureus* and streptococci, β-lactam antibiotics with activity against penicillinase-producing *S. aureus* are the usual drugs of choice.

*Indications for Initial IV Therapy* Lesion spreading rapidly, systemic response is prominent (chills, fever, of ≥37.8°C), clinically significant coexisting conditions (immunocompromise, neutropenia, asplenia, preexisting edema, cirrhosis, cardiac failure, renal insufficiency). See Table 22-5.

*Oral Therapy* In healthy persons with early infection in the absence of systemic symptoms and following initial IV therapy, oral antibiotics are given (Table 22-6).

In immunocompetent hosts: treat gram-positive cocci (*S. aureus*, GAS). In diabetics, greater range of potential pathogens, especially arising in diabetic ulcers: *S. aureus*, GAS, enterococci; gram-negative aerobes (*Proteus, Klebsiella, Enterobacter, Acinetobacter*). *P. aeruginosa*; anaerobes (*Bacterioides, Peptococcus*).

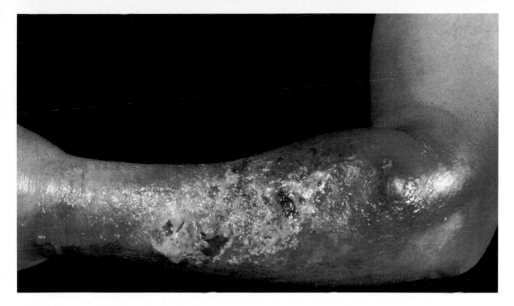

**FIGURE 22-23 Cellulitis of arm: *S. aureus*** *Cellulitis with abscess formation and blistering occurred as a puncture wound infection in a construction-site worker. The lower arm had to be debrided down to the facia and grafted.*

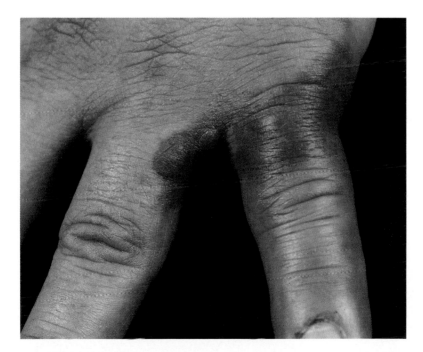

**FIGURE 22-24 Erysipeloid of hand** *A well-demarcated, violaceous, cellulitic plaque (without epidermal changes of scale or vesiculation) on the dorsa of the hand and fingers, occurred following cleaning fish; the site was somewhat painful, tender, and warm.*

**TABLE 22-5   Initial Treatment for Cellulitis at Specific Sites or Particular Exposures**

| Variable | Bacterial Spp. to Consider | Standard Antimicrobial Therapy | Alternative Antimicrobial Agent |
|---|---|---|---|
| Buccal cellulitis | *H. influenzae* | Ceftriaxone (1–2 g/d IV) | Meropenem or imipenem-cilastatin |
| Limb-threatening diabetic foot ulcer | Aerobic gram-negative bacilli | Ampicillin-sulbactam (3 g IV q6h) | Meropenem or imipenem-cilastin clindamycin + a broad-spectrum fluoroquinolone (ciprofloxacin or levofloxacin); metronidazole + fluoroquinolone or ceftriaxone |
| Human bites | Oral anaerobes | Amoxicillin-clavulanate (500 mg PO q8h) | Penicillin + a cephalosporin |
| Dog and cat bites | *P. multocida* etc; see "Etiology" | Amoxicillin-clavulanate (500 mg PO q8h) | Moxifloxacin + clindamycin |
| Exposure to salt water at site of abrasion or laceration | *V. vulnificus* | Doxycycline (200 mg IV initially, followed by 100–200 mg/d IV in 2 divided doses. Give along with antimicrobial agents for common pathogens) | Cefotaxime; ciprofloxacin |
| Exposure to fresh water at site of abrasion or laceration or after therapeutic use of leeches | *Aeromonas* spp. | Ciprofloxacin (400 mg IV q12h) or ceftazidime + gentamycin | Meropenem or imipenem-cilastin |
| Working as butcher, fish or clam handler, veterinarian | *E. rhusiopathiae* | Amoxicillin (500 mg PO q8H for mild skin infections; penicillin G (12 million–20 million U IV daily) for bacteremic infections or endocarditis | Ciprofloxacin or cefotaxime or imipenem-cilastatin |

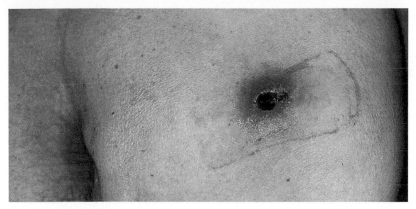

A

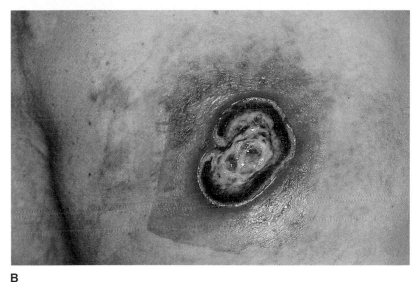

B

**FIGURE 22-25   Ecthyma gangrenosum of buttock: *P. aeruginosa*   A.** *An extremely painful, infarcted area with surrounding erythema present for 5 days on the buttock of a neutropenic HIV-infected male. This primary cutaneous infection was associated with bacteremia.* **B.** *Two weeks later, the lesion had progressed to a large ulceration. The patient died 3 months later of* P. aeruginosa pneumonitis *associated with chronic neutropenia.*

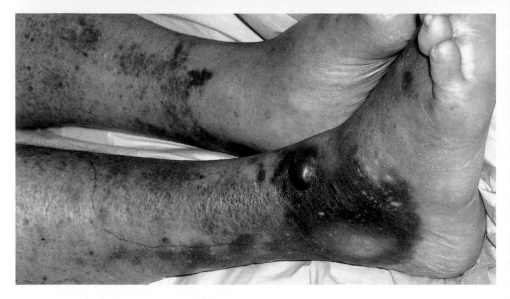

**FIGURE 22-26   Cellulitis of legs: *V. vulnificus*** *Bilateral hemorrhagic plaques and bullae on the legs, ankles, and feet of an older diabetic with cirrhosis. Unlike other types of cellulitis in which microorganisms enter the skin locally, that which is caused by* V. vulnificus *usually follows a primary enteritis with bacteremia and dissemination to the skin.*

**TABLE 22-6   Antimicrobial Treatment for a Usual Case of Cellulitis***

| Initial Treatment | Subsequent Treatment |
|---|---|
| Cefazolin, 1.0 g IV q6–8h or | Dicloxacillin, 0.5 g PO q6h or<br>Cephradine, 0.5 g PO q6h or<br>Cephalexin, 0.5 g PO q6h or<br>Cefadroxil, 0.5–1.0 g PO q12–24 h |
| Nafcillin, 1.0 g IV q4–6 h or | Same as above |
| Ceftriaxone, 1.0 g IV Q24h or | Same as above |
| Cefazolin, 2.0 g IV qd, plus probenecid (1.0 g PO qd) | Same as above |
| If MRSA is suspected or patient is highly allergic to penicillin: | |
| Vancomycin, 1.0–2.0 g IV qd *or* | Linezolid, 0.6 g PO q12h |
| Linezolid, 0.6 g IV q12h | Same as above |

*Doses given are for adults; patients should be switched to oral therapy when they are afebrile and skin findings begin to resolve (after 3–5 days). The total duration of treatment should be ≥7–14 days, depending on the rate of response. Treatment should last longer in cases with associated abscesses, tissue necrosis, or underlying skin process (e.g., infected ulcer).

# WOUND INFECTIONS    ■  ◗ → ●

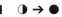

Wounds are characterized by loss of the integrity of the skin and provide a portal of entry for infection. All wounds are colonized by bacteria. Wound infection (purulence, erythema, warmth, tenderness) must be diagnosed on clinical and cultural grounds and treated appropriately.

## CLASSIFICATION OF WOUNDS

I. Chronic ulcers
  A. Arterial insufficiency
  B. Venous insufficiency
  C. Neuropathic ulcers/diabetes mellitus
  D. Pressure ulcers (bedsores)
II. Trauma
III. Bites
  A. Animal
  B. Human
IV. Surgical wounds
  A. Class I/clean
  B. Class II/clean-contaminated
  C. Class III/contaminated
  D. Class IV/dirty-infected
V. Burn wounds
  A. Burn wound impetigo
  B. Open burn–related surgical wound infection
  C. Burn wound cellulitis
  D. Invasive infection in unexcised burn wounds

## EPIDEMIOLOGY AND ETIOLOGY

**Etiology**  MRSA is currently the most common pathogen isolated in wounds cultured in hospital environment. MSSA, *Streptococcus*, and *Pseudomonas* spp. are also commonly isolated. Others: *E. coli, Enterococcus* spp., *Proteus* spp., CoNS, fungi, vancomycin-resistant enterococci, other enterobacteriaceae, *Klebsiella* spp. Anaerobes may constitute more than one-third of antimicrobial isolates.

For *human, dog, and cat bites*, see page 603.

**Predisposing Factors**  *General factors*: Age, obesity, malnutrition; endocrine/metabolic factors; hypoxia, anemia; malignant disease; immunosuppression. *Local factors*: Necrotic tissue, foreign bodies, tissue ischemia, hematoma formation, poor surgical technique. *Microbial contamination*: Type/virulence of organism; size of bacterial inoculum, antibiotic resistance.

**Risk Factors**
Surgical wound infection is up to 10 times more likely among patients who harbor *S. aureus* in nares. The vast majority of postoperative wound infections are caused by a strain of *S. aureus* that was present in nares before surgery. Presurgical clearance of carriage with topical or systemic antibiotics decreases incidence of postoperative staphylococcal infection. Postoperative infection: prolonged operative time, diabetes, obesity, chronic lung disease, male sex, treatment with glucocorticoids, social deprivation.

**Nosocomial Infections**  Hospital-acquired or health care–associated infections (most commonly surgical wound infections) are the most common complication affecting hospitalized patients. 5 to 10% of patients admitted to acute care hospitals acquire one or more infections (2 million patients annually in the United States), resulting in 90,000 deaths.

**Definition of Surgical Wound Infection**
*Types of Surgical Wound Infections*  Surgical site infection, superficial incisional infection, deep incisional infections, organ space infections.
*Surgical site infections must fulfill the following criteria:*

• Infection must occur within 30 days of surgery
• Infection must involve only the skin and subcutaneous tissue
• There must be at least one of the following:
  Purulent discharge from a superficial infection
  Organisms isolated from aseptically obtained wound culture
• Must be at least one of the following signs of infection:
  Pain or tenderness
  Localized swelling
  Redness or heat

## PATHOGENESIS

Wounds are initially colonized by skin flora or introduced organisms. In some cases, these organisms proliferate, causing a host inflammatory response defined as infection. Skin and soft tissue infections (SSTIs) include superficial conditions, such as erysipelas, cellulitis, folliculitis, and furuncles, as well as deeper infections, such as abscesses, necrotizing fasciitis, myositis, and gas gangrene.

## HISTORY

**Symptoms** Local infection: tenderness, purulent drainage. Invasive infection: malaise, anorexia, sweats; fever, chills.

## CLINICAL FINDINGS

**Skin Findings** Purulent drainage, erythema, warmth, induration, tenderness.
**Systemic Findings** Sepsis syndrome (fever, hypotension).
**Types of Surgical Infections** Superficial infection of wound, impetigo/ecthyma (Fig. 22-14), cellulitis (Fig. 22-23), erysipelas, soft tissue abscess (Fig. 22-15), necrotizing soft tissue infections, tetanus.

## DIFFERENTIAL DIAGNOSIS

Allergic contact dermatitis (e.g., topical antibiotic such as neomycin), herpes zoster; herpes simplex, pyoderma gangrenosum, vasculitis, peripheral vascular disease (infarction), disseminated intravascular coagulation (DIC) (purpura fulminans), warfarin necrosis.

## LABORATORY EXAMINATIONS

**Direct Microscopy** Gram's stain of exudate, pus, bulla fluid, aspirate, or touch preparation may show bacteria.

**Culture and Sensitivities** Indications: wounds with classic signs of infection [purulent drainage, signs of inflammation (erythema, increased warmth, induration, tenderness)]. Specimens: exudates and necrotic tissue.

## DIAGNOSIS

Because all open wounds become colonized with microorganisms, diagnosing infection relies on the clinical characteristics of the wound. Wounds with classic signs of infection. Gram's stain of exudates helpful initially. Cultures are definitive.

## MANAGEMENT

Although all wounds require treatment, only infected lesions require antimicrobial therapy.
**Prevention of Wound Infection** *Exogenous* Sterilization of instruments, sutures, etc.; positive pressure ventilation; laminar air flow; exclusion of staff with infections.
*Endogenous* Skin preparation; antibiotic prophylaxis, good surgical technique.
**Wound Care** Adjunctive treatments include weight off-loading, topical agents, special dressings, control of edema, revasculaturization.
**Surgical Debridement** Treating infected wounds often requires surgical procedures (e.g., debridement), especially for deep or necrotic wounds. Adjunctive treatments: weight off-loading, topical agents, special dressings, control of edema, revasculaturization. Modern burn wound therapy centered on early excision and closure of the wound.
**Antimicrobial Therapy** Virtually all infected wounds require antimicrobial therapy. See Table 22-6.
*Topical Antimicrobial Therapy* May be sufficient for superficial lesions.

# NECROTIZING SOFT TISSUE INFECTIONS    □    ●

Necrotizing soft tissue infection (STI) is characterized by rapid progression of infection with extensive necrosis of subcutaneous tissues and overlying skin. Clinical variants of necrotizing STIs differ with the causative organism, the anatomic location of the infection, and predisposing conditions. Correct diagnosis is imperative in understanding pathogenesis and deciding on the appropriate antimicrobial and surgical therapies.

*When skin necrosis is not obvious, diagnosis must be suspected if there are signs of severe sepsis* (accelerated heart or respiratory rates, oliguria, mental confusion) and/or some of the following local symptoms/signs: severe spontaneous pain, indurated edema, bullae, cyanosis, skin pallor, absence of lymphangitis, skin hypesthesia, crepitation, muscle weakness, foul smell of exudates. *Risk factors for necrotizing fasciitis* (NF): local lesion of skin or mucous membrane (acute or chronic disease, trauma, surgery), diabetes, arteriopathy, alcoholism, obesity, immunosuppression, use of nonsteroidal anti-inflammatory drugs (NSAIDs).

## CLINICAL VARIANTS

### NF Caused by GAS (Rarely, Groups B, C, or G)

Often begins deep at site of nonpenetrating minor trauma (bruise, muscle strain); GAS may be seeded to this site during transient bacteremia or reach the deep fascia from a cutaneous infection or penetrating trauma. May develop at the site of an injury (minor trauma, laceration, needle puncture, or surgical incision) on an extremity but can occur in postoperative abdominal incisions. Myonecrosis occurs concomitantly in 50% of NF cases.

Streptococcal necrotizing myositis occurs as a primary myositis. Myositis and myonecrosis are part of the *streptococcal TSS* GBS have caused a similar process postpartum secondary to infected episiotomy incisions and in adult diabetics unrelated to obstetric complications. Most cases occur in otherwise healthy persons, often in children and the elderly.

Initially, findings of acute cellulitis (local redness, edema, heat, and pain in the involved area), typically occur on an extremity. Characteristic findings appear within 36 to 72 h after onset: the involved area becomes dusky blue in color; vesicles or bullae appear containing initially yellowish, then red-black fluid. Infection spreads rapidly along fascial planes resulting in extensive necrotic sloughs (Fig. 22-27). Bullae rupture, and extensive, sharply demarcated cutaneous gangrene develops. At this point the area may be numb, and the black necrotic eschar (Fig. 22-28) with surrounding irregular border of erythema resembles a third-degree burn. The eschar sloughs off by the end of 1 week to 10 days. Peripheral areas of involvement develop about the initial site of infection.

Fever and other constitutional symptoms are prominent as the inflammatory process extends rapidly over the next few days. Streptococcal TSS occurs with GAS, GBS, GCS, GGS. Metastatic abscesses may occur as a consequence of bacteremia, resembling purpura fulminans but then evolving to dark-colored blebs containing streptococci. Secondary thrombophlebitis is common, but lymphangitis and lymphadenitis are not.

## DIFFERENTIAL DIAGNOSIS

Factitial ulcers, pyoderma gangrenosum, purpura fulminans (disseminated intravascular coagulation), calciphylaxis, ischemic necrosis (atherosclerosis obliterans, thromboembolism), fixed drug eruption, warfarin necrosis, heparin necrosis, pressure ulcer, amebic (*Entamoeba histolytica*) skin gangrene after bowel surgery, brown recluse spider bite.

## MANAGEMENT

**Surgical Debridement**    Requires early and complete surgical debridement of necrotic tissue in combination with high-dose antimicrobial agents.

**Antimicrobial Therapy**    See Table 22-6.

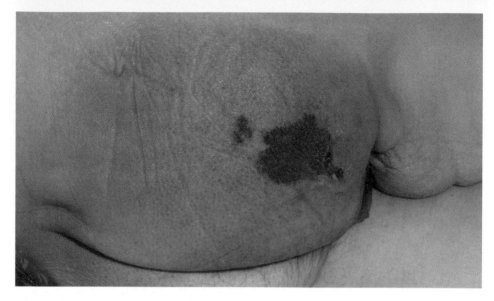

**FIGURE 22-27   Necrotizing fasciitis of buttock**   *Erythematous, edematous plaque involving the entire buttock with rapidly progressive area of necrosis.*

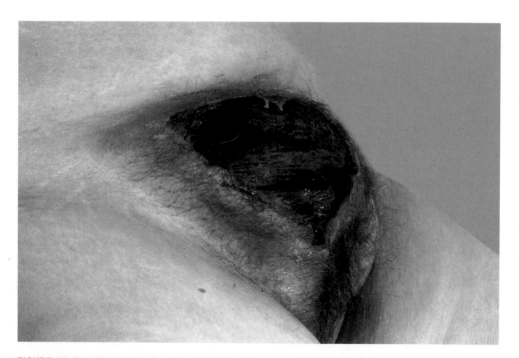

**FIGURE 22-28   Necrotizing fasciitis of pubic region**   *Extension of cellulitis from the pelvis to the lower abdomen with extensive necrosis.*

# ACUTE LYMPHANGITIS   ▯ ◑

Acute lymphangitis is an inflammatory process involving the subcutaneous lymphatic channels. It is due most often to GAS but occasionally may be caused by *S. aureus*; rarely, soft tissue infections with other organisms, such as *P. multocida*, or herpes simplex virus may be associated with acute lymphangitis.

## HISTORY

**Portal of Entry**   Break in skin, wound, an infected blister, *S. aureus* paronychia.

**Local Symptoms**   Pain and/or erythema proximal to break in the skin.

**Systemic Symptoms**   May occur either before any evidence of infection is present at the site of inoculation or after the initial lesion has subsided. May be more prominent than expected from degree of local pain and erythema.

## PHYSICAL EXAMINATION

**Skin Findings**   Red linear streaks and palpable lymphatic cords, which may be up to several centimeters in width, extend from the local lesion toward the regional lymph nodes (Figs. 22-29 and 22-30), which are usually enlarged and tender. Acute sporotrichoid lymphangitis can occur with *S. aureus* or GAS infection. Breakdown of overlying skin and ulceration occur in course of bacterial lymphangitis; rare in the antibiotic era.

## DIFFERENTIAL DIAGNOSIS

**Linear Lesions on Upper Extremities**   Phytoallergic contact dermatitis (poison ivy or oak), phytophotodermatitis (berloque dermatitis), superficial thrombophlebitis.

***Subacute Sporotrichoid Lymphangitis*** *Sporotrix schenkii, Nocardia brasiliensis, M. marinum, Leishmania* spp. are the most common pathogens.

## LABORATORY FINDINGS

**Culture**   Isolate *S. aureus* or GAS from portal of entry.

## DIAGNOSIS

The combination of a peripheral lesion with proximal tender/painful red linear streaks leading toward regional lymph nodes is diagnostic of lymphangitis.

## COURSE AND PROGNOSIS

Bacteremia with metastatic infection in various organs may occur.

## MANAGEMENT

See Table 22-2.

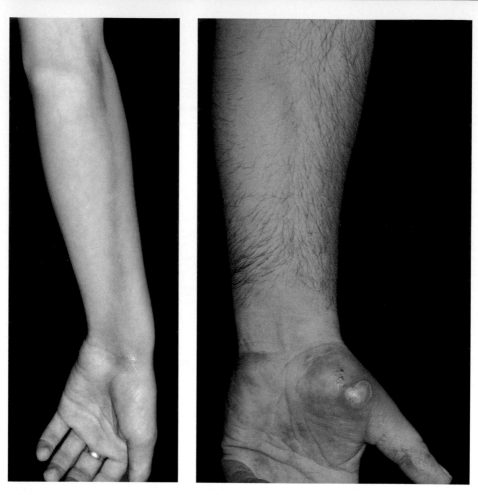

**FIGURE 22-29  (Left)    Acute lymphangitis of forearm: *S. aureus***   *A small area of cellulitis on the volar wrist with a tender linear streak extending proximally up the arm; the infection spreads from the portal of entry within the superficial lymphatic vessels.*

**FIGURE 22-30  (Right)    Acute lymphangitis of forearm: HSV**   *Primary herpes simplex virus infection of the palm with lymphangitis of the forearm.*

# GRAM-POSITIVE INFECTIONS ASSOCIATED WITH TOXIN PRODUCTION (INTOXICATIONS)

*S. aureus*, group A streptococcus (GAS), *B. anthracis*, *Corynebacterium diphtheriae*, and *Clostridium tetani* produce toxins that have local mucocutaneous and systemic effects. The clinical syndromes caused by these toxins include: staphylococcal scalded-skin syndrome (SSSS), staphylococcal toxic shock syndrome (TSS), staphylococcal food poisoning (enterotoxin), scarlet fever (SF), streptococcal TSS, anthrax, diphtheria, and tetanus.

Staphylococcal toxins include toxic shock syndrome toxin 1 (TSST-1), exfoliative (or epidermolytic) toxins (ETs), and staphylococcal enterotoxins (SEs). ET-A is responsible for the pathogenic changes of the SSSS. These toxins bind directly to desmoglein-1, a desmosomal cadherin, which results in interdesmosomal splitting and causes blistering and denudation by disruption of the epidermal granular cell layer. TSS is associated with production of TSST-1, SE-B, and SE-C.

Certain strains of GAS produce a pyrogenic exotoxin, i.e., erythrogenic toxin, which causes scarlet fever and is involved in the pathogenesis of streptococcal TSS.

Superantigens bind directly to MHC class II molecules on the surface of antigen-presenting cells and can stimulate >10% of T cells (conventional antigen can stimulate 1 in 1 million cells). Massive T cell stimulation results in release of interleukins 1 and 2, tumor necrosis factor, and interferon-γ. Staphylococcal superantigens include SEs, TSST-1, and some ETs.

## STAPHYLOCOCCAL SCALDED-SKIN SYNDROME    □  ◑ → ●

SSSS is a toxin-mediated epidermolytic disease characterized by erythema and widespread detachment of the superficial layers of the epidermis, resembling scalding; it occurs mainly in newborns and infants <2 years. Severity ranges from a localized form, bullous impetigo, to a generalized form with extensive epidermolysis and desquamation. The clinical spectrum of SSSS includes generalized form (generalized scalded-skin syndrome), localized form (bullous impetigo), and abortive form (scarlitiniform variant).
*Synonym*: Ritter's disease.
*Note*: Toxic epidermal necrolysis (TEN) is not associated with staphylococcal infection but is most often an adverse cutaneous drug reaction.

## EPIDEMIOLOGY AND ETIOLOGY

**Age of Onset**    Most common in neonates during first 3 months of life. Infants and young children <5 years. Rare in adults.
**Etiology**    *S. aureus* of phage group 2 (types 71 and 55), which produces exfoliative toxins A and B (ET-A and ET-B). Site of ET production: purulent conjunctivitis, otitis media omphalitis, occult nasopharyngeal infection; bullous impetigo.
**Risk Factors**    Age <5 years. Adults: renal failure, systemic immunosuppression.

## PATHOGENESIS

In newborns and infants, *S. aureus* colonizes nose, conjunctivae, or umbilical stump with or without causing clinically apparent infection, producing ETs that are transported hematogenously to the skin. In bullous impetigo, ET is produced in impetigo lesion. Specific antistaphylococcal antibody, metabolic differences, or the greater ability to localize, metabolize, and excrete in individuals >5 years probably accounts for decreased incidence of SSSS with older age. At times purulent conjunctivitis, otitis media, or occult nasopharyngeal infection occurs at site of toxin production. ET causes acantholysis and intraepidermal cleavage within the stratum granulosum. Local effects of the ET result in bullous impetigo, but with absorption of the toxin, a mild scarlatiniform rash accompanying the bullous lesions may appear. Conversely, local effects of the toxin may be absent, with systemic absorption resulting in a staphylococcal SF syndrome. More extensive epidermal damage is characterized by sloughing of superficial epidermis in SSSS. Healing occurs spontaneously in 5 to 7 days.

## HISTORY

**Skin Symptoms**    SSSS: early erythematous areas are very tender.

## PHYSICAL EXAMINATION

**Skin Lesions**
***Localized Form***    See "Bullous Impetigo" (p. 588). Intact flaccid purulent bullae, clustered. Rupture of the bullae results in moist red and/or crusted erosive lesions. Lesions are often clustered in an intertriginous area.
***Generalized Form***    ET-induced changes: micromacular scarlatiniform rash (staphylococcal SF syndrome) or diffuse, ill-defined erythema (Fig. 22-31) and a fine, stippled, sandpaper appearance occur initially. In 24 h, erythema deepens in color and involved skin becomes tender. Initially periorificially on face, neck, axillae, groins; becoming more widespread in 24 to 48 h. Initial erythema and later sloughing of superficial layers of epidermis are most pronounced periorificially on face and in flexural areas on neck, axillae, groins, antecubital area, back (pressure points). With epidermolysis, epidermis appears wrinkled and can be removed by gentle pressure (skin resembles wet tissue paper) (Nikolsky's sign) (Fig. 22-31). In some infants, flaccid bullae occur. Unroofed epidermis forms erosions with red, moist base. Desquamation occurs with healing (Fig. 22-33).
**Mucous Membranes**    Uninvolved in SSSS.
**General Examination**    Possible low-grade fever. Irritable child, pain.

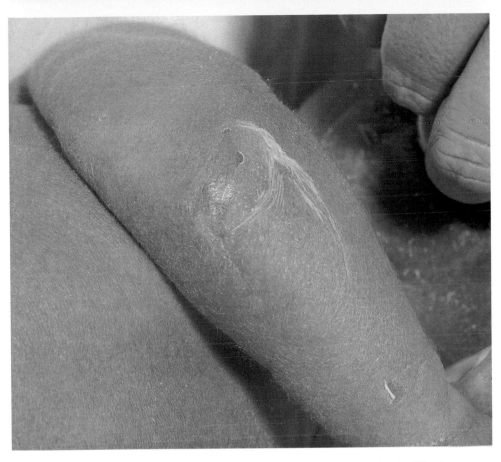

**FIGURE 22-31  Staphylococcal scalded-skin syndrome**  *The skin of this infant is diffusely erythematous; gentle pressure to the skin of the arm has sheared off the epidermis, which folds like tissue paper.*

## DIFFERENTIAL DIAGNOSIS

Drug-induced TEN, TSS, Kawasaki's syndrome.

## LABORATORY EXAMINATIONS

**Direct Microscopy** *Gram's Stain* Bullous impetigo: pus in bullae, clumps of gram-positive cocci within PMN. SSSS: gram-positive cocci only at colonized site, not in areas of epidermolysis.

**Bacterial Culture** Bullous impetigo: *S. aureus* isolated from involved site. SSSS: *S. aureus* only at site of infection (i.e., site of toxin production)—umbilical stump, ala nasi, nasopharynx, conjunctivae, external ear canal, stool. *S. aureus* is not recovered from sites of sloughing skin or bullae.

**Dermatopathology** Intraepidermal cleavage with splitting occurring beneath and within stratum granulosum.

## DIAGNOSIS

Clinical findings confirmed by bacterial cultures.

## COURSE AND PROGNOSIS

In late phases of SSSS, and in an accelerated manner, after adequate antibiotic treatment, the superficially denuded areas heal in 3 to 5 days associated with generalized desquamation in large sheets of skin (Figs. 22-32 and 22-33); there is no scarring. Death can occur in neonates with extensive disease.

## MANAGEMENT

**Prophylaxis** Prevent spread of toxigenic *S. aureus* in neonatal care units.

**General Care** Hospitalization is recommended for neonates and young children, especially if skin sloughing is extensive and parental compliance questionable. Discharge home when significant improvement is apparent. If case is mild and home care reliable, children can be treated with oral antibiotic.

**Topical Therapy** Baths or compresses for debridement of necrotic superficial epidermis. Topical antimicrobial agents for impetigo lesions: mupirocin ointment, bacitracin, or silver sulfadiazine ointment.

**Systemic Antimicrobial Therapy** See Table 22-2.

**Adjunctive Therapy** Replace significant water and electrolyte loss intravenously in severe cases.

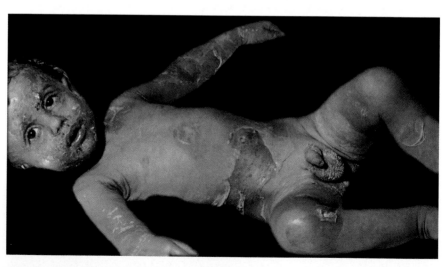

**FIGURE 22-32   Staphylococcal scalded-skin syndrome** *In this infant, painful, tender, diffuse erythema was followed by generalized epidermal sloughing and erosions.* S. aureus *had colonized the nares with perioral impetigo, the site of exotoxin production.*

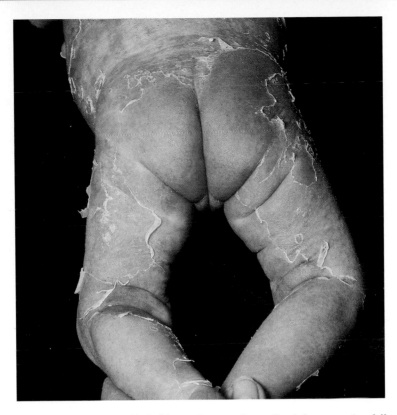

**FIGURE 22-33   Staphylococcal scalded-skin syndrome**   *Generalized desquamation following SSSS in an infant.*

# STAPHYLOCOCCAL TOXIC SHOCK SYNDROME    □   ●

Staphylococcal TSS is an acute toxin-mediated illness caused by toxin-producing *S. aureus*, characterized by rapid onset of fever, hypotension, generalized skin and mucosal erythema, organ hypoperfusion/multisystem failure, and desquamation during early convalescence. Staphylococcal TSS occurs in the setting of menstrual (MTSS) and nonmenstrual (NMTSS) patterns.

Group A streptococcus (GAS) produces streptococcal TSS, which can be indistinguishable from staphylococcal TSS.

## EPIDEMIOLOGY AND ETIOLOGY

**Age of Onset** MTSS: 23 years (mean age); NMTSS: 27 years (mean age).

**Sex** Prior to 1984, >99% of cases were in females; after 1984, equal sex distribution.

**Race** In the United States, 97% of MTSS in whites; 87% of NMTSS in whites.

**Etiology** *S. aureus* producing TSST-1. GAS infections causing streptococcal TSS.

*Site of TSST-1 Production Mentrual-associated:* Use of vaginal tampon of high absorbency. *Nonmenstrual-associated:* Nonsurgical wounds (burns, skin ulcers, cutaneous and ocular injuries, insect bites) and surgical wounds; superinfection of varicella; postpartum infections; vaginal nonmenstrual origin (contraceptive sponge, contraceptive diaphragm); superinfection after influenza or acute sinusitis.

*Streptococcal TSS* Diabetes mellitus, peripheral vascular disease.

**Underlying Disorders** NMTSS can occur secondary to a wide variety of primary *S. aureus* infections as well as secondary infection of underlying dermatoses.

## PATHOGENESIS

*S. aureus* multiplies in foreign body, minor wound infection, or mucosal surface, elaborating the TSST-1 and staphylococcal enterotoxin B. These toxins are absorbed and act as superantigens on T cells, which causes secretion of massive amounts of cytokines. Cytokines result in the clinical syndrome of fever, hypotension, rash, organ hypoperfusion/multiorgan failure. The individual must be colonized or infected with toxigenic strain of *S. aureus* and must lack a protective level of antibody to the toxin made by that strain. >90% of adults have antibodies to TSS toxins.

## HISTORY

**Incubation Period** Shorter in NMTSS. After surgical procedure, <4 days.

**Symptoms** Recurrent symptoms in MTSS in untreated cases; tampon use. Sudden onset of fever, hypotension. Tingling sensation in hands and feet. Maculopapular eruption, pruritic. Generalized myalgias, muscle tenderness and weakness; headache, confusion, disorientation, seizures; profuse diarrhea; dyspnea.

## PHYSICAL EXAMINATION

### Skin Lesions

Generalized scarlatiniform erythroderma, most intense around infected area. Macular eruption (see "Scarlet Fever," page 626). Edema, extensive generalized, nonpitting; most marked on face (Fig. 22-34), hands, feet. One week after onset of skin lesions, desquamation begins with scaling of skin of torso, face, and extremities, followed by desquamation of palms, soles, digits.

*NMTSS* Look for cutaneous site of infection/colonization.

*Streptococcal TSS* Cellulitis, necrotizing fasciitis, puerperal sepsis, varicella in children, and rarely asymptomatic streptococcal pharyngitis.

**Mucous Membranes** Look for forgotten or retained vaginal tampon. Intense erythema and injection of bulbar conjunctivae (Fig. 22-34) and mucous membranes of mouth, tongue, pharynx, vagina, tympanic membranes. Strawberry tongue. Subconjunctival hemorrhages. Ulcerations of mouth, vagina, esophagus, bladder.

**General Findings** Fever. Organ hypoperfusion results in renal and myocardial dysfunction, fluid overload, and adult respiratory distress syndrome (ARDS). Late complications include peripheral gangrene, muscle weakness, lingering asthenia, neuropsychiatric dysfunction.

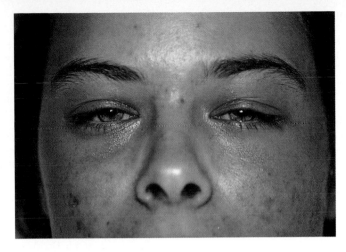

**FIGURE 22-34   Toxic shock syndrome**   *Erythema of the bulbar conjunctivae associated with facial erythema and edema in a female with menstrual TSS.*

## DIFFERENTIAL DIAGNOSIS

**Toxin-Mediated Infections**   SSSS, scarlet fever, GAS TSS, Kawasaki's disease.

**Erythema + Multisystem disease**   Streptococcal TSS, SSSS, Kawasaki syndrome, Rocky Mountain spotted fever (RMSF), leptospirosis, meningococcemia, gram-negative sepsis, exanthematous viral syndromes; severe adverse drug reactions (Stevens-Johnson syndrome, TEN).

## LABORATORY EXAMINATIONS

**Direct Microscopy**   *Gram's Stain*   Vaginal, wound exudate: many leukocytes and gram-positive cocci in clusters.

**Culture**   Vaginal, wound exudate, foreign body: TSST-1-producing *S. aureus.* Streptococcal TSS: GAS recovered from blood or primary site of infection.

**Biopsy**   Confluent epidermal necrosis, vacuolar alteration of dermal-epidermal junction, subepidermal vesiculation, little or no inflammatory infiltrate in dermis.

## DIAGNOSIS

TSS clinical case definition [Centers for Disease Control and Prevention (CDC)]:

1.  *Fever:* Temperature ≥38.9°C (102°F).
2.  *Rash:* Diffuse macular erythroderma ("sunburn" rash)
3.  *Hypotension:* Systolic blood pressure (BP) ≤90 mmHg (adults) or less than fifth percentile for age (children <16 years of age); or orthostatic hypotension (orthostatic drop in diastolic BP by 15 mmHg, orthostatic dizziness, or orthostatic syncope)
4.  *Involvement of at least three of the following organ systems:*
    a.  Gastrointesinal (vomiting or diarrhea at onset of illness)
    b.  Muscular (severe myalgias or serum creatine phosphokinase level at least twice the upper limit of normal)
    c.  Mucous membranes (vaginal, oropharyngeal, conjunctival hyperemia)
    d.  Renal (BUN or creatinine level at least twice upper limit of normal or pyuria)
    e.  Hepatic
    f.  Hematologic (thrombocytopenia)
    g.  Central nervous system
5.  *Desquamation:* 1 to 2 weeks after onset of illness (typically palms/fingers, soles/toes)
6.  *Evidence against alternative diagnosis:* Negative results of cultures of blood, throat, or CSF (if performed); no rise in titers of antibody to the agents of RMSF, leptospirosis, and rubeola (if obtained)

## COURSE AND PROGNOSIS

Diagnosis of NMTSS is often delayed because of the wide variety of clinical settings and associated symptomatology. Complications: refractory hypotension, ARDS, cardiomyopathy, arrhythmias, encephalopathy, acute renal failure, metabolic acidosis, liver necrosis, disseminated intravascular coagulation. Recurrence of untreated MTSS is possible. Antibiotic therapy and discontinuance of tampons significantly reduce risk. Recurrences after NMTSS are rare. Among cases reported to CDC (1985 to 1994), case fatality rate was 2.5% for menstrual cases, and 6.4% for nonmenstrual cases.

Streptococcal TSS: associated with mortality rate of 25 to 50%.

## MANAGEMENT

**Local Infection** Remove potentially foreign bodies. Drain and irrigate infected sites.
**Systemic Antimicrobial Therapy** (See Table 22-1.) IV antistaphylococcal antibiotic. Clindamycin, 900 mg IV q8h. Nafcillin or oxacillin, First-generation cephalosporin. Vancomycin for MRSA.
**Adjunctive Therapy** Aggressive monitoring and management of specific organ system failure (i.e., management of fluid, electrolyte, metabolic, and nutritional needs). Methylprednisolone for severe cases.

---

## SCARLET FEVER     □  

Scarlet fever (SF) is an acute infection of the tonsils, skin, or other sites by an exotoxin-producing strain of GAS, associated with a characteristic toxigenic exanthem.

## EPIDEMIOLOGY AND ETIOLOGY

**Age of Onset** Children.
**Incidence** Much less than in the past.
**Etiology** Usually group A β-hemolytic *S. pyogenes* (GAS). Uncommonly, ET-producing *S. aureus*.

## PATHOGENESIS

Production of streptococcal pyrogenic exotoxins A, B, or C depends on the presence of a temperate bacteriophage. The development of SF rash may reflect hypersensitivity reaction requiring prior exposure to toxin. Strain of *S. aureus* can synthesize an ET, producing a scarlatiniform exanthem.

## HISTORY

**Incubation Period** Rash appears 1 to 3 days after onset of infection.
**Exposure** Household member(s) may be a streptococcal carrier.

## PHYSICAL EXAMINATION

### Skin Lesions
***Site of GAS Infection*** Pharyngitis; tonsillitis. Infected surgical or other wound. Impetiginous skin lesion.
***Exanthem*** Finely punctate erythema is first noted on the upper part of the trunk (Fig. 22-35); may be accentuated in skin folds such as neck, axillae, groin, antecubital and popliteal fossae

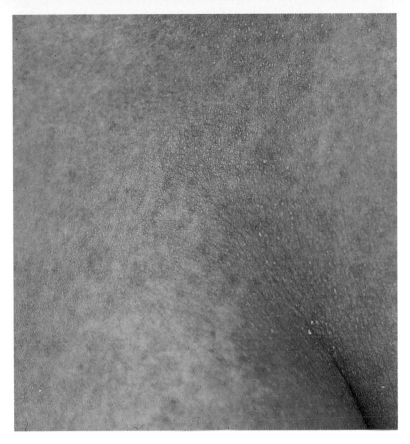

**FIGURE 22-35    Scarlet fever: exanthem**    *Finely punctated erythema has become confluent (scarlatiniform); petechiae can occur and have a linear configuration within the exanthem in body folds (Pastia's line).*

(Pastia's lines). Palms/soles usually spared. Face becomes flushed but with a perioral pallor. Initial punctate lesions become confluently erythematous, i.e., scarlatiniform. Linear petechiae (Pastia's sign) occur in body folds. Intensity of the exanthem varies from mild to moderate erythema confined to the trunk due to an extensive purpuric eruption.

*Petechiae* Scattered petechiae occur (Rumpel-Leede test for capillary fragility positive).

*Desquamation* Exanthem fades within 4 to 5 days and is followed by brawny desquamation on the body and extremities and by sheetlike exfoliation on the palms and soles. In subclinical or mild infections, exanthem and pharyngitis may pass unnoticed. In this case patient may seek medical advice only when exfoliation on the palms and soles is noted.

**Mucous Membranes** *Site of GAS Infection* Acute follicular or membranous tonsillitis. May be asymptomatic or mild and go undetected.

*Enanthem* Pharynx beefy red. Tongue initially is white with scattered red, swollen papillae (white strawberry tongue) (Fig. 22-36). By the fourth or fifth day, the hyperkeratotic membrane is sloughed, and the lingular mucosa appears bright red (red strawberry tongue) (Fig. 22-36). Punctate erythema and petechiae may occur in the palate.

**General Examination** Patient may appear acutely ill with high fever, headache, nausea, vomiting. Anterior cervical lymphadenitis associated with pharyngitis/tonsillitis.

**Variant** Streptococcal TSS: toxemia, organ failure, and a scarlatiniform rash associated with GAS cellulitis.

## DIFFERENTIAL DIAGNOSIS

**Generalized Exanthem** Staphylococcal SF (pharyngitis, tonsillitis, strawberry tongue, and palatal enanthem not seen), staphylococcal or streptococcal TSS, Kawasaki's syndrome, viral exanthem, adverse drug eruption.

## LABORATORY EXAMINATIONS

**Direct Microscopy** *Gram's Stain* Gram-positive cocci in chain (GAS) or clusters (*S. aureus*) identified in smear from infected wound or impetiginized skin lesion.

**Rapid Direct Antigen Tests (DATs)** Used to detect GAS antigens in throat swab specimens.

**Culture** Isolate GAS or *S. aureus* on culture of specimen from throat or wound.

## DIAGNOSIS

Clinical findings confirmed by detecting streptococcal antigen in a rapid test and/or culturing GAS from throat or wound.

## COURSE AND PROGNOSIS

Production of pyrogenic exotoxins does not alter the course of the GAS infection. In some cases, GAS may enter the bloodstream with resultant high fever and marked systemic toxicity (toxic scarlet fever) and consequent metastatic foci of infection. Suppurative complications of GAS infection include peritonsillar cellulitis, peritonsillar abscess, retropharyngeal abscess; otitis media, acute sinusitis; suppurative cervical lymphadenitis.

Nonsuppurative sequelae of streptococcal infections, i.e., acute rheumatic fever, acute glomerulonephritis, and erythema nodosum, may follow if the infection goes untreated. The incidence of acute rheumatic fever has markedly decreased during the past two decades.

## MANAGEMENT

**Symptomatic Therapy** Aspirin or acetaminophen for fever and/or pain.

**Systemic Antimicrobial Therapy** *Penicillin is the drug of choice* because of its efficacy in prevention of rheumatic fever. Goal is to eradicate GAS throat carriage.

| | |
|---|---|
| Penicillin G benzathine | 1.2 million units IM (adults); 600,000 units IM [Children <130 kg (<60 lb)] |
| Penicillin V | 250 mg PO qid for 10 days |

*For penicillin-allergic patients:*

| | |
|---|---|
| Erythromycin estolate | 20 to 40 mg/kg per day |
| Erythromycin ethylsuccinate | 40 mg/kg per day |
| Azithromycin | See Table 22-2 |
| Clarithromycin | See Table 22-2 |
| Cephalosporin (for those who cannot tolerate oral erythromycin) | See Table 22-2 |

**Follow-Up** Reculture of throat recommended for individuals with history of rheumatic fever or if a family member has history of rheumatic fever.

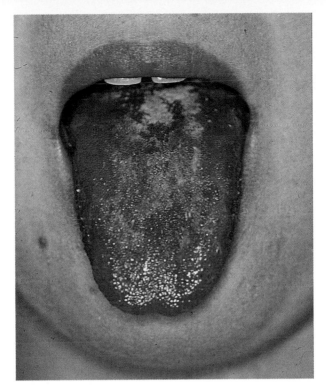

**FIGURE 22-36    Scarlet fever: white and red strawberry tongue**    *Bright red tongue with prominent papillae on the fifth day after onset of group A streptococcal pharyngitis in a child. The white patches at the back of the tongue represent residua of the initial white strawberry tongue.*

## CUTANEOUS ANTHRAX          □   ●

Cutaneous anthrax is a bacterial zoonosis caused by endospores of *Bacillus anthracis*, which enter the body through cutaneous abrasions, inhalation (woolsorters' disease), or ingestion. Typically presents as a black eschar surrounded by edema and purple vesicles. Cutaneous anthrax accounts for 95% of anthrax cases in the United States.
*Synonym*: Malignant pustule.

## EPIDEMIOLOGY AND ETIOLOGY

**Etiology**   *B. anthracis*, a nonmotile, gram-positive, aerobic rod 1.2 to 10 μm in length and 0.5 to 2.5 μm in width. Spores can remain dormant in soil for decades. Anthrax spores have been developed as a biologic weapon.

**Occupation**   Farmers, herders; slaughterhouse and textile workers.

**Transmission**   Zoonosis of mammals, especially herbivores. Human infections result from contact with contaminated wild and domestic animals (herbivores, i.e., cattle, sheep, goats, camels, antelopes) or animal products (hides, hair, wool, bone, meal). Human-to-human transmission does not occur. Recent bioterrorism (2001) in the United States resulted in cases of both cutaneous and inhalation anthrax.

**Geography**   "Anthrax zones": soil rich in organic matter and dramatic changes in climate (abundant rainfall followed by prolonged drought). Most common in agricultural regions where it occurs in animals: South/Central America, Southern/Eastern Europe, Asia, Africa, the Caribbean, Middle East.

   Recent outbreaks in Zimbabwe (1979 to 1980), Paraguay (1987). Accidental release of weapons-grade anthrax spores in Sverdlovsk (1979) resulted in 66 deaths.

## PATHOGENESIS

Introduced endospores are phagocytosed by macrophages, carried to regional lymph nodes, and germinate inside the macrophages and become vegetative bacteria. The vegetative bacilli are released from macrophages, multiply in the lymphatic system, and enter the bloodstream, causing massive septicemia, associated with production of edema and lethal exotoxins. Low-level germination occurs at the primary site, resulting in local edema and necrosis. Gastrointestinal anthrax follows ingestion of endospore-contaminated meat from diseased animals.

## HISTORY

Occupational exposure to animals or animal products. Incubation period is 1 to 10 days (in recent bioterrorism attack); usually no prodrome.

## PHYSICAL EXAMINATION

### Skin Lesions

Cutaneous anthrax is characterized by a black eschar at the site(s) of inoculation (Fig. 22-37*A*, *B*). Nondescript, painless, pruritic papule appearing 3 to 5 days after introduction of endospores. Within 24 to 35 h, evolves to vesicle(s) ± hemorrhage + necrosis. Vesicles rupture to form depressed ulcers, often with local edema, ultimately forming dry eschars (1 to 3 cm). Satellite lesions can form in a sporotrichoid pattern proximally on edematous extremity (Fig. 22-37B). Edema more extensive on head/neck.

*Distribution*   Head, neck, extremities.

**Mucous Membranes**   Oropharyngeal anthrax can occur following ingestion of contaminated meat, presenting with cervical edema and local lymphadenopathy, with dysphagia and respiratory difficulties.

**General Findings**   Possible fever and/or other systemic signs. Pain is not a feature of cutaneous anthrax. Fever in cutaneous anthrax usually indicates superinfection of the cutaneous lesion with streptococci or staphylococci. Lymph nodes in adjacent area may enlarge.

**Variants**   Inhalation anthrax, gastrointestinal anthrax.

## DIFFERENTIAL DIAGNOSIS

Cutaneous anthrax should be considered in any patient with a *painless* ulcer with vesicles, edema, without regional lymphadenopathy, and a history of exposure to animals or animal products.

**Painless, Blackened, Necrotic Eschar ± Regional Lymphadenopathy**   Brown recluse spider bite, ecthyma, ulceroglandular tularemia, accidental vaccinia, necrotic herpes simlex infection, orf, glanders.

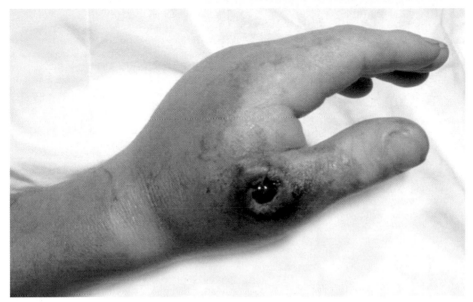

A

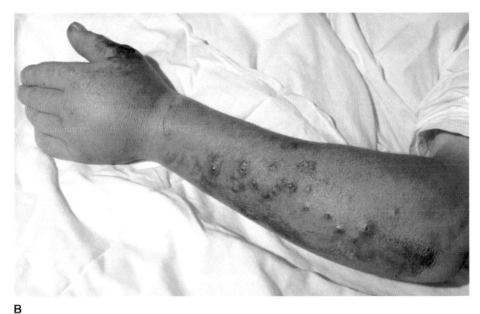

B

**FIGURE 22-37    Cutaneous anthrax**   *A. A black eschar with a central hemorrhagic ulceration on the thumb associated with massive edema of the hand. **B.** A nodular lymphangitis extending proximally from the primary lesion on the thumb.*

## LABORATORY EXAMINATIONS

**Cultures** Gram's stain and culture recommended; prior antibiotic treatment rapidly renders the site culture negative. Gentle sampling with a moist, sterile cottontip applicator is preferred; the rate of positive cultures is about 65%. Expressing eschar fluid is not recommended because it can cause dissemination of the pathogen. Blood cultures with systemic anthrax are always positive.

**Biopsy** Biopsy edge of lesion; examine by silver staining and immunohistochemical testing. May facilitate systemic dissemination.

**Dermatopathology** Nonsuppurative necrosis and massive edema with lymphocytic infiltrates. Gram's stain of tissue shows bacilli in subcutis.

## DIAGNOSIS

Isolation of *B. anthracis* from blood, skin lesions, or respiratory secretions or by measuring specific antibodies in blood of persons with suspected symptoms.

## COURSE AND PROGNOSIS

About 20% of untreated cases of cutaneous anthrax result in death; 80% of cases are self-limiting and usually resolve without scarring. Pain in cutaneous anthrax usually indicates streptococcal or straphylococcal secondary infection. 10% of cases of cutaneous anthrax progress to systemic anthrax. Malignant edema is a rare complication, usually involving the head and neck and manifested by severe edema, induration, multiple bullae, and shock. Inhalation anthrax is nearly always fatal.

## MANAGEMENT

Cutaneous anthrax can be self-limited, but antibiotic therapy is recommended. *Drug of choice*: Ciprofloxacin, 400 mg IV q12h, or doxycycline, 100 mg IV q12h, is optimal. *Alternatives*: None. Surgery for excision of eschar is contraindicated.

**Anthrax Vaccine** Indicated for persons at risk for exposure to anthrax spores: laboratory personnel working with *B. anthracis*, persons who work with imported animal hides/fur if exposure to anthrax is possible, veterinarians who travel to endemic areas, military personnel deployed to area with high risk of exposure. Protection against inhalation anthrax has not been tested. Animals are immunized in endemic regions.

**Postexposure Prophylaxis** Doxycycline, 100 mg bid, or ciprofloxacin, 500 mg bid, for 8 weeks. Amoxicillin (tid) for children and lactating women.

## CUTANEOUS DIPHTHERIA  □  ◑

Cutaneous diphtheria (CD) is a localized *Corynebacterium diphtheriae* infection, caused by toxicogenic and nontoxicogenic strains. Diphtheria toxin causes myocarditis, polyneuritis, and other toxic systemic effects. Respiratory diphtheria is usually caused by toxicogenic (*tox*+) strains. Cutaneous diphtheria is frequently caused by nontoxicogenic (*tox*− ) organisms.

## TETANUS  □  ◑

Tetanus is a neurologic disorder, characterized by increased muscle tone and spasms caused by tetanospasmin, a powerful protein toxin elaborated by *Clostridium tetani*. *C. tetani* spores survive in soil for years. Vegetative cells produce tetanospasmin, which mediates binding to nerve-cell receptors and entry into these cells and blocks neurotransmitter release. Tetanus affects nonimmunized persons, partially immunized persons, or fully immunized individuals who fail to maintain adequate immunity with booster doses of vaccine.

Globally, tetanus is common in areas where soil is cultivated, in rural areas, in warm climates, during summer months, and among males. Without immunization, tetanus occurs predominantly in neonates and other young children (490,000 neonates died of tetanus worldwide in 1994). Site of infection: an acute injury (puncture wound, laceration, abrasion; the injury is usually trivial); secondary infection of breaks in skin [injecting drug use ("skin popping")]; skin ulcers, gangrene, frostbite, burns, surgical wounds, childbirth, abortion; superinfection (abscesses, middle-ear infection). Risk behavior: farming, gardening, and other outdoor activities.

Spores germinate in wounds with low oxidation-reduction potential (devitalized tissue, foreign bodies, or active infection); *C. tetani* does not evoke inflammation. Toxin released in the wound binds to peripheral motor neuron termi-nals, enters the axon, and is transported to the nerve-cell body in the brainstem and spinal cord by retrograde intraneuronal transport. In local tetanus, only the nerves supplying the affected muscles are involved. Generalized tetanus occurs when toxin released in the wound enters the lymphatics and bloodstream and is spread widely to distant nerve terminals; the blood-brain barrier blocks direct entry into the central nervous system.

### CLINICAL MANIFESTATIONS

*Generalized tetanus* Increased muscle tone and generalized spasms: trismus or lockjaw; dysphagia; grimace/sneer (risus sardonicus); arched back (opisthotonus); apnea or laryngospasm. Autonomic dysfunction.

*Neonatal tetanus* Occurs as generalized form; usually fatal if untreated. Occurs in children of inadequately immunized mothers.

*Local tetanus* Manifestations restricted to muscles near the wound.

*Cephalic tetanus* Follows head injury or ear infection. Trismus and dysfunction of one or more cranial nerves.

*No specific skin lesions.*

# INFECTIVE ENDOCARDITIS, SEPSIS, AND SEPTIC SHOCK

Infective endocarditis (IE), sepsis, and septic shock are very serious systemic infections with high associated morbidity and mortality rates. Clinical findings are often acute in onset and relatively nonspecific in nature. Cutaneous findings, however, may be extremely helpful in making the correct diagnosis. Early recognition of clinical findings, diagnosis, and initiation of therapy increase the likelihood of a positive outcome.

## INFECTIVE ENDOCARDITIS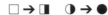

Infective endocarditis (IE) is charactized by proliferation of microorganisms on the endocardium of the heart. A vegetation forms at the site of IE, a mass of fibrin, platelets, microcolonies of microorganisms, and few inflammatory cells. IE occurs most commonly on heart valves (native or prosthetic); also on the low-pressure side of a ventricular septum at a defect site, on mural endocardium, or on cardiac devices. *Infective endarteritis* occurs in arteriovenous shunts, arterioarterial shunts, and coarctation of the aorta.

## EPIDEMIOLOGY AND ETIOLOGY

**Incidence** Subacute bacterial endocarditis (SBE) is now much less common because of the decreased incidence of rheumatic heart disease; the incidence is increasing in the elderly and in injecting drug users, and with prosthetic valve use.

**Temporal Evolution of Disease** *Acute endocarditis* rapidly damages cardiac structures, hematogenously seeds extracardiac sites, and may progress to death in a few weeks. SBE causes structural damage slowly, rarely causes metastatic infection, and is gradually progressive unless complicated by a major embolic event or ruptured mycotic aneurysm.

**Etiology** Varies with native valve IE, prosthetic valve IE, and endocarditis in injection drug users. IE is more often due to gram-positive than gram-negative bacteria, possibly because of differences in adherence to damaged valves or because of differences in their susceptibility to serum-induced killing.

*Community-acquired native valve IE*: Mouth, skin, and upper respiratory tracts are the respective primary portals for the viridans streptococci, staphylococci, and HACEK organisms (*Haemophilus, Actinobacillus, Cardiobacterium, Eikenella, Kingella*). GI tract: *Streptococcus bovis*. GU tract: enterococci.

*Nosocomial native valve IE*: Associated with bacteremia arising from intravascular catheters; less commonly, nosocomial wound and GU infection. IE complicates 6 to 25% of episodes of catheter-associated *S. aureus* bacteremia.

*Prosthetic valve IE*: 1 to 5% of cases of IE. Onset within 2 months of valve surgery associated with intraoperative contamination or postoperative bacteremia: coagulase-negative staphylococci (CoNS), *S. aureus*, facultative gram-negative bacilli, diphtheroids, fungi. Onset 2 to 12 months after surgery: nosocomial CoNS; 85% are MRSA. Onset >12 months after surgery: similar to community-acquired native valve IE, i.e., streptococci, HACEK.

*IE in injection drug users (IDU)*: Incidence increase. 60 to 80% of patients have no known preexisting valve lesions. Pathogen usually originates in skin: *S. aureus. P. aeruginosa,* and fungi. Tricuspid valve (>50% of cases): *S. aureus*, usually MSRA. Left-sided valve (aortic 25%; mitral 20%): *P. aeruginosa, Candida* spp.. Polymicrobial. Others: *Bartonella, Salmonella, Listeria.*

**Transmission** During transient bacteremia: dental procedures, injection drug user various infections, induced abortions, intrauterine contraceptive devices, temporary transvenous pacemakers, percutaneous intravenous catheter lines, endoscopic procedures.

**Groups at Risk**   IDUs (median age, 30 to 40 years) (estimated risk for IE in United States, 2 to 5% per year), elderly people with valve sclerosis, patients with intravascular prostheses, those exposed to nosocomial disease, and those undergoing hemodialysis.

**Nosocomial Endocarditis**   Frequently associated with catheters and medicosurgical procedures. Mortality >50%. In 1999, 37% of cases caused by CoNS.

**Hemodialysis**   Two to three times more common in hemodialysis than peritoneal dialysis patients. >50% of cases due to *S. aureus.*

## PATHOGENESIS

Bacterial adherence to damaged valves, which occurs during transient bacteremia, is the primary event. Bacteria grow within the cardiac lesion(s), with local extension and cardiac damage. Subsequently, septic embolization occurs to skin, kidney, spleen, brain, etc. Microulcerations and local inflammation (resembling arteriosclerosis) occur in degenerative valve lesions (occur in up to 25% of patients >40 years). IDUs, injecting impure materials; prior IE can damage right-sided valves. *S. aureus* is most likely to invade cardiac tissue, resulting in abscess formation. Circulating immune complexes may result in glomerulonephritis, arthritis, or various mucocutaneous manifestations of vasculitis.

## HISTORY

**Symptoms**   Fever (80 to 90%), chills/sweats (40 to 75%), anorexia/weight loss/malaise (25 to 50%), myalgias/arthralgias (15 to 30%), back pain (7 to 15%).

## PHYSICAL EXAMINATION

**General Findings**   Heart murmur (80 to 85%), new/worsened regurgitant murmur (80 to 85%), arterial emboli (10 to 40%), splenomegaly (15 to 50%), neurologic manifestations (20 to 40%). IDUs: 50% of cases are limited to tricuspid valve; pulmonary findings include cough, pleuritic chest pain, pulmonary infiltrates. Consider IE in any patient with fever and heart murmur.

**Skin Lesions (Table 22-7)**   Peripheral manifestations occur in 2 to 5% (Fig. 22-38).

### Embolic Lesions

*Osler's Nodes*   Palpable, tender, and almost always in the pulp of the fingers distally and occasionally on the toes. Red, hemorrhagic and infarcted. Occasionally white center. In acute IE (*S. aureus*), may be more inflammatory than in SBE. In SBE (e.g., virideans strep), lesions usually more vasculitic than septic.

*Janeway Lesions*   Red, macular, papular, infarctive, nontender, and almost always on the palms or soles; usually part of the vasculitis of SBE (Fig. 22-38).

*Septic Embolism*   Painful, hemorrhagic macules, papules, or nodules (Fig. 22-30), usually acral location.

*Subungual Splinter Hemorrhages* Septic embolic phenomenon. Linear in the *middle* of the nailbed in acute IE (see Section 30). (Distal hemorrhages are traumatic.) Common in acute *S. aureus* IE.

*Petechial Lesions*   Small, nonblanching, reddish-brown macules. Occur on extremities, upper chest, mucous membranes [conjunctivae (Fig. 22-39), palate]. Occur in crops. Fade after a few days (20 to 40%).

*Roth Spots* Retinitis septica—a white spot in the retina close to the optic disk, often surrounded by hemorrhages; also seen in pernicious anemia, leukemia.

*Clubbing of Fingers* Occurs after prolonged course of untreated SBE (15 to 20%).

*Gangrene of Extremities* Secondary to embolization.

*Pustular Petechiae, Purulent Purpura* With *S. aureus.*

## DIFFERENTIAL DIAGNOSIS

**Fever with Skin Lesions**   Meningococcemia, disseminated intravascular coagulation, acute rheumatic fever, marantic endocarditis, systemic lupus erythematosus (SLE) with cardiac involvement, systemic vasculitis, dysproteinemia, atrial myxoma, organizing left atrial thrombus, atheromatous embolism.

## LABORATORY EXAMINATION

**Imaging**   Echo-Doppler study demonstrates vegetations, acute severe mitral or aortic regurgitation. Evidence of septic pulmonary emboli suggests tricuspid valve IE. Systemic embolization can occur from aortic or mitral valve.

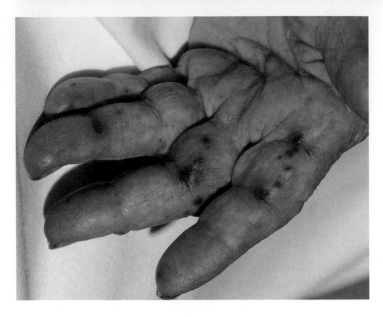

**FIGURE 22-38   Infective endocarditis, acute: Janeway lesions** *Hemorrhagic, infarcted papules on the volar fingers in a patient with* S. aureus *endocarditis.*

## DIAGNOSIS

Modified Duke criteria for diagnosis of infective endocarditis (IE) are based on both microbiologic data and echocardiographic imaging.[1]

### *Diagnosis*

Definite
    Pathology or bacteriology of vegetations, major emboli, or intracardiac abscess specimen, *or*
    Two major criteria, *or*
    One major criterion and three minor criteria, *or*
    Five minor criteria

Possible
    One major and one minor criteria, *or*
    Three minor criteria
Rejected
    Firm alternative diagnosis, *or*
    Resolution of syndrome after ≤4 days of antibiotherapy, *or*
    No pathologic evidence at surgery or autopsy after ≥4 days of antibiotherapy
    Does not meet criteria mentioned above.

## COURSE AND PROGNOSIS

Acute course in IE is common with β-hemolytic streptococci, *S. aureus*, pneumococcal infection;

---

### TABLE 22-7   Cutaneous Manifestations and Characteristics of Infective Endocarditis

| Cutaneous Manifestations | Palpation | Morphologic Findings |
| --- | --- | --- |
| Osler's node | Tender | Erythematous papules and nodules with white centers; may necrose |
| Janeway lesions | Nontender | Hemorrhagic papules |
| Splinter hemorrhages | Nontender | Subungual hemorrhagic streaks |

[1] See P Moreillon, Y-A Que: Lancet 363:139, 2004.

also, *Staphylococcus lugdunensis* and entero-cocci in some cases. Subacute typically occurs in IE caused by viridans streptococci, entero-cocci, CoNS, HACEK. Course varies with the underlying cardiac disease and baseline health of the patient, as well as with the complications that occur. Complications: congestive heart fail-ure, stroke, other systemic embolizations, sep-tic pulmonary embolization. Aortic valve involvement has higher risk of death or need for surgery. In HIV-infected IDUs, mortality rises inversely to the CD4 count.

## MANAGEMENT

**Prophylaxis** Identify patients at risk, proce-dures that might provoke bacteremia, and the most effective prophylactic regimen. Balance between risk of adverse effects of prophylaxis and of developing disease.

**Treatment** Depends on multidisciplinary ap-proach, involving specialists in infectious dis-ease, cardiologists, and cardiac surgeons.[1] Cure of IE requires eradication of all microbes from vegetation(s). Microbicidal drug regimens must produce high enough concentrations for long enough duration to sterilize vegetation(s).

**Antimicrobial Therapy** Appropriate IV antibi-otic therapy, depending on the sensitivity of the infecting organism.

**Surgery** Most common indication, congestive heart failure. Valve replacement.

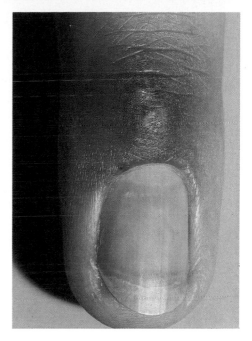

**FIGURE 22-39   Septic vasculitis associated with bacteremia** *Dermal nodule with hemorrhage and necrosis on the dorsum of a finger. This type of lesion occurs with bacteremia (e.g.,* S. aureus, gonococcus) *and fungemia (e.g.,* Candida tropicalis).

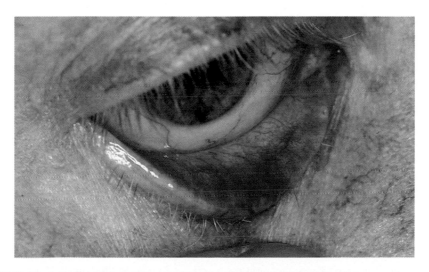

**FIGURE 22-40   Infective endocarditis, acute: subconjunctival hemorrhage** *Submucosal hemorrhage of the lower eyelid in an elderly diabetic with enterococcal endocarditis; splinter hemorrhages in the midportion of the nail bed and Janeway lesions were also present on the volar fingers. Infection followed urosepsis.*

# SEPSIS AND SEPTIC SHOCK

Sepsis and septic shock are manifestations of host response to invading microbes. *Sepsis* is the inflammatory response to microbial invasion, manifesting with fever or hypothermia, tachypnea, and tachycardia; early sepsis is usually reversible. *Severe sepsis* (microbes move from a local site to invade the bloodstream) occurs when counterregulatory control mechanisms are overwhelmed and dysfunction of major organs may supervene. Septic shock is characterized by hypotension as well as organ dysfunction, with significant risk of death.

## EPIDEMIOLOGY AND ETIOLOGY

**Age of Onset** For *N. meningitidis* (NM), highest incidence in children aged 6 months to 3 years (peak, 6 to 12 months); lowest in persons >20 years.

**Incidence** In the United States; 750,000 cases annually, with 210,000 deaths. Two-thirds of cases occur in patients hospitalized for other illnesses. Increasing incidence in the United States attributable to aging population, with increasing longevity of patients with chronic diseases.

**Etiology** See Table 22-8.

**Risk Groups** Those with influenza A virus infection; absence of spleen or functional asplenia; alcoholism; complement deficiency, especially impaired alternative pathway activation.

**Risk Factors** Widespread use of antimicrobial agents, glucocorticoids, indwelling catheters, mechanical devices, mechanical ventilation.

**Gram-negative Bacillary Bacteremia** Diabetes mellitus, lymphoproliferative disease, cirrhosis, burns, invasive procedures or devices, treatment with drugs that cause neutropenia.

**Gram-positive Bacteremia** Vascular catheterization, presence of indwelling mechanical devices, burns, IDU.

**Fungemia** Immunosuppressed patients with neutropenia, often after broad-spectrum antimicrobial therapy.

**Risk Factors for Severe Sepsis in Patients with Bacteremia** Age (>50 years) and primary pulmonary, abdominal, or neuromeningeal site of infection.

## PATHOGENESIS

Septic response triggered when microorganisms spread from skin or GI tract into contiguous tissues. Localized infection may then lead to bacteremia or fungemia. Microbes can also be introduced into bloodstream directly from such routes as venous access lines. In some cases, however, no primary site of infection is apparent. Septic response occurs when invading microbes have circumvented host's innate and acquired immune defenses. Lipopolysaccharide (LPS) (endotoxin) is the most potent gram-negative bacterial signal molecule. Septic response involves complex interaction among microbial signal molecules, leukocytes, humoral mediators, and vascular endothelium. Many of the characteristics of sepsis (fever, tachycardia, tachypnea, leukocytosis, myalgias, somnolence) are produced by release of tumor necrosis factor (TFN) $\alpha$. Intravenous fibrin deposition, thrombosis, and disseminated intravascular coagulation (DIC) are important features of septic response. C5a and other products of complement activation may promote neutrophil reactions such as chemotaxis, aggregation, degranulation, and oxygen-radical production. The underlying mechanism of tissue damage is widespread vascular endothelial injury, with fluid extravasation and microthrombosis that decrease oxygen and substrate utilization by affected tissues. Nitric oxide is a mediator of septic shock.

## HISTORY

The majority of patients experience septic response superimposed on underlying illness and primary infection. Fever may be absent in neonates, the elderly, those with uremia, and alcoholics.

## PHYSICAL EXAMINATION

### Skin Lesions
**Skin / Soft Tissue Infection as Source of Sepsis** Cellulitis, pustules, bullae, hemorrhagic lesions. Hematogenously disseminated toxins can result in diffuse cutaneous reactions such as erythema.

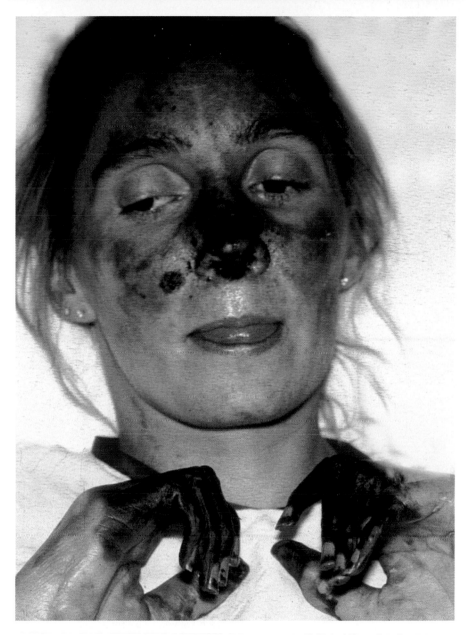

**FIGURE 22-41   Septic shock: ischemic necrosis of acral sites**   *Capnocytophaga canimorsus sepsis (dog bite) with prolonged hypotension and hypoperfusion resulted in infarction of fingers and nose.*

**TABLE 22-8   Definitions Used to Describe the Condition of Patients with Sepsis**

| | |
|---|---|
| Bacteremia | Presence of bacteria in the blood, as evidenced by positive blood cultures. |
| Septicemia | Presence of microbes or their toxins in blood. |
| Systemic inflammatory response syndrome (SIRS) | Two or more of the following conditions: (1) fever (oral temperature >38°C) or hypothermia (<36°C); (2) tachypnea (>24 breaths/min); (3) tachycardia (heart rate >90 beats/min); (4) leukocytosis (>12,000/$\mu$L), leukopenia (<4,000/$\mu$L), or >10% bands. May have an infectious or a noninfectious etiology. |
| Sepsis | SIRS that has a proven or suspected microbial etiology. |
| Severe sepsis (similar to "sepsis syndrome") | Sepsis with one or more signs of organ dysfunction (such as metabolic acidosis, acute encephalopathy, oliguria, hypoxemia, or disseminated intravascular coagulation) or hypotension. |
| Septic shock | Sepsis with hypotension (arterial blood pressure of <90 mmHg systolic or 40 mmHg less than patient's normal blood pressure) that is unresponsive to fluid resuscitation, along with organ dysfunction (see severe sepsis). |
| Refractory septic shock | Septic shock that lasts for >1 h and does not respond to fluid or pressor administration. |
| Multiple-organ dysfunction syndrome (MODS) | Dysfunction of more than one organ, requiring intervention to maintain homeostasis. |

source: Adapted from American College of Chest Physicians/Society of Critical Care Medicine Consensus Conference Committee.

**Nonspecific Cutaneous Findings**   Often subtle. Acrocyanosis, ischemic necrosis of peripheral tissues (most commonly digits), associated with hypotension (Fig. 22-41), DIC (see Section 18).
**Specific Skin Lesions**   *Petechiae* Cutaneous/oropharyngeal location suggests meningococcal infection; less commonly *H. influenzae*. In patient with tick bite living in endemic area, Rocky Mountain spotted fever.
***Ecthyma Gangrenosum*** See Fig. 22-25A, B. *P. aeruginosa* most commonly; also *Aeromonas hydrophila*.
***Hemorrhagic Bullous Lesions*** *Vibrio vulnificus* in patient (diabetes mellitus, liver disease) with history of eating raw oysters (Fig. 22-26); *Capnocytophaga canimorsus* or *C. cynodegmi* following dog bite (Fig. 22-41).
***S. aureus*** Soft tissue infection (Fig. 22-23).
***Generalized Erythema*** *S. aureus*, group A streptococcus (GAS) with toxic shock syndrome.

**General Examination**
**Fever**   May be absent in neonates, elderly patients, persons with uremia, alcoholism.
**GI Manifestations**   Nausea, vomiting, diarrhea, ileus; stress ulcer. Liver; cholestatic jaundice; hepatocellular/canalicular dysfunction. Prolonged hypotension: acute hepatic injury; ischemic bowel necrosis.
**Less Common Manifestations**   Arthritis (5 to 10%), pneumonia, sinusitis, otitis media, conjunctivitis, endophthalmitis, endocarditis, pericarditis, urethritis, endometritis.

**DIFFERENTIAL DIAGNOSIS**

**Sepsis and Shock**   Acute bacteremia and endocarditis, acute "hypersensitivity" vasculitis, enteroviral infections, RMSF, TSS.

## LABORATORY EXAMINATIONS

**Direct Microscopy**   Examine skin/mucosal surfaces. Gram stain of material from primary site of infection or from infected cutaneous lesions. In overwhelming infection (pneumococcal sepsis in splenectomized patient or fulminant meningococcemia), microorganisms can be seen in buffy coat. In meningococcemia, scrapings from nodular lesions show gram-negative diplococci.

**Hematology**   Leukocytosis with left shift, thrombocytopenia; later, leukopenia. Neutrophils contain toxic granules, Döhle bodies, cytoplasmic vacuoles.

**Clotting Studies**   Prolonged thrombin time, decreased fibrinogen, presence of D-dimers.

**Chemistry**   Hyperbilirubinemia, increased creatinine.

**Cultures**   *Blood* Obtain at least two blood samples (from different venipuncture sites) for culture. Gram-negative bacteremia is low grade; multiple blood cultures or prolonged incubation of cultures may be necessary. *S. aureus* grows rapidly and is most easily detectable. Negative blood cultures may reflect prior antibiotic administration, slow-growing or fastidious organisms, or absence of microbial invasion of bloodstream. Acute meningococcemia, NM in nearly 100%; meningitis, one-third positive.

*Skin/Soft Tissue* Obtain cultures from sites of possible cutaneous infection.

*Cerebrospinal Fluid (CSF) Culture* Acute meningococcemia, usually positive.

*Culture of Lesional Skin Biopsy Specimen* Up to 85%.

## DIAGNOSIS

Definitive etiologic diagnosis requires isolation of microorganism from blood or local site of infection.

## COURSE AND PROGNOSIS

Ventilation-perfusion mismatching produces adult respiratory distress syndrome (ARDS). Severe decrease in systemic vascular resistance results in generalized maldistribution of blood flow, functional hypovolemia, diffuse capillary leakage of intravascular components. Cardiac output may intially be elevated; subsequent cardiac dysfunction common. Renal failure occurs due to hypotension and capillary injury. Platelet counts low in patients with DIC; low counts reflect diffuse endothelial injury. Approximately 25 to 35% of patients with severe sepsis and 40 to 45% of those with septic shock die within 30 days; others die within the ensuing 5 months.

## MANAGEMENT

Requires urgent measures to treat local infection, provide hemodynamic and respiratory support, and eliminate offending organism. Outcome depends on underlying disease.

**Prevention**   Reduce number of invasive procedures, limit use of indwelling vascular and bladder catheters, reduce incidence and duration of profound neutropenia (<500 neutrophils/mL), aggressively treat localized nosocomial infections.

**Surgery**   Removal or drainage of focal source of infection is essential.

**Antimicrobial Therapy**   In the absence of an obvious source of infection, antimicrobial regimen differs in the following types of patients: immuncompetent adult, neutropenic patient, splenectomized patient, injecting drug user, HIV-infected patient. Any febrile patient with a petechial rash should be considered to have NM infection; blood culture should be obtained; treatment begun without awaiting confirmation.

**Antibiotic Therapy of Sepsis Due to Other Microbes**   Depends on the sensitivity of the infecting organism (see Table 22-2).

**Hemodynamic, Respiratory, Metabolic Support** Primary goal is to restore adequate oxygen and substrate delivery to tissues. Adequate fluids should be infused to treat intravascular volume depletion. Adrenal insufficiency should be considered in patients with refractory hypotension, fulminant meningococcemia, prior glucocorticoid use, disseminated tuberculosis, HIV disease. Ventilator therapy is indicated for progressive hypoxia, hypercapnia, neurologic deterioration, respiratory muscle failure.

# MENINGOCOCCAL DISEASE    □   ●

*Neisseria meningitidis* (NM) colonizes mucosa and is capable of causing a broad spectrum of clinical syndromes: meningococcal meningitis, meningococcal bacteremia, meningococcemia, respiratory tract infection, focal infection, and chronic meningococcemia. Meningococcal meningitis, meningococcal bacteremia, and meningococcemia are associated with high morbidity and mortality and are often accompanied by characteristic hemorrhagic cutaneous findings.

## EPIDEMIOLOGY

**Age of Onset** For NM, highest incidence is in children ages 6 months to 3 years (peak, 6 to 12 months) (protective antibodies have not yet developed). Increasing in adolescents and young adults; 28% of cases are in 12- to 29-year olds.

**Incidence** In the United States 2500 to 3000 cases annually.

**Transmission** Person-to-person through inhalation of droplets of aerosolized infected nasopharyngeal secretions; direct or indirect oral contact.

**Season** Highest incidence in midwinter, early spring; lowest in midsummer.

**Demography** Worldwide. Occurs in epidemics or sporadically. Major outbreaks reported in Africa, China, South America. African savannah from Ethiopia to east of Senegal: "meningitis belt."

**Risk Factors** Only a minority of nasopharyngeal isolates cause invasive disease. Black race, low socioeconomic status, military recruits, college freshmen living in dormitories. Persons with deficiency of antibody-dependent complement-mediated immune lysis, functional/anatomical asplenia, properdin deficiency, deficiency of terminal complement components, HIV disease, tobacco smoke, viral upper respiratory infections (URIs) are most susceptible.

## ETIOLOGY

NM is a gram-negative, encapsulated coccus; 13 serovars. Confined to humans; natural habitat is nasopharynx. Nasopharyngeal carrier rate: in nonepidemic periods, 10%; in closed populations, up to 60 to 80%. Carriage persists for a few months. Invasive infection usually occurs within first few days of carriage, before development of protective antibodies. *Worldwide*: serogroups A, B, C account for most cases; *America, Europe*: most outbreaks caused by serogroups B, C; *Asia/Africa*: A, C. *The United States, Sweden, Israel*: also have group Y.

### Infectious Syndromes Associated with Meningococcal Disease

Meningococcal meningitis
Meningococcal bacteremia
    Meningococcemia (purpura fulminans and
    Waterhouse-Friderichsen syndrome
Respiratory tract infection
    Pneumonia
    Epiglottitis
    Otitis media
Focal infection
    Conjunctivitis
    Septic arthritis
    Urethritis
    Purulent pericarditis
Chronic meningococcemia

## PATHOGENESIS

Fulminant meningococcemia is the most rapidly lethal form of septic shock experienced by humans. It differs from most other forms of septic shock by the prominence of hemorrhagic skin lesions (petechiae, purpura) and the consistent development of DIC. Extremely high blood levels of both proinflammatory mediators [TNF, interleukin (IL) 1, interferon, IL-8] and anti-inflammatory mediators (IL-1 receptor antagonist, soluble IL-1 receptors, soluble TNF receptors, and IL-10).

## HISTORY

**Acute Meningococcemia** In most cases, nasopharyngeal infection is subclinical; mild URI symptoms occasionally develop. Spiking fever, chills, arthralgia, myalgia. Stupor, hemorrhagic lesions, hypotension may be evident within a few hours of onset of symptoms in fulminant meningococcemia.

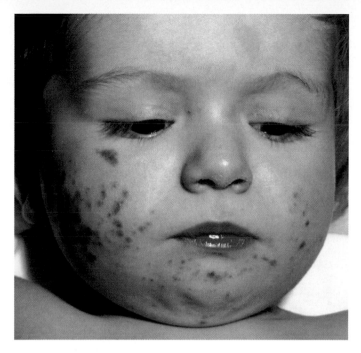

**FIGURE 22-42   Acute meningococcemia: early exanthem**   *Discrete, pink-to-purple macules and papules as well as purpura on the face of this young child. These lesions represent early disseminated intravascular coagulation with its cutaneous manifestation, purpura fulminans.*

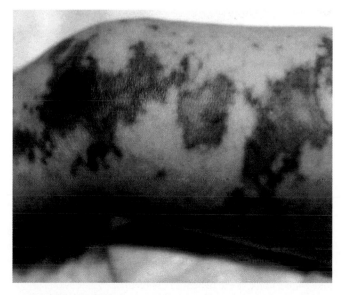

**FIGURE 22-43   Acute meningococcemia: purpura fulminans**   *Maplike, gray-to-black areas of cutaneous infarction of the leg in a child with NM meningitis and disseminated intravascular coagulation with purpura fulminans.*

## PHYSICAL EXAMINATION

Some patients (10 to 30%) with meningococcal disease have both meningococcemia and meningitis.

### Skin Lesions

*Early Exanthem* Occurs soon after onset of disease in 75% of cases; pink, 2- to 10-mm macules/papules, sparsely distributed on trunk/lower extremities as well as face, palate, conjunctivae (Fig. 22-42).

*Later Lesions* Petechiae appear in center of macules. Lesions become hemorrhagic within hours. In severe cases, petechiae may become confluent and develop into hemorrhagic bullae with extensive ulcerations. *Fulminant*: purpura, ecchymoses, and confluent, often bizarre-shaped grayish to black necrosis (purpura fulminans) associated with DIC in fulminant disease (Fig. 22-43).

### General Examination

High fever, tachypnea, tachycardia, mild hypotension. Patient appears acutely ill with marked prostration.

*Meningitis* 50 to 88% of patients with meningococcemia develop meningitis. Sudden onset of fever, signs of meningeal irritation (headache; stiffness of neck; altered mental status; agitated, maniacal behavior). Signs of increased intracranial pressure (bulging fontanelle in infant).

*Fulminant Meningococcemia* More rapid progression/overwhelming character. Occurs in 10 to 20% of cases of meningococcal disease; characterized by development of shock, DIC, hypotension, peripheral vasoconstriction with cold cyanotic extremities, and multiorgan failure. Peripheral gangrene may occur, requiring amputation in those who survive.

*Complications* Intercurrent infections, CNS damage. Patients who recover may have necrosis of skin, distal extremities, tips of ears/nose.

*Less Common Manifestations* Arthritis (5 to 10%), pneumonia, sinusitis, otitis media, conjuctivitis, endophthalmitis, endocarditis, pericarditis, urethritis, endometritis.

## DIFFERENTIAL DIAGNOSIS

**Acute Meningococcemia and Meningitis** Gonococcemia, infectious endocarditis, acute hypersensitivity, vasculitis, enteroviral infections, RMSF, endemic typhus.

## LABORATORY EXAMINATIONS

**Direct Microscopy** Pus from nodular lesions shows gram-negative diplococci. In fulminant meningococcemia, NM can be seen in buffy coat. In 85% of cases of meningitis, NM can be seen in CSF.

**Clotting Studies** Prolonged thrombin time, decreased fibrinogen, presence of D-dimers.

**Cultures** *Blood* Acute meningococcemia, NM in nearly 100%; meningitis, one-third positive.

*CSF* Acute meningococcemia, usually positive.

## DIAGNOSIS

Definitive etiologic diagnosis requires isolation of microorganism from blood or local site of infection.

## COURSE AND PROGNOSIS

Case fatality rate for fulminant meningococcemia is 20 to 40%; for meningococcal meningitis, 3 to 10%. In Africa, mortality is 10%, but many patients die before reaching hospital. In 1996, an epidemic in the meningitis belt reported 160,000 cases with 16,000 deaths.

## MANAGEMENT

**Immunization** <20% of NM isolates from associated disease belong to serogroups for which vaccines are available: A, C, W-135, Y.

**Prophylaxis of Contacts of Primary Cases** Rifampin, minocycline, or ciprofloxacin.

**Antimicrobial Therapy** Any febrile patient with a petechial rash should be considered to have NM infection; blood culture should be obtained and treatment begun without awaiting confirmation.

*Acute Meningococcemia* Third-generation cephalosporin: cefotaxime (2 g IV q8h) or ceftriaxone (1 g IV q12h). *Alternative*: Penicillin G (4 million U IV q4h). *Chloramphenicol* in penicillin-allergic individuals.

**Hemodynamic, Respiratory, Metabolic Support** Primary goal is to restore adequate oxygen and substrate delivery to tissues. Adequate fluids should be infused to treat intravascular volume depletion.

# GRAM-NEGATIVE INFECTIONS

## BARTONELLA INFECTIONS   □   ◑

*Bartonella* spp. are tiny gram-negative bacilli that can adhere to and invade mammalian cells such as endothelial cells and erythrocytes. Clinical syndromes caused by *Bartonella* (Table 22-9) include cat-scratch disease (CSD), bacillary angiomatosis (BA), endocarditis, Oroya fever, and verruga peruana; manifestations vary with the immune status of the host. *B. henselae* produces two entirely different pathologic reactions, depending on the immune status of the host, i.e., CSD or BA.

*Oroya fever* and *verruga peruana* are caused by *B. bacilliformis*, which is transmitted by the bite of the sandfly *Phlebotomus* in Andean valleys. The initial presentation is of a severe febrile illness associated with profound anemia, with significant morbidity and mortality. Verruga peruana appears after convalescence from acute Oroya fever, presenting as red-purple cutaneous lesions, tiny to sessile to large, pedunculated, and nodular; these lesions resemble the angiomatous lesions of bacillary angiomatosis or Kaposi's sarcoma.

*Trench fever* is caused by *B. quintana* and *B. henselae*, presenting as a febrile systemic illness with prolonged bacteremia. There are no cutaneous manifestations.

**TABLE 22-9   Clinical Syndromes Caused by *Bartonella* Species**

| Clinical Syndrome | Causative *Bartonella* |
|---|---|
| Oroya fever | *B. bacilliformis* |
| Verruga peruana | *B. bacilliformis* |
| Trench fever | *B. quintana, B. henselae* |
| Endocarditis (*Bartonella* bacteremic syndrome) | *B. quintana, B. henselae, B. elizabethae* |
| Cat-scratch disease | *B. henselae* |
| Cutaneous bacillary angiomatosis | *B. quintana, B. henselae* |
| Peliosis hepatitis (liver involvement) | *B. quintana, B. henselae* |
| Parenchymal bacillary peliosis (liver and spleen involvement) | *B. quintana, B. henselae* |

## CAT-SCRATCH DISEASE

CSD is a benign, self-limited zoonotic infection characterized by a primary skin or conjunctival lesion after cat scratches or contact with a cat; subsequently, there are acute to subacute tender regional lymphadenopathy and systemic symptoms.
*Synonyms*: Cat-scratch fever, benign lymphoreticulosis, nonbacterial regional lymphadenitis.

## EPIDEMIOLOGY AND ETIOLOGY

**Age of Onset**  Most patients <21 years in the United States.

**Sex**  Males > females.

**Incidence**  20,000 cases annually in the United States, of whom 2000 are hospitalized.

**Transmission**  History of cat contact in 90% of cases; of these individuals, 75% have history of scratch, bite, or lick. Blood cultures of kittens are frequently positive for *B. henselae*. Adult cats are blood culture–negative but are *B. henselae*–seropositive. Familial cases may occur shortly after addition of a kitten to the household. Fleas transmit infection between cats. Whether infection to humans can be transmitted by flea bite is unknown.

**Season**  Late fall, winter, or early spring in cooler climates; July and August in warmer climates. Worldwide.

**Etiology**  *B. henselae*.

## PATHOGENESIS

*B. henselae* causes granulomatous inflammation in healthy individuals (CSD)and angiogenesis in immuncompromised persons.

## HISTORY

**Incubation Period**  Primary lesion at bite/ scratch site: 2 weeks after inoculation (range, 1 to 8 weeks); occurs in about half of cases. Regional lymphadenopathy: 5 to 50 days after inoculation.

**Prodrome**  Mild fever and malaise occur in fewer than half the patients. Chills, general aching, and nausea are infrequently present.

## PHYSICAL EXAMINATION

### Skin Lesions

**Primary**  Innocuous-looking, small (1.5 cm) papule, vesicle, or pustule 3 to 5 days after inoculation; may ulcerate; skin color pink to red; firm, at times tender (Fig. 22-44). Residual linear cat scratch. *Distribution*: exposed skin of head, neck, extremities. Uncommonly: urticaria, transient maculopapular eruption, vesiculopapular lesions, erythema nodosum.

**Mucous Membranes**  If portal of entry is the conjunctiva, 3- to 5-mm whitish-yellow granulation on palpebral conjunctiva associated with tender preauricular and/or cervical lymphadenopathy (Parinaud's oculoglandular syndrome).

### General Examination

Most patients do not have fever. Systemic symptoms common: malaise, anorexia, weight loss.

**Regional Lymphadenopathy**  (Fig. 22-45) Evident within a few days to a few weeks after inoculation; primary lesion, if present, has usually resolved by the time lymphadenopathy occurs. Nodes are usually solitary, moderately tender, freely movable. Involved lymph nodes: epitrochlear, axillary, pectoral, cervical. Nodes may suppurate. Generalized lymphadenopathy or involvement of the lymph nodes of more than one region is unusual.

**Other**  Encephalitis (seizures, coma in children), meningitis, transverse myelitis, pneumonitis, thrombocytopenia, osteomyelitis, granulomatous hepatitis, abscesses in liver or spleen, disseminated infection.

## DIFFERENTIAL DIAGNOSIS

**Regional Lymphadenopathy, Distal Cutaneous Lesion**  Suppurative bacterial lymphadenitis, atypical mycobacteria, sporotrichosis, tularemia, toxoplasmosis, infectious mononucleosis, tumors, sarcoidosis, lymphogranuloma venereum, coccidioidomycosis.

**Other Cat-Associated Infections**  *Pasteurella multocida* bite infection, *Capnocytophaga* (DF-2) spp. bite infection, sporotrichosis, *Microsporum canis* dermatophytosis, *Toxocara cata* (larva migrans), *Dirofilaria repens* subcutaneous nodules.

## LABORATORY EXAMINATIONS

**Hematology**  WBC usually normal; ESR commonly elevated.

**Dermatopathology**  Granulomatous inflammation with stellate necrosis. Demonstration of small, pleomorphic bacilli in Warthin-Starry–stained sections of primary skin lesion, conjunctiva, or lymph nodes.

**Culture**  Isolation of *B. henselae* from lymph node aspirates is seldom possible, perhaps because the strains of *Bartonella* causing CSD are more fastidious than those that cause bacteremia or because the lymph node aspirates contain few viable bacteria.

**Serology**  Antibodies to *B. henselae* usually positive ≥1:64.

**Polymerase Chain Reaction (PCR)**  *B. henselae* 16S ribosomal genes with specific oligonucleotide primers (not available commercially).

## DIAGNOSIS

Suggested by regional lymphadenopathy developing over a 2- to 3-week period in an individual with cat contact and a primary lesion at the

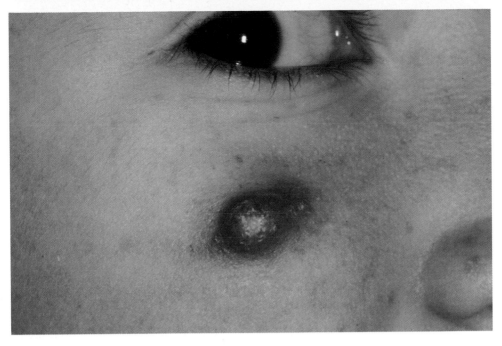

**FIGURE 22-44   Bartonellosis: cat-scratch disease with primary lesion**   *Erythematous nodule of the cheek of a 9-year-old girl at the site of cat-scratch. Diagnosis was made on the histological findings of the excised specimen.*

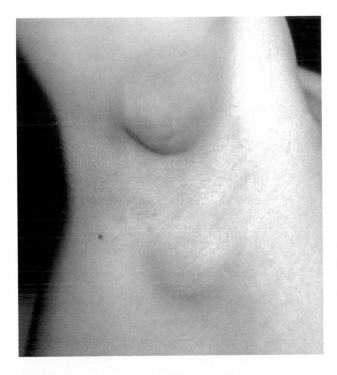

**FIGURE 22-45   Bartonellosis: cat-scratch disease with axillary adenopathy**   *Acute, very tender, axillary lymphadenopathy in a child; cat scratches were present on the dorsum of the ipsilateral hand. (Courtesy of Howard Heller, MD.)*

site of contact; confirmed by identification of *B. henselae* from tissue or serodiagnosis.

## COURSE AND PROGNOSIS

Self-limiting, usually within 1 to 2 months. Uncommonly, prolonged morbidity with persistent high fever, suppurative lymphadenitis, severe systemic symptoms. May be confused with lymphoma. Uncommonly, cat-scratch encephalopathy occurs. Antibiotic therapy has not been very effective in altering the course of the infection.

## MANAGEMENT

Symptomatic in most cases.

**Antimicrobial Therapy**　Azithromycin PO, 500 mg on day 1, 250 mg on days 2 to 5 [for adults >45.5 kg (>100 lb)] effective. Ciprofloxacin, doxycycline may be effective.

**Surgery**　Occasionally, surgical drainage of suppurative node is indicated.

## BACILLARY ANGIOMATOSIS　　□　◐

Bacillary angiomatosis (BA) is a systemic infection caused by *Bartonella* spp., occurring nearly exclusively in HIV-infected individuals. It is characterized by cutaneous vascular tumors resembling Kaposi's sarcoma and symptomatic multisystemic infection, most commonly involving the liver (peliosis hepatitis) and/or spleen (parenchymal bacillary peliosis). Incidence has markedly diminished in treated HIV disease.

## EPIDEMIOLOGY AND ETIOLOGY

**Etiology**　*B. henselae* and *B. quintana* (agent of trench fever). In immunocompetent individuals, *B. henselae* is also the agent of CSD. *B. henselae* infections associated with cat and flea exposure; *B. quintana* infection associated with exposure to body lice (*Pediculus humanis corporis*).

**Reservoir**　*B. henselae* frequently causes asymptomatic bacteremia in kittens, which has been documented by isolation of the organism by blood cultures or anti-*B. henselae* antibodies. The reservoir for *B. quintana* is unknown.

**Transmission**　(See also "Cat-Scratch Disease.") Associated with exposure to young cats infested with fleas (*Ctenocephalides felis*); a large proportion of cats have *B. henselae* bacteremia. Presumably enters percutaneously through minor breaks in the epidermis (scratches or bites). The role of the cat flea in transmission to humans is unclear. *B. quintana* is probably transmitted by ectoparasites (mites, lice).

**Risk Factors**　BA occurs almost exclusively in HIV-infected individuals with advanced immunodeficiency. It is uncommon in individuals who are immunocompetent, immunocompromised for other reasons, or organ transplant recipients.

## PATHOGENESIS

*Bartonella* spp. cause vascular proliferation (angiogenesis), histologically resembling Kaposi's sarcoma: *B. bacilliformis* causes verruga peruana, *B. henselae* and *B. quintana* cause bacillary angiomatosis. *B. henselae* is associated with hepatosplenic disease (peliosis hepatitis) and lymph nodes. *B. quintana* is associated with bony and subcutaneous lesions.

## HISTORY

Incubation period unknown, but probably days to weeks. Association with a kitten. Patients with localized infection may be free of systemic symptoms. Those with more widespread disseminated infection have fever, malaise, weight loss.

**Cutaneous BA**　Lesions may be painful, in contrast with Kaposi's sarcoma lesions, which are not painful.

**Disseminated BA**　Skin lesions usually absent. Presents with nausea, vomiting, diarrhea, fever, chills. Bony lesions may cause focal bone pain.

## PHYSICAL EXAMINATION

### Skin Lesions
Papules or nodules resembling angiomas (red, bright red, violaceous, or skin-colored) (Fig.

22-46); up to 2 to 3 cm in diameter; usually situated in dermis with thinning or erosion of overlying epidermis surrounded by a collarette of scale. Pyogenic granuloma–like lesions (Fig. 22-46). Subcutaneous nodules, 1 to 2 cm in diameter, resembling cysts. Uncommonly, abscess formation. Papules/nodules range from solitary lesions to >100 and, rarely, >1000. Firm, nonblanching. Lesions may be nontender or painful, a finding not seen in nodular lesions of Kaposi's sarcoma.

***Distribution*** Any site, but palms and soles are usually spared. Occasionally, lesions occur at the site of a cat scratch. A solitary lesion may present as dactylitis.

***Mucous Membranes*** Angioma-like lesions of lips and oral mucosa. Laryngeal involvement with obstruction.

### Systemic Findings

Infection may spread hematogenously or via lymphatics to become systemic, commonly involving the liver and spleen (hepatosplenomegaly, liver abscesses, necrotizing splenitis, hepatic/splenic necrotizing granulomata). Lesions may also occur in the heart (cardiac lesions, endocarditis), bone marrow, lymph nodes, muscles, soft tissues, and CNS (brain abscess, aseptic meningitis, encephalopathy).

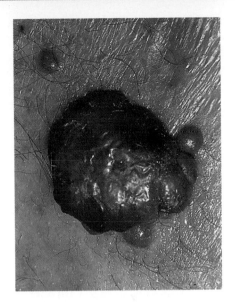

**FIGURE 22-46   Bartonellosis: bacillary angiomatosis** *3- to 5-mm cherry hemangioma-like papules and a larger pyogenic granuloma-like nodule on the shin of a male with advanced HIV disease. Subcutaneous nodular lesions were also present.*

### DIFFERENTIAL DIAGNOSIS

**Multiple Cutaneous Angiomatous Papules/Nodules in HIV disease**   Kaposi's sarcoma, pyogenic granuloma, epithelioid (histiocytoid) angioma, cherry angioma, sclerosing hemangioma, disseminated cryptococcosis.

### LABORATORY EXAMINATIONS

**Dermatopathology**   Lobular vascular proliferations composed of plump "epithelioid" endothelia. Neutrophils scattered throughout the lesion, especially around eosinophilic granular aggregates, which are masses of bacteria (visualized by Warthin-Starry staining or electron microscopy).

**Liver Biopsy**   Associated with higher morbidity and mortality rates in that the lesions are vascular tumors. Dilated capillaries or multiple blood-filled cavernous spaces; myxoid stroma containing an admixture of inflammatory cells and granular clumps (*Bartonella*).

**Culture**   *Bartonella* can be isolated from lesional skin biopsy specimens, blood, or other infected tissues on endothelial-cell monolayer.

**PCR**   Detects *Bartonella* DNA in tissue.

**Chemistry**   Bacillary peliosis hepatitis associated with elevated γ-glutamyltransferase, alkaline phosphatase.

**Serology**   Anti-*Bartonella* antibodies detected by indirect fluorescent-antibody testing (detected by the CDC). Also, enzyme immunoassay for detection of IgG antibodies to *B. henselae*.

**Imaging**   Lesions can be visualized by conventional radiographs and nuclear imaging. Lesions regress with appropriate therapy. CT scan shows hepatomegaly, ±splenomegaly.

### DIAGNOSIS

Clinical findings confirmed by demonstration of *Bartonella* bacilli on silver stain of lesional biopsy specimen or culture or antibody studies.

### COURSE AND PROGNOSIS

Course variable. In some individuals, lesions regress spontaneously. Untreated systemic infection causes significant morbidity and mortality. With effective antimicrobial therapy, lesions resolve within 1 to 2 weeks. As with other infections occurring in HIV disease, relapse may occur and require lifelong secondary prophylaxis. Azithromycin given for *Mycobacterium avium* complex (MAC) prophylaxis seems to prevent BA as well. BA does not occur in HIV-infected individuals effectively treated with highly active antiretroviral therapy (HAART).

## MANAGEMENT

**Prevention**   HIV-infected individuals should avoid contact with cats, especially kittens, to minimize the risk for acquiring BA, as well as toxoplasmosis.

**Antimicrobial Therapy**   Given for 3 to 12 weeks. A Jarisch-Herxheimer type reaction may occur shortly after beginning therapy. Cutaneous BA can be treated with oral antibiotics:

- Erythromycin 500 mg PO qid *or*
- Doxycycline 100 mg PO bid *or*
- Ciprofloxacin 750 mg PO bid *or*
- Azithromycin 500 mg PO qd

Peliosis hepatitis should be treated with IV antibiotic.

**Secondary Prophylaxis**   Lifelong maintenance if relapses occur in the setting of advance immunodeficiency.

---

## TULAREMIA   □

---

Tularemia is an acute infection transmitted by handling flesh of infected animals, by the bite of insect vectors, by inoculation of conjunctiva, by ingestion of infected food, or by inhalation; it manifests as six patterns: ulceroglandular, oculoglandular, typhoidal, pulmonary. *Synonyms*: Rabbit fever, deerfly fever.

## EPIDEMIOLOGY AND ETIOLOGY

**Age of Onset/Sex**   Young males.

**Etiology**   *Francisella tularensis*, a pleomorphic gram-negative coccobacillus.

**Occupation**   Rabbit hunters, butchers, cooks, agricultural workers, trappers, campers, sheep herders and shearers, mink ranchers, muskrat farmers, laboratory technicians.

**Transmission**   (1) Small abrasion or puncture wound, bites of infected deerflies/ticks; (2) conjunctival inoculation; (3) ingestion of infected meat; (4) inhalation. Animal reservoir—rabbits, foxes, squirrels, skunks, muskrats, voles, beavers. Insect vectors—ticks (*Ixodes, Dermacentor*), body lice, deerfly.

**Season**   Greatest frequency in summer (tick season) and rabbit-hunting season.

**Geography**   Throughout northern hemisphere. United States: midwest in summer; east of Mississippi in winter.

**Clinical Syndromes**   Ulceroglandular, glandular, pulmonary, oropharyngeal, oculoglandular, typhoidal.

## PATHOGENESIS

After inoculation, *F. tularensis* reproduces and spreads through lymphatic channels to lymph nodes and bloodstream.

## HISTORY

**Incubation Period**   2 to 10 days.

**Symptoms**   Prodrome: headache, malaise, myalgia, high fever. About 48 h after inoculation, pruritic papule develops at the site of trauma or insect bite followed by enlargement of regional lymph nodes.

## PHYSICAL EXAMINATION

### Skin Lesions

At inoculation site: erythematous tender papule evolving to a vesicopustule, enlarging to crusted ulcer with raised, sharply demarcated margins (96 h) (Fig. 22-47). Depressed center that is often covered by a black eschar (chancri-

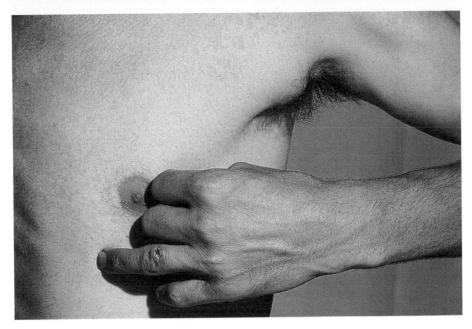

**FIGURE 22-47   Tularemia: primary lesion and regional adenopathy**   *A crusted ulcer at the site of inoculation is seen on the dorsum of the left ring finger with associated axillary lymph node enlargement (chancriform syndrome). The infection occurred after the patient killed and skinned a rabbit.*

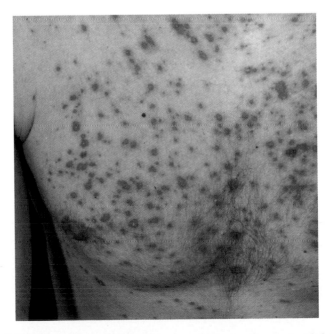

**FIGURE 22-48   Tularemia: erythema multiforme**   *An exanthem on the chest with features of erythema multiforme syndrome, a hypersensitivity to* Francisella tularensis.

form). Primary lesion on finger/hand at site of trauma/insect bite; groin/axilla after tick bite. After bacteremia, exanthem (trunk and extremities) with macules, papules, petechiae; erythema multiforme (Fig. 22-48); erythema nodosum.

**Mucous Membranes** In oculoglandular tularemia, *F. tularensis* is inoculated into conjunctiva, causing a purulent conjunctivitis with pain, edema, congestion. Small yellow nodules occur on conjunctivae and ulcerate.

### General Findings
Fever to 41°C.

**Regional Lymph Nodes** As the ulcer develops, nodes enlarge and become tender (chancriform syndrome) (Fig. 22-47). If untreated, become suppurating buboes. Lung consolidation, splenomegaly, generalized lymphadenopathy, hepatomegaly may occur.

**Variants** "Typhoidal" form occurs with ingestion of *F. tularensis*, resulting in ulcerative or exudative pharyngotonsillitis with cervical lymphadenopathy. Tularemic pneumonia occurs after bacteremia or inhalation of *F. tularensis*.

## DIFFERENTIAL DIAGNOSIS

**Inoculation Site** Furuncle, paronychia, ecthyma, anthrax, *Pasteurella multocida* infection, sporotrichosis, *Mycobacterium marinum* infection.

**Tender Regional Adenopathy** Herpes simplex virus lymphadenitis, plague, cat-scratch disease, melioidosis or glanders, lymphogranuloma venereum.

## LABORATORY EXAMINATIONS

**Cultures** Routine culture media do not support the growth of *F. tularensis* from clinical specimens.

**Serology** Diagnosis usually confirmed by demonstrating a fourfold rise in acute and convalescent *F. tularensis* antibody titers.

## DIAGNOSIS

Clinical diagnosis in a patient with chancriform syndrome with appropriate animal exposure or insect exposure and systemic manifestations. Disease in pneumonic presentation has "flulike" symptomatology and is fatal if unrecognized.

## COURSE AND PROGNOSIS

Untreated, mortality rate for ulceroglandular form is 5%; for typhoidal and pulmonary forms, 30%.

## MANAGEMENT

**Prevention** Avoid contact with wild rabbits. In tick-infested areas, wear tight wristbands and pants tucked into boots to prevent tick attachment. Inspect for ticks at day's end. Vaccine in development. Wear rubber gloves when handling or processing wild rabbits.

**Drug of Choice** Streptomycin, 1 to 2 g/d for 7 to 10 afebrile days, is most effective at cure and prevention of relapse.

**Alternatives** Gentamycin, tetracycline, chloramphenicol effect lower cure rate and higher relapse rates.

## CUTANEOUS *PSEUDOMONAS AERUGINOSA* INFECTIONS     ▣ ◑

*P. aeruginosa* is ubiquitous in our environment and is an opportunistic pathogen in compromised tissues. Hospitalized compromised individuals become colonized with the organism. Local invasion can follow colonization of any mucocutaneous site with local wound infection, soft tissue infection, and subsequent hematogenous dissemination. Ecthyma gangrenosum (EG) is the necrotizing soft tissue infection that occurs after local tissue invasion or bacteremic seeding, associated with blood vessel invasion, septic vasculitis, vascular occlusion, and infarction of tissue.

## EPIDEMIOLOGY AND ETIOLOGY

**Etiology**  *P. aeruginosa* is a small, aerobic gram-negative bacillus; motile by a single polar flagellum. Half of all clinical isolates produce blue-green pigments pyocyanin and pyoverdin. *P. pseudomallei* causes melioidosis, a tropical disease of humans and mammals with significant morbidity.

**Ecology**  *P. aeruginosa* is widespread in nature, inhabiting water, soil, plants, and animals, preferring moist environments. Carriage rate is low in healthy individuals. Colonizes skin, external ear, upper respiratory tract, and/or large bowel in those who are naturally or iatrogenically compromised, have received antimicrobial therapy, and/or been exposed to a hospital environment.

**Transmission**  Most infections are hospital acquired. Pseudomonal carriage increases with length of hospital stay and antibiotic administration. Transmitted to patients via hands of hospital personnel or via fomites. Entry sites for bacteremia at breaks in mucocutaneous barriers: sites of trauma, foreign bodies (IV or urinary catheter), aspiration/aerosolization into respiratory tract, decubitus or skin ulcers, thermal burns.

**Risk Factors for Invasive Infection**  *P. aeruginosa* is primarily a nosocomial pathogen—the fourth most commonly isolated—accounting for 10% of all hospital-acquired infections. Risk factors include hospitalization; immunocompromise; granulocytopenia; use of cancer chemotherapy, glucocorticoids, recent antibiotic therapy; catheters (IV, urethral); cancer; debilitation; mucosal ulceration; cystic fibrosis.

## PATHOGENESIS

Most infections are both invasive and toxigenic. Infection occurs in three stages: (1) bacterial attachment and colonization, (2) local invasion and damage of tissue, and (3) disseminated systemic disease. Infection may stop at any stage.

*P. aeruginosa* rarely causes disease in the healthy host. Infections occur when (1) normal cutaneous or mucosal barriers have been breached or bypassed (e.g., burn injury, penetrating trauma, surgery, endotracheal intubation, urinary bladder catheterization, IV drug abuse); (2) when immunologic defense mechanisms have been compromised (e.g., by chemotherapy-induced neutropenia, hypogammaglobulinemia, extremes of age, diabetes mellitus, cystic fibrosis, cancer, HIV disease); (3) when protective function of normal bacterial flora has been disrupted by broad-spectrum antimicrobial therapy; or (4) when a patient has been exposed to reservoirs associated with hospital environment.

Blood vessel and bloodstream invasion, dissemination, systemic inflammatory-response syndrome (SIRS) (sepsis syndrome), multiorgan dysfunction, and, ultimately, death may follow localized infection. The organism and/or its products may cause tissue injury at primary and secondary sites of infection; release of systemically acting toxins or inflammatory mediators of infected host may contribute directly or indirectly to SIRS.

## CLINICAL SYNDROMES

**Nail Colonization**  *P. aeruginosa* grows within a biofilm on the undersurface of onycholytic nails, e.g., psoriasis, onychomycosis; the under surface of the nail plate has a surface green discoloration that can easily be abraded (see Section 30, Fig. 30-4).

**Folliculitis**  *P. aeruginosa* can infect multiple hair follicles in healthy individuals after aqueous exposure in hot tubs ("hot-tub folliculitis," see Fig. 29-23) or physiotherapy pools, presenting as multiple follicular pustules on the trunk (see Section 29). The infection is self-limited.

**Toe Webspace Infection**   Intertrigo of toe webspaces. Webspace(s) macerated, moist with green color (see Section 23); usually in setting of hyperhidrosis, ± macerated interdigital tinea pedis, ± erythrasma, ± keratoderma.

**Primary and Secondary Pyoderma**   *P. aeruginosa* can cause primary infection of hair follicles or small breaks in skin, or secondary infections of sites of trauma, burn injury, inflammatory dermatoses, ulcers. With deeper invasion, necrotizing infection (due to blood vessel invasion and occlusion) occur, i.e., EG. These pyodermas have a typical blue-green exudate and characteristic fruity odor. In thermal burn injury, black, dark brown, or violaceous discoloration of burn eschar may occur.

**External Otitis**   "Swimmer's ear." Moist environment of external auditory canal provides medium for superficial infection, presenting as pruritus, pain, discharge; usually self-limited. Malignant external otitis occurs in elderly diabetics most commonly; may progress to deeper invasive infection.

## INVASIVE INFECTIONS

**Ecthyma Gangrenosum**   Begins as an erythematous macule (cutaneous ischemic lesion that quickly evolves to an infarction) (see Fig. 22-25*A*, *B*). The epidermis overlying the ischemic area may slough with formation of erosion/ulcer. EG usually occurs as a solitary lesion but may occur as a few lesions. EG can occur as a complication of primary or secondary pyoderma or of bacteremia. Initially erythematous, progressing to hemorrhagic bluish (so-called gunmetal gray). Fully evolved EG: blackish central necrosis with erythematous halo. Lesions usually tender, but may be painless. Most common sites: axillae, groin, perianal; may occur anywhere, including lip and tongue.

*Differential Diagnosis*   Other conditions that produce skin lesions by direct involvement of blood vessels such as vasculitis, cryoglobulinemia, fixed drug eruption, pyoderma gangrenosum.

*Cultures*   In most cases, *P. aeruginosa* can be cultured from both blood and ecthymatous skin lesions. However, EG can remain a localized cutaneous infection, not accompanied by systemic infection; in this case, only culture of exudate or biopsy specimen from the lesion is positive for *P. aeruginosa*.

*Dermatopathology*   Vasculitis without thrombosis; paucity of neutrophils at site of infection; bacilli found in media and adventitia but usually not in intima, of vessel.

*Diagnosis*   Clinical suspicion confirmed by blood and skin exudate/biopsy specimen culture.

*Course and Prognosis*   The heterogeneity of infections accounts for substantial differences in short-term and long-term prognosis. Prognosis depends on prompt restoration of altered immunity, usually on correction of neutropenia. When occurring as a local infection in the absence of bacteremia, prognosis is much more favorable.

**Bacteremia, General**   May be associated with SIRS; fever, tachypnea, tachycardia, prostration, hypotension. Predisposing conditions: hematologic malignancies, HIV disease, neutropenia, diabetes, severe burns. Common primary sites of infection: skin, soft tissues, urinary tract, GI tract, lungs, intravascular foci. EG develops in small minority of patients. Also, multiple subcutaneous nodules can occur following bacteremia.

**Endocarditis**   Left-sided infections present with embolic phenomena: large emboli, ecthyma gangrenosum, Osler's nodes (see Figs. 22-38 and 22-40).

**Gastrointestinal Infection**   "Rose" spotlike lesions: erythematous macules and/or papules on trunk as in typhoid fever; occur with *Pseudomonas* infection of GI tract, i.e., diarrhea, headache, high fever (Shanghai fever).

## MANAGEMENT OF INVASIVE INFECTIONS

**Correct Predisposing Factors**   White cell transfusion or granulocyte colony-stimulating factor for granulocytopenia.

**Antimicrobial Therapy**   Antibiotic and dosage are adjusted according to sensitivities and results of cultures.

**Surgery**   After control of infection, areas of infarction should be debrided.

# MYCOBACTERIAL INFECTIONS

Mycobacteria are rod-shaped or coccobacilli identified by the property of acid-fastness, a characteristic associated with the composition of their cell walls. Mycobacterial infections are classified as *tuberculosis, leprosy* (Hansen's disease), and *infections due to nontuberculous mycobacteria* (NTM). They cause infections in select populations globally.

*M. tuberculosis* complex, (consisting of *M. tuberculosis, M. bovis,* and *M. africanum*) are pathogenic in otherwise healthy individuals; however, tuberculosis is much more florid in immunocompromised hosts. *M. leprae* causes disease in humans exclusively. Otherwise healthy individuals become infected with this mycobacterium; clinical manifestations vary tremendously according to the host's immune response to the organism. NTM exist in the environment; identification in human tissue, unlike *M. tuberculosis* or *M. leprae,* is not a sine qua non of etiology of a disorder.

## EPIDEMIOLOGY

With the advent of HIV disease, tuberculosis and NTM infections have been brought to the forefront of clinical medicine. Concurrent HIV and *M. tuberculosis* infections can result in severe infections; disseminated infections with NTM are extremely common in advanced HIV disease.

---

## LEPROSY

Leprosy is a chronic granulomatous disease caused by *M. leprae,* principally acquired during childhood/young adulthood. Skin, peripheral nervous system, upper respiratory tract, eyes, and testes are the major sites of involvement. Clinical manifestations, natural history, and prognosis of leprosy are related to the host response, and the various types of leprosy (tuberculoid, lepromatous, etc.) represent the spectra of the host's immunologic response (cell-mediated immunity).

*Synonym*: Hansen's disease.

## CLINICOPATHOLOGIC CLASSIFICATION OF LEPROSY

(Based on clinical, immunologic, and bacteriologic findings)

**Tuberculoid (TL)**   Localized skin involvement and/or peripheral nerve involvement; few organisms are present in the skin biopsies.

**Lepromatous (LL)**   Generalized involvement including skin, upper respiratory mucous membrane, the reticuloendothelial system, adrenal glands, and testes; many bacilli are present in tissue.

**Borderline (or "Dimorphic") (BL)**   Has features of both tuberculoid and lepromatous leprosy. Usually many bacilli present, varied skin lesions: macules, plaques; progresses to TL or regresses to LL.

**Indeterminate and Transitional Forms**   (See "Pathogenesis," below)

## EPIDEMIOLOGY AND ETIOLOGY

**Age of Onset**   Incidence rate peaks at 10 to 20 years; prevalence peaks at 30 to 50 years.

**Sex**   Males > females.

**Race**   There appears to be an inverse relationship between the skin color and the severity of the disease; in the black African, susceptibility is high, but there is predominance of milder forms of the disease, i.e., TL vis-à-vis LL.

**Etiology** *M. leprae* is an obligate intracellular acid-fast bacillus; reproduces maximally at 27°C to 30°C. The organism cannot be cultured in vitro. Infects skin and cutaneous nerves (Schwann cell basal lamina). In untreated patients, only 1% of organisms are viable. Grows best in cooler tissues (skin, peripheral nerves, anterior chamber of eye, upper respiratory tract, and testes), sparing warmer areas of the skin (axilla, groin, scalp, and midline of back).

**Hosts** Humans are the main reservoirs of *M. leprae*. Wild armadillos (Louisiana) as well as mangabey monkeys and chimpanzees are naturally infected with *M. leprae*; armadillos can develop lepromatous lesions.

**Transmission** Mode of transmission is uncertain; possible transmission includes nasal droplet infection, contact with infected soil, insect vectors. The sneeze from an untreated LL patient may contain $10^{10}$ organisms. 20% of asymptomatic individuals in endemic areas may have *M. leprae* in the nose, identified by PCR. Portals of entry of *M. leprae* are poorly understood but include inoculation via skin (bites, scratches, small wounds, tattoos) or inhalation into nasal passages or lungs.

**Demography** Disease of developing world: 600,000 new cases annually; 1.5 to 8 million total cases worldwide. >80% of cases occur in India, China, Myanmar, Indonesia, Brazil, Nigeria. In the United States: 4000 cases, 100 to 200 new cases annually; most cases are in immigrants from Mexico, Southeast Asia, Philippines, Caribbean and in California, Texas, New York, and Hawaii. Associated with poverty, rural residence, and HIV disease. Most individuals have natural immunity and do not develop disease.

**Predisposing or Risk Factors** (1) Residence in an endemic area, (2) having a blood relative with leprosy, (3) poverty (malnutrition?), and (4) contact with affected armadillos.

## PATHOGENESIS

The clinical spectrum of leprosy depends exclusively on variable limitations in the host's capability to develop effective cell-mediated immunity (CMI) to *M. leprae*. The organism is capable of invading and multiplying in peripheral nerves and infecting and surviving in endothelial and phagocytic cells in many organs. Subclinical infection with leprosy is common among residents in endemic areas. Presumably the subclinical infection is handled readily by the host's CMI response. Clinical expression of leprosy is the development of a granuloma; and the patient may develop a "reactional state," which may occur in some form in >50% of certain groups of patients. The granulomatous spectrum of leprosy consists of (1) a high-resistance tuberculoid response (TT), (2) a low- or absent-resistance lepromatous pole (LL), (3) a dimorphic or borderline region (BB) and two intermediary regions: (4) borderline lepromatous (BL), and (5) borderline tuberculoid (BT). In order of decreasing resistance, the spectrum is TT, BT, BB, BL, LL.

**Immunologic Responses** Immune responses to *M. leprae* can produce several types of reactions associated with a sudden change in the clinical status.

*Lepra Type 1 Reactions (Downgrading and Reversal Reactions)* Individuals with BT and BL develop inflammation within existing skin lesions. Downgrading reactions occur before therapy; reversal reactions occur in response to therapy. Type 1 reactions can be associated with low-grade fever, new multiple small "satellite" maculopapular skin lesions, and/or neuritis.

*Lepra Type 2 Reactions (Erythema Nodosum Leprosum, ENL)* Seen in half of LL patients, usually occurring after initiation of antilepromatous therapy, generally within the first 2 years of treatment. Massive inflammation with erythema nodosum–like lesions.

*Lucio's Reaction* Individuals with diffuse LL develop shallow, large polygonal sloughing ulcerations on the legs. The reaction appears to be either a variant of ENL or secondary to arteriolar occlusion. The ulcers heal poorly, recur frequently, and may occur in a generalized distribution. Generalized Lucio's reaction is frequently complicated by secondary bacterial infection and sepsis.

## HISTORY

**Incubation Period** 2 to 40 years (most commonly 5 to 7 years).

**Onset** Insidious and painless; first affects the peripheral nervous system with persistent or recurrent painful paresthesias and numbness without any visible clinical signs. At this stage there may be transient macular skin eruptions; blister, but lack of awareness of trauma.

**Systems Review** Neural involvement leads to muscle weakness, muscle atrophy, severe neuritic pain, and contractures of the hands and feet.

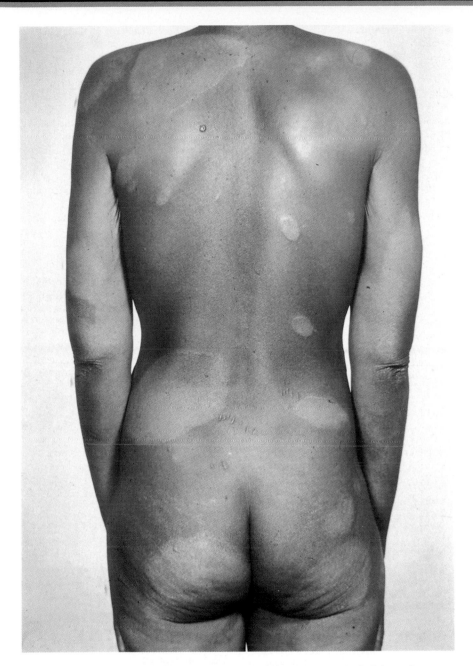

**FIGURE 22-49   Leprosy: tuberculoid type**   *Well-defined, hypopigmented, slightly scaling, anesthetic macules and plaques on the posterior trunk.*

*Lepra Type 1 Reactions* Acute or insidious tenderness and pain along affected nerve(s), associated with loss of function.

## PHYSICAL EXAMINATION

### Tuberculoid Leprosy (TT, BT)
*Skin* Most common form in India, Africa. Few well-defined hypopigmented hypesthetic macules (Fig. 22-49) with raised edges and varying in size from a few millimeters to very large lesions covering the entire trunk. Erythematous or purple border and hypopigmented center. Sharply defined, raised; often annular; enlarge peripherally. Central area becomes atrophic/depressed. Advanced lesions are anesthetic, devoid of skin appendages (sweat glands, hair follicles). Any site including the face. *TT*: Lesions may resolved spontaneously; not associated with lepra reactions. *BT*: Does not heal spontaneously; type 1 lepra reactions may occur.
*Nerve Involvement* May be a thickened nerve on the edge of the lesion; large peripheral nerve enlargement frequent (ulnar). Skin involvement is absent in *neural leprosy*. Test pinprick, temperature, vibration.

### Borderline BB Leprosy
*Skin* Lesions are intermediate between tuberculoid and lepromatous and are composed of macules, papules, and plaques (Figs. 22-50 and 22-51). Anesthesia and decreased sweating are prominent in the lesions.

### Lepromatous Leprosy (LL, BL)
*Skin* Skin-colored or slightly erythematous papules/nodules (Fig. 22-52). Lesions enlarge; new lesions occur and coalesce. Later: symmetrically distributed nodules, raised plaques, diffuse dermal infiltrate, which on face results in loss of hair (lateral eyebrows and eyelashes) and leonine facies (lion's face). *Diffuse lepromatosis*, occurring in western Mexico, Caribbean, presents as diffuse dermal infiltration and thickened dermis.
*Distribution of Lesions* Bilaterally symmetric involving earlobes, face, arms, and buttocks, or less frequently the trunk and lower extremities. Tongue: nodules, plaques, or fissures.
*Nerve Involvement* More extensive than in TT.

### Reactional States
Immunologically mediated inflammatory states, occurring spontaneously or after initiation of therapy.

*Lepra Type 1 Reactions* Downgrading and reversal reactions. Occur in borderline disease. Skin lesions become acutely inflamed, associated with edema and pain; may ulcerate: Edema most severe on face, hands, and feet.
*Lepra Type 2 Reactions (ENL)* Occur in near LL. 90% of cases occur after initiation of therapy. Present as painful red skin nodules arising superficially and deeply, in contrast to true erythema nodosum; lesions form abscesses or ulcerate. Lesions occur most commonly on face and extensor limbs.
*Lucio's Reaction* Occurs only in patients from Mexico/Caribbean with diffuse LL. Presents as irregularly shaped erythematous plaques; lesions may resolve spontaneously or undergo necrosis with ulceration.

### General Findings
*Extremities* Sensory neuropathy, plantar ulcers, secondary infection; ulnar and peroneal palsies, Charcot joints.
*Nose* Chronic nasal congestion, epistaxis; destruction of cartilage with saddle-nose deformity.
*Eyes* Cranial nerve palsies, lagophthalmus, corneal insensitivity. In LL, anterior chamber can be invaded with uveitis, glaucoma, cataract formation. Corneal damage can occur secondary to trichiasis and sensory neuropathy, secondary infection, and muscle paralysis.
*Testes* May be involved in LL with resultant hypogonadism.
*Amyloidosis* Secondary with hepatic/renal abnormalities.

## DIFFERENTIAL DIAGNOSIS

**Hypopigmented Lesions with Granulomas**   Sarcoidosis, leishmaniasis, lupus vulgaris, NTM infection, lymphoma, syphilis, yaws, granuloma annulare, necrobiosis lipoidica.

## LABORATORY EXAMINATIONS

**Slit-Skin Smears** A small skin incision is made; the site is then scraped to obtain tissue fluid from which a smear is made and examined after Ziehl-Neelsen staining. Specimens are usually obtained from both earlobes and two other active lesions. The bacterial index (BI) is computed as shown in Table 22-10. Negative BIs are seen in paucibacillary cases, treated cases, and cases examined by an inexperienced technician.

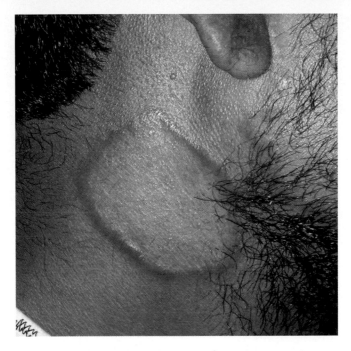

**FIGURE 22-50   Leprosy: borderline-type**   *Annular tan-pink plaque on the neck with similar lesion on the adjacent cheek. Peripheral sensory nerves were palpable on the neck. (Courtesy of Atul Taneja, MD.)*

**Nasal Smears or Scrapings**   No longer recommended.

**Culture**   *M. leprae* has not been cultured in vitro; however, it does grow when inoculated into the mouse foot pad. Routine bacterial cultures to rule out secondary infection.

**PCR**   *M. leprae* DNA detected by this technique makes the diagnosis of early paucibacillary leprosy and identifies *M. leprae* after therapy.

**Dermatopathology**   TL shows epithelioid cell granulomas forming around dermal nerves; acid-fast bacilli are sparse or absent. LL shows an extensive cellular infiltrate separated from the epidermis by a narrow zone of normal collagen. Skin appendages are destroyed. Macrophages are filled with *M. leprae*, having abundant foamy or vacuolated cytoplasm (lepra cells or Virchow cells).

## DIAGNOSIS

Made if one or more of the cardinal findings are detected: patient from endemic area, skin lesions characteristic of leprosy with diminished or loss of sensation, enlarged peripheral nerves, finding of *M. leprae* in skin or, less commonly, other sites.

## COURSE AND PROGNOSIS

After the first few years of drug therapy, the most difficult problem is management of the changes secondary to neurologic deficits—contractures and trophic changes in the hands and feet. This requires a team of health care professionals: orthopedic surgeons, hand surgeons, podiatrists, ophthalmologists, neurologists, physical medicine and rehabilitation professionals. Uncommonly, secondary amyloidosis with renal failure can complicate long-standing leprosy. Lepra type 1 reactions last 2 to 4 months in individuals with BT and up to 9 months in those with BL. Lepra type 2 reactions (ENL) occur in 50% of individuals with LL and 25% of those with BL within the first 2 years of treatment. ENL may be complicated by uveitis, dactylitis,

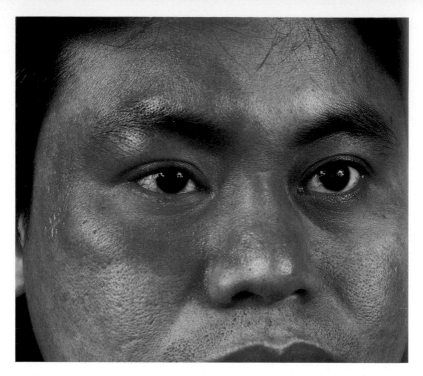

**FIGURE 22-51   Leprosy: borderline-type**  *Well-demarcated, infiltrated, erythematous plaque on the periorbital region. The initial diagnosis was erysipelas, which did not respond to antibiotic treatment.*

arthritis, neuritis, lymphadenitis, myositis, orchitis. Lucio's reaction or phenomenon occurs secondary to vasculitis with subsequent infarction.

## MANAGEMENT

General principles of management:

- Eradicate infection with antilepromatous therapy (Table 22-11).
- Prevent and treat reactions.
- Reduce the risk of nerve damage.
- Educate patient to deal with neuropathy and anesthesia.
- Treat complications of nerve damage.
- Rehabilitate patient into society.

Management involves a broad multidisciplinary approach including orthopedic surgery, ophthalmology, and physical therapy.

### Therapy of Reactions

***Lepra Type 1 Reactions*** *Prednisone*, 40 to 60 mg/d; the dosage is gradually reduced over a 2- to 3-month period. Indications for prednisone: neuritis, lesions that threaten to ulcerate, lesions appearing at cosmetically important sites (face).

***Lepra Type 2 Reactions (ENL)*** *Prednisone*, 40 to 60 mg/d, tapered fairly rapidly; *thalidomide* for recurrent ENL, 100 to 300 mg/d.

***Lucio's Reaction***  Neither prednisone nor thalidomide is very effective, *Prednisone*, 40 to 60 mg/d, tapered fairly rapidly.

**Systemic Antimicrobial Agents**  Secondary infection of ulcerations should be identified and treated with appropriate antibiotics to prevent deeper infections such as osteomyelitis.

**Orthopedic Care**  Splints should be supplied to prevent contractures of denervated regions. Careful attention to foot care to prevent neuropathic ulceration.

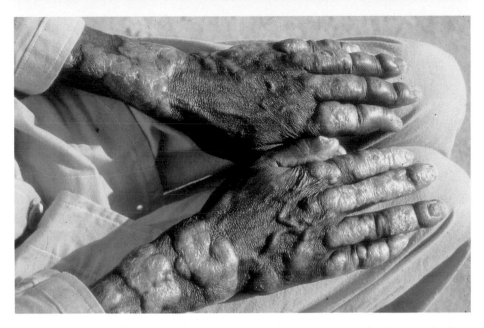

**FIGURE 22-52 Leprosy: lepromatous type** *Nodules and thick plaques on the dorsa on the fingers, wrists, and forearms, with hypopigmentation of the overlying skin. Note the symmetry of involvement and loss of tissue of several fingertips.*

**TABLE 22-10 Bacterial Index (BI)—Ridley's Logarithmic Scale**

| | |
|---|---|
| 0 | No bacteria in 100 fields (oil immersion) |
| 1+ | 1–10 bacteria in 100 fields |
| 2+ | 1–10 bacteria in 10 fields |
| 3+ | 1–10 bacteria in an average field |
| 4+ | 10–100 bacteria in an average field |
| 5+ | 100–1000 bacteria in an average field |
| 6+ | Many clumps of bacteria (>1000) in an average field |

**TABLE 22-11 Antimicrobial Regimens Recommended for Treatment of Leprosy in Adults**

| Form of Leprosy | More Intensive Regimen | WHO-Recommended Regimen (1982) |
|---|---|---|
| Tuberculoid (paucibacillary) | Dapsone (100 mg/d) for 5 years | Dapsone (100 mg/d, unsupervised) *plus* rifampin (600 mg/month supervised) for 6 months |
| Lepromatous (multiibacillary) | Rifampin (600 mg/month) for 3 years *plus* dapsone (100 mg/d) indefinitely | Dapsone (100 mg/d) *plus* clofazimine (50 mg/d, unsupervised); and rifampin (600 mg) *plus* clofazimine (300 mg) monthly (supervised) for 1 year |

## CUTANEOUS TUBERCULOSIS　　□　◑

Cutaneous tuberculosis (CTb) is highly variable in its clinical presentation, depending on the immunologic status of the patient and the route of inoculation of mycobacteria into the skin. In most cases, the organism reaches the skin via lymphatic or hematogenous spread; inoculation cutaneous tuberculosis does occur.
*Synonyms of tuberculosis*: Phthisis, consumption.

## CLASSIFICATION OF CUTANEOUS TUBERCULOSIS

### Exogenous Infection

- Primary inoculation tuberculosis (PIT): via percutaneous inoculation, occurs at inoculated site in nonimmune host.
- Tuberculosis verrucosa cutis (TVC): via percutaneous inoculation, occurs at inoculated site in individual with prior tuberculosis infection.

### Endogenous Spread

- Lupus vulgaris (LV)
- Scrofuloderma (SD)
- Metastatic tuberculosis abscess (MTA)
- Acute miliary tuberculosis (AMT)
- Orificial tuberculosis (OT)

### Tuberculosis due to BCG Immunization

## EPIDEMIOLOGY AND ETIOLOGY

Predisposing factors for tuberculosis include poverty, crowding, HIV infection. The type of clinical lesion depends on the route of cutaneous inoculation and the immunologic status of the host. Cutaneous inoculation results in a tuberculous chancre in the nonimmune host but TVC in the immune host. Modes of endogenous spread to skin include the following: direct extension from underlying tuberculous infection, i.e., lymphadenitis or tuberculosis of bones and joints, results in SD; lymphatic spread to skin, results in LV; hematogenous dissemination, results in AMT, LV, or MTA.

**Age of Onset**　AMT more common in infants and adults with advanced immunodeficiency. PIT more common in infants. SD more common in adolescents, elderly. LV affects all ages.

**Sex**　LV more common in females. TVC more common in males.

**Race**　Tuberculosis in blacks; in general, less favorable prognosis than in whites.

**Occupation**　TVC: previously in physicians, medical students, and pathologists as verruca necrogenica, anatomist's wart, postmortem wart; in butchers and farmers from *Mycobacterium bovis*.

**Etiology**　The obligate human pathogenic mycobacteria: *M. tuberculosis*, *M. bovis*, and occasionally, bacillus Calmette-Guérin (BCG).

**Incidence**　CTb has declined steadily worldwide, paralleling the decline of pulmonary tuberculosis. Always rare in the United States compared with Europe. Incidence of various types of CTb varies geographically; LV, SD most common types in Europe; LV, verrucous lesions more common in tropics; TVC a common type in Third World countries. Recently, the incidence of CTb has been increasing, often associated with HIV disease.

**Route of Cutaneous Infection**　May be exogenous, by autoinoculation, or endogenous.

**Tuberculosis in HIV Disease**　Tuberculosis is the most common opportunistic infection occurring in HIV-infected individuals who reside in developing nations; CTb has been reported in these individuals. The problem of multidrug resistance is also common in these persons.

## PATHOGENESIS

The clinical lesions occurring in the skin depend on whether the host has had prior infection with *M. tuberculosis*, and therefore delayed hypersensitivity to the organism, and the inoculation route and mode of spread.

## PHYSICAL EXAMINATION

**Primary Inoculation Tuberculosis**　Initially, papule occurs at the inoculation site 2 to 4 weeks after the wound. Lesion enlarges to a painless ulcer, i.e., a tuberculous chancre (up to 5 cm) (Fig. 22-53), with shallow granular base and multiple tiny abscesses or may be covered

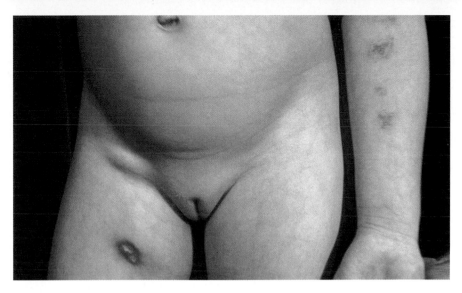

**FIGURE 22-53    Primary inoculation tuberculosis**    *A large, ulcerated nodule at the site of* Mycobacterium. tuberculosis *inoculation on the right thigh associated with inguinal lymphadenopathy. The erythematous papules on the left forearm occurred at the site of tuberculin testing.*

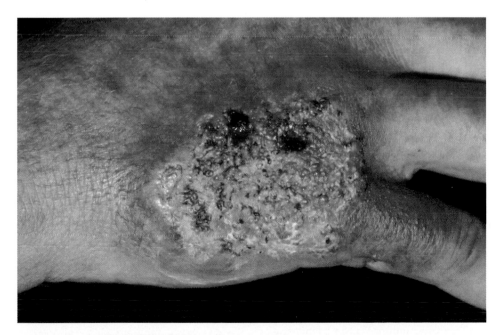

**FIGURE 22-54    Tuberculosis verrucosa cutis**    *Crusted and hyperkeratotic plaque arising at the site of inoculation in an individual previously infected with* M. tuberculosis. *There is no associated lymphadenopathy.*

by thick crust. Undermined margins; older ulcers become indurated with thick crusts. Deeper inoculation results in subcutaneous abscess. Most common on exposed skin at sites of minor injuries. Oral lesions occur after ingestion of bovine bacilli in nonpasteurized milk; in the past, lesions in male babies have occurred on the penis after ritual circumcision. Intraoral inoculation results in ulcers on gingiva or palate. Regional lymphadenopathy occurs within 3 to 8 weeks.

**Tuberculosis Verrucosa Cutis**  Initial papule with violaceous halo. Evolves to hyperkeratotic, warty, firm plaque (Fig. 22-54). Clefts and fissures occur from which pus and keratinous material can be expressed. Border often irregular. Lesions are usually single, but multiple lesions occur. Most commonly on dorsolateral hands and fingers. In children, lower extremities, knees. No lymphadenopathy.

**Lupus Vulgaris**  Initial flat papule is ill defined and soft and evolves into well-defined, irregular plaque (Fig. 22-55). Reddish-brown: diascopy (i.e., the use of a glass slide pressed against the skin) reveals an "apple jelly" (i.e., yellowish-brown) color. The consistency is characteristically soft; if the lesion is probed, the instrument breaks through the overlying epidermis. Surface is initially smooth or slightly scaly but may become hyperkeratotic. Hypertrophic forms result in soft tumorous nodules. Ulcerative forms present as punched-out, often serpiginous ulcers surrounded by soft, brownish infiltrate. Usually solitary, but several sites may occur. Most lesions on the head and neck, most often on nose and ears or scalp. Lesions on trunk and extremities rare. Disseminated lesions after severe viral infection (measles) (*lupus postexanthematicus*). Involvement of underlying cartilage but not bone results in its destruction (ears, nose). Scarring is prominent, and, characteristically, new brownish infiltrates occur within the atrophic scars.

**Scrofuloderma**  Firm subcutaneous nodule that initially is freely movable; the lesion then becomes doughy and evolves into an irregular, deep-seated node or plaque that liquefies and perforates (Fig. 22-56). Ulcers and irregular sinuses, usually of linear or serpiginous shape, discharge pus or caseous material (Fig. 22-57). Edges are undermined, inverted, and dissecting subcutaneous pockets alternating with soft, fluctuating infiltrates and bridging scars. Most often occurs in the parotidal, submandibular, and supraclavicular regions; lateral neck; SD most often results from

continuous spread from affected lymph nodes or tuberculous bones (phalanges, sternum, ribs) or joints.

**Metastatic Tuberculosis Abscess**  Also called *tuberculous gumma*. Subcutaneous abscess, nontender, "cold," fluctuant. Coalescing with overlying skin, breaking down and forming fistulas and ulcers. Single or multiple lesions, often at sites of previous trauma.

**Acute Miliary Tuberculosis**  Exanthem. Disseminated lesions are minute macules and papules or purpuric lesions. Sometimes vesicular and crusted. Removal of crust reveals umbilication. Disseminated on all parts of the body, particularly the trunk.

**Orificial Tuberculosis**  Small yellowish nodule on mucosa breaks down to form painful circular or irregular ulcer (Fig. 22-58) with undermined borders and pseudomembranous material, yellowish tubercles, and eroded vessels at its base. Surrounding mucosa swollen, edematous, and inflamed. Since OT results from autoinoculation of mycobacteria from progressive tuberculosis of internal organs, it is usually found on the oral, pharyngeal (pulmonary tuberculosis), vulvar (genitourinary tuberculosis), and anal (intestinal tuberculosis) mucous membranes. Lesions may be single or multiple, and in the mouth most often occur on the tongue, soft and hard palate, or lips. OT may occur in a tooth socket after tooth extraction.

## DIFFERENTIAL DIAGNOSIS

**Primary Inoculation Tuberculosis**  Chancriform syndrome: primary syphilis with chancre, catscratch disease, sporotrichosis, tularemia, *M. marinum* infection.

**Tuberculosis Verrucosa Cutis**  Verruca vulgaris, *M. marinum* infection, pyoderma, blastomycosis, chromomycosis, bromoderma, hypertrophic lichen planus, squamous cell carcinoma (SCC).

**Lupus Vulgaris**  Sarcoidosis, lymphocytoma, lymphoma, chronic cutaneous lupus erythematosus, tertiary syphilis, leprosy, blastomycosis, lupoid leishmaniasis, pyodermas.

**Scrofuloderma**  Invasive fungal infections, sporotrichosis, nocardiosis, actinomycosis, tertiary syphilis, acne conglobata, hidradenitis suppurativa.

**Metastatic Tuberculosis Abscess**  Panniculitis, invasive fungal infections, hidradenitis, tertiary syphilis.

**Orificial Tuberculosis**  Aphthous ulcers, histoplasmosis, syphilis, SCC.

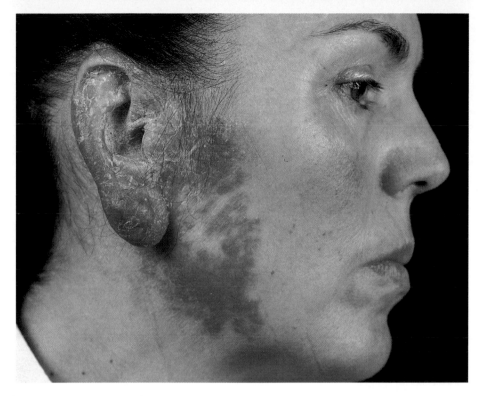

**FIGURE 22-55   Lupus vulgaris**   *Reddish-brown plaque, which on diascopy exhibits the diagnostic yellow-brown apple-jelly color. Note nodular infiltration of the earlobe, scaling of the helix, and atrophic scarring in the center of the plaque.*

## LABORATORY EXAMINATIONS

**Dermatopathology**   PIT: initially nonspecific inflammation; after 3 to 6 weeks, epithelioid cells, Langhans' giant cells, lymphocytes, caseation necrosis. AMT: nonspecific inflammation and vasculitis. All other forms of CTb show more or less typical tuberculous histopathology; TVC is characterized by massive pseudoepitheliomatous hyperplasia of epidermis and abscesses. Mycobacteria are found in PIT, SD, AMT, MTA, and OT but only with difficulty or not at all in LV and TVC.

**Culture**   Yields mycobacteria also from lesions of LV and TVC.

**PCR**   Can be used to identify *M. tuberculosis* DNA in tissue specimens.

**Skin Testing**   PIT: Patient converts from intradermal skin test negative to positive during the first weeks of the infection. AMT: usually negative. SD, MTA, and OT: may be negative or positive depending on state of immunity. LV and TVC: positive.

## DIAGNOSIS

Clinical, histologic findings, confirmed by isolation of *M. tuberculosis* on culture or by PCR.

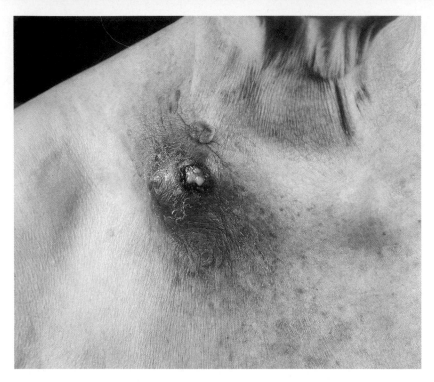

**FIGURE 22-56    Scrofuloderma: clavicle area**    *Large abscess near the clavicular head, which on pressure extrudes pus and caseous material. A tuberculous lymphadenitis undergoes necrosis with abscess formation, subsequently draining to the skin surface.*

## COURSE AND PROGNOSIS

The course of CTb is quite variable, depending on the type of cutaneous infection, amount of inoculum, extent of extracutaneous infection, age of the patient, immune status, and therapy. PIT: without treatment, usually resolves within 12 months, with some residual scarring. Rarely, LV develops at site of PIT. Tuberculosis due to BCG immunization: depends on general state of immunity. It may assume appearance and course of PIT, LV, or SD; in the immunocompromised it may lead to MTA or AMT.

## MANAGEMENT

Only PIT and TVC limited to the skin. All other patterns of CTb are associated with systemic infection that has disseminated secondarily to the skin. As such, therapy should be aimed at

achieving a cure, avoiding relapse, and preventing emergence of drug-resistant mutants.

**Antituberculous Therapy**    Prolonged antituberculous therapy with at least two drugs is indicated for all cases of CTb except for TVC that can be excised. Isoniazid (5 mg/kg daily) and rifampin (600 mg/g daily), supplemented with ethambutol (25 mg/kg daily), streptomycin (10-15 mg/kg daily), or pyrazinamide (15-30 mg/kg daily) in the initial phases. Isoniazid and rifampin for at least 9 months; can be shortened to 6 months if four drugs are given during the first 2 months.

**FIGURE 22-58 (Opposite page, bottom)    Orificial tuberculosis: lips**    *A large, very painful ulcer on the lips of this patient with advanced cavitary pulmonary tuberculosis.*

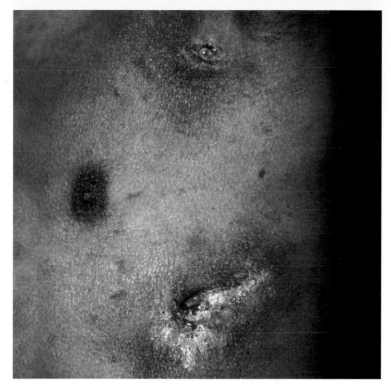

**FIGURE 22-57 Scrofuloderma: lateral chest wall.** *Two ulcers on the chest wall and axilla are associated with underlying sinus tracts.*

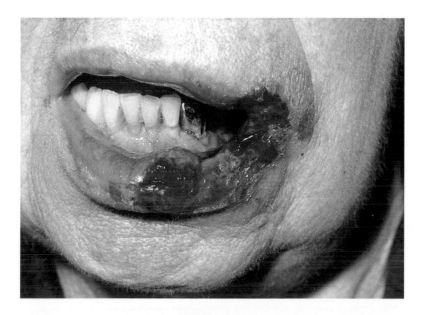

**FIGURE 22-58**

# CUTANEOUS NONTUBERCULOUS MYCOBACTERIAL INFECTIONS

Nontuberculous mycobacteria (NTM) (non-*M. tuberculosis*, non-*M. leprae*), e.g., *Mycobacterium marinum*, *M. ulcerans*, and *M. fortuitum* complex, occur naturally in the environment. They are capable of causing primary cutaneous infections at sites of inoculation in otherwise healthy individuals. These infections typically remain localized but can disseminate in the compromised host. Diagnosis has been made on detection of mycobacteria histochemically or by culture on specific media. New molecular techniques based on DNA amplification accelerate diagnosis, identify common sources of infection, and reveal new types of NTM, while new antibiotics, such as the macrolides, the rifamycins, and the fluoroquinolones, offer improved options for treatment and prevention.
*Synonyms*: Atypical mycobacteria, mycobacteria other than tuberculosis (MOTT)

## CLASSIFICATION OF NTM

The original classification of NTM depended on speed of growth, morphology, and pigmentation of colonies on solid media as well as biochemi-cal reactions. Currently, however, molecular probes are used for rapid identification of the most important species in a positive culture (Table 22-12); hybridization of the probe to specific sequences of the mycobacteria.

## *MYCOBACTERIUM MARINUM* INFECTION

*M. marinum* infection follows traumatic inoculation during fish tank exposure; it is characterized by inflammatory verrucous or crusted lesion(s) at the inoculation site and extension to lymphatics (sporotrichoid) and deeper tissues.
*Synonym*: Fish tank granuloma.

## EPIDEMIOLOGY AND ETIOLOGY

**Age of Onset**   Second to fourth decades.
**Sex**   Males > females.
**Etiology**   *M. marinum.*
**Exposure**   Tropical fish tanks; lesions usually on dominant hand. Chlorination has reduced transmission in swimming pools.

## HISTORY

**Incubation Period**   Variable: usually 1 week to 2 months after inoculation.
**Duration of Lesions**   Weeks to months.

**Symptoms**   Commonly asymptomatic. Possible local tenderness; limitation of movement if lesion over a joint; with deeper extension, pain.

## PHYSICAL EXAMINATION

### Skin Lesions
Inoculation site: papule(s) enlarging to inflammatory, red to red-brown nodule or plaque 1 to 4 cm in size on dominant hand. Surface of lesions may be hyperkeratotic/verrucous (Fig. 22-59). May become ulcerated: superficial crust, granulation tissue base, ±serosanguineous or purulent discharge. In some cases,

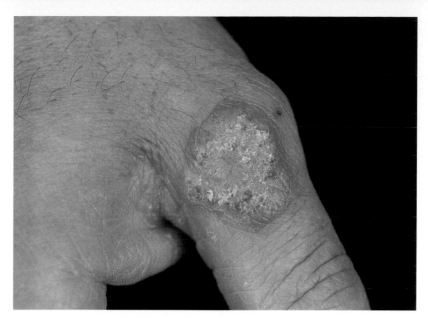

**FIGURE 22-59   *M. marinum* infection ("fish-tank" granuloma)**   *A red-violet, verrucous plaque on the dorsum of the thumb of a fish-tank hobbyist arose at the site of an abrasion.*

small satellite papules, draining sinuses, fistulas may develop. Usually solitary, over bony prominence. More extensive soft tissue infection may occur, with osteomyelitis, in the immunocompromised host. Atrophic scarring follows spontaneous regression or successful therapy.

***Sporotrichoid Pattern*** Deep-seated nodules in a linear configuration on hand and forearm exhibit sporotrichoid spread. Boggy inflammatory reaction may mimic bursitis, synovitis, or arthritis about the elbow, wrist, or interphalangeal joints.

***Disseminated Infection*** Rare. May occur in immunocompromised host.

**Lymph Nodes**   Regional lymphadenopathy uncommon.

## DIFFERENTIAL DIAGNOSIS

**Solitary Verrucous/Ulcerated Lesion on Extremity** Verruca vulgaris, sporotrichosis, blastomycosis, erysipeloid, tularemia, tuberculosis verrucosa cutis, nocardiosis, leishmaniasis, syphilis, yaws, iododerma, bromoderma, foreign-body response to sea urchin or barnacle, benign or malignant skin tumors.

**Sporotrichoid Lesion**   Staphylococcal or group A streptococcal lymphangitis, sporotrichosis, tularemia, leishmaniasis, nocardiosis, actinomycosis.

## LABORATORY EXAMINATIONS

**Skin Tests**   Intradermal tuberculin test (PPD-S) often positive.

**Skin Biopsy**   Suggestive but not pathognomonic. Older lesions: more typical tuberculoid architecture is developed with epithelioid cells and Langhans' giant cells. Acid-fast stain demonstrates *M. marinum* only in approximately 50% of cases.

**Direct Microscopy**   *Smears of exudate or pus:* Acid-fast bacilli can be demonstrated in some cases.

**Culture**   *M. marinum* grows at 32°C (but not at 37°C) in 2 to 4 weeks. Early lesions yield numerous colonies; lesions ≥3 months older generally yield few colonies.

## DIAGNOSIS

History of trauma in an aqueous environment, clinical findings, confirmed by isolation of *M. marinum* on culture.

**TABLE 22-12    The Most Important Nontuberculous Mycobacteria**

| Mycobacterial Species | Disseminated Infections | Localized Infections | |
|---|---|---|---|
| | | Lung | Lymphadenitis |
| M. abscessus | — | — | — |
| M. avium | Typical in AIDS with CD4 + count of <50/μL; rare in other immunodeficiencies | See M. intracellulare | In children (rare) |
| M. celatum | AIDS (rare) | Rare | — |
| M. chelonae | Rare | — | — |
| M. fortuitum | Rare | Rare | — |
| M. genavense | Typical in AIDS | — | Rare |
| M. gordonae | Rare | — | — |
| M. haemophilum | Typical in AIDS and other immunodeficiencies | — | — |
| M. intracellulare | See M. avium | Cavities in CF or COPD[†]; lingular infection in normal hosts | In children (rare) |
| M. kansasii | In AIDS (rare) | Typical, resembling tuberculosis | Rare |
| M. malmoense | Rare | Rare | — |
| M. marinum | Rare | — | — |
| M. scrofulaceum | Rare | Rare | Typical |
| M. simiae | In AIDS (rare) | Rare | — |
| M. szulgai | — | Rare | — |
| M. xenopi | Rare | Rare | — |

[*]Or azithromycin.
[†]CF, cystic fibrosis; COPD, chronic obstructive pulmonary disease.
[‡]Or minocycline.

SOURCE: Data are from J Clin Microbiol 31:1882, 1993 (335 strains) and the Mycobacteriology Laboratory of the University Hospital in Geneva (1993–1994, 313 strains, Dr. P. Rohner).

## COURSE AND PROGNOSIS

Most usually benign and self-limited but can remain active for a prolonged period. Single papulonodular lesions resolve spontaneously within 3 months to 3 years, whereas sporotrichoid form can persist for years. In the immunocompromised host, more extensive deep infection can occur.

**Localized Infections**

| Skin and Soft Tissue | Contaminant/ Commensal | Recommended Therapy | Percentage of Strains |
|---|---|---|---|
| Typical, linked to surgery | Typical | Debridement; clarithromycin, clofazimine, amikacin | <1 |
| In disseminated infection (rare) | Typical in sputum and feces | Clarithromycin,* ethambutol, rifabutin | 30–50 |
| — | — | See *M. avium* | <1 |
| Typical, linked to surgery | Typical | See *M. abscessus* | <1 |
| Typical | Typical | Amikacin, ciprofloxacin, sulfonamides, clofazimine, clarithromycin | 1 |
| — | — | See *M. avium* | 5 |
| Rare | Typical | — | 10–30 |
| Typical in AIDS | — | See *M. avium* | <1 |
| See *M. avium* | Possible in sputum | See *M. avium* | 4–8 |
| Rare | Possible in sputum | Rifampin, isoniazid, ethambutol, clarithromycin, sulfonamides | 2–4 |
| — | — | See *M. avium* | 1–4 |
| Typical | — | Trimethoprim-sulfamethoxazole‡ | 1 |
| — | — | See *M. avium* | 1 |
| — | Possible | See *M. avium* | 1 |
| Typical | — | Rifampin, isoniazid, ethambutol | <1 |
| — | Typical | See *M. avium* | 10–20 |

## MANAGEMENT

**Prophylaxis** Wear waterproof gloves when working in fish tank.

**Antibiotics** Drug of first choice: clarithromycin and either rifampin or ethambutol for 1 to 2 months after lesion(s) have resolved (3 to 4 months). Susceptibility testing is not routinely recommended and should be reserved for cases of treatment failure.

**Surgical Debridement** May be required for deep tissue involvement, especially in immunocompromised host. If lesion is small it should be excised.

## MYCOBACTERIUM ULCERANS INFECTION

*M. ulcerans* infection occurs at sites of traumatic inoculation, usually the legs, resulting in large to gigantic deep painless ulcerations, occurring in tropical regions of Africa and Australia. *Synonyms*: Buruli ulcer (Africa), Bairnsdale ulcer (Australia).

### EPIDEMIOLOGY AND ETIOLOGY

**Age of Onset**   Children, young adults.
**Sex**   Females > males.
**Transmission**   Inoculation probably via pricks and cuts from plants, occurring in wet, marshy, or swampy sites.
**Demography**   The tropics; most infections in Africa and Australia.
**Etiology**   *M. ulcerans.* An environmental habitat for the organism has not been established.

### PATHOGENESIS

A secreted polyketide toxin, mycolactone, is responsible for tissue damage. Schistosomiasis may be a risk factor by driving the host immune response towards a predominantly $T_H2$ pattern, away from a $T_H1$-preponderant protection against mycobacterial infection.

### HISTORY

**Incubation Period**   Approximately 3 months.
**Symptoms**   The early nodule at site of trauma and subsequent ulceration are usually painless.

### PHYSICAL EXAMINATION

#### Skin Lesions
A painless subcutaneous swelling occurs at the site of inoculation. Lesion enlarges and ulcerates. The ulcer extends into the subcutaneous fat, and its margin is deeply undermined (Fig. 22-60). Ulcerations may enlarge to involve an entire extremity. Legs more commonly involved (sites of trauma). Any site may be involved. Soft tissue and bony involvement can occur.

#### General Findings
Fever, constitutional findings are usually absent. Regional lymph nodes usually not enlarged.

### DIFFERENTIAL DIAGNOSIS

**Subcutaneous Induration**   Panniculitis, phycomycosis, nodular vasculitis, pyomyositis.
**Large Cutaneous Ulceration**   Blastomycosis, sporotrichosis, nocardiosis, actinomycosis, mycetoma, chromomycosis, pyoderma gangrenosum, basal cell carcinoma, squamous cell carcinoma, necrotizing soft tissue infections.

### LABORATORY EXAMINATIONS

**Bacterial Culture**   Rule out secondary bacterial infection.
**Mycobacterial Culture**   *M. ulcerans* grows optimally at 32° to 33°C.
**PCR**   Reported to be effective.
**Dermatopathology**   Necrosis originates in the interlobular septa of the subcutaneous fat. Ulceration is surrounded by granulation tissue with giant cells but no caseation necrosis or tubercles. Acid-fast bacilli are always demonstrable.

### DIAGNOSIS

Clinical findings confirmed by isolation of *M. ulcerans* from lesional skin biopsy specimen.

### COURSE AND PROGNOSIS

Because of delay in diagnosis and treatment, lesions are often extensive at presentation. Ulcerations tend to persist for months to years. Spontaneous healing occurs eventually in many patients. Ulceration and healing can be complicated by scarring, contracture of the limb, and lymphedema. Malnutrition and anemia delay healing.

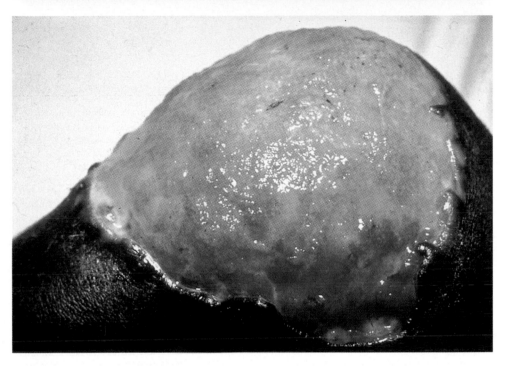

**FIGURE 22-60   *M. ulcerans* infection (buruli ulcer)**   *A huge ulcer with a clean base and under-mined margins extends into the adipose tissue of a Ugandan child. (Courtesy of M. Dittrich, MD.)*

## MANAGEMENT

**Symptomatic**   In that *M. ulcerans* prefers cooler temperatures, application of heat to the involved site has been reported to be effective. Improve nutritional status.

**Surgery**   Excision of the infected tissue, usually followed by grafting, is effective.

**Antimycobacterial Drug Therapy**   Often ineffective.

## *MYCOBACTERIUM FORTUITUM* COMPLEX INFECTION

*Mycobacterium fortuitum* complex (MFC) organisms cause infections at sites of inoculation, either surgical, injection, or traumatic, characterized by wound infections occurring several weeks after the insult. Cutaneous infection accounts for 60% of MFC infections.

## EPIDEMIOLOGY AND ETIOLOGY

**Age of Onset**    Children, young adults.
**Sex**    Females > males.
**Etiology**    MFC organisms include *M. fortuitum*, *M. chelonae*, and *M. abscessus*.
**Demography**    *M. chelonae* is predominantly in Europe; *M. abscessus*, in United States and Africa.
**Natural Reservoirs**    The organisms are widely distributed in soil, dust, and water. Can be isolated from tap water, municipal water supplies, moist areas in hospitals, contaminated biologicals, aquariums, domestic animals, marine life.
**Transmission**    Inoculation via traumatic puncture wounds or surgical procedures/injections. Silicone injections. Whirlpool footbaths in nail salons.

## HISTORY

**Incubation Period**    Usually within 1 month (range 1 week to 2 years).
**History**    Surgical wound infections follow augmentation mammaplasty, median sternotomy, and percutaneous catheterizations.
**Symptoms**    Infection presents as a painful traumatic or surgical wound infection.

## PHYSICAL EXAMINATION

**Skin Lesions**
Cold postinjection abscesses. Traumatic wound infections present as dark red, infiltrated nodule, ±abscess formation, ±drainage of serous exudate (Fig. 22-61). Linear lesions, commonly at incision sites. Traumatic infection occurs more commonly on the extremities. Surgical infections occur in scars of median sternotomy and augmentation mammaplasty. Foot baths associated with furunculosis. In immunocompromised

individuals, infection can disseminate hematogenously to skin (multiple recurring abscesses on the extremities) and joints.

**General Findings**
Other primary MFC infections include pneumonitis, osteomyelitis, lymphadenitis, postsurgical endocarditis.

## DIFFERENTIAL DIAGNOSIS

**Traumatic and Postoperative Wound Infection**
*S. aureus* and group A streptococcus infections, various other bacteria, foreign-body reaction, allergic contact dermatitis to topically applied agent, *C. albicans* infection, *Aspergillus* spp. infection.

## LABORATORY EXAMINATIONS

**Bacterial Culture**    Rule out secondary bacterial infection.
**Mycobacterial Culture**    MFC organisms can usually be isolated on primary culture in 2 to 30 days.
**Dermatopathology**    Polymorphonuclear microabscesses and granuloma formation with foreign-body-type giant cells (dimorphic inflammatory response) are seen. Necrosis is often present without caseation. Acid-fast bacilli can be seen within microabscesses.

## DIAGNOSIS

Clinical findings confirmed by isolation of MFC from lesional skin biopsy specimen.

## COURSE AND PROGNOSIS

The infection becomes chronic unless treated with antimycobacterial therapy, ±surgical debridement.

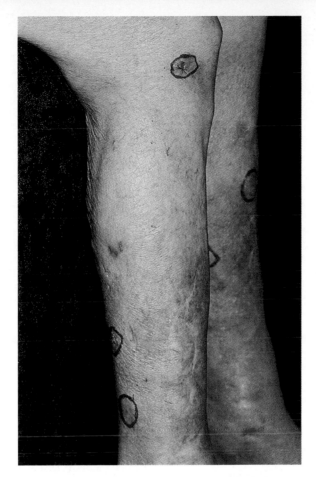

**FIGURE 22-61**  *M. chelonae* **infection**  *Edema, erythematous nodules, scars on the lower legs of an 83-year-old female, who was treated with oral glucocorticoids for asthma.*

## MANAGEMENT

**Antimycobacterial Chemotherapy**  May respond to ciprofloxacin.
**Surgery**  Debridement with delayed closure is effective for localized infections.

# LYME BORRELIOSIS ■ ◑

Lyme borreliosis (LB) is a complex, multisystem disease caused by the spirochete *Borrelia burgdorferi,* which is transmitted to humans by the bite of an infected ixodid tick. There are three stages of LB: stage 1 is localized; stage 2 (untreated stage 1) is disseminated; stage 3 is persistent infection, developing months or years later. The clinical findings associated with each stage are listed in Table 22-13.

## EPIDEMIOLOGY AND ETIOLOGY

**Etiology** Three are groups of *B. burgdorferi* organisms known as *B. burgdorferi* sensu lato. In North America, most causative strains are group 1. In Europe and Asia, the most common strains isolated are group 2 (*B. garinii*) and group 3 (*B. afzelii*) as well as group 1. Clinical variations of disease occurring in North America, Europe, and Asia may be related to differences in the various causative strains. *B. burgdorferi* has been identified in 19 of the United States.

| *Borrelia Burgdorferi* Sensu Lato Spp. | Geographic Range |
|---|---|
| *B. burgdorferi* sensu stricto | North America, Europe |
| *B. garinii* | Europe, Asia |
| *B. afzelli* | Europe, Asia |

**Vector** Infected nymphal tick of genus *Ixodes*: *I. dammini* (*I. scapularis,* deer tick, Fig. 22-62), *I. pacificus, I. ricinus* (sheep tick), *I. persulcatus.*

**Animal Hosts** White-footed mouse preferred host for immature larval and nymphal *I. dammini*. White-tailed deer, the preferred host in the adult stage of *I. dammini*, are not involved in the life cycle of the spirochete but are critical to the survival of the tick.

**Transmission** Ticks cling to vegetation; are most numerous in brushy, wooded, or grassy habitats; not found on open sandy beaches, *B. burgdorferi* is transmitted to humans after biting and feeding of nymphs or, less commonly, adult ticks. Transmission to humans occurs in association with hiking, camping, or hunting trips and with residence in wooded or rural areas.

**Season** In the midwestern and eastern United States, late May through early fall (80% of early LB begins in June and July). In the Pacific Northwest, January through May.

**Risk for Exposure** Strongly associated with prevalence of tick vectors and proportion of those ticks that carry *B. burgdorferi*. In the northeastern United States with endemic disease, the infection rate of the nymphal *I. scapularis* tick with *B. burgdorferi* is commonly 20 to 35%. Risk associated with hiking, camping, or hunting trips and with residence in wooded or rural area

**Distribution** Worldwide, primarily in temperature climates. Correlates closely with geographic ranges of ixodid ticks. *I. scapularis* is the vector in the northeastern United States (Massachusetts to Maryland); midwestern states (Wisconsin, Minnesota). *I. pacificus* is the vector in the western states (California, Oregon). *I. ricinus* is the vector in Europe and Asia (Great Britain to Scandanavia to European Russia). *I. persulcatus*, in Eastern Europe, China, and Japan.

**Incidence** LB is the most common vector-borne infection in the United States, with >10,000 cases annually.

## PATHOGENESIS

After inoculation into the skin as the tick feeds, spirochetes replicate and migrate outward, producing the EM lesion, and invade vessels, spreading hematogenously to other organs. The spirochete has a particular trophism for tissues of the skin, nervous system, and joints. The organism persists in affected tissues during all stages of the illness. The immune response to the spirochete develops gradually. Specific IgM antibody peak between the third and sixth weeks after disease onset. The specific IgG response develops gradually over months. Proinflammatory cytokines, TNF-$\alpha$, and IL-1$\beta$ are produced in affected tissues.

## HISTORY

**Incubation Period** EM: 3 to 32 days after tick bite. Cardiac manifestations: 35 days (3 weeks to >5 months after tick bite). Neurologic manifestions: average 38 days (2 weeks to months) after tick bite. Rheumatologic manifestions: 67 days (4 days to 2 years) after bite.

**Prodrome** With disseminated infection (stage 2), malaise, fatigue, lethargy, headache, fever,

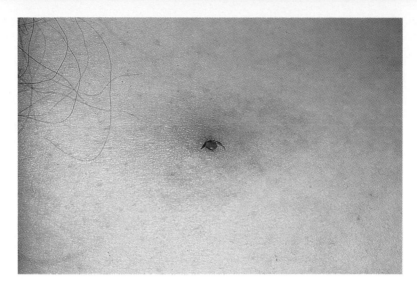

**FIGURE 22-62   Deer tick (*Ixodes scapularis*) feeding** *A nymph with its mouth parts attached to skin with surrounding erythema; this inflammation is a response to the bite itself and is not necessarily indicative of infection. Transmission of* Borrelia burgdorferi *usually occurs only after prolonged attachment and feeding (>18 h).*

**TABLE 22-13   Staging of LYME Borreliosis**

| Stage | Clinical Findings |
| --- | --- |
| Early infection: stage 1 (localized infection) | Erythema migrans (EM)<br>Lymphocytoma |
| Early infection: stage 2 (disseminated infection) | Systemic sysmptoms (fever, chills, myalgia, headaches, weakness, photophobia)<br>Secondary EM<br>Carditis<br>Meningitis, cranial neuritis, radiculoneuropathy<br>Arthralgia/myalgia |
| Late infection: stage 3 (persistent infection) | Arthritis<br>Encephalomyelitis<br>Acrodermatitis chronica atrophicans (ACA) |

chills, stiff neck, arthralgia, myalgia, backache, anorexia, sore throat, nausea, dysesthesia, vomiting, abdominal pain, photophobia.

**History** Ixodid tick bites are asymptomatic. Most LB patients are aware of a preceding tick bite. Removal of the pinhead-sized tick within 18 h of attachment may preclude transmission. EM may be associated with burning sensation, itching, or pain. Only 75% of patients with LB exhibit EM. Joint complaints more common in North America. Neurologic involvement more common in Europe. With persistent disease, chronic fatigue.

## PHYSICAL EXAMINATION

### Skin Findings

**Stage 1 Localized Infection** *Erythema Migrans* Initial erythematous macule or papule enlarges within days to form an expanding annular lesion with a distinct red border and partially clearing middle, i.e., a migrating erythema, at the bite site (Figs. 22-63 and 22-64). Maximum median diameter is 15 cm (range 3 to 68 cm). Center may become indurated, vesicular, or necrotic. The expanding lesion may have several rings of varying shades of red (targetoid or bull's eye). At times, concentric rings form. When occurring on the scalp, only a linear streak may be evident on the face or neck. Multiple EM lesions are seen with multiple bite sites (Fig. 22-65). Most common sites: thigh, groin, axilla. Less common: central hemorrhagic vesiculation or necrosis, lymphangitic streaks. Hypersensitivity to various tick antigens, other pathogens, and outer borrelial surface proteins occur in some individuals. As EM evolves, postinflammatory erythema or hyperpigmentation, transient alopecia, and desquamation may occur. 25% of patients do not exhibit EM lesion.

*Borrelial Lymphocytoma* Mainly seen in Europe. Usually arises at the site of tick bite. Some patients have a history of EM; others may show concomitant EM located around or near the lymphocytoma. Usually presents as a solitary bluish-red nodule (Fig. 22-66) or plaque. Sites of predilection: earlobe (children), nipple/areola (adults), areola, scrotum; 3 to 5 cm in diameter. Usually asymptomatic.

*Other Cutaneous Findings* Malar rash, diffuse urticaria, subcutaneous nodules (panniculitis).

**Stage 2 Disseminated Infection** *Secondary Lesions* Present in 17 to 50% of patients with early disseminated LB in North America; more common in Europe. Lesions range in number from 2 to >100 and thus may present as rash. Secondary lesions resemble EM but are smaller, migrate less, and lack central induration and may be scaly (Fig. 22-67). Lesions occur at any site except the palms and soles; can become confluent. When face, hands, feet are involved, mild swelling can occur.

**Stage 3 Persistent Infection: Acrodermatitis Chronica Atrophicans (ACA)** Associated with *B. afzelii* infection in Europe and Asia. More common in elderly women.

*Early Inflammatory Phase (Months to Years)* Initially, diffuse or localized violaceous erythema, usually on one extremity, accompanied by mild to prominent edema (Fig. 22-68), most commonly involving the extensor surfaces and periarticular areas. Asymptomatic dull red infiltrated plaques arise on the extremities, more commonly on lower legs than forearms, which slowly extend centrifugally over several months to years, leaving central areas of atrophy.

*Endstage* Skin becomes atrophic, veins and subcutaneous tissue become prominent, easily lifted and pushed into fine accordion-like folds, i.e., "cigarette paper" or "tissue paper" skin (Fig. 22-69). Lesions may be single or multiple.

*Sclerotic or Fibrotic Plaques and Bands* Localized fibromas and plaques are seen as subcutaneous nodules around the knees and elbows (Fig. 22-70); may involve the joint capsule with subsequent limitation of movement of joints in hands, feet, or shoulders. Fibrotic/sclerotic band along ulna is pathognomonic ("ulnar band").

**General Findings** See Table 22-13.
**Stage 1** None.
**Stage 2 (Disseminated Infection)** Fever: in adults, low-grade; in children, may be high and persistent. Regional lymphadenopathy, generalized lymphadenopathy.

*Neurologic Involvement* Occurs in 10 to 20% of untreated LB cases, 1 to 6 weeks (or longer) after the tick bite. Manifested as meningitis (excruciating headache, neck pain), subtle encephalitic signs (sleep disturbances, difficulty concentrating, poor memory, irritability, emotional liability, dementia), cranial neuritis (including bilateral facial palsy), motor or sensory radiculoneuropathy, mononeuritis multiplex, or myelitis. In the United States, most common presentation is fluctuating symptoms of meningitis accompanied by facial palsy and peripheral radiculoneuropathy. In Europe and Asia, the first sign is character-

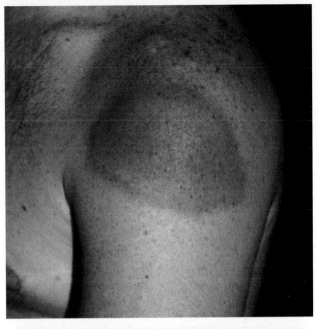

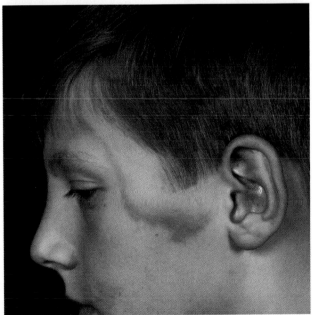

**FIGURE 22-63  (Top)    Lyme borreliosis: erythema migrans on shoulder**   *Solitary erythematous plaque with a expanding raised annular margin on the shoulder at the site of an asymptomatic tick bite.*


**FIGURE 22-64  (Bottom)    Lyme borreliosis: erythema migrans on scalp and face**   *Serpiginous erythematous lesion on the face, represents the margin of a large lesion that began on the scalp.*

istically radicular pain followed by CSF pleo-cytosis (Bannwarth's syndrome); meningeal and encephalitic signs are often absent. Early neurologic manifestations usually resolve within months; chronic neurologic disease may occur later.

***Cardiac Involvement*** Occurs in 8% of un-treated cases, usually within 4 weeks, Mani-fested by fluctuating degrees of atrioventricular block, myopericarditis, and left ventricular dys-function. Usually transient and not associated with long-term sequelae.

***Musculoskeletal Involvement*** Common. Migra-tory pain in joints, tendons, bursae, muscles, or bones. Pain lasts hours or days, affecting one or two locations at a time.

**Stage 3 (Persistent Infection)**    Fever: in adults, low-grade; in children, may be high and pre-sistent. Regional lymphadenopathy, generalized lymphadenopathy.

***Chronic Neuroborreliosis*** May become apparent months or years after onset of latent infection. Less common than arthritis. Most common presentation is subtle encephalopathy (altered memory, mood, or sleep), ofter accompanied by axonoal polyneuropathy (distal paresthesias, spinal radicular pain). Prolonged course resem-bles that of tertiary syphilis.

***Arthritis*** More common in United States, oc-curing in 60% of untreated cases. Characterized by intermittent attacks of oligoarticular arthritis in large joints (especially knees), lasting weeks to months. In a small percentage of cases, in-volvement of large joints (usually one or both knees) becomes chronic and may lead to de-struction of cartilage and bone.

## DIFFERENTIAL DIAGNOSIS

**EM**    Insect bite (annular erythema cause by ticks, mosquitoes, Hymenoptera), epidermal dermatophytoses, allergic contact dermatitis, herald patch of pityriasis rosea, granuloma annulare, early inflammatory morphea, cel-lulitis, urticaria, erythema multiforme, ery-thema annulare centrifugum, involuting psoriasis lesion, lichen simplex chronicus, fixed drug eruption.

**Secondary Lesions**    Secondary syphilis, pityra-sis rosea, erythema multiforme, urticaria.

**Lymphocytoma**    Insect bite reaction, pseudolym-phoma, cutaneous lymphoma.

**ACA**    Arterial insufficiency of the lower leg, venous insufficiency with stasis dermatitis, ve-nous thrombosis/thrombophlebitis.

**Fibrotic Nodules**    Rheumatic nodules, gouty tophi, erythema nodosum.

## LABORATORY EXAMINATIONS

**Skin Biopsy**    *EM* Deep and superficial perivas-cular and interstitial infiltrate containing lym-phocytes and plasma cells with some degree of vascular damage (mild vasculitis or hypervas-cular occlusion). Spirochetes can be demon-strated in up to 40% of EM biopsy specimens. *ACA.* Early, perivascular inflammatory infil-trate with plasma cells and dermal edema. Sub-sequently, infiltrate broadens to a dense middermal bandlike infiltrate. Ultimately, epi-dermal and dermal atrophy, dilated dermal blood vessles, plasma cell infiltrate, elastin and collagen defects.

**Serology**    The CDC recommends a two-step approach in which samples are first tested by enzyme-linked immunosorbent assay (ELISA) and equivocal or positive results are then tested by Western blotting. During the first month of infection, both IgM and IgG re-sponses to the spirochete should be deter-mined, preferably in both acute- and convalescent-phase serum samples. Approxi-mately 20 to 30% of patients have a positive response detectable in acute-phase samples; about 70 to 80% have positive response during convalescence (2 to 4 weeks later). After that time, the great majority of patients continue to have a positive IgG antibody response, and a single test (that for IgG) is usually sufficient. According to current criteria adopted by the CDC, an IgM Western blot is considered posi-tive if two of the following three bands are present: 23, 39, and 41 kDa.

Positive serology indicates past infection. It does not distinguish between an abortive infec-tion, a successfully treated past infection, or an active infection.

**Culture**    *B. burgdorferi* can be isolated from lesional skin biopsy specimen on modified Bar-bour-Stoenner-Kelly medium.

**PCR**    Detects *B. burgdorferi* DNA in lesional skin biopsy specimen, blood, or joint fluid. May be the preferred confirmatory laboratory test.

## DIAGNOSIS

CDC surveillance criteria:

- *Early LB*: Made on characteristic clinical findings in a person living in or having visited an endemic area; does not require laboratory confirmation.
- *Late LB*: Confirmed by specific serologic tests.

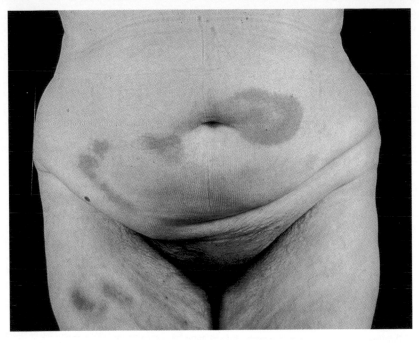

**FIGURE 22-65   Lyme borreliosis: erythema migrans with multiple lesions**   *Three erythematous plaques with central clearing on the lower abdomen and thigh at multiple tick-bite sites.*

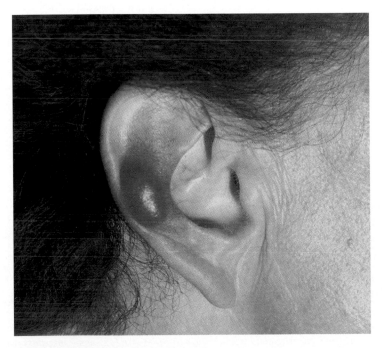

**FIGURE 22-66   Lyme borreliosis: lymphocytoma cutis**   *Solitary, red-purple nodule on the characteristic site of the ear.*

- *ACA*: Made on clinical findings confirmed by lesional biopsy.

## COURSE AND PROGNOSIS

Untreated EM and secondary lesions fade in median time of 28 days, but the range is from 1 day to 14 months. Both EM and secondary lesions can fade and recur during this time. However, after adequate treatment, early lesions resolve within several days, and late manifestations are prevented. Late manifestations identified early usually clear after adequate antibiotic therapy; however, delay in diagnosis may result in permanent joint or neurologic disabilities.

ACA shows little response to adequate antibiotic therapy once atrophy has supervened. Adequately treated patients have declining titers of anti-*B. burgdorferi* antibody within 6 to 12 months.

## MANAGEMENT

### Prophylaxis

- Avoid known habitats of *I. scapularis* and *I. pacificus* (United States). Other preventive measures include wearing long pants and long-sleeved shirts, tucking pants into socks.
- Apply tick repellents containing *N, N*-diethyl-*m*-toluamide ("DEET") to clothing and/or exposed skin.
- Check regularly for ticks and promptly remove any attached ticks.
- Acaricides containing permethrin kill ticks on contact and can provide further protection when applied to clothing.
- After a recognized tick bite, the risk of infection with *B. burgdorferi* is low, and antibiotic prophylaxis is not routinely indicated. Therapy with amoxicillin or doxycycline for 10 days may be given to prevent Lyme disease in the following circumstances: Tick engorged (feeding for >24h), Ixodes nymph from a hyperendemic area, pregnancy, immunocompromised status, follow-up difficult, patient anxious.
- Temperature of >38°C may represent human granulocytic ehrlichiosis or basbesiosis transmitted with tick bite.

**Immunization**  Immunization for prophylaxis of LB is now available for those at high risk of infection with the lyme vaccine LYMErix. It contains recombinant outer-surface protein A.
**Antimicrobial Treatment**  See Fig. 22-71.

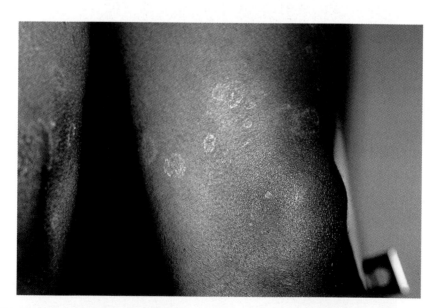

**FIGURE 22-67   Lyme borreliosis: secondary lesions**  *Multiple, small, scaling lesions on the thighs. The lesions result from spirochetemia from the primary bite size (erythema migrans) with resultant disseminated infection. These lesions are analogous to the papulosquamous lesions that occur in secondary syphilis.*

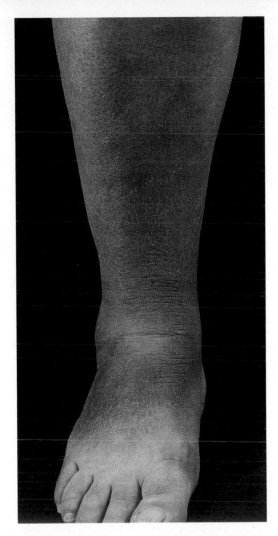

**FIGURE 22-68   Lyme borreliosis: acrodermatitis chronica atrophicans: early**   *Ill-defined, violaceous erythema and edema of the leg and foot. Onset is usually several months after primary infection and is often accompanied by symptoms of peripheral sensory neuropathy.*

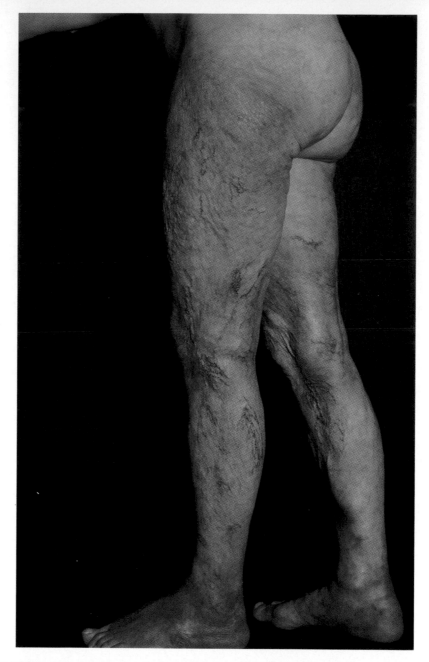

**FIGURE 22-69   Lyme borreliosis: acrodermatitis chronica atrophicans: endstage**   *Advanced atrophy of the epidermis and dermis with associated violaceous erythema of legs and feet; the visibility of the superficial veins is striking.*

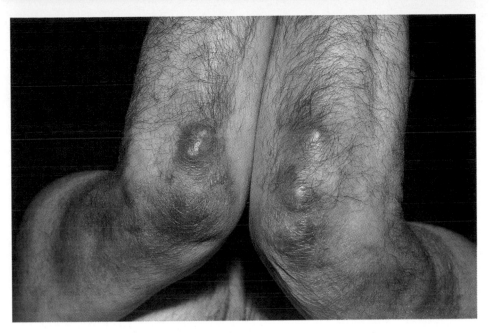

**FIGURE 22-70 Lyme borreliosis: acrodermatitis chronica atrophicans, fibrotic nodules** *Multiple, large, subcutaneous, fibrotic, violaceous nodules with surrounding erythema on the elbows.*

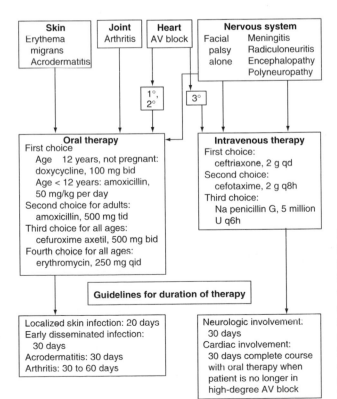

**FIGURE 22-71 Algorithm for the treatment of the various acute or chronic manifestations of Lyme borreliosis.** Relapse may occur with any of these regimens, and a second course of treatment may be necessary. AV, atrioventricular. [AC Steere: Chap. 157 in *Harrison's Principles of Internal Medicine*, 16e, D Kasper et al (eds). New York, McGraw-Hill, 2005.]

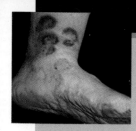
# CUTANEOUS FUNGAL INFECTIONS

Numerous fungi are capable of superficially invading the epidermis and adnexae (hair/hair follicles and nail apparatus) and mucosal sites (oropharynx, anogenitalia). These fungi are commensural organisms that frequently colonize normal epithelium, and include the dermatophytes, *Candida* spp, and *Malassezia* spp. Infections can extend more deeply in the immunocompromised host.

Deeper, chronic cutaneous fungal infections, such as mycetoma, chromomycosis, and sporotrichosis, arise after inoculation in some individuals. Systemic fungal infections, most commonly with a primary lung infection, can disseminate hematogenously to multiple organ systems, including the skin. Disseminated candidiasis commonly arises in the gastrointestinal tract. These infections occur most often in the immunocompromised host.

## SUPERFICIAL FUNGAL INFECTIONS

Superficial fungal infections are the most common of all mucocutaneous infections, often caused by overgrowth of transient or resident flora associated with a change in the microenvironment of the skin. The fungi causing these infections are of three genera: dermatophytes, *Candida* spp., and *Malassezia furfur*. Dermatophytes can infect any keratinized epithelium, hair follicles, and nail apparatus. *Candida* spp. require a warm humid environment. *M. furfur* require a humid microenvironment and lipids for growth.

*Trichosporon* spp. are yeasts that cause piedra, superficial infections (*T. cutaneum, T. asteroides*), and invasive trichosporonosis in the immunocompromised host (*T. asahii*). *Piedra* is an asymptomatic superficial fungal infection of the hair shaft. *White piedra* (pubic, axillary, beard, and eyebrow/eyelash hair; *T. inkin*) is more common in temperate and semitropical regions: Southern United States; South America, Asia, Europe, Japan. *Black piedra* (scalp hair; *T. ovoides*) is most common in tropical regions (high temperature, humidity: South America, Southeast Asia), presenting as darkly pigmented, firmly attached nodules (up to a few millimeters) on the hair shaft ± hair breakage. Invasive trichosporonosis is an emerging opportunistic infection (associated with neutropenia); dissemination occurs to skin (erythematous or purpuric tender papules), lungs, kidneys, and spleen.

*Tinea nigra* is a superficial fungal infection of the stratum corneum caused by *Hortaea* (*Exophiala* or *Phaeoannellomyces*) *werneckii*, occurring more commonly in tropical climates. Direct inoculation onto the skin from contact with decaying vegetation, wood, or soil seems to be the form of acquisition. Tinea nigra presents as brown to black nonscaly macule(s) with well-defined borders (Fig. 23-1) that resemble silver nitrate stains, arising on the palm and sole. Diagnosis is made on direct microscopy, visualizing abundant branching septate hyphae.

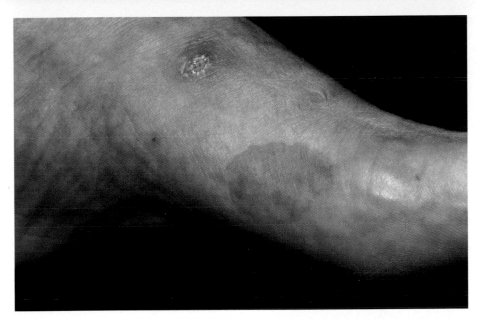

**FIGURE 23-1  Tinea nigra**  *Uniformly tan macule on the plantar foot, present for several years. KOH preparation showed hyphae.*

## DERMATOPHYTOSES   ■

Dermatophytes are a unique group of fungi capable of infecting nonviable keratinized cutaneous structures including stratum corneum, nails, and hair (Image 23-1). The term *dermatophytosis* denotes an infection caused by dermatophytes. It can be further specified according to the tissue mainly involved: *epidermomycosis* (epidermal dermatophytosis), *trichomycosis* (dermatophytosis of hair and hair follicles), or *onychomycosis* (dermatophytosis of the nail apparatus). Since differ ent anatomical structures are involved, epidermomycosis, trichomycosis, and onychomycosis clinically look different. The pathogenesis of epidermomycosis vs trichomycosis leading to different clinical manifestations is schematically depicted in Image 23-1. The term *tinea* is best used for dermatophytoses and is modified according to the anatomic site of infection, e.g., tinea pedis. "Tinea" versicolor is called *pityriasis versicolor* outside of the United States; it is not a dermatophytosis but rather an infection caused by the yeast *Malassezia*.

### EPIDEMIOLOGY AND ETIOLOGY

**Age of Onset**  Children have scalp infections (*Trichophyton, Microsporum*), and young adults have intertriginous infections. The incidence of onychomycosis is correlated directly with age; in the United States, up to 50% of individuals age 75 years have onychomycosis.

**Race**  Adult blacks are said to have a lower incidence of dermatophytosis. Tinea capitis is more common in black children.

**Etiology** Three genera of dermatophytes: *Trichophyton*, *Microsporum*, and *Epidermophyton*. More than 40 species are currently recognized; approximately 10 spp. are common causes of human infection. *T. rubrum* is the most common cause of epidermal dermatophytosis and onychomycosis in industrialized nations. Currently, 70% of the U.S. population experience at least one episode of *T. rubrum* infection (usually tinea pedis). *T. rubrum* is indigenous to Southeast Asia, the Australian outback, and western Africa. Visitors/colonizers from Europe and North America became infected in these areas, developing tinea pedis and onychomycosis; these conditions did not occur in natives, who were barefoot or wore open moccasins. These visitors/colonizers and soldiers (World Wars I and II, and the Vietnam conflict) brought *T. rubrum* to North America and Europe. Soldiers wearing occlusive boots in tropical climates developed "jungle rot"—extensive tinea pedis with secondary bacterial infection. Presently, *T. rubrum* infection can be acquired by contact with contaminated floors (homes, health clubs, athletic locker rooms, or hotel rooms). The etiology of tinea capitis in children varies geographically. In North America and Europe, *T. tonsurans* is the most common cause, having replaced *M. audouinii*. In Europe, Asia, and Africa, *T. violaceum*. In U.S. adults, *T. rubrum* is the most common cause of dermatophytic folliculitis.

**Demography** Some species have a worldwide distribution; others are restricted to particular continents or regions. However, *T. concentricum*, the cause of tinea imbricata, is endemic to the South Pacific and parts of South America. *T. rubrum* was endemic to Southeast Asia, western Africa, and Australia but now occurs most commonly in North America and Europe.

**Transmission** Dermatophyte infections can be acquired from three sources: most commonly from another person [usually by fomites, less so by direct skin-to-skin contact (tinea gladiatorum)], from animals such as puppies or kittens, and least commonly from soil. Based on their ecology, dermatophytes are also classified as follows:

> *Anthropophilic*: Person-to-person transmission by fomites and by direct contact. *Trichophyton* spp.: *T. rubrum*, *T. mentagrophytes* (var. *interdigitale*), *T. schoenleinii*, *T. tonsurans*, *T. violaceum*. *Microsporum audouinii*. *Epidermophyton floccosum*.
>
> *Zoophilic*: Animal-to-human by direct contact or by fomites. *Trichophyton* spp.: *T. equinum*, *T. mentagrophytes* (var. *mentagrophytes*), *T. verrucosum*. *M. canis*.
>
> *Geophilic*: Environmental. *Microsporum* spp.: *M. gypseum*, *M. nanum*.

**Predisposing Factors** Atopic diathesis for *T. rubrum* infections. *Immunosuppressed patients* have a higher incidence and more

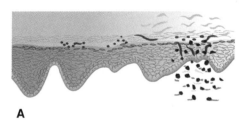

A

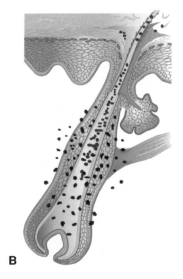

B

**IMAGE 23-1** *The pathogenesis of epidermomycosis (A) and trichomycosis (B) are different because they involve different structures leading to different clinical manifestations. In epidermomycosis, dermatophytes (red dots and lines) within the stratum corneum not only disrupt the horny layer and thus lead to scaling but also elicit an inflammatory response (the black dots symbolize inflammatory cells), which then may manifest as erythema, papulation, and even vesiculation. On the other hand, in trichomycosis the hair shaft is involved (red dots) resulting in the destruction and breaking off of the hair. If the dermatophyte infection extends farther down into the hair follicle, it will elicit a deeper inflammatory response (black dots) and this will manifest as deeper inflammatory nodules, follicular pustulation, and abscess formation. (See also Fig. 23-21.)*

intractable dermatophytoses. With topical immunosuppression (i.e., with prolonged application of topical glucocorticoids), there can be marked modification in the usual banal character of dermatophytosis (tinea incognito); this is especially true of the face, groin, and hands. In immunocompromised patients, abscesses and granulomas may occur (Majocchi's granuloma).

## CLASSIFICATION

In vivo, dermatophytes grow only on or within keratinized structures and, as such, involve the following:

- *Dermatophytoses of keratinized epidermis (epidermal dermatophytosis, epidermomycosis)*: Tinea facialis, tinea corporis, tinea cruris, tinea manus, tinea pedis.
- *Dermatophytoses of nail apparatus (onychomychosis)*: Tinea unguium (toenails, fingernails). Onychomycosis (here it is a more inclusive term, including nail infections caused by dermatophytes, yeasts, and molds).
- *Dermatophytoses of hair and hair follicle (Trichomycosis)*: Dermatophytic folliculitis, Majocchi's (trichophytic) granuloma, tinea capitis, tinea barbae.

## PATHOGENESIS

Dermatophytes synthesize keratinases that digest keratin and sustain existence of fungi in keratinized structures. Cell-mediated immunity and antimicrobial activity of polymorphonuclear leukocytes restrict dermatophyte pathogenicity.

- *Host factors that facilitate dermatophyte infections*: atopy, topical and systemic glucocorticoids, ichthyosis, collagen vascular disease
- *Local factors favoring dermatophyte infection*: sweating, occlusion, occupational exposure, geographic location, high humidity (tropical or semitropical climates)

The clinical presentation of dermatophytoses depends on several factors: site of infection, immunologic response of the host, species of fungus. Dermatophytes (e.g., *T. rubrum*) that initiate little inflammatory response are better able to establish chronic infection. Organisms such as *M. canis* cause an acute infection associated with a brisk inflammatory response and spontaneous resolution. In some individuals, infection can involve the dermis, as in kerion and Majocchi's granuloma.

## LABORATORY EXAMINATIONS

### Direct Microscopy   (Fig. 23-2)
*Sampling Skin*: Collect scale with a no. 15 scalpel blade, edge of a glass microscope slide, brush (tooth or cervical brush). Scales are placed on center of microscope slide, swept into a small pile, and covered with a coverslip.

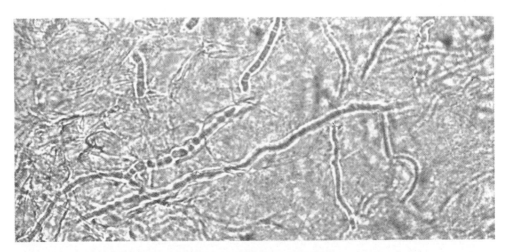

**FIGURE 23-2  Potassium hydroxide (KOH) preparation**  *Multiple, septated, tube-like structures (hyphae or mycelia) and spore formation in scales from an individual with epidermal dermatophytosis. In contrast, KOH preparation in candidiasis shows elongated yeast forms (pseudohyphae) without true septations. (Compare with Fig. 23-23.)*

Recent application of cream/ointment or powder often makes identification of fungal element difficult/impossible.

*Nails*: Keratinaceous debris is collected with a no. 15 scalpel blade or small curette. Distal lateral subungual onychomycosis (DLSO): debride from the undersurface of nail of most proximally involved site; avoid nail plate. Superficial white onychomycosis (SWO): superficial nail plate. Proximal subungual onychomycosis (PSO): undersurface of proximal nail plate; obtain sample by using a small punch biopsy tool, boring through involved nail plate to undersurface; obtain keratin from undersurface.

*Hair*: Remove hairs by epilation of broken hairs with a needle holder or forceps. Place on microscope slide and cover with glass coverslip. Skin scales from involved hairy site can be obtained with a brush (tooth or cervical).

***Preparation of Sample*** *Potassium hydroxide 5 to 20% solution* is applied at the edge of coverslip. Capillary action draws solution under coverslip. The preparation is gently heated with a match or lighter until bubbles begin to expand, clarifying the preparation. Excess KOH solution is blotted out with bibulous or lens paper.

Condenser should be "racked down." Epidermal dermatophytosis: positive unless patient is using antifungal therapy. DLSO: 90% of cases positive. Variations of KOH with fungal stains: Swartz-Lampkins stain, chlorazol black E stain. ***Microscopy*** Dermatophytes are recognized as septated, tubelike structures (hyphae or mycelia) (Fig. 23-2).

**Wood's Lamp** Hairs infected with *Microsporum* spp. fluoresce. Greenish. Darken room and illuminate affected site with Wood's lamp. Coral red fluorescence of intertriginous site confirms diagnosis of erythrasma.

**Fungal Cultures** Specimens collected from scaling skin lesions, hair, nails. Scale and hair from the scalp are best harvested with tooth or cervical brush; the involved scalp is brushed vigorously; keratinaceous debris and hairs then placed into fungal culture plate. Culture on Sabouraud's glucose medium. Repeat cultures recommended monthly

**Dermatopathology** DLSO: periodic acid–Schiff (PAS) or methenamine silver stains are more sensitive than KOH preparation or fungal culture in identification of fungal elements in DLSO.

## MANAGEMENT

| | |
|---|---|
| **Prevention** | Apply powder containing miconazole or tolnaftate to areas prone to fungal infection after bathing. |
| **Topical antifungal preparations** | *These preparations may be effective for treatment of dermatophytoses of skin but not for those of hair or nails.* |
| | Preparation is applied bid to involved area optimally for 4 weeks including at least 1 week after lesions have cleared. |
| | Apply at least 3 cm beyond advancing margin of lesion. |
| | These topical agents are comparable. Differentiated by cost, base, vehicle, and antifungal activity. |
| Imidazoles | Clotrimazole (Lotrimin, Mycelex) |
| | Miconazole (Micatin) |
| | Ketoconazole (Nizoral) |
| | Econazole (Spectazole) |
| | Oxiconizole (Oxistat) |
| | Sulconizole (Exelderm) |
| Allylamines | Naftifine (Naftin) |
| | Terbinafine (Lamisil) |
| Naphthionates | Tolnaftate (Tinactin) |
| Substituted pyridone | Ciclopirox olamine (Loprox) |

## MANAGEMENT (*CONTINUED*)

| | |
|---|---|
| **Systemic antifungal agents** | *For infections of keratinized skin*: use if lesions are extensive or if infection has failed to respond to topical preparations.<br>*Usually required for treatment of tinea capitis and tinea unguium.* Also may be required for inflammatory tineas and hyperkeratotic moccasin-type tinea pedis. |
| Terbinafine | 250-mg tablet. Allylamine. Rarely, nausea; dyspepsia, abdominal pain, loss of sense of taste. Most effective oral antidermophyte antifungal; low efficacy against other fungi. |
| Azole/imidazoles | Itraconazole and ketoconazole have potential clinically important interactions when administered with astemizole, calcium channel antagonists, cisapride-coumadin, cyclosporine, oral hypoglycemic agents, phenytoin, protease inhibitors, tacrolimus, terfenadine, theophylline, trimetrexate, and rifampin. |
| Itraconazole | 100-mg capsules; oral solution (10 mg/mL): Intravenous. Triazole. Needs acid gastric pH for dissolution of capsule. Rarely, ventricular arrhythmia when coadministered with terfenadine/astemizole. Raises levels of digoxin and cyclosporine. Approved for onychomycosis in the United States. |
| Fluconazole | 100-, 150-, 200-mg tablets; oral suspension (10 or 40 mg/mL); 400 mg IV. |
| Ketoconazole | 200-mg tablets. Needs acid gastric pH for dissolution of tablet. Take with food or cola beverage; antacids and $H_2$ blockers reduce absorption. The most hepatotoxic of azole drugs; hepatotoxicity occurs in an estimated one of every 10,000–15,000 exposed persons. Rarely, ventricular arrhythmia when coadministered with terfenadine/astemizole. Not approved for treatment of dermatophyte infections in the United States. |
| Griseofulvin | *Micronized*: 250- or 500-mg tablets; 125 mg/teaspoon suspension. *Ultramicronized*: 165- or 330-mg tablets. Active only against dermatophytes; less effective than triazoles. Adverse effects include headache, nausea/vomiting, photosensitivity; lowers effect of crystalline warfarin sodium. *T. rubrum* and *T. tonsurans* infection may respond poorly. Should be taken with fatty meal to maximize absorption. In children, CBC and LFTs recommended if risk factors for hepatitis exist or treatment lasts longer than 3 months. |

*Note*: CBC, Complete blood count; LFTs, liver function tests.

## DERMATOPHYTOSES OF EPIDERMIS

Epidermal dermatophytoses are the most common dermatophytic infection; they may be followed/accompanied by dermatophytic infection of hair/hair follicles and/or the nail apparatus. *Synonyms*: Ringworm, epidermomycosis.

## TINEA PEDIS   ■

Tinea pedis is a dermatophytic infection of the feet, characterized by erythema, scaling, maceration, and/or bulla formation. In most cases of epidermal dermatophytosis, the infection occurs initially on the feet, and, in time, spreads to sites such as the inguinal area (tinea cruris), trunk (tinea corporis), hands (tinea manuum). Tinea pedis often provides breaks in the integrity of the epidermis through which bacteria such as *Staphylococcus aureus* or group A streptococcus (GAS) can invade, causing localized infection or spreading infections such as cellulitis or lymphangitis.
*Synonym*: Athlete's foot.

## EPIDEMIOLOGY

**Age of Onset**   Late childhood or young adult life. Most common, 20 to 50 years.
**Sex**   Males > females.
**Predisposing Factors**   Hot, humid weather; occlusive footwear; excessive sweating.
**Transmission**   Walking barefoot on contaminated floors. Arthrospores can survive in human scales for 12 months.

## HISTORY

**Duration**   Months to years. Often, prior history of tinea pedis, tinea unguium of toenails. May flare if in hot climate.
**Skin Symptoms**   Asymptomatic frequently. Pruritus. Pain with secondary bacterial infection.

## PHYSICAL EXAMINATION

### Skin Lesions
*Interdigital Type*   Two patterns: (1) dry scaling (Fig. 23-3); and (2) maceration, peeling, fissuring of toe webs (Fig. 23-4). Hyperhidrosis common. Most common site: between fourth and fifth toes. Infection may spread to adjacent areas of feet.

*Moccasin Type*   Well-demarcated erythema with minute papules on margin, fine white scaling, and hyperkeratosis (Figs. 23-5 and 23-6) (confined to heels, soles, lateral borders of feet). *Distribution*: Sole, involving area covered by a ballet slipper. One or both feet may be involved with any pattern; bilateral involvement more common.
*Inflammatory/Bullous Type*   Vesicles or bullae filled with clear fluid (Fig. 23-7). Pus usually indicates secondary *S. aureus* infection or group A streptococcus. After rupturing, erosions with ragged ringlike border. May be associated with "id" reaction (autosensitization or dermatophytid). *Distribution*: Sole, instep, webspaces.
*Ulcerative Type*   Extension of interdigital tinea pedis onto dorsal and plantar foot. Usually complicated by bacterial infection.

## DIFFERENTIAL DIAGNOSIS

**Interdigital Type**   Erythrasma, impetigo, pitted keratolysis, *Candida* intertrigo, *Pseudomonas aeruginosa* webspace infection.
**Moccasin Type**   Psoriasis vulgaris, eczematous dermatitis (dyshidrotic, atopic, allergic contact), pitted keratolysis, various keratodermas.

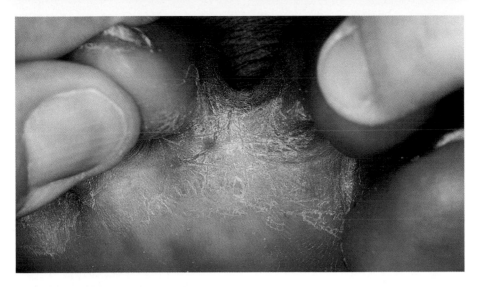

**FIGURE 23-3   Tinea pedis: interdigital dry type**   *The interdigital space between the toes shows erythema and scaling; the toenail is thickened, indicative of associated distal subungual ony-chomycosis.*

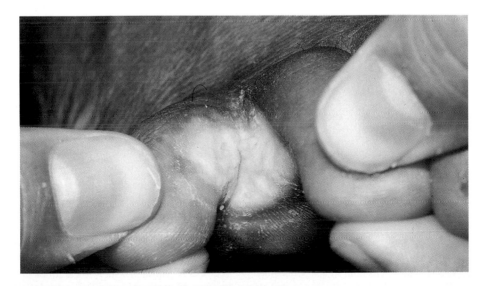

**FIGURE 23-4   Tinea pedis: interdigital macerated type**   *The webspace between the fourth and fifth toes is hyperkeratotic and macerated in a black individual with plantar keratoderma and hyper-hidrosis. The greenish hue is caused by* Pseudomonas aeruginosa *superinfection of this moist inter-triginous site. Erythrasma also occurs in the setting of moist intertriginous sites and may occur concomitantly with interdigital tinea pedis and/or* Pseudomonas *intertrigo.*

## CLASSIFICATION

| Type | Clinical Features | Etiology |
|---|---|---|
| Interdigital (acute and chronic) | Most common type; frequently over-looked | *T. rubrum* most common cause of chronic tinea pedis; *T mentagrophytes* causes more inflammatory lesions |
| | Two patterns: dry and moist with maceration | |
| Dry | Scaling of webspace, may be erosive | *T. rubrum* |
| Moist (macerated) | Hyperkeratosis of webspace with maceration of stratum corneum | *T. mentagrophytes* |
| Moccasin (chronic hyperkeratotic or dry) | Keratoderma | Most often caused by *T. rubrum*, especially in atopic individuals; also *Epidermophyton floccosum* |
| Inflammatory or bullous (vesicular) | Blisters in nonoccluded skin | Least common type; usually caused by *T. mentagrophytes* var. *mentagrophytes* (granular). Resembles an allergic contact dermatitis |
| Ulcerative | An extension of interdigital type into dermis due to maceration and secondary (bacterial) infection | *T. rubrum, E. floccosum, T. mentagrophytes, C. albicans* |
| Dermatophytid | Presents as a vesicular eruption of the fingers and/or palmar aspects of the hands secondary to inflammatory tinea pedis. A combined clinical presentation also occurs. *Candida* and bacteria (*Staphylococcus aureus*, group A *Streptococcus, Pseudomonas aeruginosa*) may cause superinfection. | *T. mentagrophytes, T. rubrum* |

**Inflammatory/Bullous Type**   Bullous impetigo, allergic contact dermatitis, dyshidrotic eczema, bullous disease.

## LABORATORY EXAMINATIONS

**Direct Microscopy**   (Fig. 23-2). In bullous type, examine scraping from the inner aspect of bulla roof for detection of hyphae.

*Wood's Lamp* Negative fluorescence usually rules out erythrasma in interdigital infection. Erythrasma and interdigital tinea pedis may coexist.

*Culture Fungal*: Dermatophytes can be isolated in 11% of normal-appearing interspaces and 31% of macerated toe webs. *Candida* spp. may be copathogens in webspaces. *Bacterial*: In individuals with macerated interdigital space,

*S. aureus, P. aeruginosa*, and diphtheroids are commonly isolated. *S. aureus* and GAS can cause superinfection.

## DIAGNOSIS

Demonstration of hyphae on direct microscopy, isolation of dermatophyte on culture.

## COURSE AND PROGNOSIS

Tends to be chronic, with exacerbations in hot weather. May provide portal of entry for lymphangitis or cellulitis, especially in patients whose leg veins have been used for coronary artery bypass surgery and have chronic low-grade edema of leg. Without secondary prophylaxis, recurrence is the rule.

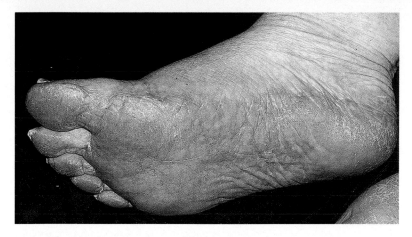

**FIGURE 23-5    Tinea pedis: moccasin type**    *Fairly sharply marginated erythema of the plantar foot with a mild keratoderma associated with distal/lateral subungual onychomycosis, typical of* T. rubrum *infection.*

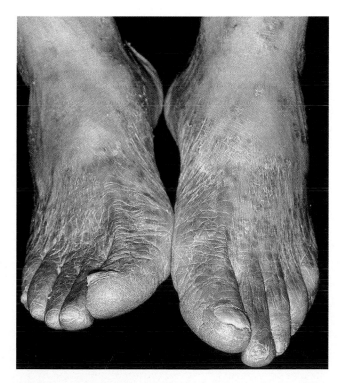

**FIGURE 23-6    Tinea pedis: moccasin type**    *Hyperkeratosis and scaling of the dorsa of the feet occurring on the portion of the foot covered by a moccasin; note the associated distal/lateral subungual onychomycosis, typical of* T. rubrum *infection.*

# MANAGEMENT

**Prevention**                          Use of shower shoes while bathing at home or in public
                                        facility. Washing feet with benzoyl peroxide bar directly
                                        after shower. Diabetics and those who have undergone
                                        coronary artery bypass with harvesting of leg veins are
                                        especially subject to secondary bacterial infection
                                        (impetiginization, lymphangitis, cellulitis).

**Special considerations by type of infection**

Macerated interdigital                  Acute: Burow's wet dressings; Castellani's paint.
                                        Chronic: aluminum chloride hexahydrate 20% bid to
                                        reduce sweating.

Moccasin                                Most difficult to eradicate. Many patients have a minor
                                        defect in cell-mediated immune response: stratum
                                        corneum thick, making it difficult for topical antifungal
                                        agents to penetrate, often associated with tinea unguium,
                                        a source of reinfection of skin. Keratolytic agent (salicylic
                                        acid, lactic acid, hydroxy acid) with plastic occlusion
                                        useful in reducing hyperkeratosis. Nail reservoir must be
                                        eradicated to cure moccasin-type infection.

Inflammatory/bullous                    Acutely, use cool compresses. If severe, systemic
                                        glucocorticoids are indicated.

**Antifungal agents**

Topical                                 See Dermatophytoses, page 690. Apply to all affected sites
                                        twice daily. Treat for 2–4 weeks.

Systemic                                Indicated for extensive infection, for failures of topical
                                        treatment, or for those with tinea unguium and moccasin-
                                        type tinea.

Terbinafine                             250 mg qd for 14 days

Itraconazole                            200 mg bid for 7 days *or*
                                        200 mg qd for 14 days

Fluconazole                             150–200 mg qd for 4–6 weeks

**Secondary prophylaxis**               Important in preventing recurrence of interdigital and
                                        moccasin types of tinea pedis. Daily washing of feet
                                        while bathing with benzoyl peroxide bar is effective and
                                        inexpensive. Antifungal powders, alcohol gels.

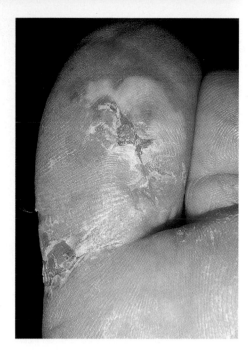

**FIGURE 23-7    Tinea pedis: bullous type**    *Ruptured vesicles, bullae, erythema, and erosion on the plantar aspect of the great toe. Hyphae were detected on KOH preparation obtained from the roof of the inner aspect of the bulla. In some cases, superficial white onychomycosis may also be seen with this* T. mentagrophytes *infection.*

## TINEA MANUUM

Tinea manuum is a chronic dermatophytosis of the hand(s), often unilateral, most commonly on the dominant hand, and usually associated with tinea pedis.

### HISTORY

**Duration**    Months to years.
**Skin Symptoms**    Frequently symptomatic. Pruritus. Pain if secondarily infected or fissured. *Dyshidrotic type*: Episodic symptoms of pruritus.

### PHYSICAL EXAMINATION

**Skin Lesions**
Well-demarcated scaling patches, hyperkeratosis and scaling confined to palmar creases, fissures on palmar hand (Fig. 23-8). Borders well demarcated; central clearing. Often extends onto dorsum of hand with follicular papules, nodules, pustules with dermatophytic folliculitis.
***Dyshidrotic Type***    Papules, vesicles, bullae (uncommon on the margin of lesion) on palms and lateral fingers, similar to lesions of bullous tinea pedis.
***Secondary Changes***    Lichen simplex chronicus, prurigo nodules, impetiginization.
***Distribution***    Diffuse hyperkeratosis of the palms with pronounced involvement of palmar creases or patchy scaling on the dorsa and sides

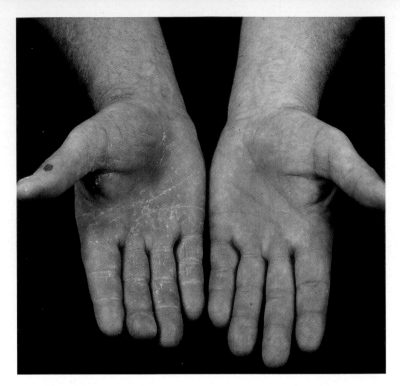

**FIGURE 23-8   Tinea manuum**   *Erythema and scaling of the right hand, which was associated with bilateral tinea pedum; the "one-hand, two-feet" distribution is typical of epidermal dermatophytosis of the hands and feet. In time, distal/lateral subungual onychomycosis occurs on the fingernails.*

of fingers; 50% of patients have unilateral involvement (Fig. 23-8). Usually associated with tinea pedis, tinea cruris. If chronic, often associated with tinea unguium of fingernails.

## DIFFERENTIAL DIAGNOSIS

**Erythema/Scaling Hands**   Atopic dermatitis, lichen simplex chronicus, allergic contact dermatitis, irritant contact dermatitis, psoriasis vulgaris, squamous cell carcinoma in situ.

## COURSE

Chronic, does not resolve spontaneously. After treatment, recurs unless onychomycosis of fingernails, feet, and toenails is eradicated. Fissures and erosions provide portal of entry for bacterial infections.

## MANAGEMENT

**Prevention**   Must eradicate tinea unguium of fingernails as well as toenails; also tinea pedis and tinea cruris, otherwise, tinea manuum will recur.

**Antifungal Agents**   *Topical*   See "Dermatophytoses," page 690. Failure common.

*Systemic*   Because of thickness of palmar stratum corneum, and especially if associated with tinea unguium of fingernails, tinea manuum is impossible to cure with topical agents. Oral agents eradicate dermatophytoses of hands, feet, and nails:

> *Terbinafine*: 250 mg qd for 14 days
> *Itraconzole*: 200 mg qd for 7 days
> *Fluconazole*: 150 to 200 mg qd for 2 to 4 weeks

> *Note*: Eradication of fingernail onychomycosis requires longer use.

## TINEA CRURIS  ■  ◑

Tinea cruris is a subacute or chronic dermatophytosis of the groin, pubic regions, and thighs. *Synonym*: "Jock itch."

### EPIDEMIOLOGY AND ETIOLOGY

**Age of Onset**   Adult.
**Sex**   Males > females.
**Etiology**   *T. rubrum*, *T. mentagrophytes*.
**Predisposing Factors**   Warm, humid environment: tight clothing worn by men; obesity. Chronic topical glucocorticoid application.

### HISTORY

**Duration**   Months to years. Often, history of long-standing tinea pedis and prior history of tinea cruris.

**Skin Symptoms**   Usually none. In some persons, pruritus causes patient to seek treatment.

### PHYSICAL EXAMINATION

#### Skin Lesions
Usually associated with tinea pedis, tinea unguium of toenails. Large, scaling, well-demarcated dull red/tan/brown plaques (Fig. 23-9). Central clearing. Papules, pustules may be present at margins. Treated lesions: lack scale; postinflammatory hyperpigmentation in darker-skinned persons. In atopics, chronic scratching

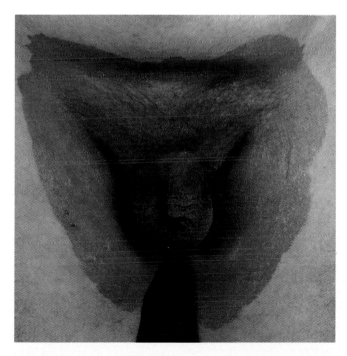

**FIGURE 23-9   Tinea cruris**   *Confluent, erythematous, scaling plaques on the medial thighs, inguinal folds, and pubic area. The margins are slightly raised and sharply marginated. Erythrasma should be ruled out by Wood's lamp examination.*

may produce secondary changes of lichen simplex chronicus.

***Distribution*** Groins and thighs (Fig. 23-9); may extend to buttocks. Scrotum and penis are rarely involved.

## DIFFERENTIAL DIAGNOSIS

**Erythema/Scaling in Groins** Erythrasma, intertrigo, *Candida* intertrigo, inverse-pattern psoriasis, pityriasis versicolor, Langerhans' cell histiocytosis.

## MANAGEMENT

**Prevention** After eradication of tinea cruris, tinea pedis, and tinea unguium, reinfection can be minimized by wearing shower shoes when using a public or home (if family members are infected) bathing facility; using antifungal powders; benzoyl peroxide wash.

**Antifungal Agents** *Topical* See "Dermatophytoses," page 690.

*Systemic* If recurrent, if dermatophytic folliculitis is present, or if it has failed to respond to adequate topical therapy. See "Tinea Manuum."

---

## TINEA CORPORIS

---

Tinea corporis refers to dermatophyte infections of the trunk, legs, arms, and/or neck, excluding the feet, hands, and groin.

## EPIDEMIOLOGY AND ETIOLOGY

**Age of Onset** All ages.

**Occupation** Animal (large and small) workers.

**Etiology** *T. rubrum* most commonly: *M. canis*. *T. tonsurans* in parents of black children with tinea capitis.

**Transmission** Autoinoculation from other parts of the body, i.e., from tinea pedis and tinea capitis. Contact with animals or contaminated soil.

**Geography** More common in tropical and subtropical regions.

**Predisposing Factors** Most commonly, infection is spread from dermatophytic infection of the feet (*T. rubrum*, *T. mentagrophytes*). Infection can also be acquired from an active lesion of an animal (*T. verrucosum*, *M. canis*) or rarely, from soil (*M. gypseum*).

## HISTORY

**Incubation Period** Days to months.

**Duration** Weeks to months to years.

**Symptoms** Often asymptomatic. Mild pruritus.

## PHYSICAL EXAMINATION

### Skin Lesions

Small (Figs. 23-10, 23-11) to large (Fig. 23-12), scaling, sharply marginated plaques with or without pustules or vesicles, usually at margins. Peripheral enlargement and central clearing (Fig. 23-11) produces annular configuration with concentric rings or arcuate lesions; fusion of lesions produces gyrate patterns. Single and occasionally scattered multiple lesions. Bullae. Granulomatous lesions (Majocchi's granuloma). Psoriasiform plaques (Fig 23-12). Verrucous lesions. Lesions of zoophilic infection (contracted from animals) are more inflammatory, with marked vesiculation and crusting at margins, bullae.

## DIFFERENTIAL DIAGNOSIS

**Well-Demarcated Scaling Plaque(s)** Allergic contact dermatitis, atopic dermatitis, annular erythemas, psoriasis, seborrheic dermatitis, pityriasis rosea, pityriasis alba, pityriasis versicolor, erythema migrans, subacute lupus erythematosus, mycosis fungoides.

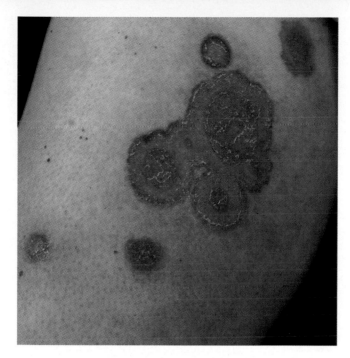

**FIGURE 23-10    Tinea corporis** *Inflammatory annular plaques, becoming confluent on the medial thigh. This type of inflammatory lesion is seen with zoophilic dermatophytic infection and with topical glucocorticoid use.*

## LABORATORY EXAMINATIONS

See "Direct Microscopy," page 689, and culture.

## MANAGEMENT

**Antifungal Agents**    See "Dermatophytoses," page 690, for topical therapy. See "Tinea Manuum," page 698, for systemic antifungal therapy.

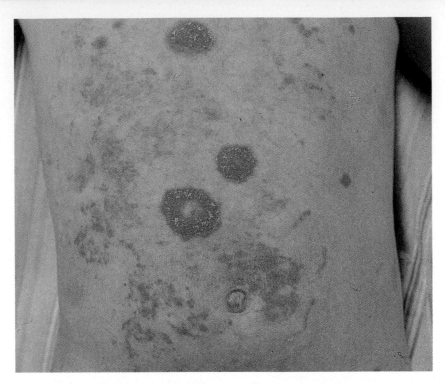

**FIGURE 23-11    Tinea corporis: acute and subacute**   *Multiple, bright red, sharply marginated lesions with only minimal scaling of several weeks' duration on the trunk of a child. Three lesions are more inflammatory and thicker.* Microsporum canis *was isolated on fungal culture, which had been contracted from a pet guinea pig.*

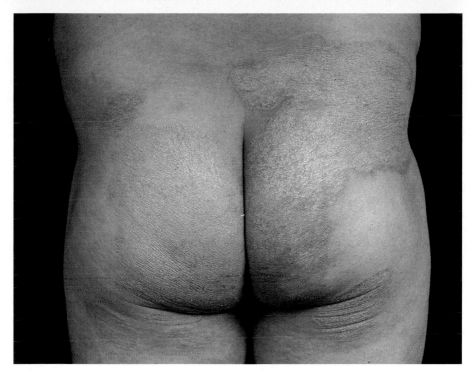

**FIGURE 23-12   Tinea corporis: chronic**   *Sharply marginated, hyperpigmented plaques of many months' duration on the back, buttocks, and thighs. The lesions have a psoriasiform appearance. Associated tinea cruris and tinea pedis are usually present.*

## TINEA FACIALIS

Tinea facialis is dermatophytosis of the glabrous facial skin, characterized by a well-circum-scribed erythematous patch; it is more commonly misdiagnosed than any other dermatophy-tosis.
*Synonym*: Tinea faciei.

## EPIDEMIOLOGY AND ETIOLOGY

**Age of Onset**   More common in children.
**Etiology**   *T. tonsurans* associated with tinea capitis in black children and their parents. *T. mentagrophytes*, *T. rubrum* most commonly; also *M. audouinii*, *M. canis*.
**Predisposing Factors**   Animal exposure, chronic topical application of glucocorticoids.

## HISTORY

**Skin Symptoms**   Most commonly asymptomatic. At times, pruritus and photosensitivity.

## PHYSICAL EXAMINATION

### Skin Lesions
Well-circumscribed macule to plaque of variable size; elevated border and central regression (Fig. 23-13). Scaling is often minimal (Fig. 23-14) but can be pronounced. Pink to red. In black patients, hyperpigmentation. Any area of face but usually not symmetric.

## DIFFERENTIAL DIAGNOSIS

**Scaling Facial Patches**   Seborrheic dermatitis, contact dermatitis, erythema migrans, lupus erythematosus, polymorphous light eruption, phototoxic drug eruption, lymphocytic infiltrate.

## LABORATORY EXAMINATIONS

See "Dermatophytoses," page 689 and culture.

## MANAGEMENT

**Antifungal Agents**   See "Dermatophytoses," page 690, for topical therapy. See "Tinea Manuum,'" page 698, for systemic antifungal therapy.

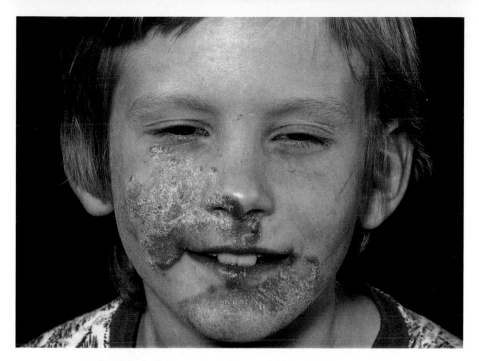

**FIGURE 23-13   Tinea facialis**   *Sharply marginated, erythematous, scaling, and crusted plaques on the face of a child. Note asymmetry.*

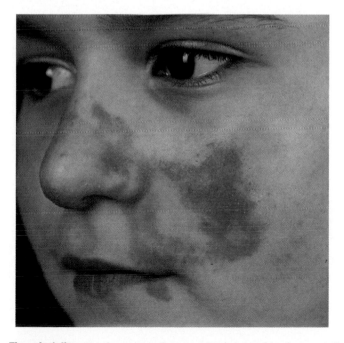

**FIGURE 23-14   Tinea facialis**   *Erythematous plaque with a geographic shape; scaling is minimal but adequate for KOH preparation.*

## TINEA INCOGNITO

Tinea incognito is an epidermal dermatophytosis, often associated with dermatophytic folliculitis, that occurs after the topical application of a glucocorticoid preparation to a site colonized or infected with dermatophyte. It usually occurs when an inflammatory dermatophytosis is mistaken for psoriasis or an eczematous dermatitis (Fig. 23-15). Lesions are usually aymptomatic but may be very pruritic or even painful. Involved sites often have exaggerated features of epidermal dermatophytoses, being a deep red or violaceous with follicular papules or pustules. Epidermal atrophy caused by chronic glucocorticoid application may be present. Systemic antifungal therapy may be indicated due to deep involvement of the hair apparatus.

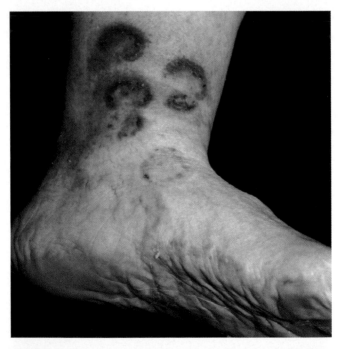

**FIGURE 23-15    Tinea incognito**   *Arcuate red plaques on the medial ankle in a patient who had applied a fluorinated glucocorticoid cream. Moccasin-type tinea pedis is apparent on the plantar foot.*

# DERMATOPHYTOSES OF HAIR

Dermatophytes are capable of invading hair follicles and hair shafts, causing dermatophytic trichomycosis (tinea capitis, tinea barbae, and dermatophytic folliculitis). Two types of hair involvement are seen (Image 23-2).

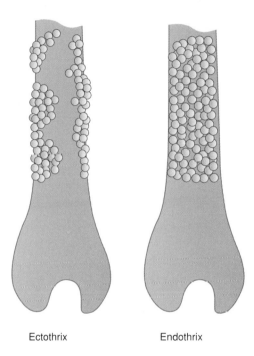

**IMAGE 23-2   Dermatophytic folliculitis.**
*Ectothrix type: mycelia and arthroconidia are seen on the surface of the hair follicle (extrapilary). Endothrix type: hyphae and arthroconidia occur within the hair shaft (intrapilary)*

Ectothrix                    Endothrix

## TINEA CAPITIS

Tinea capitis, predominantly a disease of preadolescent children, is a dermatophytic trichomycosis of the scalp. Clinical presentations vary widely, ranging from mild scaling and broken-off hairs to severe, painful inflammation with painful, boggy nodules that drain pus and result in scarring alopecia.
*Synonyms*: Ringworm of the scalp, tinea tonsurans.

### EPIDEMIOLOGY AND ETIOLOGY

**Age of Onset**   Toddlers and school-age children. Most common at 6 to 10 years of age; less common after age 16. In adults it occurs most commonly in a rural setting.
**Race**   Much more common in blacks than in whites.

**Etiology/demography**   Varies from country to country and from region to region; species change in time due to immigration. Infections can become epidemic in schools and institutions, especially with overcrowding. Random fungal cultures in urban study revealed a 4% positive rate and a 12.7% positive rate among black children.

*United States and Western Europe* 90% of cases of tinea capitis caused by *T. tonsurans*; less commonly, *M. canis*. Formerly, most cases were caused by *M. audouinii*. Less commonly, *M. gypseum*, *T. mentagrophytes*, *T. rubrum*.

*Eastern and Southern Europe, North Africa* *T. violaceum*.

**Transmission**   Person-to-person, animal-to-person, via fomites. Spores are present on asymptomatic carriers, animals, or inanimate objects.

**Risk Factors**   For favus (see below): debilitation, malnutrition, chronic disease.

## CLASSIFICATION

**Ectothrix Infection**   Invasion occurs outside hair shaft. Hyphae fragment into arthroconidia, leading to cuticle destruction. Caused by *Microsporum* spp. (*M. audouinii* and *M. canis*) (Image 23-2).

**Endothrix Infection**   Infection occurs within hair shaft without cuticle destruction (Image 23-2). Arthroconidia found within hair shaft. Caused by *Trichophyton* spp. (*T. tonsurans* in North America; *T. violaceum* in Europe, Asia, parts of Africa).

*"Black Dot" Tinea Capitis*   Variant of endothrix resembling seborrheic dermatitis.

*Kerion*   Variant of endothrix with boggy inflammatory plaques.

*Favus*   Variant of endothrix with arthroconidia and airspaces within hair shaft. Very uncommon in western Europe and North America. In some parts of the world (Middle East, South Africa), however, it is still endemic.

## PATHOGENESIS

**Noninflammatory Lesions**   Invasion of hair shaft by the dermatophytes, principally *M. audouinii* (child-to-child, via barber, hats, theater seats), *M. canis* (young pets-to-child and then child-to-child), or *T. tonsurans*. Inflammatory lesions: *T tonsurans*, *M. canis*, *T. verrucosum*, and others. Spores enter through breaks in hair shaft or scalp to cause clinical infection. Scalp hair traps fungi from the environment or fomites. Asymptomatic colonization is common. Trauma assists inoculation. Dermatophytes initially invade stratum corneum of scalp, which may be followed by hair shaft infection. Spread to other hair follicles then occurs. Eventually, infection regresses with or without an inflammatory response. Clinical appearance varies with type of hair invasion, level of host resistance, degree of inflammatory host

response: few dull gray, broken-off hairs with little scaling to severe painful inflammatory mass covering entire scalp. Partial hair loss with inflammation in all cases. Kerion is associated with a high degree of hypersensitivity to fungal hapten. Two types of hair invasion:

- *Microsporum* types: (1) Small-spored ectothrix; hair shaft is invaded in mid-follicle. Intrapilary hyphae grow inward toward hair bulb. Secondary extrapilary hyphae burst, growing over surface of hair shaft. (2) Large-spored ectothrix have similar arrangement.
- *Trichophyton* types: (1) Large-spored ectothrix (in chains); arthrospores spherical, arranged in straight chains, confined to external surface of hair shaft. Spores are all larger than those of small-spored *Microsporum* ectothrix. (2) Entothrix type; intrapilary hyphae fragment into arthroconidia within hair shaft, making it fragile, with subsequent breakage close to scalp surface.

## HISTORY

**Duration of Lesions**   Weeks to months.

**Skin Symptoms**   In patients with inflammatory tinea capitis, pain, tenderness, and/or alopecia. With noninflammatory infection, scaling, scalp pruritus, diffuse or circumscribed alopecia, or occipital or posterior auricular adenopathy.

## PHYSICAL EXAMINATION

Skin lesions and Hair Changes

*Small-Spored Ectothrix Tinea Capitis*   "Gray patch" tinea capitis (Fig. 23-16). Partial alopecia, often circular in shape, showing numerous broken-off hairs, dull gray from their coating of arthrospores. Inflammation minimal. Fine scaling with fairly sharp margin. Hair shaft becomes brittle, breaking off at or slightly above scalp. Small patches coalesce, forming larger patches. Inflammatory response minimal, but massive scaling. Several or many patches, randomly arranged may be present. *M. audouinii*, *M. ferrugineum*, *M. canis* infections show green fluorescence with Wood's lamp.

*Endothrix Tinea Capitis*

   *"Black dot" tinea capitis:* Broken-off hairs near surface give appearance of "dots" (Fig. 23-17) (swollen hair shafts) in dark-haired patients. Dots occur as affected hair breaks at surface of scalp. Tends to be diffuse and poorly circumscribed. Low-grade

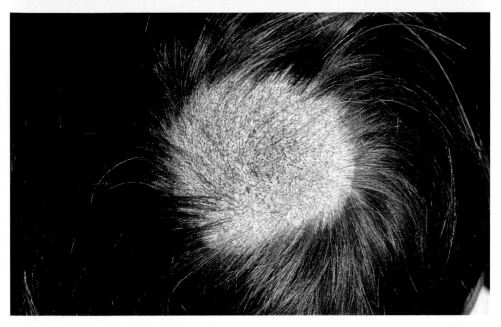

**FIGURE 23-16   Tinea capitis: "gray patch" type**   *A large, round, hyperkeratotic plaque of alopecia due to breaking off of hair shafts close to the surface, giving the appearance of a mowed wheat field on the scalp of a child. Remaining hair shafts and scales exhibit a green fluorescence when examined with a Wood's lamp.* Microsporum canis *was isolated on culture.*

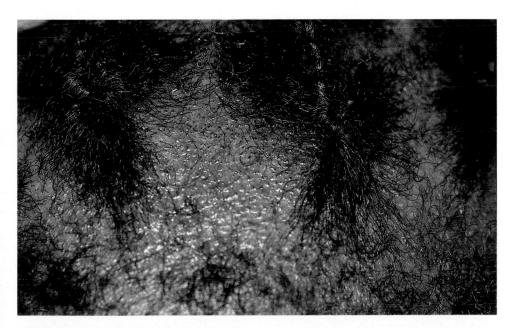

**FIGURE 23-17   Tinea capitis: "black dot" variant**   *A subtle, asymptomatic patch of alopecia due to breaking off of hairs on the frontal scalp in a 4-year-old black child. The lesion was detected because her infant sister presented with tinea corporis.* Trichophyton tonsurans *was isolated on culture.*

folliculitis may be present. Resembles seborrheic dermatitis, chronic cutaneous lupus erythematosus. Usually caused by *T. tonsurans, T. violaceum.* Onychomycosis also occurs in 2 to 3% of cases.

*Kerion*: Inflammatory mass in which remaining hairs are loose. Characterized by boggy, purulent, inflamed nodules and plaques (Fig. 23-18). Usually extremely painful; drains pus from multiple openings, like honeycomb. Hairs do not break off but fall out and can be pulled without pain. Follicles may discharge pus; sinus formation; mycetoma–like grains. Thick crusting with matting of adjacent hairs. A single plaque is usual, but multiple lesions may occur with involvement of entire scalp. Frequently, associated lymphadenopathy is present. Usually caused by zoophilic (*T. verrucosum, T. mentagrophytes* var. *mentagrophytes*) or geophilic species. Heals with scarring alopecia.

*Agminate folliculitis*: Less severe inflammation than kerion with sharply defined, dull red plaques studded with follicular pustules. Caused by zoophilic species.

*Favus*: Early cases show perifollicular erythema and matting of hair. Later, thick yellow adherent crusts (scutula) composed of skin debris and hyphae that are pierced by remaining hair shafts (Fig. 23-19). Fetid odor. In treatment, cutaneous atrophy, scar formation, and scarring alopecia. Caused by *T. schoenleinii.* Shows little tendency to clear spontaneously.

## DIFFERENTIAL DIAGNOSIS

**"Gray Patch" Tinea Capitis**  Seborrheic dermatitis, psoriasis, atopic dermatitis, lichen simplex chronicus, alopecia areata.

**"Black Dot" Tinea Capitis**  Seborrheic dermatitis, psoriasis, seborrhiasis, atopic dermatitis, lichen simplex chronicus, chronic cutaneous lupus erythematosus, alopecia areata.

**Kerion**  Cellulitis, furuncle, carbuncle.

**Favus**  Impetigo, ecthyma, crusted scabies.

## LABORATORY EXAMINATIONS

**Wood's Lamp**  Should be performed in any patient with scaling scalp lesions or hair loss of undetermined origin. *T. tonsurans*, the most common cause of tinea capitis in the United States, does not fluoresce. *M. canis* and *M. audouinii*, which previously were the most common causes of tinea capitis, could be diagnosed by Wood's lamp examination, by bright green hair shafts with ectothrix infection.

**Direct Microscopy**  Specimens should include hair roots and skin scales. Pluck hairs and use toothbrush to gather specimens. Skin scales contain hyphae and arthrospores. *Ectothrix*: arthrospores can be seen surrounding the hair shaft in cuticle. *Endothrix*: spores within hair shaft. *Favus*: loose chains of arthrospores and airspaces in hair shaft.

**Fungal Culture**  With brush-culture technique, a dry toothbrush or brush used for cervical Pap testing is rubbed over area of scale or alopecia; bristles are then inoculated into fungal medium. A wet cotton swab can also be rubbed in affected area, which is then implanted into medium. The cotton-tipped swab from a bacterial culturette, moistened with tap water, can also be used to collect the specimen and sent to a commercial laboratory. Growth of dermatophytes usually seen in 10 to 14 days.

*Endothrix  T. tonsurans, T. violaceum, T. soudanense,* and *T. schoenleinii.*

*Ectothrix  Microsporum* spp., *T. mentagrophytes, T. verrucosum.*

*Favus  T. schoenleinii,* most commonly; also *T. violaceum, M. gypseum.*

**Bacterial Culture**  Rule out bacterial superinfection, usually *S. aureus* or group A streptococcus.

**FIGURE 23-19 (Opposite page, bottom)  Tinea capitis: favus** *Extensive hair loss with atrophy, scarring, and so-called scutula, i.e., yellowish adherent crusts present on the scalp; remaining hairs pierce the scutula.* Trichophyton schoenleinii *was isolated on culture.*

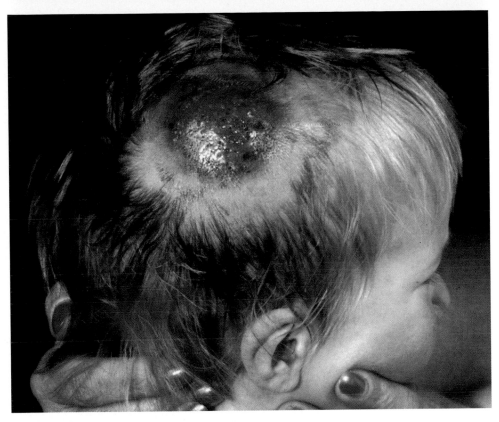

**FIGURE 23-18  Kerion**  *An extremely painful, boggy, purulent inflammatory nodule on the scalp of this 4-year-old child. The lesion drains pus from multiple openings and there is retroauricular, tender lymphadenopathy. Infection was due to* T. verrucosum *contracted from an infected rabbit.*

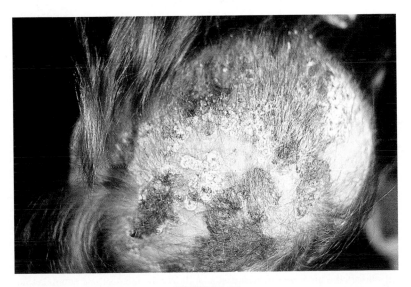

**FIGURE 23-19**

## MANAGEMENT

| | |
|---|---|
| **Prevention** | Important to examine home and school contacts of affected children for asymptomatic carriers and mild cases of tinea capitis. Ketoconazole or selenium sulfide shampoo may be helpful in eradicating the asymptomatic carrier state. |
| **Topical antifungal agents** | Topical agents are ineffective in management of tinea capitis. Duration of treatment should be extended until symptoms have resolved and fungal cultures negative. |
| **Oral antifungal agents** | Griseofulvin is considered the drug of choice in the United States. Short-term terbinafine, itraconazole, and fluconazole have been shown to be comparable in efficacy and safety to griseofulvin. |
| Griseofulvin | **Pediatric Dose**<br>• Microsized: 15 mg/kg per day; maximum 500 mg/d<br>• Ultramicrosized: 10 mg/kg per day<br>Treatment duration: at least 6 weeks to several months; better absorption with fatty meal.<br>**Adult Dose**<br>• "Gray patch" tinea capitis: 250 mg bid for 1 or 2 months<br>• "Black dot" tinea capitis: longer treatment and higher doses continued until KOH and cultures are negative<br>*For kerion*:<br>250 mg bid for 4–8 weeks, hot compresses; antibiotics for accompanying staphylococcal infection |
| Terbinafine | 250 mg qd. Reduce dosing according to weight in pediatric patients. |
| Itraconazole | 100-mg capsules or oral solution (10 mg/mL). Treatment duration: 4 to 8 weeks.<br>**Pediatric Dose** 5 mg/kg per day<br>**Adult Dose** 200 mg/d |
| Fluconazole | 100-, 150-, 200-mg tablets; oral solution (10 mg/mL, 40 mg/mL). 6–8 mg/kg per day. Treatment duration: 3–4 weeks (in some cases 2).<br>**Pediatric Dose** 6 mg/kg per day<br>Daily for 2 weeks; repeat at 4 weeks if indicated<br>**Adult Dose** 200 mg/d |
| Ketoconazole | 200-mg tablets. Treatment duration: 4–6 weeks.<br>**Pediatric Dose** 5 mg/kg per day<br>**Adult Dose** 200–400 mg/d |
| **Adjunctive therapy** | |
| Prednisone | 1 mg/kg per day for 14 days for children with severe, painful kerion. |
| Systemic antibiotics | For secondary *S. aureus* or group A streptococcus infection, erythromycin, dicloxacillin, or cephalexin |
| **Surgery** | Drain pus from kerion lesions. |

## COURSE

Chronic untreated kerion and favus, especially if secondarily infected with *S. aureus*, result in scarring alopecia. Regrowth of hair is the rule if treated with systemic antifungal agents. Favus may persist until adulthood. Radiotherapy was used to treat tinea capitis in the 1930s and 1940s; the incidence of nonmelanoma skin cancer is increased fourfold in these individuals.

## TINEA BARBAE  □  ◐

Tinea barbae is a dermatophytic trichomycosis involving the beard and moustache areas, closely resembling tinea capitis, with invasion of the hair shaft.
*Synonym*: Ringworm of the beard.

### EPIDEMIOLOGY AND ETIOLOGY

**Age of Onset**   Adult.
**Sex**   Males only.
**Etiology**   *T. verrucosum, T. mentagrophytes* var. *mentagrophytes*, most commonly. May be acquired through animal exposure. *T. rubrum* an uncommon cause.
**Predisposing Factors**   More common in farmers.

### HISTORY

**Skin Symptoms**   Pruritus, tenderness, pain.

### PHYSICAL EXAMINATION

**Skin Lesions**
Pustular folliculitis (Fig. 23-20), i.e., hair follicles surrounded by red inflammatory papules or pustules, often with exudation and crusting. Involved hairs are loose and easily removed. With less follicular involvement, there are scaling, circular, reddish patches in which hair is broken off at the surface. Papules may coalesce to inflammatory plaques topped by pustules. Kerion: boggy purulent nodules and plaques as with tinea capitis (Fig. 23-21). Beard and moustache areas, rarely, eyelashes, eyebrows.
**Systemic Findings**   Regional lymphadenopathy, especially if of long duration and if superinfected.

### DIFFERENTIAL DIAGNOSIS

**Beard Folliculitis**   *S. aureus* folliculitis, furuncle, carbuncle, acne vulgaris, rosacea, pseudofolliculitis.

### LABORATORY EXAMINATIONS

See "Tinea Capitis," page 710.

### MANAGEMENT

**Topical Agents**   Ineffective.
**Systemic Agents**   See "Tinea Capitis," page 712.

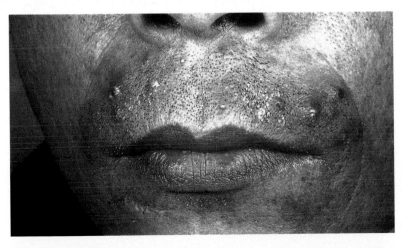

**FIGURE 23-20   Tinea barbae**   *Scattered, discrete follicular pustules and papules in the moustache area, easily mistaken for* S. aureus *folliculitis.*

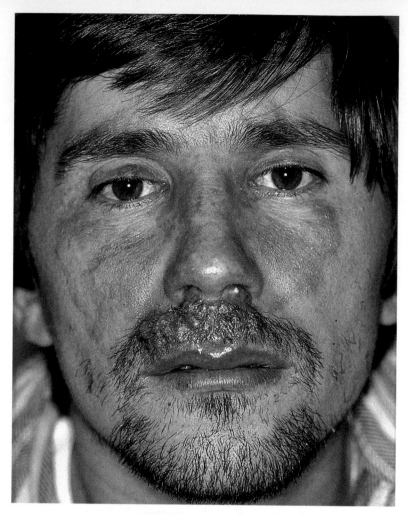

**FIGURE 23-21   Tinea barbae and tinea facialis**   *Confluent, painful papules, nodules, and pustules on the upper lip. Epidermal dermatophytosis (tinea facialis) with sharply marginated erythema and scaling is present on the cheeks, eyelids, eyebrows, and forehead.* Trichophyton mentagro-phytes *was isolated on culture. In this case, the organism caused two distinct clinical patterns (epidermal involvement, tinea facialis versus follicular inflammation, tinea barbae), depending on whether glabrous skin or hairy skin was infected. (See also Image 23-1.)*

## DERMATOPHYTIC FOLLICULITIS

See "Infectious Folliculitis" in Section 29.

## MAJOCCHI'S GRANULOMA ■ ◐

Majocchi's granuloma (MG) (dermatophytic granuloma) is a dermatophytic folliculitis, with foreign-body granuloma occurring in response to dermatophytes in the dermis, especially in the immunocompromised host. Clinically, folliculocentric papules and pustules arise within an area of epidermal dermatophytosis such as tinea incognito (Fig. 23-22).

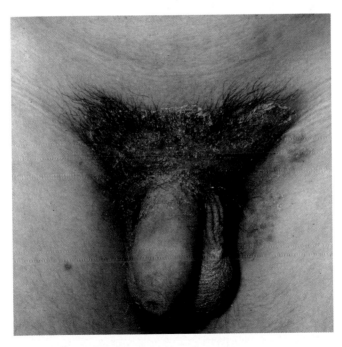

**FIGURE 23-22  Dermatophytic folliculitis: Majocchi's granuloma**  *Epidermal dermatophytosis of the pubic and inguinal area with inflammatory nodules associated with infection of the hair follicle.*

# CANDIDIASIS

Candidiasis is most frequently caused by the yeast *Candida albicans*, and less often by other *Candida* spp. Superficial infections of mucosal surface (oropharynx, genitalia) are common in otherwise healthy individuals; infections of the esophagus and/or tracheobronchial tree occur in the setting of significant immunocompromise. Cutaneous candidiasis occurs at moist occluded skin. Acute candidemia occurs in immunocompromised individuals, usually after invasion of the gastrointestinal tract or from intravenous catheters.
*Synonyms*: Candidosis, moniliasis.

## EPIDEMIOLOGY AND ETIOLOGY

**Etiology**    *C. albicans*, an oval yeast varying in size (2 to 6 μm by 3 to 9 μm). Polymorphism is displayed as yeast forms, budding yeast, pseudohyphae, and true hyphae. Besides *C. albicans*, >100 species of the genus have been identified, most of which are neither commensal nor pathogenic for humans. Other pathogenic species, usually in the setting of immunocompromise, include: *C. tropicalis*, *C. parapsilosis*, *C. guilliermondii*, *C. krusei*, *C. pseudotropicalis*, *C. lusitaneae*, *C. glabrata*.
**Ecology**    *C. albicans* and other species frequently colonize the gastrointestinal (GI) tract. Colonization may occur during birthing from the birth canal, during infancy, or later. Oropharyngeal colonization is present in approximately 20% of healthy individuals, the rate being higher in hospitalized patients. Fecal colonization is higher than oral, with a rate of 40 to 67%; the rate increases after treatment with antibacterial agents. Serologic and skin test studies indicate that a significant proportion of those not colonized have been exposed to *Candida* in the past. Antibiotic therapy increases the incidence of carriage, the number of organisms present, and the chances for tissue invasion. Approximately 13% of women are colonized vaginally with *C. albicans*; antibiotic therapy, pregnancy, oral contraception, and intrauterine devices increase the incidence of carriage. *C. albicans* may transiently colonize the skin but is not one of the permanent flora and is seldom recovered from skin of normal individuals. Usually endogenous infection. With balanitis, *Candida* may be transmitted from sexual partner.
**Age of Onset**    The young and old are more likely to be colonized.
**Host Factors**    Immunocompromise, diabetes mellitus, obesity, hyperhidrosis, heat, maceration, polyendocrinopathies, systemic and topical glucocorticoids, chronic debilitation.
**Immunologic Factors**    Reduced cell-mediated immunity is the most significant factor. Decreased specific anti-*Candida* IgA salivary antibody may be a factor. Defects in neutrophil or macrophage functions are factors in invasive candidiasis.

## LABORATORY EXAMINATIONS

**Direct Microscopy**    KOH preparation visualizes pseudohyphae and yeast forms (Fig. 23-23).
**Culture**    *Fungal* Identifies species of *Candida*; however, the presence in culture of *C. albicans* does not make the diagnosis of candidiasis; *Candida* is a normal inhabitant of the GI tract. Identifying *Candida* in the absence of symptoms should not lead to treatment, because 10 to 20% of normal women harbor *Candida* spp. and other yeasts in the vagina. Sensitivities to antifungal agents can be performed on isolate in cases of recurrent infection.
*Bacterial* Rule out bacterial superinfection.

## CLASSIFICATION

See Table 23-1

## MANAGEMENT

**Oral Antifungal Agents**    Indicated for infections resistant to topical modalities of therapy.
*Fluconazole* Tablets: 50, 100, 150, 200 mg. Oral suspension: 50 mg/5 mL. Parenteral: for injection or IV infusion.
*Itraconazole* Capsules: 100 mg. Oral solution: 10 mg/mL.
*Ketoconazole* Tablets: 200 mg.

**TABLE 23-1    Classification of Candidiasis**

| Type | Site | Clinical presentation |
|---|---|---|
| Occluded site (where occlusion and maceration create warm, moist microecology) | Body folds | Axillae, inframammary, groin, intergluteal, abdominal panniculus<br>Webspace: hands (erosio interdigitale blastomycetica), feet<br>Angular cheilitis; often associated with oropharyhgeal candidiasis |
| | Genital | Balanitis, balanoposthitis<br>Vulvitis, vulvovaginitis |
| | Occluded skin | Under occlusive dressing, under cast, back in hospitalized patient |
| | Folliculitis | Back; in hospitalized patient |
| | Area occluded under diaper | Diaper dermatitis |
| Nail apparatus | Paronychium | Chronic paronychia |
| | Nail plate | Onychia |
| | Hyponychium | Onycholysis |
| Chronic mucocutaneous | Extensive, multiple or 20 nail | Individuals with congenital immunologic (T cell defects) or endocrinologic disorders (hypoparathyroidism, hypoadrenalism, hypothyroidism, diabetes mellitus) develop persistent or recurrent mucosal, cutaneous, and/or paronychial/ nail infections. |
| Genitalia | Vulva, vagina; preputial sac | Erythema, erosions, white plaques of candidal colonies |
| Mucosal | Oropharynx | Thrush; atrophic candidiasis; hyperplastic candidiasis |
| | Esophagus | Inflamed, eroded plaques |
| | Trachea, bronchi | Inflamed, eroded plaques |
| Candidemia | Skin, viscera | Skin: erythematous papules, ± hemorrhage |

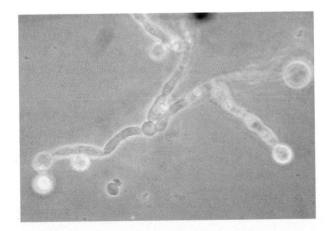

**FIGURE 23-23   *Candida albicans*: KOH preparation** *Budding yeast forms and sausage-like pseudohyphal forms.*

## CUTANEOUS CANDIDIASIS

Cutaneous candidiasis occurs in moist, occluded cutaneous sites; many patients have predisposing factors.

## HISTORY

**Intertrigo**   Erythema. Pruritus, tenderness, pain.
**Occluded Skin**   Under occlusive dressing, under cast, on back in hospitalized patient.
**Diaper Dermatitis**   Irritability, discomfort with urination, defecation, changing diapers.

## PHYSICAL EXAMINATION

### Skin Lesions
**Intertrigo**   Initial pustules on erythematous base become eroded and confluent. Subsequently, fairly sharply demarcated, polycyclic, erythematous, eroded patches with small pustular lesions at the periphery (satellite pustulosis).
*Distribution*   Inframammary (Fig. 23-24), axillae, groins (Fig. 23-25), perineal, intergluteal cleft (Fig. 23-26).
**Interdigital**   Erosio interdigitalis blastomycetica. Initial pustule becomes eroded, with formation of superficial erosion or fissure, surrounded by thickened white skin (Fig. 23-27). May be associated with *Candida* onychia or paronychia.
*Distribution*   On hands, usually between third and fourth fingers (Fig. 23-27); on feet, similar presentation as interdigital tinea pedis.
**Diaper Dermatitis**   Erythema, edema with papular and pustular lesions; erosions, oozing, collarette-like scaling at the margins of lesions

involving perigenital and perianal skin, inner aspects of thighs and buttocks (Fig. 23-28).
**Follicular Candidiasis**   Small, discrete pustules in ostia of hair follicles.

## DIFFERENTIAL DIAGNOSIS

**Intertrigo/Occluded Skin**   Nonspecific intertrigo, streptococcal intertrigo, inverse pattern psoriasis, erythrasma, dermatophytosis, pityriasis versicolor.
**Diaper Dermatitis**   Atopic dermatitis, psoriasis, irritant dermatitis, seborrheic dermatitis.
**Folliculitis**   Bacterial (*S. aureus, P. aeruginosa*) folliculitis, *Pityrosporum* folliculitis, acne.

## LABORATORY EXAMINATIONS

See "Candidiasis," page 716.

## DIAGNOSIS

Clinical findings confirmed by direct microscopy or culture.

## MANAGEMENT

See Table 23-2.

**FIGURE 23-25 (Left)   Cutaneous candidiasis: intertrigo**   *Erythematous papules with a few pustules, becoming confluent on the medial thigh. The lesions occurred during a holiday trip to the Caribbean.*

**FIGURE 23-26 (Right)   Cutaneous candidiasis: intertrigo**   *Vesicles, pustules, and papules becoming confluent on the perineum and perianal area. The patient had successfully undergone a bone marrow transplantation 4 weeks before the appearance of the cutaneous lesions. The initial impression by the oncologist was that the lesions were reactivated herpes simplex; KOH preparation and cultures confirmed the diagnosis of* Candida *intertrigo.*

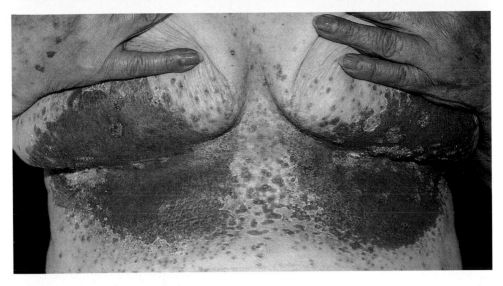

**FIGURE 23-24   Cutaneous candidiasis: intertrigo**   *Small peripheral "satellite" papules and pustules that have become confluent centrally, creating a large eroded area in the submammary region.*

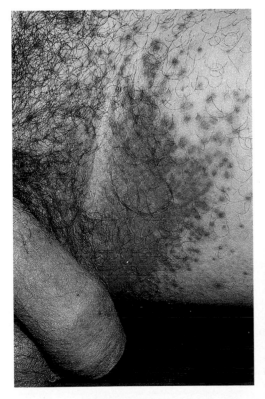

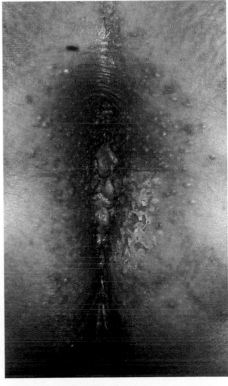

**FIGURE 23-25**

**FIGURE 23-26**

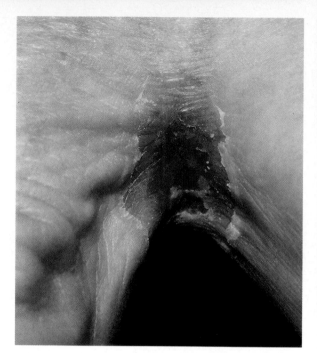

**FIGURE 23-27    Cutaneous candidiasis: interdigital intertrigo**    *Erythematous eroded webspace of the hand; several other webspaces were also involved in this elderly, obese, diabetic female.*

**TABLE 23-2    Management of Cutaneous Candidiasis**

| | |
|---|---|
| **Prevention** | Keep intertriginous areas dry (often difficult). |
| | Washing with benzoyl peroxide bar may reduce *Candida* colonization. |
| | Powder with miconazole applied daily. |
| **Topical treatment** | |
| Castellani's paint | Brings almost immediate relief of symptoms, i.e., candidal paronychia. |
| Glucocorticoid preparation | Judicious short-term use speeds resolution of symptoms. |
| **Topical antifungal agents** | Antifungal preparation: Nystatin, azole, or imidazole cream bid or more often with diaper dermatitis. Tolnaftate not effective for candidiasis. Terbinafine may be effective. |
| Nystatin cream | Effective for *Candida* only; not effective for dermatophytosis. |
| Azole creams | Effective for candidiasis, dermatophytosis, and pityriasis versicolor. |
| **Oral antifungal agents** | Eliminate bowel colonization. Azoles treat cutaneous infection. |
| Nystatin (suspension, tablet, pastille) | Not absorbed from the bowel. Eradicates bowel colonization. May be effective in recurrent candidiasis of diaper area, genitals, or intertrigo. |
| **Systemic antifungal, agents** | See Candidiasis, page 716. |

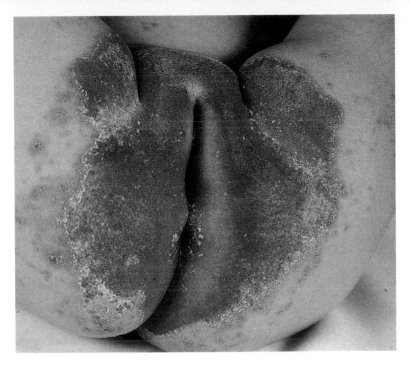

**FIGURE 23-28    Candidiasis: diaper dermatitis** *Confluent erosions, marginal scaling, and "satel-lite pustules" in the area covered by a diaper in an infant. Atopic dermatitis or psoriasis also occurs in this distribution and may be concomitant.*

## OROPHARYNGEAL CANDIDIASIS

Candidiasis of the oropharyngeal mucosa (OPC) occurs with minor variations of host factors such as antibiotic therapy, glucocorticoid therapy (topical or systemic), age (very young, very old) as well as with significant immunocompromise. Esophageal and/or tracheobronchial candidiasis may be associated with OPC and always occurs in the setting of advanced immunocompromise. *Candida* can invade through eroded mucosa, with resultant candidemia.

### EPIDEMIOLOGY AND ETIOLOGY

**Etiology**    *C. albicans*, one of the resident flora of the mouth, overgrows in association with various local or systemic factors. In some cases, an exogenous infection. After chronic antifungal therapy, especially with advanced immunocompromise, fluconazole-resistant strains of *Candida* spp. can evolve and cause infection resistant to oral/intravenous azole therapy.

**Incidence**    Although a number of risk factors exist (see below) and almost obligatory involvement occurs in immunocompromised patients, the vast majority of mucosal candidiasis occurs in otherwise healthy individuals.

*HIV Disease* OPC occurs in 50% of HIV-infected patients and 80 to 95% of those with AIDS: 60% relapse within 3 months after treatment. Esophageal candidiasis occurs in 10 to 15% of individuals with AIDS.

*Bone Marrow Transplant Recipients* 30 to 40% develop superficial mucosal candidiasis; occurs in otherwise healthy individuals.

**CDC Surveillance Case Definition for AIDS** Candidiasis of the esophagus, trachea, bronchi, or lungs is an AIDS-defining condition if the patient has no other cause of immunodeficiency and is without knowledge of HIV antibody status.

## CLASSIFICATION

**Superficial Mucosal Candidiasis** May be associated with mild to moderate impairment of cell-mediated immunity.

*Oropharyngeal Candidiasis* Pseudomembranous candidiasis (thrush); erythematous (atrophic) candidiasis; candidal leukoplakia (hyperplastic candidiasis); angular cheilitis.

**Deep Mucosal Candidiasis** Occurs in states of advanced immunocompromise: esophageal candidiasis, tracheobronchial candidiasis, both of which are AIDS-defining conditions. Bladder.

## HISTORY

**Symptoms** *Oropharynx* Asymptomatic. Burning or pain on eating spices/acidic foods, diminished taste sensation. Cosmetic concern about white curds on tongue. Odynophagia. In HIV disease, may be the initial presentation; OPC is a clinical marker for disease progression, first noted when CD4+ cell count is 390/μL.

*Esophagus* Asymptomatic. Occurs when CD4+ cell count is low (<200/μL) and is an AIDS-defining condition. Dysphagia. Odynophagia, resulting in difficulty eating and malnutrition.

## PHYSICAL EXAMINATION

### Mucosal Lesions

**Type** *Pseudomembranous Candidiasis (Thrush)* (Figs. 23-29 and 23-30) White-to-creamy plaques on any mucosal surface; vary in size from 1 to 2 mm to extensive and widespread; removal with a dry gauze pad leaves an erythematous or bleeding mucosal surface.

*Erythematous (Atrophic) Candidiasis* Smooth, red, atrophic patches (Figs. 23-30 and 23-31); may be associated with thrush.

*Candidal Leukoplakia* White plaques that cannot be wiped off but regress with prolonged anticandidal therapy.

*Angular Cheilitis* Erythema, fissuring, i.e., intertrigo at the corner of mouth (Figs. 23-29 and 23-31).

**Distribution** *Thrush*: dorsum of tongue, buccal mucosa, hard/soft palate, pharynx extending down into esophagus and tracheobronchial tree. *Erythematous (atrophic) candidiasis*: hard/soft palate, buccal mucosa, dorsal surface of tongue. *Leukoplakia*: buccal mucosa, tongue, hard palate.

### General Findings

**Invasive Candidiasis** In individuals with severe prolonged neutropenia; *Candida* can invade into submucosa and blood vessels with subsequent hematogenous dissemination to skin and viscera. Candidemia also occurs in the setting of prolonged catheterization.

## DIFFERENTIAL DIAGNOSIS

**Pseudomembranous Candidiasis (Thrush)** Oral hairy leukoplakia, condyloma acuminatum, geographic tongue, hairy tongue, lichen planus, bite irritation.

**Atrophic (Erythematous) Candidiasis** Lichen planus.

## LABORATORY EXAMINATIONS

See "Candidiasis," page 716.

**Endoscopy** Documents esophageal and/or tracheobronchial candidiasis.

## DIAGNOSIS

Clinical suspicion confirmed by KOH preparation of scraping from mucosal surface.

## COURSE AND PROGNOSIS

Most cases respond to correction of the precipitating cause (e.g., use of inhaled glucocorticoids). Topical agents effective in most cases. Clinical resistance to antifungal agents may be related to patient noncompliance, severe immunocompromise, drug-drug interaction (rifampin-fluconazole). Between 30 and 40% of bone marrow transplant recipients develop superficial mucosal candidiasis; 10 to 25% develop deep invasive candidiasis, of whom one-fourth die from the infection and others go on to develop chronic visceral candidiasis.

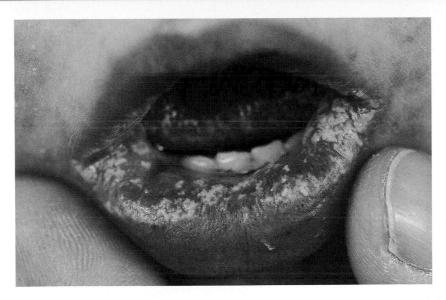

**FIGURE 23-29   Oral candidiasis: thrush**   *White curdlike material on the mucosal surface of the lower lip of a child; the material can be abraded off with gauze (pseudomembranous), revealing underlying erythema.*

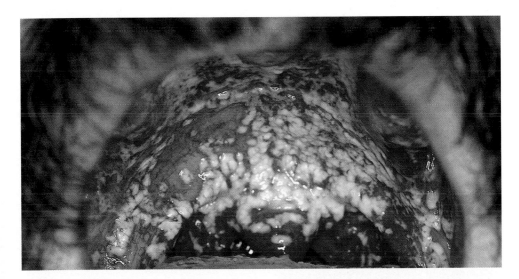

**FIGURE 23-30   Oral candidasis: thrush**   *Extensive cottage cheese-like plaques, colonies of* Candida *that can be removed by rubbing with gauze (pseudomembranous), on the palate and uvula of an individual with advanced HIV disease. Patches of erythema between the white plaques represent erythematous (atrophic) candidiasis. Involvement may extend into the esophagus and be associated with dysphagia.*

In HIV disease, oropharyngeal and esophageal candidiasis have been reported with primary HIV infection. In later HIV disease [without the use of highly active antiretroviral therapy (HAART)], OPC is nearly universal; esophageal infection occurs in 10 to 20% of patients. Relapse after topical or systemic treatment is expected. Virtually all HIV-infected individuals with CD4+ cell counts of $100/\mu L$ harbor oral *Candida*; chronic suppressive therapy is associated with changes in mouth flora rather than eradication.

## MANAGEMENT

**Topical Therapy**   These preparations are effective in the immunocompetent individual but relatively ineffective with decreasing cell-mediated immunity.

*Nystatin*   Oral tablets, 100,000 units qid dissolved slowly in the mouth, are the most effective preparation. The oral suspension, 1 to 2 teaspoons, held in mouth for 5 min and then swallowed may be effective.

*Clotrimazole*   Oral tablets (troche), 10 mg, one tablet 5 times daily may be effective.

**HIV Disease**   Responds to topical and/or systemic therapy; however, recurrence is the rule. May become refractory to intermittent therapy, requiring daily chemoprophylaxis with either topical or systemic treatment. Increase dose with resistant disease.

*Fluconazole*   200 mg PO once followed by 100 mg/d for 2 to 3 weeks, then discontinue. Increase the dose to 400 to 800 mg in resistant infection. Also available in IV form.

*Itraconazole*   Capsules or oral solution. 100 mg PO qd or bid for 2 weeks. Increase dose with resistant disease.

*Ketoconazole*   200 mg PO qd to bid for 1 to 2 weeks.

**Fluconazole-Resistant Candidiasis**   Defined as clinical persistence of infection after treatment with fluconazole, 100 mg/d PO for 7 days. Occurs most commonly in HIV-infected individuals with CD4+ cell counts $<50/\mu L$ who have had prolonged fluconazole exposure. Chronic low-dose fluconazole treatment (50 mg/d) facilitates emergence of resistant strains; 50% of resistant strains sensitive to itraconazole. Amphotericin B for severe resistant disease. New liposomal preparations are effective and less toxic. Recurrence is the rule; maintenance therapy is often required.

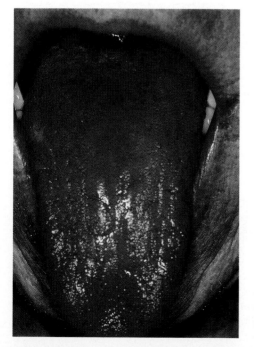

**FIGURE 23-31   Oral candidiasis: atrophic with angular cheilitis**   *The surface of the tongue is atrophic and shiny; an intertrigo is present at the angles of the lips. The patient is diabetic; anogenital candidiasis is also present.*

## GENITAL CANDIDIASIS   ■

Genital candidiasis occurs on the mucosa (nonkeratinized epithelium) of the vulva, vagina, and preputial sac of the penis. Infection usually represents overgrowth of colonizing infection rather than arising from exogenous source.

### EPIDEMIOLOGY AND ETIOLOGY

**Etiology**   >20% of normal women have vaginal colonization with *Candida. C. albicans* accounts for 80 to 90% of genital isolates.

**Incidence**   Most vaginal candidiasis (VC) occurs in the normal population. 75% of women experience at least one episode of VC during their lifetime, and 40 to 45% experience two or more episodes. Often associated with vulvar candidiasis, i.e., vulvovaginal candidiasis (VVC). A small percentage of women (probably <5%) experience recurrent VVC (RVVC).

**Risk Factors**   Usually none. Pregnancy. Usually sexually active, but also in sexually inactive, young, elderly. Uncircumcised.

**Transmission**   In neonatal OPC, *C. albicans* is acquired from the genital tract of mother. To males from colonized sexual partners.

### HISTORY

**Symptoms**   *Vulvitis/ Vulvovaginitis* Onset often abrupt, usually the week before menstruation; symptoms may recur before each menstruation. Pruritus, vaginal discharge, vaginal soreness, vulvar burning, dyspareunia, external dysuria.

*Balanoposthitis, Balanitis* Burning, itching, redness.

### PHYSICAL EXAMINATION

**Mucosal Lesions**

*Vulvitis* Erosions, pustules, erythema (Fig. 23-32), swelling, removable curdlike material.

*Vulvitis/Vulvovaginitis* Vaginitis with white discharge; vaginal erythema and edema; white plaques that can be wiped off on vaginal and/or cervical mucosa. Often associated with VC and candidal intertrigo of inguinal folds and perineum. Subcorneal pustules at periphery with fringed, irregular margins. In chronic cases, vaginal mucosa glazed and atrophic.

*Balanoposthitis, Balanitis* Glans and preputial sac: papules, pustules, erosions (Fig. 23-33). Maculopapular lesions with diffuse erythema. Edema, ulcerations, and fissuring of prepuce, usually in diabetic men; white plaques under foreskin.

### DIFFERENTIAL DIAGNOSIS

**VC/ VVC**   Trichomoniasis (caused by *T. vaginalis*), bacterial vaginosis (caused by replacement of normal vaginal flora by an overgrowth of anaerobic microorganisms and *Gardnerella vaginalis*), lichen planus, lichen sclerosus et atrophicus.

**Balanoposthitis**   Psoriasis, eczema.

### LABORATORY EXAMINATIONS

See "Candidiasis," page 716.

### DIAGNOSIS

Clinical suspicion confirmed by KOH preparation of scraping from mucosal surface.

### COURSE AND PROGNOSIS

**RVVC**   Defined as three or more episodes of symptomatic VVC annually. Affects a small proportion of women (<5%). The natural history and pathogenesis of RVVC are poorly understood. The majority of women with RVVC have no apparent predisposing conditions.

### MANAGEMENT

**VC/VVC**   *Topical Therapy* Azoles/imidazoles are more effective than nystatin and result in relief of symptoms and negative cultures among 80 to 90% of patients after therapy is completed.

***Recommended Regimens*** Single-dose regimens probably should be reserved for cases of uncomplicated mild to moderate VVC. Multiday regimens (3- to 7-day) are the preferred treatment for severe or complicated VVC.

Butoconazole: 2% cream 5 g intravaginally for 3 days *or*

Clotrimazole: 1% cream 5 g intravaginally for 7 to 14 days *or*
100-mg vaginal tablet for 7 days *or*
100-mg vaginal tablet, two tablets for 3 days *or*
500-mg vaginal tablet, one tablet in a single application *or*

Miconazole: 2% cream 5 g intravaginally for 7 days *or*
200-mg vaginal suppository, one suppository for 3 days *or*
100-mg vaginal suppository, one suppository for 7 days *or*

Tioconazole: 6.5% ointment 5 g intravaginally in a single application *or*

Terconazole: 0.4% cream 5 g intravaginally for 7 days *or*
0.8% cream 5 g intravaginally for 3 days *or*
80-mg suppository, one suppository for 3 days

Fluconazole: 150 mg PO as a single dose

**RVVC**    Weekly dosing with the following may be effective:

Clotrimazole: 500-mg vaginal tablet, one tablet in a single application *or*
Fluconazole: 150 mg PO as a single dose
Itraconazole: 100 mg PO bid

**Balanitis, Balanoposthitis**    Azole cream bid. Treat sexual partner if recurrent.
***Systemic Treatment***    See page 724.

## CANDIDIASIS OF THE NAIL APPARATUS

See "Disorders of the Nail Apparatus," Section 30.

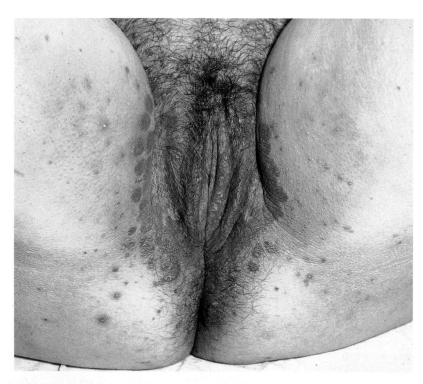

**FIGURE 23-32    Candidiasis: vulvitis**    *Psoriasiform, erythematous lesions becoming confluent on the vulva with erosions and satellite pustules on the thighs.*

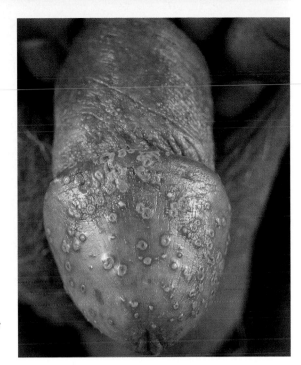

**FIGURE 23-33 Candidiasis: balanoposthitis** *Multiple, discrete pustules on the glans penis and inner aspect of the foreskin (the preputial sac).*

## CHRONIC MUCOCUTANEOUS CANDIDIASIS ☐ ●

Chronic mucocutaneous candidiasis (CMC) is characterized by persistent/recurrent *Candida* infections of the oropharynx, skin, and nail apparatus (Figs. 23-34 and 23-35), usually associated with underlying immunocompromise and onset in infancy or early childhood. Oropharyngeal candidiasis is refractory to conventional therapy, relapsing after successful therapy; chronic infection results in hypertrophic (leukoplakic) candidiasis. Cutaneous candidiasis manifests as intertrigo or widespread infection of the trunk and/or extremities; lesions become hypertrophic in chronic untreated cases. Infection of the nail apparatus is universal with chronic paronychia, nail plate infection, and eventually total nail dystrophy. Many patients also have dermatophytosis and cutaneous warts.

Six types of CMC have been defined: (1) chronic oral candidiasis; (2) chronic candidiasis with endocrinopathy; (3) chronic candidiasis without endocrinopathy; (4) chronic localized mucocutaneous candidiasis; (5) chronic diffuse candidiasis; and (6) chronic candidiasis with thymoma.

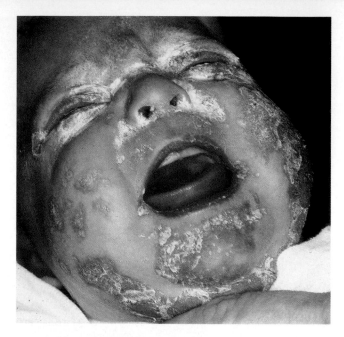

**FIGURE 23-34 Mucocutaneous candidiasis** *Persistent candidiasis in an immunocompromised infant manifesting as erosions covered by scales and crusts, oropharyngeal candidiasis, and widespread infection of the trunk.*

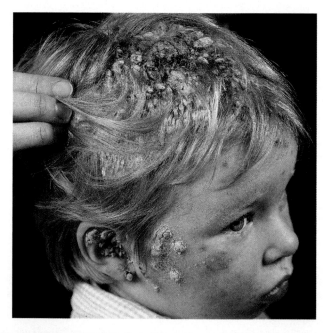

**FIGURE 23-35 Mucocutaneous candidiasis** *This 3-year-old child with hypothyroidism had oral thrush, intertriginous candidiasis, warty hyperkeratoses, and crusts on the scalp and face; and also, candidal onychomycosis. The warty growths shown in the photo consisted of dried pus, serum, and pure cultures of* Candida.

## ACUTE CANDIDEMIA

See "Systemic Fungal Infections with Dissemination to Skin," below.

## PITYRIASIS VERSICOLOR  ■  ○

Pityriasis (tinea) versicolor (PV) is a chronic asymptomatic scaling epidermomycosis associated with the superficial overgrowth of the hyphal form of *Malassezia furfur*, characterized by well-demarcated scaling patches with variable pigmentation, occurring most commonly on the trunk.

### EPIDEMIOLOGY AND ETIOLOGY

**Etiology**  *M. furfur* (previously known as *Pityrosporum ovale, P. orbiculare*) is a lipophilic yeast that normally resides in the keratin of skin and hair follicles of individuals at puberty and beyond. It is an opportunistic organism, causing pityriasis versicolor and *Malassezia* folliculitis and is implicated in the pathogenesis of seborrheic dermatitis. *Malassezia* infections are not contagious; rather, overgrowth of resident cutaneous flora occurs under certain favorable conditions.

**Age of Onset**  Young adults. Less common when sebum production is reduced or absent; tapers off during fifth and sixth decades.

**Predisposing Factors**  High temperatures/relative humidity, oily skin, hyperhidrosis, hereditary factors, glucocorticoid treatment, and immunodeficiency. Application of oils such as cocoa butter predisposes young children to PV.

**Season**  Temperate zones, appears in summertime, affecting 2% of population; may regress during cooler months; in physically active individuals, may persist year round. Subtropical and tropical zones: year around in 20%.

### PATHOGENESIS

*Malassezia* changes from the blastospore form to the mycelial form under the influence of predisposing factors. Dicarboxylic acids formed by enzymatic oxidation of fatty acids in skin surface lipids inhibit tyrosinase in epidermal melanocytes and thereby lead to hypomelanosis. The enzyme is present in the organism.

### HISTORY

**Duration of Lesions**  Months to years.
**Skin Symptoms**  Usually none. Occasionally, mild pruritus. Individuals with PV usually present because of cosmetic concerns about the blotchy pigmentation.

### PHYSICAL EXAMINATION

Skin Lesions
Macules, sharply marginated (Figs. 23-36 through 23-38), round or oval in shape, varying in size. Fine scaling is best appreciated by gently abrading lesions with a no. 15 scalpel blade or the edge of a microscope slide. Treated or burned-out lesions lack scale. Some patients have findings of *Malassezia* folliculitis and seborrheic dermatitis. In untanned skin, lesions are light brown. On tanned skin, white. In dark-skinned individuals, dark brown macules. Brown of varying intensities and hues (Fig. 23-36); off-white macules (Figs. 23-37 and 23-38). Some PV lesions are red (Fig. 23-38). In time, individual lesions may enlarge, merge, forming extensive geographic areas.

**Distribution**  Upper trunk, upper arms, neck, abdomen, axillae, groins, thighs, genitalia. Facial, neck, and/or scalp lesions occur in patients applying creams/ointments or topical glucocorticoid preparations.

## DIFFERENTIAL DIAGNOSIS

**Hypopigmented PV**  Vitiligo, pityriasis alba, postinflammatory hypopigmentation, tuberculoid leprosy.

**Scaling Lesions**  Tinea corporis, seborrheic dermatitis, pityriasis rosea, guttate psoriasis, nummular eczema.

## LABORATORY EXAMINATIONS

**Direct Microscopic Examination of Scales Prepared with KOH**  Scale is best obtained with two microscope slides, using one to raise scale and move it onto the other. The harvested scale is moved into a small pile in the center of the slide and covered with a coverslip. KOH solution (15 to 20%) is added at the edge of the coverslip; the slide is gently heated and examined. Filamentous hyphae and globose yeast forms, termed *spaghetti and meatballs*, are seen (Fig. 23-39).

**Wood's Lamp**  Blue-green fluorescence of scales; may be negative in individuals who have showered recently because the fluorescent chemical is water soluble. Vitiligo appears as depigmented, white, and has no scale.

**Dermatopathology**  Budding yeast and hyphal forms in the most superficial layers of the stratum corneum, seen best with PAS stain. Variable hyperkeratosis, psoriasiform hyperplasia, chronic inflammation with blood vessel dilatation.

## DIAGNOSIS

Clinical findings, confirmed by positive KOH preparation findings.

## COURSE AND PROGNOSIS

Infection persists for years if predisposing conditions persist. Dyspigmentation persists for months after infection has been eradicated.

## MANAGEMENT

| | |
|---|---|
| **Topical agents** | |
| Selenium sulfide (2.5%) lotion or shampoo | Apply daily to affected areas for 10 to 15 min, followed by shower, for 1 week |
| Ketoconazole shampoo | Applied same as selenium sulfide shampoo |
| Azole creams (ketoconazole, econazole, micronazole, clotrimazole) | Apply qd or bid for 2 weeks |
| Terbinafine 1% solution | Apply bid for 7 days |
| **Systemic therapy** (None of these agents is approved for use in PV in the United States) | |
| Ketoconazole | 400 mg stat (take 1 h before exercise) |
| Fluconazole | 400 mg stat |
| Itraconazole | 400 mg stat |
| **Secondary prophylaxis** | Ketoconazole shampoo once or twice a week |
| | Selenium sulfide (2.5%) lotion or shampoo |
| | Salicylic acid/sulfur bar |
| | Pyrithione zinc (bar or shampoo) |
| | Ketoconazole 400 mg PO monthly |

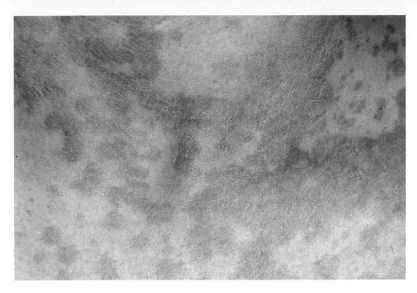

**FIGURE 23-36   Pityriasis versicolor**   *Sharply marginated brown macules on the trunk. Fine scale was apparent when the lesions were abraded with the edge of a microscope slide.*

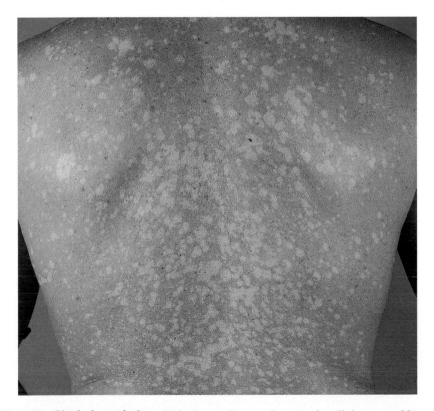

**FIGURE 23-37   Pityriasis versicolor**   *Multiple, small-to-medium-sized, well-demarcated hypopigmented macules on the back of a tanned individual with white skin.*

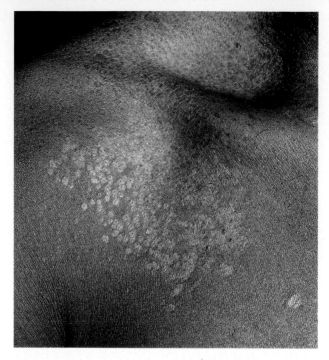

**FIGURE 23-38   Pityriasis versicolor**   *Follicular, hypopigmented macules on the upper chest of an individual with black skin.*

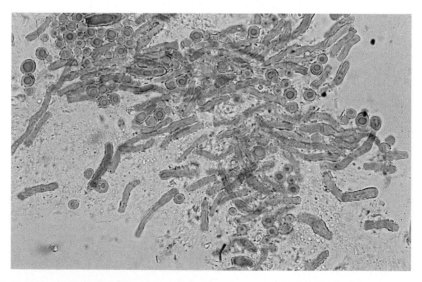

**FIGURE 23-39   *Malassezia furfur*. KOH preparation**   *Round yeast and elongated pseudohyphal forms, so-called "spaghetti and meatballs."*

# INVASIVE FUNGAL INFECTIONS

Invasive fungal infections can arise by deeper extension of local cutaneous infections (myce-toma, chromomycosis, and sporotrichosis) or by dissemination of a primary pulmonary infec-tion to the skin or mucosa (cryptococcosis, blastomycosis, histoplasmosis, coccidioidomycosis). Locally invasive fungal infections can occur in otherwise healthy individuals; in the setting of immunocompromise, these infections can disseminate systemically. Many individuals with dis-semination of fungal infections to the skin do have underlying immunocompromise.

## SUBCUTANEOUS MYCOSES

Subcutaneous mycoses include a heterogeneous group of fungal infections that develop at the site of transcutaneous trauma. Infection slowly evolves as the etiologic agent survives and adapts to the adverse host tissue environment. The diagnosis rests on clinical presentation, histopathology, and culture of the etiologic agents. Mycetoma, chromomycosis, and sporotri-chosis, are considered here.

## MYCETOMA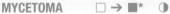

Mycetoma is a chronic suppurative infection originating in subcutaneous tissue, characterized by the presence of grains, which are tightly clumped colonies of the causative agent. Painless swelling, woody induration, and sinus tracts that discharge pus intermittently are characteristic. Systemic symptoms do not develop, and spreading to distant sites in the body does not take place. Variants: botryomycosis (caused by bacteria), actinomycetoma (caused by Actinomyc-etales organisms), eumycetoma (caused by true fungi).
*Synonyms*: Madura foot, maduromycetoma.

### EPIDEMIOLOGY AND ETIOLOGY

**Age of Onset**   20 to 50 years.
**Sex**   90% of patients are males.
**Occupation**   Rural inhabitants: Agricultural workers and laborers exposed to soil in tropical and subtropical regions.
**Transmission**   Cutaneous inoculation (thorn prick, wood splinter, stone cut) of organism, com-monly with soil or plant debris, into foot or hand.
**Etiology/Demography**   The predominant agent varies with the locality. Fungi isolated from soil except *Actinomyces israelii*. Tropical and sub-tropical climate supports growth of organisms. In Central/South America, 90% of cases caused by *Nocardia brasiliensis*. In Africa, *M. mycetomatis* is common cause. Most commonly seen in India,

Mexico, Nigeria, Saudi Arabia, Senegal, Somalia, Sudan, Venezuela, Yemen, Zaire. Causative agent forms dense colonies, i.e., grains.
**Risk Factors**   Poor hygiene, walking barefoot, necrotic injured tissue, diminished nutrition.

### PATHOGENESIS

Pathogens live in soil and enter through breaks in the skin. Only organisms that can survive at body temperature can produce mycetoma. In-fection begins in skin and subcutaneous tissues, extending into fascial planes, destroying con-tiguous tissues.

### HISTORY

**Incubation Period**   Lesion occurs at inoculation site weeks to years after trauma.

* Depending on geography.

**Duration of Lesion** Lesions may continue to expand for decades.

**Symptoms** Relatively few, with little pain, tenderness, or fever.

## PHYSICAL EXAMINATION

### Skin Lesions

Primary lesion: papule/nodule at inoculation site. Swelling increases slowly. Epidermis ulcerates and pus-containing granules (grains) drain. *Granules* are microbial colonies, small (<1 to 5 mm). Skin surrounding portals of fistula drainage is heaped up (Fig. 23-40). Infection spreads to deeper tissues, into fascia, muscle, bone. Tissue becomes greatly distorted. Old mycetoma characterized by healed scars and draining sinuses.

*Palpation* Usually not tender; pus drains on pressure. Central clearing gives older lesions an annular shape.

*Distribution* Unilateral on the leg, foot, hand. Uncommonly on torso, arm, head, thigh, buttock.

**General Findings** Fever with secondary bacterial infection. Regional lymphadenopathy occasionally. Osteomyelitis of contiguous bone may occur.

## ETIOLOGY AND CLASSIFICATION OF MYCETOMA-LIKE CLINICAL PRESENTATION WITH GRAIN FORMATION

| Type of Mycetoma | Etiologic Agents |
|---|---|
| **Botryomycosis** Caused by true bacteria. Not a true mycetoma. | Most common: *Staphylococcus aureus* Also: *S. epidermidis, Pseudomonas aeruginosa, Escherichia coli, Bacteroides* spp., *Proteus* spp., *Streptococcus* spp. |
| **Actinomycetoma (actinomycotic mycetoma)** Caused by Actinomycetales organisms | *Actinomyces: cause mycetoma and actinomycosis (cervical, thoracic, abdominal)* *Nocardia: cause mycetoma, lymphocutaneous infection (sporotrichoid pattern), superficial skin infections, disseminated infection with skin involvement* *Actinomadura* *Streptomyces* |
| **Eumycetoma (eumycotic mycetoma)** Caused by true fungi | Most common: *Pseudallescheria boydii, Madurella grisea, M. mycetomatis* Also: *Phialophora jeanselmei, Pyrenochaeta romeroi, Leptosphaeria senegaliensis, Curvularia lunata, Neotestudina rosatti, Aspergillus nidulans or flavus, Acremonium* spp., *Fusarium* spp., *Cylindrocarpon* spp., *Microsporum audouinii* |

## DIFFERENTIAL DIAGNOSIS

### Chronic Draining Subcutaneous Inflammatory Mass(es)
Osteomyelitis, botryomycosis, chromoblastomycosis, blastomycosis, bacterial pyoderma, foreign-body granuloma

## LABORATORY EXAMINATIONS

**Smear of Pus from Lesion Granules** Medlar bodies (Table 23-3) visualized on KOH preparation as microbial colonies (see below).

**Dermatopathology** Pseudoepitheliomatous hyperplasia of epidermis. Grains are found in purulent foci surrounded by fibrosis and mononuclear cell inflammatory cell response.

**Culture** Isolate organism. Secondary bacterial infection common.

**Imaging** CT scan and echosonography define the extent of involvement. X-ray of bone shows multiple osteolytic lesions (cavities), periosteal new bone formation.

## DIAGNOSIS

Clinical suspicion confirmed by demonstration of grains in pus and/or by visualization of Medlar bodies on smear of pus or lesional biopsy specimen, and/or isolation of organism on culture. Medlar bodies (granules, grains) are

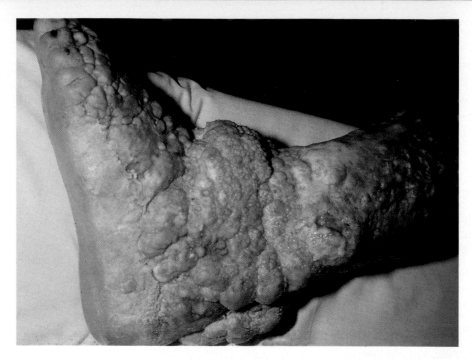

**FIGURE 23-40    Eumycotic mycetoma**    *The foot, ankle, and leg are grossly distorted with edema and confluent subcutaneous nodules, cauliflower-like tumors, and ulcerations.*

white, black to gray, pinpoint globular grains that can be seen and felt in pus. Can be crushed on slide. They represent globular colonies of organism (Table 23-3).

## COURSE AND PROGNOSIS

Mycetoma runs a relentless course over many years, destroying contiguous fascia and bone. Actinomycetoma usually enlarges more rapidly than eumycetoma. Secondary bacterial infections and relapse after antifungal or antibiotic therapy common.

## MANAGEMENT

Individuals are advised to seek medical attention early.

**Surgery**    Smaller lesions can be cured by surgical excision. More extensive lesions often recur after incomplete excision.

**Medicosurgical Approach**    Bulk reduction surgery is performed; amputation/disarticulation avoided. Causative agent identified, and effective antimicrobial agent given.

**Systemic Antimicrobial Therapy**    Usually continued for 10 months.

***Botryomycoses***    Antimicrobial agents according to sensitivities of isolated organism.

***Actinomycotic Mycetoma***    May respond to prolonged chemotherapy of streptomycin combined with either dapsone or trimethoprim-sulfamethoxazole.

***Eumycetoma***    Rarely responds to chemotherapy. Some cases caused by *M. mycetomatis* may respond to ketoconazole or itraconazole.

**TABLE 23-3    Color Grains in Mycetoma and Associated Organisms**

| Color of Grain | Organism |
| --- | --- |
| Black | *Madurella mycetomatis* |
| | *M. grisea* |
| | *Leptosphaeria senegalensis* |
| White | *Pseudallescheria boydii* |
| | *Acremonium* spp. |
| | *Nocardia brasiliensis* |
| | *N. asteroides* |
| White to yellow | *N. caviae* |
| Pink, white, | *Actinomyces israelii* |
| to cream | *Actinomadura madurae* |
| Red | *A. pelletieri* |

## CHROMOMYCOSIS ■* ◑

Chromomycosis is a chronic localized invasive fungal infection of skin and subcutaneous tissues, caused by pigmented (dematiaceous or dark-walled) fungi. Verrucous plaques usually occur on the leg or foot.
*Synonym*: Chromoblastomycosis. One of the phaeohyphomycoses.

### EPIDEMIOLOGY AND ETIOLOGY

**Age of Onset** 20 to 60 years.
**Sex** Males > females.
**Etiology** Dematiaceous fungi, characterized by melanin in mycelial walls. *Fonsecaea pedrosoi* (most commonly); also *F. compacta, Phialophora verrucosa, Cladosporium carrionii, Rhinocladiella aquaspersa, Botryomyces caespitosus*.
**Risk Groups** Agricultural workers, mine workers, those exposed to soil while barefoot in tropical and subtropical regions. May progress more rapidly in the immunocompromised host.
**Transmission** Cutaneous inoculation. Autoinoculation to other sites may occur. Transmission to other individuals does not occur.
**Demography** Fungi isolated from soil and vegetation, preferring regions with >2.5 m (> 100 in) of rainfall per year and mean temperatures from 12° to 24°C.

### HISTORY

**Duration of Lesion** Lesions may continue to expand for decades.
**Symptoms** Relatively few, with little pain, tenderness, or fever. Patients usually present with secondary infection, cosmetic disfigurement, lymphedema.

### PHYSICAL EXAMINATION

#### Skin Lesions
Initial lesion: single scaling nodule at site of traumatic implantation (Fig. 23-41). Later (months to years), new crops of nodules appear. Subsequently, expanding verrucous plaques with central clearing and islands of normal skin between verrucous macules. Large cauliflower-like lesions often form, which, in some cases, may become pedunculated. Surface of verrucous lesion: pustules, small ulcerations, "black

* Depending on geography.

dots" of hemopurulent material, friable granulation tissue that bleeds easily is common. Extension occurs via lymphatic spread or via autoinoculation. Chronic lesions may be 10 to 20 cm in diameter, enveloping calf or foot. In areas of long-standing infection; lymphedema of involved extremity (elephantiasis).
*Arrangement* Smaller lesions coalesce to form large verrucous masses. Central clearing gives older lesions an annular shape.
*Distribution* Unilateral on the leg, foot. Also, hand, thorax.

### DIFFERENTIAL DIAGNOSIS

**Large Verrucous Plaques** Blastomycosis, tuberculosis verrucosa cutis, mycetoma, sporotrichosis, nontuberculous mycobacterium infection, lepromatous leprosy, foreign-body granuloma, pyoderma gangrenosum, squamous cell carcinoma.

### LABORATORY EXAMINATIONS

**Smear of Pus from Lesion** Medlar bodies (see below) visualized on 10 to 20% KOH preparation as black dots. Hyphal forms can be seen in crusts, pus, exudate.
**Dermatopathology** Warty granuloma: pseudoepitheliomatous hyperplasia, hyperkeratosis, intraepidermal abscesses containing inflammatory cells and Medlar bodies. Medlar bodies (also known as sclerotic bodies, "copper pennies") are small brown fungal forms, which are round with thick bilaminate walls, 4 to 6 μm in diameter; occur singly or in clusters; all etiologic agents appear identical in tissue. Older lesions show dense fibrosis in and around granulomas.
**Culture** Organism in Sabouraud's glucose agar shows velvety green to black, restricted, slow-growing colonies. Agents grow very slowly, requiring 4 to 6 weeks for identification.

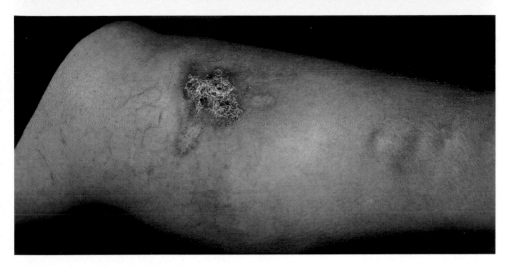

**FIGURE 23-41  Chromomycosis**  *Hyperkeratotic and crusted plaque with old scars on the leg had been present for several decades.*

## DIAGNOSIS

Clinical suspicion confirmed by visualization of Medlar bodies on smear of pus or lesional biopsy specimen and/or isolation of organism on culture.

## COURSE AND PROGNOSIS

Secondary bacterial infections and recurrence after oral triazole therapy are common. Late complication is squamous cell carcinoma arising within verrucous area.

## MANAGEMENT

**Adjunctive Therapy**  Application of heat may be helpful in that lesions arise at cooler acral sites.

**Surgery**  Smaller lesions can be cured by surgical excision.

**Systemic Antifungal Therapy**  *Amphotericin B*: is not usually effective at usual dosing.

**Oral Antifungal Agents**  Treatment is usually continued for at least 1 year. The response is highly variable.

> *Terbinafine*, 250 mg/d
> *Itraconazole*, 200 to 600 mg/d
> *Ketoconazole*, 400 to 800 mg/d

## SPOROTRICHOSIS

Sporotrichosis commonly follows accidental inoculation of the skin and is characterized by ulceronodule formation at the inoculation site, chronic nodular lymphangitis, and subcutaneous swelling. In the immunocompromised host, disseminated infection can occur from the skin involvement or pulmonary infection.

## EPIDEMIOLOGY AND ETIOLOGY

**Etiology**  *Sporothrix schenckii*, a dimorphic fungus, living as a saprophyte on plants in many areas of the world. The tissue form is an oval, cigar-shaped yeast.

**Sex**  Males > females, especially disseminated disease.

**Occupation**  Occupation exposure important: gardeners, farmers, florists, lawn laborers, agricultural workers, forestry workers, paper manufacturers, gold miners, laboratory workers. In Uruguay, 80% of cases occur after a scratch by an armadillo.

**Transmission**  Commonly, subcutaneous inoculation by a contaminated sharp object (rose or barberry thorn, barb, wood splinter) or from sphagnum moss, straw, marsh hay, soils. Rarely, inhalation, aspiration, or ingestion causes systemic infection. Most cases isolated. Epidemics do occur. Cutaneous sporotrichosis in cats has been transmitted to humans.

**Demography**  Ubiquitous, worldwide. More common in temperate, tropical zones.

**Risk Factors**  *For localized disease*: diabetes mellitus, alcoholism. *For disseminated disease*: risk factors for localized disease as well as HIV infection, carcinoma, hematologic and lymphoproliferative disease, immunosuppressive therapy.

## PATHOGENESIS

After subcutaneous inoculation, *S. schenckii* grows locally. Infection can be limited to the site of inoculation (*plaque sporotrichosis*) or extend along the proximal lymphatic channels (*lymphangitic sporotrichosis*). (Other infections have similar lymphatic involvement, the pattern being referred to as *sporotrichoid* or resembling *lymphatic sporotrichosis*.) Spread beyond an extremity is rare; hematogenous dissemination from the skin remains unproven. The portal for extracutaneous sporotrichosis (e.g., osteoarticular) is unknown but is probably the lung.

## HISTORY

**Incubation Period**  3 weeks (range, 3 days to 12 weeks) after trauma or injury to site of lesion. Lesions are relatively asymptomatic, painless. Afebrile.

## PHYSICAL EXAMINATION

### Skin Lesions

**Plaque Sporotrichosis**  Subcutaneous papule, pustule, or nodule appears at inoculation site several weeks after inoculation. Surrounding skin is pink to purplish. In time, skin becomes fixed to deeper tissues. Painless indurated ulcer (Fig. 23-42) may occur, resulting in sporotrichoid chancre. Border ragged and not sharply demarcated. Draining lymph nodes become swollen and suppurative. Crusted ulcers, ecthymatous, verrucous plaques, pyoderma gangrenosum–like, infiltrated papules and plaques may also occur.

**Lymphangitic Sporotrichosis**  Follows lymphatic extension of local cutaneous type (Fig. 23-43). Proximal to local cutaneous lesion, intervening lymphatics become indurated, nodular, thickened.

**Disseminated Sporotrichosis**  (Fungus disseminates hematogenously to skin, as well as joints, eyes, and meninges.) Crusted nodules, ulcers. Widespread.

*Distribution*  Primary lesion most common on dorsum of hand or finger with chronic nodular lymphangitis up arm. Fixed cutaneous—face in children, upper extremities in adults. Disseminated sporotrichosis: widespread lesions, usually sparing palms, soles.

**General Examination**  *Lungs*  Pulmonary sporotrichosis presents as a single cavitary upper-lobe lesion.

*Joints*  Swelling, painful joint(s) (hand, elbow, ankle, knee), often in the absence of skin lesion. Draining sinuses may occur over joints, bursae. *Hematogenous dissemination* results in skin,

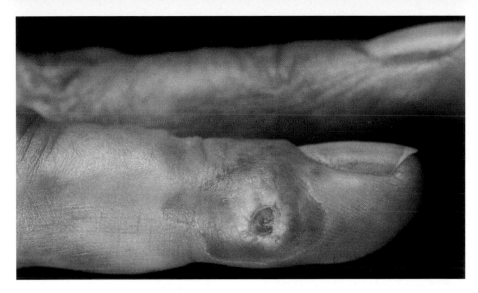

**FIGURE 23-42   Sporotrichosis: chancriform type**   *An ulcerated nodule at the site of inoculation on the finger was associated with regional axillary lymphadenopathy.*

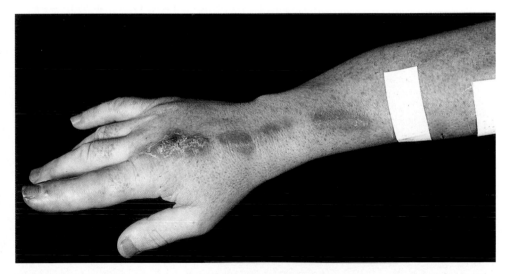

**FIGURE 23-43   Sporotrichosis: chronic lymphangitic (sporotrichoid) type**   *An erythematous papule at the site of inoculation on the index finger with a linear arrangement of erythematous dermal and subcutaneous nodules extending proximally in lymphatic vessels of the dorsum of the hand and arm.*

bone, muscle, joint, visceral, CNS (chronic meningitis) lesions.

## DIFFERENTIAL DIAGNOSIS

**Plaque Sporotrichosis** Cutaneous tuberculosis, nontuberculous mycobacterial infection, tularemia, cat-scratch disease, primary syphilis, bacterial pyoderma, foreign-body granuloma, inflammatory dermatophytoses, blastomycosis, chromomycosis, mycetoma, leishmaniasis.
**Chronic Nodular Lymphangitic Sporotrichosis** *"Common" Infecting Agents* Mycobacterium marinum, *Nocardia brasiliensis, Leishmania brasiliensis, Francisella tularensis.*

## LABORATORY EXAMINATIONS

**Touch Preparation** In disseminated sporotrichosis (usually with advanced HIV disease), KOH solution added to smear from lesional skin biopsy specimen helps visualize multiple yeast forms.
**Gram's Stain** In disseminated sporotrichosis (usually with advanced HIV disease), smear from crusted lesion shows multiple yeast forms.
**Dermatopathology** Granulomatous, Langerhans-type giant cells, pyogenic microabscesses. Organisms usually rare, difficult to visualize. In the immunocompromised host, yeast appear as myriads of 1- to 3-$\mu$m by 3- to 10-$\mu$m cigar-shaped forms.
**Culture** Organism usually isolated within a few days from lesional biopsy specimen.

## DIAGNOSIS

Clinical suspicion and isolation of organism on culture.

## COURSE AND PROGNOSIS

Shows little tendency to resolve spontaneously. Responds well to therapy, but a significant percentage relapse after completion of therapy. Disseminated infection in HIV-infected individuals responds poorly to all forms of therapy.

## MANAGEMENT[1]

### Oral Antifungal Agents
> *Itraconazole*: 200 to 600 mg qd. Very effective for lymphocutaneous infection; not as effective for bone/joint and pulmonary infection.
> *Fluconazole*: 200 to 400 mg/d reported to be effective.
> *Ketoconazole*: 400 to 800 mg/d reported to be effective.
> *Terbinafine* 1000 mg/d reported to be effective.
> *Saturated solution of potassium iodide*: 4.5 to 9 mL/d for adults effective for lymphocutaneous infection; less effective than oral antifungal agents. Adverse events: GI disturbance, acneiform rash.

**Intravenous Therapy** *Amphotericin B.* For those with pulmonary or disseminated infection or who are unable to tolerate oral therapy for lymphocutaneous disease.

[1]Kauffman CA et al: Clin Infect Dis 30:684, 2000.

# SYSTEMIC FUNGAL INFECTIONS WITH DISSEMINATION TO SKIN

Pulmonary fungal infections, i.e., cryptococcosis, histoplasmosis, blastomycosis, coccidioidomycosis, and penicillinosis, can be disseminated systemically to skin and multiple organs. Dissemination occurs most often in the immunocompromised host. Cutaneous lesions often provide the opportunity for early diagnosis by lesional biopsy.

## DISSEMINATED CRYPTOCOCCOSIS

Cryptococcosis is a systemic mycosis, having primary pulmonary infection and occasional hematogenous dissemination to the meninges and skin. Dissemination occurs commonly in advanced HIV disease.
*Synonyms*: Torulosis, European blastomycosis.

## EPIDEMIOLOGY AND ETIOLOGY

**Etiology**   *Cryptococcus neoformans*, a yeast, serotypes A, B, C, D causing infection in humans. Serotypes A and D designated *C. neoformans* var. *neoformans*: serotypes B and C, *C. neoformans* var. *gattii*. In tissue, encapsulated yeastlike fungi (3.5 to 7.0 μm in diameter). Bud connected to parent cell by narrow pore. Capsule thickness variable. The source of transmission to humans in unknown.
**Age of Onset**   More common over the age of 40 years.
**Sex**   Males > females, 3:1.
**Incidence**   Globally, cryptococcosis (usually meningitis) is the most common invasive mycosis in HIV disease, occurring in 6 to 9% of HIV-infected individuals in the United States and 20 to 30% in Africa. Incidence is also high in Europe and South America. Currently, in the industrialized nations, the incidence is much less due to immune reconstitution. In untreated HIV disease, cutaneous dissemination occurs in 10 to 15% of cryptococcosis cases.
**Risk Factors**   HIV disease, solid-organ transplantation, glucocorticoid therapy, sarcoidosis, lymphoma, diabetes mellitus.
**Demography**   Worldwide, ubiquitous. Distribution of serotype varies in geographic areas.

## PATHOGENESIS

*C. neoformans* may be inhaled in dust and cause a primary pulmonary focus of infection that tends to resolve spontaneously. Reactivation of latent infection in the immunocompromised host may result in hematogenous dissemination to meninges, kidneys, and skin; 10 to 15% of patients have skin lesions.

## HISTORY

Occurs in the setting of advanced HIV disease. Cutaneous lesions: usually asymptomatic. CNS: headache most common symptom (80%), mental confusion, impaired vision for 2 to 3 months. Lungs: pulmonary symptoms uncommon.

## PHYSICAL EXAMINATION

### Skin Lesions
Papule(s) or nodule(s): with surrounding erythema that occasionally break down and exude a liquid, mucinous material. Can present as a solitary nodule in otherwise healthy individuals. Molluscum contagiosum–like lesions commonly occur in HIV-infected patients (Fig. 23-44). Acneiform. *Cryptococcal cellulitis:* mimics bacterial cellulitis, i.e., red, hot, tender, edematous plaque on extremity; possibly multiple noncontiguous sites. In HIV disease, lesions occur most commonly on face/scalp.
*Oral Mucosa*   Occur in <5% of patients, presenting as nodules/ulcers.
**General Findings**   Meningoencephalitis. In HIV disease, cryptococcosis tends to be widespread with fungemia and infection of meninges, lungs, bone marrow, genitourinary

tract including prostate, and skin. In HIV disease, hepatomegaly and splenomegaly.

## DIFFERENTIAL DIAGNOSIS

**Widespread Papular Eruption in Immunocompromised Patient** Molluscum contagiosum, disseminated histoplasmosis acne, sarcoidosis, pyoderma.

## LABORATORY EXAMINATIONS

**Dermatopathology** Gelatinous reactions show numerous organisms in aggregates with little inflammatory response. Granulomatous reactions show tissue reaction with histiocytes, giant cells, lymphoid cells, and fibroblasts: areas of necrosis; organisms are present in smaller numbers. Capsules stain with mucicarmine stain, differentiating *C. neoformans* from *B. dermatitidis*.

**Touch Preparation** Lesional skin biopsy specimen or scrapings from skin lesion smeared on microscope slide examined with KOH to identify *C. neoformans*.

**CSF** With meningitis, encapsulated budding yeast is seen with India ink preparations in 40 to 60% of cases, lymphocytic pleocytosis, elevated protein, decreased glucose. Intracranial pressure may be moderately to extremely elevated.

**Imaging** X-ray findings of chest variable.

**Culture** CSF. Lesional skin biopsy specimen. In HIV disease, cryptococcosis tends to be widespread, with cultures positive in blood, sputum, bone marrow, and urine. If *C. neoformans* isolated from lesional skin biopsy specimen, extent of disease should be determined by examination of CSF, bone marrow, sputum, urine, and prostate fluid.

**Cryptococcal Antigens** Sensitive and specific. Detect in CSF, serum, urine. Useful in following response to therapy and in formulating prognosis.

## DIAGNOSIS

Confirmed by skin biopsy and fungal cultures.

## COURSE AND PROGNOSIS

In HIV disease in the absence of immune reconstitution, cryptococcal meningitis relapses in 30% of cases after amphotericin B therapy; lifelong secondary prophylaxis with fluconazole reduces relapse rate to 4 to 8%.

## MANAGEMENT

**Primary Prophylaxis** In some centers, fluconazole is given to HIV-infected individuals with low CD4+ cell counts; the incidence of disseminated infection is reduced, but there is no effect on the mortality rate.

**Therapy of Meningitis** Amphotericin B for 2 to 4 weeks in uncomplicated cases and for 6 weeks in complicated cases. Fluconazole (alternative).

**Infection Limited to Skin** Fluconazole, 400 to 600 mg/d. Itraconazole (alternative), 400 mg/d.

**Secondary Prophylaxis** In HIV disease (without immune reconstitution), lifelong secondary prophylaxis is given. Fluconazole, 200 to 400 mg/d; itraconazole (alternative), 200 to 400 mg/d.

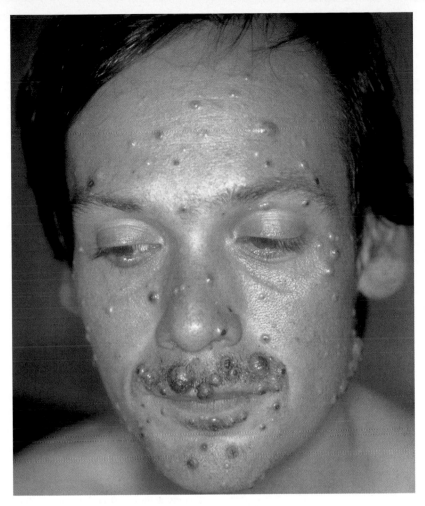

**FIGURE 23-44  Cryptococcosis: disseminated**  *Multiple, skin-colored papules and nodules on the face in an HIV-infected idividual represent dissemination of pulmonary cryptococcosis hematogenously to skin; meninges are also a common site of infection after fungemia. The lesions are easily mistaken for molluscum contagiosum, which occurs commonly in HIV disease. (Courtesy of Loïc Vallant, MD.)*

## HISTOPLASMOSIS    ■

Histoplasmosis is a common pulmonary mycosis that can disseminate hematogenously, presenting with involvement of mucous membranes, skin, and reticuloendothelial organs (liver, bone marrow, and spleen).
*Synonyms*: Darling's disease, cave disease, Ohio Valley disease.

## EPIDEMIOLOGY AND ETIOLOGY

**Etiology**    *Histoplasma capsulatum*, an unencapsulated dimorphic fungus. In Africa, *H. capsulatum* var. *duboisii*. The fungus grows well in soil enriched with bird or bat guano.

**Age of Onset**    For disseminated infection, very old and very young.

**Transmission**    Inhalation of spores in soil contaminated with bird or bat droppings. Those at risk: farmers, construction workers, children, others involved in outdoor activities (cave exploration). Acute pulmonary histoplasmosis may occur in outbreaks in individuals with occupational or recreational exposure.

**Risk Factors for Dissemination**    Immunosuppressed host (HIV infection, post-organ transplant, lymphoma, leukemia, chemotherapy), advanced age. Occurs in advanced HIV disease when CD4+ cell count is very low.

**Incidence**    Common opportunistic infection in HIV-infected individuals in highly endemic regions such as Indiana. Early in the HIV epidemic, first cases of histoplasmosis were in immigrants from the endemic foci in the Caribbean Islands who developed AIDS while living in New York or California; disease presented as reactivation of latent foci of infection. In cities such as Indianapolis and Kansas City, 20 to 25% of patients with HIV disease have primary histoplasmosis. Incidence also increased in HIV disease in South America.

**Demography**    North America: eastern and central United States, especially Ohio/Mississippi River valleys; in some areas, 80% of residents are histoplasmin-positive. Caribbean Islands. Equatorial Africa.

## PATHOGENESIS

In HIV disease, can present as either primary histoplasmosis or reactivation of latent infection.

## HISTORY

**Incubation Period**    For acute pulmonary infection, 5 to 18 days. For disseminated infection, 2 months. In severe forms of infection, presentation may be acute, resembling septicemia with associated disseminated intravascular coagulopathy.

**Acute Primary Infection**    90% of patients asymptomatic; if large numbers of spores inhaled, influenza-like syndrome may occur (fever 38.3°C, chills, night sweats, cough, headache, fatigue, myalgia).

**Disseminated Infection**    Chronic disease syndrome. In HIV disease, can present as widely disseminated infection with symptoms of sepsis, adrenal insufficiency, diarrheal illness, or colonic mass.

## PHYSICAL EXAMINATION

### Skin Lesions

*Acute Pulmonary Histoplasmosis*    Cutaneous lesions represent hypersensitivity reactions to *Histoplasma* antigen(s): Erythema nodosum, erythema multiforme–like lesions.

*Disseminated Histoplasmosis to Skin*    Lesions caused by tissue infection. Historically, lesions of mucous membranes much more common than those on skin. However, in HIV infection, 10% of patients with disseminated histoplasmosis have cutaneous lesions; in renal transplant patients, 4 to 6%. Erythematous necrotic or hyperkeratotic papules and nodules (Fig. 23-45); erythematous macules; folliculitis, pustules, acneiform ulcers; vegetative plaques; panniculitis; erythroderma; chronic ulcers. Diffuse hyperpigmentation with Addison's disease secondary to adrenal infection.

*Mucous Membranes*    Common site of involvement; nodules, vegetations, painful ulcerations of soft palate, oropharynx, epiglottis, nasal vestibule.

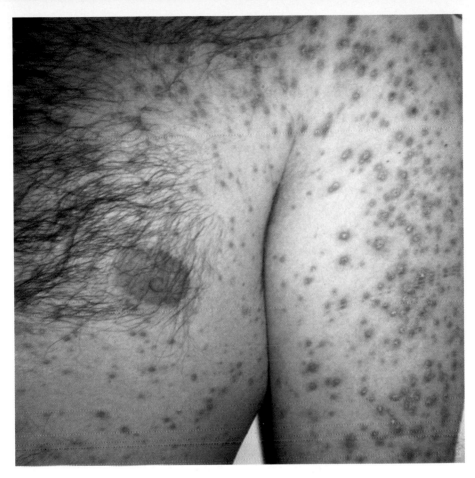

**FIGURE 23-45   Histoplasmosis, disseminated**   *Multiple, erythematous, scaling papules on the trunk and upper arm occurred during a 2-week period and mimicked acute guttate psoriasis in an individual with HIV disease. The cutaneous lesions occurred after reactivation of pulmonary infection and fungemia. Multiple yeast-like* H. capsulatum *were demonstrated within macrophages in a lesional skin biopsy specimen. (Courtesy of J. D. Fallon, MD.)*

*General Examination*   Disseminated disease: hepatosplenomegaly, lymphadenopathy, meningitis.

## DIFFERENTIAL DIAGNOSIS

**Disseminated Disease**   Miliary tuberculosis, disseminated coccidioidomycosis or cryptococcosis, leishmaniasis, lymphoma.

## LABORATORY EXAMINATIONS

**Dermatopathology**   Identify *H. capsulatum* in

tissue by size and staining. Differentiate from *Coccidioides immitis, Blastomyces dermatitidis, Leishmania donovani, Toxoplasma gondii*.

**Smear**   *H. capsulatum* can be identified by smears obtained from touching lesional skin biopsy specimen to microscope slide (touch preparation); also sputum or bone marrow aspirate, stained with Giemsa's stain.

**Culture**   Identify *H. capsulatum* from biopsy specimens of skin, oral lesions, bone marrow, sputum, lung biopsy specimen, blood, urine, lymph node, liver.

**Antigen Detection**   If positive, must be confirmed by culture or histopathology.

**Bone Marrow Aspiration**  *H. capsulatum* can be visualized in those with disseminated infection.

**Imaging**  Chest x-ray: interstitial infiltrates and/or hilar adenopathy (acute).

## DIAGNOSIS

Clinical suspicion, confirmed by culture of organism.

## COURSE AND PROGNOSIS

Primary infection resolves spontaneously in most cases. Untreated chronic cavitary pulmonary infection or progressive disseminated form has a very high mortality rate, 80% of patients dying within 1 year. Prognosis linked to underlying

condition. Chronic maintenance often required. With itraconazole therapy, cure rate 80%.

## MANAGEMENT

**Prevention**  When any material contaminated with bird or bat guano is to be disturbed in an area of endemic histoplasmosis, personal protective equipment should be used during recreational or occupational exposure.

**Systemic Antimycotic Therapy**  Non-life-threatening infections and for those unable to tolerate amphotericin B: Itraconazole, 400 mg bid PO for 12 weeks; *or* fluconazole, 800 mg qd PO for 12 weeks. Life-threatening and meningeal infection: Amphotericin B given IV.

**Secondary Prophylaxis**  In HIV disease without immune restoration, itraconazole, 200 mg/d, *or* fluconazole, 400 mg/d for life.

---

## NORTH AMERICAN BLASTOMYCOSIS    □ →

Blastomycosis is a chronic systemic mycosis characterized by primary pulmonary infection, which in some cases is followed by hematogenous dissemination to skin and other organs. *Synonyms*: Gilchrist's disease, Chicago disease.

## EPIDEMIOLOGY AND ETIOLOGY

**Etiology**  *Blastomyces dermatitidis*, a dimorphic fungus. In tissue, a yeast 10 μm in diameter with 1-μm-thick cell wall: pore of bud is wide.

**Age of Onset**  Young, middle-aged.

**Sex**  Males > females, 10:1.

**Transmission**  Most cases are isolated. Occupations at risk: outdoor vocation or avocation (farm workers, manual laborers). However, currently, many individuals infected during leisure activities: fishing, hunting, camping, hiking in areas of high endemicity.

**Demography**  Uncommon in any locality. Most cases occur in the southeastern, central, and mid-Atlantic areas of the United States. Rarely occurs in Africa, Mexico, Central America, South America.

## PATHOGENESIS

*B. dermatitidis* infection acquired from inhalation of dust from soil, decomposed vegetation, or rotting wood. Asymptomatic primary pulmonary infection usually resolves spontaneously. Hematogenous dissemination may occur to skin, skeletal system, prostate, epididymis, or mucosa of nose, mouth, or larynx. Reactivation may occur within lung or in sites of dissemination. Risk factors for dissemination: T cell dysfunction: advanced HIV disease.

## HISTORY

**Incubation Period**  Depends on size of inoculum and immune status. Estimated median, 45 days.

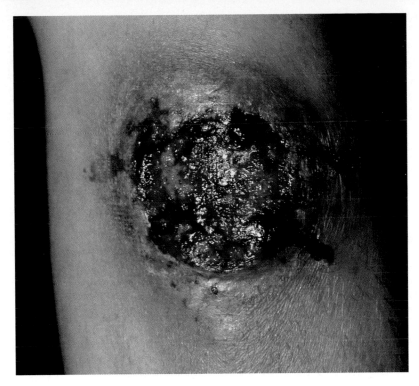

**FIGURE 23-46  North American blastomycosis: disseminated**  *Ulcerated, inflammatory plaque with surrounding erythema, edema, and fibrosis on the leg results from dissemination from pulmonary blastomycosis via blood to skin. The lesion must be differentiated from pyoderma gangrenosum. (Courtesy of Elizabeth M. Spiers, MD.)*

**Symptoms**  Primary pulmonary infection: usually asymptomatic: flulike or resembles bacterial pneumonitis. Chronic pulmonary infection: fever, cough, night sweats, weight loss. Cutaneous ulcers often painless.

## PHYSICAL EXAMINATION

### Skin Lesions
**Primary Infection**  Accompanied or followed by erythema nodosum or erythema multiforme.

**Disseminated Infection to Skin**  Initial lesion, inflammatory nodule that enlarges and ulcerates (Fig. 22-46); subcutaneous nodule, many small pustules on surface. Subsequently, verrucous/crusted plaque with sharply demarcated serpiginous borders. Peripheral border extends on one side, resembling a one-half to three-quarter moon. Pus exudes when crust is lifted. Central healing with thin geographic atrophic scar.

***Distribution***  Usually symmetrically on trunk but also face, hands, arms, legs; multiple lesions in one-half of patients.

**Mucous Membranes**  25% of patients have oral or nasal lesions, and one-half of those have contiguous skin lesions. Laryngeal infection.

**General Examination**  *Lungs* Infiltrates, miliary, cavitary lesions.

***Bones***  50% involvement; osteomyelitis in thoracolumbar vertebrae, pelvis, sacrum, skull, ribs, long bones. May extend to form large subcutaneous abscess: may occur in conjunction with cutaneous ulcer; septic arthritis and sinus tracts to skin can develop.

## DIFFERENTIAL DIAGNOSIS

**Verrucous Skin Lesion**   Squamous cell carcinoma, pyoderma gangrenosum, tumor stage of mycosis fungoides, ecthyma, tuberculosis verrucosa cutis, actinomycosis, nocardiosis, mycetoma, syphilitic gumma, granuloma inguinale, leprosy, bromoderma.

## LABORATORY EXAMINATIONS

**Direct Examination**   KOH preparation of pus or respiratory tract secretions shows large (8- to 15-μm), single, budding cells with a thick "double-contoured" wall and a wide pore of attachment. Specific diagnosis can be made with antibodies to *B. dermatitidis* antigens.

**Culture**   Of sputum, pus from skin lesion or biopsy, prostatic secretions.

**Dermatopathology**   Pseudoepitheliomatous hyperplasia. Budding yeast with thick walls and broad-based buds in microabscess in dermis visualized by silver stain or PAS stain. Mucicarmine stain differentiates *B. dermatitidis* from *Cryptococcus neoformans*.

**Imaging**   Acute (primary) infection shows pneumonitis, hilar lymphadenopathy. With chronic pulmonary infection, x-ray findings highly variable.

## DIAGNOSIS

Clinical suspicion, confirmed by culture of organism from skin biopsy, sputum, pus, urine.

## COURSE AND PROGNOSIS

Most primary pulmonary blastomycosis cases are asymptomatic, self-limited. Cutaneous infection usually occurs months or years after primary pulmonary infection. Skin most common site of extrapulmonary infection, followed by bones, prostate, and meninges; rarely, adrenals and liver. Before amphotericin B, mortality rate in individuals with disseminated infection was 80 to 90%. Cure rate with itraconazole, 95%.

## MANAGEMENT

**Prevention**   Because of the widespread extent of *B. dermatitidis* in endemic regions, avoidance is not possible.

**General Care**   Patients with mild to moderate acute pulmonary blastomycosis can often be followed without antifungal therapy, especially if the patient is improving at time of diagnosis. Patients with meningitis or acute respiratory distress syndrome are best treated in hospital with IV amphotericin B.

**Intravenous Amphotericin B**   In life-threatening infections: *amphotericin B*, 120 to 150 mg/week with a total dose of 2 g in adults. New liposomal preparations are less toxic. After initial improvement, therapy can be continued on an outpatient basis, three times weekly.

**Oral Antifungal Therapy**   In those whose infection is non-life-threatening and/or those unable to tolerate amphotericin B: Itraconazole, 200 to 400 mg/d for >2 months; ketoconazole (alternative), 800 mg/d.

---

## DISSEMINATED COCCIDIOIDOMYCOSIS

---

Coccidioidomycosis is a systemic mycosis characterized by primary pulmonary infection that usually resolves spontaneously. Subsequently, it can disseminate hematogenously and result in chronic, progressive, granulomatous infection in skin, lungs, bone, meninges.
*Synonyms*: San Joaquin Valley fever, valley fever, desert fever.

## EPIDEMIOLOGY AND ETIOLOGY

**Etiology**   *Coccidioides immitis*, a dimorphic fungus. This mold grows in soil in arid areas of the western hemisphere.

**Race**   Blacks, Filipinos.

**Sex**   Risk of dissemination greater in males, pregnant females.

**Incidence**   Greatly increased in southern California during the past few years. Approximately

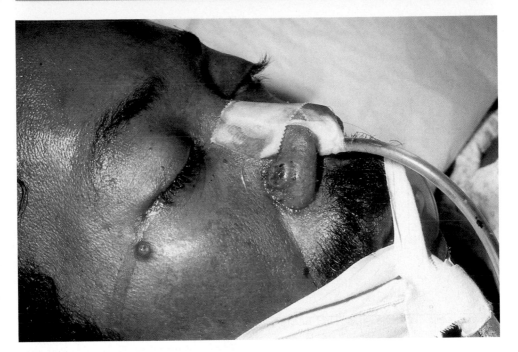

**FIGURE 23-47  Coccidioidomycosis: disseminated** *Ulcerated and crusted nodules on the cheek and nose in an individual with pulmonary coccidioidomycosis with dissemination to the skin. (Courtesy of Francis Renna, MD.)*

100,000 cases in the United States per year; most asymptomatic. In endemic areas: infection rates, measured by skin test reactivity, may be 16 to 42% or higher by early adulthood. Occurs in up to 25% of HIV-infected individuals in highly endemic regions such as Arizona or Bakersfield, CA.

**Acquisition**  Inhalation of arthroconidia is followed by primary pulmonary infection. Rarely, percutaneous.

**Risk Factors**  Nonwhite, pregnancy, immunosuppression, HIV infection with low CD4+ cell counts.

**Demography**  Regions endemic for *C. immitis* include: southern California (San Joaquin Valley), southern Arizona, Utah, New Mexico, Nevada, southwestern Texas; adjacent areas of Mexico; Central and South America. Primary pulmonary coccidioidomycosis occurs in individuals living in these regions (endemic) or in visitors to the regions (nonendemic).

**Classification**  Asymptomatic infection, febrile illness (valley fever), acute self-limited pulmonary coccidioidomycosis, disseminated coccidioidomycosis (cutaneous, osteoarticular, meningeal).

## PATHOGENESIS

Spores inhaled, resulting in primary pulmonary infection that is asymptomatic or accompanied by symptoms of coryza. Failure to develop cell-mediated immunity is associated with disseminated infection and relapse after therapy.

## HISTORY

**Incubation Period**   1 to 4 weeks.

**Symptoms**   About 40% of persons infected with *C. immitis* become symptomatic. With primary pulmonary infection, influenza- or grippe-like illness with fever, chills, malaise, anorexia, myalgia, pleuritic chest pain. With disseminated infection, headache, bone pain. In HIV disease, clinical presentation is quite variable: focal pulmonary lesions, meningitis, focal disseminated lesions, or widespread disease. In HIV disease, usually presents when CD4+ cell count is <200/μL; the lower the CD4+ cell count, the more diffuse and widespread the mycosis.

## PHYSICAL EXAMINATION

### Skin Lesions

**Primary Infection**   Toxic erythema (diffuse erythema, morbilliform, urticaria); erythema nodosum.

**Hematogenous Dissemination to Skin**   Initially, papule evolving with formation of pustules, plaques, nodules (Fig. 23-47); abscess formation, multiple draining sinus tracts, ulcers; subcutaneous cellulitis; verrucous plaques; granulomatous nodules; scars. Central face (Fig. 23-47), especially nasolabial fold—preferential site; extremities.

**Primary Cutaneous Inoculation Site (Rare)** Nodule eroding to ulcer. May have sporotrichoid lymphangitis, regional lymphadenitis.

**General Examination** *Bone*   Osteomyelitis. Psoas area produces draining abscess.

*CNS*   Signs of meningitis.

## DIFFERENTIAL DIAGNOSIS

**Disseminated Papules/Pustules**   Warts, furuncles, ecthyma, rosacea, lichen simplex chronicus, prurigo nodularis, blastomycosis, cryptococcosis, tuberculosis. In HIV-infected patient: may resemble folliculitis, molluscum contagiosum.

## LABORATORY EXAMINATIONS

**Dermatopathology**   Granulomatous inflammation; spores in tissue.

**Culture**   Pus, biopsy specimen grows organism on Sabouraud's medium.

## DIAGNOSIS

Detection of *C. immitis* sporangia containing typical sporangiospores in sputum/pus; culture; skin biopsy.

## COURSE AND PROGNOSIS

About 40% of persons infected with *C. immitis* become symptomatic. Disseminated disease is rare in immunocompetent persons but occurs at a higher rate in the United States among blacks, Filipinos, pregnant women, and immunosuppressed persons, particularly those with HIV infection. Most infected residents of endemic areas heal spontaneously. Meningeal infection difficult to cure. The incidence of relapse of pulmonary or dissemiated infection is relatively high. In HIV disease without immune reconstitution, mortality rate is 43%; 60% mortality rate with diffuse pulmonary disease; relapse rate very high.

## MANAGEMENT

**Systemic Antifungal Therapy**   *Non-Life-Threatening Infection*   Fluconazole, 200 to 400 mg/d, *or* itraconazole.

*Life-Threatening Infection*   Amphotericin B deoxycholate.

**Secondary Prophylaxis**   Lifelong therapy for meningeal infection may be required and is required in HIV disease.

## Acute Candidemia   ❒ ●

Candidemia is caused by *Candida albicans* and non-*albicans* species; it is the fifth most common cause of nosocomial bloodstream infections in the United States. Risk factors include neutropenia, immunocompromise, perforation of GI tract, mucosal damage due to cytotoxic agents used for cancer chemotherapy, intravenous drug use, and third-degree burns. Candidemia usually occurs in febrile neutropenic patients, presenting with small erythematous cutaneous papules (Fig. 23-48), which may become necrotic. On lesional skin biopsy, *Candida* yeast forms are visualized in the dermis. The differential diagnosis includes *Malassezia* folliculitis, which occurs on the trunk of healthy individuals. Candidemia has high associated morbidity and mortality.

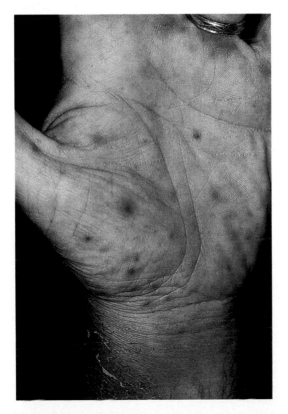

**FIGURE 23-48   Invasive candidiasis with candidemia**   *Multiple, erythematous papules on the hand of a febrile patient with granulocytopenia associated with treatment of acute myelogenous leukemia. The usual source of the infection is the gastrointestinal tract.* Candida tropicalis *was isolated on blood culture; candidal forms were seen on lesional skin biopsy.*

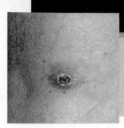

# RICKETTSIAL INFECTIONS

The Rickettsiae are a family of gram-negative coccobacilli and short bacilli, characterized by their obligate localization and persistence within eukaryotic cells, movement through mammalian reservoirs, and transmission by insect vectors. Except for louse-borne typhus, humans are incidental hosts. Rickettsioses are classified into five groups (Table 24-1); an exanthem is a major clinical and diagnostic feature of the first group, i.e., the spotted fevers.

## SPOTTED FEVERS     □  ◑ → ●

The spotted fevers include Rocky Mountain spotted fever (RMSF), tick typhus, and rickettsialpox and are characterized by an exanthem and fever. All, except for rickettsialpox, are transmitted to humans by the bite of ixodid ticks. Clinically, the spectrum of severity of clinical findings is broad, ranging from mild symptoms of general malaise and an exanthem to life-threatening illness. RMSF is covered in a separate section.

### EPIDEMIOLOGY AND ETIOLOGY

**Age of Onset** More common in children and young adults, related to out-of-doors activities.
**Sex** Males > females.
**Etiology, Geographic Distribution** See Table 24-2. The rickettsiae causing the spotted fevers are collectively referred to as the *spotted fever group* (SFG).
**Transmission** All except rickettsialpox (transmitted by mite bite) are transmitted by ixodid tick bite.
**Season** Mediterranean spotted fever (MSF) occurs mainly in warmer summer months (July, August, September) when ticks are feeding.

### PATHOGENESIS

Rickettsiae reproduce within endothelial cells at the bite site; the subsequent injury results in dermal and epidermal necrosis and perivascular edema, which presents clinically as a papule that evolves to a crusted ulcer at the bite site (tâche noire, or eschar). Rickettsiae then seed from this site both into blood and systemically. In severe cases, disseminated vascular infection occurs, with meningoencephalitis and

vascular lesions in kidneys, lungs, gastrointestinal (GI) tract, liver, pancreas, heart, spleen, and skin.

### HISTORY

**Incubation Period** Range, 3 to 14 days (mean, 7 days) after the tick bite.
**Prodrome** Nonspecific.
**Travel History** Recent travel to endemic region.
**History of Tick Bite** Often not elicited in that the rickettsiae are transmitted by tiny immature larvae and nymphs.
**Symptoms** Onset is sudden in 50% of patients. Most common: headache, fever; also chills, myalgias, arthralgias, malaise, anorexia.

### PHYSICAL EXAMINATION

#### Skin Lesions
**Types** *RMSF* See "Rocky Mountain Spotted Fever," below.
*Tâche Noire* An inoculation eschar: papule forms at the bite site and evolves to a painless, black-crusted ulcer with a red areola (resembles a cigarette burn) (Fig. 24-1) in 3 to 7 days. Occurs in all spotted fevers except RMSF.

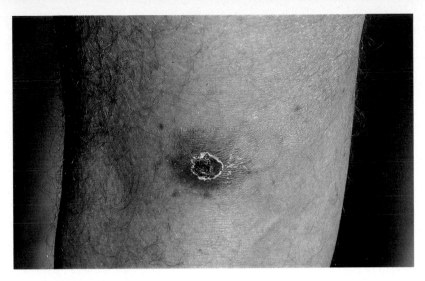

**FIGURE 24-1    Rickettsialpox: tâche noire**    *A crusted, ulcerated papule (eschar) with a red halo resembling a cigarette burn at the site of a tick bite.*

**TABLE 24-1    Classification of Groups of Rickettsial Infections and Clinical Features**

| Groups of Rickettsial Infections | Cutaneous Findings |
|---|---|
| Tick- and gamasid mite–borne spotted fever group (SFG) | Exanthem is a major clinical and diagnostic feature |
| Flea- and louse-borne typhus group rickettsial disease | |
| Flea-borne typhus (endemic murine) | Maculopapular rash occurring on the extremities and trunk, sparing the face, palms, and soles, in 13% of patients |
| Louse-borne typhus | Generalized maculopapular rash, sparing the face, palms, and soles, possibly becoming petechial and confluent |
| Chigger-borne scrub typhus | Eschar at site of chigger feeding (<50% of cases); maculopapular rash may occur, but seldom observed |
| Ehrlichiosis | Rash in ≤5% at onset |
| Q fever | Rare |

**Table 24-2   Etiology and Geographic Distribution of Spotted Fevers**

| Disease in Humans | Etiology | Distribution |
|---|---|---|
| **Rocky Mountain spotted fever** | *Rickettsia rickettsii* | Western hemisphere |
| **Tick typhus** | | Primarily Mediterranean countries (southern Europe below 45th parallel), all of Africa, India, southwestern and southcentral Asia |
| Mediterranean spotted fever (fièvre boutonneuse, Marseilles fever), Kenya tick typhus, Israeli spotted fever, Indian tick typhus, Astrakhan spotted fever | *R. conorii* | Mediterranean islands and surrounding lands; Africa |
| African tick-bite fever | *R. africae* | Central, eastern, southern Africa |
| Siberian (North Asian) tick typhus | *R. sibirica* | Siberia, Mongolia, northern China |
| Queensland tick typhus | *R. australis* | Australia |
| Flinders Island spotted fever | *R. honei* | Flinders Island (near Tasmania) |
| Japanese/Oriental spotted fever | *R. japonica* | Japan |
| **Rickettsialpox** | *R. akari* | United States, Russia, South Africa, Korea, Europe |

*Tick Typhus* About 3 to 4 days after appearance of the tâche noire, an erythematous maculopapular eruption appears on the forearms and subsequently becomes generalized, involving the face, palms/soles. The density of the eruption heightens during the next few days. In severe cases, the lesions may become hemorrhagic.

*Rickettsialpox* About 2 to 3 days after the onset of symptoms, a papulovesicular eruption appears. The initial lesions are erythematous papules (2 to 10 mm in diameter) (Fig. 24-2). Papules evolve to vesicles and then heal after crust formation.

**Distribution** Similar pattern of spread and distribution in all spotted fevers—trunk, extremities, face (centrifugal)—except RMSF, which first appears at wrists and ankles and spreads centripetally.

**General Findings** Conjunctivitis, pharyngitis, photophobia. CNS symptoms (confusion, stupor, delirium, seizures, coma) common in RMSF but not seen in other spotted fevers.

**Lymph Nodes** Nodes proximal to tâche noire are usually enlarged and nontender.

## DIFFERENTIAL DIAGNOSIS

**Tick Typhus** Viral exanthems, drug eruption.
**Rickettsialpox** Varicella, pityriasis lichenoides et varioliformis acuta (PLEVA), viral exanthems, disseminated gonococcal infection.

## LABORATORY EXAMINATIONS

**Skin Biopsy** *Rickettsialpox* Basal layer of epidermis shows vacuolar degeneration; vesiculation is subepidermal. Superficial and mid-dermal neutrophilic and mononuclear cell infiltrate are present.

**Direct Immunofluorescence** Rickettsiae can be detected in lesional biopsy specimens from site of tick bite and cutaneous lesions; also in circulating endothelial cells and various tissues obtained postmortem.

**Polymerase Chain Reaction** Detects rickettsial DNA in skin lesions.

**Serodiagnosis** Various tests are available. Antirickettsial therapy usually blunts antibody responses. Demonstration of antibodies to SFG rickettsiae by microimmunofluorescence, latex agglutination, enzyme immunoassay, Western blot, or complement fixation. Enzyme-linked immunosorbent assay (ELISA) (IgM capture assays) among the most sensitive.

**Culture** Not available as a routine test. Rickettsiae can be cultured in the guinea pig and in a shell vial cell culture system.

**FIGURE 24-2   Rickettsialpox: exanthem**   *Multiple, erythematous papules and pustules, some with central hemorrhage and crusting, on the back after hematogenous dissemination of* R. akari *from the tick bite site.*

## DIAGNOSIS

Epidemiologic and clinical findings with identification of a tâche noire confirmed by demonstration of rickettsiae by immunohistologic techniques in lesional skin biopsy specimens and/or serology. In an endemic area, patients presenting with fever, rash, and/or a skin lesion consisting of a black necrotic area or a crust surrounded by erythema should be considered to have one of the rickettsial spotted fevers.

## COURSE AND PROGNOSIS

In France and Spain, the mortality rate ranges from 1.4 to 5.6%, similar to that of RMSF. Spotted fevers are usually milder in children. Morbidity and mortality rates are higher (up to 50%) in individuals with diabetes mellitus, cardiac insufficiency, alcoholism. In rickettsialpox, clinical symptoms are usually mild, morbidity and mortality are uncommon; in untreated cases, symptoms resolve in 2 to 3 weeks.

## MANAGEMENT

**Prevention** Control host animals and vectors.
**Antirickettsial Therapy** Specific antirickettsial therapy abbreviates the length and severity of illness, i.e., spotted fevers, tick typhus, and rickettsialpox.
***Drug of Choice*** Doxycycline, 100 mg PO bid for 1 to 5 days.
***Alternatives*** Ciprofloxacin, 750 mg PO bid for 5 days, *or* chloramphenicol, 500 mg PO qid for 7 to 10 days, *or* josamycin (in pregnancy), 3 g/d PO for 5 days.

## ROCKY MOUNTAIN SPOTTED FEVER    □    ●

Rocky Mountain spotted fever, the most severe of the rickettsial spotted fevers, is characterized by sudden onset of fever, severe headache, myalgia, and a characteristic acral exanthem; it is associated with significant morbidity and mortality rates.

### EPIDEMIOLOGY AND ETIOLOGY

**Age of Onset** Incidence of infection highest in 5- to 9-year-old children.
**Etiology** *Rickettsia rickettsii* (*RR*)
**Transmission** Through bite of infected tick; inoculation through abrasions contaminated with tick feces or tissue juices. Reservoirs and vectors: wood tick *Dermacentor andersoni* in western United States; dog tick *D. variabilis* (4% infected with rickettsiae, most often with nonpathogenic species, i.e., *R. montana, R. belli*) in eastern two-thirds of United States and Canada; *Rhipicephalus sanguineus* in Mexico; and *Amblyomma cajennense* in Mexico and Central and South America. Patient either lives in or has recently visited an endemic area, *but only 60% have knowledge of a recent tick bite during the 2 weeks before onset of illness.* Exposure to ticks occurs in tick-infested areas or in association with dogs who bring the dog tick into the patient's yard and home.
**Season** Cases occur mainly in the spring in northern areas. In warmer southern states, most cases occur April 1 to September 30. The longest season and greatest number of wintertime cases occur farther south.
**Demography** Occurs only in the western hemisphere. In the United States, highest incidence: Oklahoma, North Carolina, Virginia, Maryland, Georgia, Michigan, Alaska, Montana, South Dakota. Rarely occurs in the Rocky Mountain region. Also documented in Canada, Mexico, Costa Rica, Panama, Columbia, Brazil. Travelers to the western hemisphere may import RMSF.
**Incidence** In the United States, 600 cases of RMSF are reported to the Centers for Disease Control and Prevention (CDC) annually. The actual incidence is probably significantly higher. Four states (North Carolina, Oklahoma, Tennessee, South Carolina) account for 48% of United States cases. Incidence highest in 5- to 9-year-old children.

### PATHOGENESIS

Inoculation usually requires >6 h feeding, after which *RR* are released from the salivary glands. After inoculation of *RR* into the dermis, initial local replication of *RR* occurs in endothelial cells and is followed by hematogenous and lymphatic dissemination. Organisms spread throughout the body and attach to the vascular endothelial cells, the principal target. Foci infected by *RR* enlarge as rickettsiae spread from cell to cell, forming a network of contiguously infected endothelial cells in the microcirculation of the dermis, and to multiple organs and tissues. Focal infection of vascular smooth muscle causes a generalized vasculitis. Patients with severe infection of brain and lungs have a high mortality rate. Increased vascular permeability results in edema, hypovolemia, hypotension, ischemia, gangrene. Rash results from extravasation of blood after vascular necrosis.

### HISTORY

**Incubation Period** Range, 3 to 14 days (mean, 7 days) after the tick bite.
**Prodrome** Anorexia, irritability, malaise, chilliness, and feverish feeling.
**History of Tick Bite** Given in only 60% of cases.
**Symptoms** Onset of symptoms is usually abrupt with fever (94%), severe headache (86%), generalized myalgia (especially the back and leg muscles; 83%), a sudden shaking rigor, photophobia, prostration, nausea with occasional vomiting, all within the first 2 days. However, onset is at times less striking. Symptoms are similar to those of many acute infectious diseases, making specific diagnosis difficult during the first few days. On first day of illness, only 14% of patients have characteristic rash; during first 3 days, 49% of patients have rash. In 20% of cases, rash appears only on day 6 or after. In 13% of cases, no rash is detected (spotless RMSF).

## PHYSICAL EXAMINATION

**General Findings** Initially during first 3 days, nonspecific symptoms: fever, headache, malaise, myalgia, vomiting, anorexia. Subsequently, fever to 40°C. Hypotension, shock later in course. Hepatomegaly, splenomegaly, GI hemorrhage, encephalitis (altered consciousness, confusion, lethargy, stupor, delirium, coma), cranial nerve palsy, incontinence, renal failure, and secondary bacterial infections of the lung, middle ear, and parotid gland may occur.

### Variants

> *Spotless fever*: 13% of cases. Associated with higher mortality rate because diagnosis is overlooked.
> *Abdominal syndrome*: Can mimic acute abdomen, acute cholecystitis, acute appendicitis.
> *Thrombotic thrombocytopenic purpura.*

### Skin Lesions

Day 1 of illness, 14% have rash; day 3, 49%. Initially, few small, pink macules. Temporal evolution of the rash is extremely helpful in the diagnosis. Extensive cutaneous necrosis due to disseminated intravascular coagulation (DIC) or hypotension rare.

*Types* Early lesions, 2 to 6 mm, pink, blanchable macules (Figs. 24-3 and 24-4). In 1 to 3 days, evolve to deep red papules (Fig. 24-5). In 2 to 4 days, become hemorrhagic, no longer blanchable. Local edema. Rarely, on eschar (round crusted ulcer associated with an acute *RR* infection) is present at the site of the tick bite. Necrosis of the skin and underlying structures. With DIC or prolonged hypotension, skin infarcts (gangrene) occur.

*Distribution* Characteristically, rash begins *on wrists* (Fig. 24-3), forearms, and ankles (Fig. 24-4) and somewhat later on palms and soles. Within 6 to 18 h, rash spreads centripetally to the arms, thighs, trunk (Fig. 24-5), and face. The hemorrhagic rash involving the palms and soles occurs in 36 to 82% of cases and appears after the fifth day of illness in 43%. Necrosis occurs in acral extremities and scrotum.

## DIFFERENTIAL DIAGNOSIS

Usually of a tick-exposed patient who presents between May and September with a 1- to 3-day history of fever, headache, myalgia, malaise:

• *Without Rash* influenza, enteroviral infection, infectious mononucleosis, viral hepatitis, leptospirosis, typhoid fever, gram-negative or positive sepsis, ehrlichiosis, murine typhus, rickettsialpox.

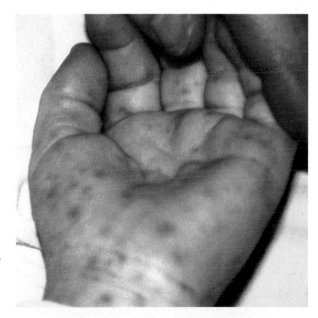

**FIGURE 24-3  Rocky Mountain spotted fever: early** *Erythematous and hemorrhagic macules and papules appeared initially on the wrists of a young child.*

- **With Rash** rubeola, rubella, meningococcemia, disseminated gonococcal infection, toxic shock syndrome, drug hypersensitivity, thrombocytopenic purpura, Kawasaki syndrome, vasculitis.

## LABORATORY EXAMINATIONS

**Skin Biopsy** Necrotizing vasculitis: *RR* can at times be demonstrated within the endothelial cells by immunofluorescence or immunoenzyme staining techniques.

**Direct Immunofluorescence** Specific *RR* antigen within endothelial cells 70% sensitive; 100% specific. Treatment with antirickettsial drugs within 48 h reduces sensitivity.

**Serodiagnosis** Indirect immunofluorescence assay (IFA) can be used to measure both IgG and IgM anti-*R. rickettsii* antibodies. Fourfold rise in titer between acute and convalescent stages is diagnostic, with a titer of $\geq 64$ detectable between 7 and 10 days after onset of illness.

## DIAGNOSIS

Clinical and epidemiologic considerations more important than a laboratory diagnosis in early RMSF. Suspect in febrile children, adolescents, and men >60 years of age—particularly those who reside in or have traveled to the southern Atlantic states and south-central states from May through September and participated in outdoor activity. Diagnosis must be made clinically and confirmed later. Only 3% of patients with RMSF present with the triad of rash, fever, and history of a tick bite during the first 3 days of illness.

## COURSE AND PROGNOSIS

Death is associated with older age, delay in diagnosis and delay in treatment or no treatment, treatment with chloramphenicol (compared with tetracycline). Untreated (before the availability of effective antibiotics), the fatality rate was 23%; treated, 3% (6% if >40 years of age). Fatality rate: 1.5% with known tick bite but 6.6% if no known tick exposure. Fulminant RMSF is defined as a fatal disease whose course is unusually rapid (i.e., 5 days from onset to death) and is usually characterized by early onset of neurologic signs and late or absent rash. In 1990, the case-fatality rate was 8% for individuals <20 years of age and 6.8% for those >20 years. In uncomplicated cases, defervescence usually occurs within 48 to 72 h after initiation of therapy.

## MANAGEMENT

**Prevention** Avoid tick bites: protective clothing, tick repellants. After possible exposure, inspect for ticks. (see "Lyme Borreliosis" in Section 22).

**Antirickettsial Therapy** Specific antirickettsial therapy should be initiated as soon as the diagnosis is susptected clinically.

**Drug of Choice** Doxycycline (except for pregnant patients, history of allergy to doxycycline), 200 mg/d PO or IV in two divided doses for adults. Tetracycline, 25 to 50 mg/kg per day in four divided doses.

**Alternative** Chloramphenicol, 50 to 75 mg/kg per day in four divided doses.

**Supportive Therapy** For acute problems of shock, acute renal failure, respiratory failure, prolonged coma.

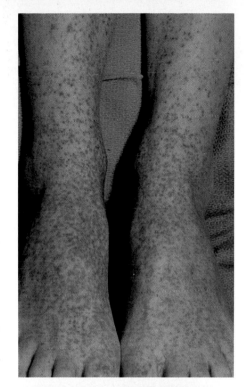

**FIGURE 24-4   Rocky Mountain spotted fever: early**
*Erythematous and hemorrhagic macules and papules appeared initially on the ankles of an adolescent.*

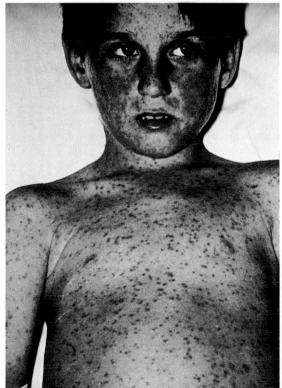

**FIGURE 24-5   Rocky Mountain spotted fever: late** *Disseminated hemorrhagic macules and papules on the face, neck, trunk, and arms on the fourth day of febrile illness in an older child. The initial lesions were noted on the wrists and ankles, subsequently extending centripetally.*

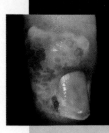

# VIRAL INFECTIONS OF SKIN AND MUCOSA

Viral infections of skin and mucosa produce a wide spectrum of clinical manifestations. Viruses such as human papillomavirus (HPV) and molluscum contagiosum virus (MCV) colonize the epidermis of most individuals without causing any clinical lesions. Benign epithelial proliferations, i.e., warts and molluscum, occur in some, are transient, and eventually resolve without therapy. In immunocompromised individuals, however, these lesions may become extensive, persistent, and refractory to therapy. Viruses that cause febrile illness with exanthems are usually self-limited, with primary infection conveying lifetime immunity. The eight human herpesviruses often have asymptomatic primary infection but are characterized by lifelong latent infection. In the setting of immunocompromise, these viruses can become active and cause disease with significant morbidity and mortality rates.

## POXVIRUS INFECTIONS

The poxvirus family is a diverse group of epitheliotropic viruses that infect both humans and animals. The genera of poxviruses that infect humans include orthopoxvirus, parapoxvirus, molluscipoxvirus, and yatapoxvirus (Table 25-1). Only smallpox virus (SPV) and molluscum contagiosum virus (MCV) cause natural disease in humans; other poxviruses are associated with zoonotic infections. SPV and monkeypox virus typically cause systemic disease with rash; other poxviruses cause localized skin lesions.

Poxviruses are the largest of all animal viruses and have a double-strand DNA genome. They are the only DNA viruses that replicate in cytoplasm, where accumulated viral particles form eosinophilic inclusions, or Guarnieri bodies, visible by light microscopy (200 to 400 μm). Poxviruses appear as brick-shaped or oval virus particles by electron microscopy. The nucleosome contains double-strand DNA, which is surrounded by a membrane. The outer surface of the lipoprotein bilayer has surface tubules that are randomly arranged and give the virion its characteristic textured appearance.

Smallpox, or variola, has been eradicated as a naturally occurring infection. Cowpox is an infection of cattle and is caused by cowpox virus.

The origins of vaccinia virus, which is used to immunize humans against smallpox, are uncertain. It may be derived from variola virus, cowpox virus, or be a hybrid of the two. MCV colonizes the skin of many healthy individuals, causing molluscum contagiosum, self-limited epidermal proliferations that resolve spontaneously. Human orf and milker's nodules are zoonotic infections that can sometimes occur in exposed humans. Other poxviruses that are zoonoses in animal hosts (monkeys, cows, buffalo, sheep, goats) can also infect humans.

Poxviruses cause toxic effects on cells, which result in cell rounding and clumping, degeneration of cell architecture, and production of cytoplasmic vacuoles. Different poxviruses are capable of producing a localized, self-limited infection by inoculation to the skin (e.g., orf) or a fulminant systemic disease (e.g., variola). The same virus can affect different species in different ways.

**TABLE 25-1   Poxviruses That Infect Humans* and Cause Disease**

| Genus and Species (Disease) | Primary Reservoir | Geographic Region | Mode of Transmission | Protection Provided by Vaccination |
|---|---|---|---|---|
| **Orthopoxvirus** | | | | |
| Cowpox | Rodents | Europe, Africa, central/northern Asia | Direct contact | Yes |
| Monkeypox | Rodents | West/central Africa | Direct contact, Respiratory droplets | Yes Yes |
| Vaccinia | Unknown | | Direct contact | |
| Variola (smallpox) | Humans | U.S., Russia | Direct contact, Respiratory droplets | Yes |
| **Yatapoxvirus** | | | | |
| Tanapox | Nonhuman primates | Kenya, Zaire | Direct contact | No |
| Yabapox | Nonhuman primates | Central Africa | Direct contact | No |
| **Parapoxvirus** | | | | |
| Pseudocowpox (milker's nodules and paravaccinia) | Ungulates | Worldwide | Direct contact | No |
| Bovine papular stomatitis (milker's nodules) | Ungulates (humans) | U.S., Canada, Africa, Australia, New Zealand, Great Britain, Europe | Direct contact | No |
| Orf (Human orf) | Ungulates (humans) | North America, Europe, New Zealand | Direct contact | No |
| Sealpox | Seals | North Sea, Pacific Ocean, Atlantic Ocean | Direct contact | No |
| **Molluscipoxvirus** | | | | |
| Molluscipox (molluscum contagiosum) | Humans | Worldwide | Direct contact | No |

*Poxviruses that do not infect humans include camelpox and sheep and goat lumpy skin disease complex.

## MOLLUSCUM CONTAGIOSUM     ■  ○ → ◑

Molluscum contagiosum (MC) is a self-limited epidermal viral infection, characterized clinically by skin-colored papules that are often umbilicated, occurring in children and sexually active adults. In HIV-infected individuals, however, numerous large mollusca often arise on the face, causing significant cosmetic disfigurement.

### EPIDEMIOLOGY AND ETIOLOGY

**Etiology**   Molluscum contagiosum virus (MCV), a poxvirus, with 30% homology with smallpox virus. Types MCV-1 and MCV-2. The virus has not been cultivated. Not distinguishable from other poxviruses by electron microscopy. In many healthy adults, the epidermis and infundibulum of hair follicle are colonized by MCV.

**Age, Sex**   Children; sexually active adults; males > females.

**Risk Factors**   HIV-infected individuals may have hundreds of small mollusca or giant mollusca on the face.

**Transmission**   Skin-to-skin contact.

**Classification by Risk Groups**   *Children*   Mollusca commonly occur on exposed skin sites. Child-to-child transmission relatively low. Resolve spontaneously. Usually caused by MCV-1. *Sexually Active Adults* Occur in genital region. Virus transmitted during sexual activity. Resolve spontaneously. *HIV-Infected Individuals* Most commonly occur on the face, spread by shaving. Without aggressive therapy, mollusca enlarge. Spontaneous regression does not occur. Usually caused by MCV-2. With response to highly active antiretroviral therapy (HAART), lesions often resolve.

### PATHOGENESIS

A subclinical carrier state of MCV probably exists in many adults. Unique among poxviruses, MCV infection results in epidermal tumor formation; other human poxviruses cause a necrotic "pox" lesion. Rupture and discharge of the infectious virus-packed cells occur in the umbilication/crater of the lesion.

### HISTORY

**Duration of Lesions**   In the normal host, mollusca usually persist up to 6 months and then undergo spontaneous regression. In HIV-infected individuals without HAART, mollusca persist and proliferate even after aggressive local therapy.

**Skin Symptoms**   Usually none. Cosmetic disfigurement. Concern about having a transmissible infection. Painful if secondarily infected.

### PHYSICAL EXAMINATION

#### Skin Lesions

Papules (1 to 2 mm), nodules (5 to 10 mm) (rarely, giant) (Figs. 25-1 and 25-2). Pearly white or skin-colored. Round, oval, hemispherical, umbilicated (Fig. 25-1). Isolated single lesion; multiple, scattered discrete lesions; or confluent mosaic plaques. Most larger mollusca have a central keratotic plug, which gives the lesion a central dimple or umbilication, best observed after light liquid nitrogen freeze. Gentle pressure on a molluscum causes the central plug to be extruded. Autoinoculation is apparent in that mollusca are clustered at a site such as the axilla. Host immune response to viral antigen results in an inflammatory halo around MC, i.e., "MC dermatitis," which usually heralds spontaneous regression; purulence may occur.

In HIV-infected males who shave, mollusca can be confined to the beard area. Hundreds of lesions occur in HIV-infected patients (Fig. 25-3). Mollusca undergoing spontaneous regression have an erythematous halo. In dark-skinned individuals, significant postinflammatory hyperpigmentation after treatment or spontaneous regression may occur.

**Distribution**   Any site may be infected, especially axillae, antecubital, popliteal fossae, crural folds. In children: genital lesions occur via autoinoculation. In atopic dermatitis, MC may be widespread. In adults with sexually transmitted MC: groins, genitalia, thighs, lower abdomen. Multiple facial MC suggest HIV infection. MC can occur in the conjunctiva, causing a unilateral conjunctivitis.

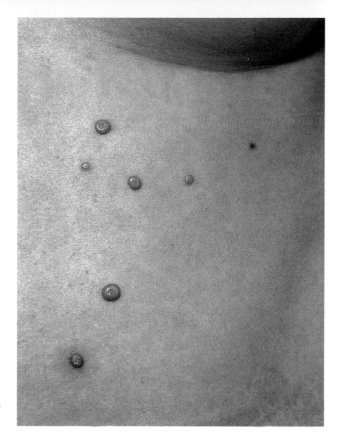

**FIGURE 25-1    Molluscum contagiosum: trunk**   *Discrete, solid, skin-colored papules, 1 to 2 mm in diameter, with central umbilication on the chest of an adolescent female. The lesion with an erythematous halo is undergoing spontaneous regression.*

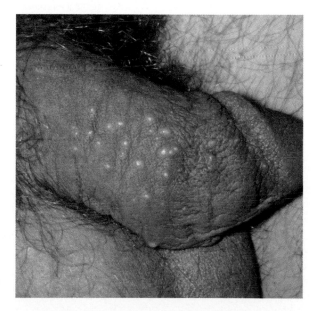

**FIGURE 25-2    Molluscum contagiosum: penis**   *Multiple, small glistening pink papules on the penile shaft.*

## DIFFERENTIAL DIAGNOSIS

**Multiple Small Mollusca**   Flat warts, condylomata acuminata, syringoma, sebaceous hyperplasia.

**Large Solitary Molluscum**   Keratoacanthoma, squamous cell carcinoma, basal cell carcinoma, epidermal inclusion cyst.

**Multiple Facial Mollusca in HIV-Infected Individual**   Disseminated invasive fungal infection, i.e., cryptococcosis, histoplasmosis, coccidioidomycosis, penicillinosis.

## LABORATORY EXAMINATIONS

**Smear of Keratotic Plug**   Direct microscopic examination of Giemsa-stained central semisolid core reveals "molluscum bodies" (inclusion bodies).

**Dermatopathology**   Epidermal cells contain large intracytoplasmic inclusion bodies, i.e., molluscum bodies, that appear as single, ovoid eosinophilic structures in lower cells of stratum malpighii. Molluscum bodies contain large numbers of maturing virions. Epidermis grows down into dermis. Infection also occurs in epithelium and follicle.

## DIAGNOSIS

Usually made on clinical findings. Biopsy lesion in HIV-infected individual if disseminated invasive fungal infection is in the differential diagnosis.

## COURSE AND PROGNOSIS

In healthy individuals, MC resolves spontaneously without scarring, but may take up to 2 years. In HIV-infected individuals, mollusca often progress even with aggressive therapies, creating significant cosmetic disfigurement, especially by facial lesions. In HIV-infected individuals successfully treated with HAART, mollusca either do not occur or resolve after several months. Recurrence of mollusca usually indicates failure of HAART.

## MANAGEMENT

| | |
|---|---|
| **Prevention** | Avoid skin-to-skin contact with individual having mollusca. HIV-infected individuals with mollusca in the beard area should be advised to minimize shaving facial hair or grow a beard. |
| **Supportive therapy** | In immunocompetent children and sexually active adults, mollusca regress spontaneously; painful aggressive therapy is not indicated. |
| **Treatment of lesions** | |
|   Topical patient-directed therapy | 5% imiquimod cream applied hs 3 times per week for up to 1–3 months. |
|   Clinician-directed therapy (office) | These procedures are painful and traumatic, especially for young children. EMLA cream applied to lesions 1 h before therapy may reduce/eliminate pain. |
|     Curettage | Small mollusca can be removed with a small curette with little discomfort or pain. |
|     Cryosurgery | Freezing lesions for 10–15 s is effective and minimally painful, using either a cotton-tipped applicator or liquid nitrogen spray. |
|     Electrodesiccation | For mollusca refractory to cryosurgery, especially in HIV-infected individuals with numerous and/or large lesions, electrodesiccation or laser surgery is the treatment of choice. Large lesions usually require injected lidocaine anesthesia. Giant mollusca may require several cycles of electrodesiccation and curettage to remove the large bulk of lesions; these lesions may extend through the dermis into the subcutaneous fat. |

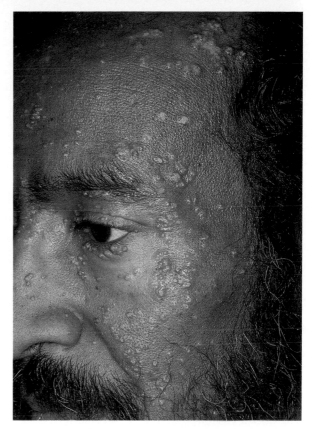

**FIGURE 25-3    Molluscum contagiosum in advanced HIV disease**
*Discrete and confluent skin-colored umbilicated papules on the face of a 52-year-old black male; note the periorbital clustering. The image is from 1990, before effective antiretroviral therapy. The lesions recurred and progressed after aggressive cryo- and electrosurgery.*

# HUMAN ORF

Human orf is a parapoxvirus infection that normally occurs in ungulates but occurs in humans exposed to the virus; it is characterized by nodular lesions on exposed cutaneous sites. *Synonym*: Ecthyma contagiosum.

## EPIDEMIOLOGY

**Synonyms of Animal Infection**   Sheep-pox, lip scab of sheep, scabby mouth, sore mouth, contagious pustular dermatosis, infectious pustular dermatitis.

**Disease in Animals**   Ungulates (sheep, goats, yaks, deer, etc.). Virus survives for many months on fences, feeding basins, and surfaces in barns. Only newborn lambs lacking viral immunity are susceptible. In lambs, orf is manifested as erythematous, exudative nodules around mouth that heal spontaneously in about a month, producing permanent immunity; lesions may become superinfected.

**Transmission to Humans**   Humans are infected either by inoculation of virus by direct contact with lambs (bottle feeding) or indirectly via fomites (knives, shears, barbed wire, feeding troughs, barn doors, fences, etc.). Human-to-human infection does not occur.

**Incidence**   Most common in farmers, veterinarians, sheep shearers exposed to infected ungulates.

**Season**   Usually in springtime (when lambs are born) and season (Easter) of slaughter of lambs and sheep.

**Demography**   Occurs worldwide with epidemics in Norway and other parts of Europe, New Zealand; rare in North America.

## PHYSICAL EXAMINATION

### Skin Lesions

Initially, one to four papule(s) to nodule(s) to plaque(s) on the hand(s); may appear very edematous to vesicular to bullous. Lesions average 1.6 cm in diameter.

The infection goes through six clinical stages, each lasting 6 days:

- Stage 1: Macule to papule, pink to red
- Stage 2: Target lesion: nodule with red center (Fig. 25-4), white middle ring, and red periphery
- Stage 3: Acute exudative nodule
- Stage 4: Regenerative dry nodule covered by a thin crust with black dots
- Stage 5: Papillomatous
- Stage 6: Regressive with dry crust (Fig. 25-5)

**Distribution**   Exposed sites (hands, arms, legs, face); most common site is dorsum of right index finger.

**Other Findings**   Ascending lymphangitis and lymphadenopathy may occur. Bacterial superinfection may occur. More extensive infection may occur in the immunocompromised host.

## DIFFERENTIAL DIAGNOSIS

Milker's nodules, anthrax, tularemia, primary inoculation tuberculosis, atypical mycobacteria infection, syphilitic chancre, sporotrichosis, pyogenic granuloma.

## LABORATORY EXAMINATION

**Electron Microscopy**   Biopsy of lesional skin shows characteristic brick-shaped viral particles 200 to 380 nm in length.

## DIAGNOSIS

Clinical findings with the appropriate history.

## COURSE

Resolves spontaneously in 4 to 6 weeks, healing without scar formation. Erythema multiforme-like eruptions have been reported in human orf. Widespread lesions spread by autoinoculation may occur in atopic dermatitis. Lesion may be large and fail to regress in chronic lymphocytic leukemia. In humans, lasting immunity is conferred by infection.

## MANAGEMENT

Antiviral agents are not effective. Treat bacterial superinfection; manage pain.

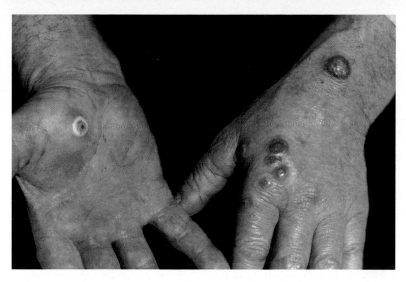

**FIGURE 25-4    Human orf: multiple lesions on hands**    *Stage 2: Multiple blisters with target/iris patterns in lesions on the hands of a sheep herder.*

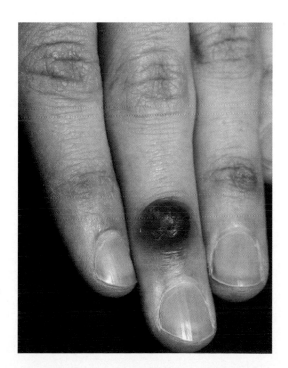

**FIGURE 25-5    Human orf: finger**    *Stage 6: Crusted regressing nodule on middle finger; lesion on index finger has resolved. Lesions arose 10 days after Greek Easter and was associated with killing a lamb.*

## MILKER'S NODULES     □   ◑

Milker's nodules (MN) are cutaneous infections caused by parapoxviruses, which normally infect cattle and only accidentally cause infection in humans. They are characterized clinically by nodular lesions on exposed cutaneous sites.
*Synonym*: Milker's node.

### EPIDEMIOLOGY AND ETIOLOGY

**Etiology**   Parapoxvirus (pseudocowpox virus), similar to that which causes orf.
**Synonyms of Animal Infection**   Paravaccinia, bovine papular stomatitis.
**Disease in Animals**   Papular lesions occur on muzzles/oral cavity of calves and on teats of cows.
**Transmission to Humans**   Contact with bovine lesions or teat cups of milking machines.
**Incidence**   Most common in dairy farmers.
**Risk Factors**   New milkers, young people, vacation milkers, veterinary students who have contact with mouths of cows (feeding or endotracheal tubes).
**Demography**   Worldwide

### PHYSICAL EXAMINATION

**Skin Lesions**
Clinical findings and course are similar to human orf. Clinically, lesions can present as solitary red-purple nodules (Fig. 25-6) or, less commonly, as multiple cherry-red papules and nodules, arising at site of inoculation.
*Distribution*   Usually on exposed sites such as hands; may occur in burn wounds.
**Other Findings**   Lymphadenopathy.

### DIFFERENTIAL DIAGNOSIS

Human orf, smallpox vaccination site, staphylococcal abscess, herpes simplex virus infection, anthrax, tularemia, primary inoculation tuberculosis, atypical mycobacteria infection, syphilitic chancre, sporotrichosis, pyogenic granuloma.

### LABORATORY EXAMINATION

See "Human Orf," above.

### DIAGNOSIS

Diagnosis is usually made on history of bovine exposure and clinical findings.

### COURSE

Self-limited.

### MANAGEMENT

Antiviral agents are not effective; treatment should be directed at treatment of bacterial superinfection and pain management.

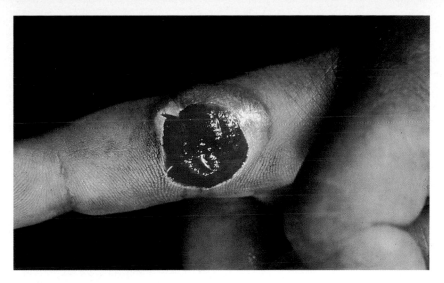

**FIGURE 25-6   Milker's nodule: finger**   *A single beefy eroded nodule on the finger of a dairy farmer at the site of inoculation.*

## SMALLPOX ☐ ●

Smallpox is an acute exanthematous disease caused by infection with poxvirus variolae. It is characterized by a severe 3-day prodromal illness and a generalized rash spreading centrifugally with rapidly successive papules, vesicles, pustules, umbilication, and crusting within 14 days. Epidemics have occurred in all populations, resulting in hundreds of millions of deaths. *Synonyms*: Variola, variola major, variola minor (alastrim).
http://www.bt.cdc.gov/agent/smallpox/overview/disease-facts.asp
http://www.who.int/ emc/diseases/smallpox/Smallpoxeradication.html

### EPIDEMIOLOGY AND ETIOLOGY

The last cases of endemic smallpox occurred in 1977; eradication of the disease was declared in 1980.

**Etiology**   Variola virus of the family Poxviridae, genus Orthopoxvirus [includes vaccinia (smallpox vaccine), monkeypox virus, other animal poxviruses]. Humans are the only host of variola. No longer exists naturally but is maintained in research laboratories and may be used as a bioterrorism weapon. DNA virus that replicates in cell cytoplasm.

**Occupation**   Laboratory workers.

**Susceptibility**   Few persons in the general population in the United States under age 30 have been vaccinated; all such persons are susceptible to smallpox. Some persons born before 1972 and vaccinated may still be protected; may have milder disease if exposed and less likely to transmit infection.

**Transmission**   Respiratory-droplet nuclei (most likely from patients with severe disease or who are coughing); contaminated clothing/bedding. Less transmissible than measles, chickenpox, influenza. Secondary attack rates among unvaccinated contacts, 37 to 88%. Maximal transmissibity: from onset of enanthema through first 7 to 10 days of rash.

**Season**    Winter, early spring (endemic).

**Classification of Clinical Types of Variola**

- *Variola major* ("ordinary"): 90% of cases, 30% mortality
- *Variola minora* (*alastrim*; modified-type): 2% of cases, occurring in unvaccinated persons and in 25% of previously vaccinated persons
- *Variola sine eruptione*: occurs in previously vaccinated contacts or in infants with maternal antibodies
- *Smallpox with flat lesions*: case fatality 97% among unvaccinated persons
- *Hemorrhagic smallpox*: near 100% case fatality rate

## PATHOGENESIS

Enters the respiratory tract, seeding mucous membranes, passing rapidly into local lymph nodes. After a brief period of viremia, latent period of 4 to 14 days occurs, during which the virus multiples in the reticuloendothelial system. Another brief period of viremia precedes prodrome, during which mouth/pharynx are infected. Virus invades capillary endothelium of dermal layer in skin, resulting in skin lesions. Virus is abundant in skin and oropharyngeal lesions in early illness. Acquired immunity via cytotoxic T cells and B cells. Neutralizing antibodies appear during first week of illness. Correlation between humoral antibodies and protection from smallpox is not certain. Death ascribed to toxemia, associated with immune complexes, and to hypotension. Infection with smallpox confers lifelong immunity.

## HISTORY

**Incubation Period**    7 to 17 days (mean, 10 to 12).

**Prodrome**    2 to 3 days. Sudden onset of severe headache, backache, fever ($\pm$40°C); subsides over 2 to 3 days. A prodomal maculopapular or petechial rash occurring in a "swimming-trunk" distribution has been reported.

## PHYSICAL EXAMINATION

**Skin Lesions**
Small red macules evolve to papules (2 to 3 mm) over 1 to 2 days; in 1 to 2 more days,

papules become vesicles (2 to 5 mm). Papules evolve to pustules (4 to 6 mm) 4 to 7 days after onset of rash (Fig. 25-7*A*, *B*), remain 5 to 8 days, and are followed by umbilication and crusting (Fig. 25-7*C*). Lesions are generally all at the same stage of development. Palm/soles lesions persist longest. Pockmarks/pitted scars occur in 65 to 85% of severe cases, especially on the face. Bacterial superinfections present as abscesses, cellulitis.

***Distribution***    Initial lesions on face and extremities, then gradually become disseminated. Peripheral/centrifugal distribution.

**Mucous Membranes**    Enanthema (tongue, mouth, oropharynx) precedes exanthem by a day.

**General Findings**    Variants: Panophthalmitis, keratitis, secondary infection of eye (1%). Arthritis in children (2%). Encephalitis (<1%)

## DIFFERENTIAL DIAGNOSIS

Severe chickpox (varicella where lesions are in different stages of development), human monkeypox (patients often have lymphadenopathy), tanapox, hand-foot-and-mouth disease (coxsackievirus A-16), insect bites, widespread molluscum contagiosum in HIV disease, adverse cutaneous drug eruption (bullous), secondary syphilis. Historically, smallpox has been confused with chickenpox, syphilis, and measles.

## LABORATORY EXAMINATIONS

**Specimens**    Skin lesions (papular, vesicular, pustular fluid; crusts); blood samples; tonsillar swabbings.

**Polymerase Chain Reaction (PCR)**    For orthopoxvirus genes, PCR identfies variola virus.

**Cultures**    Virus isolated on live cell cultures; DNA of orthopoxvirus identified.

**Serology**    Does not differentiate among orthopoxvirus species. Newer methods detect IgM responses.

**Dermatopathology**    Vaccinia replicates in basal epithelium, causing a local cellular reaction. In papular stage, capillary dilatation and edema of papillary dermis.

**Electron Microscopy**    Brick-shaped virus seen in clinical specimens.

## DIAGNOSIS

An illness with acute onset of fever >38.3°C (101°F) followed by a rash characterized by firm, deep-seated vesicles or pustules in the

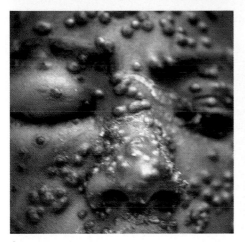

**A**

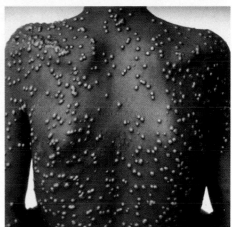

**B**

same stage of development without other apparent cause.

### Laboratory Criteria for Confirmation

- PCR identification of variola DNA in a clinical specimen, *or*
- Isolation of smallpox (variola) virus from a clinical specimen [World Health Organization (WHO) Smallpox Reference Laboratory or laboratory with appropriate reference capabilities] *plus* variola PCR confirmation.

## MANAGEMENT

In United States, possible smallpox should be reported to state health officials; diagnosis confirmed in a Biological Safety Level 4 laboratory where staff members have been vaccinated. State officials contact Centers for Disease Control and Prevention (CDC) (770-488-7100). CDC informs WHO Department of Communicable Disease Surveillance and Response Unit.

**Immunization** Vaccination against smallpox not performed in the United States since 1972 and in the rest of world since 1982. A large population of susceptible persons exists. The U.S. military is immunized against smallpox. Since the threat of bioterrorism in 2001, selected health care personnel have been vaccinated in the United States.

If an outbreak does occur, prompt recognition and vaccination would be important. Vaccination begun 2 to 3 days after exposure offers substantial protection.

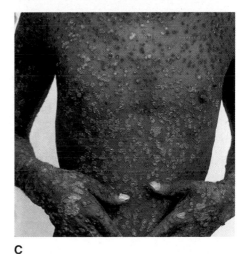

**C**

**FIGURE 25-7 Smallpox: variola major** *A. Multiple pustules becoming confluent on the face. **B.** Multiple pustules on the trunk, all in the same stage of development. **C.** Multiple crusted healing lesions on the trunk, arms, hands.*

**Precautions** Suspect case should be managed in negative-pressure room. Strict respiratory and contact isolation imperative.

**Drug of Choice** There is no treatment approved by the U.S. Food and Drug Administration (FDA) for orthoviruses. Cidofovir may be effective.

**Bacterial Superinfection** Usually *Staphylococcus aureus* or group A streptococcus. (See also "Bacterial Infections.)

# COWPOX, MONKEYPOX, TANAPOX

Cowpox, monkeypox, and tanapox are zoonotic infections, accidentally transferred to humans from animal hosts. They rarely cause human infections in developed nations. When human infections do occur, the differential diagnosis includes infections associated with bioterrorism, i.e, smallpox, anthrax, tularemia, plague. Identification of poxvirus can be made from skin-lesion tissue viral culture, PCR, immunohistologic analysis (IHC), or electron-microscopic (EM) methods.

## COWPOX

Zoonosis of cats, cows, rodents, and occasionally humans. Jenner used cowpox isolate for vaccination. Reservoir: cats (most common source for human infection), small rodents (voles, mice). Source of outbreaks in cows is unknown. Demography: occurs in Europe and in countries of the former Soviet Union. Disease in cows: pustules on teats. Disease in cats: blisters at sites of bites/scratches. Disease in humans: painful papule(s), which evolve to vesicles to umbilicated pustules (surrounded by edema/erythema) to eschar or ulcer. Multiple lesions occur on hands/face, which resolve in 3 to 4 weeks. Lymphadenopathy is common. Lesions may be extensive in atopic dermatitis. Incidence may have increased due to discontinuation of smallpox immunization and increased numbers of immunocompromised hosts.

## MONKEYPOX

Zoonosis of captive primates and rodents; human cases in Africa and recently in midwestern United States. Transmission: to humans from pet prairie dogs via open wound or scratch or bites: person-to-person transmission may occur. Incubation period: 4 to 24 days (median 15). Human illness is characterized by fever, drenching sweats, and severe chills, with skin lesions that evolve from papules to vesicopustules to serous-to-hemorrhagic crusts. Lesions occur on skin, conjunctivae, and buccal mucosa. Regional lymphadenopathy can occur.

## TANAPOX

Zoonosis of African nonhuman primates and humans. Transmission to humans: unknown; possibly by mosquitoes that have fed on infected monkeys. Disease in humans: febrile illness with 1 to 10 pruritic, indurated, ± umbilicated papules that become necrotic with red halo; occur on exposed sites. Lymphadenopathy is common.

# VACCINIA

Vaccination against smallpox consists of the introduction of vaccinia virus into the outer layers of intact skin. Local multiplication of virus occurs, and in some instances regional lymphadenopathy and systemic symptoms ensue. The infection is a local one; it heals by scarring and is limited by host response. Complications of vaccination include allergic reaction to a component of vaccine, bacterial superinfection, or persistent/spread of local vaccinia infection. *Synonym*: Cowpox.

http://www.bt.cdc.gov/training/smallpoxvaccine/reactions/sitemap.htm

## EPIDEMIOLOGY AND ETIOLOGY

**Etiology** Vaccinia virus, related to cowpox virus (see "Cowpox," above). The origin of the strains of vaccinia virus currently used for vaccination is unknown. Infection with cowpox virus confers immunity to smallpox.

**Age, Sex** Most reactions occur after first (primo) vaccination.

**Season** Superinfection occurs more often in warm weather.

**Transmission** Iatrogenic inoculation. Inadvertent transmission: autoinoculation, transmission to another person. Bioterrorism is of recent concern.

## PATHOPHYSIOLOGY

**Normal Reaction** Vaccinia replicates in the basal layer and disseminates from cell to cell, causing necrosis and formation of fluid-filled vesicles. Initial spread of virus is slowed by innate antiviral mechanisms, and, by the second week, the cell-mediated immune response begins to eliminate infected cells. Neutrophils, macrophages, and lymphocytes infiltrate the inoculation site, forming a confluent pustule and releasing cytokines and chemokines that cause hyperemia and edema in surrounding tissues. Clinical manifestations may include malaise and other mild constitutional symptoms; fever; and tender, enlarged axillary lymph nodes. Local "satellite" pustules that resolve along with the primary lesion may occur. Limited viremia occurs in some vaccines. The inflammatory process peaks 10 to 12 days after vaccination and begins to resolve by day 14, with shedding of the scab by day 21. This sequence of events, which simulates the development of a smallpox pock, is known as a "take" reaction. A successful take is required for the development of anti-vaccinia antibody and cell-mediated responses.

## Adverse Reactions (Complications)

Bacterial superinfection
Abnormal viral replication
Altered reactivity or "allergy" to some viral component.

## VACCINATION

**Contraindications** Because of adverse reactions, mandatory vaccination in the general population of the United States was discontinued in 1972 because the risk of complications outweighed the threat of endemic smallpox. Since that time, the number of immunocompromised persons has increased markedly because of the spread of HIV infection and increased numbers of patients receiving immunosuppressive medications. These persons are at risk for progressive vaccinia. (See also "Management," below.)

**Vaccine** Inoculation against smallpox is performed using vaccinia, a related Orthopoxvirus. The vaccine currently available in the United States, Dryvax (Wyeth), is obtained from pustules on inoculated calves. Nearly all side effects can be predicted from the unusual nature of smallpox vaccination, which essentially employs a small circle of skin as a "culture plate" in which to grow vaccinia virus. Newer vaccines will be produced on cell culture. Two attenuated vaccine strains have been developed and tested: modified vaccinia Ankara (MVA) and a Japanese strain (LC16m8).

**Method** Vaccine is administered with the use of a bifurcated needle, which is dipped into reconstituted vaccine. 15 assertive jabs into the dermis of the upper deltoid are given in an area with a diameter of about 0.5 cm; a small amount of blood should appear at the vaccination site within 20 to 25 s.

## CLASSIFICATION OF COMPLICATIONS OF VACCINIA VIRUS

Before 1972 in the United States, the risk of complication from vaccination was 1254 per 1 million vaccinations. Children under the age of 5 who were undergoing primary vaccination had the highest rates of complications. The case fatality rate was 1 per 1 million primary vaccinations; in 1968, there were nine vaccine-associated deaths.

**Noninfectious Rashes** Erythema multiforme-like; macular ("toxic eruption"); maculopapular; vesicular; urticarial. Most common 7 to 14 days after primovaccination or earlier after revaccination.

**Noninfectious Immune-Mediated** Encephalitis (meningoencephalitis syndrome), pericarditis/myocarditis.

**Bacterial Superinfection** Group A streptococcus (GAS); *S. aureus*, mixed; tetanus. Uncommon. Vaccine may not be sterile. Infections occur more often in persons with nasal colonization by *S. aureus* or oropharyngeal colonization with GAS. Contamination from soil or dung may result in tetanus. Other factors: trauma to site, maceration, manipulation of site.

**Accidental Inoculation** Virus usually remains localized at site of implantation but may be transposed to normal or abnormal skin/mucosa (burns, pyoderma, exanthem, eczema, other dermatitides, mucosal, corneal) elsewhere on the body or to another person. May occur in vaccinated or from vaccinated individual.

**Congenital Vaccinia** Vaccination during pregnancy may result in dissemination of infection to fetus. Infant may be stillborn or develop lesions shortly after birth.

**Generalized Vaccinia** Benign, becoming malignant with progression (see below). Usually occurs in a healthy individual whose antivaccinal antibody response is delayed but adequate. Almost always benign, with normal-healing primary vaccination. Viremic lesions are self-limited, usually occurring in one crop.

**Progressive Vaccinia (Vaccinia Gangrenosa, Vaccinia Necrosa, Disseminated Vaccinia)** Incidence during universal vaccination: 1 per million vaccines in general population. Characterized by relentless outward spread of infection from vaccination site and eventual dissemination to other areas of the body. Occurs only in persons with defective cellular immune function. *Congenital immunodeficiency*: severe, combined immunodeficiency. *Acquired immunodeficiency*: HIV disease, organ transplant recipient, chronic immunosuppression (e.g., connective tissue disorders), hypogammaglobulinemia, dysglobulinemia, malignancies (chronic lymphatic leukemia, lymphoma). Course is chronic and progressive, spreading deep into tissues and causing necrosis and osteomyelitis with bacterial superinfection, leading to death weeks or months after vaccination.

## PHYSICAL EXAMINATION

### Skin Lesions

**Normal Vaccination Reaction** 6 to 8 days after vaccination, loculated pustule (Jennerian pustule) 1 to 2 cm in diameter develops at site (Fig. 27-8). Central crusting begins and spreads peripherally over 3 to 5 days. Local edema and a dark crust remain until the third week. Other reactions are classified as equivocal, and another vaccination is required.

**Noninfectious Rashes** Erythema multiforme-like; macular, maculopapular, vesicular, or urticarial. Usually diffuse. Vesicular form may be difficult to distinguish from generalized vaccinia. Intense erythema usually surrounds vaccination site (which is normal in all other respects).

**Bacterial Superinfection** Presents as enlarging crusted inoculation site (impetigo or ecthyma). Must differentiate from progressive vaccinia. Gram stain of exudates shows gram-positive cocci.

**Accidental Inoculation** Keratitis may follow conjunctival inoculation. Inoculation on site of eczematous (atopic) dermatitis may result in progressive vaccinia infection (*eczema vaccinatum*); similar infection may also occur in burns, lichen simplex chronicus, dermatitis herpetiformis, pemphigus, herpes simplex lesions, and varicella. Mucosal inoculation may occur in conjunctiva (keratitis), mouth, vagina, airway, etc.

**Generalized Vaccinia** Multiple disseminated lesions, borne from the site of primary vaccination, via bloodstream, to distant skin sites.

**Progressive Vaccinia (Vaccinia Gangrenosa, Vaccinia Necrosa)** Presumptive diagnosis is made if vaccination shows no evidence of normal resolution within 2 weeks; initial vesicles form on normal skin, without surrounding erythema or edema. Vesicles fail to transform to pustules by the end of the first week. The vaccination site fails to heal and continues to enlarge, forming a shallow ulcer with central necrosis and raised edges containing vesicles.

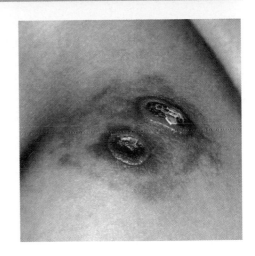

**FIGURE 25-8  Vaccination site: shoulder** *Two edematous pustules with surrounding erythema (Jennerian pustules) on the seventh day after inoculation.*

**General Findings**  Immune-mediated disorders: Encephalitis, pericarditis/myocarditis, hemolytic anemia.

## DIFFERENTIAL DIAGNOSIS

### Nonhealing/Expanding Lesion at Vaccination Site
Abnormally large vaccination lesion (unusually strong take reaction) or bacterial superinfection with GAS or *S. aureus* (both of which are accompanied by an increased (rather than diminished) inflammatory response; progressive vaccinia (slow pace of development, minimal inflammatory response); generalized vaccinia (numerous additional pocks appear along with the primary lesion); and eczema vaccinatum (multiple areas of spreading infection appear soon after vaccination or close contact with a recent vaccinee).

## LABORATORY EXAMINATIONS

**Culture**  Detects GAS and *S. aureus.*
**Dermatopathology**  Vaccinia replicates in basal epithelium, causing a local cellular reaction.

## DIAGNOSIS

Clinical history, physical examination, and clinical course. Persistence of virus can be confirmed by culturing vaccinia virus from the skin lesions.

## COURSE AND PROGNOSIS

**Normal Vaccination Reaction**  A Jennerian pustule is classified as a major reaction, indicating successful primary vaccination; successful revaccination is indicated by palpable inflammation at 6 to 8 days. A successful vaccination confers full immunity to smallpox in >95% of persons for 5 to 10 years; successful revaccination probably provides protection for ≥10 to 20 years. Reactions other than a Jennerian pustule are classified as equivocal, and another vaccination is required.
**Progressive Vaccinia**  In infants who completely lack cellular immune function: lethal.

Infection in adults with acquired immunodeficiency, many resolved if treated with vaccinia immunoglobulin (VIg).

## MANAGEMENT

**Contraindication to Vaccination**  If in doubt, don't vaccinate. Any abnormality of skin in vaccinated individual or in contacts: eczema, burns, lichen simplex chronicus, pyodermas. Any immunologic defect/disorder, any hematologic disorders involving white blood cells, any inflammatory lesions of periorbital structures, GAS or *S. aureus* carrier states, any acute febrile illness, exposure to or incubation of exanthematous disease, family history of febrile convulsions or of postvaccinal encephalitis.
**VIg**  Available from the CDC through state health departments for treatment of severe complications. May be beneficial in management of accidental inoculation, eczema vaccinatum, generalized vaccinia. Response of progressive vaccinia not well documented. Administered IM 0.6 mL/kg.
**Antiviral Drug**  Cidofovir is protective against orthopoxvirus in animals.
**Immunomodulators**  The TH1 cytokines interleukin 2 and interferon stimulate orthopoxvirus clearance. Local or systemic treatment with immunomodulators that potentiate a TH1 response could help suppress vaccinia infection in immunodeficient patients.
**Immunosuppression**  Tapering or discontinuation of immunosuppressive therapies if patients are iatrogenically immunosuppressed.
**Myopericarditis**  High-dose glucocorticoids.

# HUMAN PAPILLOMAVIRUS INFECTIONS

Human papillomaviruses (HPV) are very widespread-to-ubiquitous in humans, causing sub-clinical infection or a wide variety of benign clinical lesions on skin and mucous membranes. They also have a role in the oncogenesis of cutaneous and mucosal premalignancies [squamous cell carcinoma (SCC) and SCC in situ (SCCIS)] and malignancies (invasive SCC). More than 150 types of HPV have been identified and are associated with various clinical lesions and diseases (Table 25-2).

Three clinical manifestations of cutaneous HPV infections occur commonly in the general population: common warts, plantar warts, and flat warts. Common warts represent approximately 70% of all cutaneous warts, occurring in up to 20% of all school-age children. Plantar warts are common in older children and young adults, accounting for 30% of cutaneous warts. Flat warts occur in children and adults, accounting for 4% of cutaneous warts. Common in butchers, meat packers, and fish handlers are butcher's warts. Oncogenic HPV can cause SCCIS and invasive SCC in immunocompromised hosts, especially in those with HIV disease, solid organ transplant recipients, and those with epidermodysplasia verruciformis (EDV).

The most common presentation of mucosal HPV infection is condyloma acuminatum (genital wart), which is the most prevalent sexually transmitted disease (see Section 27). Some HPV types have a major etiologic role in the pathogenesis of in situ as well as invasive SCC of the anogenital epithelium. During delivery, maternal genital HPV infection can be transmitted to the neonate, resulting in anogenital warts or recurrent respiratory papillomatosis (RRP) after aspiration of the virus into the upper respiratory tract.

## ETIOLOGY

Papillomaviruses are double-stranded DNA viruses of the papovavirus class which infect most vertebrate species with exclusive host and tissue specificity. They infect squamous epithelia of skin and mucous membranes. Clinical lesions induced by HPV and its natural history are largely determined by HPV type. HPV are normally grouped according to their pathologic associations and tissue specificity—either cutaneous or mucosal. The 23 mucosal-associated HPV can be further subgrouped according to their risk of malignant transformation. New types of HPV are defined as possessing <90% homology to known types in six specified early and late genes.

## HUMAN PAPILLOMAVIRUS: CUTANEOUS INFECTIONS　　■　○ → ◑

Certain human HPV types commonly infect keratinized skin. Cutaneous warts are a discrete benign epithelial hyperplasia with varying degrees of surface hyperkeratosis manifested as minute papules to large plaques; lesions may become confluent, forming a mosaic. The extent of lesions is determined by the immune status of the host.
*Synonym*: Verruca, myrmecia.

## EPIDEMIOLOGY AND ETIOLOGY

**Etiology**　See Table 25-2.
**Transmission**　Skin-to-skin contact. Minor trauma with breaks in stratum corneum facilitates epidermal infection. Contagion occurs in groups—small (home) or large (school gymnasium).

## TABLE 25-2    Correlation of Human Papillomavirus Type with Disease

| Disease | Associated HPV Types |
|---|---|
| Plantar warts | 1,[*] 2,[†] 4, 63 |
| Myrmecia | 60 |
| Common warts | 1,[*] 2,[*] 4, 26, 27, 29, 41,[†] 57, 65, 77 |
| Common warts of meat handlers | 1, 2,[*] 3, 4, 7,[*] 10, 28 |
| Flat warts | 3,[*] 10,[*] 27, 38, 41,[†] 49, 75, 76 |
| Intermediate warts | 10,[*] 26, 28 |
| Epidermodysplasia verruciformis | 2,[*] 3,[*] 5,[*†] 8,[*†] 9,[*] 10,[*] 12,[*] 14,[*†] 15,[*] 17,[*†] 19, 20,[†] 21, 22, 23, 24, 25, 36, 37, 38,[†] 47, 50 |
| Condyloma acuminatum | 6,[*] 11,[*] 30,[†] 42, 43, 44, 45,[†] 51,[†] 54, 55, 70 |
| Intraepithelial neoplasias | |
|   Unspecified | 30,[†] 34, 39,[†] 40, 53, 57, 59, 61, 62, 64, 66,[†] 67, 69, 71 |
|   Low-grade | 6,[*] 11,[*] 16,[†] 18,[†] 31,[†] 33,[†] 35,[†] 42, 43, 44, 45,[†] 51,[†] 52,[†] 74 |
|   High-grade | 6, 11, 16,[*†] 18,[*†] 31,[†] 33,[†] 34, 35,[†] 39,[†] 42, 44, 45,[†] 51,[†] 52,[†] 56,[†] 58,[†] 66,[†] |
| Bowen's disease | 16,[*†] 31,[†] 34 |
| Bowenoid papulosis | 16,[*†] 34, 39,[†] 42, 45,[†] 55 |
| Cervical carcinoma | 16,[*†] 18,[*†] 31,[†] 33,[†] 35,[†] 39,[†] 45,[†] 51,[†] 52,[†] 56,[†] 58,[†] 66,[†] 68, 70 |
| Laryngeal papillomas | 6,[*] 11[*] |
| Focal epithelial hyperplasia of Heck | 13,[*] 32[*] |
| Conjunctival papillomas | 6,[*] 11,[*] 16[*†] |
| Others | 6, 11, 16,[†] 30,[†] 33,[†] 36, 37, 38,[†] 41,[†] 48,[†] 60, 72, 73 |

[*]Most common associations.
[†]High malignant potential.

NOTE: Additional information on new HPV types can be found on the HPV Sequence Data Base through the Internet (*hpv-web.lanl.gov*).

SOURCE: From RC Reichman, in E Braunwald, AS Fauci, DL Kasper, SL Hauser, DL Lango, JL Jameson (eds): *Harrison's Principles of Internal Medicine*, 15th ed. New York, McGraw-Hill, 2001.

**Other Factors** Immunocompromise, such as occurs in HIV disease or after iatrogenic immunosuppression with solid organ transplantation, is associated with an increased incidence of and more widespread cutaneous warts. Occupational risk associated with meat handling. **Inheritance** EDV: most commonly autosomal recessive.

## HISTORY

**Duration of Lesions** Warts often persist for several years if not treated.
**Symptoms** Cosmetic disfigurement. Plantar warts act as a foreign body and can be quite painful during normal daily activities such as walking if located over pressure points. More aggressive therapies such as cryosurgery often result in much more pain than that caused by the wart itself. Bleeding, especially after shaving.

## PHYSICAL EXAMINATION

### Skin Lesions
***Verruca Vulgaris (Common Warts)*** Firm papules, 1 to 10 mm or rarely larger (Fig. 25-9), hyperkeratotic, clefted surface, with vegetations (Fig. 25-10). Palmar lesions disrupt the normal line of fingerprints. Return of fingerprints is a sign of resolution of the wart. Characteristic "red or brown dots" (Figs. 25-9 and 25-10) are better seen with hand lens and are pathognomonic, representing thrombosed capillary loops. Isolated lesion, scattered discrete lesions. Annular at sites of prior therapy. Occur at sites of trauma: hands, fingers, knees. Butcher's warts: large cauliflower-like lesions on hands of meat handlers. Filiform warts have relatively small bases, extending out with elongated cap (Fig. 25-11).

*Verruca Plantaris (Plantar Warts)* Early small, shiny, sharply marginated papule (Fig. 25-12) → plaque with rough hyperkeratotic surface, studded with brown-black dots (thrombosed capillaries). As with palmar warts, normal dermatoglyphics are disrupted. Return of dermatoglyphics is a sign of resolution of the wart. Warts heal without scarring. Therapies such as cryosurgery and electrosurgery can result in lifelong scarring at treatment sites. Tenderness may be marked, especially in certain acute types and in lesions over sites of pressure (metatarsal head). Confluence of many small warts results in a mosaic wart (Fig. 25-9). "Kissing" lesion may occur on opposing surface of two toes. Plantar foot, often solitary but may be three to six or more. Pressure points, heads of metatarsal, heels, toes.

*Verruca Plana (Flat Warts)* Sharply defined, flat papules (1 to 5 mm); "flat" surface; the thickness of the lesion is 1 to 2 mm (Fig. 25-13). Skin-colored or light brown. Round, oval, polygonal, linear lesions (inoculation of virus by scratching). Lesions that arise after trauma may have a linear arrangement. Occur on face, beard area, dorsa of hands, shins.

*Epidermodysplasia Verruciformis* Flat-topped papules. Pityriasis versicolor-like lesions, particularly on the trunk. Color: skin-colored, light brown, pink, hypopigmented. Lesions may be numerous, large, and confluent. Seborrheic keratosis-like and actinic keratosis-like lesions. SCC, in situ and invasive. Lesions often become confluent, forming large maplike areas. Linear arrangement after traumatic inoculation. *Distribution:* face, dorsa of hands, arms, legs, anterior trunk. Premalignant and malignant lesions arise most commonly on face.

**HIV Disease, Iatrogenic Immunosuppression** HPV-induced warts are common and may be difficult to treat successfully. Some have atypical histologic features and may progress into SCC.

## DIFFERENTIAL DIAGNOSIS

**Verruca Vulgaris** Molluscum contagiosum, seborrheic keratosis, actinic keratosis, keratoacanthoma, SCCIS, invasive SCC.
**Verruca Plantaris** Callus, corn (keratosis) have no thrombosed capillary loops, exostosis.
**Verruca Plana** Syringoma (facial), molluscum contagiosum.
**Epidermodysplasia Verruciformis** Pityriasis versicolor, actinic keratoses, seborrheic keratoses, SCC, basal cell carcinoma.

## LABORATORY EXAMINATION

**Dermatopathology** Acanthosis, papillomatosis, hyperkeratosis. Characteristic feature is foci of vacuolated cells (koilocytosis), vertical tiers of parakeratotic cells, foci of clumped keratohyaline granules.

## DIAGNOSIS

Usually made on clinical findings. In the immunocompromised host, HIV-induced SCC at periungual sites or anogenital region should be ruled out by lesional biopsy.

## COURSE AND PROGNOSIS

In immunocompetent individuals, cutaneous HPV infections usually resolve spontaneously, without therapeutic intervention. In immunocompromised individuals, cutaneous HPV infections may be very resistant to all modalities of therapy. In EDV, disease starts at 5 to 7 years of age; lesions appear progressively, becoming widespread in some. 30 to 50% of individuals with EDV develop malignant cutaneous lesions on areas of skin exposed to sunlight.

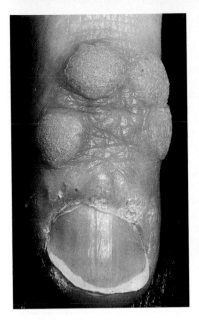
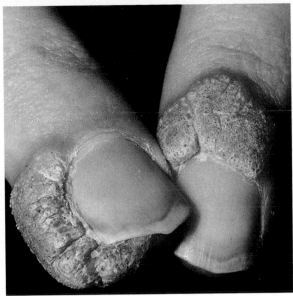

**FIGURE 25-9  (Left)   Verruca vulgaris: periungual**  *Hyperkeratotic papules located periungually on the dorsum of a finger. Similar lesions were present on all fingers of both hands. All modalities of therapy had failed. The warts resolved with microinjections of bleomycin. Note, black and brown dots.*

**FIGURE 25-10  (Right)   Verruca vulgaris in an immunocompromised individual**  *Large, very thick, fissured, painful periungual and subungual warts are present on two fingers of a 20-year-old male treated with immunosuppressive drugs after renal transplantation. Similar lesions were also present on multiple toes.*

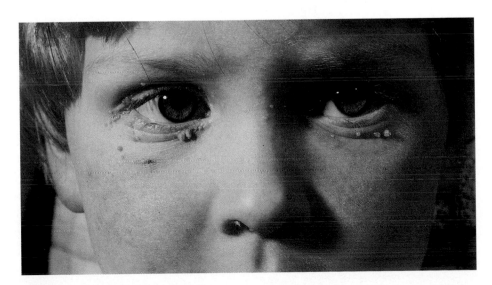

**FIGURE 25-11   Filiform warts**  *Multiple, elongated keratotic papules on the face of a child; note the clustering on the eyelids.*

## MANAGEMENT

| | |
|---|---|
| **Goal** | Aggressive therapies, which are often quite painful and may be followed by scarring, are usually to be avoided because the natural history of cutaneous HPV infections is for spontaneous resolution in months or a few years. Plantar warts that are painful because of their location warrant more aggressive therapies. |
| **Patient-initiated therapy** | Minimal cost; no/minimal pain. |
| For small lesions | 10–20% salicylic acid and lactic acid in collodion. |
| For large lesions | 40% salicylic acid plaster for 1 week, then application of salicylic acid–lactic acid in collodion. |
| Imiquimod cream | At sites that are not thickly keratinized, apply half-strength 3 times per week. Persistent warts may require occlusion. Hyperkeratotic lesions on palms/soles should be debrided frequently; Imiquimod used alternately with a topical retinoid such as tararotene topical gel may be effective. |
| Hyperthermia for verruca plantaris | Hyperthermia with hot water (113°F) immersion for 1/2 to 3/4 h two or three times weekly for 16 treatments is effective in some patients. |
| **Clinician-initiated therapy** | Costly, painful. |
| Cryosurgery | If patients have tried home therapies and liquid nitrogen is available, light cryosurgery using a cotton-tipped applicator or cryospray, freezing the wart and 1 to 2 mm of surrounding normal tissue for approximately 30 s, is quite effective. Freezing kills the infected tissue but not HPV. Cryosurgery is usually repeated about every 4 weeks until the warts have disappeared. Painful. |
| Electrosurgery | More effective than cryosurgery, but also associated with a greater chance of scarring. EMLA cream can be used for anesthesia for flat warts. Lidocaine injection is usually required for thicker warts, especially palmar/plantar lesions. |
| $CO_2$ laser surgery | May be effective for recalcitrant warts, but no better than cryosurgery or electrosurgery in the hands of an experienced clinician. |
| Surgery | Single, nonplantar verruca vulgaris:curettage after freon freezing; surgical excision of cutaneous HPV infections is not indicated in that these lesions are epidermal infections. |

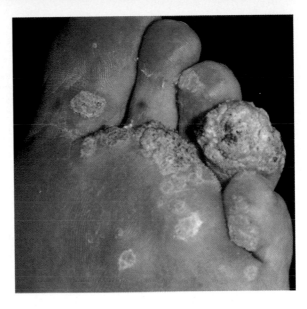

**FIGURE 25-12   Verruca plantaris**
*Confluent, skin-colored, verrucous papules, forming a mosaic, disrupting the normal dermatoglyphics of the plantar foot. The thrombosed capillaries (brown dots) differentiate the lesion from a corn (an often painful, translucent, yellowish, keratotic granule) and a callus (a poorly demarcated, hyperkeratotic plaque with normal dermatoglyphics at pressure sites). The patient had some degree of immunocompromise associated with prior non-Hodgkin's lymphoma. Warts nearly resolved with oral acitretin.*

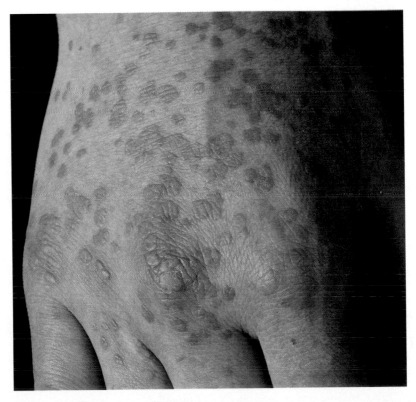

**FIGURE 25-13   Verruca plana (flat warts)**   *Flat-topped, pink papules with sharp margination and minimal hyperkeratosis on the dorsa of the hands and fingers.*

## INFECTIOUS EXANTHEMS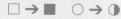

An infectious exanthem (IE) is a generalized cutaneous eruption associated with a primary systemic infection; it is often accompanied by oral mucosal lesions, i.e., an enanthema. IEs are most commonly caused by viral agents but can also be associated with bacterial, rickettsial, and parasitic infections. Certain IEs have fairly characteristic morphology; in many cases an accurate diagnosis cannot be made on the basis of morphology alone. Historic factors may be helpful, including season, disease contacts, immunizations, previous exanthematous illnesses, and associated prodromal symptoms.

### EPIDEMIOLOGY AND ETIOLOGY

**Age of Onset** Usually <20 years.
**Etiology** *Viral* Rubella virus, attenuated rubella virus in vaccine; paramyxovirus (measles); parvovirus B19 (erythema infectiosum); rhinovirus; respiratory syncytial virus; adenoviruses; herpesviridae: cytomegalovirus (CMV), Epstein-Barr virus (EBV), human herpesvirus 6 and 7 (exanthem subitum, roseola infantum); enteroviruses [e.g., coxsackieviruses, echo virus (eruptive pseudoangiomatosis)]; flavivirus (dengue); hepatitis B virus; HIV (acute symptomatic HIV syndrome); orbivirus (Colorado tick fever); reoviruses; rotaviruses.
*Bacterial* Group A streptococcus (scarlet fever); *S. aureus* (toxic shock syndrome); *Legionella*, *Leptospira*, *Listeria*, meningococci.

*Mycoplasmal*
*Rickettsial* Rocky Mountain spotted fever, other spotted fevers, rickettsialpox, murine and epidemic typhus.
*Miscellaneous* *Mycoplasma pneumoniae*, *Strongyloides*, *Toxoplasma*, *Treponema pallidum*.
**Transmission** Respiratory, food, sexual, blood.
**Season** Enterovirus infections, summer months.
**Geography** Worldwide.

### PATHOGENESIS

Skin lesions may be produced by the direct effect of microbial replication in infected cells, the host response to the microbe, or the interaction of these two phenomena.

### HISTORY

**Incubation Period** Usually <3 weeks; hepatitis B virus, several months.
**Prodrome** Fever, malaise, coryza, sore throat, nausea, vomiting, diarrhea, abdominal pain, headache.

### PHYSICAL EXAMINATION

Skin Lesions
*Scarlitiniform* Erythema. Diffuse to generalized. May be more prominent in body folds. May be associated with erythema of oropharynx and/or genitalia. Desquamation may occur with resolution of exanthem.
*Exanthematous [Morbilliform (Measles-Like)]* Erythematous macules and/or papules (Fig. 25-14); less frequently, vesicles, petechiae, Usually central, i.e., head, neck, trunk, proximal extremities. Diffuse erythema of cheeks, i.e., "slapped cheek" with erythema infectiosum.
*Vesicular* Initially, vesicles with clear fluid; may evolve to pustules. In a few days to a week, roof of vesicle sloughs, resulting in erosions. In varicella, lesions are disseminated and may involve oropharynx. In hand-foot-and-mouth disease, vesicles/erosion occur in oropharynx; painful linear vesicles on palms/soles.
*Mucous Membranes* Koplik's spots in measles; microulcerative lesions in herpangina due to coxsackievirus A (Fig. 25-15); palatal petechiae in mononucleosis syndrome of EBV or CMV; conjunctivitis.
**General Examination** Lymphadenopathy, hepatomegaly, splenomegaly.

### DIFFERENTIAL DIAGNOSIS

**Exanthematous Eruption** Drug eruption, systemic lupus erythematosus, Kawasaki's syndrome.

### LABORATORY EXAMINATIONS

**Cultures** If practical.
**Serology** Acute and convalescent titers most helpful in specific diagnosis.

### DIAGNOSIS

Usually made on history and clinical findings.

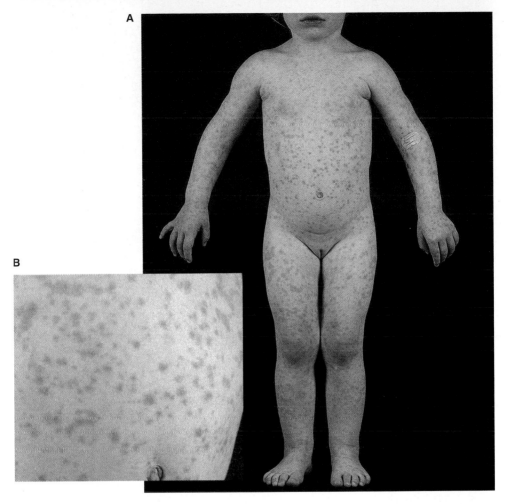

**FIGURE 25-14   Infectious exanthem**   *Disseminated, erythematous macules and papules, typical of the cutaneous changes with many acute infections. The eruption must be differentiated from an exanthematous (morbilliform) drug eruption.* **A.** *Typical distribution of lesions on the trunk and extremities.* **B.** *Closeup of pink macules and papules becoming confluent in some areas.*

## COURSE AND PROGNOSIS

Usually resolves in <10 days. Patients with primary EBV or CMV infection very often develop an exanthematous eruption if given ampicillin or amoxacillin.

## MANAGEMENT

Symptomatic.
**Antimicrobial Therapy**   Specific antimicrobial therapy when available.

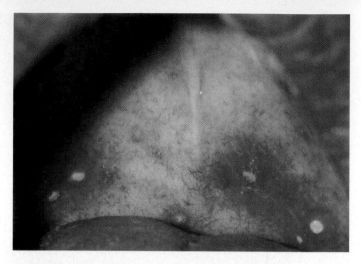

**FIGURE 25-15    Infectious enanthem: herpangina**    *Multiple, small vesicles and erosions with erythematous halos on the soft palate; some taste buds on the posterior tongue are inflamed and prominent.*

RUBELLA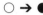

Rubella is a viral infection of children and adults with a characteristic exanthem and lymphadenopathy. Many infections are subclinical. Rubella virus infecting a pregnant female, while causing a benign illness in the mother, may result in the congenital rubella syndrome with serious chronic fetal infection and malformation. Childhood immunization is highly effective at preventing infection.
*Synonyms*: German measles, "3-day measles."

## EPIDEMIOLOGY AND ETIOLOGY

**Age of Onset**    Before widespread immunization, children <15 years. Currently, young adults.
**Etiology**    *Rubella virus*, an RNA togavirus, member of *Rubivirus* genus. Attenuated rubella virus used in immunization can cause an illness with rubella-like rash, lymphadenopathy, and arthritis.
**Occupation**    Young adults in hospitals, colleges, prisons, prenatal clinics.
**Transmission**    Inhalation of aerosolized respiratory droplets; moderately contagious; 10 to 40% of cases asymptomatic; period of infectivity from end of incubation period to disappearance of rash.

**Risk Factors**    Lack of active immunization, lack of natural infection. After immunization began in 1969, incidence has decreased by 99%.
**Season**    Before 1969, epidemics in the United States every 6 to 9 years, occurring in spring.
**Geography**    Worldwide. Marked reduction in incidence in developed countries after immunization.

## HISTORY

**Incubation Period**    14 to 21 days.
**Prodrome**    Usually absent, especially in young children. In adolescents and young adults:

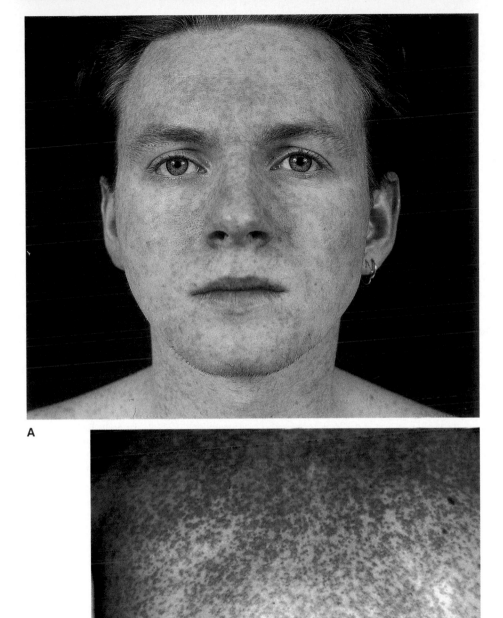

**FIGURE 25-16   Rubella**   *A.   Erythematous macules and papules appearing initially on the face and spreading inferiorly to the trunk and extremities, usually within the first 24 h. Postauricular and posterior cervical lymph nodes were enlarged. Lesions becoming confluent on the cheeks while clearing on the forehead. B. Truncal lesions appear 24 h after onset of facial lesions.*

anorexia, malaise, conjunctivitis, headache, low-grade fever, mild upper respiratory tract symptoms.
**History**    Arthralgia, especially in adult women after immunization.
**Immune Status**    In women, rubella-like illness frequently follows administration of attenuated live rubella virus.

## PHYSICAL EXAMINATION

### Skin Lesions
Pink macules, papules (Fig. 25-16*A*). Initially on forehead, spreading inferiorly to face, trunk, and extremities during first day. By second day, facial exanthem fades. By third day, exanthem fades completely without residual pigmentary change or scaling. Trunkal lesions may become confluent, creating a scarlatiniform eruption (Fig. 25-16*B*).
*Mucous Membranes*    Petechiae on soft palate (*Forchheimer's sign*) during prodrome (also seen in infectious mononucleosis).
**General Examination**    *Lymph nodes*: Enlarged during prodrome. Postauricular, suboccipital, and posterior cervical lymph nodes enlarged and possibly tender. Mild generalized lymphadenopathy may occur. Enlargement usually persists for 1 week but may last for months. *Spleen*: May be enlarged. *Joints*: Arthritis in adults; possible effusion. Arthralgia, especially in adult women after immunization.

## DIFFERENTIAL DIAGNOSIS

**Exanthem**    Other infectious exanthems, adverse drug eruption, scarlet fever, erythema infectiosum, enteroviral infection.
**Exanthem with Arthritis**    Acute rheumatic fever, rheumatoid arthritis, erythema infectiosum.

## LABORATORY EXAMINATIONS

**Serology**    Acute and convalescent rubella antibody titers show fourfold or greater rise.
**Culture**    Virus can be isolated from throat, joint fluid aspirate.

## DIAGNOSIS

Clinical diagnosis; can be confirmed by serology.

## COURSE AND PROGNOSIS

In most persons, rubella is a mild, inconsequential infection. However, when rubella occurs in a pregnant woman during the first trimester, the infection can be passed transplacentally to the developing fetus. Approximately half of infants who acquire rubella during the first trimester of intrauterine life will show clinical signs of damage from the virus. Manifestations of the *congenital rubella syndrome* are congenital heart defects, cataracts, microphthalmia, deafness, microcephaly, hydrocephaly.

## MANAGEMENT

**Prevention**    Rubella is preventable by immunization. Previous rubella should be documented in young women; if antirubella antibody titers are negative, rubella immunization should be given.
**Acute Infection**    Symptomatic.

## MEASLES   □ → ■*   ◑ → ●*

Measles is a highly contagious childhood viral infection characterized by fever, coryza, cough, conjunctivitis, pathognomonic enanthem (Koplik's spots), and an exanthem. Significant morbidity and mortality occur in acute and chronic course. Childhood immunization is highly effective at preventing infection.
*Synonyms*: Rubeola, morbilli.

### EPIDEMIOLOGY AND ETIOLOGY

**Age of Onset**   Before measles immunization: 5 to 9 years of age in the United States. In developing countries, up to 45% of cases occur before the age of 9 months.
**Etiology**   Measles virus, member of RNA genus *Morbillivirus* and family Paramyxoviridae.
**Incidence**   No longer endemic in the United States; cases result from international importation. *Worldwide:* hyperendemic in many developing nations, resulting in 800,000 deaths annually.
**Risk Factors**   After immunization began in 1963, incidence has decreased by 98%. Current outbreaks in the United States occur in inner-city unimmunized preschool-age children, school-age persons immunized at an early age, and imported cases. Most outbreaks are in primary or secondary schools, colleges or universities, day-care centers.
**Transmission**   Spread by respiratory droplet aerosols produced by sneezing and coughing. Infected persons contagious from several days before onset of rash up to 5 days after lesions appear. Attack rate for susceptible contacts >90 to 100%. Asymptomatic infection rare.
**Season**   Before widespread use of vaccine, epidemics occurred every 2 to 3 years in late winter to early spring.
**Demography**   No longer endemic in Americas. Hyperendemic in Africa, with half a million deaths annually.

### PATHOGENESIS

Virus enters cells of respiratory tract, replicates locally, spreads to local lymph nodes, and disseminates hematogenously to skin and mucous membranes. Viral replication also occurs on skin and mucosa. Modified measles, a milder form of the illness, may occur in individuals with preexisting partial immunity induced by active or passive immunization. Persons deficient in cellular immunity are at high risk for severe measles.

### HISTORY

**Incubation Period**   10 to 15 days.
**Prodrome**   Fever, malaise; upper respiratory symptoms (coryza, hacking barklike cough), photophobia, conjunctivitis with lacrimation, malaise, fever, periorbital edema. As exanthem progresses, systemic symptoms subside.

### PHYSICAL EXAMINATION

#### Skin Lesions
***Exanthem***   On the fourth febrile day, erythematous macules and papules. Appear on forehead at hairline, behind ears; spread centrifugally and inferiorly to involve the face, trunk (Fig. 25-17), extremities, palms/soles, reaching the feet by third day. Initial discrete lesions may become confluent, especially on face (Fig. 25-18), neck, and shoulders. Lesions gradually fade in order of appearance, with subsequent residual yellow-tan stain or faint desquamation. Exanthem resolves in 4 to 6 days.
***Mucous Membranes (Enanthem)***   *Oropharynx/Koplik's spots*: Pathognomonic. Appear before exanthem. Cluster of tiny bluish-white spots on red background, appearing on or after second day of febrile illness, on buccal mucosa opposite premolar teeth. Also: entire buccal/inner labial mucosa may be inflamed; lips red. *Bulbar conjunctivae*: conjunctivitis.
**General Examination**   Generalized lymphadenopathy, diarrhea, vomiting, splenomegaly common. Otherwise unremarkable.
#### Variants
***Modified Measles***   Milder clinical findings with preexisting partial immunity.

* In Africa.

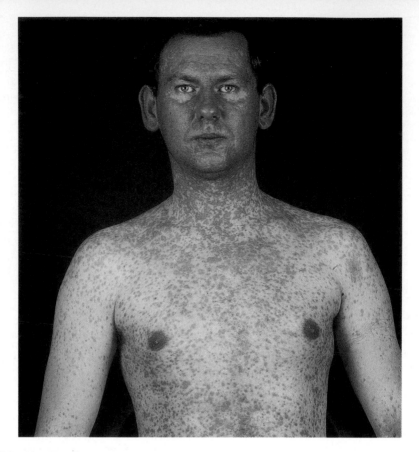

**FIGURE 25-17   Measles**   *Erythematous flat papules, first appearing on the face and neck where they become confluent, spreading to the trunk and arms in 2 to 3 days where they remain discrete. In contrast, rubella also first appears initially on the face but spreads to the trunk in 1 day. Koplik's spot on the buccal mucosa were also present.*

***Atypical Measles*** Occurs in individuals immunized with formalin-inactivated measles vaccine, subsequently exposed to measles virus. Exanthem begins peripherally and moves centrally; can be urticarial, maculopapular, hemorrhagic, and/or vesicular. Systemic symptoms can be severe.

***Measles in Immunocompromised Host*** Rash may not occur. Pneumonitis, encephalitis more common.

**DIFFERENTIAL DIAGNOSIS**

**Disseminated Maculopapular Eruption**   Drug eruption, other viral exanthems (e.g., rubella), scarlet fever. Kawasaki syndrome, infectious mononucleosis, toxoplasmosis, *M. pneumoniae* infection.

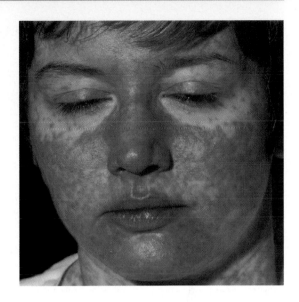

**FIGURE 25-18   Measles: face** *Erythematous papules have become confluent on the face on the fourth day.*

## LABORATORY EXAMINATIONS

**Cytology**   Multinucleated giant cells in secretions.

**Cultures**   Isolate virus from blood, urine, pharyngeal secretions.

**Measles Antigen**   Detect in respiratory secretions by immunofluorescent staining.

**Serology**   Demonstrates fourfold or greater rise in measles titer.

**PCR**   Detects genomic sequences of measles virus RNA in serum, throat swabs, and CSF.

## DIAGNOSIS

Clinical diagnosis, at times, confirmed by serology.

## COURSE AND PROGNOSIS

Self-limited infection in most patients. Mortality rate: in the United States, 0.3%; in developing countries, 1 to 10%. Sites of complications: respiratory tract, CNS, GI tract. Complications more common in malnourished children, the unimmunized, and those with congenital immunodeficiency and leukemia. Acute complications (9.8% of cases): otitis media, pneumonia (bacterial or measles), diarrhea, measles encephalitis (1 in 800 to 1000 cases), thrombocytopenia. In unimmunized HIV-infected children, fatal measles pneumonia has occurred without rash. Chronic complication: subacute sclerosing panencephalitis.

## MANAGEMENT

**Prevention**   Prophylactic immunization. The goal of eliminating indigenous measles transmission in the United States is based on four components: (1) maintaining high coverage with a single dose of measles-mumps-rubella (MMR) vaccine among preschool-age children, (2) achieving coverage with two doses of MMR for all school and college attendees, (3) enhancing surveillance and outbreak response, and (4) increasing efforts to develop and implement strategies for global measles elimination.

**Acute Infection**   Symptomatic.

**Secondary Bacterial Infections**   Administration of appropriate antibiotics.

## HAND-FOOT-AND-MOUTH DISEAS        □   ○

Hand-foot-and-mouth disease (HFMD) is a systemic infection caused by coxsackievirus A16, characterized by ulcerative oral lesions and a vesicular exanthem on the distal extremities in association with mild constitutional symptoms.

### EPIDEMIOLOGY AND ETIOLOGY

**Age of Onset**   <10 years but also young and middle-age adults.

**Etiology**   Enterovirus (picornavirus group, single-strand RNA, unenveloped). Commonly: coxsackievirus A16, enterovirus 71. Also coxsackieviruses A4–7, A9, A10, B2, and B5.

**Season**   Epidemic outbreaks every 3 years. In temperate climates, outbreaks during warmer months (late summer, early fall).

**Transmission**   Highly contagious, spread from person to person by oral-oral and fecal-oral routes.

### PATHOGENESIS

Enteroviral implantation in the GI tract (buccal mucosa and ileum) leads to extension into regional lymph nodes, and 72 h later a viremia occurs with seeding of the oral mucosa and skin of the hands and feet.

### HISTORY

**Incubation Period**   3 to 6 days.

**Prodrome**   12 to 24 h of low-grade fever, malaise, and abdominal pain or respiratory symptoms.

**Symptoms**   Frequently 5 to 10 *painful* ulcerative oral lesions, leading to refusal to eat in children. Few to 100 cutaneous lesions appear together or shortly after the oral lesions and may be asymptomatic or *tender* and *painful*.

### PHYSICAL EXAMINATION

#### Skin Lesions

Lesions begin as 2- to 8-mm *macules* or *papules* that quickly evolve to *vesicles*. Lesions on palms and soles usually do not rupture (Fig. 25-20). At other cutaneous sites, vesicles can rupture, with formation of *erosions* and *crusts*. Lesions heal without scarring. Early papules, pink to red.

Vesicles have clear fluid with a watery appearance or yellowish hue. Cutaneous lesions have a characteristic "linear" shape on the palms and soles. Characteristically, lesions arise on palms and soles, especially on sides of fingers, toes, and buttocks.

*Mucosal Lesions*   5- to 10-mm, small, punched-out painful ulcers preceded by macules → grayish vesicles, arising on the hard palate, tongue, buccal mucosa (Fig. 25-19).

**General Findings**   Typically, HFMD is accompanied by low-grade fever, malaise, and a sore mouth. In some patients, it may be associated with high fever, severe malaise, diarrhea, and joint pains. Enterovirus 71 infections may have associated CNS (aseptic meningitis, encephalitis, meningoencephalitis, flaccid paralysis), and lung involvement.

### DIFFERENTIAL DIAGNOSIS

A sudden outbreak of oral and distal extremity lesions is pathognomonic for HFMD. However, if only the oral lesions are present, the differential diagnosis would include HSV infection, aphthous stomatitis, herpangina, erythema multiforme, adverse drug reaction.

### LABORATORY EXAMINATIONS

**Histopathology**   Epidermal reticular degeneration leads to an intraepidermal vesicle filled with neutrophils, mononuclear cells, and proteinaceous eosinophilic material. The dermis reveals a perivascular mixed cell infiltrate. Electron microscopy: Intracytoplasmic particles in crystalline array characteristic of coxsackie viral infections.

**Serology**   In acute serum, neutralizing antibodies may be detected but disappear rapidly. In convalescent serum, elevated titers of complement-fixing antibodies are found.

**Tzanck Preparation**   Negative for both multinucleated giant cells and inclusion bodies.

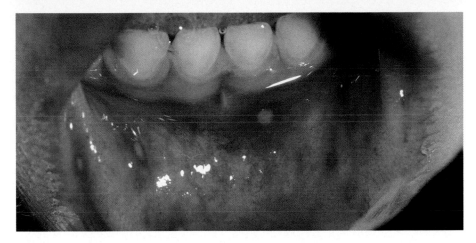

**FIGURE 25-19   Hand-foot-and-mouth disease**   *Multiple, superficial erosions and small, vesicular lesions surrounded by an erythematous halo on the lower labial mucosa; the gingiva is normal. In primary herpetic gingivostomatitis, which presents with similar oral vesicular lesions, a painful gingivitis usually occurs as well.*

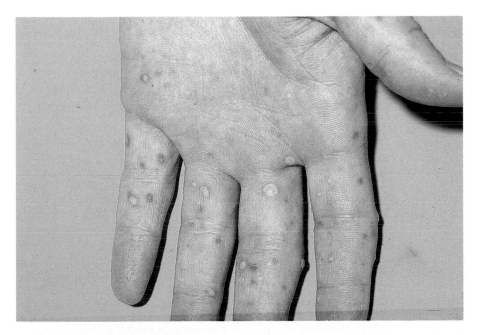

**FIGURE 25-20   Hand-foot-and-mouth disease**   *Multiple, discrete, small, vesicular lesions on the fingers and palms; similar lesions were also present on the feet. Some vesicles are typically linear.*

**Viral Culture** Virus may be isolated from vesicles, throat washings, and stool specimens.

## DIAGNOSIS

Usually made on clinical findings.

## COURSE AND PROGNOSIS

Most commonly, HFMD is self-limited, and a rise in serum antibodies eliminates the viremia in 7 to 10 days. A few cases have been more prolonged or recurrent. Serious sequelae rarely occur; however, coxsackievirus has been implicated in cases of myocarditis, meningoencephalitis, aseptic meningitis, paralytic disease, and a systemic illness resembling rubeola. Enterovirus 71 infections have higher morbidity/mortality rates due to CNS involvement and pulmonary edema. Infection acquired during the first trimester of pregnancy may result in spontaneous abortion.

## MANAGEMENT

Symptomatic treatment, including topical application of dyclonine HCl solution or lidocaine gel, may reduce oral discomfort.

# HERPANGINA

Herpangina is caused by coxsackievirus A1–6, 8, 10, 22; also coxsackie group B (strains 1–4). echoviruses, and other enteroviruses. It usually affects children <5 years and is prevalent in late summer and early fall in temperate climates. The symptoms are a sudden onset of fever, malaise, headache, anorexia, dysphagia, and sore throat. The enanthem consists of 1- to 2-mm gray-white papules/vesicles that evolve to ulcers with red halos, and diffuse pharyngeal hyperemia (see Fig. 25-15). These are distributed on the anterior tonsillar pillars, soft palate, uvula, and tonsils. Herpangina usually lasts 4 to 6 days, and its course is self-limited.

# ERYTHEMA INFECTIOSUM   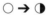

Erythema infectiosum (EI) is a childhood exanthem associated with primary human parvovirus B19 (HPV B19) infection, characterized by edematous erythematous plaques on the cheeks ("slapped cheeks") and an erythematous lacy eruption on the trunk and extremities. *Synonym*: Fifth disease.

## EPIDEMIOLOGY AND ETIOLOGY

**Age of Onset** All ages, but more common in young. Up to 60% of adolescents and adults are seropositive for anti-HPV B19 IgG. Symptomatic rheumatic involvement is more common in adults.

**Etiology** Parvovirus, a small single-strand, unenveloped DNA virus. Human infection caused by HPV B19.

**Sex** Symptomatic illness with arthralgias more common in adult women.

**Season** Occurs year round; outbreaks in schools in late winter, early spring.

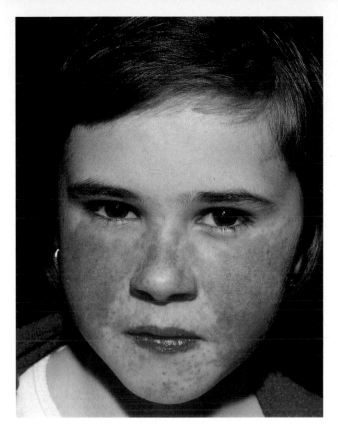

**FIGURE 25-21   Erythema infectiosum**   *Diffuse erythema and edema of the cheeks with "slapped cheek" facies in a child.*

**Transmission**   Virus presents in respiratory tract during the viremic stage of HPV B19 infection and spreads via droplet aerosol. Secondary attack rate among close contacts, 50%.

## PATHOGENESIS

Viremia develops 6 days after intranasal inoculation of B19 into volunteers who lack serum antibodies to the virus. Nonspecific symptoms occur during this time. IgM and then IgG antibodies develop after a week and clear viremia. Significant bone marrow depression can occur at this time. The exanthem begins 17 to 18 days after inoculation and may be accompanied by arthralgia and/or arthritis; these findings are mediated by immune complexes. In compromised hosts, B19 can destroy erythroid precursor cells, causing severe aplastic crisis in adults and hydrops fetalis in the fetus.

## HISTORY

**Incubation**   4 to 14 days.
**Contacts**   Exposure to classmates or siblings with EI.
**Symptoms**   20 to 60% of individuals are symptomatic; remainder asymptomatic.
*Children*   Prodrome of fever, malaise, headache, coryza 2 days before rash. Headache, sore throat, fever, myalgias, nausea, diarrhea, conjunctivitis, cough may coincide with rash. Uncommonly arthralgias. Pruritus is variably present.

*Adults* Constitutional symptoms more severe, with fever, adenopathy, arthritis/arthralgias involving small joints of hand, knees, wrists, ankles, feet. Numbness and tingling of fingers. Pruritus ± rash; rash usually absent in adults.

## PHYSICAL EXAMINATION

### Skin Lesions
Edematous, confluent plaques on malar face ("slapped cheeks") (nasal bridge, periorbital regions spared) (Fig. 25-21); lesions fade over 1 to 4 days. Nonfacial lesions, appearing after facial lesions: erythematous macules and papules that become confluent, giving a lacy or reticulated appearance (Fig. 25-22); lesions fade in 5 to 9 days. Less commonly, morbilliform, confluent, circinate, annular. Rarely, purpura, vesicles, pustules, palmoplantar desquamation. Reticulated rash may recur.
*Distribution* Face. Extensor surface of extremities, trunk, neck: confluent macules/papules. In adults with rash, "slapped cheeks" usually absent, reticulated macules on extremities.
*Other Findings* HPV B19 also reported to cause papular-purpuric "gloves and socks" syndrome.
*Mucosal Lesions* Uncommonly, enanthem with glossal and pharyngeal erythema; red macules on buccal and palatal mucosa.
**General Findings** *Adults*: More constitutional symptoms (fever, adenopathy, arthritis), especially women; often no rash. *Joints*: Arthralgia and/or arthritis in 10% of children; typically involving large joints.

## DIFFERENTIAL DIAGNOSIS

**Children with Erythema Infectiosum** Childhood exanthems—rubella, measles, scarlet fever, erythema subitum, enteroviral infection, *Haemophilus influenzae* cellulitis, adverse cutaneous drug reaction.
**Adults with Arthritis** Lyme arthritis, rheumatoid arthritis, rubella.

## LABORATORY EXAMINATIONS

**Serology** Demonstration of IgM anti-HPV B19 antibodies or IgG seroconversion. Demonstration of HPV B19 in serum.

**Electron Microscopy** Infected erythroid precursor cells show parvovirus-like particles.
**Hematology** During aplastic crisis: absence of reticulocytes, falling hemoglobin, hypoplasia or aplasia of erythroid series in bone marrow.

## DIAGNOSIS

Usually made on clinical findings.

## COURSE AND PROGNOSIS

**Erythema Infectiosum** "Slapped cheeks" are noted first, fading over 1 to 4 days. Then, reticulated rash appears on the trunk, neck, and extensor extremities. Eruption lasts 5 to 9 days but characteristically can recur for weeks or months, triggered by sunlight exposure, exercise, temperature change, bathing, emotional stress.
**Arthralgias** Self-limited, lasting 3 weeks; but may persist for several months or years.
**Aplastic Crisis** In patients with chronic hemolytic anemias (sickle cell anemia, hereditary spherocytosis, thalassemias, pyruvate kinase deficiency, autoimmune hemolytic anemia), transient aplastic crisis may occur, manifested by worsening anemia, fatigue, pallor.
**Fetal B19 Infection** Intrauterine infection may be complicated by nonimmune fetal hydrops secondary to infection of RBC precursors, hemolysis, severe anemia, tissue anoxia, high-output heart failure. Risk <10% after maternal infection.
**Immunocompromised Host** Prolonged chronic anemia associated with persistent lysis of RBC precursors. At risk: HIV disease, congenital immunodeficiencies, acute leukemia, organ transplants, systemic lupus erythematosus, infants less than 1 year. Responds to intravenous immunoglobulin (IVIg).

## MANAGEMENT

Symptomatic.

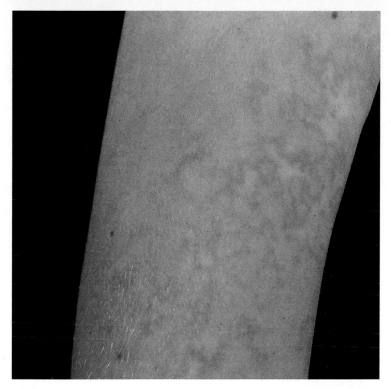

**FIGURE 25-22 Erythema infectiosum** *Discrete, erythematous macules with ring formation on the upper arm.*

## GIANOTTI-CROSTI SYNDROME ☐ ○

The exanthem occurs in children 1 to 6 years old, presenting as discrete, nonpruritic, erythematous, monomorphic papules on the face, buttocks, and extensor surfaces of the extremities. Typically, the trunk is spared. Duration is 2 to 3 weeks. It is associated with various viral infections including hepatitis B virus, EBV, CMV, coxsackievirus A16, parainfluenza virus, etc. *Synonym*: Papular acrodermatitis of childhood.

# HUMAN HERPESVIRUSES

Human herpesviruses (HHVs) (family Herpesviridae) are defined by the architecture of the virion, which has a core containing a linear double-stranded DNA and an icosahedral capsid 100 to 110 nm in diameter composed of 162 capsomers with an envelope containing viral glycoprotein spikes on the surface. Worldwide, 60 to 90% of the population is infected with one or more HHVs. Eight HHVs have been identified: herpes simplex virus (HSV)-1 (HHV-1), HSV-2 (HHV-2), varicella-zoster virus (VZV, or HHV-3), Epstein-Barr virus (EBV, or HHV-4), cytomegalovirus (CMV, or HHV-5), HHV-6, HHV-7, HHV-8 (Kaposi sarcoma–associated virus). Primary HHV infections are usually asymptomatic with the exception of VZV, which nearly always presents with symptomatic varicella. After primary infection, HHVs remain latent in neural or lymphoid cells and reactivate if an adequate immune response does not exist.

HHVs are categorized into three groups: alpha-, beta-, and gammaherpesvirinae (Table 25-3). *Alphaherpesvirinae* [HSV-1, HSV-2, VZV (HHV-3)] are characterized by a variable host range, relatively short reproductive cycle, rapid spread in culture, rapid destruction of infected cells, and latent infection primarily, but not exclusively, of sensory ganglia.

*Betaherpesvirinae* [CMV (HHV-5)] have a restricted host range and spread slowly in cultures. *Gammaherpesvirinae* [EBV (HHV-4), HHV-6, HHV-7, HHV-8, and herpesvirus saimiri] are lymphotropic, specific for either T or B lymphocytes. The HHV-8 DNA sequences are closely homologous to minor capsid and tegument protein genes of gammaherpesvirinae EBV and herpesvirus saimiri.

**TABLE 25-3    Human Herpesviruses and Associated Diseases in Immunocompetent and Immunocompromised Individuals**

| Human Herpesvirus | Disease in Immunocompetent Individuals | Disease in Immuno-compromised Individuals | Management |
|---|---|---|---|
| Herpes simplex virus-1(HSV-1) (HHV-1) | Primary infection often asymptomatic<br>Primary herpetic gingivostomatitis<br>Herpes labialis<br>Herpetic whitlow<br>Aseptic meningitis<br>HSV encephalitis | Widespread local infection<br>Chronic ulcers<br>Disseminated cutaneous infection<br>Disseminated visceral infection | Immunization: vaccine promising<br>Antiviral agents<br>Acyclovir<br>Valacyclovir<br>Famciclovir<br>Foscarnet |
| Herpes simplex virus-2 (HSV-2) (HHV-2) | Primary infection often asymptomatic<br>Herpes genitalis, primary and recurrent<br>Herpetic whitlow<br>Aseptic meningitis | Widespread local infection<br>Chronic ulcers<br>Disseminated cutaneous infection<br>Disseminated visceral infection | Immunization: vaccine promising<br>Antiviral agents<br>Acyclovir<br>Valacyclovir<br>Famciclovir<br>Foscarnet |
| Varicella-zoster virus (VZV) (HHV-3) | Primary infection nearly always symptomatic<br>Varicella (primary infection)<br>Herpes zoster | Disseminated cutaneous infection<br>Disseminated visceral infection<br>Chronic herpes zoster<br>Chronic ecthymatous VZV infection | Immunization: vaccine available<br>Antiviral agents<br>Acyclovir<br>Valacyclovir<br>Famciclovir<br>Foscarnet |

*(continued)*

**TABLE 25-3   (Continued)**

| Human Herpesvirus | Disease in Immunocompetent Individuals | Disease in Immunocompromised Individuals | Management |
|---|---|---|---|
| Epstein-Barr virus (EBV) (HHV-4) | Primary infection often asymptomatic<br>EBV mononucleosis (primary EBV infection)<br>Nasopharyngeal carcinoma<br>Burkitt's lymphoma<br>Post-transplantation lymphoma<br>T cell lymphoma, and other lymphomas | Lymphoma<br><br><br><br><br><br><br><br><br>??? | Antiviral agents<br>Acyclovir<br>Ganciclovir<br><br><br><br><br><br><br>??? |
| Cytomegalovirus (CMV) (HHV-5) | Primary infection often asymptomatic<br>CMV mononucleosis (primary CMV infection) | Retinitis<br>Pneumonitis<br>Colitis<br><br><br>Oral hairy leukoplakia | Immunization: vaccine promising<br>Antiviral agents<br>Ganciclovir<br>Foscarnet<br>Cidofovir<br>Immunization: none |
| Human herpesvirus-6 (HHV-6) | Primary infection often asymptomatic<br>Exanthem subitum | <br><br>??? | <br><br>??? |
| Human herpesvirus-7 (HHV-7) | Primary infection often asymptomatic<br>Exanthem subitum | | <br><br>??? |
| Human herpesvirus-8 (HHV-8) | Primary infection may present with fever and *mobiliform rash*<br>Kaposi's sarcoma | Kaposi's sarcoma<br>Body cavity–lymphoma in HIV-infected individuals | |

## HERPES SIMPLEX VIRUS INFECTION ■ ○ → ●

Herpes simplex virus (HSV) infection, whether first-symptomatic or recurrent, may "typically" present clinically with grouped vesicles arising on an erythematous base on keratinized skin or mucous membrane. Most HSV infections are "atypical," with patch(es) of erythema, small erosions, fissures, or subclinical lesions that shed HSV. Once an individual is infected, HSV persists in sensory ganglia for the life of the patient, recurring with lessening in immunity. In healthy individuals, recurrent infections are asymptomatic or minor, resolving spontaneously or with antiviral therapy. In the immunocompromised host, mucocutaneous lesions can be extensive, chronic, or disseminate to skin or viscera.

*Synonyms*: Herpes, herpes simplex, cold sore, fever blister, herpes febrilis, herpes labialis, herpes gladiatorum, scrum pox, herpetic whitlow, genital herpes, herpes progenitalis.

## EPIDEMIOLOGY AND ETIOLOGY

**Age of Onset** Most commonly young adults; range, infancy to senescence.

**Etiology** HSV-1, HSV-2.

- Labialis: HSV-1 (80 to 90%), HSV-2 (10 to 20%).
- Urogenital: HSV-2 (70 to 90%), HSV-1 (10 to 30%).
- Herpetic whitlow: <20 years of age usually HSV-1; >20 years of age, usually HSV-2.
- Neonatal: HSV-2 (70%), HSV-1 (30%).

**Transmission** Most transmission occurs when persons shed virus but lack lesions. Usually skin-skin, skin-mucosa, mucosa-skin contact. Herpes gladiatorum transmitted by skin-to-skin contact in wrestlers. Increased HSV-1 transmission associated with crowded living conditions and lower socioeconomic status.

**Precipitating Factors for Recurrence** Approximately one-third of persons who develop herpes labialis will experience a recurrence; of these, one-half will experience at least two recurrences annually. Usual factors for herpes labialis: skin/mucosal irritation (UV radiation), altered hormonal milieu (menstruation), fever, common cold, altered immune states, site of infection (genital herpes recurs more frequently than labial).

**Immunocompromising Factors Predisposing to HSV Reactivation** HIV infection, malignancy (leukemia/lymphoma), transplantation (bone marrow, solid organ), chemotherapy, systemic glucocorticoids, other immunosuppressive drugs, radiotherapy.

## PATHOGENESIS

Primary HSV infection occurs through close contact with a person shedding virus at a peripheral site, mucosal surface, or secretion. HSV is inactivated promptly at room temperature; aerosol or fomitic spread unlikely. Infection occurs via inoculation onto susceptible mucosal surface or break in skin. After exposure of skin sites to HSV, the virus replicates in parabasal and intermediate epithelial cells, causing lysis of infected cells, vesicle formation, and local inflammation. After primary infection at inoculation site, HSV ascends peripheral sensory nerves and enters sensory (trigeminal, cervical, or lumbosacral) or autonomic nerve root (vagal) ganglia, where latency is established. Retrograde transport of HSV among nerves and establishment of latency are not dependent on viral replication in skin or neurons; neurons can be infected in the absence of symptoms. Latency can occur after both symptomatic and asymptomatic primary infection.

Periodically, HSV may reactivate from its latent state and virus particles then travel along sensory neurons to skin and mucosal sites to cause recurrent disease episodes (Image 25-1). Recurrent mucocutaneous shedding can be associated with or without (asymptomatic shedding) lesions; virus can be transmitted to a new host when shedding occurs. Recurrences usually occur in the vicinity of the primary infection; may be clinically symptomatic or asymptomatic.

## CLINICAL MANIFESTATIONS

Mucocutaneous HSV infections can be classified as follows:

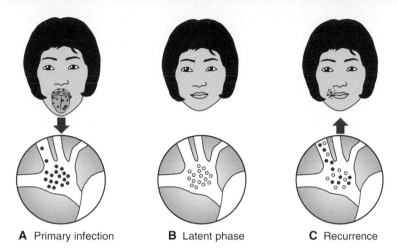

**A** Primary infection          **B** Latent phase          **C** Recurrence

**IMAGE 25-1   Herpes labialis   A.** *With primary HSV infection, virus replicates in the oropharyn-geal epithelium, ascends peripheral sensory nerves into the trigeminal ganglion. **B.** HSV persists in a latent phase within the trigeminal ganglion for the life of the individual. **C.** Various stimuli initiate reactivation of latent virus, which then descends sensory nerves to the lips or perioral skin, resulting in recurrent herpes labilis.*

Primary infection
   Primary herpetic gingivostomatitis
   Primary genital herpes
   Primary infection at other inoculation sites
   Neonatal HSV infection
   Widespread cutaneous herpes associated
      with cutaneous immunocompromise
   Primary herpes in systemically immuno-
      compromised host

Recurrent infection
   First symptomatic infection
   Herpes labialis
   Herpes genitalis
   Recurrent herpes at other sites
   Recurrent widespread cutaneous herpes
      associated with cutaneous immunocom-
      promise
   Recurrent herpes in systemically immuno-
      compromised host
   Chronic herpetic ulcers
Disseminated HSV infection
   Disseminated cutaneous HSV infection
   Disseminated visceral HSV infection, cu-
      taneous involvement

HSV infections of the peripheral sensory nerv-ous system can be classified as follows:

Trigeminal nerve
   Gingivostomatitis
   Recurrent cold sores
   Corneal infections

Facial resurfacing
   HSV gladiatorum

7th cranial nerve
   Facial paralysis
   HSV gladiatorum

Cervical and thoracic sensory nerves
   Herpetic whitlow
   Nipple infection
   HSV gladiatorum

Lumbosacral sensory nerves
   Genital herpes

Complications
   Eczema herpeticum
   Erythema multiforme

## LABORATORY EXAMINATIONS

**Direct Microscopy**   *Tzanck Smear* (Fig. 25-23). Optimally, fluid from intact vesicle is smeared thinly on a microscope slide, dried, and stained with either Wright's or Giemsa's stain. Positive, if acantholytic keratinocytes or multinucleated giant acantholytic keratinocytes are detected. Positive in 75% of early cases, either primary or recurrent.
***Antigen Detection*** Monoclonal antibodies, spe-cific for HSV-1 and HSV-2 antigens, detect and differentiate HSV antigens on smear from lesion.

**Dermatopathology** Ballooning and reticular epidermal degeneration, acantholysis, and intraepidermal vesicles; intranuclear inclusion bodies, multinucleate giant keratinocytes; multilocular vesicles. Immunoperoxidase techniques can be used to identify HSV-1 and HSV-2 antigens in formalin-fixed tissue samples.

**Cultures** Positive HSV cultures from involved mucocutaneous site or tissue biopsy specimens.

**Serology** Antibodies to glycoprotein (g)G1 and (g)G2 detect and diffentiate past HSV-1 and HSV-2 infections. Primary HSV infection can be documented by demonstration of seroconversion.

Recurring herpes can be ruled out if seronegative for HSV antibodies.

**Polymerase Chain Reaction (PCR)** To determine HSV-DNA sequences in tissue, smears, or secretion.

## DIAGNOSIS

Clinical suspicion confirmed by viral culture or antigen detection. Cultures should be used for diagnosing first-episode infections since antibodies to (g)H1 or (g)G2 may take 2 to 6 weeks to develop.

## MANAGEMENT

| | |
|---|---|
| **Prevention** | Skin-to-skin contact should be avoided during outbreak of cutaneous HSV infection. |
| **Topical Antiviral Therapy** | Approved for herpes labialis; minimal efficacy. |
| Acyclovir 5% ointment | Apply q3h, 6 times daily for 7 days. Approved for initial genital herpes and limited mucocutaneous HSV infections in immunocompromised individuals. |
| Penciclovir 1% Cream | Apply q2h while awake for recurrent orolabial infection in immunocompetent individuals. |
| **Oral Antiviral Therapy** | Currently, anti-HSV agents are approved for use in genital herpes Presumably, similar dosing regimens are effective for nongenital infections. Drugs for oral HSV therapy include acyclovir, valacyclovir, and famciclovir. Valacyclovir, the prodrug of acyclovir, has a better bioavailability and is nearly 85% absorbed after oral administration. Famciclovir is equally effective for cutaneous HSV infections. |
| *First episode* | Antiviral agents more effective in treating primary infections than recurrences. |
| Acyclovir | 400 mg tid or 200 mg 5 times daily for 7–10 days |
| Valacyclovir | 1 g bid for 7–10 days |
| Famciclovir | 250 mg tid for 5–10 days |
| *Recurrences* | Most episodes of recurrent herpes do not benefit from pulse therapy with oral acyclovir. In severe recurrent disease, patients who start therapy at the beginning of the prodrome or within 2 days after onset of lesions may benefit from therapy by shortening and reducing severity of eruption; however, recurrences cannot be prevented. |
| Acyclovir | 400 mg PO tid for 5 days *or* 800 mg PO bid for 5 days |
| Valacyclovir | 500 mg bid for 5 days *or* 2 g bid for day 1, then 1 g bid on day 2 |
| Famciclovir | 125 mg bid for 5 days |
| *Chronic suppression* | Decreases frequency of symptomatic recurrences and asymptomatic HSV shedding. After 1 year of continuous daily suppressive therapy, acyclovir should be discontinued to determine the recurrence rate. |
| Acyclovir | 400 mg bid |
| Valacyclovir | 500–1000 mg qd |
| Famciclovir | 250 mg bid |
| *Mucocutaneous disease in immunocompromised individuals* | Neither the need for nor the proper increased dosage of acyclovir has been established conclusively. Patients with herpes who do not respond to the recommended dose of acyclovir may require a |

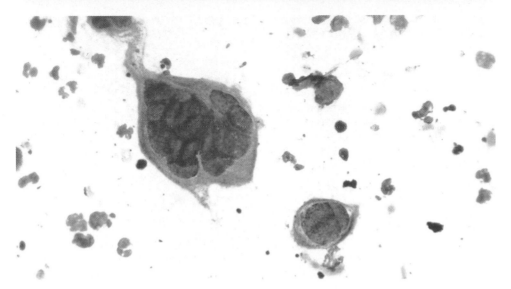

**FIGURE 25-23  Herpes simplex virus: positive Tzanck smear**  *A giant, multinucleated keratinocyte on a Giemsa-stained smear obtained from a vesicle base. Compare size of the giant cell to that of neutrophils also seen in this smear. Another smaller multinucleated acantholytic keratinocyte is seen as well as acantholytic keratinocytes. Identical findings are present in lesions caused by varicella-zoster virus.*

|  |  |
|---|---|
|  | higher oral dose of acyclovir, IV acyclovir, or be infected with an acyclovir-resistant HSV strain, requiring IV foscarnet. The roles of valacyclovir and famciclovir are not yet established. |
| Acyclovir | 5 mg/kg IV q8h for 7–14 days *or* 400 mg 5 times daily: for 7–14 days |
| Oral valacyclovir *or* famciclovir | Reduces the necessity for IV acyclovir therapy. |
| *Neonatal* |  |
| Acyclovir | 20 mg/kg IV q8h for 14–21 days |
| *Acyclovir resistance* | Extremely rare in immunocompetent host. Usually occurs in immunocompromised individuals with large herpetic lesions with high HSV viral load. Resistant HSV strains are thymidine-kinase deficient. Alternative drugs: foscarnet, cidofovir. In HIV-infected patients, chronic HSV infections are mucocutaneous, rarely invasive. |
| Foscarnet | 40 mg/kg IV q8h for 14–21 days |
| Imiquimod cream | May be effective. |
| *HIV infections* | Lesions caused by HSV are relatively common among HIV-infected persons. For severe disease, IV acyclovir therapy may be required. If lesions persist among patients undergoing acyclovir treatment, resistance to acyclovir should be suspected. |
| Acyclovir | Intermittent or suppressive therapy with oral acyclovir may be needed. 400 mg PO 3–5 times daily may be useful. Therapy should continue until clinical resolution is attained. |
| Foscarnet | For severe disease caused by proven or suspected acyclovir-resistant strains, hospitalization should be considered. Foscarnet, 40 mg/kg body weight q8h until clinical resolution is attained. Appears to be the best available treatment. |

## NONGENITAL HERPES SIMPLEX VIRUS INFECTION

Nongenital HSV infection, whether primary or recurrent, is often asymptomatic. Lesions may present as group vesicles on an erythematous base or as a recurrent erythematous plaque ± erosions. *Synonyms*: Herpes, herpes simplex, cold sore, fever blister, herpes febrilis, herpes labialis, herpes gladiatorum, scrum pox, herpetic whitlow.
For genital HSV infection, see Section 27.

### HISTORY

**Incubation Period**    2- to 20-day (average 6) incubation period for primary infection.

**Systems Review**   *Primary Herpes* Many individuals with primary HSV infection are either asymptomatic or have only trivial symptoms. Symptomatic primary herpes, which is uncommon, is characterized by vesicles at the site of inoculation associated with regional lymphadenopathy, at times accompanied by fever, headache, malaise, myalgia. It peaks within the first 3 to 4 days after onset of lesions, resolving during the subsequent 3 to 4 days. Primary herpetic gingivostomatitis is the most common symptom complex accompanying primary HSV infection in children; in young women, primary herpetic vulvovaginitis (see also Section 27).

*Recurrent Herpes* Prodrome of tingling, itching, or burning sensation usually precedes any visible skin changes by 24 h. Systemic symptoms are usually absent.

### PHYSICAL EXAMINATION

**Primary Herpes**   *Skin Findings* Erythema often noted initially, followed soon by grouped, often umbilicated vesicles, which may evolve to pustules (Fig. 25-24); these become eroded as the overlying epidermis sloughs. Erosions may enlarge to ulcerations, which may be crusted or moist. These epithelial defects heal in 2 to 4 weeks, often with resultant postinflammatory hypo- or hyperpigmentation, uncommonly with scarring. The area of involvement may be circumferential around the mouth. Location: oropharyngeal, labial, perioral; distal fingers; other sites.

*Mucous Membranes* Oral mucosa usually involved only in primary HSV infection with vesicles that quickly slough to form erosions (Fig. 25-24) at any site in the oropharynx, scanty to numerous; gingivitis with gingival tenderness,

edema, violaceous color. Sialorrhea. Severe pain. Conjunctival and corneal autoinoculation may occur; regional lymphadenopathy.

**Recurrent Herpes**   Grouped vesicles on erythematous base—erosions and crusts (Figs. 25-25 and 25-26). Documented and recurrent intraoral HSV is uncommon.

### *Specific Features of HSV Infections of Different Sensory Nerves: Trigeminal Nerve*

*Cold sores*: Reactivation of HSV-1 causes cutaneous and mucocutaneous manifestations: *recurrent facial herpes/cold sores* (Figs. 25-25 and 25-26). Usually preceded by prodromal symptoms (tingling, pain, burning sensation, itching) due to early viral replication at sensory nerve endings and in epidermis/mucosa. Affect 20 to 40% of adults. Severe recurrences may complicate laser-resurfacing surgery.

*Ocular HSV infections*: Recurrent keratitis is a major cause of corneal scarring and visual loss, resulting from direct viral cytopathic effect and immune-mediated response. Continuous suppression therapy is recommended.

*Herpetic facial paralysis*: Reactivation of geniculate ganglion infection implicated in pathogenesis of idiopathic facial palsy (Bell's palsy). HSV-1 shedding detected in 40% of cases. Inflammation plays a major role in pathogenesis; glucocorticoids may be effective.

*HSV gladiatorum*: Transmission occurs during contact sports (wrestling, rugby, football). Also occurs in cervical or lumbosacral dermatomes. Prophylaxis may prevent recurrence.

### *Cervical and Thoracic Sensory Nerves Infections*

*Herpetic whitlow*: Prior to "Universal Precautions," occurred in health care profes-

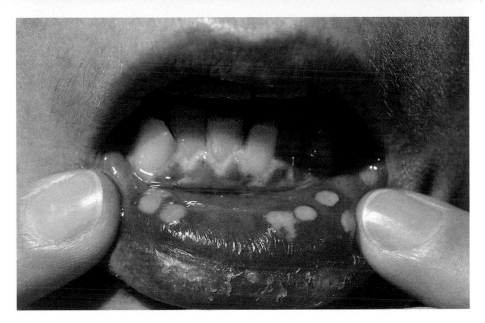

**FIGURE 25-24   Herpes simplex virus infection: primary gingivostomatitis**   *Multiple, very painful erosions on the lower labial mucosa with erythema and edema of the gingiva; fibrin deposits on teeth and gingiva. Fever and tender submandibular lymphadenopathy were also present.*

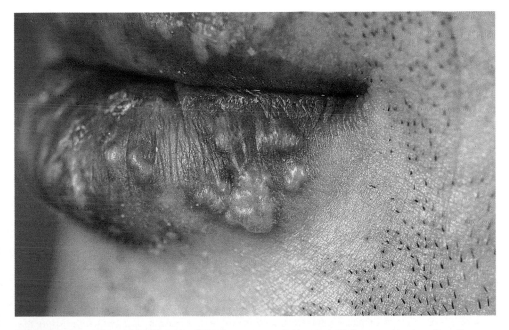

**FIGURE 25-25   Herpes simplex virus infection: recurrent herpes labialis**   *Grouped and confluent vesicles with an erythematous rim on the lips, 24 h after onset of symptoms.*

sionals, especially dental personnel. Associated with painful neuritis in the affected finger and forearm (Fig. 25-27). May last for ≥3 weeks.

*HSV infection of the nipple*: Related to transmission of HSV from infant to mother during breast feeding.

*HSV infections of the lumbosacral sensory nerves*: When lumbosacraal ganglia become infected subsequent to anogenital herpes, recurrent lesions can occur on genitalia as well as buttocks, thighs, perianal mucosa. Perianal herpes does not necessarily imply direct anal inoculation of HSV. Symptomatic herpes in the sacral dermatome may be accompanied by asymptomatic HSV reactivation/shedding from genital mucosa. Recurrent itching, burning, blistering, erythema below the waist should be regarded as genital HSV infection until proven otherwise.

### Complications of HSV Infections of Peripheral Sensory Nervous System

*Eczema herpeticum*: Usually follows autoinoculation of HSV (most commonly orolabial herpes) to atopic dermatitis (see "Herpes Simplex Virus: Widespread Cutaneous Infection Associated with Cutaneous Immunocompromise," below).

*Erythema multiforme*: In some individuals with recurrent HSV infections, erythema multiforme may occur with each recurrence (Fig. 25-28). (See "Erythema Multiforme," Section 7.)

**General Findings**　Fever may be present during symptomatic primary herpetic gingivostomatitis.
***Regional Lymphadenopathy*** May be firm, nonfluctuant, tender; usually unilateral.
***CNS*** Signs of aseptic meningitis: headache, fever, nuchal rigidity, CSF pleocytosis with normal sugar content and positive HSV CSF culture.

### DIFFERENTIAL DIAGNOSIS

**Primary Intraoral HSV Infection**　Aphthous stomatitis, hand-foot-and-mouth disease, herpangina, erythema multiforme.
**Recurrent Lesion**　Fixed drug eruption.

### LABORATORY EXAMINATIONS

See page 799.

### DIAGNOSIS

Clinical suspicion confirmed by Tzanck smear, viral culture, or antigen detection.

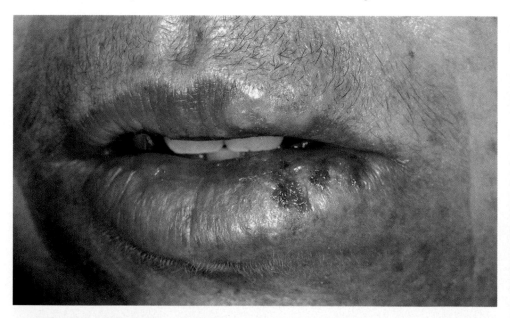

**FIGURE 25-26　Herpes simplex virus infection: recurrent herpes labialis**　*Edema with crusting of the lips that followed sun exposure, 48 to 72 h after onset of symptoms; vesiculation is present but difficult to detect because of confluence of lesions. In some cases, crusting is the only finding.*

**FIGURE 25-27  Herpes simplex virus infection: herpetic whitlow**  *Painful, grouped, confluent vesicles on an erythematous edematous base on the distal finger were the first (and presumed primary) symptomatic infection.*

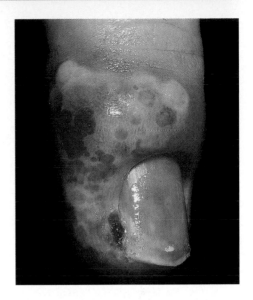

## COURSE AND PROGNOSIS

Recurrences of HSV tend to become less frequent with the passage of time. Eczema herpeticum (see also page 808) may complicate various dermatoses. Patients with immunodeficiency may experience (1) cutaneous and (2) systemic dissemination of HSV and chronic herpetic ulcers (see also page 808). Erythema multiforme may complicate each episode of recurrent herpes, occurring 1 to 2 weeks after an outbreak.

## MANAGEMENT

See page 800.

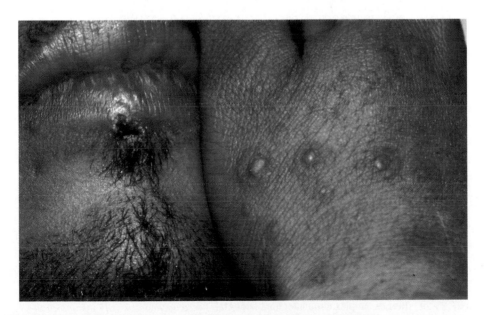

**FIGURE 25-28  Herpes simplex virus infection: recurrent erythema multiforme**  *Recurrent herpes labialis associated with irislike edematous papules on the dorsum of the hand.*

## NEONATAL HERPES SIMPLEX VIRUS INFECTION

Neonatal HSV infection occurs via three routes: (1) in utero infection, (2) intrapartum, and (3) postnatal acquisition. The mother is the most common source of infection. There is usually no evidence of shedding at the time of delivery. Shedding also occurs from uterine cervix. The majority of infections are caused by HSV-2; HSV-1 is more virulent in the newborn and associated with higher morbidity and mortality rates. 70% of infants with neonatal HSV infection are born to mothers with asymptomatic genital herpes; 70% of cases occur in the first-born child. Eruption occurs on the mucous membranes (Fig. 25-29) or on the intact skin at inoculation sites (such as monitoring sensors) (Fig. 25-30). Disseminated HSV infection in neonates is difficult to diagnose in that up to 70% of infants have no mucocutaneous lesions. IV acyclovir therapy is mandatory in these cases.

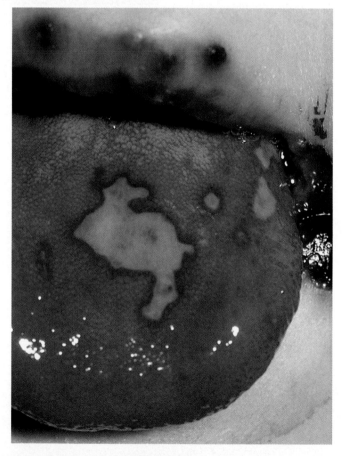

**FIGURE 25-29   Herpes simplex virus infection: neonatal**   *Vesicles and crusted erosions on the upper lip and large geographic ulcerations of the tongue were the clinical findings in this neonate with herpetic gingivostomatitis.*

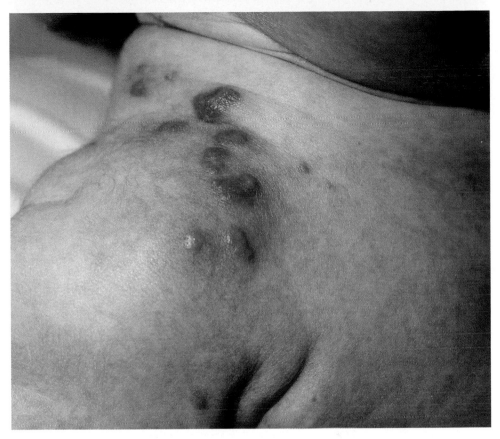

**FIGURE 25-30  Herpes simplex virus infection: neonatal** *Grouped and confluent vesicles with underlying erythema and edema on the shoulder of a newborn infant, arising at the inoculation site.*

## MANAGEMENT

**Prophylaxis**  Many experts recommend serotesting for HSV-1 and HSV-2 at the first prenatal visit. Infants born to women who asymptomatically shed HSV have reduced birth weight and increased prematurity. Acyclovir suppressive therapy at the end of pregnancy probably (but not documented) reduces the risk of transmission to the neonate.

*Pregnancy*  The safety of systemic acyclovir for pregnant women and the fetus has not yet been established, although acyclovir appears to be completely safe in last months of pregnancy. Acyclovir, valacyclovir, and famciclovir are active only in cells with active viral infection. If

HSV is acquired late in pregnancy, cesarean section is indicated.

**Perinatal Infections**  Most mothers of infants who acquire neonatal herpes lack histories of clinically evident genital herpes. The risk for transmission to the neonate from an infected mother appears highest among women with first-episode genital herpes near the time of delivery and is low ($<3\%$) among women with recurrent herpes. The results of viral cultures during pregnancy do not predict viral shedding at the time of delivery, and such cultures are not routinely indicated.

**Antiviral Therapy**  Acyclovir, 20 mg/kg IV q8h for 14 to 21 days.

## HERPES SIMPLEX VIRUS: WIDESPREAD CUTANEOUS INFECTION ASSOCIATED WITH CUTANEOUS IMMUNOCOMPROMISE  ◻ ●

Widespread HSV cutaneous infection in underlying dermatoses occurs most commonly in atopic dermatitis (eczema herpeticum) and is characterized by widespread vesicles and erosions; it may occur as a primary or recurrent infection.
*Synonym*: Kaposi's varicelliform eruption.

## EPIDEMIOLOGY AND ETIOLOGY

**Age of Onset**   Children > adults.
**Etiology**   HSV-1 > HSV-2.
**Transmission**   Commonly from parental herpes labialis to altered epidermis.
**Risk Factors**   Most commonly, atopic dermatitis; more serious infections occur in erythrodermic atopic dermatitis. Also, Darier's disease, thermal burns, pemphigus vulgaris, bullous pemphigoid, ichthyosis vulgaris, cutaneous T cell lymphoma (mycosis fungoides), Wiscott-Aldrich syndrome.

## PATHOGENESIS

See "Herpes Simplex Virus Infection," page 798.

## HISTORY

Primary eczema herpeticum often associated with fever, malaise, irritability. When recurrent, history of prior similar lesions; systemic symptoms less severe. Primary skin disease may be pruritic; onset of eczema herpeticum associated with pain and tenderness. Lesions begin in abnormal skin and may extend peripherally for several weeks during the primary infection or secondary eruption.

## PHYSICAL EXAMINATION

**Skin Lesions**
Umbilicated vesicles evolving into "punched-out" erosions (Fig. 25-31). Vesicles are first confined to eczematous skin and are, in contrast to primary or recurrent HSV eruptions, not grouped but disseminated. Common sites: face, neck, trunk. May later spread to normal-appearing skin. Erosions may become confluent, producing large denuded areas (Fig. 25-32). Successive crops of new vesiculation may occur.

**General Examination**   Primary infection may be associated with fever and lymphadenopathy.

## DIFFERENTIAL DIAGNOSIS

**Widespread Vesiculopustules/Erosions**   Varicella, disseminated VZV infection, disseminated (systemic) HSV infection, wound infection (staphylococcal, pseudomonal, *Candida*), eczema vaccinatum.

## LABORATORY EXAMINATIONS

See pages 799 and 800.

## DIAGNOSIS

Clinical, confirmed by detection of HSV on culture or antigen detection.

## COURSE AND PROGNOSIS

Primary episode of eczema herpeticum runs its course with resolution in 2 to 6 weeks. Recurrent episodes tend to be milder and not associated with systemic symptoms. Systemic dissemination can occur, especially in immunocompromised patients; reported mortality rates range from 10 to 50%. Widely distributed cutaneous HSV infection in burn patients can be difficult to detect clinically.

## MANAGEMENT

**Management of Underlying Dermatosis**   For atopic dermatitis, see "Eczema/Dermatitis," Section 2.
**Antiviral Therapy**   See "Herpes Simplex Virus Infection," page 800.
**Antibacterial Therapy**   Treat associated bacterial infection. See "Bacterial Infections Involving the Skin," Section 22.

**FIGURE 25-31   Herpes simplex virus infection: eczema herpeticum on face**   *Confluent and discrete crusted erosions associated with erythema and edema of the face of a female with atopic dermatitis.*

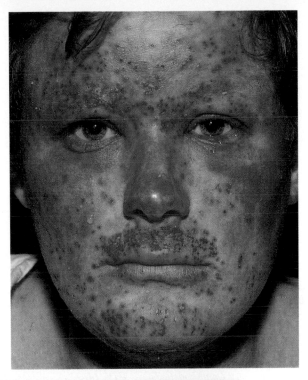

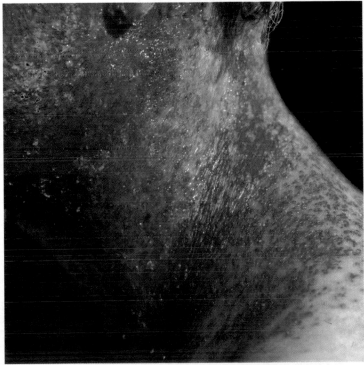

**FIGURE 25-32   Herpes simplex virus infection: eczema herpeticum on neck**   *Confluent crusted erosions with peripheral vesicle on neck and face in the setting of atopic dermatitis.*

## HERPES SIMPLEX VIRUS: INFECTIONS ASSOCIATED WITH SYSTEMIC IMMUNOCOMPROMISE   ▢ ◑ → ●

HSV in the host with systemic immunocompromise may cause (1) local infection with extensive cutaneous involvement (e.g., eczema herpeticum), (2) chronic herpetic ulcers, or (3) widespread systemic infection (widespread mucocutaneous lesions as well as systemic infection).

## EPIDEMIOLOGY

**Incidence**   Rising due to an increasing population of immunocompromised individuals: 80% in bone marrow transplant recipients, 65% in solid organ transplant recipients, 60% in those with lymphoma, 55% in those with leukemia, and 25% in individuals with HIV disease. Incidence of symptomatic outbreaks has decreased markedly because of the primary prophylaxis of HSV-seropositive immuncompromised individuals with oral antiviral drugs.

**Risk Factors**   *Immunodeficiency: HIV Infection* Frequency and duration increase sharply as CD4+ T cell count falls to <50/μL. In most HIV-infected individuals, frequency, duration, and severity of HSV outbreaks similar to those in immunocompetent individuals; however, asymptomatic shedding is increased. Disseminated cutaneous and visceral HSV infections are less common than in other immunocompromised states. *CDC Surveillance Case Definition for AIDS*: HSV infection causing a mucocutaneous ulcer that persists longer than 1 month, or HSV infection causing bronchitis, pneumonitis, or esophagitis for any duration in a patient older than 1 month, is an AIDS-defining condition if the patient has no other cause of immunodeficiency and is without knowledge of HIV antibody status. Immune restoration with HAART has markedly reduced the incidence of serious HSV infections.

*Leukemia/Lymphoma* HSV reactivation typically occurs during induction or reinduction within 20 days in individuals with latent HSV infection.

*Bone Marrow Transplantation (BMT)* HSV reactivation occurs within the first 5 weeks after BMT (median, day 8 posttransplantation). Untreated, 3% of patients die from disseminated HSV infection.

*Chemotherapy* For solid organ or BMT, congenital or acquired cellular immune defects.

Cytotoxic cancer chemotherapy, glucocorticoid therapy.

*Other* Autoimmune diseases, malnutrition; rarely, pregnancy. Radiotherapy. Instrumentation such as nasogastric tube in debilitated patient associated with HSV esophagitis.

## PATHOGENESIS

60 to 80% of HSV-seropositive transplant recipients and patients undergoing chemotherapy for hematologic malignancies will experience reactivation of HSV. After viremia, disseminated cutaneous or visceral HSV infection may occur. Factors determining whether severe localized disease, cutaneous dissemination, or visceral dissemination will occur are not well defined.

## HISTORY

**General**   Patients often hospitalized with underlying condition or disease.

**Skin Symptoms**   Tender and painful mucocutaneous ulcers.

*Recurrent herpetic lesion*: Mild pain in ulcers.
*Chronic herpetic ulcers*: Mild to moderate pain.
*Herpetic whitlow*: Severe pain.
*Oropharyngeal ulcers*: Oral pain on eating.
*Esophageal ulcers*: Retrosternal pain and/or painful swallowing (odynophagia) and/or dysphagia.
*Anorectal ulcers*: Perianal/anal ulcers are usually quite painful. Anorectal ulcers are associated with pain, constipation, pain on defecation, discharge, tenesmus, and at times, sacral radiculopathy, impotence, neurogenic bladder.
*Mucocutaneous dissemination:* Fever.

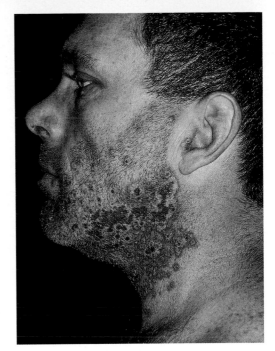

**FIGURE 25-33   Herpes simplex virus infection: primary infection in HIV disease**   *Confluent vesicles and erosions with underlying erythema and edema (5 to 6 days' duration) in the beard area of a 35-year-old HIV-infected male (CD4 cell count, 400/mL). Gingivostomatitis and acute lymphadenopathy were also present, with onset 5 days after orogenital sex.*

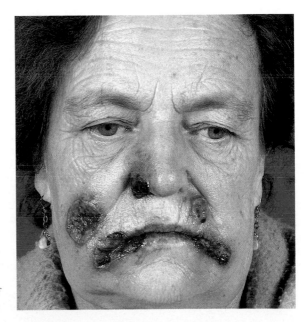

**FIGURE 25-34   Herpes simplex virus infection: chronic ulcer in an immunocompromised host**   *Multiple, slowly spreading, deep ulcers with central necrosis and hemorrhagic crusts on the lips, cheeks, and nose of a female with leukemia.*

**Visceral Dissemination**  Fever, deterioration of clinical status.

## PHYSICAL EXAMINATION

### Skin Lesions

*Primary Infection* Local infection may be widespread on the face (Fig. 25-33), oropharynx, anogenital region with initial vesiculation followed by crusted erosions. Without antiviral therapy, lesions may persist to become chronic herpetic ulcers.

*Recurrent Herpetic Lesions* In most immunocompromised individuals, lesions appear as in the immunocompetent host. However, outbreaks may present with recurrent lesions (grouped crusts, erosions, ulcers) in a much larger area of involvement than usual. In HIV-infected individuals, large, necrotic, eroded lesions may appear over a period of a few days without apparent vesicle formation.

*Chronic Herpetic Ulcers* Recurrent lesions enlarge over weeks to months, forming large ulcers, 10 to 20 cm in diameter (Fig. 25-34). Margins may be slightly rolled, hyperplastic. Coalescence of ulcerations may result in linear ulcers in intergluteal cleft or inguinal fold. Base of ulcer may be crusted or moist. Painful on palpation. Perianal and/or rectal > genital > orofacial > digital (Fig. 25-35A). Uncommonly, ulcer on face and perineum simultaneously.

*Oropharyngeal Ulcers* Large ulcerations occur on the hard palate, often at the site of dental extraction. Linear ulcerations occur on the tongue (Fig. 25-B).

*Esophageal Ulcers* Usually associated with oropharyngeal herpetic ulcer and swallowing HSV-infected saliva. Esophagoscopy: mucosal erosions/ulceration.

*Genital, Perineal, Perianal, Anorectal Ulcers* Acute ulceration of the vulva penis (Fig. 25-36) scrotum, and/or perineum may become chronic ulcers unless effectively treated. In individuals infected with acyclovir-resistant HSV, ulcerations do not respond to usual antiviral therapies. Anal ulcers usually occur via enlargement of perianal ulcers. Herpetic proctitis: sigmoidoscopy shows friable mucosa and ulcerations.

*Mucocutaneous Dissemination* Disseminated (nongrouped) vesicles and pustules often hemorrhagic with inflammatory halo; quickly rupture, resulting in "punched-out" erosions. Lesions may be necrotic and then ulcerate (Fig. 25-37). Ulcers may become confluent with polycyclic well-demarcated borders; edges may be slightly raised, rolled.

*Infarctive Skin Lesions* If complicated by purpura fulminans.

*Mucous Membranes* Oropharyngeal erosion: necrotizing gingivitis, palatal ulcers, glossitis.

**General Examination**  Oropharyngeal infection can occur in the absence of external facial lesions. HSV esophagitis, tracheobronchitis, and focal pneumonitis can be local infection associated with spread by aspirated or swallowed secretions. Diffuse interstitial pneumonitis can be a manifestation of hematogenous infection. HSV pneumonitis often results from endogenous reactivation. Widespread visceral involvement (liver, lungs, adrenals, GI tract, CNS) can occur in immunocompromised individuals.

### Variations with Specific States of Immunocompromise

**Leukemia/Lymphoma**  HSV infection is often atypical, with extensive lesions on lips or nasolabial skin; oropharyngeal infection manifested as necrotic gingival papillae, intraoral ulcerations that mimic thrush, or mucositis from chemotherapy or radiotherapy.

**HIV Disease**  HSV reactivation is usually local, with chronic herpetic ulcers on the face or anogenital region. HSV esophagitis may coexist with candidal esophagitis. Persistent perianal herpes and herpetic proctitis. Disseminated visceral disease is uncommon.

## DIFFERENTIAL DIAGNOSIS

**Chronic Herpetic Ulcers**  Chronic VZV infection, wound infection, ecthyma, ecthyma gangrenosum, pressure ulcer, deep mycotic (cryptococcal, histoplasmal, blastomycotic, coccidioidal) ulcer.

**Oropharyngeal Ulcers**  Aphthous ulcers, lymphoma, histoplasmosis with oral ulcer.

**Esophageal Ulcers**  CMV ulcers, aphthous (idiopathic) ulcers, *Candida* esophagitis, histoplasmosis with esophageal ulcer.

**Anorectal Ulcers**  HPV-induced squamous cell carcinoma, Crohn's disease; amebiasis, chronic rectal abuse of ergot alkaloids.

**Mucocutaneous Dissemination**  VZV infection (varicella, disseminated herpes zoster), eczema herpeticum, eczema vaccinatum, disseminated vaccinia in immunosuppressed patients.

## LABORATORY EXAMINATIONS

See pages 799 and 800.
**Urinalysis**  Hematuria due to HSV cystitis.

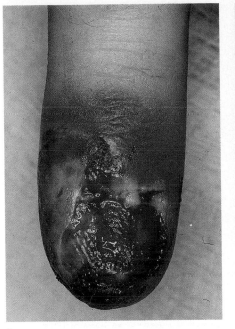
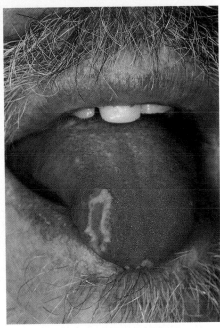

A                                                                    B

**FIGURE 25-35   Herpes simplex virus infection: chronic ulcers in HIV disease**   *The patient with advanced HIV disease presented to the surgical service with subacute ulceration of the distal finger (A). He was treated with debridement and intravenous antibiotic. When seen by the dermatology service, chronic ulcers were also noted on the tongue (B) and left nares. All lesions resolved with oral acyclovir with minimal scarring.*

## DIAGNOSIS

Clinical suspicion confirmed by Tzanck smear, positive HSV antigen detection, or isolation of HSV on viral culture.

## COURSE AND PROGNOSIS

In most immunocompromised individuals with reactivation of HSV, clinical manifestations differ little from infections in healthy hosts. In renal transplant recipients, HSV is excreted in throat washings of 80% of patients shortly after grafting; two-thirds of those excreting HSV develop lesions shortly after excretion is detected. In some immunocompromised individuals, however, large ulcerations can persist for weeks to years. Herpetic ulcers provide a break in the epithelium, facilitating superinfection with bacteria or fungi.

When widespread, HSV may disseminate to liver, lungs, adrenals, GI tract, CNS. Visceral spread can be complicated by disseminated intravascular coagulation, which has a very high mortality rate. Factors determining whether severe localized disease, cutaneous involvement, or visceral dissemination will occur in an individual are not well defined. Disseminated HSV infection with visceral involvement in neonates has a 50 to 80% mortality rate if untreated.

In HIV disease, individuals successfully treated with HAART usually experience reduction in frequency and severity of HSV recurrences. Chronic herpetic ulcers that fail to

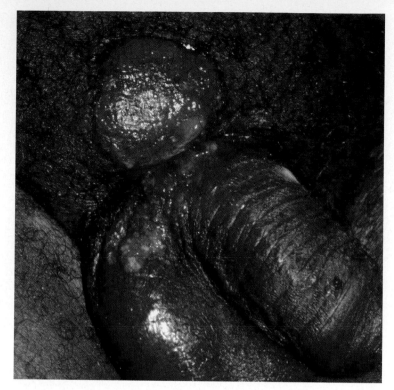

**FIGURE 25-36    Herpes simplex virus infection: chronic ulcer in HIV disease**    *Chronic ulcers and ulcerated tumor on the penis and pubic area caused by acyclovir-resistant HSV. Lesions resolved with topical cidofovir.*

respond to acyclovir should be evaluated promptly for the presence of resistant virus. Infection with acyclovir-resistant strains results in chronic, progressive ulcerations that persist and/or continue to enlarge despite oral and IV acyclovir treatment. These ulcers can enlarge to 20 to 30 cm in diameter and are associated with major morbidity and pain.

## MANAGEMENT

**Prevention**    *Acyclovir prophylaxis* for seropositive patients undergoing bone marrow transplantation, induction therapy for leukemia, or solid organ transplantation: acyclovir, 5 mg/kg IV q8h or 400 mg PO tid, from the day of conditioning, induction, or transplantation for 4 to 6 weeks suppresses both HSV and VZV reactivation. Also oral valacyclovir, famciclovir.
**Systemic Antiviral Therapy**    See "Herpes Simplex Virus Infection," pages 800 and 801.

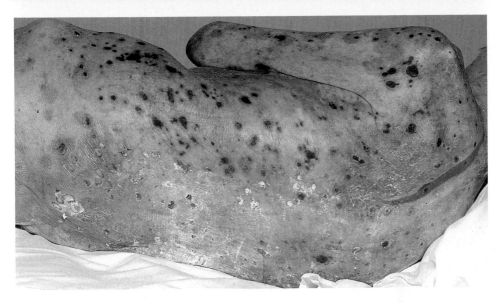

**FIGURE 25-37   Herpes simplex virus infection: disseminated in an immunocompromised host**
*Disseminated erosion, ulcerations, vesicles with hemorrhagic crusts and necrotic bases in an individual with advanced lymphoma. Patients often have infection of lungs, liver, and brain.*

## VARICELLA-ZOSTER VIRUS INFECTIONS    ■   ◑ → ●

Varicella-zoster virus (VZV) is a human herpesvirus that infects 98% of adult populations. Primary VZV infection (varicella or chickenpox) is nearly always symptomatic and characterized by disseminated pruritic vesicles. During primary infection, VZV establishes lifelong infection in sensory ganglia. When immunity to VZV declines, VZV reactivates within the nerve cell, traveling down the neuron to the skin, where it erupts in a dermatomal pattern [herpes zoster (HZ), or shingles]. In the immunocompromised host, primary and reactivated VZV infection is often more severe, associated with higher morbidity rates and some mortality.

## EPIDEMIOLOGY AND ETIOLOGY

**Age of Onset**   90% of cases occur in children <10 years, <5% in persons older than 15 years.

**Etiology**   VZV, a herpesvirus. Structurally similar to other herpesviruses: lipid envelope surrounding nucleocapsid with icosahedral symmetry, a total diameter of approximately 150 to 200 nm, centrally located double-stranded DNA with a molecular weight of 80 million.

**Transmission**   Airborne droplets as well as direct contact; indirect contact uncommon. Patients are contagious several days before exanthem appears and until last crop of vesicles. Crusts are not infectious. VZV can be aerosolized from skin of individuals with herpes zoster, which is about one-third as contagious as varicella, causing varicella in susceptible contacts.

**Season**   In metropolitan areas in temperate climates, varicella epidemics occur in winter and spring.

## PATHOGENESIS

In varicella, VZV is thought to enter through mucosa of upper respiratory tract and oropharynx, followed by local replication and primary viremia; VZV then replicates in cells of reticuloendothelial system with subsequent secondary viremia and dissemination to skin and mucous membranes. Localization of VZV in the basal cell layer is followed by virus replication, vacuole formation, ballooning degeneration of epithelial cells, and accumulation of edema fluid. Second episodes of varicella have been documented but are rare. During the course of varicella, VZV passes from the skin lesions to the sensory nerves, travels to the sensory ganglia, and establishes latent infection.

In HZ, humoral and cellular immunity to VZV established with primary infection ebbs naturally or because of an underlying cause of immunocompromise, resulting in VZV replication in sensory ganglia. VZV then travels down the sensory nerve, resulting in initial dermatomal pain followed by skin lesions. Since the neuritis precedes the skin involvement, pain appears before the skin lesions are visible. The locations of pain are varied and relate directly to the ganglion where VZV has emerged from latency to active infection. Prodromal symptoms may appear initially in the trigeminal, cervical, thoracic, lumbar, or sacral dermatome. Postherpetic neuralgia (PHN) is caused by reflex sympathetic dystrophy.

## LABORATORY EXAMINATIONS

**VZV Antigen Detection**   Smear of vesicle fluid or scraping from ulcer base/margin is made on a glass microscope slide. Direct fluorescent antibody (DFA) test detects VZV-specific antigens. Sensitive and specific method for identifying VZV-infected lesions. Higher yield than VZV cultures.

**Viral Cultures**   Isolation of virus on viral culture (human fibroblast monolayers) from vesicular skin lesions, biopsy specimens, corneal scraping, and CSF is possible but more difficult than for HSV. Distinctive cytopathic effects usually appear in 3 to 10 days. Vesicle fluid can be cultured.

**Tzanck Smear**   Cytology of fluid or scraping from base of vesicle or pustule shows both giant and multinucleated acantholytic epidermal cells (as does that of HSV infections) (see Fig. 23-23). Cytologists and dermatopathologists are most experienced in interpretation of smear.

**Serology**  Seroconversion documents primary VZV infection.
**Dermatopathology**  Lesional skin or visceral biopsy specimen shows multinucleated giant epithelial cells indicating HSV-1, HSV-2, or VZV infection. Immunoperoxidase stains specific for HSV-1, HSV-2, or VZV antigens can identify the specific herpesvirus.

## VARICELLA    ■

Varicella is the highly contagious primary infection caused by varicella-zoster virus. It is characterized by successive crops of pruritic vesicles that evolve to pustules, crusts, and at times, scars. This infection is often accompanied by mild constitutional symptoms; the primary infection occurring in adulthood may be complicated by pneumonia and encephalitis.
*Synonym*: Chickenpox.

### EPIDEMIOLOGY

**Age of Onset**  See page 816.
**Incidence**  3 to 4 million cases in the United States annually.
**Transmission**  See page 816.
**Season**  See page 816.

### HISTORY

**Incubation Period**  14 days (range, 10 to 23 days).
**Prodrome**  Characteristically absent or mild. Uncommon in children, more common in adults: headache, general aches and pains, severe backache, malaise. Exanthem appears within 2 to 3 days.
**History**  Exposure at day care, school, to older sibling; relative with zoster.
**Skin Symptoms**  Exanthem usually quite pruritic.

### PHYSICAL EXAMINATION

**Skin Lesions**
In most children, illness begins with appearance of exanthem, vesicular lesions evident in successive crops. Often single, discrete lesions or scanty in number in children and much more dense in adults. Initial lesions are *papules* (often not observed) that may appear as *wheals* and quickly evolve to *vesicles* and initially appear as small "drops of water" or "dewdrops on a rose petal" (Fig. 25-38), superficial and thin-walled with surrounding

erythema. Vesicles become umbilicated and rapidly evolve to *pustules* and *crusts* over an 8- to 12-h period. With subsequent crops, all stages of evolution may be noted simultaneously, i.e., papules, vesicles, pustules, crusts.
**Distribution**  First lesions begin on face (Fig. 25-38) and scalp, spreading inferiorly to trunk (Fig. 25-39) and extremities; most profuse in areas least exposed to pressure, i.e., back between shoulder blades, flanks, axillae, popliteal and anticubital fossae; density highest on trunk and face, less on extremities; palms and soles usually spared.
Crusts fall off in 1 to 3 weeks, leaving a pink, somewhat depressed base. Characteristic punched-out permanent scars may persist. Uncommonly, hemorrhage into pustular lesion occurs in otherwise healthy children, i.e., *hemorrhagic varicella*. Complicated by superinfection by staphylococci or streptococci; impetigo, furuncles, cellulitis, and gangrene may occur.
**Mucous Membranes**  Vesicles (not often observed) and subsequent shallow erosions (2 to 3 mm) most common on palate but also occur on mucosa of nose, conjunctivae, pharynx, larynx, trachea, GI tract, urinary tract, vagina.
**General Examination**  Low-grade fever. Vesicopustules may occur in respiratory, GU, and GI tracts.
**Pneumonitis**  Occurs with increased frequency in immunocompromised individuals of all ages and in immunocompetent adolescents and adults. 3 to 16% of healthy adults with varicella have radiologic evidence of VZV pneumonitis (diffuse interstitial lobular infiltrate); one-third

of these will have respiratory symptoms. More frequent/severe in pregnancy. Prior to antiviral therapy, morbidity/mortality was high.

*CNS* Most commonly, varicella with cerebellar ataxia and encephalitis.

### Variants
**Bacterial Superinfection**   Most commonly, *S. aureus* or group A streptococcus can cause impetigo, ecthyma, cellulitis, necrotizing fasciitis, or toxic shock syndrome in varicella lesions.

**"Malignant" Varicella**   Immunosuppressed or glucocorticoid-treated individuals may develop pneumonitis, hepatitis, encephalitis, disseminated intravascular coagulation, and purpura fulminans. Continued VZV replication and dissemination result in prolonged high-level viremia, more extensive rash, longer period of new vesicle formation.

### DIFFERENTIAL DIAGNOSIS

**Widespread Vesicles/Crusts**   Disseminated HSV infection, cutaneous dissemination of zoster, eczema herpeticum, eczema vaccinatum, disseminated vaccinia in immunosuppressed patients (smallpox vaccination still given in the U.S. military), rickettsialpox, enterovirus infections, bullous form of impetigo.

### LABORATORY EXAMINATIONS

See "Varicella-Zoster Virus Infections," page 816.

**Bacterial Cultures**   Rule out superinfection with *S. aureus* or group A streptococcus.

**Serology**   Seroconversion, i.e., fourfold or greater rise in VZV titers.

### DIAGNOSIS

Usually made on clinical findings alone.

### COURSE AND PROGNOSIS

In healthy children, the course is self-limited; however, a mortality rate of 1 per 50,000 cases in the United States is reported (100 deaths annually in the 3 to 4 million cases). 6500 hospitalizations annually (United States) for varicella. The most common complication of varicella in children <5 years is bacterial (*S. aureus*, group A streptococcus) superinfection; severe infection of pox can occur with bacteremia. In children 5 to 11 years of age, the most common complications are varicella encephalitis and Reye's syndrome.

In adults, prodromal symptoms are common and may be severe; exanthem may last for a week or more, with prolonged period of recovery. Primary varicella pneumonia, which presents 1 to 6 days after appearance of rash, is relatively common in adults, with 16% of adults showing x-ray evidence of pneumonitis; however, only 4% have clinical signs of pneumonitis. VZV encephalitis may also complicate varicella in adults. Less common complications of varicella include viral arthritis, uveitis, conjunctivitis, carditis, inappropriate antidiuretic hormone syndrome, nephritis, and orchitis. The mortality rate in adults is 15 per 50,000 cases; 25% of varicella-associated deaths occur in adults.

Maternal varicella during the first trimester of pregnancy may result in fetal varicella syndrome (limb hypoplasia, eye and brain damage, skin lesions) in 2% of exposed fetuses. Women with varicella occurring during pregnancy have a 10% risk for severe VZV pneumonitis. Neonatal varicella has higher associated incidence of pneumonitis and encephalitis than occurs in older children.

Immunocompromised or glucocorticoid-treated patients with varicella may manifest dissemination, hepatitis, encephalitis, and hemorrhagic complications. If varicella occurs at an early age when maternal antibody is still present, an individual can have a second episode of varicella. In HIV-infected patients, reactivation of VZV may result in chronic painful ecthymatous varicella.

In immunocompromised individuals, VZV hepatitis and pneumonitis are relatively common and are associated with significant mortality.

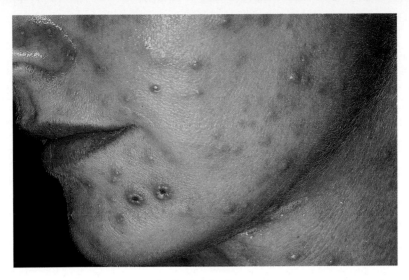

**FIGURE 25-38    Varicella-zoster virus infection: varicella**    *Multiple, very pruritic, erythematous papules, vesicles ("dewdrops on a rose petal"), and crusted papules on erythematous, edematous bases on the face and neck of a young female. The spectrum of lesions, arising over 7 to 10 days, is typical of varicella.*

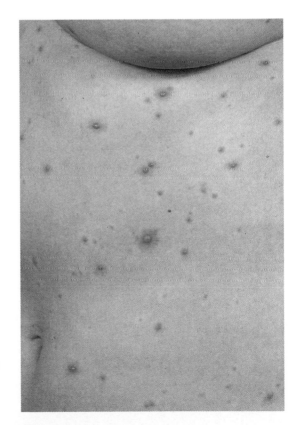

**FIGURE 25-39    Varicella-zoster virus infection: varicella**    *Multiple papules and vesicles on erythematous bases in a random pattern of dissemination on the trunk. Note different stages of evolution of individual lesions.*

## MANAGEMENT

**Prevention**
Immunization

VZV immunization is now available (Varivax) and is 80% effective in preventing symptomatic primary VZV infection. 5% of newly immunized children develop rash. Those at high risk for varicella, who should be immunized, include: normal VZV-negative adults, children with leukemia, and immunocompromised individuals (immunosuppressive treatment, HIV infection, cancer). VZV vaccine results in both cell-mediated immunity and antibody production against the virus. Immunization with VZV vaccine may boost humoral and cell-mediated immunity and decrease the incidence of zoster in populations with declining VZV-specific immunity.

**Symptomatic therapy**
Lotions | Directed at reducing pruritus.
Oral antihistamines | Application gives short-term relief of pruritus.
Caution re antipyretic agents | Antipyretic administration is of concern because of a possible link between aspirin and Reye's syndrome in children with varicella.

**Antiviral agents**
Otherwise healthy patients | If begun within 24 h after onset of varicella, decreases the severity of varicella and reduces secondary cases.

Acyclovir | 20 mg/kg (800 maximum) qid for 5 days
Valacyclovir | Effective but not an approved use; dosing same as for herpes zoster.

Famciclovir | Effective but not an approved use; dosing same as for herpes zoster.

VZV infection (varicella or zoster) in immunocompromised patients
Acyclovir | 10 mg/kg IV q8h for 7 days

Acyclovir-resistant | 40 mg/kg IV q8h for 7 days
Foscarnet

**Treatment of bacterial superinfection**
Mupirocin ointment | Directed at *S. aureus* and/or group A streptococcus.
Oral antibiotics | Applied twice daily to lesions.
See Table 22-1.

## HERPES ZOSTER   ■

Herpes zoster (HZ) is an acute dermatomal infection associated with reactivation of VZV and is characterized by unilateral pain and a vesicular or bullous eruption limited to a dermatome(s) innervated by a corresponding sensory ganglion. The major morbidity is postherpetic neuralgia (PHN).
*Synonym*: Shingles.

## EPIDEMIOLOGY

**Age of Onset**   More than 66% are >50 years of age; 5% of cases in children <15 years.

**Incidence**   In the United States, nearly 100% of adults are seropositive for anti-VZV antibodies by the third decade of life and are thus at risk for reactivation of latent VZV. More than 500,000 cases of HZ annually. Cumulative lifetime incidence: 10 to 20%. In one cohort, 5% of individuals with HZ were HIV-infected and 5% had cancer. Recurrent HZ <1% of cases. Occurs in 25% of HIV-infected individuals, an eight times higher incidence than the general population, ages 20 to 50 years; 7 to 9% of renal and cardiac transplant recipients. Recurrent HZ more common in immunocompromised individuals. Immunization to VZV in childhood will alter the epidemiology of HZ.

**Risk Factors**   Most common factor is diminishing immunity to VZV with advancing age, with most cases occurring in those ≥55 years. However, in most cases triggering factors are not known. Malignancy; immunosuppression, especially from lymphoproliferative disorders and chemotherapy; radiotherapy. HIV-infected individuals have an eightfold increased incidence of HZ.

**Pathogenesis**   In varicella passes VZV from lesions in the skin and mucosa via sensory fibers centripetally to sensory ganglia. In the ganglia the virus establishes latent infection lasting for life. Reactivation occurs in those ganglia in which VZV has achieved the highest density and is triggered by immunosuppression, trauma, tumor, or irradiation (see risk factors). Reactivated virus can no longer be contained. Virus multiplies and spreads antidromically down the sensory nerve to the skin/mucosa where it produces the characteristic vesicles (Image 25-2).

**Classification**   HZ manifests in three distinct clinical stages: prodromal, active, and chronic.

## HISTORY

**Duration of Symptoms**   Prodromal stage: neuritic pain or paresthesia precedes for 2 to 3 weeks (84% of cases). Acute vesiculation: 3 to 5 days. Crust formation: days to 2 to 3 weeks. PHN: months to years. Acute pain is that preceding or accompanying the dermatomal rash. Chronic pain or PHN is that persisting after the lesions have healed or persisting 4 weeks after the onset of lesions, regardless of degree of healing.

**Skin Symptoms**   *Prodromal Stage* Pain (stabbing, pricking, sharp, boring, penetrating, lancinating, shooting), tenderness, paresthesia (itching, tingling, burning, freeze-burning) in the involved dermatome precedes the eruption. Allodynia: heightened sensitivity to mild stimuli.

*Active Vesiculation* Skin lesions may be pruritic but in themselves are not painful.

*Zoster Sine Zoster* Nerve involvement can occur without cutaneous zoster.

*Abdominal Zoster* Presents with severe abdominal (or chest pain) that may precede rash by hours to days.

*Chronic Stages* PHN, described as "burning," "ice-burning," "shooting," or "lancinating," can persist for weeks, months, or years after the cutaneous involvement has resolved.

**Constitutional Symptoms**   Prodromal stage and active vesiculation: flulike symptoms such as headache, malaise, fever. Chronic stages: depression is very common in individuals with PHN.

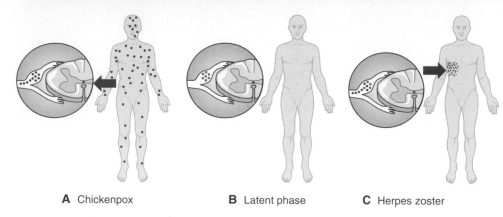

**A** Chickenpox     **B** Latent phase     **C** Herpes zoster

**IMAGE 25-2   Varicella and herpes zoster** *A. During primary VZV infection (varicella or chickenpox), virus infects sensory ganglia. **B.** VZV persists in a latent phase within ganglia for the life of the individual. **C.** With diminished immune function, VZV reactivates within sensory ganglia, descends sensory nerves, and replicates in skin.*

## PHYSICAL EXAMINATION

### Skin Lesions
Papules (24 h) → vesicles-bullae (Fig. 25-40) (48 h) → pustules (96 h) → crusts (7 to 10 days). New lesions continue to appear for up to 1 week. Necrotic and gangrenous lesions sometimes occur. Erythematous, edematous base (Fig. 25-40) with superimposed clear vesicles, sometimes hemorrhagic. The vesicle-bulla is oval or round, may be umbilicated. Some scarring is very common after healing of HZ.
*Distribution* Unilateral, dermatomal (Image 25-3; Figs. 25-41, 25-42). Two or more contiguous dermatomes may be involved (Fig. 25-41). Noncontiguous dermatomal zoster is rare. Hematogenous dissemination to other skin sites in 10% of healthy individuals.
*Site of Predilection* Thoracic (>50%), trigeminal (10 to 20%) (Fig. 25-43), lumbosacral and cervical (10 to 20%).
**Mucous Membranes** Vesicles and erosions occur in mouth, vagina, and bladder depending on dermatome involved.
**General Examination** *Lymphadenopathy* Regional nodes draining the area are often enlarged and tender.
*Sensory or Motor Nerve Changes* Detectable by neurologic examination. Sensory defects (temperature, pain, touch) and (mild) motor paralysis, e.g., facial palsy.

*Eyes* In ophthalmic zoster, nasociliary involvement of VI (ophthalmic) branch of the trigeminal nerve occurs in about one-third of cases and is heralded by vesicles on the side and tip of the nose (Fig. 25-43). Complications include uveitis, keratitis, conjunctivitis, retinitis, optic neuritis, glaucoma, proptosis, cicatricial lid retraction, and extraocular muscle palsies. Acute retinal necrosis (rapidly progressive herpetic retinal necrosis) is more common in the immunocompromised host
*Delayed Contralateral Hemiparesis* Occurs weeks to months (mean, 7 weeks) after an episode of HZ involving the first division of the trigeminal nerve (V-1). Typical presentation is headache and hemiplegia occurring in a patient with recent history of HZ ophthalmicus. Arteriogram shows inflammation, narrowing, and thrombosis of proximal branches of anterior or middle cerebral artery. Pathogenesis: direct VZV invasion of cerebral arteries by extension along intracranial branches of V-1, resulting in inflammation of internal carotid artery or one of its branches on the side ipsilateral to rash.

## DIFFERENTIAL DIAGNOSIS

**Prodromal Stage/Localized Pain** Can mimic migraine, cardiac or pleural disease, an acute abdomen, or vertebral disease.
**Dermatomal Eruption** Zosteriform HSV infection, phytoallergic (poison ivy, poison oak)

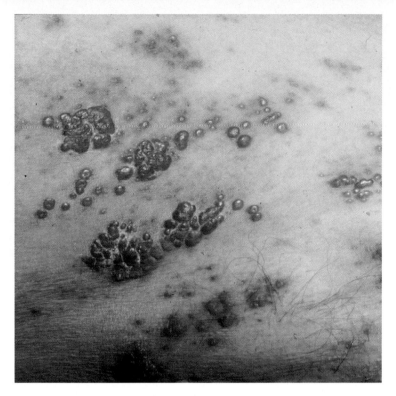

**FIGURE 25-40   Varicella-zoster virus infection: herpes zoster with cluster of grouped vesicles**
*Grouped and confluent vesicles surrounding erythema on the chest wall.*

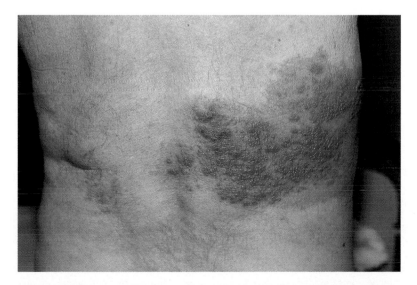

**FIGURE 25-41   Varicella-zoster virus infection: herpes zoster in T8 to T10 dermatomes**   *Typical grouped vesicles and pustules with erythema and edema of three contiguous thoracic dermatomes on the posterior chest wall.*

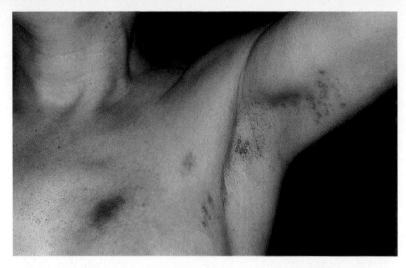

**FIGURE 25-42    Varicella-zoster virus infection: herpes zoster in dermatomes**   *Grouped and confluent papules, vesicles, and crusted erosions arising in the fourth left cervical dermatome in a healthy 41-year-old female. Pruritus and a burning sensation accompanied the clinical findings. The involvement is relatively mild and can be mistaken for other dermatoses, such as allergic contact dermatitis.*

contact dermatitis, erysipelas, bullous impetigo, necrotizing fasciitis.

## LABORATORY EXAMINATIONS

See "Varicella-Zoster Virus Infections," page 816.
**Electrocardiogram**   In prodromal stage with individuals with chest pain, rule out ischemic heart disease.
**Imaging**   In prodromal stage, rule out organic, pleural, pulmonary, or abdominal disease.

## DIAGNOSIS

**Prodromal Stage**   Suspect HZ in older or immunocompromised individual with unilateral pain.
**Active Vesiculation**   Clinical findings usually adequate; may be confirmed by Tzanck test and possible DFA or viral culture to rule out HSV infection.
**PHN**   By history and clinical findings.

## COURSE AND PROGNOSIS

In immunocompetent host, rash usually resolves in 2 to 3 weeks. Complications can be local: hemorrhage, gangrene: or general: meningoencephalitis, cerebral vascular syndromes, cranial nerve syndromes [trigeminal (ophthalmic) branch (HZ ophthalmicus), facial and auditory nerves (Ramsay Hunt syndrome)], peripheral motor weakness, transverse myelitis, visceral involvement (pneumonitis, hepatitis, pericarditis/myocarditis, pancreatitis, esophagitis, enterocolitis, cystitis, synovitis), cutaneous dissemination, and superinfection of skin lesions.

The course in HIV-infected patients and renal and cardiac transplant recipients is usually uncomplicated without significant dissemination. Dissemination generally occurs 6 to 10 days after onset of localized lesions and is most often limited to cutaneous involvement. In immunosuppressed individuals, visceral dissemination can occur, involving CNS, lung, heart, and GI tract. The risk of PHN is 40% in

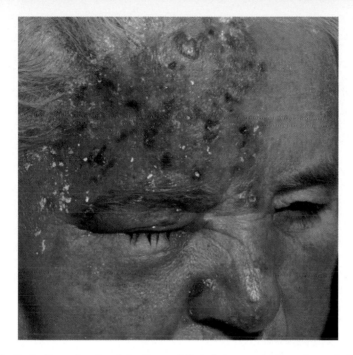

**FIGURE 25-43   Varicella zoster virus infection: ophthalmic herpes zoster**   *Crusted ulcerations and vesicles on the right forehead and periorbital area in the ophthalmic branch of the trigeminal nerve; marked facial edema is also present. Vesicles on the tip of the nose indicates nasociliary involvement. Hutchinson's rule: involvement of the nasociliary nerve suggests that eye involvement may occur.*

patients >60 years. In one large follow-up study, PHN was present 1 month after onset of the rash in 60%, by 3 months there was some pain in 24%, and by 6 months 13% of the patients still had pain. The highest incidence of PHN is in ophthalmic zoster. Dissemination of zoster—≥20 lesions outside the affected or adjacent dermatomes—occurs in up to 10% of patients, usually in immunosuppressed patients. Motor paralysis occurs in 5% of patients, especially when the virus involves the cranial nerves.

Pain with HZ is associated with neural inflammation, nerve infection during the acute reactivation, and neural inflammation and scarring with PHN.

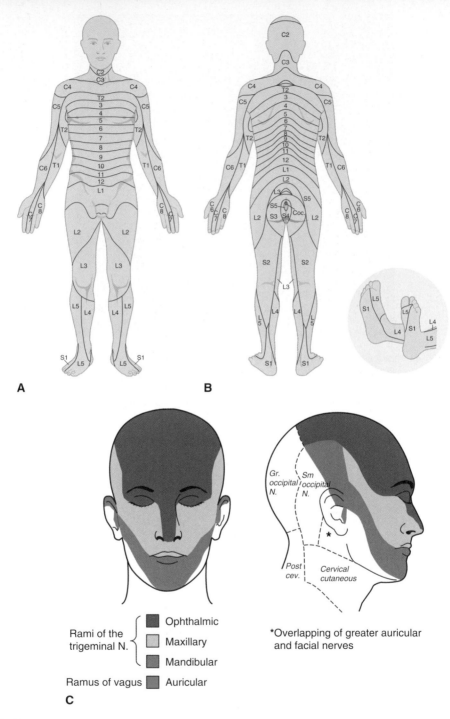

**IMAGE 25-3**   **Dermatomes**   *The cutaneous fields of peripheral nerves.*

## MANAGEMENT

| | |
|---|---|
| **Prevention** | |
| Immunization | Immunization with VZV vaccine may boost humoral and cell-mediated immunity and decrease the incidence of zoster in populations with declining VZV-specific immunity. |
| **Goals of management** | Relieve constitutional symptoms; minimize pain; reduce viral shedding; prevent secondary bacterial infection; speed crusting of lesions and healing; ease physical, psychological, emotional discomfort; prevent viral dissemination or other complications; prevent or minimize PHN. |
| **Antiviral therapy** | In individuals at high risk for reactivation of VZV infection, oral acyclovir can reduce the incidence of HZ. In prodromal stage: begin antiviral agent if diagnosis is considered likely; analgesics. With active vesiculation: antiviral therapy begun $\leq$72 h accelerates healing of skin lesions, decreases the duration of acute pain, and may decrease the frequency of PHN when given in adequate dosage. |
| Acyclovir | 800 mg PO qid for 7–10 days. The 50% viral inhibitory concentration of acyclovir is three to six times higher for VZV than for HSV in vitro, and drug dose must be increased appropriately. The bioavailability of acyclovir is only 15 to 30% of the orally administered dose. For ophthalmic zoster and HZ in the immunocompromised host, acyclovir should be given intravenously. Acyclovir hastens healing and lessens *acute* pain if given within 48 h of the onset of the rash. |
| Valacyclovir | 1000 mg PO tid for 7 days, 70 to 80% bioavailable. |
| Famciclovir | 500 mg PO tid for 7 days, 77% bioavailable. Reduce dose in individuals with diminished renal function. |
| *Acyclovir-resistant VZV* | Foscarnet |
| *Immunosuppressed patients* | IV acyclovir and recombinant interferon $\alpha$-2a to prevent dissemination of HZ is indicated. |
| **Supportive therapy for acute HZ** | |
| Constitutional symptoms | Bed rest, NSAIDs. |
| Sedation | Pain often interferes with sleep. Sleep deprivation and pain commonly result in depression. Doxepin, 10 to 100 mg hs, is an effective agent. |
| Oral glucocorticoids | Prednisone given early in the course of HZ relieves constitutional symptoms but has not been proven to reduce PHN. |
| Dressings | Application of moist dressings (water, saline, Burow's solution) to the involved dermatome is soothing and alleviates pain. |
| Pain management | Early control of pain with narcotic analgesics is indicated; failure to manage pain can result in failure to sleep, fatigue, and depression: Best to begin with more potent analgesics and then reduce potency as pain lessens. |
| **Chronic stages (PHN)** | |
| Pain management | Pain is that of reflex sympathetic dystrophy. |
| | Severe prodromal pain or severe pain on the first day of rash is predictive of severe PHN. Gabapentin: 300 mg tid. Tricyclic antidepressants such as doxepin, 10 to 100 mg PO hs. Capsaicin cream every 4 h. Topical anesthetic such as EMLA or 5% lidocaine patch for allodynia. Nerve block to area of allodynia. Analgesics. |

## VARICELLA-ZOSTER VIRUS INFECTIONS IN THE IMMUNOCOMPROMISED HOST  ☐ ●

In immunocompromised individuals, VZV infections can be more severe in primary infections (varicella) and reactivated infections (HZ). In individuals with varicella, cutaneous and visceral involvement can be more severe. In those with HZ, the infection may involve several contiguous dermatomes, have more extensive cutaneous necrosis, have wide hematogenous dissemination to mucocutaneous structures as well as to the viscera, and often be associated with high morbidity and mortality rates.

### EPIDEMIOLOGY

**Incidence**  Population of immunocompromised individuals is increasing. Most cases of recurrent HZ occur in immunocompromised individuals.

**Risk Factors**  Immunosuppression, especially from lymphoproliferative disorders, and cancer chemotherapy.

Visceral dissemination of varicella: children undergoing cancer chemotherapy; solid organ and bone marrow transplant recipients; HIV infection; certain cell-mediated immunodeficiency disorders of childhood.

HZ: often the first sign of HIV infection, preceding oral candidiasis and oral hairy leukoplakia by 1 year. Visceral dissemination of HZ: Hodgkin's disease (risk of developing zoster is 13 to 15% compared with 7 to 9% for non-Hodgkin's lymphoma patients and 1 to 3% for patients with solid tumors).

### CLASSIFICATION OF VZV INFECTION IN THE IMMUNOCOMPROMISED HOST

- Primary varicella with visceral dissemination
- HZ with cutaneous dissemination
- HZ with visceral and cutaneous dissemination
- Reactivated VZV with hematogenous dissemination but without HZ
- HZ with persistent dermatomal infection
- Chronic cutaneous VZV infection after hematogenous dissemination

### HISTORY

**Skin Symptoms**  Symptoms of varicella and zoster. Chronic cutaneous VZV infections following hematogenous dissemination are often associated with significant lesional pain requiring narcotic analgesia for pain management.

**Constitutional Symptoms**  Visceral dissemination usually accompanied by fever.

### PHYSICAL EXAMINATION

**Skin Lesions**

***Varicella and Cutaneous Dissemination of Reactivated VZV Infection***  (See "Varicella," page 817.) Reactivated VZV without HZ with dissemination cannot be distinguished clinically from varicella (Fig. 25-44).

***Herpes Zoster***  In HIV disease and leukemia, involvement of several contiguous dermatomes is common (Fig. 25-45).

***Herpes Zoster with Cutaneous Dissemination***  A variable number of vesicles or bullae are seen at any mucocutaneous site, which evolve into crusted erosions. Lesions are disseminated and range from a few to hundreds. The condition thus appears clinically as zoster plus varicella.

***Herpes Zoster with Persistent Dermatomal Infection***  Papules and nodules, which can become hyperkeratotic or verrucous, persisting in a dermatomal pattern (single or multiple contiguous) after an outbreak of zoster (Fig. 25-46). Chronic ulcers can persist for months (Fig. 25-47).

***Chronic Cutaneous VZV Infection After Hematogenous Dissemination***  Lesions on the palms or soles may present initially as bullae. Continual appearance of vesicles/bullae in a dermatomal or generalized distribution. Dissemination can occur without dermatomal HZ. Chronic lesions present as nodules, ulcers, crusted nodules/ulcers (ecthymatous). Postinflammatory hyper- or hypopigmentation.

**Systemic Findings**  *Eyes*  In HIV disease, retinal VZV infection (acute retinal necrosis) can occur in the absence of apparent conjunctival or cuta-

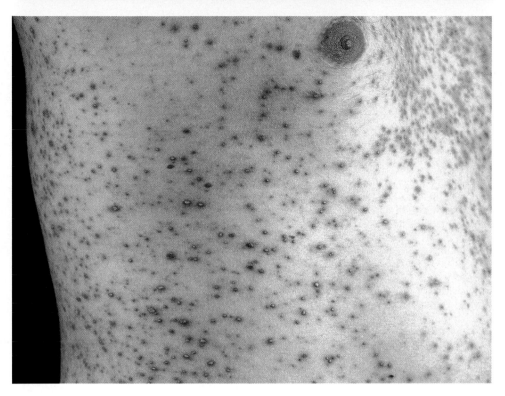

**FIGURE 25-44    Varicella-zoster virus infection: disseminated cutaneous, in an immunocompromised patient**    *Hundreds of vesicles and pustules on erythematous bases of the trunk of a patient with lymphoma. Note the absence of grouping of lesions seen in herpes simplex or herpes zoster. The eruption is indistinguishable from varicella and must be differentiated from disseminated HSV infection.*

neous involvement with subsequent loss of vision. Bilateral involvement in one-third of cases with subsequent loss of vision. VZV optic neuritis is rare.

*CNS* In HIV disease, VZV is the etiologic agent of up to 2% of CNS disease (encephalitis, polyneuritis, myelitis, vasculitis).

## DIFFERENTIAL DIAGNOSIS

**Primary Varicella with Visceral Dissemination** Pneumonia must be distinguished from *Pneumocystis carinii* pneumonia associated with varicella.

**Herpes Zoster with Cutaneous Dissemination** Zosteriform HSV infection with dissemination.

**Herpes Zoster with Visceral and Cutaneous Dissemination** Zosteriform HSV infection with dissemination. Pneumonia must be distinguished from *P. carinii* pneumonia associated with varicella.

**Herpes Zoster with Persistent Dermatomal Infection** Chronic zosteriform HSV infection. Hypertrophic scars or keloids.

**Chronic Cutaneous VZV Infection After Hematogenous Dissemination** Ecthyma, ecthyma gangrenosum, disseminated mycobacterial infection, deep fungal infection, syphilis.

## LABORATORY EXAMINATIONS

See "Varicella-Zoster Virus Infection," page 816.
**Antiviral Sensitivities** When isolated, VZV from cultured lesion can be tested for sensitivity to acyclovir and other antiviral agents.

**Bacterial Culture** Rule out secondary bacterial infection, most commonly caused by S. *aureus* or group A streptococcus.
**Chemistries** Abnormalities of liver function tests with VZV hepatitis.

## COURSE AND PROGNOSIS

Approximately 2 to 35% of children with varicella who are undergoing cancer chemotherapy experience visceral dissemination; the associated mortality rate is 7 to 30%. Dissemination is more common in those with a peripheral blood lymphocyte count of $<500/\mu L$.

**Children with Varicella** Visceral involvement most commonly affects lungs; less often, liver and brain. Varicella pneumonia occurs 3 to 7 days after onset of skin lesions; can progress rapidly over a few days or remain indolent with gradual improvement over 2 to 4 weeks. Neurologic complications present 4 to 8 days after onset of rash; associated with poor prognosis.

**Adults with HZ** In HIV-infected adults, recurrent episodes occur in same or different dermatome(s); disseminated zoster infrequent. Between 15 and 30% of patients with Hodgkin's disease experience significant dissemination (most often cutaneous). Mortality rates for disseminated zoster much lower than for children with disseminated varicella. PHN does not appear to be more common in immunocompromised individuals than in the general population.

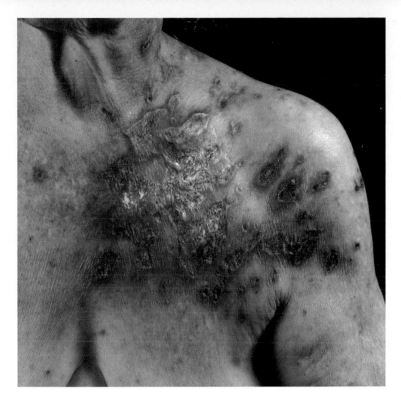

**FIGURE 25-45 Varicella-zoster virus infection: necrotizing herpes zoster** *Confluent, crusted ulcerations on an inflammatory base in several contiguous dermatomes in an elderly male with leukemia.*

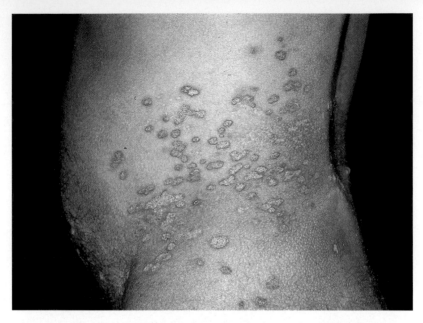

**FIGURE 25-46    Varicella-zoster virus infection: chronic herpes zoster in HIV disease**   *Discrete and confluent hyperkeratotic plaques in several contiguous dematomes persistent for 2 years in a male with advanced untreated HIV disease. The lesions were minimally symptomatic.*

**FIGURE 25-47   Varicella-zoster virus infection: chronic ulcers** *Two large, deep ulcers, present for 6 months, on the lower leg of a 31-year-old male with advanced HIV disease. A severe neuritis pain accompanied the ulcers. There was an associated transverse myelitis. The ulcers and myelitis resolved with oral famciclovir and highly active antiretroviral therapy (HAART). Chronic suppression with oral famciclovir was continued for 3 years; when discontinued, V2 herpes zoster occurred in 5 days in spite of a high CD4 cell count.*

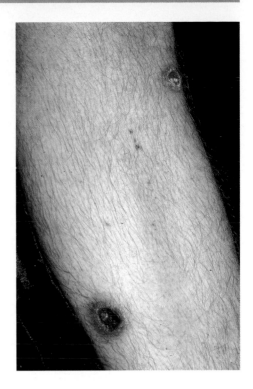

## MANAGEMENT

| | |
|---|---|
| **Prevention** | |
| Immunization | VZV immunization is available and is 80% effective in preventing symptomatic primary VZV infection. About 5% of newly immunized children develop rash. Those at high risk for varicella who should be immunized include normal adults, children with leukemia, neonates, and immunocompromised individuals (immunosuppressive treatment, HIV infection, cancer). |
| Antiviral agents for VZV- and/or HSV-seropositive individuals Undergoing BMT | |
| Acyclovir | 400 mg PO bid, from the day of conditioning, induction, or transplantation for 4 to 6 weeks, suppresses both HSV and VZV reactivation. |
| **Systemic antiviral therapy** | Oral acyclovir, valacyclovir, famciclovir may be effective in some patients. |
| In individuals with mild to moderate immunocompromise | High-dose oral acyclovir, 800 mg five times daily for 7 days, hastens healing and lessens *acute* pain if given within 48 h of the onset of the rash. Large controlled studies in patients over 60 years of age have not, however, demonstrated any effect on the incidence and severity of *chronic* postherpetic neuralgia of high-dose oral acyclovir. A recent preliminary study of older patients (age 60) demonstrated a reduced frequency of persistent pain when IV acyclovir, 10 mg/kg q8h for 5 days, was given within 4 days of the onset of the pain or within 48 h after the onset of the rash. |
| In individuals with advanced immunocompromise | IV acyclovir or recombinant interferon $\alpha$-2a to prevent dissemination of HZ is indicated. |

# HUMAN HERPESVIRUS-6 AND -7 INFECTIONS   □

Exanthema subitum (ES) (sudden rash) is a childhood exanthem associated with primary human herpesvirus type 6 (HHV-6) and HHV-7 infection, characterized by the sudden appearance of rash as high-fever lysis in a healthy-appearing infant.
*Synonym*: Roseola infantum.

## EPIDEMIOLOGY AND ETIOLOGY

**Age of Onset**   6 to 24 months.
**Etiology**   HHV-6 (variants -6A and -6B) and HHV-7. They share genetic, biologic, and immunologic features; primary T cell tropic. At birth, most children have passively transferred anti-HHV-6 and-7 IgG. Primary infection is acquired via oropharyngeal secretions. HHV-6 antibodies reach a nadir at 4 to 7 months and increase throughout infancy. By 12 months, two-thirds of children become infected, with peak antibody levels reached at 2 to 3 years of age. Similarly, HHV-7 antibodies reach nadir at 6 months, with level peaking at 3 to 4 years of age. Latent infection may persist for the lifetime of the individual.

## PATHOGENESIS

Pathogenesis of ES rash is not known.

## HISTORY

**Incubation Period**   5 to 15 days.
**Prodrome**   High fever ranging from 38.9° to 40.6°C. Remains consistently high, with morning remission, until the fourth day, when it falls precipitously to normal, coincident with the appearance of rash. Infant remarkably well despite high fever. Asymptomatic primary HHV-6 and HHV-7 infection is common.
**Symptoms**   Usually absent.

## PHYSICAL EXAMINATION

### Skin Lesions
Small blanchable pink macules and papules, 1 to 5 mm in diameter (Fig. 25-48). Lesions may remain discrete or become confluent.
*Distribution* Trunk and neck.

**General Findings**   Absent in presence of high fever. Febrile seizures are common.

## DIFFERENTIAL DIAGNOSIS

**Morbilliform Exanthem**   See "Infectious Exanthems," page 782.

## LABORATORY EXAMINATIONS

**Serology**   Demonstration of IgM anti-HHV-6 or anti-HHV-7 antibodies or IgG seroconversion.
**Other**   Viral culture and isolation from peripheral blood mononuclear cells. Demonstration of HHV-6 or HHV-7 DNA by PCR.

## DIAGNOSIS

Usually made on clinical findings.

## COURSE AND PROGNOSIS

Course self-limited with rare sequelae. In some cases, high fever may be associated with seizures. Intussusception associated with hyperplasia of intestinal lymphoid tissue and hepatitis have been reported. As with other HHV infections, HHV-6 and HHV-7 persist throughout the life of the patient; however, clinical manifestations associated with HHV-6 and HHV-7 reactivation have not yet been identified. An infant with HHV-6 ES may experience a second clinical syndrome, HHV-7 ES, and vice versa.

## MANAGEMENT

Symptomatic.

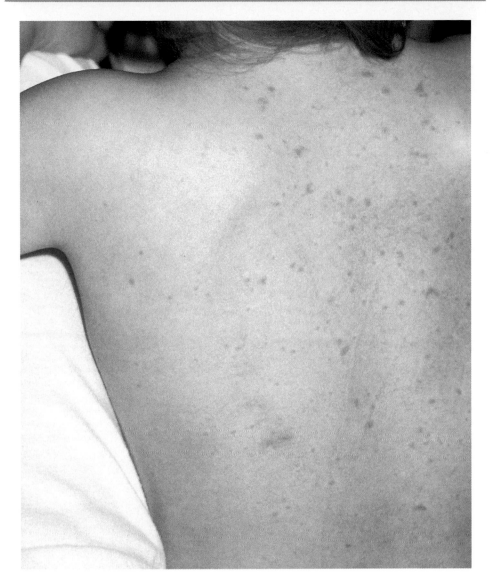

**FIGURE 25-48   Exanthema subitum**   *Multiple, blanchable macules and papules on the back of a febrile child, which appeared as the temperature fell (Courtesy of Karen Wiss, MD.)*

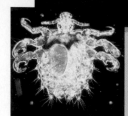

# INSECT BITES AND INFESTATIONS

Insect bite reactions, pediculosis, and scabies are common in temperate climates. Infestations are much more prevalent in semitropical and tropical climates, affecting residents and travelers. Infestations to be considered include cutaneous larva migrans, myiasis, tungiasis, cutaneous leishmaniasis, dengue fever, rickettsial spotted fevers, African trypanosomiasis, Buruli ulcer, gnathostomiasis.

## CUTANEOUS REACTIONS TO ARTHROPOD BITES

Cutaneous reactions to arthropod bites (CRAB) are inflammatory and/or allergic reactions, characterized by an intensely pruritic eruption at the bite sites hours to days after the bite, manifested by solitary or grouped urticarial papules, papulovesicles, and/or bullae that persist for days to weeks; patients are often unaware of having been bitten. In some cases, systemic symptoms may occur, ranging from mild to severe, with death occurring from anaphylactic shock. Arthropod bites are also the method of transmission of many systemic infections and infestations.

### EPIDEMIOLOGY

**Season**   Summer in temperate climates.
**Etiology**   5 of 9 classes of arthropods cause local and systemic reactions associated with their bites: Arachnida, Chilopoda, Diplopoda, Crustacea, Insecta.

### Arthropods That Infest, Bite, or Sting

I.   Arachnida (four pairs of legs): mites, ticks, spiders, scorpions
   A.  Acarina
      1. Mites: follicle (*Demodex*), food, fowl, grain, harvest, murine, scabies (*Sarcoptes*)
      2. Ticks
   B.  Araneae: spiders
   C.  Scorpionida
II.  Chilopoda and Diplopoda: centipedes, millipedes
III. Insecta (three pairs of legs)

A.  Anoplura: lice (*Phthirius* and *Pediculus*)
B.  Coleoptera: beetles
C.  Diptera: mosquitoes, black flies, midges (punkies, no seeums, sand flies), Tabandae (horseflies, deerflies, clegs, breeze flies, greenheads, mango flies); botflies, *Callitroga americana, Dermatobia hominis,* phlebotomid sand flies, tsetse flies
D.  Hemiptera: bedbugs, kissing bugs
E.  Hymenoptera: ants, bees, wasps, hornets
F.  Lepidoptera: caterpillars, butterflies, moths
G.  Siphonaptera: fleas, chigoe or sand flea

### Arthropod-Borne Infections and Infestations

Scrub typhus, endemic (murine) typhus, Lyme borreliosis, babesiosis, ehrlichiosis, spotted fever groups, Q fever, tick-borne encephalitis, malaria, filariasis, onchocerciasis (river blindness), tularemia, leishmaniasis, loiasis, cutaneous myiasis, trypanosomiasis (sleeping sickness, Chagas' disease), bubonic plague.

**Geographic Distribution**  Worldwide.

## PATHOGENESIS

**Mites**  Produce pruritus and/or allergic reactions through salivary proteins deposited during feeding. Harvest mites (chiggers) may present as intense pruritus on the ankles, legs, belt line; mites usually fall off after feeding or may be scratched off. In nonsensitized individuals, 1 to 2 mm pruritic papules are seen. In sensitized individuals, CRAB may be papular urticaria, vesiculation, or granulomatous reaction with fever and lymphadenopathy.

**Ticks**  Reactions include foreign body reactions, reactions to salivary secretions, reactions to injected toxins, and hypersensitivity reactions. Tick paralysis is caused by a toxin secreted in the saliva of the tick.

**Spiders**  Brown recluse spider (*Loxosceles reclusa*) bite causes reactions ranging from mild urticaria to full-thickness necrosis (*loxoscelism*). "Widow" spiders (*Latrodectus*) inject a venom that contains a neurotoxin (α-latrotoxin) producing reactions at the bite site as well as varying degrees of systemic toxicity.

**Scorpion**  Venom also contains a neurotoxin that can cause severe local and systemic reactions.

**Blister Beetles**  Contain the chemical cantharidin, which produces blister when the beetle is crushed on the skin.

**Black Flies**  Bites produce local reactions as well as black fly fever, characterized by fever, headache, nausea, generalized lymphadenitis.

**Nonbiting Flies**  Flies commonly feed on open wounds, exudates, and skin ulcers and may deposit eggs at these sites, resulting in wound myiasis. Fly larvae can burrow into injured or normal skin, invading through the epidermis into the dermis, resulting in furuncular myiasis. In some cases, larvae move about the subcutis (migratory myiasis), mimicking the pattern of cutaneous larva migrans.

**Bedbugs**  Nocturnal feedings produce a linear arrangement of papular urticaria.

**Hymenoptera**  Bees, hornets, wasp bites can produce painful stings and anaphylaxis in the sensitized individual.

**Caterpillars and Moths**  Hairs can produce local irritant and allergic reactions.

**Fleas (Cat, Dog, Bird)**  Bites tend to cause more local reactions than human flea bites.

**Chigoe or Sand Fleas**  (*Tunga penetrans*) Recently impregnated female flea penetrates skin of a human host, burrows into epidermis to dermal-epidermal junction, where she feeds on blood drawn from host vessels in superficial dermis. Enlargement of the buried flea to 5 to 8 mm causes local pain in the infested skin. Mature eggs (150 to 200) are extruded singly from a terminal abdominal orifice during a period of 7 to 10 days. The female dies shortly after egg extrusion, and the infested tissues collapse around it; ulcerations can occur at the site. Inflammation and secondary infection can arise if parts of the flea are retained in the tissue.

## HISTORY

**Incubation Period**  CRAB appears minutes to days after the bite.

**Duration of Lesions**  Days, weeks, months.

**Skin Symptoms**  Pruritus, pain at bite site. Systemic symptoms with systemic reaction.

## PHYSICAL EXAMINATION

### Skin Findings

***Erythematous Macules*** Occur at bite sites and are usually transient.

***Papular Urticaria*** Persistent (>48 h) urticarial papules (Figs. 26-1 to 26-5), often surmounted by a vesicle, usually <1 cm. Excoriations and excoriated urticarial papules, vesicles. Crusted painful lesions, usually purulent, may represent impetigo, ecthyma, or cutaneous diphtheria. Excoriated or secondarily infected lesions may heal with hyper- or hypopigmentation and/or raised or depressed scars, especially in more darkly pigmented individuals.

***Bullous Lesions*** Tense bullae with clear fluid on a slightly inflamed base. Excoriation results in large erosion.

***Tick Bites*** Attach and feed painlessly. Secretions can produce local reactions (Fig. 26-6), febrile illness, paralysis. Soft ticks attached for >1 h produce erythematous macular lesions up to 2 to 3 cm in diameter. Induration, necrosis, and tick granulomas may develop. Erythema migrans occurs as an enlarging plaque occurring at site of Ixodes tick bite, characteristic of Lyme borreliosis (see Section 22); lymphocytoma cutis also occurs at tick bite sites.

***Spiders*** Brown recluse and black widow bites can result in mild local urticarial reactions to

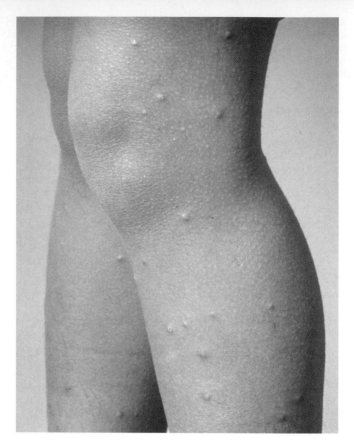

**FIGURE 26-1   Papular urticaria: flea bites**   *Multiple, very pruritic, urticaria-like papules at the sites of flea bites on the knees and legs of a child; these persistent urticaria-like papules are usually <1 cm in diameter and may have a vesicle on the top. When scratched, they exhibit erosions or crusts.*

full-thickness skin necrosis, associated with a maculopapular exanthem, fever, headache, malaise, arthralgia, nausea/vomiting.

### Diptera

*Mosquitoes:* Bites usually present as papular urticaria on exposed sites; reactions can be urticarial, eczematous, or granulomatous.

*Black flies:* Anesthetic is injected, resulting in painless initial bite; may subsequently become painful with itching, erythema, and edema. Black fly fever characterized by fever, nausea, generalized lymphadenitis.

*Midges:* Bites produce immediate pain with erythema at bite site with 2- to 3-mm papulovesicles, followed by indurated nodules (up to 1 cm) persisting for many months.

*Tabandae:* Bites painful with papular urticaria; rarely associated anaphylaxis.

*Botfly:* Larvae penetrate skin or are deposited on open wounds producing cutaneous myiasis. Larvae may be fixed or migrate resembling larva migrans *C. americana* most common in United States.

*D. hominis* in tropical regions causes furuncular myiasis, painful lesions that resemble pyogenic granuloma or abscess; a pruritic papule develops at the site, slowly enlarging over several weeks into a domed nodule (resembles a furuncle) with a central pore (Fig. 26-7) through which the posterior end of the larvae intermittently protrudes.

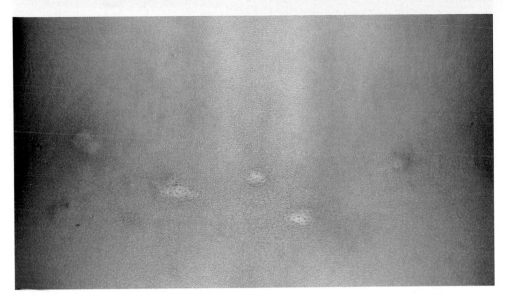

**FIGURE 26-2   Papular urticaria: bedbug bites**   *Pruritic, urticaria-like papules at the sites of bedbug bites on the lower back at the waist. Bedbugs* (Cimex lectularius) *share human domains, residing in crevices of floors and walls, in beddings, and in furniture. They usually feed only once a week and less often in cold weather. Bedbugs can travel long distances in search of a human host and can survive for 6 to 12 months without feeding. Bite reactions occur on exposed sites such as the face, neck, arms, and hands, with two to three lesions in a row ("breakfast, lunch, dinner"). In previously unexposed individuals, bite sites appear as erythematous, pruritic macules. In sensitized individuals, intensely pruritic papules, papular urticaria, or vesicles/bullae may arise at the bite sites. Changes secondary to scratching include excoriations, eczematous dermatitis, and secondary infections.*

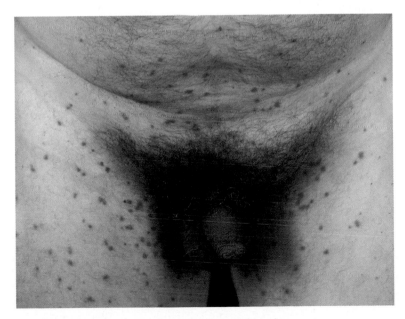

**FIGURE 26-3   Papular urticaria: mites**   *Multiple papular urticaria at bite sites of mite* Trombicula *in the bathing trunk area. Mites fall off vegetation into clothing; multiple bites are often followed by papular urticarial reactions.*

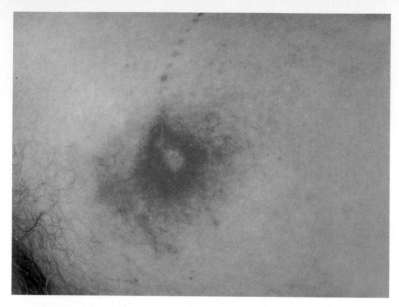

**FIGURE 26-4  Urticarial plaque: spider**   *Urticaria plaque on the upper medial arm on day after a spider bite.*

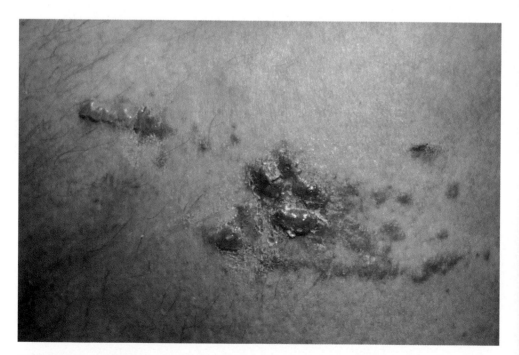

**FIGURE 26-5  Immunologic IgE-mediated contact urticaria: pine processionary caterpillar**   *Linear edematous papules and vesicles occurred on the exposed arm shortly after exposure to* Thaumetopoea pitycampa *in a pine forest.*

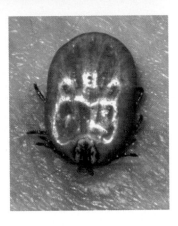

**FIGURE 26-6    Dermacentor variabilis feeding**    *The tick has been attached for 24 h; it is the vector of Rocky Mountain spotted fever.*

*House flies:* Larvae deposited into any exposed skin site (ear, nose, paranasal sinuses, mouth, eye, anus, and vagina) or at any wound site (leg ulcers, ulcerated squamous and basal cell carcinomas, hematomas, umbilical stump) and grow into maggots, which can be seen on surface of wound (Fig. 26-8); although repulsive for the patient, maggots are very effective at debriding nonviable tissue and debris.

**Hemiptera**    Bedbug bites produce papular urticaria that have a characteristic linear array. Reduvid (kissing bugs, assassin bugs, conenosed bugs) bites usually present as papular urticaria; severe reactions can produce necrosis and ulceration resembling spider bites.

**Fleas**    Papular pruritic urticaria (Fig. 26-2) at exposed bite site.

*Tungiasis:* Papule or vesicle (6 to 8 mm in diameter) with central black dot produced by posterior part of the flea's abdominal segments. As eggs mature and abdomen swells, papule becomes a white, pea-sized nodule. With

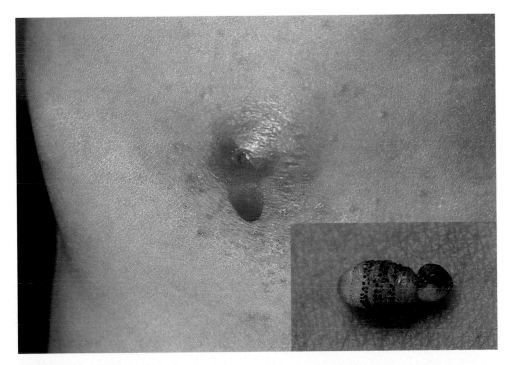

**FIGURE 26-7    Furuncular myiasis**    *A pruritic papule at the site of deposition of a botfly larva, slowly enlarging over several weeks into a domed nodule (resembles a furuncle). The lesion has a central pore through which the posterior end of the larva intermittently protrudes and thus respires. The larva (inset) can be induced to exit the lesion by occluding it with petrolatum or fat.*

intralesional hemorrhage, it becomes black (Fig. 26-9). With severe infestation, nodules and plaques with a honeycombed appearance. If lesions are squeezed, eggs, feces, and internal organs are extruded through pore. Sites: feet, especially under toenails, between toes, plantar aspect of the feet, sparing weight-bearing areas; in sunbathers, any area of exposed skin.

*Hymenoptera* Stings by female bee, hornet, or wasp from modified ovipositor (stinger apparatus) produces immediate burning/pain, followed by intense, local, erythematous reaction with swelling and urticaria. Severe systemic reactions occur in individuals who are sensitized (0.4 to 0.8%), with angioedema/generalized urticaria and/or respiratory insufficiency from laryngeal edema or bronchospasm and/or shock. Fire ants and harvester ants produce local skin necrosis and systemic reactions to sting; bite reaction begins as an intense local inflammatory reaction that evolves to a sterile pustule.

*Lepidoptera* Contact with hairs of caterpillars/moths can produce burning/itching sensation, papular urticaria, irritation due to histamine release, allergic contact dermatitis (Fig. 26-5), and /or systemic reactions. Wind-borne hairs can cause keratoconjunctivitis.

**Systemic Findings**   Systemic findings may occur associated with toxin or allergy to substance injected during bite. Many varied systemic infections can be injected during bite.

## DIFFERENTIAL DIAGNOSIS

**Bite Site Reactions (Erythematous Papules, Blisters)**   Allergic contact dermatitis, especially to plants such as poison ivy or poison oak.
**Furuncular Myiasis/Tungiasis**   *Staphylococcus aureus* paronychia, *Candida* paronychia, cercarial dermatitis, scabies, fire ant bite, folliculitis.
**Cutaneous Necrosis**   Necrotizing soft tissue infection, vascular insufficiency, adverse cutaneous drug reaction.

## LABORATORY EXAMINATIONS

**Dermatopathology** *Bite Site Reactions* In acute phase, variable epidermal necrosis, spongiosis, parakeratosis with plasma exudate; dermal inflammatory infiltrate extends into deep dermis in a wedge-shaped pattern, surrounding vessels with some extension into dermal collagen. The dermal infiltrate is mixed, composed of eosinophils, neutrophils, lymphocytes, and histiocytes. Eosinophils are usually prominent;

neutrophils may predominate in reactions to fleas, mosquitoes, fire ants, and brown recluse spiders. Bullae form secondary to marked edema. Insect parts are rarely seen except in scabies and in tick bites where removal is incomplete.

In chronic phase, lesions result from retained arthropod parts or hypersensitivity. Chronic lesions can appear as a pseudolymphoma.

**Infection at Bite Site** In infestations such as leishmaniasis, the pathogen can be demonstrated in the lesional biopsy specimen by special stains.

**Bacterial Culture**   Rule out secondary infection with *S. aureus* or group A streptococcus (GAS). Rule out systemic infection.

**Serology**   Rule out systemic infection/infestation.

## DIAGNOSIS

Clinical diagnosis, at times confirmed by lesional biopsy.

## COURSE AND PROGNOSIS

Excoriation of CRAB commonly results in secondary infection of the eroded epidermis by GAS and/or *S. aureus* causing impetigo or ecthyma. This is especially common in humid tropical climates. Less common is secondary infection with *Corynebacterium diphtheriae*, with resultant cutaneous diphtheria (see page 633). Streptococcal skin infections are, at times, complicated by glomerulonephritis.

## MANAGEMENT

**Prevention**   Avoid contact with arthropods. Apply insect repellent such as diethyltoluamide (DEET) to skin. Apply permethrin spray [Permanone (United States)] to clothing. Use passive measures such as screens, nets, clothing. Treat flea-infested cats and dogs; spray household with insecticides (e.g., malathion, 1 to 4% dust) with special attention to baseboards, rugs, floors, upholstered furniture, bed frames, mattresses, and cellar.

**Larvae in Skin**   Tungiasis: remove flea with needle, scalpel, or curette, attempting to remove all flea parts; oral thiabendazole (25 mg/kg per day) or albendazole (400 mg/d for 3 days) effective for heavy infestations. Furuncular myiasis: suffocate larvae by covering the larvae with petrolatum; remove the following day when

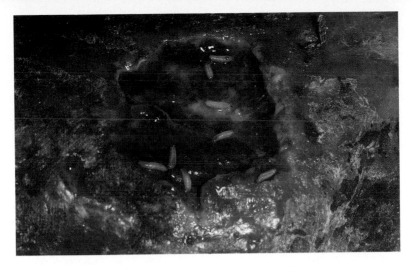

**FIGURE 26-8    Wound myiasis**    *Multiple larvae or maggots of the housefly are seen in a chronic stasis ulcer on the ankle. The leg had been treated with Castellani's paint and Unna boot for 1 week. When the dressing was removed, the maggots were visible; the base of the ulcer was red and clean, having been debrided by the maggots.*

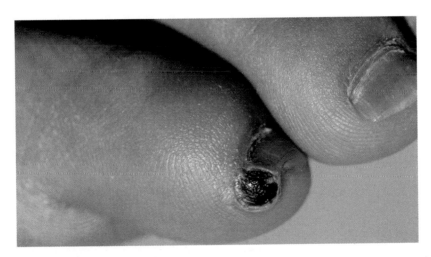

**FIGURE 26-9    Tungiasis**    *A necrotic, periungual papule with surrounding erythema on the lateral margin of the fifth toe; the larva is visualized by removing the overlying crust.*

dead. Oral ivermectin has been used as primary prophylaxis in animals.

**Glucocorticoids**    Potent topical glucocorticoids given for a short time are helpful for intensely pruritic lesions. In some cases, a short tapered course of oral glucocorticoids can be given for extensive CRAB that are persistent.

**Antimicrobial Agents    *Secondary Infection***    Antibiotic treatment with topical agents such as mupirocin ointment or antistaphylococcal/antistreptococcal agents if secondary infection is present.

***Systemic Infection/Infestation***    Treat with appropriate antimicrobial agent.

# PEDICULOSIS  

Pediculosis, or louse infestation, is an infestation of sucking lice that lay their eggs on hair shafts or in seams of clothing. Two species of bloodsucking lice of the order Anoplura have evolved to be obligate ectoparasites of humans: *Pediculus humanus* and *Pthirius pubis*. The two variants of *Pediculus,* the head louse and the body louse, are similar morphologically but distinct in ecologic niches on the body and the clinical manifestations of infestation. The body louse may have evolved from the head louse after humans began to wear clothes.

## EPIDEMIOLOGY AND ETIOLOGY

**Etiology**   Lice are 1 to 3 mm long, are flattened dorsoventrally, and have three pairs of legs that end in powerful claws of a diameter adapted to the region colonized. The female lives for 1 to 3 months; it dies in <24 h when separated from the host (head lice). A female louse lays up to 300 eggs (nits) during her lifetime. Nits are <1 mm in diameter and, when viable, are opalescent. Nits are deposited on hair shafts emerging from the skin and hatch 6 to 10 days after laying, giving rise to nymphs that become adults in 10 days. Empty egg cases remain on the hair shaft after hatch; demonstration of empty egg cases away from the skin is not diagnostic of active infestation.

**Incidence**   Hundreds of millions of cases worldwide annually.

**Transmission**   Most commonly by direct contact between individuals or indirectly by contact with bedding, brushes, or clothing, according to species. Pediculosis and scabies may coexist in the same individual.

**Associated Infections**   *Scabies, Head and Crab Lice S. aureus*, GAS: Excoriation may become secondarily infected. Infection can extend, resulting in cellulitis, lymphangitis, and/or bacteremia.

## SYMPTOMS

Pruritus occurs in a variable proportion. Excoriations can become secondarily infected.

## MANAGEMENT

**Topically Applied Insecticides**   Ideally, should have 100% activity against louse and egg. Malathion kills all lice after 5 min of exposure, and >95% of eggs fail to hatch after 10 min of exposure. Synthetic pyrethroids, syner-gized pyrethrins, and malathion are most efficacious and safe. Lotion preparations are preferred; creams, foams, gels are also available.

**Recommended Regimen**   *Permethrin*   Synthetic pyrethroid. Over-the-counter 1% products: Nix. 5% product: Elimite is prescription. Product applied to infested area(s) and washed off after 10 min. Not totally ovicidal; has residual activity; in that the incubation period of louse eggs is 6 to 10 days, should be reapplied in 7 to 14 days.

*Pyrethrin and Piperonyl Butoxide*   Pyrethrins derived from extract of chrysanthemums. Products: RID Mousse, RID shampoo, A-200, R and C, Pronta, Clear Lice System.

*Malathion*   0.5% in 78% isopropyl alcohol (Ovide). Applied to involved site for 8 to 12 h; binds to hair providing residual protection. Indicated in lindane-resistant cases. Should not be used in children younger than 6 months.

**Alternative Regimen**   *Pyrethrins with Piperonyl Butoxide*   Applied to scalp and washed off after 10 min.

*Lindane*   1% shampoo applied for 4 min and then thoroughly washed off. (Not recommended for pregnant or lactating women.) Not totally ovicidal and lacks residual activity; in that the incubation period of louse eggs is 6 to 10 days, the agents should be reapplied in 7 to 14 days. Retreatment may be necessary if lice are found or eggs are observed at the hair-skin junction.

*Ivermectin*   0.8% lotion or shampoo.

**Systemic Therapy**   *Oral Ivermectin* 200 µg/kg; repeat on day 10 to kill emerging nymphs.

**Acquired Resistance to Insecticides**   Occurs worldwide, mainly to pyrethrins and pyrethroids; also to malathion. If resistance is suspected, an alternative agent should be used. Other alternatives include newer insecticides and oral ivermectin in cases of resistance to both pyrethroids and malathion.

# PEDICULOSIS CAPITIS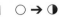

Pediculosis capitis is an infestation of the scalp by the head louse, which feeds on the scalp and neck and deposits its eggs on the hair; presence of head lice is associated with few symptoms but much consternation.

## EPIDEMIOLOGY AND ETIOLOGY

**Etiology**   The subspecies *Pediculus humanus capitis.* Sesame seed size, 1 to 2 mm. Feed every 4 to 6 h. Move by grasping hairs close to scalp; can crawl up to 23 cm/day. Lice lay nits within 1 to 2 mm of scalp. Nits are ova within chitinous case. Young lice hatch within 1 week, passing through nymphal stages, growing larger and maturing to adults over a period of 1 week. One female can lay 50 to 150 ova during a 16-day lifetime. Survive only for a few hours off scalp.

**Vector of Infection**   Head louse is not a vector of infectious disease.

**Sex, Age of Onset**   Girls > boys. 3 to 11 years, but all ages.

**Predisposing Factors**   School-age children and their mothers. More common in warmer months.

**Race**   In United States, more common in whites than blacks; claws have adapted to grip cylindrical hair; hair pomade may inhibit infestation. In Africa, pediculosis capitis is relatively uncommon; however, lice easily grip non-cylindrical hair.

**Transmission**   Shared hats, caps, brushes, combs; head-to-head contact. Epidemics in schools; classrooms are the main source of infestations. Head lice can survive off the scalp for up to 55 h.

**Incidence**   Most common pediculosis. Estimated that 6 to 12 million persons in the United States are infested annually. Bordeaux, France: up to 49% of schoolchildren. Jerusalem, Israel: 20% in 1991. Bristol, UK: 25% in 1998. Ilorin, Nigeria: 3.7% in 1987.

## HISTORY

**Skin Symptoms**   Pruritus of the back and sides of scalp. Scratching and secondary infection associated with occipital and/or cervical lymphadenopathy.

**Psychiatric Symptoms**   Some individuals exhibit obsessive compulsive disorder or delusions of parasitosis after eradications of lice and nits.

## PHYSICAL EXAMINATION

### Skin Findings

*Infestation Head lice* are identified by eye or with hand lens but are difficult to find (Fig. 26-10*A*). Most patients have a population of <10 head lice. Nits are the oval grayish-white egg capsules (1 mm long) firmly cemented to the hairs (Fig. 26-10*B*); vary in number from only a few to thousands. Nits are deposited by head lice on the hair shaft as it emerges from the follicle. With recent infestation, nits are near the scalp; with infestation of long standing, nits may be 10 to 15 cm from the scalp. In that scalp hair grows 0.5 mm daily, the presence of nits 15 cm from the scalp indicates that the infestation is approximately 9 months old. New viable eggs have a creamy-yellow color; empty eggshells are white.

### Skin Lesions

- *Bite reactions* at site of louse bites, apparent on neck. Phase I: no clinical symptoms, phase II: papular urticaria with moderate pruritus; phase III: wheals immediately following bite with subsequent delayed papules/intense itching; phase IV: smaller papules with mild pruritus. Phases related to immune sensitivity/tolerance.
- *Eczema, excoriation, lichen simplex chronicus* on occipital scalp and neck secondary to chronic scratching/rubbing.
- *Secondary impetiginization* with *S. aureus* of eczema or excoriations; may extend onto neck, forehead, face, ears.
- *Confluent, purulent mass* of matted hair, lice, nits, crusts, and purulent exudation in extreme cases.
- *Pediculid* is a hypersensitivity rash, resembling a viral exanthem.

*Sites of Predilection* Head lice nearly always confined to scalp, especially occipital and postauricular regions. Rarely, head lice infest beard or other hairy sites. Although more common with crab lice, head lice can also infest the eyelashes (*pediculosis palpebrarum*).

**Wood's Lamp** Live nits fluoresce with a pearly fluorescence; dead nits do not.

**Regional Lymph Nodes** Postoccipital lymphadenopathy secondary to impetiginization of excoriated sites.

## DIFFERENTIAL DIAGNOSIS

**Small White Hair "Beads"** Hair casts (inner root sheath remnants), hair lacquer, hair gels, dandruff (epidermal scales), black piedra (*Trichosporon ovoides*), white piedra (*T. inkin*)

**Scalp Pruritus** Impetigo, lichen simplex chronicus.

## LABORATORY EXAMINATIONS

**Microscopy** The louse or a nit on a hair shaft (Fig. 26-10*B*) can be examined to confirm the gross examination of the scalp and hair.

*Nits* 0.5-mm oval, whitish eggs. Nonviable nits show an absence of an embryo or operculum.

*Louse* Insect with six legs, 1 to 2 mm in length, wingless, translucent grayish-white body that is red when engorged with blood.

**Culture** If impetiginization is suspected, bacterial cultures should be obtained.

## DIAGNOSIS

Clinical findings, confirmed by detection of lice. Louse comb increases chances of finding lice. Nits alone are not diagnostic of active infestation. Nits within 4 mm of scalp suggests active infestation.

## MANAGEMENT

**Fomite/Environmental Control** Avoid contact with possibly contaminated items such as hats, headsets, clothing, towels, combs, hair brushes, bedding, upholstery. The environment should be vacuumed. Bedding, clothing, and head gear should be washed and dried on the hot cycle of a dryer. Combs and brushes should be soaked in rubbing alcohol or Lysol 2% solution for 1 h. Families should look for lice routinely. Many schools in the United States adhere to a "no-nit" policy before children can return after infestation.

**Pediculocide Therapy** See "Pediculosis," page 844.

**Causes of Therapeutic Failure** Misunderstanding of instructions; noncompliance; inappropriate instructions on head-lice products or from health professionals; high cost of products; misdiagnosis; psychogenic itch; incomplete ovicidal activity; inappropriate preparation (e.g., shampoo); insufficient dose-time, frequency, and/or quantity of product applied; failure to retreat; reinfestation; live eggs not removed; acquired resistance to insecticides.

**Removal of Nits** After treatment and neutral shampoo, the hair is wet-combed with a fine-toothed comb to remove nits. Complete nit removal depends on comb structure, duration/technique of combing, and thoroughness.

Overnight application of petroleum jelly or HairClean 1-2-3 may facilitate removal of nits.

**Pediculosis Palpebrarum** Apply petrolatum to lashes twice daily for 8 days, followed by removal of nits, *or* physostigmine ophthalmic preparations applied twice daily for 1 or 2 days.

**Secondary Bacterial Infection** Should be treated with appropriate doses of erythromycin *or* dicloxacillin or cephalexin.

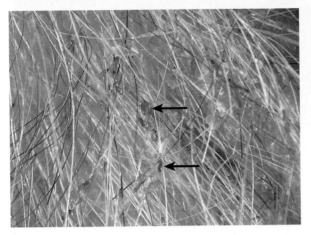

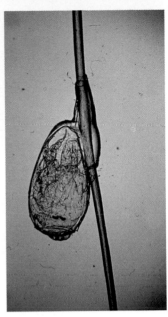

**A**

**FIGURE 26-10    Pediculosis capitis: multiple nits on scalp hair**
*A. Myriads of nits (oval, grayish-white egg capsules) are
firmly attached to the hair shafts, visualized with a lens. On
close examination these have a bottle shape.* ***B.*** *Under a
microscope, an egg with a developing head louse, attached to
a hair shaft, is seen.*

**B**

**PEDICULOSIS CORPORIS**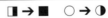

In body louse infestations, lice remain in clothing except when feeding, unable to survive more
than a few hours away from the human host.

### EPIDEMIOLOGY AND ETIOLOGY

**Etiology** *Pediculus humanus humanus.* Larger
than head louse: 2 to 4 mm; otherwise indistinguishable. Life span 18 days. Female lays 270
to 300 ova. Nits: ova within chitinous case. Nits
incubate for 8 to 10 days; nymphs mature to
adults in 14 days. Habitat: live in seams of
clothing; can survive without blood meal for up
to 3 days. Grab body hairs to feed.

**Risk Factors** Poor socioeconomic conditions,
when clothing is not changed or washed
frequently: poverty, war, natural disasters, indi-
gence, homelessness, refugee-camp populations.

**Body Lice as Vectors of Disease** Body lice transmit many infectious agents while feeding.

- *Bartonella quintana* causes *trench fever* (fever,
  myalgias, headache, meningoencephalitis,

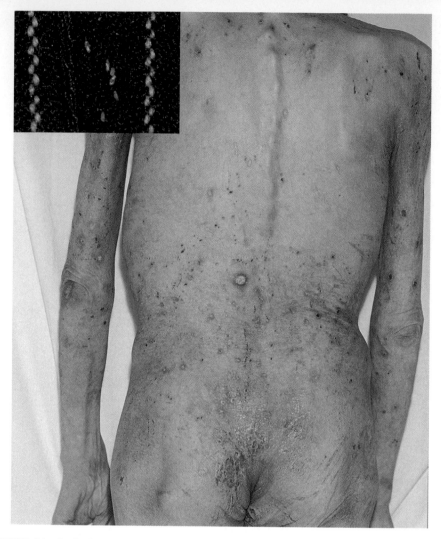

**FIGURE 26-11   Pediculosis corporis**   *Severely malnourished, ill-kept, homeless male with multiple excoriations, erosions and crusted papules, and nodules and eczematized lesions. Lice and nits are seen in the seams of clothing (inset).*

chronic lymphadenopathy, transient macu-lopapular eruption) and endocarditis. In United States, 15% of homeless persons tested had *B. quintana* bacteremia. *B. quintana* transmitted by fleas causes cat-scratch disease or bacillary angiomatosis.

- *Rickettsia prowazekii* causes *epidemic typhus*, characterized by fever, headache, rash, confusion. Large outbreaks (1995 to 1997) in Burundi, first affecting prison inmates, then >45,000 camp refugees. Small outbreak occurred in Russia in 1998. *Brill-Zinsser disease* (louse-borne relapsing fever) is recrudescence of epidemic typhus fever occurring in mild forms years after primary infection.

### PHYSICAL EXAMINATION

**Skin Findings** *Infestation* Lice and nits are found in clothing seams (Fig. 26-11). Lice grab onto body hairs to feed.

*Lesions*
- Bite reactions identical to those of head lice (see page 845).
- Eczema, excoriation, lichen simplex, secondary impetiginization, postinflammatory hyperpigmentation (Fig. 26-11).
- Clothing may be stained with louse feeds, blood/serum.

- Scabies, pediculosis corporis, and *Pulex irritans* (the human flea) can coexist.

### DIFFERENTIAL DIAGNOSIS

Atopic dermatitis, contact dermatitis, scabies, adverse cutaneous drug reaction.

### DIAGNOSIS

Lice and eggs are found in clothing seams.

### MANAGEMENT

Bedding and clothing must be systematically decontaminated.
**Hygiene Measures** Basic sanitation measures, and hygiene measures to assure changes of clean clothing, body washing, and sometimes shaving.
**Delousing** Pyrethrins/pyrethroids or malathion for 8 to 24 h is recommended in some cases. Outbreaks necessitate delousing of individuals with 1% permethrin dusting powder.
**Louse-Borne Infections** Antibiotics are indicated if louse-borne infectious disease (trench fever, epidemic typhus) exists.

## PEDICULOSIS PUBIS (PTHIRIASIS)

Pediculosis pubis is an infestation of hair-bearing regions, most commonly the pubic area but at times the hairy parts of the chest and axillae and the upper eyelashes. It is manifested clinically by mild to moderate pruritus, papular urticaria, and excoriations.
*Synonyms:* Crabs, crab lice, pubic lice.

### EPIDEMIOLOGY

**Age of Onset** Most common in young adults; range, from childhood to senescence.
**Sex** More extensive infestation in males.
**Etiology** *Pthirius pubis*, the crab or pubic louse. Size 0.8 to 1.2 mm. First pair of legs ves-tigial; other two clawed. Life span 14 days. Female lays 25 ova. Nits incubate for 7 days; nymphs mature over 14 days. Mobility: adults can crawl 10 cm/day. Prefers a humid environment; tends not to wander.
**Transmission** Close physical contact: sexual exposure [frequently coexisting with another

sexually transmitted infection (STI)]; sharing bed; possibly exchange of towels. Nonsexual transmission occurs in homeless persons who have pubic lice in hair on head and back.

## HISTORY

**Skin Symptoms**   May be asymptomatic. Mild to moderate pruritus for months. Patient may detect a nodularity to hairs (nits or eggs) while scratching. With excoriation and secondary infection, lesions may become tender and be associated with enlarged regional, e.g., inguinal, lymph node.

## PHYSICAL EXAMINATION

### Skin Findings
*Infestation Lice* appear as 1- to 2-mm, brownish-gray specks (Figs. 26-12 and 26-13) in hairy areas involved. Remain stationary for days; mouth parts embedded in skin; claws grasping a hair on either side. Usually few in number. *Nits* attached to hair appear as tiny white-gray specks (Fig. 26-13). Few to numerous. Eggs at hair-skin junction indicate active infestation.

### Skin Lesions

- *Papular urticaria* (small erythematous papules) at sites of feeding, especially periumbilical (Fig. 26-14); blisters.

- Secondary changes of *lichenification, excoriations.*
- *Secondary infection* detected in patients with significant pruritus.
- *Maculae ceruleae (taches bleues)* are slate-gray or bluish-gray macules 0.5 to 1 cm in diameter, irregular in shape, nonblanching (Fig. 26-15). Pigment thought to be breakdown product of heme affected by louse saliva.
- *Eyelash infestation* Serous crusts may be present along with lice and nits (Fig. 26-13); occasionally, edema of eyelids with severe infestation.

*Distribution* Most common in pubic and axillary areas; also, perineum, thighs, lower legs, trunk, especially periumbilical (Fig. 26-14). In hairy males: nipple areas, upper arms, rarely wrists; rarely, beard and moustache area. In children, eyelashes (Fig. 26-13) and eyebrows may be infested without pubic involvement. Maculae cerulea most common on lower abdominal wall, buttocks, upper thighs (Fig. 26-15).

**General Findings**   With secondary impetiginization, regional lymphadenopathy.

## DIFFERENTIAL DIAGNOSIS

**Infestation**   Trichomycosis pubis, white piedra
**Pruritic Dermatosis**   Atopic dermatitis, seborrheic dermatitis, tinea cruris, folliculitis, molluscum contagiosum, scabies.

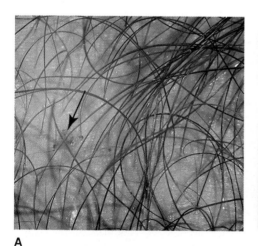

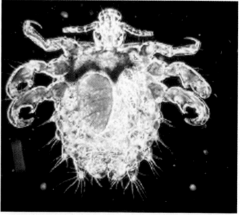

**A**                    **B**

**FIGURE 26-12   Pediculosis pubis: crab louse in pubis**   *A. A crab louse (arrow) on the skin in the pubic region. B. Under a microscope, an adult female crab louse containing an egg is seen suspended in mineral oil.*

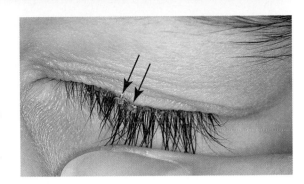

**FIGURE 26-13   Pediculosis pubis: crab lice in eyelashes of a child**   *Crab lice (arrows) and nits on the upper eyelashes of a child; this was the only site of infestation.*

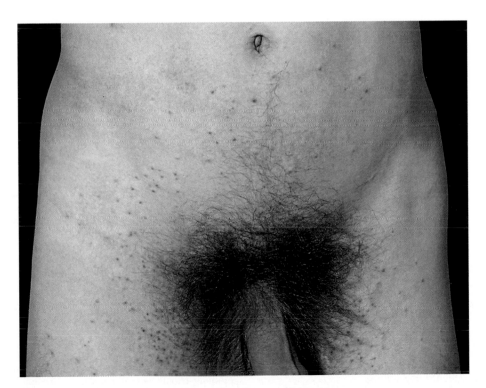

**FIGURE 26-14   Pediculosis pubis: papular urticaria**   *At this magnification only inflammatory papules (sites of crab lice bites), which are extremely pruritic, are seen on the abdomen and the inner aspects of the thighs. Closer examination reveals nits on the pubic hairs.*

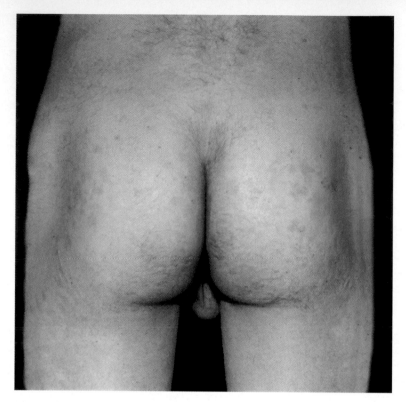

**FIGURE 26-15    Pediculosis pubis: maculae coeruleae (taches bleues)**    *Slate colored nonblanching macules on the buttocks at sites of louse bites.*

## LABORATORY EXAMINATIONS

**Microscopy**    Lice (Fig. 26-12*B*) and nits may be identified and differentiated from head/body louse with hand lens or microscope.
**Cultures**    Bacterial cultures if excoriation impetiginized.
**Serology**    Sexually transmitted. Testing for other STIs may be indicated in some individuals.

## DIAGNOSIS

Demonstration of live adult lice, nymphs, or nits in pubic area to diagnose active infestation.

## COURSE AND PROGNOSIS

Patients should be evaluated after 1 week if symptoms persist. Retreatment may be necessary if lice are found or if eggs are observed at hair-skin junction. Patients not responding to one regimen should be retreated with an alternative.

## MANAGEMENT

**Prevention**    Patient and sexual partners should be treated.
**Screening for STIs**    30% of persons with crab lice have another concurrent STI; screen for HIV disease, syphilis, gonorrhea, *Chlamydia* infection, herpes simplex, human papilloma virus infection, trichomoniasis, scabies.
**Topical Insecticides**    Hair of head/beard should be treated as well as pubic, axillary, and other body hair.
**Pediculocides**    See "Pediculosis," page 844.
**Infestation of Eyelids**    1% Permethrin or vaseline if infestation is present.
**Decontamination of Environment**    Bedding and clothing should be decontaminated (machine-washed or machine-dried using heat cycle or dry-cleaned) or removed from body contact for at least 72 h.
**Management of Sex Partner(s)**    Sex partners within last month should be treated. Screening for other STIs may be indicated.

# SCABIES   ■   ◑

Scabies is an infestation by the mite *Sarcoptes scabiei,* usually spread by skin-to-skin contact, characterized by generalized intractable pruritus often with minimal cutaneous findings. The diagnosis may be easily missed and should be considered in a patient of any age with persistent generalized severe pruritus.

*Synonym:* Chronic undiagnosed scabies is the basis for the colloquial expression, "the 7-year itch."

## EPIDEMIOLOGY AND ETIOLOGY

**Age of Onset**   Young adults (usually acquired by body contact); elderly and bedridden patients in the hospital (contact with mite-infested sheets); children (often ≤5 years). Nodular scabies more common in children.

**Etiology**   *S. scabiei* var. *hominis.* Thrive and multiply only on human skin. Mites of all developmental stages burrow/tunnel into epidermis shortly after contact, no deeper than stratum granulosum; deposit feces in tunnels. Females lay eggs in tunnels. Burrow 2 to 3 mm daily. Usually burrow at night and lay eggs during the day. Female lives 4 to 6 weeks, laying 40 to 50 eggs. Eggs hatch after 72 to 96 h. In classic scabies, about a dozen females per patient are present. In hyperkeratotic or crusted scabies, >1 million mites may be present, or up to 4700 mites/g skin.

**Incidence**   Estimated at 300 million cases/year worldwide. In the past, epidemics occurred in cycles every 15 years; the latest epidemic began in the late 1960s but has continued to the present.

**Demography**   Major public health problem in many less-developed countries. In some areas of South and Central America, prevalence is about 100%. In Bangladesh, the number of children with scabies exceeds that of children with diarrheal and upper-respiratory disease. In countries where human T cell leukemia/lymphoma virus (HTLV-I) infection is common, generalized crusted scabies is a marker of this infection, including cases of adult T cell leukemia/lymphoma.

**Transmission**   Mites transmitted by skin-to-skin contact as with sex partner, children playing, or health care workers providing care. Mites can remain alive for >2 days on clothing or in bedding; hence, scabies can be acquired without skin-to-skin contact. Patients with crusted scabies shed many mites into their environment daily and pose a high risk of infecting those around them, including health care professionals.

**Risk Factors**   In nursing homes, risk factors include age of institution (>30 years), size of institution (>120 beds), ratio of beds to health care workers (>10:1).

## PATHOGENESIS

Hypersensitivity of both immediate and delayed types occurs in the development of lesions other than burrows. For pruritus to occur, sensitization to *S. scabiei* must take place. Among persons with their first infection, sensitization takes several weeks to develop; after reinfestation, pruritus may occur within 24 h. Various immunocompromised states or individuals with neurologic disease predisposed to crusted Norwegian scabies. Infestation is usually by only approximately 10 mites. In contrast, the number of infesting mites in crusted scabies may exceed a million.

## HISTORY

Patients are often aware of similar symptoms in family members or sexual partners. Patients with crusted scabies are usually immunocompromised (HIV disease, organ transplant recipient) or have neurologic disorders (Down's syndrome, dementia, strokes, spinal cord injury, neuropathy, leprosy).

**Incubation Period**   Onset of pruritus varies with immunity to the mite: first infestation, about 21 days; reinfestation, immediate, i.e., 1 to 3 days.

**Duration of Lesions**   Weeks to months unless treated. Crusted scabies may be present for years.

**Skin Symptoms**   *Pruritus* Intense, widespread, usually sparing head and neck. Itching often interferes with or prevents sleep. Often present in family members. One-half of patients with crusted scabies do not itch.

*Rash* Ranges from no rash to generalized erythroderma. Patients with atopic diathesis scratch, producing eczematous dermatitis. Other individuals experience pruritus for many months with no rash. Tenderness of lesions suggests secondary bacterial infection.

## PHYSICAL EXAMINATION

**Skin Findings** Common cutaneous findings can be classified: lesions occurring at the sites of mite infestation, cutaneous manifestations of hypersensitivity to mite, lesions secondary to chronic rubbing and scratching, secondary infection. Variants of scabies in special hosts including those with an atopic diathesis, nodular scabies, scabies in infants/small children, scabies in the elderly, crusted (Norwegian) scabies, scabies in HIV disease, animal-transmitted scabies (zoonosis), scabies of the scalp, dyshidrosiform scabies, urticarial/vasculitis scabies, and bullous scabies.

### Lesions at Site of Infestation
**Intraepidermal Burrows** Gray or skin-colored ridges, 0.5 to 1 cm in length (Figs. 26-16 to 26-18), either linear or wavy (serpiginous), with minute vesicle or papule at end of tunnel. Each infesting female mite produces one burrow. Mites are about 0.5 mm in length. Burrows average 5 mm in length but may be up to 10 cm. In light-skinned individuals, burrows have a whitish color with occasional dark specks (due to fecal scybala). Fountain-pen ink applied to infested skin concentrates in tunnels, highlighting and marking the burrow. Blind end of burrow where mite resides appears as a minute elevation with tiny halo of erythema or as a vesicle.
*Distribution* Areas with few or no hair follicles, usually where stratum corneum is thin and soft, i.e., interdigital webs of hands > wrists > shaft of penis > elbows > feet > genitalia > buttocks > axillae > elsewhere (Image 26-1). In infants, infestation may occur on head and neck.
**Scabietic (Scabious) Nodule** Inflammatory papule or nodule (Fig. 26-19); burrow sometimes seen on the surface of a very early lesion.
**Hyperkeratosis/Crusting Psoriasiform** In areas of heavily infested crusted scabies, well-demarcated plaques covered by a very thick crust or scale (Figs. 26-20 to 26-22). Warty dermatosis of hands/feet with nail bed hyperkeratosis. Erythematous scaling eruption on face, neck, scalp, trunk.

### Cutaneous Manifestations of Hypersensitivity to Mite
**Pruritus** Some individuals experience only pruritus without any cutaneous findings.
**"Id" or Autosensitization-Type Reactions** Characterized by widespread small urticarial edematous papules mainly on anterior trunk, thighs, buttocks, and forearms.
**Urticaria** Usually generalized.
**Eczematous Dermatitis** At sites of heaviest infestation: hands, axillae (Figs. 26-20 and 26-21).

### Lesions Secondary to Chronic Rubbing and Scratching
Excoriation, lichen simplex chronicus, prurigo nodules. Generalized eczematous dermatitis. Psoriasiform lesions. Erythroderma.
**Atopy** In individuals with atopic diathesis, atopic dermatitis occurs at sites of excoriation, most commonly on the hands, webspaces of hands, wrists, axillae, areolae, waist, buttocks, penis, scrotum. In adults, the scalp, face, and upper back are usually spared; but in infants, the scalp, face, palms, and soles are involved.
**Postinflammatory Hyper- and Hypopigmentation** Especially in more deeply pigmented individuals.

### Secondary Infection
***S. aureus* or Group A Streptococcus Infection** (Fig. 26-22) Impetiginized excoriations (crusted, tender, surrounding erythema), ecthyma, folliculitis, abscess formation; lymphangitis, lymphadenitis; cellulitis; bacteremia, septicemia. Acute poststreptococcal glomerulonephritis reported associated with streptococcal impetiginization.

### Variants of Scabies in Special Hosts
**Infants/Young Children** Atypical lesions: vesicles, pustules, nodules; generalized; lesions concentrated on hands/feet/body folds. Head, palms, soles are not spared. Difficult to differentiate from infantile acropustulosis, which may be a postscabietic nonspecific reaction.
**Elderly** Altered inflammatory response may delay diagnosis. In bedridden patients, lesions may be concentrated on the back. Bullous scabies can mimic bullous pemphigoid.
**Nodular Scabies** Nodular lesions develop in 7 to 10% of patients with scabies. Nodules are 5 to 20 mm in diameter, red, pink, tan, or brown in color, smooth (Fig. 26-19). A burrow may be seen on the surface of early nodule.
*Distribution* Penis, scrotum, axillae, waist, buttocks, areolae (Image 26-1). Resolve with postinflammatory hyperpigmentation. May be

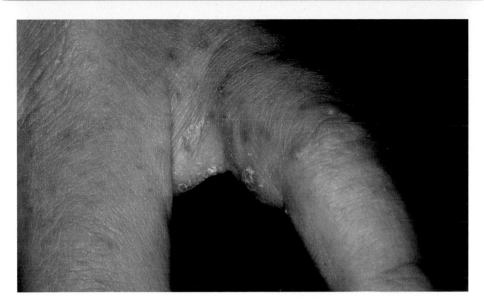

**FIGURE 26-16    Scabies: webspace**   *Papules and burrows in typical location on the finger web. Burrows are tan or skin-colored ridges with linear configuration with a minute vesicle or papule at the end of the burrow; they are often difficult to define.*

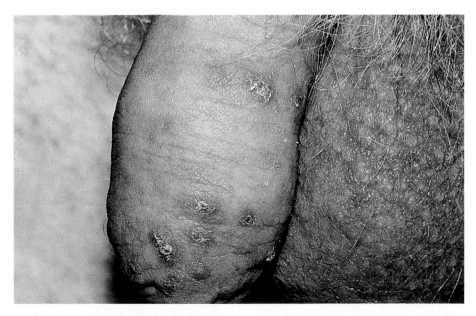

**FIGURE 26-17    Scabies**   *Multiple, crusted, and excoriated papules and burrows on the penile shaft.*

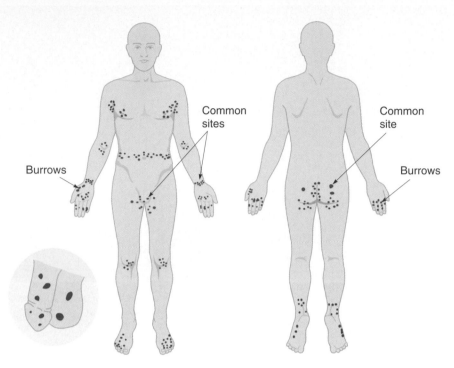

**IMAGE 26-1   Scabies: Predilection sites** *Burrows are most easy to identify on the webspace of the hands, wrists, lateral aspects of the palms. Scabietic nodules occur uncommonly, arising on the genitalia, especially the penis and scrotum, waist, axillae, and areolae.*

more apparent after treatment, as eczematous eruption resolves. Upper back, lateral edge of foot (infants). Nodules are usually countable.

**Crusted or Norwegian Scabies** Predisposing factors: glucocorticoid therapy, Down's syndrome, HIV disease, HTLV-I infection, organ transplant recipients, elderly. May begin as ordinary scabies. In others, clinical appearance is of chronic eczema, psoriasiform dermatitis (Figs. 26-21 and 26-22), seborrheic dermatitis, or erythroderma. Lesions often markedly hyperkeratotic and/or crusted.

*Distribution* Generalized (even involving head and neck in adults) or localized. Scale/crusts found on dorsal surface of hands, wrists, fingers, metacarpophalangeal joints, palms, extensor aspect of elbows, scalp, ears, soles, and toes. In patients with neurologic deficit, crusted scabies may occur only in affected limb. May be localized only to scalp, face, finger, toenail bed, or sole.

**General Findings** Lymphadenopathy in some cases.

## DIFFERENTIAL DIAGNOSIS

**Pruritus, Localized or Generalized, Rash** Adverse cutaneous drug reaction, atopic dermatitis, contact dermatitis, fiberglass dermatitis, dyshidrotic eczema, dermatographism, physical urticaria, pityriasis rosea, dermatitis herpetiformis, animal scabies, pediculosis corporis, pediculosis pubis, lichen planus, delusions of parasitosis, metabolic pruritus.

**Pyoderma** Impetigo, ecthyma, furunculosis.

**Nodular Scabies** Urticaria pigmentosa (in young child), papular urticaria (insect bites), Darier's disease, prurigo nodularis, secondary syphilis, pseudolymphoma, lymphomatoid papulosis, vasculitis.

**Crusted Scabies** Psoriasis, eczematous dermatitis, seborrheic dermatitis, erythroderma, Langerhans cell histiocytosis.

## LABORATORY EXAMINATIONS

**Microscopy** *Finding the Mite* A healthy adult

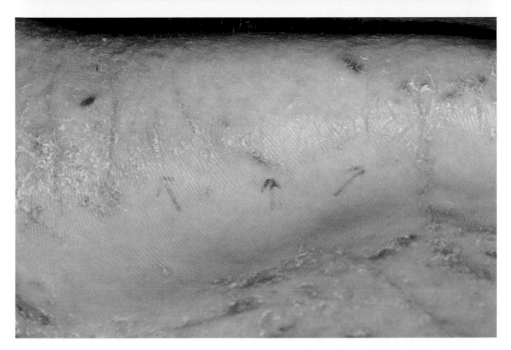

**FIGURE 26-18 Scabies** *Papules and burrows on the lateral foot; in young children, the feet and neck are often infested, sites usually spared in older individuals. In this adult case, there was massive infestation of the foot.*

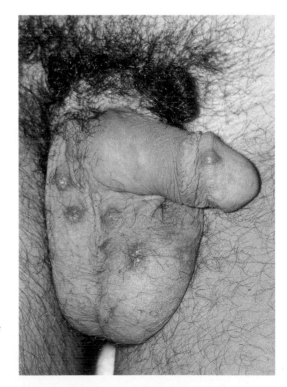

**FIGURE 26-19 Scabietic nodules: penis, scrotum** *Red-brown papules and nodules on the penis and scrotum; these lesions are pathognomonic for scabies, occurring at sites of infestation in some individuals.*

with scabies has an average of 6 to 12 adult mites infesting the body. Highest yield in identifying a mite is in typical burrows on the finger webs, flexor aspects of wrists, and penis. A drop of mineral oil is placed over a burrow, and the burrow is scraped off with a no. 15 scalpel blade and placed on a microscope slide.

***Conventional Microscopy*** A drop immersion of mineral oil is placed on the scraping, which is then covered by a coverslip. Three findings are diagnostic of scabies: *S. scabiei* mites, their eggs, and their fecal pellets (scybala) (Fig. 26-23).

***Dermoscopy*** Characteristic image of scabies, "jet-with-contrail" image.

**Dermatopathology** *Scabietic burrow:* located within stratum corneum; female mite situated in blind end of burrow. Body round, 400 $\mu$m in length. Spongiosis near mite with vesicle formation common. Eggs also seen. Dermis shows infiltrate with eosinophils. *Scabietic nodules:* dense chronic inflammatory infiltrate with eosinophils. In some cases, persistent arthropod reaction resembling lymphoma with atypical mononuclear cells. *Crusted scabies:* thickened stratum corneum riddled with innumerable mites.

**Hematology** Eosinophilia in crusted scabies.

**Cultures** *S. aureus* and GAS cause secondary infection.

## DIAGNOSIS

Clinical findings, confirmed, if possible, by microscopy (identification of mites, eggs, or mite feces). Assiduous search for burrows or papules should be made in every patient with severe generalized pruritus. Sometimes when the mite cannot be demonstrated, a "therapeutic test" will clinch the diagnosis.

## COURSE AND PROGNOSIS

**Pruritus** Often persists up to several weeks after successful eradication of mite infestation, understandable in that the pruritus is a hypersensitivity phenomenon to mite antigen(s). If reinfestation occurs, pruritus becomes symptomatic within a few days. Most cases resolve after recommended regimen of therapy. Glomerulonephritis has followed GAS secondary infection. Bacteremia and death have followed secondary *S. aureus* infection of crusted scabies in an HIV-infected patient. Delusions of parasitosis can occur in individuals who have been successfully treated for scabies or have never had scabies.

**Crusted Scabies** May be impossible to eradicate in HIV-infected individuals. Recurrence more likely to be relapse than reinfestation.

**Nodular Scabies** In treated patients, 80% resolve in 3 months but may persist up to 1 year.

## MANAGEMENT

**Principles of Treatment** Infested individuals and close physical contacts should be treated at the same time, whether or not symptoms are present. Topical agents are more effective after hydration of the skin, i.e., after bathing. Application should be to all skin sites, especially the groin, around nails, behind ears, including face and scalp. Sexual partners and close personal or household contacts within last month should be examined and treated prophylactically.

**Scabicides** Choice of scabicide based on effectiveness, potential toxicity, cost, extent of secondary eczematization, and age of patient. Permethrin is effective and safe but costs more than lindane. Lindane is effective in most areas of the world, but resistance has been reported. Seizures have occurred when lindane was applied after a bath or used by patients with extensive dermatitis. Aplastic anemia after lindane use was also reported. No controlled studies have confirmed that two applications are better than one. Clean clothing should be put on afterwards. Clothing and bedding are decontaminated by machine-washing at 60°C. Pruritus can persist for up to 1 to 2 weeks after the end of effective therapy. After that time, cause of persistent itching should be investigated.

**Recommended Regimens**

> *Permethrin 5% Cream* Applied to all areas of the body from the neck down. Wash off 8 to 12 h after application. Adverse events very low.
>
> *Lindane (γ-Benzene Hexachloride) 1% Lotion or Cream* Applied thinly to all areas of the body from the neck down; wash off thoroughly after 8 h. *Note*: Lindane should not be used after a bath or shower, and it should not be used by persons with extensive dermatitis, pregnant or lactating women, and children younger than 2 years. Mite resistance to lindane has developed in North, Central, and South America and Asia. Low cost makes lindane a key alternative in many countries.

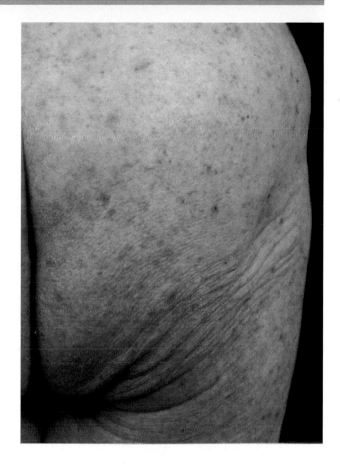

**FIGURE 26-20   Crusted scabies: buttocks**   *An eczematous dermatitis on the buttock in a chronic care facility patient. Pruritus, may be mild, and the diagnosis of scabies missed for months, during which time staff and other patients become infested.*

### Alternative Regimens

*Crotamiton 10% Cream* Applied thinly to the entire body from the neck down, nightly for 2 consecutive nights; wash off 24 h after second application.

*Sulfur 2 to 10% in Petrolatum* Applied to skin for 2 to 3 days.

*Benzyl Benzoate 10% and 25% Lotions* Several regimens are recommended: swabbing only once; two applications separated by 10 min, or two applications with a 24-h or 1-week interval. 24 h after application, preparation should be washed off and clothes and bedding changed. The compound is an irritant and can induce pruritic irritant dermatitis, especially on face and genitalia.

*Benzyl Benzoate with Sulfiram* Several regimens are recommended: swabbing only once:

*Esdepallethrine 0.63%*

*Malathion 0.5% Lotion*

*Sulfiram 25% Lotion* Can mimic effect of disulfiram; no alcoholic drinks should be consumed for at least 48 h.

*Ivermectin 0.8% Lotion*

**Systemic Ivermectin** Ivermectin, 200 g/kg PO; single dose reported to be very effective for common as well as crusted scabies in 15 to 30 days. Two to three doses, separated by 1 to 2 weeks, usually required for heavy infestation or in immunocompromised individuals. May effectively eradicate epidemic or endemic scabies in institutions such as nursing homes, hospitals, and refugee camps. Not approved by U.S. Food and Drug Administration or European Drug Agency.

**Infants, Young Children, Pregnant/Lactating Women** Permethrin or crotamiton regimens or precipitated sulfur ointment should be used with application to all body areas. Lindane and ivermectin should not be used.

**Crusted Scabies** *Scabicides* Lindane should be avoided because of risk of CNS toxicity. Multiple scabicide applications are required to all the skin. Treatment should also be directed

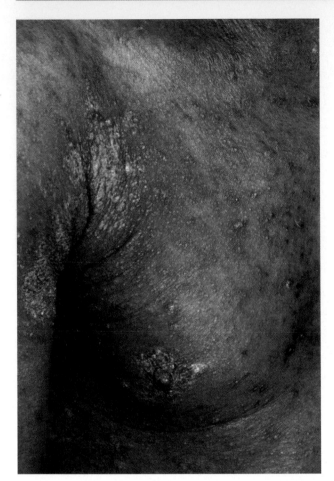

**FIGURE 26-21   Crusted scabies: chest, axilla, arm** *An eczematous dermatitis with lichen simplex chronicus in an HIV-infected male with chronic pruritus.*

at removing scale/crusts that protect mites from scabicide; nails should be trimmed. Oral ivermectin combined with topical therapy is most effective. Control of dissemination is essential and includes isolation of patient, avoidance of skin-to-skin contact, use of gloves/gowns by staff, prophylactic treatment of contacts (entire institution and visitors or family members).

*Decontamination of Environment* Bedding, clothing, and towels should be decontaminated (machine washed or machine dried using heat cycle or dry-cleaned) or removed from body contact for at least 72 h. Thorough cleaning of patient's room or residence.

**Treatment of Eczematous Dermatitis** *Antihistamines* Systemic sedating antihistamine such as hydroxyzine hydrochloride, doxepin, or diphenhydramine at bedtime.

*Topical Glucocorticoid Ointment* Applied to areas of extensive dermatitis associated with scabies.

*Systemic Glucocorticoids* Prednisone 70 mg, tapered over 1 to 2 weeks, gives symptomatic relief of severe hypersensitivity reaction.

**Postscabietic Itching** Generalized itching that persists a week or more is probably caused by hypersensitivity to remaining dead mites and mite products. Nevertheless, a second treatment 7 days after the first is recommended by some physicians. For severe, persistent pruritus, especially in individuals with history of atopic disorders, a 14-day tapered course of prednisone (70 mg on day 1) is indicated.

**Secondary Bacterial Infection** Treat with mupirocin ointment or systemic antimicrobial agent.

**Scabietic Nodules** May persist in association with pruritus for up to a year after eradication of infestation. Intralesional triamcinolone, 5 to 10 mg/mL into each lesion, is effective; repeat every 2 weeks if necessary.

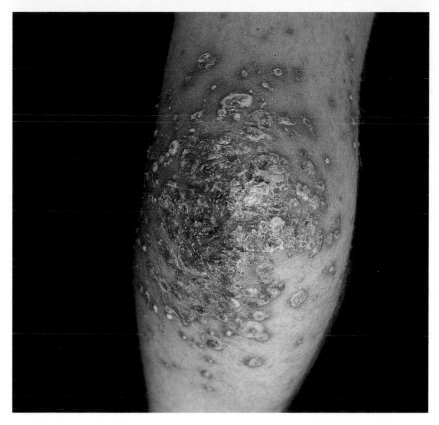

**FIGURE 26-22   Crusted scabies**   *Crusted erythematous papules becoming confluent over the elbow; numerous pustules are seen associated with secondary* S. aureus *infection.*

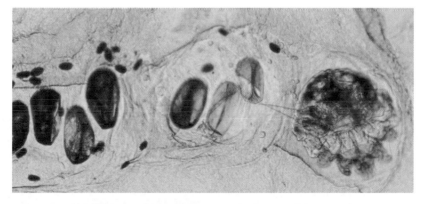

**FIGURE 26-23   Burrow with *Sarcoptes scabiei* (female), eggs, and feces**   *Under a microscope, a mite at the end of a burrow with eight eggs and smaller fecal particles obtained from a papule on the webspace of the hand.*

## CUTANEOUS LARVA MIGRANS    ◨ → ■   ◑

Cutaneous larva migrans (CLM) is a cutaneous lesion produced by percutaneous penetration and migration of larvae of various nematode parasites, characterized by erythematous, serpiginous, papular, or vesicular linear lesions corresponding to the movements of the larvae beneath the skin.

*Synonyms:* Creeping eruption, creeping verminous dermatitis, sandworm eruption, plumber's itch, duckhunter's itch.

## EPIDEMIOLOGY

**Etiology**   See Table 26-1
*CLM Ancylostoma braziliense* is most common cause in central and southeastern United States. Other penetrating nematode larvae: *A. caninum, Uncinaria stenocephala* (hookworm of European dogs), *Bunostomum phlebotomum* (hookworm of cattle).

Ova of hookworms are deposited in sand and soil in warm, shady areas, hatching into larvae that penetrate human skin. Activities and occupations that pose risk include contact with sand/soil contaminated with animal feces: playing in sandbox, walking barefoot or sitting on beach, working in crawl spaces under houses, gardeners and plumbers, farmers, electricians, carpenters, pest exterminators.

*Larva Currens* Filariform larvae of *Strongyloides stercoralis* can penetrate skin (usually on buttocks), producing similar lesions, i.e., *larva currens.*

*Other Migrating Cutaneous Parasitic Infestations* Other parasites *(Gnathostoma spinigerum, Strongyloides procyonis, Dirofilaria repens, Fasciola hepatica)* and some forms of myiasis can cause migratory skin lesions.

**Travel History**   Most common imported ectoparasite in U.S. travelers returning to the United States after holiday.

**Demographic Distribution**   Endemic in deprived communities. Tropical and subtropical areas, especially southeastern United States, Caribbean, Africa, Central/South America, Southeast Asia.

## PATHOGENESIS

Humans are aberrant, dead-end hosts who acquire the parasite from environment contaminated with animal feces. Larvae remain viable in soil/sand for several weeks. Third-stage larvae penetrate human skin and migrate up to several centimeters a day, usually between stratum germinativum and stratum corneum. Parasite induces localized eosinophilic inflam-

matory reaction. Most larvae are unable to develop further or invade deeper tissues and die after days or months. Migration to viscera causes Loeffler's syndrome.

## HISTORY

**Incubation Period**   1 to 6 days from time of exposure to onset of symptoms.
**Skin Symptoms**   Local pruritus begins within hours after larval penetration.

## PHYSICAL EXAMINATION

**Skin Lesions**
Serpiginous, thin, linear, raised, tunnel-like lesion 2 to 3 mm wide containing serous fluid (Fig. 26-24). Several or many lesions may be present depending on the number of penetrating larvae. Larvae move a few to many millimeters daily, confined to an area several centimeters in diameter. If multiple larvae are present, multiple tracts are seen.
*Distribution* Exposed sites, most commonly the feet, lower legs, buttocks, hands.
**Variant**   *Larva Currens* Caused by *S. stercoralis.* Papules, urticaria, papulovesicles at the site of larval penetration (Fig. 26-25). Associated with intense pruritus. Occurs on skin around anus, buttocks, thighs, back, shoulders, abdomen. Pruritus and eruption disappear when larvae enter blood vessels and migrate to intestinal mucosa.
**Systemic Findings**   Visceral larva migrans characterized by persistent hypereosinophilia, hepatomegaly, and frequently pneumonitis (Loeffler's syndrome). Caused by *Toxocara canis, T. cati, A. lumbricoides.*

## DIFFERENTIAL DIAGNOSIS

**Curvilinear Inflammatory Lesion**   Larva currens, migratory lesions from other parasites, phytoallergic contact dermatitis, phytophoto-

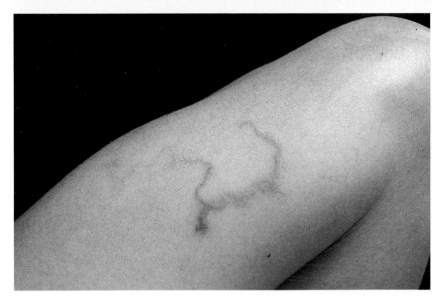

**FIGURE 26-24    Cutaneous larva migrans**    *A serpiginous, linear, raised, tunnel-like erythematous lesion outlining the path of migration of the larva. Upon palpation, it feels like a thread within the superficial layers of the skin.*

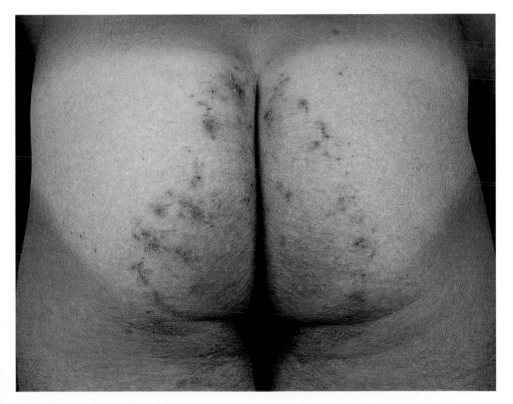

**FIGURE 26-25    Larva currens**    *Multiple, pruritic, serpiginous, inflammatory lines on the buttocks at sites of penetration of* S. stercoralis *larvae.*

**TABLE 26-1   Helminthic Causes of Migratory Dermatologic Lesions**

| Infestation | Helminth(s) | Comments |
|---|---|---|
| Cutaneous larva migrans | Primarily *Ancylostoma braziliense* and *A. caninum* | Larvae of dog/cat hookworms |
| Dracunculiasis | *Dracunculus medinensis* | Movement of worm just below dermis before eruption |
| Fascioliasis | *Fasciola hepatica* and *F. gigantica* | Migratory areas of inflammation, especially with *F. gigantica* |
| Gnathostomiasis | *Gnathostoma spinigerum* and other *Gnathostoma* species | Migratory inflammatory lesions, 1 cm/h or faster when subcutaneous |
| Hookworm | *Ancylostoma duodenale, Necator americanus, A. ceylanicum* | |
| Loiasis | *Loa loa* | Migratory inflammatory swellings; worm may be visible crossing conjunctivae |
| Paragonimiasis | Primarily *Paragonimus westermani* | Subcutaneous migratory swelling or subcutaneous nodules |
| Spirometrosis (sparganosis) | *Spirometra erinaceri, S. mansoni, S. mansonides, S. proliferum* | Subcutaneous nodules |
| Strongyloidiasis | *Strongyloides stercoralis* | Migratory, serpiginous lesions (larva currens), 5–10 cm/h |

dermatitis, erythema migrans of Lyme borreliosis, jelly fish sting, bullous impetigo, epidermal dermatophytosis, granuloma annulare, scabies, loiasis.

## LABORATORY EXAMINATIONS

**Hematology**   Peripheral eosinophilia.
**Dermatopathology**   Part of the parasite can be seen on biopsy specimens from the advancing point of the lesion(s).

## DIAGNOSIS

Clinical findings.

## COURSE

Self-limited; humans are "dead-end" hosts. Most larvae die and the lesions resolve within 2 to 8 weeks; rarely, up to 2 years.

## MANAGEMENT

**Prevention**   Avoid direct skin contact with fecally contaminated soil.
**Symptomatic Therapy**   Topical application of a glucocorticoid preparation under occlusion to lesion.
### Anthelmintic Agents
*Topical Agents Thiabendazole, ivermectin, albendazole* are effective topically.
*Systemic Agents Thiabendazole*, orally 50 mg/kg per day in two doses (maximum 3 g/d) for 2 to 5 days; also effective when applied topically under occlusion. *Ivermectin*, 6 mg bid. *Albendazole*, 400 mg/d for 3 days; highly effective.
**Cryosurgery**   Liquid nitrogen to advancing end of larval burrow.
**Removal of Parasite**   Do not attempt to extract; parasite not in visible lesion.

# WATER-ASSOCIATED INFECTIONS AND INFESTATIONS

Various organisms normally live in aqueous environments and can cause soft tissue infections after exposure: *Aeromonas hydrophila*, *Edwardsiella tarda*, *Erysipelothrix rhusiopathiae*, *Mycobacterium marinum*, *Pfisteria piscicida*, *Pseudomonas* species, *Streptococcus iniae*, *Vibrio vulnificus*, other *Vibrio* species, *Prototheca wickerhamii*. Localized cutaneous infestations, including cercarial dermatitis and seabather's eruption, can also occur after exposure to microscopic marine animals (Table 26-2).

## CERCARIAL DERMATITIS    ◧    ◑

Cercarial dermatitis (CD) (known also as swimmer's itch, clam digger's itch, schistosome dermatitis, sedge pool itch) is an acute pruritic papular eruption at the sites of cutaneous penetration by *Schistosoma cercariae* (larvae) of nonhuman schistosomes, whose usual hosts are birds and small mammals. Nonhuman schistosomes implicated: *Trichobilharzia*, *Gigantobilharzia*, *Ornithobilharzia*, *Microbilharzia*, *Schistosomatium*. Exposure can be to fresh, brackish, or salt water. Eggs produced by adult schistosomes living in animals are shed with animal feces into the environment; on reaching water, schistosome eggs hatch, releasing miracidia (fully developed larvae). Snails are the appropriate hosts for miracidia, from which they emerge as cercariae. These must penetrate the skin of a vertebrate host to continue development. Humans are dead-end hosts. Cercariae penetrate human skin, elicit an inflammatory response, and die without invading other tissues. CD occurs worldwide in areas with fresh and salt water inhabited by appropriate molluscan hosts.

CD is acquired by skin exposure to fresh/salt water infested by cercariae. Pruritus and rash begin within hours after exposure. A pruritic macular, papular, papulovesicular, and/or urticarial eruption develops at exposed sites with marked pruritus (Fig. 26-26), sparing parts of the body covered by clothing. (In contrast, seabather's eruption occurs on areas of the body covered by swimsuits.) Papular urticaria occurs at each site of penetration in previously sensitized individuals. In highly sensitized persons, lesions may progress to eczematous plaques, urticarial wheals, and/or vesicles, reaching a peak 2 to 3 days after exposure. Schistosomes capable of causing invasive disease in humans (*Schistosoma mansoni*, *S. haematobium*, *S. japonicum*) may cause a similar skin eruption shortly after penetration as well as late visceral complications. Lesions usually resolve within a week. Topical and/or systemic glucocorticoids may be indicated in more severe cases.

CD has to be distinguished from seabather's eruption (Table 26-2).

**TABLE 26-2    Comparison of Cercarial Dermatitis and Seabather's Eruption**

| Factor | Cercarial Dermatitis | Seabather's Eruption |
|---|---|---|
| Type of water | Fresh and salt | Salt |
| Body part involved | Uncovered | Covered and hairy areas |
| Geographic locale | Northern USA, Canada, Europe | Florida, Cuba |
| Etiology | Cercarial forms of schistosomes | Larval forms of marine coelenterates: *L. unquiculata*, *E. lineata* |

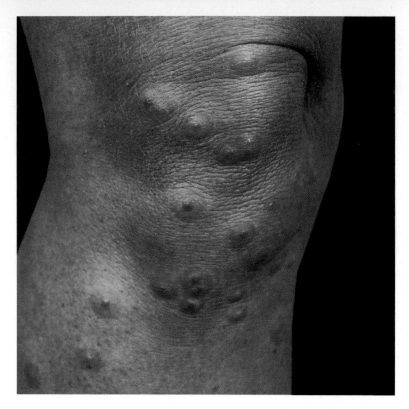

**FIGURE 26-26   Cercarial dermatitis**   *A highly pruritic papulovesicular eruption on the knees acquired after the patient waded through a slow-flowing creek.*

## SEABATHER'S ERUPTION

Seabather's eruption is caused by exposure to two marine animals: larvae of the thimble jellyfish, *Linuche unquiculatum,* in waters off the coast of Florida and in the Caribbean, and planula larvae of the sea anemone, *Edwardsiella lineata,* Long Island, NY. Nematocysts of coelenterate larvae sting the skin of hairy areas or under swimwear, presumably causing an allergic reaction. Some affected individuals recall a stinging or prickling sensation while in the water. Lesions present clinically as inflammatory papules 4 to 24 h after exposure. A monomorphous eruption of erythematous papules or papulovesicles is seen most commonly: vesicles, pustules, and papular urticaria, which may progress to crusted erosions. In comparison with cercarial dermatitis, which occurs on exposed sites, seabather's eruption occurs at sites covered by bathing apparel (Fig. 26-27) while bathing in salt water. On average, lesions persist for 1 to 2 weeks. In sensitized individuals, the eruption can become progressively more severe with repeated exposures and may be associated with systemic symptoms. Topical or systemic glucocorticoids provide symptomatic relief.

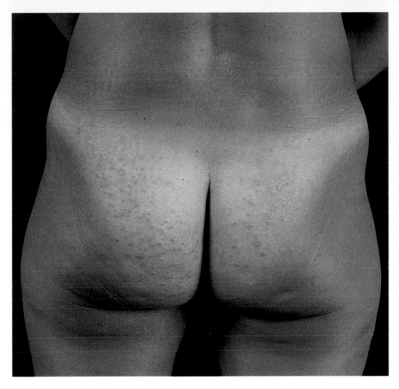

**FIGURE 26-27 Seabather's eruption** *This papulovesicular rash appeared on a swimmer while on vacation in the Caribbean. During swimming the patient experienced slight stinging in the regions covered by her bikini; later that evening she noticed the eruption. The rash is characteristically confined to the areas covered by the swimwear.*

## ENVENOMATIONS CAUSED BY CNIDARIA (JELLYFISH, PORTUGUESE MAN-OF-WAR, SEA ANEMONES, CORALS)   ◧ ◑

Cnidarian stings range from mild, self-limited irritations to extremely painful and serious injuries, depending on the toxin of the species involved and the magnitude of the enven-omation (Fig. 26-28). Stings from box jelly-fish can be fatal. In most cases jellyfish stings elicit toxic rather than allergic types of reactions.

## INJURIES CAUSED BY ECHINODERMS (SEA URCHIN, STARFISH, AND SEA CUCUMBERS)   ◧ ◑

Sea urchins have calcareous spines, which can break off in skin following a puncture wound. The spines are composed of calcium carbonate and a proteinaceous membrane; in certain species spines are venomous, causing excruci-ating pain. Immediate reactions are usually lo-calized: burning pain at wound site, tattooing from the spines, and paresthesias. Delayed reactions may be nodular or diffuse: foreign body reaction to spine fragments, delayed-type hypersensitivity, and fusiform swelling of digit with pain and loss of function. Starfish injuries are similar to those caused by sea urchins. Sea cucumbers can cause a papular contact dermati-tis caused by holothurin, a toxin secreted from cell walls.

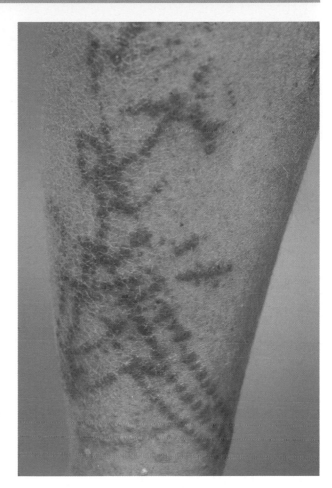

**FIGURE 26-28 Jellyfish envenomation** *Pruritic and painful papules in a linear arrangement on the leg, appearing after contact with jellyfish.*

# CUTANEOUS AND MUCOCUTANEOUS LEISHMANIASIS

Leishmaniasis is a parasitic infection caused by many species of obligate intracellular protozoa *Leishmania*, manifested clinically as four major syndromes

- Cutaneous leishmaniasis (CL) of Old World (OWCL) and New World (NWCL) types, characterized by development of single or multiple cutaneous papules at the site of a sandfly bite, often evolving into nodules and ulcers, which heal spontaneously with a depressed scar.
- Mucosal leishmaniasis (ML)
- Diffuse (anergic) cutaneous leishmaniasis (DCL)
- Visceral leishmaniasis (VL); kala-azar; post–kala-azar dermal leishmaniasis (PKDL)

*Synonyms* OWCL: Baghdad/Delhi boil or button, oriental/Aleppo sore/evil, *bouton d'Orient.* NWCL: chiclero ulcer, pian bois (bush yaws), uta. Mucosal leishmaniasis: Espundia. Visceral leishmaniasis: Kala-azar.

## EPIDEMIOLOGY

**Etiology** Clinical symptomatology, whether cutaneous, mucosal, or visceral, depends on infecting species. See Table 26-3.

**Life Cycle** *Leishmania* dimorphic. In mammalian host: amastigote (leishmanial) form—2 to 3 μm in length, oval/round, aflagellate; lives intracellularly in cells of reticuloendothelial system. In GI tract of sandfly/in culture: promastigote (leptomonad) form—10 to 15 μm in length, spindle-shaped, flagellated; extracellular. Speciation: isoenzyme patterns, kinetoplast DNA buoyant densities, specific phlebotomine vectors, monoclonal antibodies, DNA hybridization, DNA restriction endonuclease fragment analysis.

**Reservoir** Varies with geography and leishmanial species. Zoonosis involves rodents/canines. Mediterranean littoral—dogs. Southern Russia—gerbils. For *L. major,* desert rodents. For *L. tropica,* rats. For *L. infantum,* wild canines, dogs; in endemic areas of Spain, up to 20% of dogs tested harbored parasites in skin and viscera.

**Vector** Female sandflies of genus *Phlebotomus* (Old World) and genera *Lutzomyia* (New World). Breed in cracks in buildings, rubbish, rubble; rodent burrows, termite hills, rotting vegetation. Weak fliers; remain close to ground near breeding site, Ingest amastigotes while feeding on infected mammals, converting to promastigotes in the gut of the sandfly; replicate in gut.

**Transmission** Promastigotes deposited on skin of host into a small pool of blood drawn by probing sandfly.

**Prevalence** Estimated 12 million people infected worldwide; 1 million new cases annually; 350 million individuals are at risk of infection. 75,000 individuals die annually of MCL and ML.

**Demography** All inhabited continents except Australia. >90% of cases of CL occur in Afghanistan, Algeria, Iran, Iraq, Saudi Arabia, Syria, Brazil, Peru.

**OWCL** Asia Minor, Middle East (Egypt to Iran), southern Russia, China, the Mediterranean littoral, Asia, Pakistan, Afghanistan, India, Africa (Sudan, Ethiopia, Congo Basin).

**Iraq 2004:** 1000 cases OWCL in U.S. soldiers in Iraq, largest outbreak U.S. military has seen. Sandfly season: begins in April. Long incubation period. No cases of VL. Treatment: Pentostam. >1 million cases of CL reported annually, with large outbreaks currently in Sudan and Afghanistan. Availability of Pentostam is limited. Vaccine: in development; a long way off.

**ACL, MCL** Forests of South and Central America. *L. mexicana* endemic in south-central Texas.

**DCL** South America, Dominican Republic, Africa.

## PATHOGENESIS

The clinical and immunologic spectrum of leishmaniasis parallels that of leprosy. CL occurs in a host with good protective immunity. MCL occurs in those with an intense inflammatory reaction. DCL occurs with extensive and widespread proliferation of the organism in the skin but without much inflammation or tendency for visceralization. VL occurs in the host with little immune response and/or in immunosuppression. Unlike leprosy, extent and pattern are strongly influenced by the specific species of *Leishmania* involved. Additional factors that

## TABLE 26-3   Major *Leishmania* Species That Cause Disease in Humans

| Species[*] | Clinical Syndrome[†] | Geographic Distribution |
|---|---|---|
| **SUBGENUS *LEISHMANIA*** | | |
| L. donovani complex | | |
|   L. donovani | VL (PKDL, OWCL) | China, Indian subcontinent, southwestern Asia, Ethiopia,[#] Kenya, Sudan, Uganda; possibly sporadic in sub-Saharan Africa |
|   L. infantum | VL (OWCL) | China, central and southwestern Asia, Middle East, southern Europe, North Africa, Ethiopia,[#] Sudan; sporadic in sub-Saharan Africa |
|   L. chagasi | VL (NWCL) | Central and South America |
| L. mexicana complex | | |
|   L. mexicana | NWCL (DCL) | Texas, Mexico, Central and South America |
|   L. amazonensis | NWCL (ML, DCL, VL) | Panama and South America |
| L. tropica | OWCL (VL)[‡] | Central Asia, India, southwestern Asia, Middle East, Turkey, Greece, North Africa, Ethiopia,[#] Kenya, Namibia |
| L. major | OWCL[§] | Central Asia, India, southwestern Asia, Middle East, Turkey, North Africa, Sahel region of north-central Africa, Ethiopia,[#] Sudan, Kenya |
| L. aethiopica | OWCL (DCL) | Ethiopia,[#] Kenya |
| **SUBGENUS *VIANNIA*** | | |
| L. (V.) braziliensis | NWCL (ML) | Central and South America |
| L. (V.) guyanensis | NWCL (ML) | South America |
| L. (V.) panamensis | NWCL (ML) | Central America, Venezuela, Colombia, Ecuador, Peru |
| L. (V.) peruviana | NWCL[¶] | Peru (western slopes of Andes) |

[*] Species other than those listed here have been reported to infect humans.

[†] Abbreviations: VL, visceral leishmaniasis; PKDL, post–kala-azar dermal leishmaniasis; OWCL, Old World cutaneous leishmaniasis; NWCL, New World (American) cutaneous leishmaniasis; DCL, diffuse cutaneous leishmaniasis; ML, mucosal leishmaniasis. Clinical syndromes less frequently associated with the various species are shown in parentheses.

[‡] *L. tropica* also causes leishmaniasis recidivans and viscerotropic leishmaniasis.

[§] *L. major*–like organisms also cause New World cutaneous leishmaniasis.

[¶] The cutaneous leishmaniasis syndrome caused by this species is called *uta*.

[#] Cutaneous and visceral leishmaniasis also are endemic in parts of Eritrea, but the causative species have not been well established.

SOURCE: From BL Herwaldt, in DL Kasper, E Braunwald, AS Fauci, SL Hauser, DL Lango, JL Jameson (eds): *Harrison's Principles of Internal Medicine*, 16th ed, Chap. 196. New York, McGraw-Hill, 2005.

affect the clinical picture: number of parasites inoculated, site of inoculation, nutritional status of host, nature of the last non-blood meal of vector. Infection and recovery are followed by lifelong immunity to reinfection by the same species of *Leishmania*. In some cases, interspecies immunity occurs.

## HISTORY

**Incubation Period**  Inversely proportional to size of inoculum: shorter in visitors to endemic area. OWCL: *L. tropica major*, 1 to 4 weeks; *L. tropica*, 2 to 8 months; acute CL: 2 to 8 weeks or more.

**Symptoms**  Noduloulcerative lesions usually asymptomatic. With secondary bacterial infection, may become painful.

## PHYSICAL EXAMINATION

### Skin Findings

**Types of Lesions**  Primary lesions occur at site of sandfly bite, usually on exposed site.

**OWCL**  *L. major* Asia, Africa, Europe in tropical and subtropical zones; Middle East (Iran, Iraq, eastern Saudi Arabia, Jordan Valley of Israel and Jordan, Sinai Peninsula). More common in rural areas. Begins as small erythematous papule, which may appear immediately after sandfly bite but usually 2 to 4 weeks later. Papule slowly enlarges to 2 cm over a period of several weeks and assumes a dusky violaceous hue (Fig. 26-29). Eventually, lesion becomes crusted in center with a shallow ulcer and raised indurated border = vulcano sign (Fig. 26-30). In some cases, the center of the nodule becomes hyperkeratotic, forming a cutaneous horn. Small satellite papules may develop at periphery of lesion, and occasionally subcutaneous nodules along the course of proximal lymphatics. Rarely, lesions become locally invasive and extend into subcutaneous tissue and muscle. Peripheral extension usually stops after 2 months, and ulcerated nodule persists for another 3 to 6 months, or longer. The lesion then heals with a slightly depressed scar. In some cases, CL remains active with positive smears for 24 months (nonhealing chronic cutaneous leishmaniasis). The number of lesions depends on the circumstances of the exposure and extent of infection within the sandfly vector. May result in multiple lesions, up to 100 or more (Figs. 26-30 and 26-31).

*L. tropica* Southern Europe, Iran, Iraq, Middle East, southern republics of former U.S.S.R. More common in urban areas. Clinical pattern similar to that of *L. major*, although lesions caused by *L. tropica* are more apt to be solitary, more inflammatory, last longer, and be more difficult to treat.

*L. infantum* Countries bordering Mediterranean, including southern Europe and northern Africa. Lesions are similar to those in *L. major* form but duration is shorter.

*L. aethiopica* Kenya, Sudan, Ethiopia. The common form of CL in these areas is similar to CL caused by *L. major.* In approximately

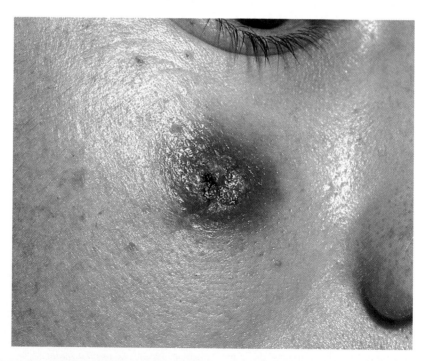

**FIGURE 26-29  Old World cutaneous leishmaniasis**  *A solitary, inflamed nodule with central necrosis and ulceration on the cheek for 1 month arising at the site of a sandfly bite.*

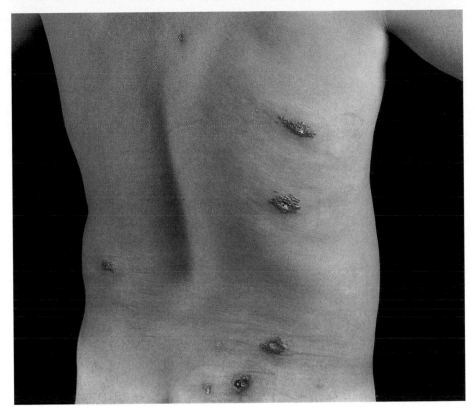

**FIGURE 26-30 Old World cutaneous leishmaniasis** *Multiple, crusted nodules on the exposed back, arising at sites of sandfly bites. Many of the lesions resemble a volcano with a central depressed center, i.e., volcano sign.*

20% of individuals, widespread skin involvement develops (DCL) that resembles lepromatous leprosy.

**NWCL** ***L. mexicana Complex*** Mexico, Central America, as far north as Texas, as far south as Brazil. Lesions develop in similar fashion to those caused by *L. major.* Small erythematous papule develops at sandfly bite site, evolving into ulcerated nodule (Fig. 26-32). Eventually lesion heals with a depressed scar. Enlarges 3 to 12 cm with raised border. Nonulcerating nodules may become verrucous. Lymphangitis, regional lymphadenopathy. Isolated lesions on hand or head usually do not ulcerate; heal spontaneously. Ear lesions may persist for years, destroying cartilage (chiclero ulcers) (Fig. 26-33). ***L. braziliensis Complex*** Clinical lesions similar to those of OWCL. Some strains can invade mucous membranes of mouth, nose, pharynx, larynx to cause MCL.

**Mucosal Leishmaniasis** Characterized by nasooropharyngeal mucosal involvement, a metastatic complication of CL. Caused by *Viannia* subgenus, typically *L. (V.) braziliensis, L. (V.) panamensis,* and *L (V.) guyanensis.* Mucosal disease usually becomes evident several years after healing of original cutaneous lesions; cutaneous and mucosal lesions can coexist or appear decades apart. Edema and inflammatory changes lead to epistaxis and coryzal symptoms. In time, nasal septum, floor of mouth, and tonsilar areas destroyed (Fig. 26-34). Results in marked disfigurement (referred to as *espundia* in South America). Death may occur due to superimposed bacterial infection, pharyngeal obstruction, or malnutrition.

**Diffuse Cutaneous Leishmaniasis** Resembles lepromatous leprosy; large number of parasites in macrophages in dermis; no visceral involvement. In Old World, occurs in 20% of individuals with leishmaniasis in Ethiopia and Sudan. In South America, attributed to a member of *L. braziliensis* complex. Presents as a single nodule, which then spreads locally, often through extension from satellite lesions, and eventually by metastasis. In time, lesions become widespread with nonulcerating nodules appearing diffusely over face, trunk. Responds poorly to treatment.

**Leishmaniasis Recidivans (LR)**　Complication of *L. tropica* infection. Dusky-red plaques with active, spreading borders and healing centers, giving rise to gyrate and annular lesions. Most commonly affects face; can cause tissue destruction and severe deformity.

**Post–Kala-Azar Dermal Leishmaniasis (PKDL)** Sequel to VL that has resolved spontaneously or during/after adequate treatment. Lesions appear $\geq 1$ y after course of therapy with macular, papular, nodular lesions, and hypopigmented macules/plaques on face, trunk, extremities. Resembles lepromatous leprosy when lesions are numerous. Develops in 20% of Indian patients treated for VL caused by *L. donovani* and in a small percentage of Ethiopian patients with VL caused by *L. aethiopica*.

**General Examination**　*Visceral Leishmaniasis* Can remain subclinical or become symptomatic, with acute, subacute, chronic course. Inapparent VL cases outnumber clinically apparent cases. Malnutrition is risk factor for clinically apparent VL. Bone marrow, liver, spleen are involved. Term *kala-azar* (Hindi for 'black fever,' some patients had gray color) refers to profoundly cachectic febrile patients with life-threatening disease. Occurs in China, India, former U.S.S.R. Middle East, east Africa through Sudan to west Africa, and South America. Patients present with fever, splenomegaly, pancytopenia, wasting.

*Viscerotrophic Leishmaniasis* Caused by *L. tropica* (typically dermotropic); recognized in U.S. soldiers who participated in Operation Desert Storm. Parasitic burdens light; nonspecific manifestations of visceral infection (fatigue, fever, GI symptoms).

*VL in HIV Disease* Relatively avirulent *Leishmania* strains can disseminate to viscera. Consider in HIV-infected patient with CD4 cell count $<200/\mu L$, travel history to leishmaniasis-endemic areas, unexplained fever, organomegaly, anemia, pancytopenia.

## DIFFERENTIAL DIAGNOSIS

**Acute CL**　Insect bite reaction, impetigo, furuncle, carbuncle, ecthyma, anthrax, orf, milker's nodule, tularemia, *M. marinum* infection, tuberculosis cutis, yaws, sporotrichosis, blastomycosis, kerion, myiasis, dracunculosis, trypanosomal chagoma or chancre, foreign body granuloma, keratoacanthoma, basal cell carcinoma, squamous cell carcinoma, metastases, lymphoma.

**Chronic CL and Relapsing CL**　Lupus vulgaris, leprosy, sarcoidosis, granuloma faciale, Jessner's lymphocytic infiltrate, lymphocytoma cutis, discoid lupus erythematosus, psoriasis, acne, rosacea, cellulitis, erysipelas, keloids, Wegener's granulomatosis, syphilitic gumma.

**ML**　Sarcoidosis, neoplasms, midline granuloma, rhinoscleroma, paracoccidioidomycosis, histoplasmosis, leprosy, syphilis, tertiary yaws.

**VL**　Tropical infectious diseases that cause fever or organomegaly (typhoid fever, miliary tuberculosis, brucellosis, malaria, tropical splenomegaly syndrome, and schistosomiasis); leukemia and lymphoma.

**PKDL**　Syphilis, yaws, leprosy.

## LABORATORY EXAMINATIONS

**Leishmanin (Montenegro) Skin Test**　Of no use in endemic areas. Negative in DCL.

**Serology**　Lacks specificity.

**Dermatopathology**　Large macrophages filled with 2- to 4-μm amastigotes (Leishman-Donovan bodies); mixed lymphocytic, plasmacytic infiltrate. In Wright- and Giemsa-stained preparations, the amastigote cytoplasm appears blue, nucleus relatively large and red; distinctive kinetoplast is rod-shaped and stains intensely red.

**Culture**　Novy-MacNeal-Nicolle medium at 22°C to 28°C for 21 days grows motile promastigotes.

**Touch Preparation**　Macrophages containing organisms: dark, slightly flattened nucleus and rod-shaped kinetoplast observed.

**Needle Aspiration**　Visualize amastigote within macrophages.

**Polymerase Chain Reaction**　Can detect different species of *Leishmania*.

## DIAGNOSIS

Clinical suspicion, confirmed by demonstrating amastigotes on smear or in skin biopsy specimen or promastigotes on culture of aspirates or tissue.

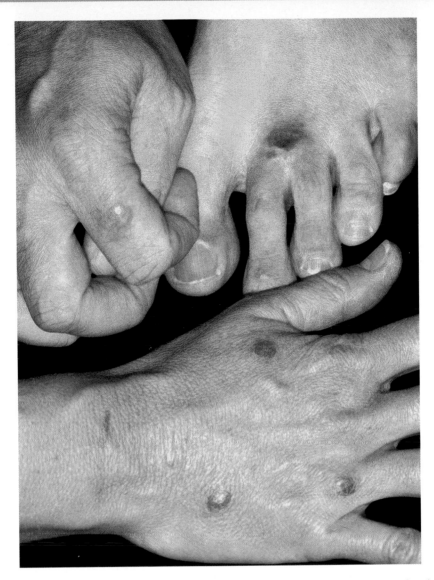

**FIGURE 26-31 Old World cutaneous leishmaniasis** *Multiple erythematous papules and nodules on the dorsa of hands and foot in a husband and wife who had been camping in Israel. A facial papule was present in the wife. All lesions resolved spontaneously within 2 to 3 months.*

**TABLE 26-4    Drug Regimens for Treatment of Leishmaniasis**[*]

| Clinical Syndrome, Drug | Route of Administration | Regimen |
|---|---|---|
| **VISCERAL LEISHMANIASIS** | | |
| First-line | | |
| Pentavalent antimony[†] | IV, IM | 20 mg $Sb^V$/kg qd for 28 days |
| Amphotericin B, lipid formulation[‡] | IV | 2–5 mg/kg qd (total: usually ~15–21 mg/kg) |
| Alternatives | | |
| Amphotericin B (deoxycholate) | IV | 0.5–1 mg/kg qod or qd (total: usually ~15–20 mg/kg) |
| Paromomycin sulfate[§] | IV, IM | 15–20 mg/kg qd for ~21 days |
| Pentamidine isethionate | IV, IM | 4 mg/kg qod or thrice weekly for ~15–30 doses |
| **CUTANEOUS LEISHMANIASIS** | | |
| First-line | | |
| Pentavalent antimony[†] | IV, IM | 20 mg $Sb^V$/kg qd for 20 days |
| Parenteral alternatives | | |
| Pentamidine isethionate | IV, IM | 3 mg/kg qod for 4 doses or 2 mg/kg qod for 7 doses |
| Amphotericin B (deoxycholate) | IV | 0.5–1 mg/kg qod or qd (total: up to ~20 mg/kg) |
| Oral alternatives | | |
| Ketoconazole | PO | 600 mg/d for 28 days[¶] |
| Itraconazole | PO | 200 mg bid for 28 days[¶] |
| Dapsone | PO | 100 mg bid for 6 weeks[¶] |
| **MUCOSAL LEISHMANIASIS** | | |
| First-line | | |
| Pentavalent antimony[†] | IV, IM | 20 mg $Sb^V$/kg qd for 28 days |
| Alternatives | | |
| B (deoxycholate) | IV | 1 mg/kg qod or qd (total: usually ~20–40 mg/kg) |
| Pentamidine isethionate | IV, IM | 2–4 mg/kg qod or thrice weekly for ≥15 doses |

[*] To maximize effectiveness and minimize toxicity, the listed regimens should be individualized according to the particularities of the case.

[†] The Centers for Disease Control and Prevention (CDC) provides the pentavalent antimonial ($Sb^V$) compound sodium stibogluconate (Pentostam; Glaxo Wellcome, PLC, United Kingdom; 100 mg $Sb^V$/mL) to U.S.-licensed physicians through the CDC Drug Service (404-639-3670). The other widely used pentavalent antimonial compound, meglumine antimonate (Glucantime; Rhône Poulenc, France; 85 mg $Sb^V$/mL), is available primarily in Spanish- and French-speaking areas of the world.

[‡] The lipid formulations of amphotericin B include liposomal amphotericin B, amphotericin B lipid complex, and amphotericin B cholesteryl sulfate. The U.S. Food and Drug Administration recently approved the following regimen of liposomal amphotericin B for immunocompetent patients: 3 mg/kg qd on days 1–5, 14, and 21, for a total of 21 mg/kg; for immunosuppressed patients, the approved regimen is 4 mg/kg qd on days 1–5, 10, 17, 24, 31, and 38, for a total of 40 mg/kg. Alternative regimens that have been proposed for immunocompetent patients include treatment on days 1–5 and 10 with 3–4 mg/kg qd for cases from Europe or Brazil, with 3 mg/kg qd for cases from Africa, and with 2–3 mg/kg qd for cases from India.

[§] Not commercially available as of this writing.

[¶] Adult dosage.

SOURCE: From BL Herwaldt, in E Braunwald, AS Fauci, DL Kasper, SL Hauser, DL Longo, JL Jameson (eds): *Harrison's Principles of Internal Medicine*, 15th ed, Chap. 215. New York, McGraw-Hill, 2001.

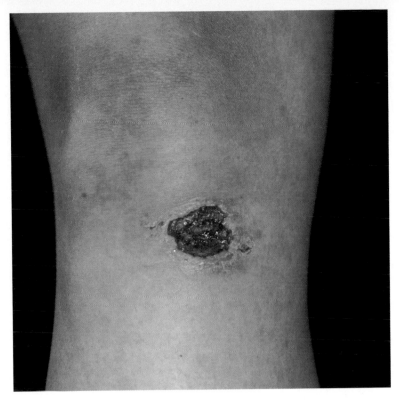

**FIGURE 26-32   New World cutaneous leishmaniasis: ulcer**  *A large ulcerated nodule developed on the right knee at the site of a sandfly bite in a 20-year-old traveler who visited Bolivia. The diagnosis was delayed and eventually made by isolating the organism on culture of skin biopsy.*

## COURSE AND PROGNOSIS

**CL**  Whether caused by *L. tropica* or *L. mexicana*, CL is self-limited. Scarring is increased by secondary bacterial infection.
**MCL**  May extend to secondary sites. Superinfection common. Death from pneumonia.
**DCL**  Progressive; refractory to treatment; cures rare.

## MANAGEMENT

**Prophylaxis**  No chemoprophylaxis for travelers exists. OWCL: Delay specific treatment until ulceration occurs, allowing protective immunity to develop, unless lesions are disfiguring, disabling, persist ± 6 months.
**Lesional Therapy**  Local injection of antimonials (Pentostam), usually at weekly intervals; up to 1 mg/kg may be injected in borders of lesions. Also cryosurgery, ultrasound-induced hyperthermia, excision, electrosurgery. Topical 15% paramomycin sulfate, 12% methylbenzethonium chloride in white paraffin twice daily for 10 days.
**Systemic Therapy**  See Table 26-4.

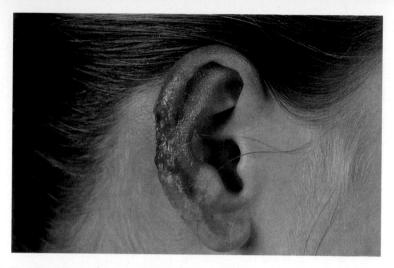

**FIGURE 26-33   New World cutaneous leishmaniasis: chiclero ulcer**   *A deep ulcer on the helix at the site of a sandfly bite. This variant typically occurs in leishmaniasis acquired in Central and South America.*

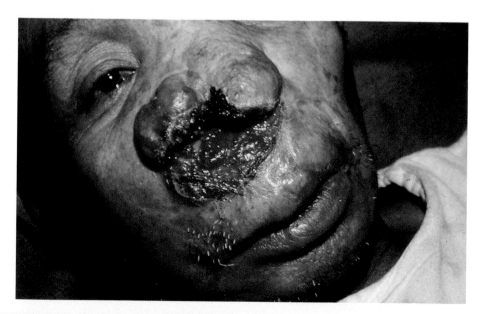

**FIGURE 26-34   Mucocutaneous leishmaniasis: espundia**   *Painful, mutilating ulceration with destruction of portions of the nose. (Courtesy of Eric Kraus, MD.)*

# TRYPANOSOMIASIS

*Trypanosoma* protozoan hemoflagellates cause chronic infestation, endemically in Central and South America and in Africa; they are associated with significant morbidity and mortality.

## AMERICAN TRYPANOSOMIASIS (AT)

AT (*Chagas' disease*) is a zoonosis caused by *T. cruzi*, which is transmitted by reduviid bugs. AT is prevalent in Central and South America, infecting 16 to 18 million people. Acute AT is usually a mild febrile illness that results from initial infection with the organism. Most infected persons remain so for life. In a minority of chronically infected patients, cardiac and gastrointestinal lesions develop that can result in serious morbidity and mortality.

### Mucocutaneous Findings of AT

- *Inoculation chagoma* An indurated area of erythema and swelling (*chagoma*), at the portal of entry, occurring 7 to 14 days after inoculation. May be accompanied by local lymphadenopathy. Parasites located within leukocytes and cells of subcutaneous tissues. These initial local signs are followed by malaise, fever, anorexia, and edema of the face and lower extremities.
- *Romaña's sign* Unilateral painless edema of palpebrae and periocular tissues. Occurs when conjunctiva is the portal of entry. Classic finding in acute AT.
- *Morbilliform, urticariform, or erythematopolymorphic eruptions* "Trypanosomides."

- *Hematogenic or metastatic chagomas* Nodule(s) caused by dissemination of infection. Hard, painful, wine-colored nodules; rarely soften or ulcerate.
- Generalized lymphadenopathy and hepatosplenomegaly may develop. Severe myocarditis may occur in acute AT; most deaths are due to heart failure.
- *Reactivation chagoma* Nodule in the immunocompromised host (HIV disease, organ transplant recipient) with AT. A cellulite-mimicking plaque.
- Chronic AT Commonly involves the heart (rhythm disturbances, cardiomyopathy, and thromboembolism) and GI tract (megaesophagus, megacolon)

---

* In endemic regions.

## HUMAN AFRICAN TRYPANOSOMIASIS (HAT)    ■<sup>*</sup>  ●

HAT is caused by the complex *T. brucei*. *T. b. gambiense* causes West African sleeping sickness, and *T. b. rhodesiense* causes East African sleeping sickness. Acquired through bites of infected tsetse flies. Nearly all cases of HAT in travelers is East African trypanosomiasis.

- *A painful trypanosomal chancre* appears in some patients at inoculation site (Fig. 26-35), 7 to 14 days after tsetse-fly bite. Occurs more commonly in travelers than in Africans. Typically 2 to 5 cm, indurated; may ulcerate; resolved in few weeks. Parasites can be seen in fluid expressed from chancre and buffy coat.
- Hemolymphatic stage (stage I disease) is marked by the onset of fever, arthralgias, malaise, localized facial edema, and moderate splenomegaly. Lymphadenopathy is prominent in *T. b. gambiense* trypanosomiasis.

- *Characteristic macular rash* occurs on the trunk in stage I.
- *Winterbottom's sign* Enlargement of the nodes of the posterior cervical triangle; cervical nodes also enlarged.
- *Pruritus and maculopapular rashes* are common.
- CNS invasion (stage II disease) is characterized by insidious development of protean neurologic symptoms. Progressive indifference and daytime somnolence develops (hence the designation "sleeping sickness").

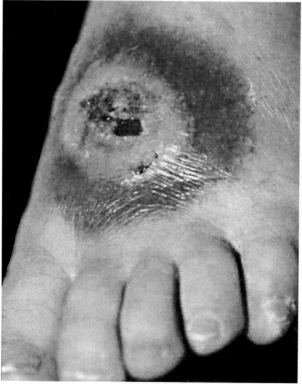

**FIGURE 26-35    Human East African trypanosomiasis: tyrpanosomal *chancre*** *A shallow ulceration was present on the dorsum of the left foot, surrounded by a ring that contained bullae and that was, in turn, surrounded by another ring, characterized by violaceous erythema and induration; the entire lesion, which was approximately 5 cm in diameter, was painful. A macular exanthem was present on the trunk. The patient was a traveler to South Africa. Trypanosoma brucei was identified in an aspirate from the ulcer. (Courtesy of Edward T. Ryan, MD. N Engl J Med 346: 2069, 2002; with permission.)*

<sup>*</sup> In endemic regions.

## CUTANEOUS AMEBIASIS

Amebiasis is caused by *Entamoeba histolytica*, which infects the GI tract and rarely skin; more prevalent in tropics and in rural areas. Skin involvement is associated with malnutrition and immunocompromise. Cutaneous amebiasis (CA) is usually a consequence of an underlying amebic abscess invading the skin. Typical sites for CA are the perianal area (extension of sigmorectal involvement) (Fig. 26-36) or abdominal wall (draining sinus from liver or colon). Penis or vulva may become infected during intercourse. Surgical wound infections may follow removal of hepatic or abdominal abscess. Remote ulcers (e.g., face) may result from autoinoculation. CA begins as an indurated pustule that evolves to a painful ragged ulcer, foul-smelling and covered with pus or necrotic debride. Without treatment, CA progressively enlarges.

Cutaneous acanthamebiasis is an infection caused by free-living *Acanthamoeba*. Primary cutaneous acanthamebiasis occurs at sites of trauma sustained in aquatic environment (streams, ponds, swimming pools). Lesions begin as indurated red/violaceous deep nodules or large pustules that soon ulcerate. Disseminated cutaneous acanthamebiasis occurs in HIV disease, presenting with multiple soft red nodules that ulcerate, possibly disseminating from nasal/sinus colonization.

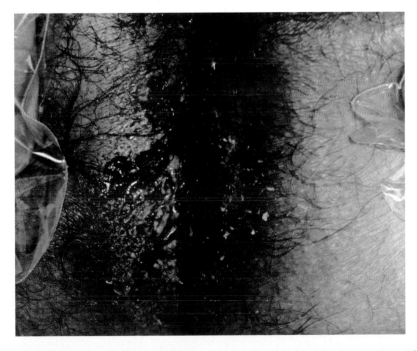

**FIGURE 26-36  Cutaneous amebiasis: perineum**  *Perineal/perianal erosion in a patient with rectal amebiasis.*

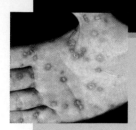

# SEXUALLY TRANSMITTED INFECTIONS

Sexually transmitted infections (STIs), caused by a broad range of pathogens (Table 27-1), have a high physical and psychosocial morbidity. The syndromes caused by these pathogens affect both the sexually active couple and neonates born to an infected mother (Table 27-2). The combination of subtle or absent symptoms and the stigma, which prevents the seeking of health care, leaves many infections undiagnosed.

Bacterial STIs such as gonorrhea, syphilis, chancroid, donovanosis, and lymphogranuloma venereum can easily be cured with antimicrobial therapy. In contrast, viral STIs, such as those caused by HIV, human papillomavirus (HPV), and herpes simplex virus 2 (HSV-2), are chronic infections, characterized by prolonged viral shedding and opportunity for infecting a sexual partner; these cannot be cured by antiviral therapy. Nearly all sexually active individuals are at risk for these viral STIs. HPV persists in the anogenital mucosa for months, years, or decades after primary infection. HSV-2 infection is chronic and lifelong. Prevention offers the best approach to managing STIs.

Many STIs can be transmitted perinatally to the neonate. In developing nations, where STIs are more common, lack of funds for health care often limit detection and treatment of STIs as well as immunizations. Syphilis can be a lifelong infection with severe long-term morbidity. Transmission of HIV to neonates occurs commonly in developing nations, where the prevalence of infection is high; antiretroviral treatment of mother and neonate markedly reduces neonatal infection. Transmission of HSV has more immediate effects on the neonate, who is more susceptible to acute visceral infection. Transmission of HPV infection to the neonate can result in anogenital condyloma, and, later in life, respiratory papillomatosis.

## LABORATORY EXAMINATIONS

All individuals being evaluated for STIs should have a culture for gonorrhea and serotesting for HIV and syphilis. Serologic testing for HPV infections is not available. Antibodies to glycoprotein (g)G1 and (g)G2 detect and differentiate past HSV-1 and HSV-2 infections. Primary HSV infection can be documented by demonstration of seroconversion. The development of nucleic-acid amplification tests heralded a new era in sensitive and diagnostic procedures for STIs. Many of these tests, however, are not commercially available or are too expensive for the populations that need them most.

## MANAGEMENT

The most effective way to prevent sexual transmission of STIs is to avoid sexual intercourse with an infected partner. Ideally, both new partners should get tested for STIs before initiating sexual intercourse. If a person chooses to have sexual intercourse with a partner whose infection status is unknown or who is infected with HIV or another STI, a new condom should be used for each act of intercourse. Condom use is not completely protective against acquisition of STI because of the presence of pathogen outside the protected skin or condom breakage. HPV or HSV infections often occur at the base of the penis or pubic area, which are not protected by condoms. Chronic suppressive therapy can reduce transmission of HSV-2. Prospects for development of a vaccine for HSV-2 and HPV are excellent. An effective HPV vaccine should reduce the incidence of anogenital cancers. Immunization for hepatitis A and B is advised to prevent transmission of these viral infections during intercourse.

## TABLE 27-1 Sexually Transmissible Pathogens and Associated Disease Syndromes

| Pathogen | Associated Disease or Syndrome |
| --- | --- |
| **Bacteria** | |
| *Neisseria gonorrhoeae* | Urethritis, epididymitis, proctitis, cervicitis, endometritis, salpingitis, perihepatitis, bartholinitis, pharyngitis, conjunctivitis, prepubertal vaginitis, prostatitis, accessory gland infection, disseminated gonococcal infection (DGI), chorioamnionitis, premature rupture of membranes, premature delivery, amniotic infection syndrome |
| *Chlamydia trachomatis* | All of the above except DGI, plus otitis media, rhinitis, and pneumonia in infants, and Reiter's syndrome |
| *Ureaplasma urealyticum* | Nongonococcal urethritis (NGU) |
| *Mycoplasma genitalium* | (?) Nongonococcal urethritis |
| *M. hominis* | Postpartum fever, salpingitis (?) |
| *Treponema pallidum* | Syphilis |
| *Gardnerella vaginalis* | Bacterial ("nonspecific") vaginosis (in conjunction with *Mycoplasma hominis* and vaginal anaerobes, such as *Mobiluncus* spp.) |
| *Mobiluncus curtisii* | Bacterial vaginosis |
| *M. mulieris* | Bacterial vaginosis |
| *Haemophilus ducreyi* | Chancroid |
| *Calymmatobacterium granulomatis* | Donovanosis (granuloma inguinale) |
| *Shigella* spp. | Shigellosis in men who have sex with men (MSM) |
| *Campylobacter* spp. | Enteritis, proctocolitis in MSM |
| *Helicobacter cinaedi* | (?) Proctocolitis; dermatitis, bacteremia in AIDS |
| *H. fenneliae* | (?) Proctocolitis; dermatitis, bacteremia in AIDS |
| **Viruses** | |
| HIV-1 and -2 | HIV disease, AIDS |
| HSV types 1 and 2 | Initial and recurrent genital herpes, aseptic meningitis, neonatal herpes |
| HPV | Condyloma acuminata; laryngeal papilloma; intraepithelial neoplasia and carcinoma of the cervix, vagina, vulva, anus, penis |
| Hepatitis A virus (HAV) | Acute hepatitis A |
| Hepatitis B virus (HBV) | Acute hepatitis B, chronic hepatitis B, hepatocellular carcinoma, polyarteritis nodosa, chronic membranous glomerulonephritis, mixed cryoglobulinemia (?), polymyalgia rheumatica (?) |
| Hepatitis C virus (HCV) | Acute hepatitis C, chronic hepatitis C, hepatocellular carcinoma, mixed cryoglobulinemia, chronic glomerulonephritis |
| Cytomegalovirus (CMV) | Heterophil-negative infectious mononucleosis; congenital CMV infection with gross birth defects and infant mortality, cognitive impairment (e.g., mental retardation, sensorineural deafness); protean manifestations in the immunosuppressed host |
| Molluscum contagiosum virus (MCV) | Genital molluscum contagiosum |
| Human T cell lymphotrophic virus (HTLV-I) | Human T cell leukemia or lymphoma, tropical spastic paraparesis |
| Human herpes virus type 8 (HHV-8) | Kaposi's sarcoma, body cavity lymphoma, multicentric Castleman's disease |

**TABLE 27-1    Sexually Transmissible Pathogens and Associated Disease Syndromes (*Continued*)**

| Pathogen | Associated Disease or Syndrome |
| --- | --- |
| **Protozoa** | |
| *Trichomonas vaginalis* | Vaginal trichomoniasis, NGU |
| *Entamoeba histolytica* | Amebiasis in MSM |
| *Giardia lamblia* | Giardiasis in MSM |
| **Fungi** | |
| *Candida albicans* | Vulvovaginitis, balanitis |
| **Ectoparasites** | |
| *Phthirus pubis* | Pubic lice infestation |
| *Sarcoptes scabiei* | Scabies |

SOURCES: Adapted from W Cates, Jr, KK Holmes, in JM Last, RB Wallace (eds): *Maxcy-Rosenau-Last, Public Health and Preventive Medicine,* 14th ed. Norwalk, CT. Appleton & Lange, 1998, pp 137–155; and KK. Holmes, HH Handsfield, in A Fauci, E Braunwald, KJ Isselbacher, JD Wilson, JB Martin, DL Kasper, SL Hauser, DL Longo (eds): *Harrison's Principles of Internal Medicine,* 14th ed. New York, McGraw-Hill, 1998.

**TABLE 27-2    Selected Syndromes and Complications of Sexually Transmitted Pathogens**

| Syndrome or Complication | Associated Sexually Transmitted Pathogen |
| --- | --- |
| **In men** | |
| HIV disease | HIV |
| Urethritis | *Neisseria gonorrhoeae, Chlamydia trachomatis,* HSV, *Ureaplasma urealyticum,* (*?*) *Mycoplasma genitalium, T. vaginalis* |
| Epididymitis | *C. trachomatis, N. gonorrhoeae* |
| Intestinal infections | |
| Proctitis | *N. gonorrhoeae,* HSV, *C. trachomatis* |
| Proctocolitis or enterocolitis | *Campylobacter* spp., *Shigella* spp., *Entamoeba histolytica,* (*?*) *Helicobacter* spp. |
| Enteritis | *Giardia lamblia* |
| **In women** | |
| HIV disease | HIV |
| Lower genitourinary tract infection | |
| Vulvitis | *Candida albicans,* HSV |
| Vaginitis | *Trichomonas vaginalis, C. albicans* |
| Vaginosis | *Gardnerella vaginalis, Mobiluncus* spp., other anaerobes, *Mycoplasma hominis* |
| Cervicitis | *N. gonorrhoeae, C. trachomatis,* HSV |
| Pelvic inflammatory disease | *N. gonorrhoeae, C. trachomatis, M. hominis,* anaerobes, group B streptococcus |
| Infertility | |
| Postsalpingitis, postobstetrical, postabortion | *N. gonorrhoeae, C. trachomatis, M. hominis* (*?*) |
| Pregnancy morbidity | Several STIs implicated in one or more of these conditions |
|   Chorioamnionitis, amniotic fluid infection, prematurity, premature rupture of membranes, preterm delivery, postpartum endometritis, ectopic pregnancy | |

**TABLE 27-2   Selected Syndromes and Complications of Sexually Transmitted Pathogens (*Continued*)**

| Syndrome or Complication | Associated Sexually Transmitted Pathogen |
|---|---|
| **In men and women** | |
| Rashes generalized, localized | *T. pallidum* |
| Neoplasia | |
| Cervical, vulvar, vaginal, anal, and penile, intraepithelial neoplasia, carcinoma | HPV |
| Hepatocellular carcinoma | HBV, HCV |
| Kaposi's sarcoma, body cavity lymphoma, Castleman's disease | HHV-8 |
| T cell lymphoma/leukemia | HTLV-I |
| Genital ulceration | HSV, *T. pallidum, Haemophilus ducreyi, Calymmatobacterium granulomatis, C. trachomatis* (LGV strains) |
| Acute arthritis with urogenital or intestinal infection | *N. gonorrhoeae, C. trachomatis, Shigella* spp., *Campylobacter* spp. |
| Hepatitis | HAV, HBV, HCV, CMV, *Treponema pallidum* |
| Genital warts | HPV |
| Molluscum contagiosum | MCV |
| Ectoparasite infestations | *Sarcoptes scabiei, Phthirus pubis* |
| Heterophil-negative mononucleosis | CMV, Epstein-Barr virus (some evidence for sexual transmission) |
| Tropical spastic paraparesis | HTLV-I |
| **In neonates and infants** | |
| Neonatal systemic infection, with potential cognitive impairment, deafness, death | Cytomegalovirus, HSV, *T. pallidum,* HIV |
| Conjunctivitis | *C. trachomatis, N. gonorrhoeae* |
| Pneumonia, (?) chronic pulmonary disease | *C. trachomatis, U. urealyticum (?)* |
| Otitis media | *C. trachomatis* |
| Sepsis, meningitis | Group B streptococcus |
| Laryngeal papillomatosis | HPV |

NOTE: For each of the above syndromes, some cases cannot yet be ascribed to any cause and must currently be considered idiopathic. "?" indicates a possible associated syndrome.

SOURCES: Adapted from W Cates, Jr, KK Holmes, in JM Last, RB Wallace (eds): *Maxcy-Rosenau-Last, Public Health and Preventive Medicine,* 14th ed. Norwalk, CT. Appleton & Lange, 1998, pp 137 155; and KK Holmes, HH Handsfield, in A Fauci, E Braunwald, KJ Isselbacher, JD Wilson, JB Martin, DL Kasper, SL Hauser, DL Longo (eds): *Harrison's Principles of Internal Medicine,* 14th ed. New York, McGraw-Hill, 1998.

# HUMAN PAPILLOMAVIRUS: MUCOSAL INFECTIONS ■

Mucosal HPV infections are the most common STIs seen by the dermatologist. When clinically symptomatic, lesions are barely visible papules to nodules to confluent masses occurring on anogenital or oral mucosa or skin, caused by a mucosal HPV type. Only 1 to 2% of HPV-infected individuals have any visibly detectable clinical lesion. HPV present in the birth canal can be transmitted to a newborn during vaginal delivery and can cause external genital warts (EGW) and respiratory papillomatosis. HPV dysplasia of the anogenital skin and mucosa ranging from mild to severe to squamous cell carcinoma (SCC) in situ (SCCIS); invasive SCC can arise within SCCIS, most commonly in the cervix and anal canal.

*Synonyms*: Condylomata acuminata, external genital warts, anogenital warts, venereal warts.

## EPIDEMIOLOGY AND ETIOLOGY

**Etiology**  HPV is a DNA papovavirus that multiplies in the nuclei of infected epithelial cells. More than 20 types of HPV can infect the genital tract: types 6, 11 most commonly; also types 16, 18, 31, 33 (see Table 25-2). Types 16, 18, 31, 33, and 35 are strongly associated with genital dysplasia and carcinoma. In individuals with multiple sexual partners, subclinical infection with multiple HPV types is common.

**Age of Onset**  Young, sexually active adults.

**Risk Factors for Acquiring HPV Infection**  Number of sexual partners/frequency of sexual intercourse; sexual partner with EGW, sexual partner's number of sexual partners, infection with other STIs.

**Transmission**  Through sexual contact: genital-genital, oral-genital, genital-anal. Microabrasions occur on epithelial surface allowing virions from infected partner to gain access to basal cell layer of noninfected partner. Digital transmission of nongenital warts probably accounts for few cases of EGW. During delivery, mothers with anogenital warts can transmit HPV to neonate, resulting in EGW and laryngeal papillomatosis in children.

**Incidence**  Most sexually active individuals are subclinically infected with HPV; most HPV infections are asymptomatic, subclinical, or unrecognized. 1% of sexually active adults (15 to 19 years of age) develop EGW. Increased manyfold during the past two decades.

**Psychosexual Impact of Genital Warts**  Public awareness of genital HPV infections is low. Few patients are aware of the role of HPV in anogenital cancer. Diagnosis of genital warts may result in fears about transmission and recurrence, sexual lifestyle changes (abstinence, caution, condoms), depression or low self-esteem, relationships becoming strained and/or breaking down, anxiety related to partner disclosure.

## PATHOGENESIS

"Low-risk" and "high-risk" HPV types both cause EGW. *HPV infection may persist for years in a dormant state and becomes infectious intermittently.* Exophytic warts are probably more infectious than subclinical infection.

*Immunosuppression* may result in new extensive HPV lesions, poor response to treatment, increased multifocal intraepithelial neoplasia. Immunosuppressed renal transplant recipients have a 17-fold greater incidence of genital HPV infection.

All HPV types replicate exclusively in host's cell nucleus. In benign HPV-associated lesions, HPV exists as a plasmid in cellular cytoplasm, replicating extrachromosomally. In malignant HPV-associated lesions, HPV integrates into host's chromosome, following a break in the viral genome (around E1/E2 region). E1 and E2 function is deregulated, resulting in cellular transformation.

# EXTERNAL GENITAL WARTS   ■

## HISTORY

**Incubation Period**   Several weeks to months to years.
**Duration of Lesions**   Months to years.
**Skin Symptoms**   Usually asymptomatic, except for cosmetic appearance. Itching, burning, bleeding, vaginal or urethral discharge, dyspareunia. Obstruction if large mass.

## PHYSICAL EXAMINATION

### Mucocutaneous Lesions
Four clinical types of genital warts occur; small papular, cauliflower-floret (acuminate or pointed) lesions (Figs. 27-1 through 27-3), keratotic warts, and flat-topped papules/plaques (most common on cervix). Lesions are skin-colored, pink, red, tan, brown. Lesions may be solitary, scattered, and isolated, or form voluminous confluent masses. In immunocompromised individuals, lesions may be huge. (Fig. 27-4) Acetic acid is helpful in visualizing lesions on the cervix and anus but is of little help in defining small EGW.
**Sites of Predilection**   *Male* Frenulum, corona, glans penis, prepuce, shaft (Fig. 27-1), scrotum.
*Female* Labia, clitoris, periurethral area, perineum, vagina (Fig. 27-2), cervix (flat lesions) (Fig. 27-5).
*Both Sexes* Perineal, perianal (Figs. 27-3 and 27-4), anal canal, rectal; urethral meatus, urethra, bladder; oropharynx.

### Laryngeal Papillomas
Relatively uncommon; associated with HPV-6 and -11. Arise most commonly on true vocal cords of larynx. Age: children <5 years of age; adults >20 years of age.

## DIFFERENTIAL DIAGNOSIS

**Papular/Nodular External Genital Lesions**   Normal anatomy (e.g., sebaceous glands, pearly penile papules, vestibular papillae), squamous intraepithelial lesions, SCCIS, invasive SCC, benign neoplasms (moles, seborrheic keratoses, skin tags, pilar cyst, angiokeratoma), inflammatory dermatoses (lichen nitidus, lichen planus), molluscum contagiosum, condylomata lata, folliculitis, scabietic nodules.

## LABORATORY EXAMINATIONS

**Acetowhitening**   Helpful in defining the extent of cervical and anal HPV infection. Acetowhitening of external genital lesions is not specific for warts. (See Appendix B.)
**Pap Smear**   All women should be encouraged to have an annual Pap smear since HPV is the major etiologic agent in pathogenesis for cancer of the cervix. Anal Pap test with a cervical brush and fixative solution is helpful in detecting anal dysplasia.
**Dermatopathology**   Biopsy is indicated if diagnosis is uncertain; the lesions do not respond to standard therapy; the lesions worsen during therapy; the patient is immunocompromised; warts are pigmented, indurated, fixed, and/or ulcerated; all suspect cervical lesions. Indicated in some cases to confirm diagnosis and/or rule out SCCIS or invasive SCC.
**Detection of HPV DNA**   Presence of HPV DNA and specific HPV types can be determined on smears and lesional biopsy specimens by in situ hybridization. However, no data support the use of type-specific HPV nucleic acid tests in the routine diagnosis or management of visible genital warts.
**Serology**   Occurrence of genital warts is a marker of unsafe sexual practices. Serologic tests for syphilis should be obtained on all patients to rule out coinfection with *Treponema pallidum, and all patients offered HIV testing.*

## DIAGNOSIS

Clinical diagnosis, occasionally confirmed by biopsy.

## COURSE AND PROGNOSIS

HPV is highly infectious, with an incubation period of 3 weeks to 8 months. Most HPV-infected individuals who develop EGW do so 2 to 3 months after becoming infected. Spontaneous regression occurs in 10 to 30% of patients within 3 months and is associated with an appropriate cell-mediated immune response. After regression, *subclinical infection may persist for life.* Recurrence may occur in individuals with normal immune function as well as with immunocompromise. Condylomata may recur due to

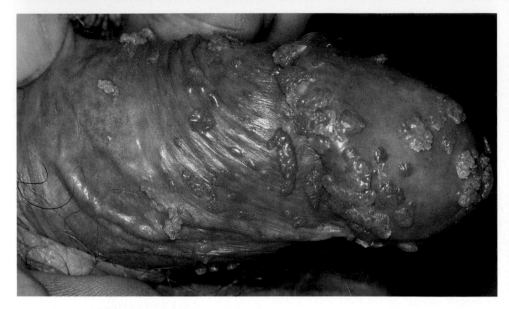

**FIGURE 27-1   Condylomata acuminata: penis**   *Multiple, soft, filiform papules, discrete with some coalescing to raspberry-like lesions, on the glans penis and prepuce.*

persistence of latent HPV in normal-appearing perilesional skin (see "Transmission," above). Recurrences more commonly result from reactivation of subclinical infection than from reinfection by a sex partner. If left untreated, genital warts may resolve on their own, remain unchanged, or grow. In placebo-treated cases, genital warts clear spontaneously in 20 to 30% of patients within 3 months.

In pregnancy, genital warts may increase in size and number, show increased vaginal involvement, and have an increased rate of secondary bacterial infection of vaginal warts. Children delivered vaginally of mothers with genital HPV infection are at risk for developing recurrent respiratory papillomatosis in later life.

The major significance of HPV infection is its oncogenicity. HPV types 16, 18, 31, and 33 are the major etiologic factors for cervical dysplasia and cervical SCC; bowenoid papulosis, in situ and invasive carcinoma of both the vulva and penis; anal SCC of homosexual/bisexual males. Treatment of external genital warts is not likely to influence the development of cervical cancer. The importance of the annual Pap test must be stressed for women with genital warts.

## MANAGEMENT

**Prevention**   Use of condoms reduces transmission to uninfected sex partners. Goal of treatment is removal of exophytic warts and amelioration of signs and symptoms—not eradication of HPV. No therapy has been shown to eradicate HPV. Treatment is more successful if warts are small and have been present for <1 year. Risk of transmission might be reduced by "debulking" genital warts. Selection of treatment should be guided by preference of patient—expensive therapies, toxic therapies, and procedures that result in scarring avoided.

**Indications for Therapy**   Cosmetic; reduce transmissibility; provide relief of symptoms; improve self-esteem.

**Primary Goal of Treating Visible Genital Warts**   Removal of symptomatic warts. Treatment can induce wart-free periods in most patients. Genital warts are often asymptomatic. No evidence indicates that currently available treatments eradicate or affect the natural history of HPV infection. Removal of warts may or may not decrease infectivity. If untreated, visible genital warts may resolve on their own, remain unchanged, or

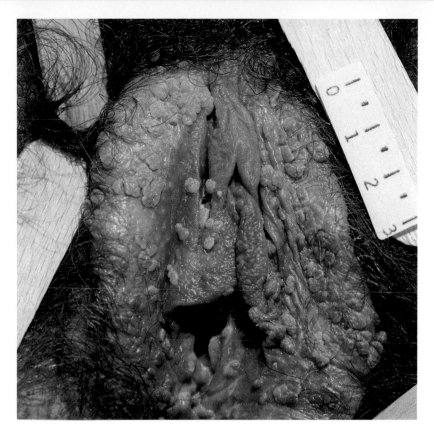

**FIGURE 27-2    Condylomata acuminata: vulva**    *Multiple, pink-brown, soft papules on the labia.*

increase in size and number. No evidence indicates that treatment of visible warts affects the development of cervical or anal cancer.

**Subclinical Genital HPV Infection (Without Exophytic Warts)**    Subclinical genital HPV infection is much more common than exophytic warts among both men and women. Infection is often indirectly diagnosed on the cervix by Pap smear, colposcopy, or biopsy and on the penis, vulva, and other genital skin by the appearance of white areas after application of acetic acid. Treatment is not indicated.

### External Genital/Perianal Warts
*Patient-Applied Agents*

*Imiquimod, 5% cream* Mechanism of action is via local cytokine release (interferon, tumor necrosis factor, interleukin). No direct antiviral activity. The cream, which is supplied in single-dose packets, is applied to the involved site by the patient, three times per week, usually at bedtime. Some patients experience local cytokine dermatitis. Treatment duration up to 16 weeks.

*Podofilox* 0.5% solution and gel. A purified and stable preparation of the active agent in podophyllin. Solution applied with a cotton swab and gel with a finger to condylomata and/or site involved (including normal-appearing skin between lesions) twice daily for 3 days, followed by 4 days of no therapy. This cycle may be repeated as necessary for a total of four cycles. Total area of treatment should not exceed 10 cm², and total volume should not exceed 0.5 mL/d. The health care provider should apply the initial treatment to demonstrate the proper application technique and identify lesions and sites to be treated. Podofilox is contraindicated during pregnancy.

### Clinician-Administered Therapy

*Cryosurgery with liquid nitrogen*   Apply with cotton swab or cryospray. Repeat weekly or biweekly. Relatively inexpensive, does not require anesthesia, and does not result in scarring.

*Podophyllin, 10 to 25%*   In compound tincture of benzoin. Limit the total volume of podophyllin solution applied to 0.5 mL or 10 cm$^2$ per session. Thoroughly wash off in 1 to 4 h. Treat <10 cm$^2$ per session. Repeat weekly if necessary. If warts persist after six applications, other therapeutic methods should be considered. Podophyllin contraindicated during pregnancy. Repeated application may cause irritation.

*Trichloroacetic acid (TCA) or bichloroacetic acid bicarbonate (BCA), 80 to 90%*   Apply only to warts: powder with talc or sodium (baking soda) to remove unreacted acid. Repeat weekly if necessary. If warts persist after six applications, other therapeutic methods should be considered.

*Surgical removal*   Either by tangential scissor excision, tangential shave excision, curettage, or electrosurgery.

*Electrodesiccation/electrocautery*   Highly effective in destruction of infected tissue and HPV. Should be attempted only by clinicians trained in the use of this modality. Electrodesiccation is contraindicated in patients with cardiac pacemakers.

*Carbon dioxide laser and electrodesiccation*   Useful in management of extensive warts, particularly for those patients who have not responded to other regimens; not appropriate for treatment of limited lesions.

### Cervical Warts

For women who have exophytic cervical warts, high-grade squamous intraepithelial lesions (SIL) must be excluded before treatment is begun. Management of exophytic cervical warts should include consultation with an expert.

### Vaginal Warts

*Cryosurgery with liquid nitrogen*   This modality is difficult due to "fog" formation, which restricts visualization of lesions.

*TCA or BCA, 80 to 90%*   Applied to warts only, powder with talc or sodium bicar-

bonate to remove unreacted acid if an excess amount is applied. Repeat weekly if necessary.

*Podophyllin, 10 to 25%*   In compound tincture of benzoin. Treated area must be dry before the speculum is removed. Treat with 2 cm$^2$ per session. Repeat application at weekly intervals. Systemic absorption is a concern.

### Urethral Meatus Warts

*Cryosurgery with liquid nitrogen*   As above.

*Podophyllin, 10 to 25%*   In compound tincture of benzoin. Treated area must be dry before contact with normal mucosa. Wash off in 1 to 2 h. Repeat weekly if necessary. If warts persist after six applications, other therapeutic methods should be considered.

### Anal Warts

Management of warts on rectal mucosa should be referred to an expert.

*Cryosurgery with liquid nitrogen*   As above.

*TCA or BCA, 80 to 90%*   Apply to warts only, powder with talc or sodium bicarbonate (baking soda) to remove unreacted acid. Repeat weekly if necessary. If warts persist after six applications, other therapeutic methods should be considered.

*Surgical removal*   As above.

### Oral Warts

*Cryosurgery with liquid nitrogen*   As above.

*Surgical removal*   As above.

**Follow-Up**   After visible warts have cleared, a follow-up evaluation is not mandatory. Patients should be cautioned to watch for recurrences, which occur most frequently during the first 3 months. Because the sensitivity and specificity of self-diagnosis of genital warts are unknown, patients concerned about recurrences should be offered a follow-up evaluation 3 months after treatment. Earlier follow-up visits may also be useful to document a wart-free state, to monitor for or treat complications of therapy, and to provide the opportunity for patient education and counseling. Women should be counseled about the need for regular cytologic screening as recommended for women without genital warts. The presence of genital warts is not an indication for cervical colposcopy.

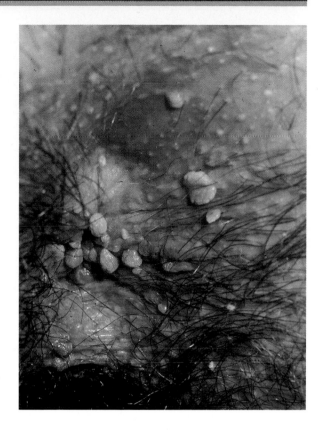

**FIGURE 27-3 Condylomata acuminata: perianal** *Typical condylomatous papules at anal orifice and perineum.*

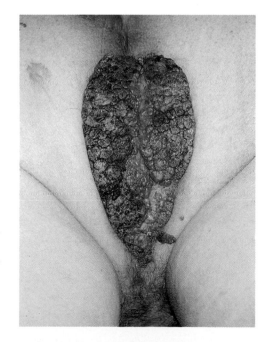

**FIGURE 27-4 Condylomata acuminata in an immunosuppressed individual** *A 21-year-old male, who underwent liver transplantation two years previously, noted the appearance of extragenital warts several months after the operation. A huge tumorous mass of condylomata on the perineum; the mass of tissue was painful and hygiene was difficult.*

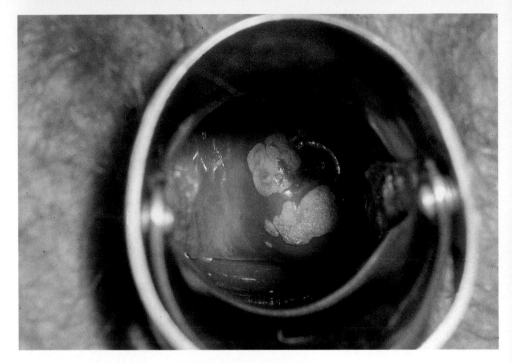

**FIGURE 27-5   Condylomata acuminata: uterine cervix**   *Sharply demarcated, whitish, flat plaques becoming confluent around the cervix.*

**Immunosuppressed Patients**   Persons who are immunosuppressed because of HIV or for other reasons may not respond as well as immunocompetent persons to therapy for genital warts and may have more frequent recurrences after treatment. SCC arising in or resembling genital warts might occur more frequently among immunosuppressed persons, requiring more frequent biopsy for confirmation of diagnosis.

**Management of Sex Partners**   Examination of sex partners is not necessary because role of re-infection is probably minimal. Most partners are probably already subclinically infected with HPV, even if no warts are visible.

## SQUAMOUS CELL CARCINOMA IN SITU AND INVASIVE SQUAMOUS CELL CARCINOMA OF THE ANOGENITAL SKIN   ■  ●

HPV infection of the anogenital epithelium can result in a spectrum of changes referred to as *squamous intraepithelial lesions* (SILs), ranging from mild dysplasia to SCCIS. Over time, these lesions can regress, persist, progress, or recur, in some cases to invasive SCC. Clinically, lesions appear as multifocal macules, papules, plaques on the external anogenital region. Lesions involving the cervix and anus have the highest risk for transformation to invasive SCC; however, lesions can transform at any site.

*Synonyms*: Vulvar intraepithelial neoplasia, penile intraepithelial neoplasm, bowenoid papulosis.

### EPIDEMIOLOGY AND ETIOLOGY

**Terminology**   The Bethesda System (National Cancer Institute) is currently used as terminology for "dysplastic" lesions caused by HPV on anogenital sites (Table 27-3). The terminology applies to both cytologic (Pap test) and histologic assessments. Intraepithelial neoplasia are designated as cervical (CIN), vulvar (VIN), penile (PIN), and anal (AIN). VIN is classified as VIN1 (mild dysplasia), VIN2 (moderate dysplasia), VIN3 (severe dysplasia or carcinoma in situ), and VIN3 differentiated type, basaloid, bowenoid (warty).

**Etiology**   HPV types 16, 18, 31, and 33 (see Table 25-2).

**Transmission**   HPV transmitted sexually. Autoinoculation. Rarely, HPV-16 transmitted from mother to newborn with subsequent development of bowenoid papulosis (BP) on penis.

**Incidence**   Marked increase during past two decades associated with increased sexual promiscuity. Cervical SCC is the second most common female malignancy worldwide, second only to breast cancer. It is the most frequent malignancy in developing countries—500,000 new cases and 200,000 deaths worldwide attributed to it annually.

**Risk Factors**   Immunocompromised state, cigarette smoking are risk factors for more dysplastic lesions and invasive SCC.

### PATHOGENESIS

HPV-16- and -18-infected cells may not be able to differentiate fully as a result of either (1) functional interference of cell cycle–regulating proteins, caused by viral gene expression (e.g., interaction between HPV-16 E6 with cellular protein p53, interaction between HPV-16 E7 with cellular protein pRB); or (2) overproduction of E5, E6, and E7. When this occurs, the host DNA synthesis continues unchecked and leads to rapidly dividing undifferentiated cells with morphologic characteristics of intraepithelial neoplasias. Accumulated chromosomal breakages, rearrangements, deletions, and other genomic mutations in these cells lead to cells with invasion capability and, ultimately, to cervical malignancy.

### HISTORY

**Duration of Lesions**   Weeks to months to years to decades.

**Incubation Period**   Months to years.

**Systems Review**   Prior history of condylomata acuminata. Female partners of males may have CIN.

### PHYSICAL EXAMINATION

#### Skin Lesions

Erythematous macules. Lichenoid (flat-topped) or pigmented papules (called *bowenoid papulosis*) (Figs. 27-6 to 27-8); may show some confluence or form plaque(s) (Fig. 27-8). Leukoplakia-like plaque. Surface usually smooth, velvety. Nodule or ulceration in field of SIL suggests invasive SCC (Figs. 27-9 and 27-10). Tan, brown, pink, red, violaceous, white. Characteristically clusters, i.e., commonly multifocal. May be solitary.

*Distribution*   Males: glans penis, prepuce (75%) (flat lichenoid papules or erythematous macules); penile shaft (25%) (pigmented papules) (Fig. 27-6). Females: labia majora and minora, clitoris (Fig. 27-7). Multicentric involvement of the cervix, vulva, perineum,

TABLE 27-3   Bethesda System for Classification of Anogenital Dysplasia

| Histologic Findings | Older Terminology/ Replaced | | Still Older Terminology |
|---|---|---|---|
| Atypical proliferating suprabasal cells present in the lower one-third of the epithelium, although cytopathic changes of HPV are full thickness | Low-grade squamous intraepithelial lesion (LSIL) | Intraepithelial 1 (IN1) | Mild dysplasia |
| Atypical proliferating suprabasal cells present in the lower two-thirds of the epithelium, although cytopathic changes of HPV are full thickness | High-grade SIL (HSIL) | IN2 and IN3 | |
| Atypical proliferating suprabasal cells present in the full thickness of the epithelium | Squamous cell carcinoma in situ (SCCIS) | Squamous cell carcinoma in situ (SCCIS) | Erythroplasia of Querat, Bowen's disease, bowenoid papulosis |
| Invasive SCC present, usually arising in a field of HSIL | Invasive SCC | Invasive SCC | |

and/or anus (Fig. 27-8) occurs not infrequently. Both sexes: inguinal folds, perineal/perianal skin (Fig. 27-8). Oropharyngeal mucosa.

*Acetowhitening* Application of 3 to 5% acetic acid to the area of involvement for 5 min may facilitate visualization of lesions on the cervix or in the anal canal.

*Other* May be associated with cervical dysplasia, CIN, cervical SCC. Rarely, SCCIS of other sites, i.e., periungual, intraoral.

## DIFFERENTIAL DIAGNOSIS

**Multiple Skin-Colored Papules ± Hyperkeratosis** External genital warts, psoriasis vulgaris; lichen planus.

**Pigmented Anogenital Macule(s)/Papule(s)** Genital lentiginosis, melanoma (in situ or invasive), pigmented basal cell carcinoma, angiokeratomas.

## LABORATORY EXAMINATIONS

**Dermatopathology** Epidermal proliferation with numerous mitotic figures, abnormal mitoses, atypical pleomorphic cells with large hyperchromatic, often clumped nuclei, dyskeratotic cells;

basal membrane intact. Koilocytosis. Recent application of podophyllin to condyloma acuminatum may cause changes similar to SCCIS.

**Southern Blot Analysis** Identifies HPV type.

**Pap Smear** Koilocytotic atypia.

**Exfoliative Cytology** Cervical Pap smears have been recommended annually for women ≥50 years of age. Cytology of the anal canal may also be helpful in management of individuals with a history of anal HPV infection, especially if immunocompromised (HIV disease, renal transplant recipients). Anal Pap tests are obtained with a cervical brush and ThinPrep solution. By the Bethesda System, these cytologic findings are reported as atypical squamous cells of undetermined significance (ASCUS), low-grade squamous intraepithelial lesion (LSIL), high-grade (SILH), and SCC.

## DIAGNOSIS

Clinical suspicion, confirmed by biopsy of lesion.

## COURSE AND PROGNOSIS

Invasive SCC develops only through well-

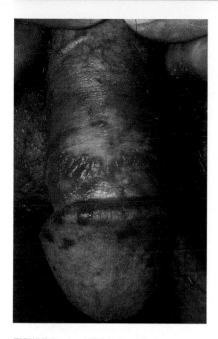

**FIGURE 27-6 HPV-induced squamous cell carcinoma in situ: penis** *Multiple, red papules, discrete and confluent, on the distal shaft and glans penis. Diagnosis is made on lesional biopsy.*

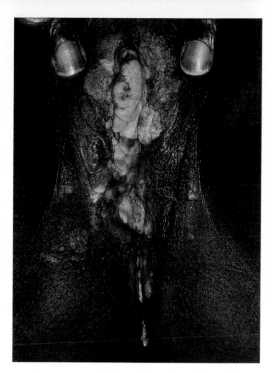

**FIGURE 27-7 HPV-induced squamous cell carcinoma in situ: vulva/perineum** *Huge verrucous lesions on the vulva and perineum recurred several times after laser surgery in an HIV-infected female; SCCIS was also present on the cervix. The vulvar lesion evolved into invasive SCC, so-called verrucous carcinoma (giant condyloma of Buschke and Lowenstein).*

defined precursor lesions. Over time, these lesions can regress, persist, recur, or progress, in some cases to invasive SCC. Natural history of CIN is best studied: progression to invasive SCC occurs in 36% of cases over a 20-year period. Rate of progression of AIN is not known but appears to be increasing. AIN may develop deep in glands and, although detected cytologically, can exist before visible lesions are detected with colposcopy. Patients with intraepithelial neoplasias, which often occurs in immunocompromised individuals, should be followed indefinitely, with monitoring by exfoliative cytology and lesional biopsy specimens.

## MANAGEMENT

**Colposcopy** A colposcope is a binocular microscope used to examine the cervix, providing magnification (6- to 40-fold) and illumination. The most common indication for colposcopy is abnormal exfoliative cytology. Acetic acid, 3 to 5%, is applied to the cervix, which causes columnar and abnormal epithelium to become edematous. Abnormal (atypical) epithelium adopts a white or opaque appearance that can be distinguished from the normal pink epithelium. Abnormal epithelium is then biopsied. Colposcopy can also be performed on individuals with abnormal anal exfoliative cytology, and biopsy specimens obtained from abnormal site(s).

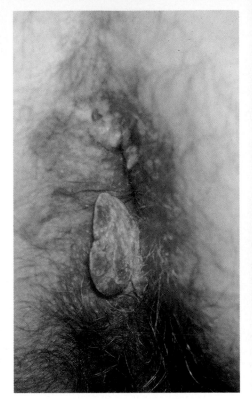

**FIGURE 27-8   HPV-induced squamous cell carcinoma in situ: perianal/perineal**   *Asymptomatic well-demarcated perianal/perineal pink plaque. The rudder-like lesion is a skin tag at the site of an old hemorrhoid. The lesions resolved with 5% imiquimod cream. Although the individual was apparently healthy, underlying immunodeficiency was present; lymphoma was diagnosed 1 year after the SCCIS was detected.*

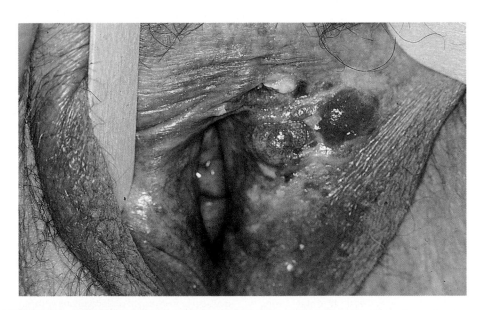

**FIGURE 27-9   HPV-induced in situ and invasive squamous cell carcinoma: vulva**   *Several red, flesh nodules (invasive SCC) arising within a white plaque (SCCIS) on the left labium.*

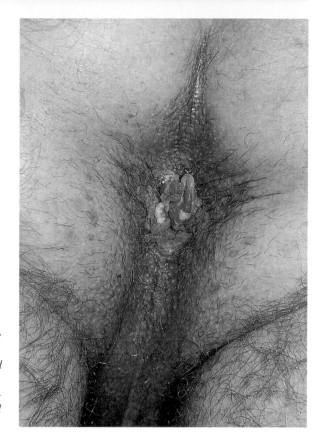

**FIGURE 27-10 HPV-induced in situ and invasive squamous cell carcinoma: perineal/perianal** *Brown perineal and perianal macules and papules (SCCIS) with a pink nodule arising at the anal verge in an HIV-infected male. The patient presented when he detected the nodule, which he thought was a hemorrhoid. Excisional biopsy of the nodule detected invasive SCC arising within SCCIS.*

**Biopsy of Lesions** In cases of documented SIL or SCCIS, biopsy specimens should be obtained from rapidly enlarging lesions, areas of ulceration or bleeding, exuberant tissue with abnormal vascularity.

**Local Therapy of SIL** The only way of possibly reducing the potential risk of invasive SCC with its morbidity and mortality is diagnosis and eradication of intraepithelial disease. Because lesions are relatively uncommon, cases are often best managed by a dermatologist with clin-ical experience in the care of these patients, an oncologic gynecologist, or a colorectal surgeon. If lesion biopsy specimens do not show early invasion, lesions can be treated medically or surgically.

**Medical Management** 5-Fluorouracil cream has been used but is difficult to use because of erosions. Imiquimod cream 5% is also effective.

**Surgical Management** Surgical excision, Mohs' surgery, electrosurgery, laser vaporization, cryosurgery.

# HERPES SIMPLEX VIRUS: GENITAL INFECTIONS     ■   ◑

Genital herpes (GH) is a chronic sexually transmitted viral infection, characterized by symptomatic and asymptomatic viral shedding. In most cases, both primary infection and recurrences are asymptomatic. When symptomatic, primary GH may present with grouped vesicles at the site of inoculation associated with significant pain and regional lymphadenopathy. When aware of GH, individuals may notice mild symptoms, uncommonly of recurring outbreaks of vesicles at the same site. Most symptoms from GH relate to the psychological stigma of having a chronic incurable and transmissible STI. (See also "Herpes Simplex Virus Infections," Section 25.) Neonates are susceptible to HSV infection when exposed perinatally, with risk of significant morbidity and mortality.

*Synonyms*: Herpes progenitalis, herpes genitalis, genital herpes simplex.

## EPIDEMIOLOGY AND ETIOLOGY

**Age of Onset**   Young, sexually active adults.

**Etiology**   HSV-2 > HSV-1. Currently in the United States, 30% of new cases of GH are caused by HSV-1.

**Prevalence**   Highly variable. Depends on many factors: country, region of residence, population subgroup, sex, age. Higher among higher risk sexual behavior groups. Higher among women than men.

Prevalence of HSV-2 seropositivity in general population:

• United States: 21%
• Europe: 8 to 15%
• Africa: 40 to 50% in 20-year-olds

Strongly associated with age, increasing from negligible levels in children <12 to as high as 80% among higher risk populations. In a given population, HSV-1 prevalence is almost always > HSV-2 prevalence.

Prevalence is highest in areas of Africa and parts of the Americas. Lower in western and southern Europe than in northern Europe and North America. Lower in Asia than other areas.

In the United States, >600,000 new infections annually; 30 million Americans are HSV-2 infected, i.e., approximately one in five adults. Older studies report the presence of antibodies to HSV-2 varies with the sexual history of the individual: nuns, 3%; middle class, 25%; heterosexuals at an STD clinic, 26%; homosexuals, 46%; lower classes, 46 to 60%; prostitutes, 70 to 80%.

**Race and Sex**   By HSV-2 seropositivity studies in the United States, more common in blacks: 3 in 5 men, 4 in 5 women; in whites: 1 in 5 men, 1 in 4 women. In whites, prevalence levels off after age 30 years. In blacks/Hispanics, prevalence continues to increase after age 30.

**Transmission**   Usually skin-to-skin contact. In most cases, 70% of transmission occurs during times of asymptomatic HSV shedding, which occurs during 1% of days when no identifiable lesion is present. Shedding rate is higher from HSV-2 than HSV-1. Transmission rate in discordant couples (one partner infected, the other not) approximately 10% per year; 25% of females become infected, compared with only 4 to 6% of males. Prior HSV-1 infection is protective; in females with anti-HSV-1 antibodies, 15% become infected with HSV-2, but in those without anti-HSV-1 antibodies, 30% become infected with HSV-2.

**Risk Factors for Transmission**   Risk increases with number of sex partners. 40% of those with 50 different partners have genital HSV infection.

**Diseases Characterized by Genital Ulcers**   In the United States, most patients with genital ulcers have GH, syphilis, or chancroid. The relative frequency varies by geographic area and patient population, but in most areas GH is the most common of these diseases. More than one of these diseases may be present among at least 3 to 10% of patients with genital ulcers. Each disease has been associated with an increased risk for HIV infection.

**Impact of GH**   The physical symptoms of GH are minor in most individuals. The major symptoms are psychological, i.e., social stigmatization and fear of harming someone through sexual intercourse.

**Pregnancy and GH**   Asymptomatic HSV shedding occurs in 0.35 to 1.4% of women in labor in the United States. 32% of pregnant women have anti-HSV antibodies. 10% of pregnant women are at risk for primary HSV-2 infection from HSV-2 infected partners. Incidence of neonatal herpes: 1 in 2000 to 1 in 15,000 births.

95% of newborns with HSV infection contract it during labor and delivery. Transmission can occur intrauterine, perinatally, or postnatally. Risk factors for neonatal HSV infection: primary GH in mother at time of delivery, absent maternal anti-HSV antibody, procedures on fetus, father with HSV infection. Treatment of mother with GH at time of delivery is an option for cesarean section (not approved).

## PATHOGENESIS

HSV infection is transmitted through close contact with a person shedding virus at a peripheral site, mucosal surface, or secretion. HSV is inactivated promptly at room temperature; aerosol or fomitic spread unlikely. Infection occurs via inoculation onto susceptible mucosal surface or break in skin. Subsequent to primary infection at inoculation site, HSV ascends peripheral sensory nerves and enters sensory or autonomic nerve root ganglia, where latency is established. Latency can occur after both symptomatic and asymptomatic primary infection. Recrudescences may be clinically symptomatic or asymptomatic.

## HISTORY

**Incubation Period** 2- to 20-day (average 6) incubation period.
**Symptoms** Only 9.2% of HSV-2 seropositive individuals are aware that symptoms are those of GH; 90.8% do not recognize symptoms of GH.
*Primary GH* Most individuals with primary infection are asymptomatic. Those with symptoms report fever, headache, malaise, myalgia, peaking within the first 3 to 4 days after onset of lesions, resolving during the subsequent 3 to 4 days. Depending on location, pain, itching, dysuria, lumbar radiculitis, vaginal or urethral discharge are common symptoms. Tender inguinal lymphadenopathy occurs during second and third weeks. Deep pelvic pain associated with pelvic lymphadenopathy. Some cases of first clinical episode of GH are manifested by extensive disease that requires hospitalization.
*Recurrent GH* New symptoms may result from old infections. Most individuals with GH do not experience "classic" findings of grouped vesicles on erythematous base. Common symptoms are itching, burning, fissure, redness, irritation

prior to eruption of vesicles. Dysuria, sciatica, rectal discomfort.
*Systemic Symptoms* Symptoms of aseptic HSV-2 meningitis can occur with primary or recurrent GH.

## PHYSICAL EXAMINATION

### Skin Lesions
Most clinical lesions are minor breaks in the mucocutaneous epithelium, presenting as erosion, "abrasions," fissures. The classically described findings are uncommon.
*Primary GH* An erythematous plaque is often noted initially, followed soon by grouped vesicles, which may evolve to pustules; these become eroded as the overlying epidermis sloughs (Fig. 27-11). Erosions are punched out and may enlarge to ulcerations, which may be crusted or moist. These epithelial defects heal in 2 to 4 weeks, often with resulting postinflammatory hypo- or hyperpigmentation, uncommonly with scarring. The area of involvement may be circumferential around the penis, or the entire vulva may be involved.
*Recurrent GH* Lesions may be similar to primary infection but on a reduced scale. Often a 1- to 2-cm plaque of erythema surmounted with vesicles (Fig. 27-12), which rupture with formation of erosions (Fig. 27-13). Heals in 1 to 2 weeks.
**Distribution** *Males* Primary infection: glans, prepuce, shaft, sulcus, scrotum, thighs, buttocks. Recurrences: penile shaft (Fig. 27-12), glans, buttocks.
*Females* Primary infection: labia majora/minora (Fig. 27-11), perineum, inner thighs. Recurrences: labia majora/minora (Fig. 27-13), buttocks.
**Anorectal Infection** Occurs in male homosexuals (often HSV-1); characterized by tenesmus, anal pain, proctitis, discharge, and ulcerations (Fig. 27-14) as far as 10 cm into anal canal.
**General Findings** *Regional Lymph Nodes* Inguinal/femoral lymph nodes enlarged, firm, nonfluctuant, tender; usually unilateral.
*Signs of Aseptic Meningitis* Fever, nuchal rigidity. Can occur in the absence of GH. Pain along sciatic nerve.

## DIFFERENTIAL DIAGNOSIS

**Anogenital Erosive(s)/Ulcer(s)** Trauma, candidiasis, syphilitic chancre, fixed drug eruption, chancroid, gonococcal erosion.

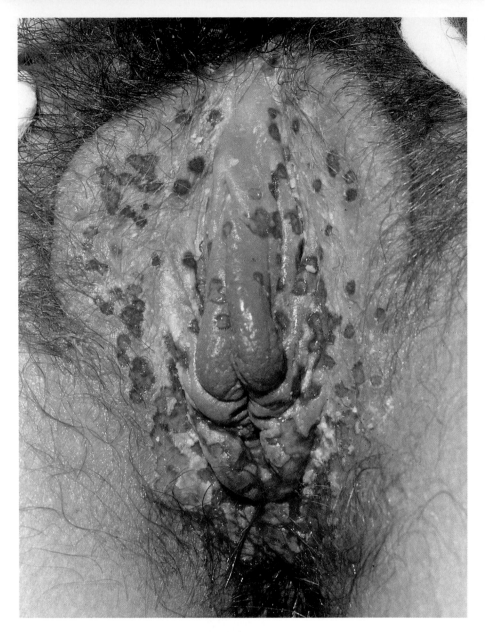

**FIGURE 27-11    Genital herpes: primary vulvar infection**    *Multiple, extremely painful, punched-out, confluent, shallow ulcers on the edematous vulva and perineum. Micturition is often very painful. Associated inguinal lymphadenopathy is common.*

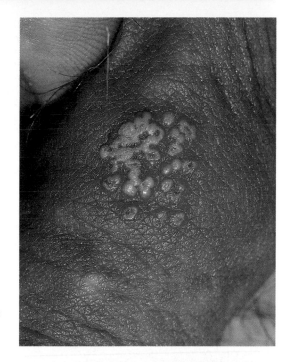

**FIGURE 27-12 Genital herpes: recurrent infection of the penis** *Group of vesicles with early central crusting on a red base arising on the shaft of the penis. This "textbook" presentation, however, is much less common than small asymptomatic erosions or fissures.*

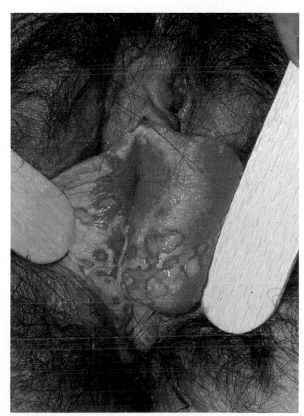

**FIGURE 27-13 Genital herpes: recurrent vulvar infection** *Large, painful erosions on the labia. Extensive lesions such as these are uncommon in recurrent genital herpes in an otherwise healthy individual.*

## LABORATORY STUDIES

See "Herpes Simplex Virus Infections," page 799.

## DIAGNOSIS

Because in most cases intermittent asymptomatic shedding is occurring and lesions are "atypical" (not grouped vesicles on erythematous base), GH must be confirmed by viral culture or direct fluorescent antibody (DFA) or serology.

## COURSE AND PROGNOSIS

GH may be recurrent and has no cure. 70% of HSV-2 infections are asymptomatic. HSV-2 GH recurs approximately six times per year; HSV-1 GH usually recurs, on the average, only once per year. Of individuals with initially symptomatic genital HSV-2 infection, almost all have symptomatic recurrences; recurrence rates are high in those with an extended first episode of infection, regardless of whether antiviral therapy is given. The rate of recurrence is 20% higher in men than women. Chronic suppressive therapy does not completely suppress viral shedding; it is reduced by 95% as detected by viral culture, and by 80% by polymerase chain reaction (PCR). Chronic suppressive therapy may reduce transmission, but this has not been documented. The incidence of primary infection with acyclovir-resistant HSV strains in individuals never exposed to acyclovir is 2.7% in the United States. Treatment of first-episode infection prevents compliations such as meningitis, radiculitis. Erythema multiforme may complicate GH, occurring 1 to 2 weeks after an outbreak.

## MANAGEMENT

See Table 27-4.

---

**TABLE 27-4   Management of Genital Herpes**

| | |
|---|---|
| **Prevention of GH** | |
| Sexual transmission | • Patients should be advised to abstain from sexual activity while lesions are present. |
| | • Use of condoms should be encouraged during all sexual exposures. |
| | • Efficacy of chronic suppressive therapy not proven. |
| | • Patients with GH should be told about the natural history of the disease, with emphasis on the potential of recurrent episodes, asymptomatic viral shedding, and sexual transmission. |
| | • Sexual transmission of HSV has been documented to occur during periods without evidence of lesions. In discordant couples, transmission usually occurs during period of asymptomatic shedding. |
| | • Risk for neonatal infection should be explained to all patients— male and female—with GH. |
| Perinatal transmission | Many experts recommend serotesting for HSV-1 and HSV-2 (Western blot) at the first prenatal visit. Infants born to women who asymptomatically shed HSV have reduced birth weight and increased prematurity. |
| **Topical antiviral therapy** | No significant efficacy. |
| **Oral antiviral therapy** | Antiviral agents provide partial control of symptoms and signs of herpes episodes when used to treat first clinical episode or when used as suppressive therapy. They neither eradicate latent virus nor affect subsequent risk, frequency, or severity of recurrences after drug is discontinued. Even after laboratory testing, at least a quarter of patients with GH have no laboratory-confirmed diagnosis. Many experts recommend treatment for chancroid and syphilis as well as GH if the diagnosis is unclear or if the patient resides in a community in which chancroid is present. |

*(Continued)*

**TABLE 27-4    Management of Genital Herpes (Continued)**

| | |
|---|---|
| First clinical episode (primary or first symptomatic) | Antiviral agents are more effective in treating primary infections than recurrences. Most effective when initiated ≤48 h after onset of symptoms. |
| Acyclovir | 400 mg tid or 200 mg 5 times daily for 7–10 days or until clinical resolution occurs. |
| Valacyclovir | 1 gm bid for 10 days. |
| Famciclovir | 250 mg bid for 10 days. |
| First clinical episode of herpes proctitis | |
| Acyclovir | 400 mg PO 5 times daily for 10 days or until clinical resolution occurs. |
| Recurrent episodes | When treatment is instituted (by patient) during the prodrome or within 2 days of onset of lesions, patients with recurrent disease experience limited benefit from therapy because the severity of the eruption is reduced. If early treatment cannot be administered, most immunocompetent patients with recurrent disease do not benefit from acyclovir treatment; and for these patients it is not generally recommended. |
| Acyclovir | 400 mg PO tid for 5 days or 800 mg PO bid for 5 days. |
| Valacyclovir | 500 mg bid for 5 days. |
| Famciclovir | 250 mg bid for 5 days. |
| Daily suppressive therapy | Reduces frequency of recurrences by at least 75% among patients with frequent (more than 6–9 per year) recurrences. Suppressive treatment with oral acyclovir does not totally eliminate symptomatic or asymptomatic viral shedding or the potential for transmission. Safety and efficacy have been documented among persons receiving daily therapy for as long as 5 years. Acyclovir-resistant strains of HSV have been isolated from some persons receiving suppressive therapy, but these strains have not been associated with treatment failure among immunocompetent patients. *After 1 year of continuous therapy, acyclovir should be discontinued to allow assessment of the patient's rate of recurrent episodes.* |
| Acyclovir | 400 mg bid. |
| Valacyclovir | 500–1000 mg/d. |
| Famciclovir | 250 mg bid. |
| Severe disease/immuno-compromise | Patients with herpes who do not respond to the recommended dose of acyclovir may require a higher oral dose of acyclovir, IV acyclovir, or may be infected with an acyclovir-resistant HSV strain, requiring IV foscarnet. The role of valacyclovir and famciclovir are not yet established. IV therapy should be provided for patients with severe disease or complications necessitating hospitalization (e.g., disseminated infection that includes encephalitis, pneumonitis, or hepatitis). |
| Acyclovir | 5 mg/kg body weight IV every 8 h for 5–7 days or until clinical resolution is attained or 400 mg PO 5 times a day for 7–14 days. |
| Oral valacyclovir *or* famciclovir | Have reduced the necessity for IV acyclovir therapy. |
| Neonatal | See "Neonatal HSV Infection," Section 25. |
| Acyclovir-resistant | See "HSV Infections," Section 25. |
| Foscarnet | 40 mg/kg IV q8h for 14–21 days. |
| Imiquimod cream 5% | May be effective. |

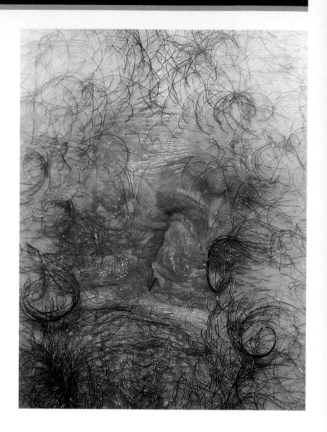

**FIGURE 27-14   Genital herpes: recurrent infection of the anus and perineum**   *Multiple, painful, sharply demarcated ulcers in an HIV-infected male.*

**Website**

American Social Health Association: *http://www.ashastd.org/hrc/helpgrp1.html*

**Keys for Health Care Providers When Discussing GH with Patients**

- Genital herpes is common and may be caused by HSV-1 or HSV-2.
- 1 person in 6 worldwide has genital herpes caused by HSV-2.
- 1 person in 5 in the United States has genital herpes.
- About 80% of infections are not recognized because of mild or absent symptoms.
- Most first presentations of herpes represent reactivation of previously latent infection rather than recently acquired primary infection.
- More than one-half of infected persons get genital herpes from a partner who does not know he or she is infected.
- Genital herpes can be transmitted by genital or oral sex (cold sores).

- Anyone with genital herpes may shed virus a few days each year without symptoms.
- Transmission of herpes can occur within committed long-term relationships and can occur through close genital or oral-genital contact in persons who have never had penetrative sex.
- People who experience a first episode will get better; lesions will heal and recurrences will usually be less severe.
- HSV-2 reactivates more frequently than HSV-1.
- Antiviral treatment can be effective, especially suppressive therapy.
- Condoms reduce the risk of transmission, but it is also advisable to avoid skin-to-skin contact when lesions are present.
- Genital herpes does not cause cervical cancer or affect fertility.
- Neonatal herpes is serious but rare.
- Women with genital herpes can have a safe pregnancy and vaginal delivery; new infections in the first or third trimester need especially close medical follow-up.

## *NEISSERIA GONORRHOEAE* INFECTIONS

Mucosal infections with *Neisseria gonorrhoeae* (gonococcus) share the clinical spectrum of *Chlamydia trachomatis*; symptoms are usually more severe with gonococcal infections. Most infections among men produce symptoms that cause them to seek curative treatment soon enough to prevent serious sequelae–but this may not be soon enough to prevent transmission to others. Many infections among women do not produce recognizable symptoms until complications [e.g., pelvic inflammatory disease (PID)] have occurred. In males, the most common presentation is an acute urethritis; in females, cervicitis. Other sites in the genitourinary tract may become infected as well as the rectum, pharynx, and conjunctiva. Both symptomatic and asymptomatic cases of PID can result in tubal scarring that leads to infertility or ectopic pregnancy. Because gonococcal infections among women are often asymptomatic, an important component of gonorrhea control continues to be the screening of women at high risk for STIs. Gonococcemia results in seeding of multiple sites, most commonly the joints and skin, resulting in DGI.

### EPIDEMIOLOGY AND ETIOLOGY

**Etiology**  *N. gonorrhoeae*, the gonococcus, a gram-negative diplococcus. Humans are the only natural reservoir of the organism. Strains that cause DGI tend to cause minimal genital inflammation. In the United States, these strains have occurred infrequently during the past decade.

**Age of Onset**  Young, sexually active. In newborns, conjunctivitis.

**Sex**  Young females; males who have sex with males. Symptomatic infection more common in males. Pharyngeal and anorectal in homosexual males.

**Race**  In the United States; highest incidence in blacks, lowest in those of Asian/Pacific Island descent.

**Transmission**  *Sexually*, from partner who either is asymptomatic or has minimal symptoms. *Neonate* exposed to infected secretions in birth canal. About 1% of patients with untreated mucosal gonococcal infection develop DGI. Gonorrhea may enhance HIV transmission.

**Co-infection**  Up to 40% of persons co-infected with *C. trachomatis*. Gonorrhea enhances transmission as well as acquisition of HIV.

**Demography**  Worldwide. In Africa, median prevalence of gonorrhea in pregnant women is 10%. Incidence of DGI varies with local incidence of DGI strains of gonococcus.

**Incidence**  Highest in developing countries. Prevalence of DGI in pregnant women: 10% in Africa; 5% in Latin America; 4% in Asia.

### PATHOGENESIS

Gonococcus has affinity for columnar epithelium; stratified and squamous epithelia are more resistant to attack. Epithelium is penetrated between epithelial cells, causing a submucosal inflammation with polymorphonuclear (PMN) leukocyte reaction with resultant purulent discharge. Strains of gonococcus that cause DGI tend to cause little genital inflammation and thereby escape detection. Most signs and symptoms of DGI are manifestations of immune-complex formation and deposition. Multiple episodes of DGI may be associated with abnormality of terminal complement component factors.

### LABORATORY STUDIES

**Gram's Stain**  Gram-negative diplococci intracellularly in PMNs in exudate (Fig. 27-15).

**Culture**  Isolation on gonococcal-selective media, i.e., chocolatized blood agar, Martin-Lewis medium, Thayer-Martin medium. Antimicrobial susceptibility testing important due to resistant strains.

***Specimen Collection Sites*** *Heterosexual men*: Urethra, oropharynx. *Homosexual men*: Urethra, rectum, oropharynx. *Women*: Cervix, rectum, oropharynx. *DGI*: Blood.

**Serologic Tests**  None available for gonorrhea. All patients should have a serologic test for syphilis and should be offered HIV testing.

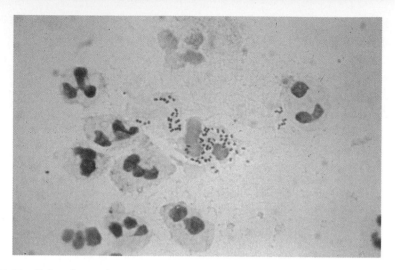

**FIGURE 27-15**   *Neisseria gonorrhoeae*: Gram's stain   *Multiple, gram-negative diplococci within polymorphonuclear leukocytes as well as in the extracellular areas of a smear from a urethral discharge.*

## MANAGEMENT

See Table 27-5, page 908. For Centers for Disease Control and Prevention (CDC) STD treatment guidelines—2002, see *http://-www.cdc.gov/mmwr/preview/mmwrhtml/rr5106 a1.htm*

## LOCALIZED INFECTION (GONORRHEA)    ■

Gonorrhea affectes mucocutaneous surfaces of the lower genitourinary tract, anus and rectum and the oropharynx. The most common presentation in males is a purulent urethral discharge. In females, cervical infection is most common and is often asymptomatic; if untreated, infection can spread to deeper structures with abscess formation and DGI.
*Synonyms*: Clap, blennorrhagia, blennorrhea.

## HISTORY

**Incubation Period**   *Males*: 90% of males develop urethritis within 5 days of exposure. *Females*: Usually >14 days when symptomatic; however, up to 75% of women are asymptomatic.

**Skin Symptoms**   *Urethra*: discharge, dysuria. *Vagina*: discharge; deep pelvic or lumbar pain. *Anus/rectum*: Copious purulent anal discharge; burning or stinging pain on defecation; tenesmus; blood in/on stool. *Oropharynx*: Mild sore throat.

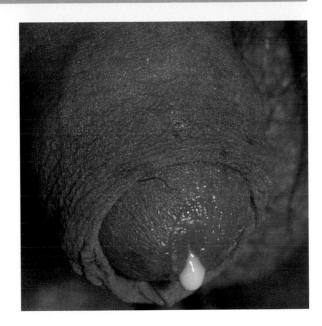

**FIGURE 27-16 Gonorrhea** *Purulent, creamy urethral discharge from the distal urethra of a male.*

## PHYSICAL EXAMINATION

**External Genitalia** *Males* Urethral discharge ranging from scanty and clear to purulent and copious (Fig. 27-16). *Edema*: meatus, prepuce, or penis. Balanoposthitis with subpreputial discharge in uncircumcised men; balanitis in circumcised men. Folliculitis or cellulitis of thigh or abdomen. *Deeper structures*: Prostatitis, epididymitis, vesiculitis, cystitis.
*Females* Periurethral edema, urethritis. Purulent discharge from cervix but no vaginitis. In prepubescent females, vulvovaginitis. Bartholin's abscess. *Deeper structures*: PID with signs of peritonitis, endocervicitis, endosalpingitis, endometritis.
**Anorectum** In females and homosexual males, proctitis with pain and purulent discharge. In female, can spread from cervicitis.
**Pharynx** Occurs secondary to oral-genital sexual exposure. In females and homosexual males, pharyngitis with erythema. Always coexists with genital infection.
**Eyes** Conjunctivitis, swollen eyelid, severe hypermia, chemosis, profuse purulent discharge; rarely, corneal ulcer and perforation. In newborn, organism is transmitted as newborn passes through birth canal. Usually occurs in the absence of genital infection, copious purulent conjunctival discharge. Can be complicated by corneal ulceration and perforation.
**General Examination** *DGI* Acral hemorrhagic pustules.

## DIFFERENTIAL DIAGNOSIS

**Urethritis** Genital herpes with urethritis, *C. trachomatis* urethritis, *Ureaplasma urealyticum* urethritis, *Trichomonas vaginalis* urethritis, Reiter's syndrome.
**Cervicitis** *C. trachomatis* or HSV cervicitis.

## LABORATORY EXAMINATIONS

See "*Neisseria gonorrhoeae* Infections," page 905.

## DIAGNOSIS

Clinical suspicion, confirmed by laboratory findings, i.e., presumptively by identifying gram-negative diplococci intracellularly in PMNs in smears, confirmed by culture.

### TABLE 27-5    Management of Uncomplicated Gonococcal Infections

**Cervix, urethra, and rectum**
  Recommended regimens
| | |
|---|---|
|     Cefixime | 400 mg orally in a single dose, *or* |
|     Ceftriaxone | 125 mg IM in a single dose, *or* |
|     Ciprofloxacin | 500 mg orally in a single dose, *or* |
|     Ofloxacin | 400 mg orally in a single dose, *or* |
|     Levofloxacin | 250 mg orally in a single dose, *plus*, if chlamydial infection is not ruled out, |
|     Azithromycin | 1 g orally in a single dose, *or* |
|     Doxycycline | 100 mg orally twice a day for 7 days. |

  Alternative regimens
| | |
|---|---|
|     Spectinomycin | 2 g in a single, IM dose, *or* |

Single-dose cephalosporin regimens
| | |
|---|---|
|     Ceftizoxime | 500 mg, administered IM, *or* |
|     Cefoxitin | 2 g, administered IM, with probenecid, 1 g orally, *or* |
|     Cefotaxime | 500 mg, administered IM. |

Single-dose quinolone regimens
| | |
|---|---|
|     Gatifloxacin | 400 mg orally, *or* |
|     Norfloxacin | 800 mg orally, *or* |
|     Lomefloxacin | 400 mg orally. |

**Pharynx**

Gonococcal infections of the pharynx are more difficult to eradicate than infections at urogenital and anorectal sites. Few antimicrobial regimens can reliably cure >90% of infections.

Although chlamydial coinfection of the pharynx is unusual, coinfection at genital sites sometimes occurs. Therefore, treatment for both gonorrhea and chlamydia is recommended.

  Recommended regimens
| | |
|---|---|
|     Ceftriaxone | 125 mg IM in a single dose, *or* |
|     Ciprofloxacin | 500 mg orally in a single dose, *plus* if chlamydial infection is not ruled out, |
|     Azithromycin | 1 g orally in a single dose, *or* |
|     Doxycycline | 100 mg orally twice daily for 7 days. |

## COURSE AND PROGNOSIS

Most infections among men produce symptoms that cause the person to seek curative treatment soon enough to prevent serious sequelae—but not soon enough to prevent transmission to others. If not treated, complications due to ascending infection occur: prostatitis—pain on defecation; epididymitis—swelling of epididymis and pain in walking; cystitis. Many infections among women do not produce recognizable symptoms until complications such as PID occur. PID, whether symptomatic or asymptomatic, can cause tubal scarring, leading to infertility or ectopic pregnancy. Because gonococcal infections among women are often asymptomatic, a primary measure for controlling gonorrhea in the United States has been screening of high-risk women. DGI more common in women with asymptomatic cervical, endometrial, or tubal infection and in homosexual men with asymptomatic rectal or pharyngeal gonorrhea.

## MANAGEMENT

See Table 27-5.

# DISSEMINATED GONOCOCCAL INFECTION

DGI is a systemic infection that follows the hematogenous dissemination of gonococcus from infected mucosal sites to skin, tenosynovium, and joints. Characterized by fever, petechial or pustular acral lesions, asymmetric arthralgias, tenosynovitis, or septic arthritis. Occasionally complicated by perihepatitis and, rarely, endocarditis or meningitis.
*Synonyms*: Gonococcemia, gonococcal arthritis–dermatitis syndrome.

## HISTORY

**Incubation Period**   7 to 30 days of mucosal infection (range, from a few days to 1 year). Varies with host factors such as menstruation, invasiveness of infecting organism.
**Prodrome**   Fever, anorexia, malaise, shaking chills, polyarthralgias (knees, elbows, distal joints).
**Other Factors**   Recurring symptoms around menses, migratory polyarthralgias.

## PHYSICAL EXAMINATION

### Skin Findings
1- to 5-mm erythematous macules evolving to hemorrhagic pustules (Fig. 27-17) within 24 to 48 h in 75% of cases. Centers at times hemorrhagic/necrotic, 5 to 40 in number. Rarely, large hemorrhagic bullae.
*Distribution* Acral (Fig. 27-17), arms more often than legs, near small joints of hands or feet. Difficult to detect in black patients; look in web spaces. Face spared.
**Mucous Membranes**   Usually asymptomatic colonization of oropharynx, urethra, anorectum, endometrium.
**General Examination**   Fever 38°C to 39°C usual. Severity varies: (1) DGI with skin lesions alone, (2) classic DGI with skin lesions and tenosynovitis, (3) DGI with septic arthritis, (4) DGI with metastatic infection at other sites.
*Tenosynovitis* Common. Single or few sites, acrally. Extensor/flexor tendons and sheaths of hands/feet. Erythema, tenderness, swelling along tendon sheath aggravated by moving tendon.
*Septic Arthritis* Joints—red, hot, tender with effusion; asymmetric. Most commonly involved:

knee, wrist, ankle, elbow, metacarpophalangeal/interphalangeal joints of hand, shoulder, hip. Usually only one to two joints involved.
*Other* Hepatitis, perihepatitis (Fitz-Hugh–Curtis syndrome), myopericarditis, endocarditis, meningitis, perihepatitis. Rarely, pneumonitis, adult respiratory distress syndrome, osteomyelitis.

## DIFFERENTIAL DIAGNOSIS

**Scant, Acral, Hemorrhagic Pustules**   Bacteremia: meningococcemia, other bacteremias, endocarditis.
**Tenosynovitis/Arthritis**   Infectious arthritis, infectious tenosynovitis, Reiter's syndrome, psoriatic arthritis, systemic lupus erythematosus.

## LABORATORY EXAMINATIONS

**Dermatopathology**   Immunofluorescence of skin lesion biopsy shows gonococci in 60%.
**Gram's Stain**   From the male urethra or cervix, may show gonococci.
**Culture**   Mucosal sites yield 80 to 90% positive cultures. Skin biopsy: ≤ 5% chance of positive culture; joint fluid, blood also low yield.

## DIAGNOSIS

Made on clinical criteria, confirmed by culture of gonococcus from mucosal sites.

## COURSE AND PROGNOSIS

Untreated, skin/joint lesions often gradually resolve; endocarditis usually fatal.

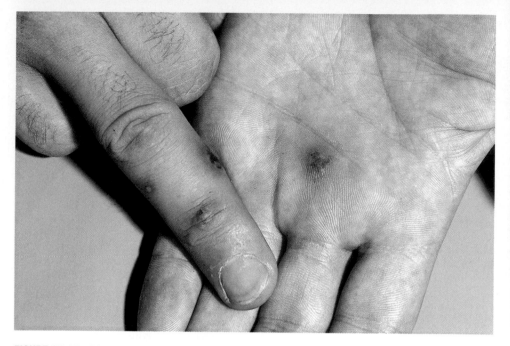

**FIGURE 27-17   Disseminated gonococcal infection**   *Hemorrhagic, painful pustules on erythematous bases on the palm and the finger of the other hand. These lesions occur at acral sites and are few in number.*

## MANAGEMENT

Recommended regimen
| | |
|---|---|
| Ceftriaxone | 1 g IM or IV every 24 h. |

Alternative regimens
| | |
|---|---|
| Cefotaxime | 1 g IV every 8 hours, *or* |
| Ceftizoxime | 1 g IV every 8 hours, *or* |
| Ciprofloxacin | 400 mg IV every 12 hours, *or* |
| Ofloxacin | 400 mg IV every 12 hours, *or* |
| Levofloxacin | 250 mg IV daily, *or* |
| Spectinomycin | 2 g IM every 12 h. |

All of the preceding regimens should be continued for 24 to 48 h after improvement begins, at which time therapy may be switched to one of the following regimens to complete at least 1 week of antimicrobial therapy:

| | |
|---|---|
| Cefixime | 400 mg orally twice daily, *or* |
| Ciprofloxacin | 500 mg orally twice daily, *or* |
| Ofloxacin | 400 mg orally twice daily, *or* |
| Levofloxacin | 500 mg orally once daily. |

# SYPHILIS    ■    ◑ → ●

Syphilis is a chronic systemic infection, characterized by the appearance of a painless ulcer or chancre at the site of inoculation, associated with regional lymphadenopathy; shortly after inoculation, syphilis becomes a systemic infection with characteristic secondary and tertiary stages (Table 27-6). During the past few years, the incidence of syphilis has increased, and the clinical course and response to standard therapy may be altered in HIV-infected patients. *Synonyms:* Lues, the great imitator. Primary syphilis, L1; secondary syphilis, L2; tertiary syphilis, L3.

## EPIDEMIOLOGY AND ETIOLOGY

**Etiology**    Venereal syphilis: *Treponema pallidum* subspecies *pallidum* (*T. pallidum*). Yaws: *T. pallidum* subspecies *pertenue*. Endemic syphilis (bejel): *T. pallidum* subspecies *endemicum.* Pinta: *T. carateum.* Subspecies identified by PCR-based methods. *T. pallidum* is a thin delicate spirochete with 6 to 14 spirals. Only natural host for *T. pallidum* is the human.

**Age of Onset**    In decreasing order: 20 to 39 years, 15 to 19 years, 40 to 49 years.

**Incidence**    Increasing in males who have sex with males (MSM).

**Race**    All races; in the United States, incidence increasing in African Americans and Hispanics.

**Sex**    Males outnumber females 2:1 to 4:1.

**Other Factors**    Until recently, nearly half of all males with syphilis in the United States were homosexual, but this percentage has decreased due to safer sexual practices. Incidence of syphilis, however, has markedly increased in minorities and is associated with exchange of sex for drugs. Associated with the increase in venereal syphilis is a marked increase in the number of cases of congenital syphilis.

## Transmission

*Sexual contact:* Contact with infectious lesion (chancre, mucous patch, condyloma latum, cutaneous lesions of secondary syphilis). 60% of contacts of persons with primary and secondary syphilis become infected.

*Congenital infection:* In utero or perinatal transmission.

*Blood products:* One-half of cases named as contacts of infectious syphilis become infected.

**Serologic Testing**    Serologic testing for syphilis (STS) has declined in the United States. Currently, testing is performed in pregnant women, persons admitted to hospitals, military inductees, persons undergoing examination in physicians' offices. Premarital testing is performed in some states.

## PATHOGENESIS

The spirochetes pass through intact mucous membrane and microscopic abrasion in skin, enter lymphatics and blood within a few hours, and produce systemic infection and metastatic foci before development of a primary lesion.

---

**TABLE 27-6    Classification of the Clinical Stages (See Image 27-1)**

| Stage | Characterization |
|---|---|
| Primary syphilis | Localized infection at site of inoculation (chancre) |
| Secondary syphilis | Disseminated infection (exanthem, maculopapules, condylomata lata) |
| Latent syphilis | No clinical signs or symptoms of infection (seropositive) |
| Early | < 1-year duration; any period between primary and secondary stage |
| Late | ≥ than 1 year since patient became infected |
| Syphilis of unknown duration | |
| Late (tertiary) syphilis | Cutaneous, vascular, neurologic findings |
| Congenital syphilis | Acquired perinatally; early and late clinical findings |

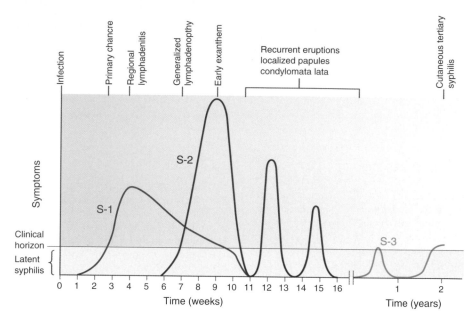

CLINICAL MANIFESTATIONS OF SYPHILIS

**IMAGE 27-1** *Clinical manifestations of syphilis. S-1, primary syphilis; S-2, secondary syphilis; S-3, tertiary syphilis. (From JL Bolognia, JL Jorizzo, RP Rapin, in Dermatology. London, New York, Philadelphia, Mosby, 2003, p. 443; with permission.*

Spirochetes divide locally, with resulting host inflammatory response and chancre formation, either a single lesion or, less commonly, multiple lesions. Cellular immunity is of major importance in healing of early lesions and control of infection ($T_H1$ type). Primary syphilis is the most contagious stage of the disease. Later syphilis is essentially a vascular disease, lesions occurring secondary to obliterative endarteritis of terminal arterioles and small arteries and by the resulting inflammatory and necrotic changes.

## LABORATORY EXAMINATIONS

**Demonstration of the Organism** *Dark-Field Examination* Simple/reliable test to demonstrate spirochete. Chancre or secondary lesion is debrided from crusts and cleaned with saline swabs and, if not primarily eroded or ulcerated, scarified with scalpel by gentle scraping, blotted until bleeding stops, and then squeezed between gloved fingers until serous fluid emerges on surface or base of ulcer. Serous exudate is removed by a glass capillary and pipetted onto microscope slide, covered with coverslip, and examined in dark-field microscope. *T. pallidum* is recognized

as a corkscrew-like organism, 5 to 20 μm in length, showing rotatory, pocket knifelike kinking and harmonica-like contractile movements. Positive in primary chancre and papular lesions of secondary syphilis, in particular condylomata lata. Unreliable in oral cavity because of the presence of saprophytic spirochetes, and negative in patients treated systemically or topically with antibiotics. Regional lymph node aspirated and aspirate examined in the dark-field microscope.
*Direct Fluorescent Antibody T. pallidum (DFA-TP) Test* Fluorescent antibodies are used to detect *T. pallidum* in exudate from lesion, lymph node aspirate, or tissue.
*PCR* Available in research laboratories.
**Serologic Tests for Syphilis** Positive in persons with any treponemal infection (venereal syphilis, endemic syphilis, yaws, pinta). Both tests always positive in secondary syphilis.
*Nontreponemal STS* Measures IgG and IgM directed against cardiolipin-lecithin-cholesterol antigen complex. Rapid plasma reagin (RPR) test (automated RPR: ART). VDRL slide test. Nonreactive in 25% of patients with primary syphilis. In early syphilis: either do fluorescent treponemal antibody-absorbed (FTA-ABS) test or repeat VDRL in 1 to 2

weeks if initial VDRL negative. Prozone phenomenon: if antibody titer high, test may be negative; must dilute serum. Becomes nonreactive or reactive in lower titers following therapy for early syphilis.

*Treponemal STS* FTA-ABS test. Agglutination assays for antibodies to *T. pallidum*: microhemagglutination assay (MHA-TP; Serodia TP-PA test). *T. pallidum* hemagglutination test (TPHA). Often remain reactive after therapy; not helpful in determining infectious status of patient with past syphilis.

*False-Positive STS* See Table 27-7. Antigen used in nontreponemal test found in other tissues; may be positive (does not exceed 1:8 dilution).

**Evaluation of Neurosyphilis** Lumbar puncture indicated in following: neurologic signs or symptoms, treatment failure, serum reagin titer $\geq$1:32, HIV seropositivity, other evidence of active syphilis (aortitis, gumma, visual hearing changes), plans to administer nonpenicillin therapy. CSF examination for pleocytosis, increased protein concentration, VDRL activity. Abnormal in 40% of early syphilis and 25% of latent infection.

**Evaluation for Syphilis in HIV Disease** STS for newly diagnosed HIV disease. CSF for all co-infected patients.

**Dermatopathology** In primary and secondary syphilis, lesional skin biopsy shows central thinning or ulceration of epidermis. Lymphocytic and plasmacytic dermal infiltrate. Proliferation of capillaries and lymphatics with endarteritis; may have thrombosis and small areas of necrosis. Dieterle stain demonstrates spirochetes.

## COURSE AND PROGNOSIS

Even without treatment, chancre heals completely in 4 to 6 weeks, the infection either becoming latent or clinical manifestations of secondary syphilis appearing. Secondary syphilis usually manifests as macular exanthem initially; after weeks, lesions resolve spontaneously and recur as maculopapular or papular eruptions. In 20% of untreated cases, up to three to four such recurrences followed by periods of clinical remission may occur over a period of 1 year. Infection then enters a latent stage, in which there are no clinical signs or symptoms of the disease. After untreated syphilis has persisted for >4 years, it is rarely communicable, except in the case of pregnant women, who, if untreated, may transmit syphilis to their fetuses, regardless of the duration of their disease. One-third of patients with untreated latent syphilis developed clinically apparent tertiary disease.

Gummas hardly ever heal spontaneously. Noduloulcerative syphilides undergo spontaneous partial healing, but new lesions appear at the periphery.

## MANAGEMENT

See Table 27-8.

**TABLE 27-7   Causes of False-Positive Reactions in Nontreponemal Serologic Tests for Syphilis**

| Cause | Rate of False-Positive Reactions, %* |
|---|---|
| **ACUTE FALSE-POSITIVE REACTION (<6 MONTHS)** | |
| Recent viral illness or immunization | 1–2 |
| Genital herpes | 4–4 |
| Human immunodeficiency virus infection | 1–4 |
| Malaria | 11 |
| Parenteral drug use | 20–25 |
| **CHRONIC FALSE-POSITIVE REACTION (≥6 MONTHS)** | |
| Aging | 9–11 |
| Autoimmune disorders | 1–20 |
| Systemic lupus erythematosus | 11–20 |
| Rheumatoid arthritis | 5 |
| Parenteral drug use | 20–25 |

*Data were collected from a variety of published reports.

SOURCE: SA Lukehart, in E Braunwald, AS Fauci, DL Kasper, SL Hauser, DL Longo, JL Jameson (eds): *Harrison's Principles of Internal Medicine*; 15th ed. New York, McGraw-Hill, 2001.

**TABLE 27-8   Recommendations for the Treatment of Syphilis**

| Stage of Syphilis | Patients without Penicillin Allergy | Patients with Confirmed Penicillin Allergy |
|---|---|---|
| Primary, secondary, or early latent | Penicillin G benzathine (single dose of 2.4 million units IM, 1.2 million units in each buttock) | Tetracycline hydrochloride (500 mg PO qid) or doxycycline (100 mg PO bid) for 2 weeks |
| Late latent (or latent of uncertain duration), cardiovascular, or benign tertiary | Lumbar puncture CSF normal: Penicillin G benzathine (2.4 million units IM weekly for 3 weeks) CSF abnormal: Treat as neurosyphilis | Lumbar puncture CSF normal: Tetracycline hydrochloride (500 mg PO qid) or doxycycline (100 mg PO bid) for 4 weeks CSF abnormal: Treat as neurosyphilis |
| Neurosyphilis (asymptomatic or symptomatic) | Aqueous penicillin G (18–24 million units/d IV, given in divided doses every 4 h) for 10–14 days *or* Aqueous penicillin G procaine (2.4 million units/d IM) plus oral probenecid (500 mg qid), both for 10–14 days | Desensitization and treatment with penicillin if allergy is confirmed by skin testing |
| Syphilis in pregnancy | According to stage | Desensitization and treatment with penicillin if allergy is confirmed by skin testing |

SOURCE: These recommendations are modified from those issued by the Centers for Disease Control and Prevention in 1998.

# PRIMARY SYPHILIS ■ ◐

## HISTORY

**Symptoms** A genital or extragenital lesion may be noted. Ulcers are usually painless unless superinfected.

**Incubation Period** 21 days (average); range, 10 to 90 days.

## PHYSICAL EXAMINATION

### Skin Lesions

*Chancre* Button-like papule that develops at the site of inoculation into a painless erosion and then ulcerates with raised border and scanty serous exudate (Figs. 27-18 and 27-19). Surface may be crusted. Size: few millimeters to 1 or 2 cm in diameter. Border of lesion may be raised. Palpation: most commonly, firm with indurated border; painless. Extragenital chancres, particularly on the fingers, may be painful. Atypically, genital chancres painful, especially if secondarily infected with *Staphylococcus aureus*. Arrangement: single lesion; less commonly, few, multiple, or kissing lesions.

*Sites of Predilection* Genital sites are most common. Male: inner prepuce (Fig. 27-18), coronal sulcus of the glans penis, shaft, base. Female: cervix, vagina, vulva (Fig. 27-19), clitoris, breast; chancres observed less frequently in women because of their location within vagina or on cervix. Extragenital chancres (Fig. 27-20): anus or rectum, mouth, lips, tongue (Fig. 27-21), tonsils, fingers (painful!), toes, breast, nipple.

**General Findings** Syphilis is a systemic infection; all patients should have a thorough clinical examination. Regional lymphadenopathy appears within 7 days. Nodes are discrete, firm, rubbery, nontender, more commonly unilateral; may persist for months.

## DIFFERENTIAL DIAGNOSIS

**Genital Erosion/Ulcer:** Genital herpes, traumatic ulcer, fixed drug eruption, chancroid, lymphogranuloma venereum.

## DIAGNOSIS

Clinical suspicion, confirmed by dark-field examination or serologically.

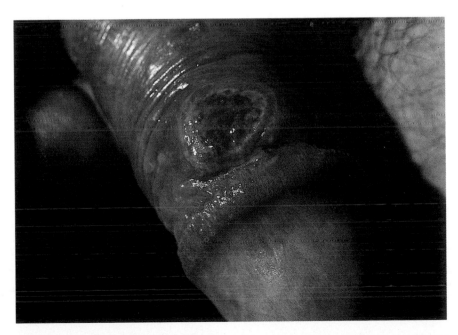

**FIGURE 27-18 Primary syphilis: penile chancre** *Large, painless ulcer on the distal shaft of the penis. On palpation, the area surrounding the ulcer is strikingly indurated. The chancre arises at the site of inoculation of* T. pallidum.

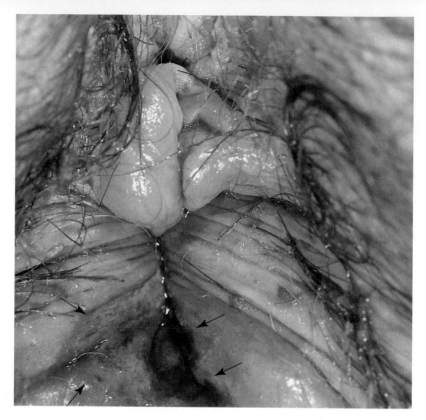

**FIGURE 27-19   Primary syphilis: vulvar chancre**   *Large, painless erosion with jagged margins on the anterior introitus.*

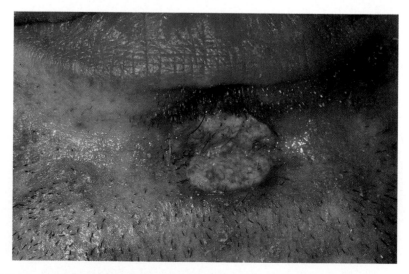

**FIGURE 27-20   Primary syphilis: extragenital chancre on chin**   *A painless ulcer on the chin at the site of inoculation of* T. pallidum *after orogenital sex.*

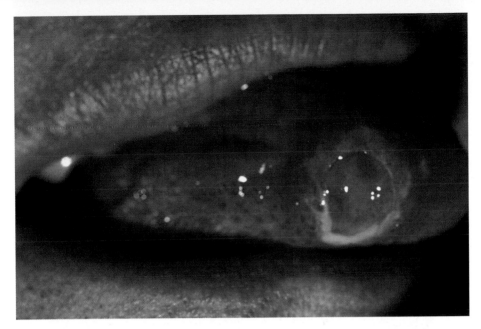

**FIGURE 27-21    Primary syphilis: extragenital chancre on tongue**   *A painful ulcer had been present on the tip of the tongue for 2 weeks. A disseminated papulosquamous eruption occurred 2 weeks later.*

## SECONDARY SYPHILIS   ■

### HISTORY

Secondary syphilis appears 2 to 6 months after primary infection; 2 to 10 weeks after appearance of the primary chancre; 6 to 8 weeks after healing of chancre. Chancre may still be present when secondary lesions appear (15% of cases). Concomitant HIV infection may alter course of secondary syphilis.

**Symptoms**   Fever, sore throat, weight loss, malaise, anorexia, headache, meningismus. Mucocutaneous lesions are asymptomatic.

**Duration of Lesions**   Weeks.

### PHYSICAL EXAMINATION

#### Skin Lesions

Macules (Fig. 27-22) and papules 0.5 to 1 cm, round to oval; pink brownish-red. *First exanthem* always macular and faint. *Later eruptions may be papulosquamous* (Figs. 27-23 to 27-25), pustular, or acneiform. Vesiculobullous lesions occur only in neonatal congenital syphilis (palms and soles). Uncommonly, lesions of secondary syphilis and chancre of primary syphilis occur concomitantly. On palpation, papules are firm; condylomata lata, soft. Shape of lesions may be annular or polycyclic, especially on face in dark-skinned individuals (Fig. 27-26). In relapsing secondary syphilis, arciform lesions. Always sharply defined except for macular exanthem. Lesions are scattered, tend to remain discrete, and usually symmetric.

*Condylomata lata*: soft, flat-topped, moist, red to pale papules, nodules, or plaques (Fig. 27-27), which may become confluent.

**Distribution**   Generalized eruption on the trunk (Fig. 27-23); localized eruptions most commonly are scaling and papular localizing, especially on the head (hairline, nasolabial, scalp), neck, palms (Fig 27-24), and soles (Fig. 27-25). Here they are often hyperkeratotic-psoriasiform. Condylomata lata (Fig. 27-27): most commonly in anogenital region and mouth; can be seen on any body

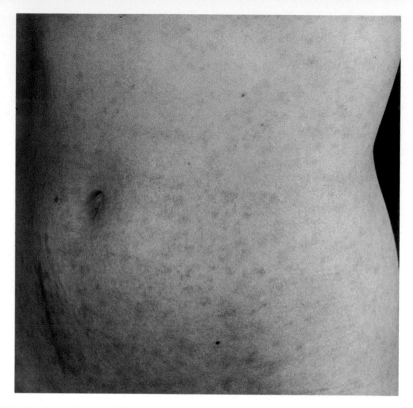

**FIGURE 27-22   Secondary syphilis: early exanthem**   *An asymptomatic morbilliform (measles-like) exanthem on the trunk associated with very early dissemination of* T. pallidum *from the site of inoculation. A chancre of primary syphilis may be coexistent with this finding.*

surface where moisture can accumulate between intertriginous surfaces, i.e., axillae or toe webs.
**Hair** (1) Diffuse hair loss, including temples and parietal scalp; (2) patchy, "moth-eaten" alopecia on the scalp and beard area; and (3) loss of eyelashes, lateral third of eyebrows.
**Mucous Membranes** *Mucous patches*, i.e., small, asymptomatic, round or oval, slightly elevated, flat-topped macules and papules 0.5 to 1 cm in diameter, covered by hyperkeratotic white to gray membrane, occurring on the oral or genital mucosa; *split papules* at the angles of the mouth.
**General Findings**   Fever. Generalized lymphadenopathy (cervical, suboccipital, inguinal, epitrochlear, axillary) and splenomegaly.
**Associated Findings** *Musculoskeletal involvement*: periostitis of long bones, particularly tibia (nocturnal pain); arthralgia; hydrarthrosis of knees or ankles without x-ray changes. *Eyes*: acute bacterial iritis, optic neuritis, uveitis.

*Meningovascular reaction*: CSF positive for inflammatory markers. *Gastrointestinal involvement*: diffuse pharyngitis, hypertrophic gastritis, hepatitis, patchy proctitis, ulcerative colitis, rectosigmoid mass). *Genitourinary involvement*: glomerulonephritis/nephrotic syndrome, cystitis, prostatitis.

## LABORATORY EXAMINATIONS

**Dermatopathology**   Epidermal hyperkeratosis; capillary proliferation with endothelial swelling; perivascular infiltration by monocytes, plasma cells, lymphocytes. Spirochete is present in many tissues including skin, eye, CSF.
**CSF**   Abnormal in 40% of patients. Spirochetes in CSF in 30% of cases.
**Liver Function**   Elevated enzymes.
**Renal Function**   Immune complex–induced membranous glomerulonephritis.

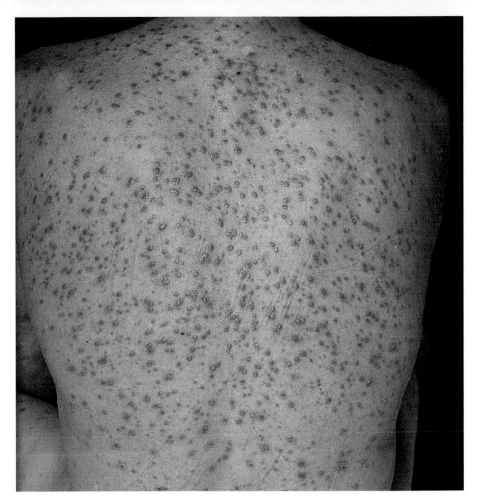

**FIGURE 27-23 Secondary syphilis: disseminated papulosquamous eruption** *Red to copper colored scaling papules of the trunk.*

## COURSE

In secondary syphilis there may be only one or several recurrent eruptions that appear after month-long asymptomatic intervals. First secondary syphilis eruption is a relatively faint exanthem, always macular, pink; lesions are ill-defined. Later lesions of early syphilis are papular, brownish, and tend to be more localized. Symptoms may last 2 to 6 weeks (4 weeks average) and may recur in untreated or inadequately treated patients. Secondary lesions subside within 2 to 6 weeks, infection entering latent stage.

## DIFFERENTIAL DIAGNOSIS

**Exanthem/Enanthem** Adverse cutaneous drug eruption (e.g., captopril), pityriasis rosea, viral exanthem, infectious mononucleosis, tinea corporis, tinea versicolor, scabies, "id" reaction, condylomata acuminata, acute guttate psoriasis, lichen planus.

## DIAGNOSIS

Clinical suspicion confirmed by dark-field examination and/or serology. Dark-field is positive in all secondary syphilis lesions except for macular exanthem.

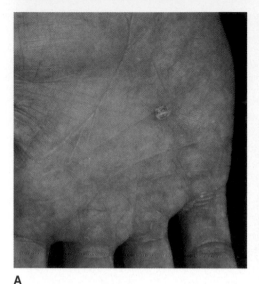
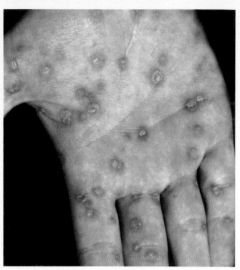

A                                                B

**FIGURE 27-24    Secondary syphilis: disseminated papulosquamous eruption on palms**    *A. A solitary keratotic papule on palm of patient in Fig. 27-21; the chancre was also present on the tongue at the time of presentation of secondary syphilis. Papulosquamous lesions were also disseminated on trunk. **B.** This is the more usual appearance of secondary syphilis in the palms: multiple psoriasiform keratotic papules.*

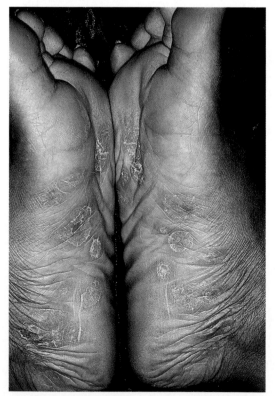

**FIGURE 27-25    Secondary syphilis: annular papulosquamous eruption on soles**    *Hyperkeratotic, scaling plaques on the plantar aspects of both feet in a 20-year-old female. Similar lesions were present on the palms, but to a lesser extent. No other clinical findings were detected.*

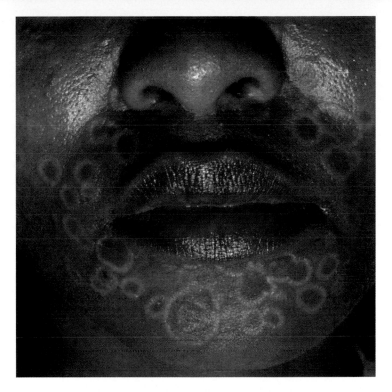

**FIGURE 27-26   Secondary syphilis: annular facial lesions**   *Annular plaques merging on the face of a South African woman. (Courtesy of Jeffrey S. Dover, MD.)*

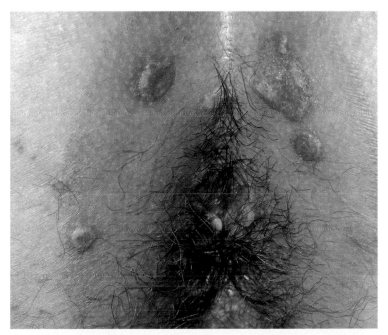

**FIGURE 27-27   Secondary syphilis: condylomata lata**   *Soft, flat-topped, moist, pink-tan papules and nodules on the perineum and perianal area. The lesions are teeming with* T. pallidum.

## LATENT SYPHILIS    ▮  ○

No clinical signs or symptoms of infection; STS positive; CSF is normal. Suspected on the basis of a history of primary or secondary lesions, history of exposure to syphilis, or delivery of an infant with congenital syphilis; can occur without prior recognized primary or secondary lesions. A previous negative STS defines the duration of latency. Early latent syphilis (<1 year) is distinguished from late latent disease (≥1 year). Latent disease does not preclude infectiousness or the development of gummatous skin lesions, cardiovascular lesions, or neurosyphilis. A pregnant woman with latent disease can infect her fetus with congenital syphilis. 70% of untreated patients never develop clinically evident tertiary syphilis. The more sensitive treponemal antibody test rarely becomes negative without treatment.

## TERTIARY/LATE SYPHILIS    ☐  ◐

### HISTORY

**Duration of Lesions**  In *untreated* syphilis, 15% of patients developed late benign syphilis, mostly skin lesions. Tertiary syphilis is now very rare. Previously, patients presenting with tertiary syphilis gave a history of lesions of 3 to 7 years' duration (range, 2 to 60 years); gumma develop by fifteenth year.

### PHYSICAL EXAMINATION

**Gumma**  Nodular or papulosquamous plaques that may ulcerate, form circles/arc. May expand rapidly causing destruction. May be indolent and heal with scarring. Solitary. Skin: any site (Fig. 27-28), especially on scalp, face (Fig. 27-29), chest (sternoclavicular), calf. Internal: skeletal system (long bones of legs), oropharynx, upper respiratory tract (perforation of nasal septum, palate), larynx, liver, stomach.

**Neurosyphilis**  *Asymptomatic Neurosyphilis* Occurs in 25% of patients with untreated late latent syphilis. Definition: Lack neurologic symptoms/signs and CSF abnormalities (mononuclear pleocytosis, increased protein concentrations, reactive VDRL slide test). 20% of patients with asymptomatic neurosyphilis progress to clinical neurosyphilis in first 10 years; risk increases with time.

*Symptomatic Neurosyphilis:* Meningeal, meningovascular, parenchymatous syphilis (general paresis, tabes dorsalis). *Meningeal syphilis*: onset of symptoms <1 year after infection; headache, nausea/vomiting, stiff neck, cranial nerve palsies, seizures, changes in mental status. *Meningovascular syphilis*: Onset of symptoms 5 to 10 years after infection; subacute encephalitis prodrome followed by stroke syndrome, progressive vascular syndrome. *General paresis*: Onset of symptoms 20 years after infection; mnemonic paresis [*p*aresis, *a*ffect, *r*eflexes (hyperactive), *e*ye (Argyll Robertson pupils), *s*ensorium (illusions, delusions, hallucinations), *i*ntellect (decrease in recent memory, orientation, calculations, judgment, insight), *s*peech]. *Tabes dorsalis*: Onset of symptoms 25 to 30 years after infection; ataxic wide-based gait and footslap, paresthesia, bladder disturbances, impotence, areflexia, loss of position, deep pain, temperature sensations (Charcot/neuropathic joints, foot ulcers), optic atrophy.

**Cardiovascular Syphilis**  Results from endarteritis obliterans of vasa vasorum. Occurs in 10% of persons with late untreated syphilis, 10 to 40 years after infection. Uncomplicated aortitis, aortic regurgitation, saccular aneurysm, coronary ostial stenosis.

### DIFFERENTIAL DIAGNOSIS

**Plaque(s) ± Ulceration ± Granulomas**  Cutaneous tuberculosis, cutaneous atypical mycobacterial infection, lymphoma, invasive fungal infections.

### DIAGNOSIS

Clinical findings, confirmed by STS and lesional skin biopsy; dark-field examination always negative; silver impregnation of histologic sections for demonstration of spirochetes only very rarely positive.

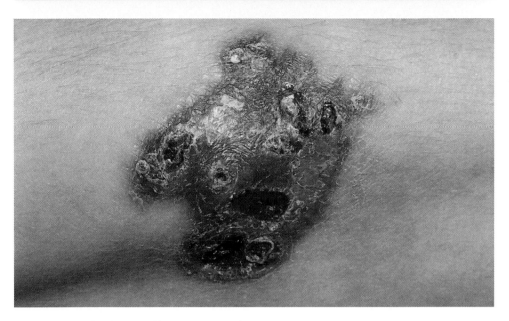

**FIGURE 27-28    Tertiary syphilis: noduloulcerative type** *Asymptomatic, red-brown, translucent, crusted, ulcerated plaque with serpiginous borders.*

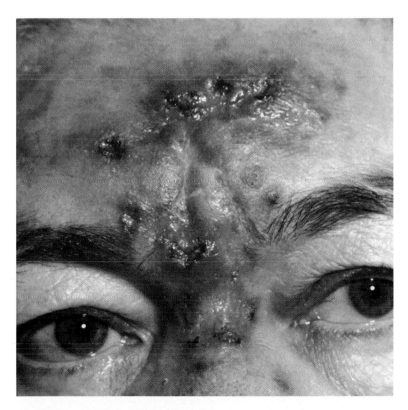

**FIGURE 27-29    Tertiary syphilis: gumma** *Large plaque on forehead and glabella with multiple ulcerations.*

HIV-infected individuals with neurosyphilis are more likely to present with uveitis or retinitis and have significantly higher RPR titers. Some, however, fail to respond immunologically to *T. pallidum* infection with antibody formation (i.e., negative STS).

## DIAGNOSIS

HIV testing is advised for all patients with syphilis. Neurosyphilis should be considered in the differential diagnosis of neurologic disease in HIV-infected persons. When clinical findings suggest syphilis but STS are negative or confusing, alternative tests such as biopsy of lesions, dark-field examination, and DFA staining of lesional material should be used.

## CONGENITAL SYPHILIS

### Transmission
During gestation or intrapartum. Risk of transmission: Early maternal syphilis, 75 to 95%; >2 years' duration, 35%.

### Pathogenesis
Lesions usually develop after fourth month of gestation, associated with fetal immunologic competence. Pathogenesis depends on immune response of fetus rather than toxic effect of spirochete. Adequate treatment before sixteenth week of pregnancy prevents fetal damage. Untreated: fetal loss up to 40%.

### Clinical Manifestations
*Early Manifestations* Appear before 2 years of age, often at 2 to 10 weeks. Infectious, resembling severe secondary syphilis in adult. Rhinitis/"snuffles" (23%); bullae, vesicles, superficial desquamation, petechiae, papulosquamous lesions, mucous patches, condylomata latum; bone changes (osteochondritis, osteitis, periostitis); hepatosplenomegaly, lymphadenopathy, anemia, jaundice, thrombocytopenia, leukocytosis.

*Late Manifestations* Appear after 2 years of age. Noninfectious. Similar to late acquired syphilis in adult. Cardiovascular syphilis. Interstitial keratitis, eighth-nerve deafness. Recurrent arthropathy; bilateral knee effusions (Clutton joints). Asymptomatic neurosyphilis in 33% of patients; clinical syphilis in 25%. Gummatous periostitis results in destructive lesions of nasal septum/palate.

*Residual Stigmata* Hutchinson teeth (centrally notched, widely spaced, peg-shaped upper central incisors; "mulberry" molars (multiple poorly developed cusps). Abnormal facies: frontal bossing, saddle nose, poorly developed maxillae, rhagades (linear scars at angles of mouth, caused by bacterial superinfection of early facial eruption). Saber shins. Nerve deafness; old chorioretinitis, optic atrophy, corneal opacities due to interstitial keratitis.

# *HAEMOPHILUS DUCREYI*: CHANCROID  □ → ■ ◑

Chancroid is an acute STI characterized by a *painful* ulcer at the site of inoculation, usually on the external genitalia, and the development of suppurative regional lymphadenopathy. Chancroid is the STI most strongly associated with increased risk for HIV transmission.
*Synonyms*: Soft chancre, ulcus molle, chancre mou.

## EPIDEMIOLOGY AND ETIOLOGY

**Etiology**  *H. ducreyi*, a gram-negative streptobacillus.
**Sex**  Young males. Lymphadenitis more common in males.
**Risk Factors**  (1) Transmission mainly heterosexual, (2) males > females 3:1 to 25:1, (3) prostitution important, (4) strongly associated with illicit drug use.
**Transmission**  Most likely during sexual intercourse with partner who has *H. ducreyi* genital ulcer. Chancroid is a cofactor for HIV transmission; high rates of HIV infection among those who have chancroid. 10% of individuals with chancroid have syphilis or genital herpes.
**Incidence**  Underreported. In 1997, 48 cases reported to U.S. Centers for Disease Control and Prevention.
**Demography**  Uncommon in industrialized nations. Endemic in tropical and subtropical developing countries, especially in poor, urban, and seaport populations.

## PATHOGENESIS

Primary infection develops at the site of inoculation (break in epithelium), followed by lymphadenitis. The genital ulcer is characterized by perivascular and interstitial infiltrates of macrophages and of CD4+ and CD8+ lymphocytes, consistent with a delayed-type hypersensitivity, cell-mediated immune response. CD4+ cells and macrophages in the ulcer may explain the facilitation of transmission of HIV in patients with chancroid ulcers.

## HISTORY

Incubation period is 4 to 7 days.

## PHYSICAL EXAMINATION

**Skin Lesions**
Primary lesion: tender papule with erythematous halo that evolves to pustule, erosion, and ulcer. Ulcer is usually quite *tender* or *painful*. Its borders are sharp, undermined, and not indurated (Figs. 27-30 and 27-31). Base is friable

with granulation tissue and covered with gray to yellow exudate. Edema of prepuce common. Ulcer may be singular or multiple, merging to form large or giant ulcers (>2 cm) with serpiginous shape.
***Distribution***  Multiple ulcers (Fig. 27-31) develop by autoinoculation. Male: prepuce, frenulum, coronal sulcus, glans penis, shaft. Female: fourchette, labia, vestibule, clitoris, vaginal wall by direct extension from introitus, cervix, perianal. Extragenital lesions: breast, fingers, thighs, oral mucosa. Bacterial superinfection of ulcers can occur.
**General Findings**  Painful inguinal lymphadenitis (usually unilateral) occurs in 50% of patients 7 to 21 days after primary lesion. Ulcer may heal before buboes occur. Buboes occur with overlying erythema and may drain spontaneously.

## DIFFERENTIAL DIAGNOSIS

**Genital Ulcer**  Genital herpes, primary syphilis, lymphogranuloma venereum (LGV), donovanosis, secondarily infected human bites, traumatic lesions.
**Tender Inguinal Mass**  Genital herpes, secondary syphilis, LGV, incarcerated hernia, plague, tularemia.

## LABORATORY EXAMINATIONS

**Gram's Stain**  Of scrapings from ulcer base or pus from bubo, usually not helpful.
**Culture**  Special growth requirements; isolation difficult. Using special media, sensitivity is no higher than 80%.
**Serologic Tests**  None available. Patients should be tested for HIV infection at time of diagnosis. Patients should also be tested 3 months later for both syphilis and HIV infection if initial results are negative.
**Dermatopathology**  May be helpful. Organism rarely demonstrated.
**PCR**  Detects *H. ducreyi* DNA sequences.

## DIAGNOSIS

Combination of painful ulcer with tender lymphadenopathy (one-third of patients) is

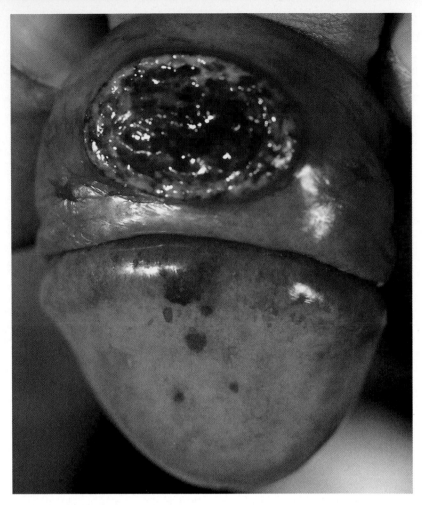

**FIGURE 27-30   Chancroid**   *Painful ulcer with marked surrounding erythema and edema. (Courtesy of Prof. Alfred Eichmann, MD.)*

suggestive of chancroid and, when accompanied by suppurative inguinal lymphadenopathy, is almost pathognomonic.

**Definitive Diagnosis**   Made by isolation of *H. ducreyi* on special culture media (not widely available). Sensitivity 80%.

**Probable Diagnosis**   Made if patient has following criteria: (1) painful genital ulcers; (2) no evidence of *T. pallidum* infection by dark-field examination of ulcer exudate or by STS performed at least 7 days after onset of ulcers; and (3) clinical presentation, appearance of genital ulcers, and lymphadenopathy, if present, are typical for chancroid and a test for HSV is negative. The combination of a painful ulcer and tender inguinal adenopathy,

which occurs in about one-third of patients, suggests a diagnosis of chancroid; when accompanied by suppurative inguinal lymphadenopathy, these signs are pathognomonic.

## COURSE AND PROGNOSIS

Patients should be reexamined 3 to 7 days after initiation of therapy. If treatment is successful, ulcers improve symptomatically within 3 days and improve objectively within 7 days after therapy is begun. If no clinical improvement is evident, diagnosis may be incorrect, co-infection with another STI agent

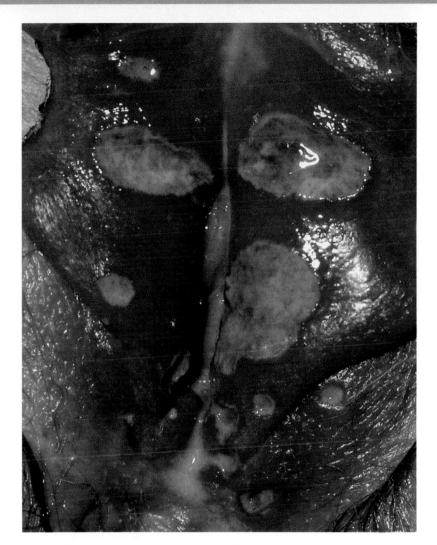

**FIGURE 27-31  Chancroid**  *Multiple, painful, punched-out ulcers with undermined borders on the vulva occurring after autoinoculation.*

exists, the patient is HIV-infected, treatment was not taken as instructed, or the *H. ducreyi* strain causing infection is resistant to the prescribed antimicrobial. The time required for complete healing is related to the size of the ulcer; large ulcers may require 14 days. Complete resolution of fluctuant lymphadenopathy is slower than that of ulcers and may require needle aspiration through adjacent intact skin—even during successful therapy. In HIV-infected persons, healing may be slower, and treatment failures may occur; longer treatment regimens may be advisable.

## MANAGEMENT

### Antimicrobial Therapy

| | |
|---|---|
| Azithromycin | 1 g PO in a single dose, *or* |
| Ceftriaxone | 250 mg IM in a single dose, *or* |
| Ciprofloxacin | 500 mg PO bid for 3 days, *or* |
| Erythromycin base | 500 mg PO qid for 7 days. |

**Management of Sex Partners**  Sex partners should be referred for evaluation and treatment.

## *CALYMMATOBACTERIUM GRANULOMATIS*: DONOVANOSIS   □

Donovanosis is a chronic, indolent, progressive, autoinoculable, ulcerative disease involving the skin and lymphatics of the genital and perianal areas.
*Synonyms*: Granuloma inguinale, granuloma venereum.

### EPIDEMIOLOGY AND ETIOLOGY

**Etiology**   *C. granulomatis*, an encapsulated intracellular gram-negative rod. Closely related to *Klebsiella* spp.
**Sex**   Young males.
**Transmission**   Usually transmitted sexually. Nonsexual transmission and autoinoculation occur.
**Geography**   Endemic foci in tropical and subtropical environments (India; Papua, New Guinea; southern Africa; central Australia; Caribbean and adjacent areas of South America). Rare in United States, Canada, Europe.

### PATHOGENESIS

Poorly understood. Mildly contagious. Repeated exposure necessary for clinical infection to occur. In most cases, lesions cannot be detected in sexual contacts.

### HISTORY

**Incubation Period**   Most lesions appear within 30 days after sexual exposure (range, 8 to 80 days).
**Travel History**   Sexual exposure in endemic area.
**Characterization**   Genital ulcers are relatively painless.

### PHYSICAL EXAMINATION

#### Skin Lesions
**Primary Lesion**   Button-like papule or subcutaneous nodule that ulcerates within a few days. Ulcers have beefy-red friable granulation tissue base with sharply defined irregular margins. Spreads by continuity or by autoinoculation of approximated skin surfaces. Anaerobic superinfection may produce pain and foul-smelling exudate. Less common complications: deep ulcerations, chronic cicatricial lesions, phimosis, lymphedema (elephantiasis of penis, scrotum, vulva), exuberant epithelial proliferation that grossly resembles carcinoma.

**Distribution**   *Males*: prepuce or glans, penile shaft, scrotum. *Females*: labia minora, mons veneris, fourchette. Ulcerations then spread by direct extension or autoinoculation to inguinal and perineal skin. Extragenital lesions occur in mouth, lips, throat, face, GI tract, and bone.
**Variants**   *Ulcerovegetative* (Fig. 27-32): Develops from the nodular variant; large, spreading, exuberant ulcers. *Nodular*: Soft, red nodules that eventually ulcerate with bright red granulating bases. *Hypertrophic*: Cauliflower- or wartlike lesions. *Sclerotic/cicatricial*: Spreading scar tissue formation associated with spread of infection.
**Late Sequela**   Squamous cell carcinoma of genital skin.
**General Findings**   Regional lymph node enlargement is uncommon. Large subcutaneous nodule may mimic a lymph node, i.e., pseudobubo.

### DIFFERENTIAL DIAGNOSIS

**Genital Ulcer(s)**   Syphilitic chancre, chancroid, chronic herpetic ulcer, LGV, cutaneous tuberculosis, cutaneous amebiasis, filariasis, SCC.

### LABORATORY EXAMINATIONS

**Culture**   The organism cannot be cultured on standard microbiologic media. Bacterial superinfection common. Co-infection with other STIs may be present.
**Touch or Crush Preparation**   Punch biopsy stained with Wright's or Giemsa's stain shows Donovan bodies in cytoplasm of macrophages. Clinical variants differ in quantity of organisms.
**Dermatopathology**   Extensive acanthosis and dense dermal infiltrate, mainly plasma cells and histiocytes. Large mononuclear cells containing cytoplasmic inclusions (Donovan bodies), i.e., *C. granulomatis*, are pathognomonic.

### DIAGNOSIS

Clinical diagnosis excluding other causes of genital ulcer(s) and identifying organism with

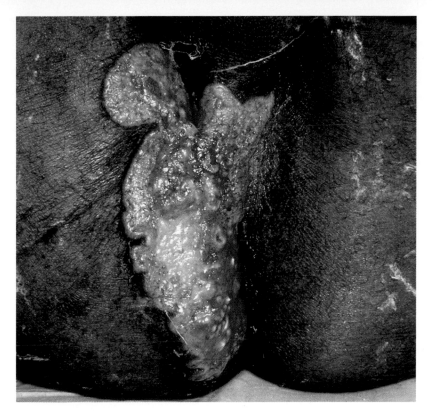

**FIGURE 27-32   Donovanosis: ulcerovegetative type**   *Extensive granulation tissue formation, ulceration, and scarring of the perineum, scrotum, and penis.*

touch preparation or crush preparation of biopsied tissue.

## COURSE AND PROGNOSIS

Little tendency toward spontaneous healing. After antibiotic treatment, lesions often heal with depigmentation of reepithelialized skin. Relapse can occur 6 to 18 months later despite effective initial therapy. Dissemination can occur to bones, particularly the spine, mimicking tuberculosis and actinomycosis.

## MANAGEMENT

**Follow-up**  Patients should be followed clinically until signs and symptoms have resolved.

### Antibiotic Therapy
Recommended regimens
  Treatment appears to halt progressive destruction of tissue, although prolonged duration of therapy often is required to enable granulation and re-epithelialization of ulcers.
  Trimethoprim-sulfamethoxazole
    One double-strength tablet bid for at least 3 weeks
Doxycycline
  100 mg bid for at least 3 weeks
Alternative regimens
  Sulfamethoxazole
    750 mg bid for at least 3 weeks
  Erythromycin base
    500 mg qid for at least 3 weeks
  Parenteral therapy
    If lesions do not respond within the first few days of therapy, the addition of an aminoglycoside (gentamicin, I mg/kg IV q8h) should be considered.

# *CHLAMYDIA TRACHOMATIS* INFECTIONS   ■ ◑

*C. trachomatis* (serovars A–K) commonly causes asymptomatic and symptomatic mucosal infections, as well invasive disease [lymphogranuloma venereum (LGV), hemorrhagic protocolitis]. These infectious syndromes resemble and must be differentiated from those caused by gonococci.

## EPIDEMIOLOGY AND ETIOLOGY

**Etiology** *C. trachomatis*, obligate intracellular bacteria. Major outer-membrane protein delineates >20 serovars (immunotypes):

*Trachoma* Serovars A, B, Ba, and C.
*Mucosal STIs* Serovars D–K (most common bacterial STIs).
*Invasive STIs* Serovars $L_1$, $L_2$, $L_3$ (in United States, $L_2$ most commonly)

**Age of Onset** Late teens, early twenties, while most sexually active.

**Incidence** Most common bacterial STI in virtually every population examined. 4 million cases in the United States annually. Prevalence in young American males: 3 to 5% in general medical settings or urban high schools; >10% in asymptomatic soldiers; 15 to 20% in heterosexual men in STD clinics. Chlamydial urethritis more common in heterosexual men and high socioeconomic status; gonococcal urethritis more common in homosexual men and indigent populations. Prevalence of cervical infection in the United States: 5% for asymptomatic college students; >10% in family planning clinics: >20% in STD clinics. LGV more common in homosexual men; persons returning from abroad (travelers, sailors, military personnel).

**Transmission** *Sexual*: *C. trachomatis* in purulent exudate is inoculated onto skin or mucosa of sexual partner and gains entry through minute lacerations and abrasions. *Perinatal*.

## SYNDROMES

- *Nongonococcal (NGU) and postgonococcal urethritis* 20 to 40% of NGU in heterosexual men are chlamydial. Also caused by *U. urealyticum, T. vaginalis,* HSV.
- *Epididymitis* Most common cause (70%) in sexually active men <35 years.
- *Reiter syndrome C. trachomatis* recovered from urethra in up to 70% of men with untreated nondiarrheal Reiter syndrome and associated urethritis. Chlamydial and other mucosal infections (*Salmonella, Shigella, Campylobacter*) thought to initiate aberrant, hyperactive immune response that produces inflammation at involved target organs in genetically (HA-B27 phenotype) predisposed individuals.
- *Proctitis* Genital immunotypes D–K (most common in the United States) or LGV immunotypes cause proctitis in homosexual men who practice receptive anorectal intercourse.
- *Mucopurulent cervicitis* Many women have no symptoms.
- *Pelvic inflammatory disease (PID)* 50% of cases of PID in the United States caused by *C. trachomatis*. Intraluminal spread results in endometritis, endosalpingitis, pelvic peritonitis. Silent salpingitis causes infertility. 75% of Fitz-Hugh–Curtis syndrome caused by *C. trachomatis.*
- *Lymphogranuloma venereum (LGV).*
- *Perinatal infections* 50 to 75% of newborns exposed to *C. trachomatis* at birth acquire infection. 50% of those infected develop clinical evidence of inclusion conjunctivitis; pneumonitis, otitis media also occur.
- *Adult inclusion conjunctivitis* Caused by exposure to infected genital secretions.
- *Trachoma* Responsible for 20 million cases of blindness worldwide. Transmitted from eye to eye via hands, flies, towels, other fomites. Incidence has decreased during past four decades.

## PATHOGENESIS

*C. trachomatis* preferentially infects columnar epithelium of genital tract, eye, and respiratory tract. Infection often persists for months or years in the absence of antimicrobial therapy. Serious sequelae often occur in association with repeated or persistent infections. Mechanism through which repeated infection elicits an inflammatory response that leads to tubal scarring and damage in the female upper genital tract unclear. Chlamydial 60-kDa heat-shock protein may induce pathologic immune response or elicit antibodies that cross-react with human heat-shock proteins. Chlamydial infections are often totally asymptomatic for months. Simultanaeous infections with gonococcus are common. Infections can persist for months or years if not treated.

## LOCALIZED *C. TRACHOMATIS* INFECTION ■

### HISTORY

*NGU* <50% of men have symptoms. Urethral discharge (whitish, mucoid), dysuria, urethral itching. *Women*: dysuria, frequency, pyuria.
*Proctitis* Mild rectal pain, mucous discharge, tenesmus, bleeding.
*Mucopurulent Cervicitis* Many women have no symptoms or slight vaginal discharge or intermenstrual bleeding.
*PID* Vaginal bleeding, lower abdominal pain, uterine tenderness without adnexal tenderness. Silent salpingitis results in fallopian tube scarring, ectopic pregnancy, and infertility.

### PHYSICAL EXAMINATION

#### Mucosal Lesions
*NGU* Meatal erythema/tenderness; exudates.
*Proctitis* On anoscopy, mild, patchy mucosa; friability, mucopurulent discharge.
*Mucopurulent Cervicitis* 30 to 50% of asymptomatic cases have changes on speculum examination. Yellow mucopurulent discharge from endocervical columnar epithelium; friable.
*PID* Endometritis, endosalpingitis, pelvic peritonitis.
Symptoms of *C. trachomatis* infection are summarized in Table 27-9A.

### DIFFERENTIAL DIAGNOSIS

*Urethritis* Gonorrhea, *U. urealyticum*, *Mycoplasma genitalium*, trichomoniasis, herpetic urethritis.

### LABORATORY EXAMINATIONS

*Direct Microscopy* Low sensitivity. DFA staining used for conjunctival smears.

*PCR* Most specific and sensitive.
*Culture* *C. trachomatis* can be cultured on tissue-culture cell lines in up to 60 to 80% of cases.
*DFA* Examine exudate for antigens.
**Antibodies to *C. trachomatis* *Enzyme-Linked Immunosorbent Assay (ELISA)*** 60 to 80% sensitive and specific; 97 to 99% in high-risk populations; sensitivities higher in cervical infection than urethritis in males.
***DNA-RNA Hybridization*** As sensitive and specific as ELISA. Chlamydial DNA in urine is diagnostic.
***Complement-Fixation (CF) Test*** Acute LGV usually has titer 1:64. Microimmunofluorescence test most sensitive and specific, identifying infecting serovar/immunotypes.
Diagnostic tests are summarized in Table 27-9B.

### COURSE AND PROGNOSIS

Absence of symptoms of *C. trachomatis* infection leaves women at risk of serious chlamydia-related morbidity through the complication of PID: recurrent PID with endogenous vaginal flora, chronic pelvic pain, ectopic pregnancy, and infertility. Gynecologic PID typically affects older women, is clinically severe, and is more likely to present to hospital. Most common cause of epididymitis in young men. Other complications: conjunctivitis, reactive arthritis, pneumonitis in neonates.

### MANAGEMENT

**Screening** Annually for sexually active women: adolescents, 20 to 25 years old, older women with risk factors (new sex partner, multiple sex partners).
**Antimicrobial Therapy** Cures infection and prevents ongoing tissue damage, although tissue reaction can result in scarring.

**TABLE 27-9A   Symptoms and Therapy of Sexually Transmitted *Chlamydia trachomatis* Infection**

| Infection | Suggestive Signs/Symptoms |
| --- | --- |
| NGU, PGU | Discharge, dysuria |
| Epididymitis | Unilateral intrascrotal swelling, pain, tenderness; fever; NGU |
| Cervicitis | Mucopurulent cervical discharge, bleeding and edema of the zone of cervical ectopy |
| Salpingitis | Lower abdominal pain, cervical motion tenderness, adnexal tenderness or masses |
| Urethritis | Dysuria and frequency without urgency or hematuria |
| Proctitis | Rectal pain, discharge, tenesmus, bleeding; history of receptive anorectal intercourse |
| Reiter's syndrome | NGU, arthritis, conjunctivitis, typical skin lesions |
| LGV | Regional adenopathy, primary lesion, proctitis, systemic symptoms |

**Recommended regimen**

| | |
| --- | --- |
| Azithromycin | 1 g PO in single dose, *or* |
| Doxycycline | 100 mg PO bid for 7 days. |

**Alternative regimens**

| | |
| --- | --- |
| Erythromycin base | 500 mg PO qid for 7 days, *or* |
| Erythromycin ethylsuccinate | 800 mg PO qid for 7 days, *or* |
| Ofloxacin | 300 mg PO bid for 7 days, *or* |
| Levofloxacin | 500 mg PO qd for 7 days. |

## TABLE 27-9B   Diagnostic Tests for Sexually Transmitted *Chlamydia trachomatis* Infection

| Presumptive Diagnosis* | Confirmatory Test of Choice |
|---|---|
| **MEN** | |
| Gram's stain with >4 neutrophils per oil-immersion field; no gonococci | Urethral culture or nonculture test for *C. trachomatis*; urine PCR or LCR for *C. trachomatis* |
| Gram's stain with >4 neutrophils per oil-immersion field; no gonococci; urinalysis with pyuria | Urethral culture or nonculture test for *C. trachomatis*; urine PCR or LCR for *C. trachomatis* |
| **WOMEN** | |
| Cervical Gram's stain with ≥20 neutrophils per oil-immersion field in cervical mucus | Cervical culture or nonculture test for *C. trachomatis*; urine PCR or LCR for *C. trachomatis* |
| *C. trachomatis* always potentially present in salpingitis for *C. trachomatis* | Cervical culture or nonculture test for *C. trachomatis*; urine PCR or LCR |
| MPC; sterile pyuria; negative routine urine culture | Urethral and cervical cultures or nonculture test for *C. trachomatis*; urine PCR or LCR for *C. trachomatis* |
| **ADULTS OF EITHER SEX** | |
| Negative gonococcal culture and Gram's stain; at least 1 neutrophil per oil-immersion field in rectal Gram's stain | Rectal culture or direct immuno-fluorescence test for *C. trachomatis* |
| Gram's stain with >4 neutrophils per oil-immersion field; lack of gonococci indicative of NGU | Urethral culture or nonculture test for *C. trachomatis* |
| None | Isolation of LGV strain from node or rectum, occasionally from urethra or cervix; LGV CF titer, ≥1:64; micro-IF titer, ≥1:512 |

*A presumptive diagnosis of chlamydial infection is often made in the syndromes listed when gonococci are not found. A positive test for *Neisseria gonorrhoeae* does not exclude the involvement of *C. trachomatis*, which often is present in patients with gonorrhea.

NOTE: CF, complement-fixing; LCR, ligase chain reaction; LGV, lymphogranuloma venereum; micro-IF, microimmunofluorescence; MPC, mucopurulent cervicitis; NGU, nongonococcal urethritis; PCR, polymerase chain reaction; PGU, postgonococcal urethritis.

SOURCE: From WE Stamm, in E Braunwald, AS Fauci, DL Kasper, SL Hauser, DL Longo; JL Jameson (eds): *Harrison's Principles of Internal Medicine*, 15th ed. New York, McGraw-Hill, 2001.

# INVASIVE *C. TRACHOMATIS* INFECTION: LYMPHOGRANULOMA VENEREUM □ ◑

Acute LGV in heterosexual men is characterized by a transient primary genital lesion followed by multilocular suppurative regional lymphadenopathy. Women, homosexual men, and—in occasional instances—heterosexual men may develop hemorrhagic proctitis with regional lymphadenitis. After a latent period of years, late complications include genital elephantiasis due to lymphatic involvement; strictures; and fistulas of penis, urethra, rectum.

## EPIDEMIOLOGY

**Sex** *Heterosexual men*: acute infection presents as inguinal syndrome. *Women/homosexual men*: Anogenitorectal syndrome most common.
**Demography** Sporadic/rare in North America, Europe, Australia, and most of Asia and South America. Endemic in East and West Africa, India, parts of southeast Asia, South America, and the Caribbean.

## PATHOGENESIS

Primarily an infection of lymphatics and lymph nodes. Lymphangitis and lymphadenitis occur in drainage field of inoculation site with subsequent perilymphangitis and periadenitis. Necrosis occurs; loculated abscesses, fistulas, and sinus tracts develop. As the infection subsides, fibrosis replaces acute inflammation with resulting obliteration of lymphatic drainage, chronic edema, and stricture. Inoculation site determines affected lymph nodes:

- Penis, anterior urethra — Superficial, deep inguinal
- Posterior urethra — Deep iliac, perirectal
- Vulva — Inguinal
- Vagina, cervix — Deep iliac, perirectal, retrocrural, lumbosacral
- Anus — Inguinal
- Rectum — Perirectal, deep iliac

## HISTORY

**Incubation Period** 3 to 12 days or longer for primary stage; 10 to 30 days (but up to 6 months) for secondary stage.
**Acute** Primary genital lesion noticed in fewer than one-third of men and rarely in women. *In heterosexual men, women*: small painless vesicle or nonindurated ulcer/papule on penis or labia/posterior vagina/fourchette; heals in a few days. *In homosexual men, women*: primary anal or rectal infection develops after receptive anal intercourse. *In women*: anal/rectal infection can spread from perineum or via pelvic lymphatics. Infection can spread from primary site of infection to regional lymphatics.
**Inguinal Syndrome** Characterized by painful inguinal lymphadenopathy beginning 2 to 6 weeks after presumed exposure. Unilateral in two-thirds of cases; palpable iliac/femoral nodes often present on same side (Fig. 27-33). Initially, nodes are discrete, but progressive periadenitis results in a matted mass of nodes that may become fluctuant and suppurative. Overlying skin becomes fixed, inflamed, thin, and eventually develops multiple draining fistulas. "Groove" sign: Extensive enlargement of chains of inguinal nodes above and below the inguinal ligament; nonspecific.

## PHYSICAL EXAMINATION

**Acute LGV** Papule, shallow erosion or ulcer, grouped small erosions or ulcers (herpetiform), or nonspecific urethritis.

*Heterosexual males* Cordlike lymphangitis of dorsal penis may follow. Lymphangial nodule (bubonulus) may rupture, resulting in sinuses and fistulas of urethra and deforming scars of penis. Multilocular suppurative lymphadenopathy.
*Females* Cervicitis, perimetritis, salpingitis may occur.
*Female and homosexual males/receptive anal intercourse* Primary anal rectal infection (hemorrhagic proctitis with regional lymphadenitis).

*Other* Erythema nodosum in 10% of cases.
**Secondary Stage *Inguinal Syndrome*** Unilateral bubo in two-thirds of cases (most common presentation) (Fig. 27-33). Marked edema and erythema of skin overlying node. One-third of inguinal buboes rupture; two-thirds slowly

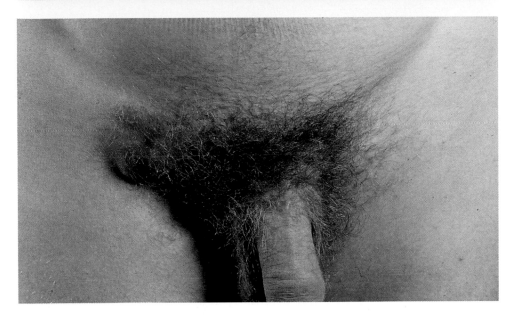

**FIGURE 27-33  Lymphogranuloma venereum** *Striking tender lymphadenopathy occurring at the femoral and inguinal lymph nodes separated by a groove made by Poupart's ligament (groove sign).*

involute. "Groove" sign: inflammatory mass of femoral and inguinal nodes separated by depression, or groove, made by Poupart's ligament. 75% of cases have deep iliac node involvement with a pelvic mass that seldom suppurates.

*Anogenitorectal Syndrome* Associated with receptive anal intercourse, proctocolitis, hyperplasia of intestinal and perirectal lymphatic tissue. Resultant perirectal abscesses, ischiorectal and rectovaginal fistulas, anal fistulas, rectal stricture. Overgrowth of lymphatic tissue results in lymphorrhoids (resembling hemorrhoids) or perianal condylomata.

*Esthiomene* Elephantiasis of genitalia, usually females, which may ulcerate, occurring 1 to 20 years after primary infection.

## DIFFERENTIAL DIAGNOSIS

**Primary Stage** Genital herpes, primary syphilis, chancroid.
**Inguinal Syndrome** Incarcerated inguinal hernia, plague, tularemia, tuberculosis, genital herpes, syphilis, chancroid, Hodgkin's disease.
**Anogenitorectal Syndrome** Rectal stricture caused by rectal cancer, trauma, actinomycosis, tuberculosis, schistosomiasis.
**Esthiomene** Filariasis, mycosis.

## LABORATORY EXAMINATIONS

See Table 27-9B.
**Imaging** MRI may show massive pelvic lymphadenopathy in women and homosexual men.
**Dermatopathology** Not pathognomonic. *Primary stage*: small stellate abscesses surrounded by histiocytes, arranged in palisade pattern. *Late stage*: epidermal acanthosis/papillomatosis; dermis—edematous; lymphatics—dilated with fibrosis and lymphoplasmocytic infiltrate.

## DIAGNOSIS

By DFA, culture, serologic tests, and exclusion of other causes of inguinal lymphadenopathy or genital ulcers.

## COURSE AND PROGNOSIS

Highly variable. Bacterial superinfections may contribute to complications. Rectal stricture is late complication. Spontaneous remission is common.

## MANAGEMENT

**Antimicrobial Therapy** A 3-week course of the antimicrobial agents recommended for acute *C. trachomatis* infections is given (page 932).

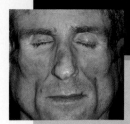

# MUCOCUTANEOUS MANIFESTATIONS OF HUMAN IMUNODEFICIENCY VIRUS DISEASE

## THE HIV EPIDEMIC

The HIV pandemic has been under way for more than 20 years, the first cases being reported in the summer of 1981. Currently, sub-Saharan Africa bears the greatest burden of the epidemic worldwide. The number of new infections is escalating in the former Soviet Union, India, and China. The epidemiology of the pandemic is ever changing, with some of the documented parameters as follows (2002):

1. 69.8 million persons already infected
2. 68 million will die from HIV disease between 2000 and 2020
3. 42 million living with HIV disease
4. 5 million new infections annually (15,000 new infections daily)
   a. > 95% of cases are in developing countries
   b. 47% are women
   c. 87% are persons ages 15 to 49 years
   d. 50% are persons ages 15 to 24 years
   e. 1700 are children under age 15 years
   f. 80% acquired by heterosexual sex
5. Spread of HIV disease continues unchecked.

In the United States, 40,000 new HIV infections have occurred annually since the 1990s. The number of annual deaths has declined sharply due to the availability of highly active antiretroviral therapy (HAART). An estimated 1 million individuals are currently infected with HIV, of whom 250,000 are unaware of their infection. Through 1999, 733,374 cumulative cases of AIDS had been reported to the Centers for Disease Control and Prevention (CDC). Early in the epidemic, homosexual men were nearly exclusively infected; today new cases of HIV infection result predominantly from injecting-drug use and heterosexual contact, with a disproportionate representation among minority populations. Women are increasingly affected. In Canada, Australia, and western Europe, the epidemiology is similar to that in the United States.

Nearly all HIV-infected individuals exhibit some dermatologic disorder attributable to progressive immunodeficiency during the course of the infection. Some disorders are highly associated with HIV infection, and their diagnosis often warrants HIV serotesting (Table 28-1).

Early diagnosis is critical in the management of HIV disease for several reasons. Given the knowledge of their HIV infection and its contagiousness, most patients will reduce or eliminate behaviors associated with transmission of HIV. Early treatment with HAART retards progression of HIV-induced immunodeficiency and, in many cases, reduces immunocompromise. In patients with low CD4+ cell counts, many of the opportunistic infections such as *Pneumocystis carinii* pneumonia (PCP) are better treated by primary prophylactic regimens before development of clinical disease.

**TABLE 28-1   Mucocutaneous Findings Associated with HIV Infection and Indications for HIV Serotesting**

| Risk for HIV Infection | Mucocutaneous Finding |
|---|---|
| High—serotesting always indicated | Acute retroviral syndrome |
| | Kaposi's sarcoma |
| | Oral hairy leukoplakia |
| | Proximal subungual onychomycosis |
| | Bacillary angiomatosis |
| | Eosinophilic folliculitis |
| | Chronic herpetic ulcers (>1 month duration) |
| | Any sexually transmitted disease |
| | Skin findings of injecting-drug use |
| Moderate—serotesting may be indicated | Herpes zoster |
| | Molluscum contagiosum: multiple facial in an adult |
| | Candidiasis: oropharyngeal, esophageal, or recurrent vulvovaginal |
| Possible—serotesting may be indicated | Generalized lymphadenopathy |
| | Seborrheic dermatitis |
| | Aphthous ulcers (recurrent, refractory to therapy) |

# ACUTE HIV-1 SYNDROME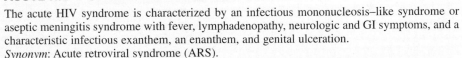

The acute HIV syndrome is characterized by an infectious mononucleosis–like syndrome or aseptic meningitis syndrome with fever, lymphadenopathy, neurologic and GI symptoms, and a characteristic infectious exanthem, an enanthem, and genital ulceration.
*Synonym*: Acute retroviral syndrome (ARS).

## EPIDEMIOLOGY AND ETIOLOGY

**Age of Onset**   Commonly in the young, but any age.

**Sex**   Currently, about equal. Heterosexual transmission is the most common mode of transmission, particularly in developing countries.

**Incubation Period**   Signs and symptoms occur within 5 to 30 days following exposure (most within 21 to 28 days).

**Etiology**   Nearly all infections are HIV-1. HIV-2 causes disease in western Africa.

**Incidence**   Shortly after becoming infected, 50 to 70% of persons experience significant symptoms.

**Transmission of HIV**   *Sexual Exposure Predominant* mode of transmission worldwide: heterosexual and homosexual contact.
*Injecting-Drug Use (IDU)* Needle sharing transmits HIV.
*Blood or Blood Products* Recipients of blood or blood products after 1978 but before 1985 were inadvertently infected with HIV. Currently, blood is screened for p24 antigen and anti-HIV antibody. Risk of HIV infection after transfusion of HIV-contaminated blood: 90 to 100%.
*Organ Transplant Recipients* Prior to HIV testing, HIV was transmitted during transplantation of solid organs, bone marrow, and corneae.

***Semen*** Occurred during artificial insemination from HIV-infected donor.

***Health Care Workers*** HIV can be transmitted by needle sticks and cuts contaminated with HIV-infected blood during medical procedures. Risk for HIV infection after puncture with HIV-contaminated blood is 0.3%.

***Perinatal Transmission*** Child born to mother with HIV infection, i.e., intrapartum, perinatally, or by breast feeding, may become infected.

**Risk Factors** Genital ulcer disease, such as genital herpes, chancroid, or syphilis, increases the risk of HIV transmission. HIV is concentrated in seminal fluid, particularly in genital inflammatory states such as other sexually transmitted diseases. HIV-infected individuals with higher viral loads may transmit the virus more efficiently. Strong association of HIV transmission with receptive anal intercourse.

## PATHOGENESIS

After primary HIV infection, billions of virions are produced and destroyed each day; a concomitant daily turnover of actively infected CD4+ cells is also in the billions. HIV infection is relatively unique among human viral infections in that, despite robust cellular and humoral immune responses that are mounted after primary infection, the virus is not cleared completely from the body (with a few exceptions). Chronic infection develops that persists with varying degrees of virus replication for a median of 10 years before an individual becomes clinically ill.

## HISTORY

Symptoms range from asymptomatic to severe requiring hospitalization (15%). One study reported symptomatic illness in 89% of acute HIV infections. The diagnosis is often missed, considered in only 25% of cases. Between 50 and 70% of recently infected individuals experience symptomatic primary infection.

**Mucocutaneous Symptoms** Cutaneous: Rash (50 to 60%). Exanthem usually appears 2 to 3 days after onset of fever, lasting 5 to 8 days; enanthem, asymptomatic; ulcers, painful in mouth and/or anogenital region. Pharyngitis (50 to 70%); oral ulcers (10 to 20%). Genital ulcers (5 to 15%).

**Systemic Symptoms** Fever (>80 to 90%), fatigue/lethargy/malaise (>70 to 90%), myalgia/arthralgia (50 to 70%), night sweats (50%), anorexia/weight loss (25%), aseptic meningitis (24%), other neurologic symptoms (encephalitis, peripheral neuropathy, myelopathy, headache, retrobulbar pain), anorexia (21%), nausea/vomiting/diarrhea (30 to 60%), lymphadenopathy.

## PHYSICAL EXAMINATION

**Skin Lesions**
Morbilliform rash, i.e., infectious exanthem (Fig. 28-1) with pink macules, papules up to 1 cm in diameter. Ulcers occur on penis and/or scrotum. Less common: urticaria. Also reported: vesicular and pustular exanthems, desquamation of palms/soles. Lesions remain discrete. Most common site of exanthem is upper thorax and collar region (100%) > face (60%) > arms (40%) > scalp, thighs (20%). Palms.

**Mucous Membranes** Pharyngitis. Enanthem, spotty, on hard and soft palate. Ulcers: 5 to 10 mm in diameter, round to oval, shallow with white bases surrounded by a red halo, arising on the tonsils, palate, and/or buccal mucosa; esophageal ulcers. Uncommonly, oral candidiasis.

***Anogenitalia*** Ulcers: prepuce of penis, scrotum, anus, anal canal.

**General Examination** ***Lymph Nodes*** Lymphadenopathy.

***Neurologic Findings*** Acute meningitis; acute reversible encephalopathy with loss of memory, alteration of consciousness, and personality change.

## DIFFERENTIAL DIAGNOSIS

**Viral Syndromes** Primary Epstein-Barr virus (EBV) infection (infectious mononucleosis) (1% of negative monospots are ARS); primary cytomegalovirus (CMV) infection; influenza; acute hepatitis A, B, and C infection; rubella.

**Other Syndromes** Streptococcal infection, toxoplasmosis (acute), early toxic shock syndromes, syphilis, Rocky Mountain spotted fever, Lyme disease.

## LABORATORY EXAMINATIONS

**Hematology** Lymphocytopenia. Elevated erythrocyte sedimentation rate (ESR).

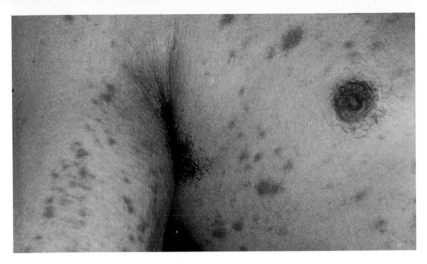

**FIGURE 28-1    Acute retroviral syndrome: exanthem**  *Discrete, erythematous macules and papules on the trunk and arm; associated findings were fever, scrotal ulcers, erythematous macules on palate, and lymphadenopathy.*

**CD4+ T Lymphocytes**  Usually dip down by several hundred (normal in adults, approximately 1000/μL), occasionally as low as 200/μL, but return to normal levels within several weeks. After a latent period, CD4+ cell levels again fall. CD4+ cell counts are used to monitor degree of immunodeficiency and response to antiretroviral therapy.

**Detection of HIV**  *Viral Load Levels (VLLs)* Usually extremely high initially. Subsequently reduced to low or undetectable levels. After a hiatus of years, the viral load eventually increases as immune function declines. Individuals with low VLLs and relatively high CD4+ cell counts are usually not treated with HAART. VLLs are used to monitor response to HAART.

*HIV Antigen* p24 antigen is detectable in serum during ARS before HIV seroconversion. Becomes undetectable after immune response. Recurs as immune function declines.

*Viral Cultures* HIV isolation from blood or CSF during ARS. Virus is undetectable after immune response. Viremia recurs as immune function declines.

**Serologic Testing**  *Acute Retroviral Syndrome* Demonstrated seroconversion of anti-HIV-1 antibodies by enzyme-linked immunosorbent assay (ELISA); confirmed by Western blot, within 3 weeks of illness. HIV-2 infection is rare in industrialized countries.

*Asymptomatic HIV Infection* HIV antibody is detectable in ≥95% of individuals within 6 months of infection. Although a negative antibody test usually means an individual is not infected, antibody tests cannot rule out infection that occurred <6 months before the test.

## DIAGNOSIS

Must have a very high level of suspicion; risk factors and physical findings critical; HIV ELISA, HIV Western blot, HIV viral load, p24 antigen, p31. Demonstrated seroconversion of anti-HIV antibodies by ELISA, confirmed by Western blot, confirms diagnosis of primary HIV infection. Established HIV infection can be confirmed by these serologic tests as well as by isolation of HIV from blood or CSF or demonstration of p24 antigen.

## COURSE AND PROGNOSIS

The spectrum of symptoms associated with primary HIV infection is broad; most individuals experience no or mild symptoms that do not prompt medical consultation. In those with symptomatic illness, the mean duration of illness in one study was 13 days (range 5 to 44 days).

Long-term illness of >2 weeks is associated with an eight times higher risk of developing AIDS within 3 years of seroconversion.

After an asymptomatic or symptomatic primary infection, HIV infection becomes latent with no clinical symptoms or findings. With disease progression and diminution of immune function, criteria for diagnosis of AIDS occur. The pace of disease progression is variable. The median time between primary HIV infection (seroconversion) and the development of AIDS among young homosexual men is >10 years (in the United States), with a range from a few months to 12 years. Most adults and adolescents infected with HIV remain symptom-free for long periods, but with viral replication occurring at a high rate. Factors that correlate with more rapid disease progression are HIV infection transmitted from someone with advanced HIV disease rather than an asymptomatic individual, older individuals (>30 years), and severe ARS. Essentially all HIV-infected individuals will eventually have symptoms related to the infection: 70 to 85% of infected adults develop symptoms and 55 to 62% develop AIDS within 12 years of seroconversion. Additional cases occur among those who have remained AIDS-free for >12 years.

## MANAGEMENT

**HIV Prevention**   *Sex Education* The most common mode of HIV transmission is during sexual intercourse. Currently, in terms of numbers of new HIV infections, female-to-male and male-to-female transmission is much more common than male-to-male. Safer sexual practices must be taught at an early age.
*Transfusions and Transplantation* Blood and blood by-products must be tested before administration. HIV infection must be ruled out in donors of any transplanted organ.
**Approved Antiretroviral Agents**   Nucleoside reverse transcriptase inhibitors (NRTIs): zidovudine, didanosine, zalcitabine, stavudine, lamivudine, abacavir, tenofovir, emtricitabine. Nonnucleoside reverse transcriptase inhibitors (NNRTIs): nevirapine, delavirdine, efavirenz. Protease inhibitors (PIs): saquinavir, rotonavir, indinavir, nelfinavir, amprenavir, lopinavir, atazanavir. Entry: enfuvirtide.
**Immune Reconstitution Reactions**   *Mycobacterium avium* complex (MAC), CMV, tuberculosis, other (hepatitis B and C), cryptococcosis, histoplasmosis, polymorphonuclear leukocytes, noninfectious "autoimmune" diseases, eosinophilic folliculitis.

# EOSINOPHILIC FOLLICULITIS   ■   ●<sup>*</sup>

Eosinophilic folliculitis (EF) is a pruritic follicular eruption of the upper trunk, face, neck, and proximal extremities occurring in advanced HIV disease and/or after initiation of HAART. EF occurring in HIV disease is different from that of Ofuji's disease, which presents commonly on the face of healthy young Asians.
*Synonym*: Eosinophilic pustular folliculitis.

## EPIDEMIOLOGY AND PATHOGENESIS

Unknown.

## HISTORY

Moderate to intense itching unrelieved by many therapies. Pruritus may be severe, especially in those with atopic diathesis, disturbing sleep. Initially, occurred in the setting of advanced HIV disease. Currently, occurs following initiation of HAART, associated with immune reconstitution syndrome.

## PHYSICAL EXAMINATION

### Skin Lesions
The primary lesions are 3- to 5-mm erythematous, edematous, follicular papules and pustules (Fig. 28-2A and 2B). Dozens or hundreds of lesions may be present, in various stages of evolution. Frequently, changes secondary to

---

*Not serious itself but an indicator of serious HIV disease.

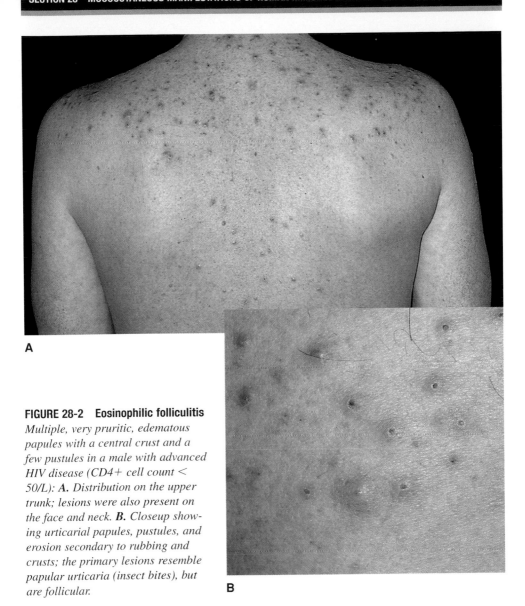

**FIGURE 28-2   Eosinophilic folliculitis**
*Multiple, very pruritic, edematous papules with a central crust and a few pustules in a male with advanced HIV disease (CD4+ cell count < 50/L): **A.** Distribution on the upper trunk; lesions were also present on the face and neck. **B.** Closeup showing urticarial papules, pustules, and erosion secondary to rubbing and crusts; the primary lesions resemble papular urticaria (insect bites), but are follicular.*

scratching/rubbing are seen: excoriations/crusting of papules/pustules; atopic dermatitis, lichen simplex chronicus, prurigo nodularis. *Secondary infections of excoriated sites:* impetiginization, furunculosis, cellulitis. Postinflammatory hyperpigmentation occurs in more darkly pigmented individuals and can be quite disfiguring.
***Distribution*** Trunk; head and neck; proximal extremities. In some individuals, lesions present only on face or on trunk.

## DIFFERENTIAL DIAGNOSIS

Allergic contact dermatitis, adverse cutaneous drug reaction, atopic dermatitis, scabies, papular urticaria (insect bites), acne vulgaris, dermatophytic folliculitis, bacterial folliculitis (*Staphylococcus aureus*), *Malassezia* folliculitis.

## LABORATORY EXAMINATIONS

**Serology**   HIV ELISA and Western blot positive.

**Cultures**   Negative for pathogenic organisms. Many patients with longstanding untreated EF have secondary colonization/infection with *S. aureus.*

**Dermatopathology**   Perifollicular and perivascular infiltrate with varying numbers of eosinophils. Epithelial spongiosis of follicular infundibulum and/or sebaceous glands associated with a mixed cellular infiltrate. Eosinophilic pustules uncommon. Special stains for bacteria, fungi, and parasites are negative.

**Hematology**   Eosinophilia. CD4+ cell count usually $<100/\mu L$.

## DIAGNOSIS

Clinical diagnosis confirmed by skin biopsy, with cultures ruling out infectious causes. A new primary lesion (follicular papule) should be marked with a pen and 2-mm punch biopsy specimen obtained.

## COURSE AND PROGNOSIS

In untreated HIV disease, the course of EF tends to be chronic and persistent. Occuring after the initiation of HAART, symptoms often persist for weeks to months if untreated.

## MANAGEMENT

Pruritus is moderate to severe, significantly affecting quality of life. Changes secondary to chronic scratching such as secondary infections and lichen simplex chronicus should also be identified and treated. The most predictably effective therapy is a short tapered course of oral glucocorticoid such as prednisone (Table 28-2).

### TABLE 28-2   Management of Eosinophilic Folliculitis

| | |
|---|---|
| **Antihistamines** | Those causing sedation are more effective for symptomatic relief of pruritus. Doxepin, 10–100 mg, is especially effective at bedtime |
| **Topical agents** | |
| Glucocorticoids | Class I (superpotent) glucocorticoids applied to affected areas produce fair to moderate improvement in pruritus and lesions. Patients using these agents on the face should be closely monitored for atrophic changes. |
| **Systemic agents** | |
| Prednisone | Initial dose of 70 mg, followed by a taper of 5–10 mg/d (14 → 7 days) provides rapid symptomatic improvement as well as resolution of EF. EF gradually recurs after completion of course. |
| Isotretinoin | 1–2 mg/kg per day (about 80 mg) very effective in causing resolution of EF. Once symptoms and skin findings have resolved, dose is reduced to 40 mg/d for 2–4 weeks and then tapered to 40 mg qod. Dosing may be discontinued in 1–2 months if symptoms do not recur. Many HIV-infected individuals treated with HAART have elevated triglyceride levels; isotretinoin can further increase triglyceride levels. |
| Itraconazole | 400 mg/d for 4 weeks reported to be effective. |
| **Phototherapy** | |
| UVB | Treatments are usually given three times a week, tapering as symptoms of EF resolve. Moderately effective. |
| Natural sunlight | Many individuals cannot tolerate natural sunlight because of treatment with photosensitizing drugs such as trimethoprim-sulfamethoxazole (Bactrim), which are photosensitizing in the UVA spectrum. |

# ORAL HAIRY LEUKOPLAKIA ■ ●

Oral hairy leukoplakia (OHL) is a benign, viral-induced hyperplasia of the oral mucosa, most commonly of the inferolateral surface of the tongue, characterized by white, corrugated plaques, occurring in patients with symptomatic HIV disease.
*Synonym*: Oral viral leukoplakia.

## ETIOLOGY AND PATHOGENESIS

Many adults have asymptomatic EBV infection of the oropharynx. EBV is thought to emerge from latency as HIV-induced immunocompromise progresses and to cause the epidermal hyperplasia.

## HISTORY

**Incubation Period** Usually 5 to 10 years after primary HIV infection.
**Symptoms** Asymptomatic, but stigmatization of HIV disease.

## PHYSICAL EXAMINATION

**Oral Mucosa** White or grayish-white, well-demarcated verrucous plaque (Fig. 28-3) with corrugated or hairy texture. Most commonly on the lateral and inferior surfaces of the tongue. Often present bilaterally, but size of plaques usually not equal. Some individuals may have oropharyngeal candidiasis and/or condyloma in addition to OHL.

## DIFFERENTIAL DIAGNOSIS

Thrush, condyloma acuminatum, geographic or migratory glossitis, lichen planus, tobacco-associated leukoplakia, mucous patch of secondary syphilis, squamous cell carcinoma (SCC) either in situ or invasive, occlusal trauma.

## LABORATORY EXAMINATIONS

**Dermatopathology** Acanthotic epithelium with hyperkeratosis, hairlike projections of keratin, areas of koilocytes (ballooned cells with clear cytoplasm). *Electron microscopy*: Herpes

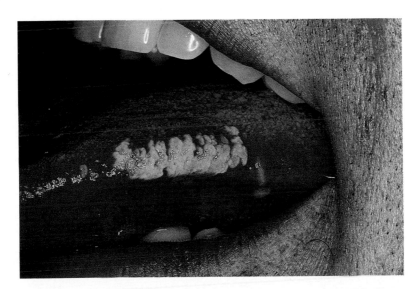

**FIGURE 28-3 Oral hairy leukoplakia** *White plaque on the lateral tongue with corduroy-like pattern. The finding is essentially pathognomonic for HIV infection and in this case, was the indication for HIV serotesting. CD4+ cell count was 223 cell/L at the time of diagnosis.*

*Not serious itself but an indicator of serious HIV disease.

viral structures in epithelial cells; positive for EBV markers.

**Cultures**   Not helpful. *Candida albicans* is commonly isolated.

### DIAGNOSIS

Clinical diagnosis. Does not rub off; does not clear with adequate anticandidal therapy.

### COURSE AND PROGNOSIS

Much less common in HIV-infected individuals treated with and responding to HAART. May also clear completely during a course of treatment with acyclovir/valaciclovir, ganciclovir, or foscarnet.

### MANAGEMENT

Reassurance that OHL is a benign viral infection is usually adequate to reduce patients' concerns, a cosmetic problem that is not precancerous.

**Topical Therapy**   Podophyllin 25% in tincture of benzoin applied to the lesion with a cotton-tipped applicator for 5 min.

**Systemic Antiviral Drugs**   Concomitant use of acyclovir, valacyclovir, famciclovir, ganciclovir, foscarnet for other indications often results in regression/clearing of OHL.

---

## ADVERSE CUTANEOUS DRUG ERUPTIONS

The incidence of adverse cutaneous drug eruptions (ACDEs) to a variety of drugs is high in HIV disease and increases with advancing immunodeficiency. Antiretroviral therapy (ART) can cause a wide spectrum of adverse reactions.

### EPIDEMIOLOGY AND ETIOLOGY

**Etiology**   Most common drugs causing ACDE: trimethoprim-sulfamethoxazole (TMP-SMX), sulfadiazine, trimethoprim-dapsone, and aminopenicillins.

**Prevalence**   Drug hypersensitivity complicated 3 to 20% of all prescriptions in those with advanced HIV disease, Up to 100 times more common than in the general population.

### PATHOGENESIS

Incidence increases with advancing immunodeficiency; may be correlated with the decline and dysregulation of immune function. After immune reconstitution by ART, some patients who had previously tolerated a drug may develop allergic cutaneous drug reactions.

### CLASSIFICATION

Drug eruptions can mimic virtually all the morphologic expressions in dermatology and must be first on the differential diagnosis in the appearance of a sudden symmetric eruption (see Section 20).

> *Exanthematous/morbilliform*: Account for 95% of ACDE in HIV disease. Between 50 and 60% of AIDS patients treated with TMP-SMX develop a morbilliform eruption 1 to 2 weeks after starting therapy.
> *Crixivan*: Retinoid dermatitis: chronic paronychia, cheilitis, pyogenic granuloma.
> *Toxic epidermal necrolysis (TEN)*: The incidence of TEN caused by sulfonamides is also increased.
> *Lipodystrophy syndrome*: See below.

### CLINICAL FINDINGS   See Section 20

### MANAGEMENT

In most cases, the implicated or suspected drug should be discontinued. In some, such as with morbilliform eruptions, the offending drug can be continued and the eruption may resolve. In cases of urticaria/angioedema or early Stevens-Johnson syndrome (SJS)/TEN, the ACDE can be life-threatening, and the drug should be discontinued.

## ACDE BY DRUG TYPE

### Antiretroviral Therapy (ART)

Drug hypersensitivity commonly occurs with the NNRTIs nevirapine, delavirdine, and efavirenz; the NRTI abacavir; and the protease inhibitor amprenavir. ART hypersensitivity is manifested by exanthematous/morbilliform eruptions (>95%); 20% of nevirapine-treated patients experience rash, most commonly an exanthematous eruption and rarely SJS, requiring drug discontinuation. Between 18 and 50% of delavirdine-treated patients experience rash. Approximately one-half of cases of ART hypersensitivity resolve despite continuation of therapy. Drug therapy should be discontinued if the following occur: mucosal involvement, blistering, exfoliation, clinically significant hepatic dysfunction, fever >39°C, or intolerable fever or pruritus. Rechallenge with abacavir has been associated with several deaths.

**Indivavir**  Has a retinoid-like effect. Cheilitis (57%); diffuse dryness and pruritus; asteatotic dermatitis on the trunk, arms, and thighs; scalp defluvium; pyogenic granulomas, single or multiple.

**Zidovudine**  (**ZVD, AZT**) Longitudinal melanonychia, brown-black longitudinal streaks in the nail plate, occur in up to 40% of those treated, more commonly in blacks than in Latinos or whites. Melanonychia are usually noted in the finger-and/or toenails within 4 to 8 weeks after initiation of therapy. Pigmented macules of mucous membranes common, occurring more commonly in more heavily melanized individuals. Diffuse hyperpigmentation mimicking primary adrenal insufficiency reported. (Melanonychia and mucocutaneous pigmentation have also been reported with administration of hydroxyurea in HIV disease.)

**Enfuvirtide**  First of a new class of antiretroviral agents for the treatment of HIV-1 infection, called *fusion inhibitors*. The most common type of ACDE is injection site reactions, occurring in up to 98% of patients. Many of these lesions are symptomatic. Lesional biopsy specimens show an inflammatory response consistent with a localized hypersensitivity reaction, resembling that of granuloma annulare and the recently described interstitial granulomatous drug reaction.

### Other Drugs

**Trimethoprim-Sulfamethoxazole**  Between 50 and 60% of those treated with IV TMP-SMX develop an exanthematous eruption (often associated with fever) 1 to 2 weeks after starting therapy (incidence 10 times greater than that in the general population). Successful desensitization has been accomplished in patients with prior exanthematous/morbilliform or urticarial reactions to TMP-SMX, sulfadiazine, and dapsone. Coadministration of glucocorticoids with TMP-SMX reduces incidence of ACDE. The occurrence of adverse reactions to TMP-SMX has also been noted to be associated with more rapid decline in CD4 cell counts. Sulfa drugs (sulfadiazine, TMP-SMX, sulfadoxine-pyrimethamine) can also cause severe bullous eruptions. Sulfa drugs are the most common cause of TEN, the incidence being 375 times higher than expected. TEN occurs most commonly in those with advanced HIV disease; 21% mortality rate.

**Oral Glucocorticoids**  Concerns: increased immunosuppression with exacerbations of opportunistic infections and neoplasms such as Kaposi's sarcoma or herpes simplex virus (HSV) infections. Prednisone is usually well tolerated and safe, especially when given for only 1 to 2 weeks.

**Foscarnet   (Trisodium   Phosphonoformate)**  Causes painful, penile erosions and/or ulcers in 30% of patients undergoing high-dose induction therapy for CMV retinitis, 7 to 24 days after starting treatment. Ulceration caused by high urinary concentration of the urinary metabolites of foscarnet. Hyperhydration reduces the risk of ulceration; in some cases, the drug must be discontinued for the ulcers to heal.

# HIV LIPODYSTROPHY SYNDROME   ⬛ ◗

Lipodystrophy (LD) is a general term used to describe varying degrees of fat redistribution (lipo-atrophy, lipohypertrophy) in different body regions. HIV lipodystrophy syndrome is characterized by (1) a *metabolic syndrome* characterized by dyslipidemia (high triglycerides, low high-density lipoprotein), insulin resistance ($\pm$ diabetes mellitus), and fat redistribution (lipohypertrophy/vis-ceral adiposity); and (2) *subcutaneous lipoatrophy*. Occurs following multidrug antiretroviral reg-imens. *Metabolic changes* are associated with increased risk for cardiovascular disease and diabetes. *Morphologic changes* are highly stigmatizing; can cause discomfort, disability, and psy-chological morbidity and reduce adherence to or discontinuation of effective ART.

## EPIDEMIOLOGY AND ETIOLOGY

**Prevalence**   LD was noted in HIV disease prior to HAART; prevalence has increased dras-tically with widespread use of HAART. More than 50% of HIV-infected patients treated with PIs (mean duration 13.9 months) had loss of facial/extremity fat and/or increase of truncal fat by clinical examination.

**Etiology**   Unknown. Occurs in HIV-infected in-dividuals who have never taken ART. Ritonavir-saquinavir combination (>indinavir or nelfinavir) most strongly associated with meta-bolic syndrome.

### Classification of Morphologic Changes

1. *Lipoatrophy* (fat depletion): correlates with stavudine use.
2. *Lipohypertrophy* (obesity or subcutaneous adiposity syndrome): related to increased caloric intake.
3. *Mixed condition* (lipoatrophy and -hyper-trophy) (fat redistribution syndrome): re-lated to an unusual side-product of effective virus control.

## PATHOGENESIS

Unknown. Factors in pathogenesis: (1) multiple drug-associated events in metabolic pathways and in different tissues; and (2) host predisposi-tion: age, genetics, HIV disease stage, inflam-matory states. Metabolic changes related to direct effects of PIs on glucose, insulin, lipids, and fat, as well as effects of HIV itself and re-lated cytokines.

Patients with lipoatrophy (significantly de-creased abdominal and mid-thigh subcutaneous fat) have elevated levels of plasma triglycerides. Those with obesity/mixed condition (increased intraabdominal fat) have elevated levels of plasma insulin and C-peptide. Use of stavudine correlates with fat wasting in both NRTI and PI groups. NRTI-associated mitochondrial toxicity leads to fat wasting. Stavudine-based regimens have a higher cumulative prevalence of lipoatro-phy than regimens based on zidovudine, aba-cavir, or tenofovir. Regimens based on nelfinavir are associated with more rapid fat loss than efavirenz. In general, thymidine-based nu-cleoside analogues have been most associated with lipoatrophy and protease inhibitor drugs most associated with the metabolic syndrome.

## HISTORY

Cosmetic disfigurement, stigmatization. Ather-osclerotic cardiovascular disease, type 2 diabetes.

## PHYSICAL EXAMINATION

### Skin Findings

Three types of altered fat distribution: periph-eral lipoatrophy, central adiposity, or a mixed presentation.

*Central Adiposity/Lipohypertrophy*   Occurs more commonly at several anatomical locations (86%) than in one location (14%). The dor-sothoracic fat pad becomes hypertrophied to a variable extent (6%) (Fig. 28-4), from mild to severe (up to 5 to 10 cm thick); can extend cir-cumferentially around the neck. Breasts may become enlarged (20%) in males and females. Abdominal girth can increase due to accumula-tion of intraabdominal fat (60%).

*Lipoatrophy*   Loss of subcutaneous fat in the face (58%) (Fig. 28-5), giving a gaunt charac-teristic appearance. The upper arms/shoulders (50%), buttocks/thighs (73%) also become de-pleted of subcutaneous fat; superficial veins are visible in these sites. There is also generalized loss of body fat.

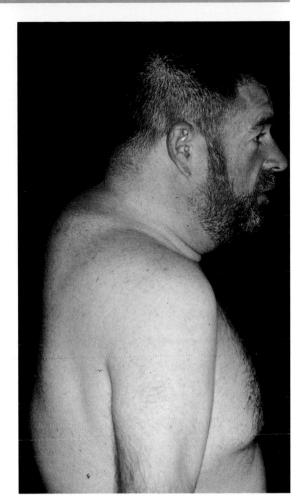

**FIGURE 28-4   HIV lipodystrophy syndrome: lipohypertrophy** *Increase in subcutaneous fat is seen on the upper back creating a "buffalo hump," neck, and breast of an otherwise thin middle-aged HIV-infected male, who is on highly active antiretroviral therapy (HAART). Liposuction of the fat had been performed two years previously, however, the lipohypertrophy recurred. Mild lipoatrophy of the cheek is also apparent.*

***Mixed Presentation*** Elements of central adiposity and lipoatrophy are present.

### DIFFERENTIAL DIAGNOSIS

**Fat Accumulation** Cushing's disease, glucocorticoid therapy, Launois-Bensaude syndrome, scleredema of diabetes mellitus.

**Lipoatrophy** Wasting of chronic disease, malnutrition.

### LABORATORY EXAMINATIONS

**Hyperlipidemia** In 74% of PI recipients; 28% in treatment-naïve patients.
**Glucose Tolerance** Impaired in 16% of PI recipients; type 2 diabetes mellitus in 7%.

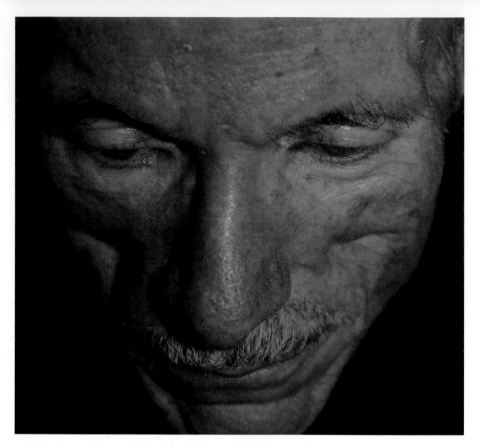

**FIGURE 28-5   HIV lipodystrophy syndrome: lipoatrophy**   *Striking loss of facial fat in a thin middle-aged HIV-infected male on highly active antiretroviral therapy (HAART). Lipohypertrophy was also present on the neck and upper central back.*

## DIAGNOSIS

Clinical diagnosis.

## COURSE AND PROGNOSIS

Lipodystrophy may progress for the first 2 years of HAART, then stabilize. Change in HAART may result in improvement of lipodystrophy.

## MANAGEMENT

For most individuals with mild to moderate lipodystrophy, changes in body habitus are not significant. However, with more severe involve-

ment, patients may request change in HAART in spite of excellent response of HIV disease.

**Metabolic Syndrome**   Changing NRTI may result in regression. Metabolic strategies: lipid-lowering strategies [fibric acids (clofibrate, fenofibrate, gemfibrozil)], insulin-sensitizing agents (metformin), strategies to change fat distribution (glitazones to increase subcutaneous fat, growth hormone to decrease visceral fat).

**Lipoatrophy**   Remains the most difficult manifestation to manage. Replacing stavudine with abacavir may result in improvement in stavudine-induced lipoatrophy. For facial lipoatrophy, various filler substances have been injected into sites in the cheeks; however, the effects are evanescent and costly.

# VARIATIONS OF COMMON MUCOCUTANEOUS DISORDERS IN HIV DISEASE

Early in the course of HIV disease when immune function is relatively intact, common dermatoses, adverse cutaneous drug eruptions, and infections present as typical clinical manifestations, have the usual course, and respond to standard therapies. However, with progressive decline in immune function, each of these characteristics of a disease can be strikingly altered. With effective management with HAART and immune reconstitution, the diseases either do not occur, resolve without specific therapy, or respond more readily to therapy.

### Kaposi's Sarcoma (KS) (See also "Kaposi's Sarcoma," Section 19)

Early in the HIV epidemic in the United States and Europe, 50% of homosexual men at the time of initial AIDS diagnosis had KS. In HIV-infected individuals, the risk for KS is 20,000 times that of the general population, 300 times that of other immunosuppressed hosts. In untreated HIV disease, KS may progress rapidly with extensive mucocutaneous and systemic involvement. KS in patients successfully treated with HAART does not occur, resolves without specific therapy other than immune reconstitution, or responds better to chemotherapies.

### Nonmelanoma Skin Cancers

As in solid organ transplant recipients, the incidence of ultraviolet light (UVL)-induced invasive SCC may be increased in HIV-infected individuals with skin phototypes I to III with much UVL exposure during early decades of life. SCC can be quite aggressive, invading locally, growing rapidly, and metastasizing by lymphatics and blood, with increased morbidity and mortality.

### Aphthous Stomatitis (See also "Aphthous Ulcers," Section 31)

Recurrent aphthous ulcerations may occur more frequently, become larger (often >1 cm), and/or become chronic with advanced HIV disease. Ulcers may be quite extensive and/or multiple, commonly involving the tongue, gingiva, lips, and esophagus, at times causing severe odynophagia with rapid weight loss. Intralesional triamcinolone and/or a 1 to 2-week tapered course of prednisone (70 to 0 mg). In resistant cases, thalidomide is an effective agent.

### *Staphylococcus aureus* Infection (See also "Impetigo and Ecthyma," "Abscess, Furuncle, and Carbuncle," and "Erysipelas and Cellulitis," Section 22)

*S. aureus* is the most common cutaneous bacterial pathogen in HIV disease. The nasal carriage rate of *S. aureus* is 50%, twice that of HIV-seronegative control groups. In most instances, *S. aureus* infections are typical, presenting as primary infections (folliculitis, furuncles, carbuncles), secondarily impetiginized lesions (excoriations, eczema, scabies, herpetic ulcer, Kaposi's sarcoma), cellulitis, or venous access device infections, all of which can be complicated by bacteremia and disseminated infection. The incidence of methicillin-resistant *S. aureus* (MRSA) infections is increasing; the severity of infections may be more severe because of delay in initiation of effective anti-MRSA therapy.

### Dermatophytoses (See also "Dermatophytoses," Section 23, and "Fungal Infections: Onychomycosis," Section 30)

Epidermal dermatophytosis in HIV-infected individuals can be extensive, recurrent, and difficult to eradicate. Proximal subungual onychomycosis, which is common in untreated HIV disease, presents as a chalky-white discoloration of the undersurface of the proximal nail plate and is an indication for HIV serotesting.

### Mucosal Candidiasis (See also "Candidiasis," Section 23)

Mucosal candidiasis affecting the upper aerodigestive tracts and/or vulvovagina is common in HIV disease. Oropharyngeal candidiasis, the most common presentation, is often the initial manifestation of HIV disease and a marker for disease progression. Esophageal and tracheobronchial candidiasis occur in advanced HIV disease and are AIDS-defining conditions. The incidence of cutaneous candidiasis may be somewhat increased. In young children with HIV disease, chronic candidal paronychia and nail dystrophy are seen frequently.

### Disseminated Fungal Infection (See also "Disseminated Cryptococcosis," "Histoplasmosis," and "Disseminated Coccidioidomycosis," Section 23)

Latent pulmonary fungal infections with *Cryptococcus neoformans, Coccidioides immitis, Histoplasma capsulatum,* and *Penicillium marneffei* can be reactivated in HIV-infected individuals and disseminated to the skin and other organs. The most common cutaneous presentation of disseminated infection is molluscum contagiosum–like lesions on the face; other lesions such as nodules, pustules, ulcers, abscesses, or a papulosquamous eruption resembling guttate psoriasis (seen with histoplasmosis) also occur.

### Herpes Simplex Virus Infection (See also "Herpes Simplex Virus: Infections Associated with Systemic Immunocompromise," Section 25)

Reactivated herpes simplex virus type 1 (HSV-1) or HSV-2 infection is one of the most common viral complications of HIV disease. Most HIV-infected persons are HSV-2 seropositive. HIV-infected persons reactivate HSV-2 on 30 to 50% of days. Most reactivation is subclinical. Perianal reactivation is particularly frequent. Frequency of HSV-2 reactivation is influenced by both CD4 cell count and viral RNA levels. With increasing immunodeficiency, early lesions present with erosions or ulcerations due to epidermal necrosis without vesicle formation. Untreated, these lesions may evolve to large, painful ulcers with raised margins. In contrast to its effect in healthy individuals, reactivated HSV in those with advanced HIV disease can cause large, chronic ulceration in the oropharynx, esophagus, and anogenitalia. HSV should be considered in the differential diagnosis of any ulcerative or crusted lesion on the face, mouth, anogenitalia, or fingers in an individual with advanced HIV disease.

### Varicella-Zoster Virus (VZV) Infection (See also "Varicella-Zoster Virus Infections in the Immunocompromised Host," Section 25)

Primary VZV infection (varicella or chickenpox) in HIV-infected individuals can be severe, prolonged, and complicated by parenchymal infection, bacterial superinfection, and death. Herpes zoster (HZ) occurs in 25% of HIV-infected persons during the course of their HIV disease, associated with modest decline in immune function. Cutaneous dissemination of HZ is relatively common; however, visceral involvement is rare. With increasing immunodeficiency, VZV infection can present clinically as chronic dermatomal verrucous lesions; one or more chronic painful ulcers or ecthymatous lesions within a dermatome; ecthymatous lesion(s), ulcer(s), or nodule(s) resembling basal cell carcinoma or SCC. Untreated, these lesions persist for months or the lifetime of the patient. HZ can be recurrent within the same dermatome(s) or in other dermatomes. VZV can cause a rapidly progressive chorioretinitis with acute retinal necrosis, often bilaterally, in the absence of any cutaneous involvement and must be differentiated from CMV chorioretinitis. Black persons with extensive HZ may experience hypertrophic or keloidal scarring as lesions heal.

### Molluscum Contagiosum (See also "Molluscum Contagiosum," Section 25)

In HIV-infected individuals, molluscum contagiosum has up to an 18% prevalence; the severity of the infection is a marker for advanced immunodeficiency. Patients may have multiple small papules or nodules or large tumors, >1 cm in diameter, most commonly arising on the face, especially the beard area, the neck, and intertriginous sites. Shaving is a major factor in the facial spread of mollusca and should be avoided if possible. Cystlike mollusca occur on the ears. Occasionally, mollusca can arise on the non-hair-bearing skin of the palms/soles.

### Human Papillomavirus (HPV) Infection (See also "Human Papillomavirus: Mucosal Infections," Section 27)

With advancing immunodeficiency, cutaneous and/or mucosal warts can become extensive and refractory to treatment. Of more concern, however, HPV-induced intraepithelial neoplasia, more recently termed *squamous intraepithelial lesion* (SIL), is a precursor to invasive SCC, arising most often on the cervix, vulva, penis, perineum, and anus. In HIV-infected females, the incidence of cervical SIL is six to eight times that of controls. The current trend toward longer median survival of patients with advanced HIV disease may lead to an increased incidence of HPV-associated neoplasia and invasive SCC in the future. SIL on the external genitalia, perineum, or anus is best managed with local therapies such as imiquimod cream, cryosurgery, electrosurgery, or laser surgery rather than with aggressive surgical excision.

### Syphilis (See also "Syphilis," Section 27)

The clinical course of syphilis in HIV-infected individuals is most often the same as in the normal host. However, an accelerated course with the development of neurosyphilis or tertiary syphilis has been reported within months of initial syphilitic infection.

# SKIN SIGNS OF HAIR, NAIL, AND MUCOSAL DISORDERS

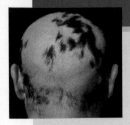

# DISORDERS OF HAIR FOLLICLES AND RELATED DISORDERS

Human hair has little vestigial function: (1) it reduces heat loss through the scalp; (2) it protects the scalp, face, and neck from UV solar radiation; and (3) it contributes to a psychological perception of beauty and attractiveness. The protective properties of hair can easily be replaced by a hat. Alteration of the "normal" quantity of hair is often associated with profound psychological impact. Loss of scalp hair is considered abnormal in many societies, associating balding with old age (androgenetic alopecia) or impaired health (chemotherapy). Excess hair on the face (hirsutism, hypertrichosis) and extremities of women is often considered unattractive. Billions of dollars are spent annually in industrialized countries to care for hair and perceived abnormalities.

## TYPES OF HAIR

*Lanugo hair* Soft fine hair that covers much of fetus; usually shed before birth.

*Vellus hair* Fine, nonpigmented hair (peach fuzz) that covers the body of children and adults; growth not affected by hormones. Beard hair in women and children is vellus.

*Intermediate hair* Shows the characteristics of vellus and terminal hairs.

*Terminal hair* Thick pigmented hair found on scalp, beard, axillae, pubic area; growth is influenced by hormones. Eyebrow/eyelash hair are terminal hairs.

## REGIONS OF THE PILOSEBACEOUS AND APOCRINE APPARATUS

*Infundibulum* Superior region extending down to the junction of the sebaceous duct with the follicle.

*Isthmus* Mid-region between the sebaceous duct and the erector pili muscle protuberance.

*Inferior region* Lower region below the erector pili muscle protuberance.

## BIOLOGY OF HAIR GROWTH

Hair growth on the scalp occurs in cycles of intermittent activity (Fig. 29-1); phases of growth are followed by periods of quiescence.

*Anagen* Phase of normal active growth

*Catagen* Brief transition phase (between anagen and telogen) during which hair growth stops.

*Telogen* Resting phase.

*Exogen* Hair shedding phase (relationship between hair shaft and base of telogen follicle)

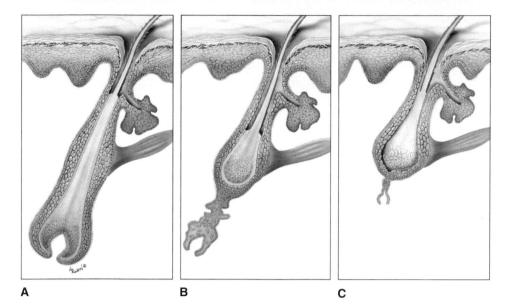

A                                    B                                    C

**FIGURE 29-1    Hair growth cycle**   *Diagrammatic representation of the changes that occur to the follicle and hair shaft during the hair growth cycle.* **A.** *Anagen (growth stage);* **B.** *Catagen (degenerative stage);* **C.** *Telogen (resting stage). (Courtesy of Lynn M. Klein, MD.)*

Duration and rate of growth of anagen phase (varying at different body sites, in different individuals, and at various ages) determine the ultimate length of hair in that area. Eyebrows, eyelashes, and axillary pubic hair: anagen phase is short; telogen phase prolonged. Scalp, beard: relatively long anagen phase. Terminal scalp hair follicles: 100,000 at birth; genetically determined to produce long, thick pigmented hairs. Vellus hairs (Latin *Vellus,* "Fleece"): present over most of the body; genetically predestined to produce hairs that are short, fine, nonpigmented.

Hair follicles can vary in size under the influence of androgens, which increase the size of hair follicles in the beard, chest, legs, and arms but decrease the size of the hair follicles in the temporal regions of the scalp; this shapes the hairline in men and many women.

The response of the hair follicle to testosterone and dihydrotestosterone (DHT) is under genetic control. DHT causes growth of the prostate, growth of terminal hair, androgenetic alopecia, and acne. Testosterone causes growth of axillary hair and lower pubic hair, as well as sex drive, growth of the phallus and scrotum, and spermatogenesis.

## LABORATORY EXAMINATIONS

**Hair Pull**   Scalp is gently pulled. Normally, three to five hairs are dislodged; shedding more hair suggests pathology.

**Trichogram**   Determines the number of anagen and telogen hairs and is made by epilating (plucking) 50 hairs or more from the scalp with a needleholder and counting the number of anagen hairs (growing hairs with a long encircling hair sheath) and the number of club or telogen hairs (resting hairs with an inner root sheath and roots usually largest at the base). Normally, 80 to 90% of hairs are in anagen phase.

**Scalp Biopsy**   Offers insight into pathogenesis of alopecia.

# HAIR LOSS: ALOPECIA

Shedding of hair is termed *effluvium* or *defluvium*, and the resulting condition is called *alopecia* (Greek alópekia, baldness). Individuals are often aware of and very concerned about subtle thinning of the hair. Disorders characterized by loss of hair are conveniently classified into *noncicatricial alopecia*, where, at least clinically, there is no sign of tissue inflammation, scarring, or atrophy of skin, and *cicatricial alopecia*, where evidence of tissue destruction such as inflammation, atrophy, and scarring is apparent.

## NONSCARRING ALOPECIA

Nonscarring alopecia can occur globally or be focal (Table 29-1). Loss of scalp hair has the most cosmetic impact on individuals.

---

### TABLE 29-1  Etiology of Hair Loss

**Diffuse (global) hair loss** (nonscarring)
  Failure of follicle production
  Hair shaft abnormality
  Abnormality of cycling (shedding)
    Telogen effluvium
    Anagen effluvium
    Loose anagen syndrome
    Alopecia areata
**Focal (patchy, localized) hair loss**
  Nonscarring
    Production decline
      Triangular alopecia
      Pattern hair loss (androgenetic alopecia)
    Hair breakage
      Trichotillomania
      Traction alopecia
      Tinea capitis
      Primary or acquired hair shaft abnormality
    Unruly hair
    Abnormality of cycling
      Alopecia areata
      Syphilis
  Cicatricial (scarring) alopecia

## ALOPECIA AREATA

*Alopecia areata* (AA) is a localized loss of hair in round or oval areas without any visible inflammation of the skin in hair-bearing areas; the most common presenting site is the scalp. *AA totalis* (AAT): total absence of terminal scalp hair. *AA universalis* (AAU): Total loss of terminal body and scalp hair. *Ophiasis*: Bandlike pattern of hair loss over periphery of scalp.

## EPIDEMIOLOGY AND ETIOLOGY

**Age of Onset**   Young adults (<25 years); children are affected more frequently.

**Sex**   Equal in both sexes, although the male:female ratio is reported to be 2:1 in Italy and Spain.

**Prevalence**   Relatively common. About 1% of the U.S. population has at least one episode of AA by age 50.

**Etiology**   Unknown. Association with other autoimmune diseases suggests an anti–hair bulb autoimmune process.

## PATHOGENESIS

An autoimmune disease; not a sign of any multisystem disease. Associated autoimmune disorders: vitiligo, familial autoimmune polyendocrinopathy syndrome (hypoparathyroidism, Addison's disease, mucocutaneous candidiasis), thyroid disease (Hashimoto's disease). Follicular damage occurs in anagen followed by rapid tranformation to telogen. White or graying hairs are frequently spared; with fulminant AA, persons may experience "going gray overnight."

## HISTORY

**Duration of Hair Loss**   Gradual over weeks to months. Patches of AA can be stable and often show spontaneous regrowth over a period of several months; new patches may appear while others resolve.

**Skin Symptoms**   Not symptomatic. Individuals are usually very concerned about hair loss and potential for continued, progressive balding.

**Associated Findings**   Hashimoto's thyroiditis, vitiligo, myasthenia gravis.

## PHYSICAL EXAMINATION

**Skin Findings**   Usually none. Possibly minimal erythema in area of hair loss.

**Hair**   Alopecia, normal-appearing skin with follicular openings present (Figs. 29-2 through 29-4). No scarring, no atrophy; occasionally, with diagnostic broken-off stubby hairs called *exclamation point hairs* (distal ends are broader than proximal ends) (Fig.29-2). With regrowth of hair, new hairs are fine, often white or gray. Alopecia often sharply defined. Scattered, discrete areas of alopecia (Fig. 29-3) or confluent with total loss of scalp hair (AAT) (Fig. 29-4), or AAU with generalized loss of body hair (including vellus hair). Sometimes hair loss in AAT may follow a diffuse (noncircumscribed) pattern.

**Sites of Predilection**   Scalp, eyebrows, eyelashes, pubic hair, beard.

**Nails**   Fine pitting ("hammered brass") of dorsal nail plate. Also: mottled lunula, trachyonychia (rough nails), onychomadesis (separation of nail from matrix).

## DIFFERENTIAL DIAGNOSIS

**Nonscarring Alopecia**   Secondary syphilis ("moth-eaten" appearance in beard or scalp), white-patch tinea capitis, trichotillomania, traction alopecia, early chronic cutaneous lupus erythematosus, androgenetic alopecia.

## LABORATORY EXAMINATIONS

**Serology**   Antinuclear antibodies (to rule out lupus erythematosus); rapid plasma reagin (RPR) test (to rule out secondary syphilis).

**KOH Preparation**   Rule out tinea capitis.

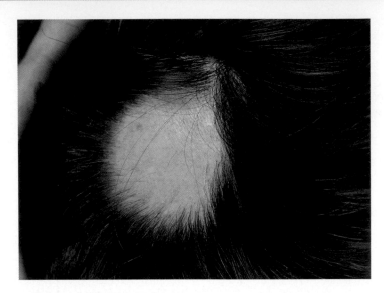

**FIGURE 29-2   Alopecia areata of scalp: solitary lesion**   *A sharply outlined portion of the scalp with complete alopecia without scaling, erythema, atrophy, or scarring. Empty follicles can still be seen on the involved scalp. The short, broken-off hair shafts (so-called exclamation point hair) appear as very short stubs emerging from the bald scalp.*

**Dermatopathology**   Peribulbar, perivascular, and outer root sheath mononuclear cell infiltrate of T cells and macrophages; follicular dystrophy with abnormal pigmentation and matrix degeneration.

## COURSE

Spontaneous remission is common in patchy AA but is less so with AAT or AAU. Poor prognosis associated with ophiasis, age of onset (<5 years with AAT or AAU have worse prognoses), association of atopy, duration of hair loss in given area.

If occurring after puberty, 80% regrow hair. AAU is rare. After first episode of AA, 33% completely regrow the hair within 1 year. Recurrences of AA, however, are frequent. Systemic glucocorticoids or cyclosporine can induce remission of AA but do not alter the course.

## MANAGEMENT

Treatment directed at inflammatory infiltrate and growth inhibitor factors produced by inflammation. No curative treatment is currently available. Treatment for AA is unsatisfactory. In many cases, the most important factor in management of the patient is psychological support from the dermatologist, family, and support groups (The National Alopecia Areata Foundation, *http://www.naaf.org/*). Individuals may prefer to wear a wig; makeup applied to eyebrows is helpful.

**Glucocorticoids**   *Topical* Superpotent agents may be effective.

***Intralesional Injection*** Few and small spots of AA can be treated with intralesional triamcinolone acetonide, 3 mg/mL, which can be very effective temporarily.

***Systemic Glucocorticoids*** Usually induce regrowth, but AA recurs on discontinuation; risks of long-term therapy therefore preclude their use.

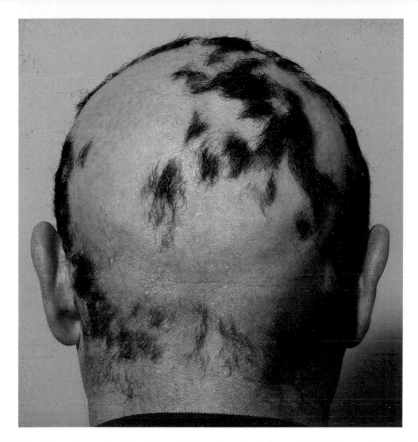

**FIGURE 29-3  Alopecia areata of scalp: multiple, extensive lesions**  *Multiple, confluent, involved sites on the scalp with "exclamation point hairs" and evidence of regrowth in some areas. Newly regrowing hairs may be fine and gray-white in color.*

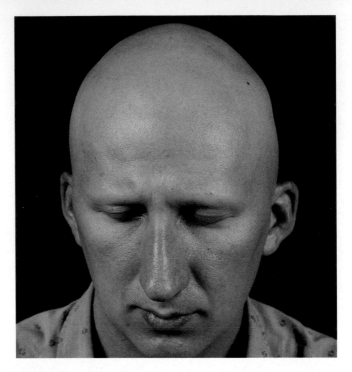

**FIGURE 29-4   Alopecia universalis**   *This patient has lost all scalp hair (alopecia totalis), eyebrows, eyelashes, beard, and all body hair (alopecia universalis), and has dystrophic ("hammered brass") nails.*

**Systemic Cyclosporine**   Induces regrowth, but AA recurs when drug is discontinued.

**Induction of Allergic Contact Dermatitis**   Dinitrochlorobenzene, squaric acid dibutylester, or diphencyprone can be used successfully, but local discomfort due to allergic contact dermatitis and swelling of regional lymph nodes poses a problem.

**Oral PUVA (Photochemotherapy)**   Variably effective, as high as 30%, and worth a trial in patients who are highly distressed about the problem. Entire body must be exposed, in that the therapy is believed to be a form of systemic immune suppression.

## ANDROGENETIC ALOPECIA

Androgenetic alopecia (AGA) is the common progressive balding that occurs through the combined effect of (1) genetic predisposition, and (2) action of androgen on scalp hair follicles. Pattern/extent of hair loss in males varies from bitemporal recession, to frontal and/or vertex thinning, to loss of all hair except that along the occipital and temporal margins ("Hippocratic wreath").

*Synonyms*: Pattern hair loss, male-pattern baldness, common baldness (males), hereditary thinning (females).

## EPIDEMIOLOGY AND ETIOLOGY

**Etiology**   Combined effects of androgen on genetically predisposed hair follicles. Genetics: (1) autosomal dominant and/or polygenic; (2) inherited from either or both parents.

**Age of Onset**   *Males*: May begin any time after puberty, as early as the second decade; often fully expressed in 40s. *Females*: Later—in about 40% occurs in the sixth decade.

**Sex**   Males >> females.

## CLASSIFICATION

Hamilton[1] classified male-pattern hair loss into stages (Fig. 29-5*A*): type I, loss of hair along the frontal margin; type II, increasing frontal hair loss as well as onset of loss on the occipital scalp (crown); and types III, IV, and V, increasing hair loss in both regions with eventual confluent and complete balding of the top of the scalp with sparing of the sides. Ludwig[2] classified hair loss in female (Fig. 29-5*B*).

## PATHOGENESIS

Testosterone is converted to DHT by $5\alpha$-reductase ($5\alpha$-R). Two isozymes of $5\alpha$-R occur: type I and type II. Type I $5\alpha$-R is localized to sebaceous glands (face, scalp), chest/back skin/liver, adrenal gland, kidney. Type II $5\alpha$-R is localized to scalp hair follicle, beard, chest skin, liver, seminal vesicle, prostate, epididymis, foreskin/scrotum. Finasteride inhibits conversion of testosterone to DHT by type II $5\alpha$-R.

Role of testosterone: (1) prenatal: internal sex organ development of male fetus; (2) postnatal: spermatogenesis, libido, muscle/bone mass. Role of DHT: (1) prenatal: external genitalia development in male fetus; (2) postnatal: scalp hair loss, prostate enlargement. Clinical features of type II $5\alpha$-R deficiency in men: ambiguous genitalia at birth, virilized at puberty; underdeveloped prostate, no enlargement with age; otherwise healthy (normal libido after puberty, normal bone/muscle mass after puberty); sparse facial/body hair; no scalp hair loss with age. In males, testosterone produced by the testes is the major androgen. In females, androstenedione and dehydroepiandrosterone sulfate are the major peripheral androgens.

In genetically predisposed individuals, DHT causes terminal follicles to transform into vellus–like follicles, which in turn undergo atrophy. During successive follicular cycles, hairs produced are of shorter length and of decreasing diameter. Conversely, androgens induce vellus-to-terminal follicle production of secondary sexual hair.

## HISTORY

**Skin Symptoms**   Most patients present with complaints of gradually thinning hair or baldness. In males (Fig. 29-6), there is a receding anterior hairline, especially in the parietal regions, which results in an M-shaped recession. Following this, a bald spot may appear on the vertex. If AGA progresses rapidly, some patients also complain of increased falling out of hair. In females, parietal and temporal recession is not usually a major feature, and effluvium follows a pattern depicted in Fig. 29-7; severe

---

[1] Hamilton: Am J Anat 71:451, 1941.
[2] Ludwig: Br J Dermatol 97:249, 1977.

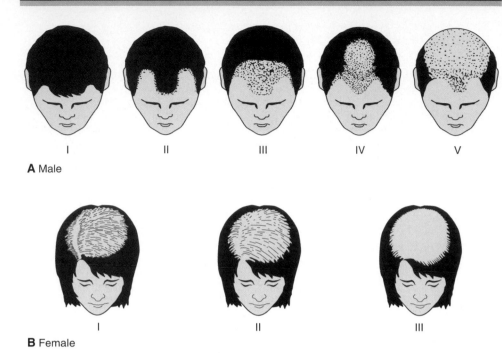

I    II    III    IV    V

**A** Male

I    II    III

**B** Female

**FIGURE 29-5    Androgenetic alopecia: patterns in males and females**    *A. Hamilton classified the severity and pattern of hair loss in males into types I to V. **B.** Ludwig classified hair loss in females into types I to III.*

thinning is not common. The cosmetic appearance of AGA is very disturbing to many persons owing to the high value that our society places on a "healthy head of hair."

**Systems Review**    In young women, manifestations of androgen excess should be sought as significant: acne, hirsutism, irregular menses, or virilization. However, most women with AGA are endocrinologically normal.

## PHYSICAL EXAMINATION

**Skin Findings**    Scalp skin is normal. In young women, look for signs of virilization (acne, excess facial or body hair, male-pattern escutcheon). With advanced AGA, scalp is smooth and shiny; orifices of follicles are barely perceptible with the unaided eye.

**Hair**    (Figs. 29-6 and 29-7) Hair in areas of AGA becomes finer in texture (shorter in length, reduced diameter). In time, hair becomes vellus and eventually atrophies completely.

***Distribution***    Males usually exhibit patterned loss in the frontotemporal and vertex areas (Fig. 29-7). The end result may be only a rim of residual hair on the lateral and posterior scalp. In these regions hair never falls out in AGA. Paradoxically, males with extensive AGA may have excess growth of secondary sexual hair, i.e., axillae, pubic area, chest, and beard. Females, including those who are endocrinologically normal, also lose scalp hair according to the male pattern, but hair loss is far less pronounced. Often hair loss is more diffuse in women following the pattern described by Ludwig [2] (Fig. 29-7).

**Systemic Findings**    In young women with AGA, look for signs of virilization (clitoral hypertrophy, acne, facial hirsutism) and, if present, rule out endocrine dysfunction.

## DIFFERENTIAL DIAGNOSIS

**Diffuse Nonscarring Scalp Alopecia**    Diffuse pattern of hair loss with alopecia areata, telogen

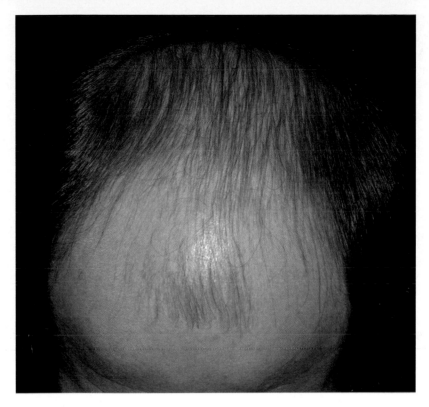

**FIGURE 29-6   Androgenetic alopecia: male**   *Loss of hair in the frontotemporal and vertex areas in a male corresponding to Hamilton types IV and V.*

defluvium, secondary syphilis, systemic lupus erythematosus, iron deficiency, hypothyroidism, hyperthyroidism, trichotillomania, seborrheic dermatitis.

### LABORATORY EXAMINATIONS

**Trichogram**   In AGA, the earliest changes are an increase in the percentage of telogen hairs.
**Dermatopathology**   Abundance of telogen stage follicles is noted, associated with hair follicles of decreasing size and eventually nearly complete atrophy.
**Hormone Studies**   In women with hair loss and evidence of increased androgens (menstrual irregularities, infertility, hirsutism, severe cystic acne, virilization), determine:

- Testosterone: total and free
- Dehydroepiandrosterone sulfate (DHEAS)
- Prolactin

**Other Studies**   Treatable causes of thinning hair should be excluded with measurement of thyroid-stimulating hormone (TSH), $T_4$, serum iron, serum ferritin, and/or total iron-binding capacity (TIBC), CBC, ANA.

### DIAGNOSIS

Clinical diagnosis is made on the history, pattern of alopecia, and family incidence of AGA. Skin biopsy may be necessary in some cases.

### COURSE

The progression of alopecia is usually very gradual, over years to decades.

### MANAGEMENT

**Oral Finasteride**   1 mg PO qd, competitively

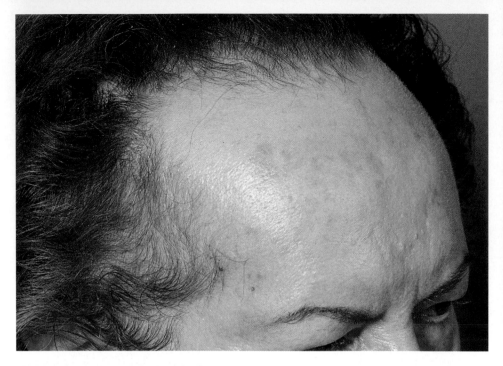

**FIGURE 29-7    Androgenetic alopecia: female**    *This woman had pronounced diffuse thining of hair on the crown, but in addition, also had thinning of the hair in the frontotemporal region of the scalp after treatment with androgens.*

inhibits type II 5α-R and thus the conversion of testosterone to DHT; this results in lower serum and scalp levels of DHT. Finasteride has no affinity for androgen receptors and therefore does not block the important actions of testosterone (growth of the phallus and scrotum, spermatogenesis, libido). Most men may begin to see first benefit in slowing hair loss as early as 3 months. After 6 months; there is a regrowth of terminal hair on the vertex and anterior mid-scalp. If the drug is stopped, however, the hair that had grown will be lost within 12 months. 2% of men taking finasteride report decrease in libido and erectile function; these effects were reversible when the drug was stopped and disappeared in two-thirds of those who continued taking finasteride.

**Topical Minoxidil**    Topically applied minoxidil, 2% and 5% solution, may be helpful in reducing rate of hair loss or in partially restoring lost hair in both males and females.

**Antiandrogens**    In women with AGA who have elevated adrenal androgens, spironolactone, cyproterone acetate, flutamide, and cimetidine bind to androgen receptors and block the action of DHT. These must not be used in men.

**Hairpiece**    Wigs, toupees, prosthetics; hair weaves.

**Surgical Treatment**

*Hair transplantation* Moving multiple punch grafts of follicles taken from androgen-insensitive hair sites (peripheral occipital and parietal hairy areas) to bald androgen-sensitive scalp areas.

*Scalp reduction/rotation flaps*

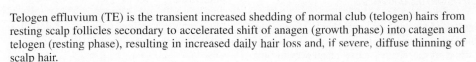

# TELOGEN EFFLUVIUM

Telogen effluvium (TE) is the transient increased shedding of normal club (telogen) hairs from resting scalp follicles secondary to accelerated shift of anagen (growth phase) into catagen and telogen (resting phase), resulting in increased daily hair loss and, if severe, diffuse thinning of scalp hair.
*Synonym*: Telogen defluvium.

## EPIDEMIOLOGY AND ETIOLOGY

**Age of Onset**   Any age.
**Sex**   More common in women due to parturition, cessation of an oral contraceptive, and "crash" dieting.
**Incidence**   Second most common cause of alopecia after androgenetic alopecia.
**Etiology**   A reaction pattern to a variety of physical or mental stressors:

  I. Endocrine
     A. Hypo- or hyperthyroidism
     B. Postpartum
     C. Peri- or postmenopausal state
 II. Nutritional
     A. Deficiency: biotin, zinc, iron, essential fatty acid
     B. Deprivation: caloric, protein
III. Drugs
     A. Antimitotic agents (dose dependent): cancer chemotherapy, benzimidazoles
     B. Antihypertensives: angiotensin-converting enzyme (ACE) inhibitors, beta blockers
     C. Anticoagulants
     D. Interferon
     E. CNS drugs: lithium, valproic acid
     F. Hormonal: oral contraceptives
     G. Retinoid effect: vitamin A excess, retinoids (isotretinoin, acitretin), indinavir
 IV. Physical stress: anemia, surgery, systemic illness
  V. Psychological stress
 VI. Idiopathic: no obvious cause is apparent in a significant number of cases.

## PATHOGENESIS

In the normal scalp, 80 to 90% of hairs are in anagen phase, 5% in catagen phase, and 10 to 15% in telogen phase; 50 to 100 hairs are shed as they are replaced daily. With telogen effluvium, many more hairs than normal are shed daily. The precipitating stimulus for TE results in a premature shift of anagen follicles into the telogen phase. Anagen phase occurs again in 3 to 4 months after the inciting event occurred. If the inciting cause is removed, shedding will resolve over the next few months as the number of hairs in telogen return to normal. Hair density may take 6 to 12 months to return to baseline. TE can become chronic with decreased hair density, always has potential for reversal, does not lead to total scalp hair loss, and rarely goes beyond 50% loss.

## HISTORY

**Skin Symptoms**   Patient presents with complaint of increased hair loss on the scalp that may be accompanied by varying degrees of hair thinning. Most individuals are anxious, fearing baldness. The patient often presents a plastic bag containing shed hair. The precipitating event precedes the telogen effluvium by 6 to 16 weeks.

## PHYSICAL EXAMINATION

**Skin Lesions**   No abnormalities of the scalp are detected.
**Hair**   (Fig. 29-8) Diffuse shedding of the scalp hair. Gentle hair pull gathers several to many club or telogen hairs.
*Distribution*   Hair loss occurs diffusely throughout the scalp and includes the sides and back of the head. If hair loss is significant enough to result in thinning of hair, alopecia is noted diffusely throughout the scalp. Short regrowing new hairs are present close to the scalp; these hairs are finer than older hairs and have tapered ends.
*Site of Predilection*   Scalp.
**Nails**   The precipitating stimulus for TE may also affect the growth of nails, resulting in

Beau's lines (see Fig. 30-32), which appear as transverse lines or grooves on the fingernail and toenail plates.

## DIFFERENTIAL DIAGNOSIS

**Increased Shedding of Scalp Hair ± Nonscarring Alopecia**   Androgenetic alopecia, diffuse-pattern alopecia areata, loose anagen syndrome, hyperthyroidism, hypothyroidism, systemic lupus erythematosus, secondary syphilis, drug-induced alopecia (Table 29-2).

## LABORATORY EXAMINATIONS

**Hair Pull**   Compared with the normal hair pull, in which 80 to 90% of hair is in the anagen phase, telogen effluvium is characterized by a reduced percentage of anagen hairs, varying with the intensity of hair shedding. See "Biology of Hair Growth" for an explanation of the hair pull.
**CBC**   Rule out iron-deficiency anemia.
**Chemistry**   Serum iron, iron-binding capacity.
**TSH**   Rule out thyroid disease.

**Serology**   Antinuclear antibodies (ANA), RPR.
**Histopathology**   No abnormality other than an increase in the proportion of follicles in telogen.

## DIAGNOSIS

Made on history, clinical findings, hair pull, and possible biopsy, excluding other causes.

## COURSE AND PROGNOSIS

Complete regrowth of hair is the rule. In postpartum TE, if hair loss is severe and recurs after successive pregnancies, regrowth may never be complete. TE may continue for up to a year after the precipitating cause.

## MANAGEMENT

No intervention is needed or required. The patient should be reassured that the process is part of a normal cycle of hair growth and shedding and that full regrowth of the hair is to be expected in most cases.

### TABLE 29-2   Drug-Induced Alopecia*

| Drugs | Features of Alopecia |
| --- | --- |
| **ACE inhibitors** | |
| Enalapril | Probable telogen effluvium |
| **Anticoagulants** | |
| Heparin | Few reports |
| Warfarin | Reported incidence ranges from 19 to 70% but is probably much lower; diffuse shedding with increased number of hairs in telogen phase. |
| **Antimitotic agents** | |
| Colchicine | Diffuse hair loss; increased number of telogen hairs |
| **Antineoplastic agents** | |
| Bleomycin | Anagen effluvium |
| Cyclophosphamide | Anagen effluvium |
| Cytarabine | Anagen effluvium |
| Dacarbazine | Anagen effluvium |
| Dactinomycin | Anagen effluvium |
| Daunorubicin | Anagen effluvium |
| Doxorubicin | Anagen effluvium |
| Etoposide | Anagen effluvium |
| Fluorouracil | Anagen effluvium |
| Hydroxyurea | Anagen effluvium |
| Ifosfamide | Anagen effluvium |
| Mechlorethamine | Anagen effluvium |
| Melphalan | Anagen effluvium |
| Methotrexate | Anagen effluvium |
| Mitomycin | Anagen effluvium |
| Mitoxantrone | Anagen effluvium |

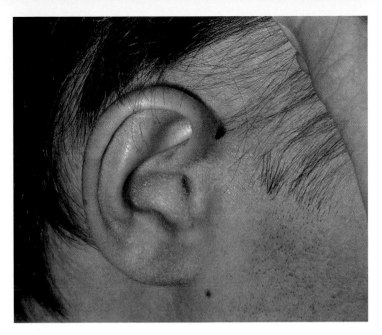

**FIGURE 29-8   Telogen effluvium**   *A clump of hair in the hand, associated with striking thinning of scalp hair. The patient was HIV-infected and experienced* Pneumocystis carinii *pneumonia 10 weeks previously. Using the fingers as shown, 30 to 40 hairs could be removed with each "hair pull."*

**TABLE 29-2   (continued)**

| Drugs | Features of Alopecia |
|---|---|
| Nitrosourea | Anagen effluvium |
| Procarbazine | Anagen effluvium |
| Thiotepa | Anagen effluvium |
| Vinblastine | Anagen effluvium |
| Vincristine | Anagen effluvium |
| **Antiparkinsonian agents** | |
| Levodopa | Probable telogen effluvium |
| **Antiseizure agents** | |
| Trimethadione | Probable telogen effluvium |
| **Beta blockers** | |
| Metoprolol | Probable telogen effluvium |
| Propranolol | Probable telogen effluvium |
| **Birth control agents** | |
| Oral contraceptives | Diffuse hair loss (telogen effluvium) 2 to 3 months after cessation of oral contraceptive |
| **Drugs used in treatment of bipolar disorders** | |
| Lithium | Probable telogen effluvium |
| **Ergot derivatives (used in treatment of prolactinemia)** | |
| Bromocriptine | Probable telogen effluvium |

**TABLE 29-2    (continued)**

| Drugs | Features of Alopecia |
|---|---|
| **H₂ blockers** | |
| Cimetidine | Onset 1 week to 11 months; probable telogen effluvium |
| **Heavy metals (poisoning)** | |
| Thallium | Diffuse shedding of abnormal anagen hair 10 days after ingestion; complete hair loss in 1 month; characteristic is pronounced hair loss on sides of head, also of lateral eyebrows. |
| Mercury and lead | Diffuse hair loss with acute and chronic exposure. |
| **Cholesterol-lowering drugs** | |
| Clofibrate | Occasionally associated with hair loss. |
| **Pesticides** | |
| Boric acid | Total scalp alopecia reported after acute intoxication; with chronic exposure hair becomes dry and falls out. |
| **Retinoids** | |
| Etretinate | Increased hair shedding and plucked telogen count; decreased duration of anagen phase. |
| Isotretinoin | Diffuse loss; probably same mechanism as above. |

\* Prepared by Suzanne Virnelli-Grevelink, M.D.

## ANAGEN EFFLUVIUM    ■ ◑

In anagen effluvium (AE), hair loss/balding is diffuse, involving entire scalp. Results from a rapid growth arrest or damage to anagen hairs that skip catagen and telogen phases and are shed. Onset is usually rapid and extensive (Fig. 29-9). In AE, abnormal anagen hairs are usually broken off. AE is caused by radiation therapy to head, drugs, systemic chemotherapy, severe protein malnutrition. Regrowth is usually rapid after discontinuation of chemotherapy.

### PATHOGENESIS

AE occurs after any insult to hair follicle that impairs its mitotic/metabolic activity. Hair loss results from exposure to cancer chemotherapeutic agents (antimetabolites, alkylating agents, mitotic inhibitors). Inhibition/arrest of cell division in hair matrix leads to thin, weakened hair shaft, susceptible to fracture with minimal trauma as well as complete failure of hair formation. hair bulb itself may be damaged, and hairs may separate at the bulb and fall out. Only actively growing anagen follicles are subject to these processes. More common and

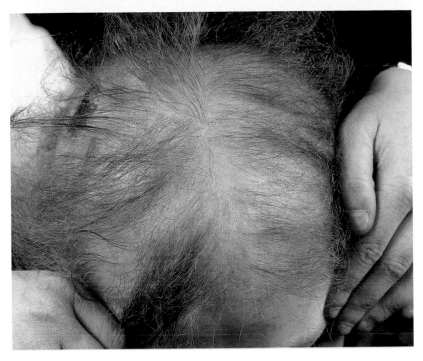

**FIGURE 29-9    Anagen efluvium**    *Massive, diffuse hair loss of the scalp following initiation of cancer chemotherapy.*

severe with combination chemotherapy than with the use of a single drug. Severity is generally dose dependent.

## ETIOLOGY

*Cancer chemotherapy*    Table 29-2.
*Intoxications*    Mercury, boric acid, thallium, colchicines.
*Deficiencies*    Severe protein deficiency.

## PHYSICAL EXAMINATION

**Skin Findings**    Scalp and other sites appear normal.

**Hair**    Breaks off or is shed at the level of the scalp. AE is usually extensive with generalized loss of scalp (Fig. 29-9), eyebrow/lashes, beard, etc.
**Nails**    Transverse banding or ridging is often seen with successive rounds of chemotherapy.

## COURSE

Regrowth of hair occurs rapidly after discontinuation of chemotherapy.

# PRIMARY CICATRICIAL ALOPECIA    ☐ ◑

Primary cicatricial (scarring) alopecia (PCA) results from damage or destruction of the hair follicles by inflammatory (usually noninfectious) or other pathologic processes; the end result is replacement of the follicular structure by fibrous tissue (Table 29-3)

### Chronic Cutaneous (Discoid) Lupus Erythematosus (CCLE)

(See Section 14) Characterized by erythema, atrophy, variable hypopigmentation, and/or follicular plugging (Fig. 29-10). CCLE may occur without other manifestations or serologic evidence of Lupus erythematosus (LE). Histology: vacuolar degeneration of basal cell layer, perivascular/periadnexal lymphoid infiltrate, increased dermal mucin, sebaceous gland loss; direct immunofluorescence usually negative.

### Lichen Planopilaris (LPP)

(See Section 7) Lichen planus (LP) associated with cicatricial scalp alopecia, resulting in scaling, atrophy, permanent hair loss. Most commonly affects middle-aged women. Distribution: most commonly parietal scalp. Symptoms/findings in scalp: follicular hyperkeratosis, pruritus, perifollicular erythema, violaceous color of scalp, scalp pain. May also affect other hair-bearing sites: groin, axilla. LP may be present on skin or mucosa. *Graham-Little syndrome*: LP-like lesions + follicular "spines"/keratosis pilaris–like lesions in areas of alopecia on scalp, eyebrows, axillary, pubic areas. *Frontal fibrosing alopecia*: frontotemporal hairline recession and eyebrow loss in postmenopausal women with perifollicular erythema; histology shows LPP. *Perifollicular erythema and follicular keratosis*: progressive scarring alopecia limited to area of pattern hair loss; overlaps with frontal fibrosing alopecia.

### Classic Pseudopelade (Brocq)

Clinically discrete, smooth, skin- or pink-colored irregularly shaped alopecia without follicular hyperkeratosis or perifollicular inflammation (Figs. 29-11 and 29-12). Begins in moth-eaten pattern with eventual coalescence into larger patches of hair loss. Histology: perifollicular/perivascular lymphocytic infiltrate in follicular infundibulum; loss of sebaceous epithelium; fibrotic streams into subcutis with interface or follicular plugging changes. Rule out other PCAs such as LPP or CCLE.

### Central Centrifugal Scarring Alopecia (CCSA)

*Synonyms*: follicular degeneration syndrome, pseudopelade (blacks), hot comb alopecia, central elliptical pseudopelade (Caucasians). Slowly progressive alopecia begins in the vertex and advances to surrounding areas. Most commonly occurs in black women. May be related to chemical processing, heat, or chronic tension on the hair. Histology early in CCSA shows lichenoid perifolliculitis; infundibula are enveloped by lymphocytes. Progressive fibrosis occurs; end-stage CCSA shows sparse perivascu-

---

**TABLE 29-3 Classification of Primary Cicatricial Alopecias**

| | |
|---|---|
| **Lymphocytic** | Chronic cutaneous (discoid) lupus erythematosus |
| | Lichen planopilaris (LPP) |
| | Classic LPP |
| | Frontal fibrosing alopecia |
| | Graham-Little syndrome |
| | Classic pseudopelade of Brocq |
| | Central centrifugal cicatricial alopecia |
| | Alopecia mucinosa |
| | Keratosis follicularis spinulosa decalvans |
| **Neutrophilic** | Folliculitis decalvans |
| | Dissecting folliculitis (cellulitis) |
| **Mixed** | Folliculitis keloidalis |
| | Folliculitis necrotica |
| | Erosive pustular dermatosis |
| **Nonspecific** | |

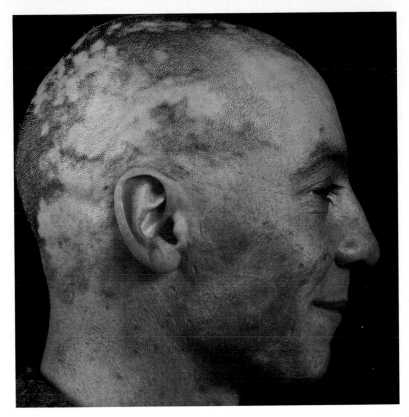

**FIGURE 29-10   Scarring alopecia of scalp and beard: chronic cutaneous lupus erythematosus**
*Active inflammatory plaques and burned out lesions with white depressed scars and scarring alopecia on scalp. Similar findings are also present in the beard area.*

lar lymphocytic infiltrates, markedly thinned lower portion of infundibulum, isthmus consequent to effects of bands of fibroplasias, foreign-body granulomatous reaction to infundibular cornified cells that lie outside follicle in dermis.

**Alopecia Mucinosa**   Characterized by erythematous plaques or flat patches without hair, occurring mainly on scalp/face. Histology: prominent follicular, epithelial/sebaceous gland mucin, perifollicular lymphohistiocytic infiltrate without concentric lamellar fibrosis. May be symptom of cutaneous T cell lymphoma.

**Keratosis Follicularis Spinulosa Decalvans (KFSD)**
Characterized by follicular hyperkeratosis, scarring alopecia of scalp, absence of eyebrows and sometimes eyelashes, severe photophobia, corneal dystrophy. X-linked disorder.

**Folliculitis Decalvans**   Characterized by bogginess or induration of scalp/beard with pustules, erosions, crusts (Fig. 29-13), scale. Staphylococcus *aureus* secondary infection common. Histology: acute suppurative folliculitis, early.

**Dissecting Folliculitis**   *Synonyms*: dissecting cellulitis, perifolliculitis abscedens et suffodiens. Characterized by initial deep inflammatory nodules, primarily over the occiput, that progress to coalescing regions of boggy scalp (Fig. 29-14). Sinus tracts may form; purulent exudates can be expressed. Race: black. *S. aureus* secondary infection common. Histology: early follicular plugging and suppurative follicular/perifollicular abscesses with mixed inflammatory infiltrate; later, foreign-body giant cells, granulation tissue, scarring with sinus tracts. Poor response to therapy.

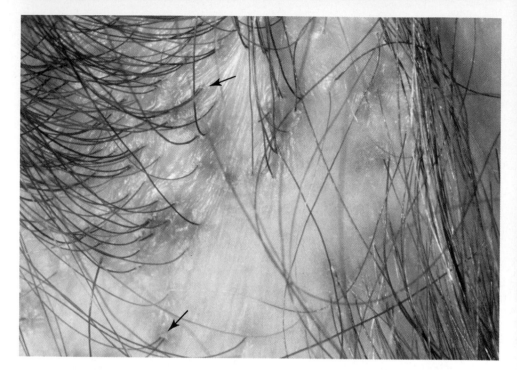

**FIGURE 29-11    Scarring alopecia of scalp: pseudopelade of Brocq caused by lichen planus**   *The scalp is smooth, shiny, devoid of hair and hair follicles in many areas; some of the remaining follicles are inflamed with perifollicular erythema and scale. Several hairs are seen emerging from a single site within the area of alopecia (arrows).*

**Follicultis Keloidalis**   *Synonym*: acne keloidalis nuchae. Occurs most commonly in black men. Usually occurs on the nape of the neck, starting with a chronic papular or pustular eruption (Fig. 29-15). Results in a spectrum of severity from small fibrotic papules to hypertrophic keloidal scar formation. Distribution: nape of the neck, occipital scalp.

**Pseudofolliculitis Barbae**   Variant or same disease as folliculitis keloidalis. Occurs commonly in black African males who shave. Related to curved hair follicles. Cut hair retracts beneath skin surface, grows, and penetrates follicular wall, causing a foreign-body reaction. Distribution: any shaved area, i.e., beard, scalp, pubic. *S. aureus* secondary infection is common (Fig. 29-16). Has been linked to a polymorphism of the keratin gene KGhf.

**Nonspecific Cicatricial Alopecia**   Idiopathic scarring alopecia with inconclusive clinical and histopathologic findings. May include end stage of a variety of PCA, e.g., LPP, folliculitis decalvans.

## LABORATORY EXAMINATION

**Scalp Biopsy**   4-mm punch biopsy including subcutaneous tissue, prepared for horizontal section. A second 4-mm punch biopsy specimen for vertical sections and direct immunofluorescence.

## MANAGEMENT

**Glucocorticoids**   Topical high-potency and intralesional glucocorticoids (e.g., triamcinolone) are the mainstay of treatment, improving symptoms and hair growth.

**Antibiotics**   A combination of clindamycin and rifampicin administered intermittently is effective in folliculitis decalvans.

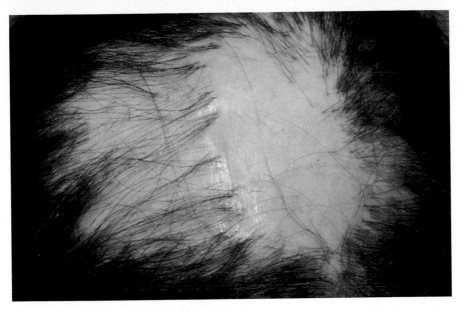

**FIGURE 29-12 Scarring alopecia of scalp: pseudopelade of Brocq** *Extensive hair loss with residual islands of hair follicles and hair. Note the absence of erythema, scale, or crust.*

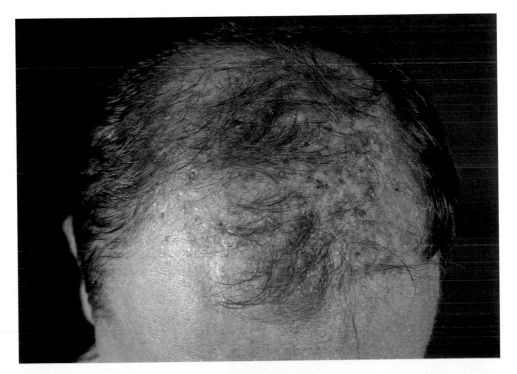

**FIGURE 29-13 Scarring alopecia of scalp: folliculitis decalvans** *Erythema, inflammatory papules, crusts, and scarring in a male who also has androgenetic alopecia.*

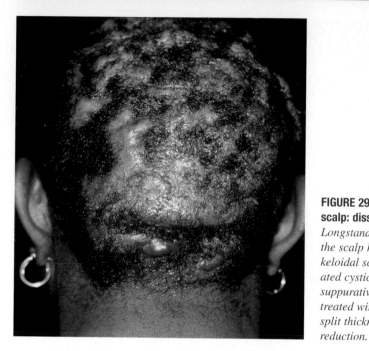

**FIGURE 29-14    Scarring alopecia of scalp: dissecting perifolliculitis** *Longstanding abscess formation of the scalp has resulted in very severe keloidal scarring. There was associated cystic acne and hidradenitis suppurativa. The scalp lesions were treated with surgical "scalping," split thickness skin grafts, and scalp reduction.*

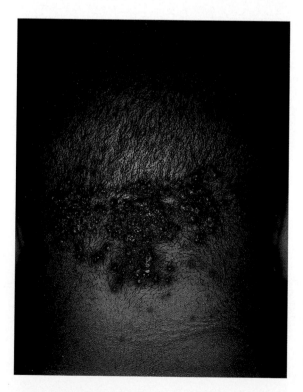

**FIGURE 29-15    Scarring alopecia of scalp: folliculitis keloidalis** *Papular scars, of 3 years' duration, becoming confluent on the occipital scalp of a black male. The condition is chronic and progressive, resulting in significant hair loss.*

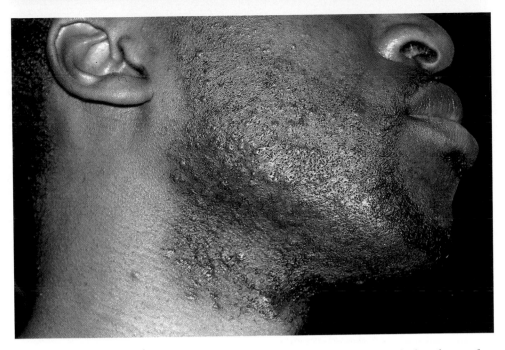

**FIGURE 29-16   Pseudofolliculitis barbae** *Multiple follicular papular scars in the beard area of a black male; the presence of follicular pustules usually is indicative of secondary* Staphylococcus aureus *folliculitis.*

## EXCESS HAIR GROWTH

Excess hair growth occurs in two patterns. *Hirsutism*: occurs in women at sites where hair is under androgen control. *Hypertrichosis*: hair density or length beyond accepted limits of normal for age, race, sex (generalized, localized; lanugo, vellus, terminal hair).

## HIRSUTISM    ■    ○

Hirsutism is excessive hair growth (women) in androgen-dependent hair patterns, secondary to increased androgenic activity. Normally only postpubescent males have terminal hair in these sites.

## EPIDEMIOLOGY AND ETIOLOGY

**Etiology**   Table 29-4.
**Risk Factors**   Familial, ethnic, and racial influences. Hirsuteness: white > black > Asian
**Prevalence in United States**   Survey of college-aged women: 25% had easily noticeable facial hair; 33% had hair along linea alba below umbilicus; 17% had periareolar hair. Series of 100 patients: 15% idiopathic, 3% late-onset congenital adrenal hyperplasia (CAH) (varies within ethnic group).

## PATHOGENESIS

Androgens promote conversion of vellus hairs to terminal hairs in androgen-sensitive hair follicles: beard area, face, chest, areolae, linea alba, lower back, buttocks, abdomen, external genitalia, inner thighs. DHT, derived from conversion of testosterone by $5\alpha$-R at the hair follicle, is the hormonal stimulus for hair growth. 50 to 70% of circulating testosterone in normal women is derived from precursors, androstenedione, and DHEA; the rest is secreted directly, mostly by the ovaries. In hyperandrogenic women, a greater percentage of androgens may be secreted directly. In women, adrenal glands secrete androstenedione, DHEA, DHEA sulfate, and testosterone; ovaries secrete mainly androstenedione and testosterone.

## HISTORY

- Family history
- Drug history
- Virilization symptoms: androgenic alopecia (female pattern hair loss), acne, deepened voice, increased muscle mass, clitoromegaly, increased libido, personality change. Relatively recent or rapid onset of symptoms and signs *not* associated with puberty.
- Other: Amenorrhea or changes in menstruation. New-onset hypertension.

## PHYSICAL EXAMINATION

**Skin Findings**   Note: acne, acanthosis nigricans, striae.
**Hair**   *Hirsutism*: (1) amount of excess hair, (2) all sites of hair, (3) evaluate progression and therapy. New growth of terminal hair (Fig. 29-17), especially on chest (Fig. 29-18), abdomen, upper back, shoulders. *Ferriman-Gallwey scale* rates hair growth in each of 11 androgen-sensitive areas (upper lip, chin, chest, upper back, lower back, upper abdomen, lower abdomen, arm, forearm, thigh, leg) from 0 (no hair growth) to 4. Score of $\geq 8$ is considered hirsutism.
**Cushing's Syndrome**   Centripetal obesity, muscle wasting (especially peripheral muscle weakness), violaceous striae.
**Pelvic Examination**   If polycystic ovary (PCO) syndrome is suspected.

**FIGURE 29-18 (Opposite page, bottom)   Hirsuitism: chest of female**   *Increased constitutional hair growth in androgen-dependent hair follicles of the presternal and periareolar regions in a female. In this case, no androgen excess was detected, the finding occurring in other female relatives. Removal of these black hairs can be done with a laser.*

**FIGURE 29-17    Hirsuitism: face of female**  *Increased hair growth in androgen-dependent hair follicles of the beard area in a female, associated with androgen excess.*

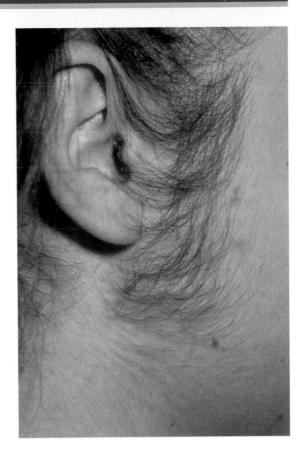

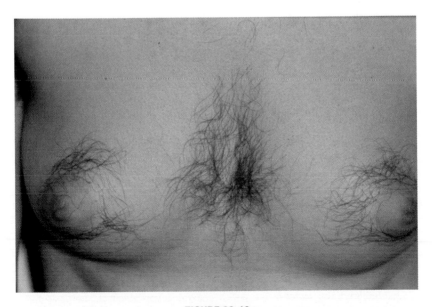

**FIGURE 29-18**

**TABLE 29-4    Etiology of Hirsutism**

**Androgen-secreting tumors** Usually associated with irregular menses/amenorrhea.
  Adrenal
    Adenoma
    Adenocarcinoma
    Ectopic ACTH-secreting tumor
  Ovarian
    Gonadal stromal tumor
    Thecoma
    Lipoid tumor
**Functional androgen excess**
  Adrenal enzyme deficiencies (congenital adrenal hyperplasia)
    Early onset 21-hydroxylase deficiency
    Late onset 21-hydroxylase deficiency
    11β-hydroxylase deficiency
    3β-dehydroxylase deficiency
  Cushing syndrome
  Polycystic ovarian disease
    With and without adrenal contribution
    Hyperthecosis
**"Idiopathic" hirsutism**
**Medication/drug-induced**

## LABORATORY EVALUATION

**Urinary 17-Ketosteroid**   Helpful in evaluating the overall amount of androgen secretion. Results checked against age-appropriate normal levels; peak levels occur at 30 years (significant decline with age thereafter).

**Oligomenorrhea/Amenorrhea**   Prolactin, Follicle-stimulating hormone (FSH) total testosterone.

**Virilization**   *Serum testosterone*: 200 ng/dL in women with ovarian or adrenal tumor. *Urinary 17-ketosteroids*: elevated adrenal androgens. *Serum DHEA sulfate*: most specific to adrenals (>90% arising in adrenals); if >800 μg/d, suggestive of adrenal tumor.

## MANAGEMENT

**Cosmetic Treatment**   *Bleaching*: hydrogen peroxide. *Temporary removal*: Shaving, waxing, chemical (Nair). *Permanent hair removal*: LASER, electrolysis.

**Endocrinology Consultation**   For suspected late-onset CAH, Cushing's syndrome, tumor.

**Systemic Antiandrogen Therapy**   *Cyproterone Acetate (CPA)* Potent progestogen. Both antiandrogen and inhibitor of secretion of gonadotropin. Decreases androgen production.

Increases testosterone clearance. Decreases 5α-R activity. Administered with cyclical estrogens to maintain regular menstruation. *Regimen*: 50 to 100 mg CPA for 10 days per cycle. *Adverse effects*: weight gain, fatigue, loss of libido, mastodynia, nausea, headache, depression. *Contraindications*: smoking, obesity, hypertension.

*Spironolactone* An antihypertensive diuretic. Decreases testosterone biosynthesis. Binds to androgen receptor. Decreases 5α-R activity.

*Regimen*: begin at 50 mg bid from day 4 through day 22 of each menstrual cycle; dose can be given as high as 100 mg bid.

*Cimetidine* $H_2$ receptor antagonist; competes for target tissue binding with androgens; less effective than spironolactone.

*Glucocorticoid* First-line therapy for classic CAH. *Regimen*: 1 mg dexamethasone qhs. For late-onset, nonclassic CAH, use antiandrogens or oral contraceptives.

*Oral Contraceptives* Suppress ovarian and adrenal androgen production by decreasing luteinizing hormone (LH) and FSH. Recommend an oral contraceptive with the lowest tolerable dose of ethinyl estradiol (30 to 35 μg) and a low dose of a progestin with low androgenic potential (<1 mg norethindrone, norgestimate, desogestrel, ethynodiol diacetate). Avoid levonorgestrel, norgestrel, and high doses of norethindrone acetate.

# HYPERTRICHOSIS

Hypertrichosis is excessive hair growth (density, length) beyond accepted limits of normal for age, race, sex in areas that are not androgen-sensitive (Fig. 29-19); may be generalized/universal or localized; may consist of lanugo, vellus, or terminal hair.

**ETIOLOGY**   See Table 29-5.

## HISTORY

**Localized Hypertrichosis**   Trauma/scar/occupation-related sites of irritation.

## PHYSICAL EXAMINATION

**Acquired Hypertrichosis Lanuginosa**   Production of lanugo hair in follicles previously producing vellus hair ("malignant down"). Hair may be > 10 cm in length in nonscalp areas. Can involve entire body, except for palms and

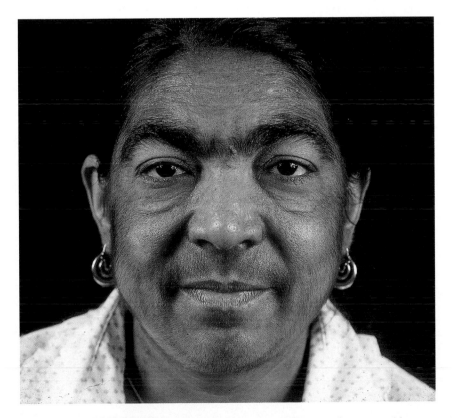

**FIGURE 29-19   Hypertrichosis of face**   *Excessive hair growth in nonandrogen-sensitive areas of the face in a female treated with cyclosporine.*

**TABLE 29-5   Etiology of Hypertrichosis**

**Universal hypertrichosis**
   Congenital/hereditary generalized hypertrichosis
   Acquired generalized hypertrichosis
      Acquired hypertrichosis lanuginosa (malignancy): Usually harbinger of malignancy; of all
        cases of reported, 98% had malignancy of the GI tract, bronchus, breast, gallbladder,
        uterus, bladder; can precede neoplastic diagnosis by several years.
      Drug-induced: minoxidil (80% of those treated), diazoxide (50%), phenytoin (occurs after
        2–3 months of treatment), cyclosporine (80%), PUVA, oral glucocorticoids, streptomycin,
        acetazolamide, oxaliazolopyrimidine, fenoterol, penicillamine
      Porphyria: porphyria cutanea tarda, hepatoerythropoietic porphyria, variegate
       porphyria, erythropoietic porphyria
      POEMS syndrome
      Juvenile dermatomyositis
      Hypothyroidism
      Acrodynia
      Malabsorption syndromes
      CNS-related problems of trauma: postencephalitis, multiple sclerosis, schizophrenia,
        head injury, hyperostosis interna, anorexia nervosa
**Localized hypertrichosis**
   Secondary to irritation, trauma, etc.
   Drug-induced: interferon, topical minoxidil, topical latanoprost

soles. Fine, downy hair covers large areas of the body. In mild types, downy hair is limited to the face; hair on previously hairless areas such as the nose and eyelids is usually noticed first. Scalp, beard, and pubic hair may not be replaced.

**Universal Hypertrichosis**  Increase of lanugo, vellus, or terminal hair.

## INFECTIOUS FOLLICULITIS    ■ ◑

Infectious folliculitis occurs in the upper portion of the hair follicle, characterized by a follicular papule, pustule, erosion, or crust at the follicular infundibulum; infection can extend deeper into the entire length of the follicle (sycosis).

### EPIDEMIOLOGY AND ETIOLOGY

**Predisposing Factors**  Shaving hairy regions such as the beard area, axillae, or legs facilitates follicular infection. Extraction of hair such as plucking or waxing. Occlusion of hair-bearing areas facilitates growth of microbes: clothing, plastic film, adhesive plaster, position (sitting occludes buttocks, lying in bed occludes back), prosthesis, natural occlusion in intertriginous sites (axillae, inframammary, anogenital). Topical climate with high temperature and relative humidity. Topical glucocorticoid preparations. Systemic antibiotic promotes growth of gram-negative bacteria. Diabetes mellitus. Immunosuppression.

**Etiology**  See Table 29-6.

### HISTORY

**Symptoms**  Duration: days; S. aureus and dermatophytic folliculitis can be chronic. Usually nontender or slightly tender; may be pruritic. Uncommonly, tender regional lymphadenitis.

### PHYSICAL EXAMINATION

#### Skin Lesions
Papule or pustule confined to the ostium of the hair follicle, at times surrounded by an erythematous halo (Figs. 29-20, 29-21). Rupture of pustule leads to superficial erosions or crusts. Scattered discrete or more frequently grouped and clustered. Usually, only a small percentage of follicles in a region is infected. Superficial infection heals without scarring, but in darkly pigmented individuals, postinflammatory hypo-and hyperpigmentation. Extension of infection can progress to abscess or furuncle formation (Fig. 29-22). In chronic folliculitis, a full range of lesions is noted. Pseudofolliculitis barbae caused by penetration of the skin by sharp tips of shaved hairs frequently complicated by S. aureus secondary infection (see Fig. 23-16).

**Distribution**  *Face*  S. aureus. Gram-negative folliculitis: resembles or may coexist with acne vulgaris. Molluscum contagiosum. Demodicidosis resembles rosacea.

*Beard Area*  S. aureus folliculitis: folliculitis (sycosis) barbae, most commonly of shaved beard area (Fig. 29-22). Dermatophytic folliculitis: tinea barbae; papulopustules may coalesce to deeply infiltrated kerion. Herpes simplex virus. Molluscum contagiosum. Demodicidosis resembles rosacea.

*Scalp*  S. aureus. Dermatophytic.

*Neck*  S. aureus in shaved area and nape of neck, occipital scalp, especially in diabetics. Pseudofolliculitis in shaved area. Keloidal folliculitis in nape of neck; follicular keloids to large nodular–tumorous keloidal masses.

*Legs*  In western nations, occurs in women who shave legs. In India, a chronic folliculitis occurs in young men, lasting for years. Pustular dermatitis atrophicans of the legs reported commonly from West Africa, usually affecting the shins, sometimes the thighs and forearms.

*Trunk*  S. aureus in axillae, especially in those who shave. *Pseudomonas aeruginosa* ("hot tub") folliculitis. *Malassezia* folliculitis. *Candida* folliculitis on the back of hospitalized patients with fever who lie in supine position.

*Buttocks*  Common site for S. aureus folliculitis. Dermatophytic.

#### Variants
**S. Aureus Folliculitis**  Can be either superficial folliculitis (infundibular) (follicular impetigo of Bockhart) (Figs. 29-20 and 29-21) or deep (sycosis) (extension beneath infundibulum) with abscess formation (Fig. 29-22). In the shaved beard area, also known as sycosis vulgaris, or barber's itch. In severe cases (lupoid sycosis), the pilosebaceous units may be destroyed and replaced by fibrous scar tissue.

**Gram-Negative Folliculitis**  Occurs in individuals with acne vulgaris treated with oral antibiotics. "Acne" typically worsens, having been in good control. Characterized by small follicular pustules and/or larger abscesses on the cheeks.

**Hot Tub Folliculitis**  Occurs on the trunk following immersion in spa water (Fig. 29-23).

**Dermatophytic Folliculitis**  Infection begins in the perifollicular stratum corneum and spreads into follicular ostia and hair shafts (see Section 23).

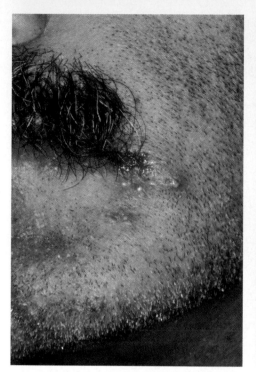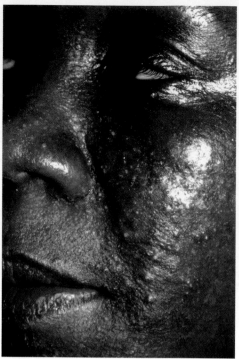

**FIGURE 29-20  (Left)    Infectious folliculitis, superficial: *S. aureus***   *Numerous follicular papules and pustules in the shaved beard area with impetigo on the angle of the lips.*

**FIGURE 29-21  (Right)    Infectious folliculitis, superficial: *S. aureus***   *Numerous follicular papules and pustules on the face of a female with advanced HIV disease.*

**TABLE 29-6    Classification of Infectious Folliculitis by Etiology**

| Infectious Agent | Organism |
| --- | --- |
| Bacterial | *S. aureus*: superficial (Bockhart's impetigo); deep (sycosis); may progress to furuncle (boil) or carbuncle formation |
| | *Pseudomonas aeruginosa* (hot-tub) folliculitis |
| | Gram-negative folliculitis |
| Fungal | Dermatophytic folliculitis: tinea capitis, tinea barbae, Majocchi's granuloma |
| | *Malassezia* folliculitis |
| | *Candida* folliculitis |
| Viral | Herpes simplex virus |
| | Varicella-zoster virus |
| | Molluscum contagiosum |
| Syphilitic | Secondary syphilis: alopecia, acneiform |
| Infestation | Demodicidosis |

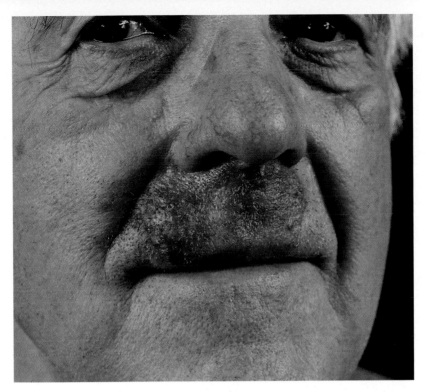

**FIGURE 29-22    Infectious folliculitis, deep (sycosis): *S. aureus*** *Confluent follicular pustules forming a tender, thick, erythematous plaque on the moustache area. The differential diagnosis includes tinea barbae with kerion formation.*

*Tinea capitis*: "gray patch" (alopecia associated with scaling of the scalp) and "black dot" (slight scaling and brittle hair breaking off at skin surface) and kerion (characterized by alopecia and an inflammatory boggy plaque); follicular involvement may not be apparent due to the more extensive involvement of the skin. Favus is characterized by suppurative and granulomatous folliculitis associated with scarring. In Majocchi's or dermatophytic granuloma, scattered papules and nodules, usually associated with tinea cruris or tinea corporis (Fig. 23-24).

***Malassezia* Folliculitis**   More common in subtropical and tropical climates. Pruritic, monomorphic eruption characterized by follicular papules and pustules on the trunk, most often on the back (Fig. 29-25), upper arms, and less often on the neck and face; excoriated papules. Absence of comedones differentiates it from acne vulgaris (see Section 23).

***Candida albicans***   Occurs in sites of occluded skin such as the back of a hospitalized febrile patient or under plastic dressing, especially if topical glucocorticoid preparations are used. Large follicular pustules (see Section 23).

**Herpetic Folliculitis**   Occurs predominantly in the beard area (viral sycosis) in men. Characterized by follicular vesicles and later crusts (Fig. 29-26).

**Molluscum Sycosis**   Presents as umbilicated skin-colored papules in a follicular and perifollicular distribution over the beard area.

**Syphilitic Folliculitis**   Manifested by dull red papules; may be arranged in oval groups (corymbiform syphilis). Nonscarring alopecia of the scalp and beard.

**Demodicidosis**   Clinical presentation: perifollicular scaling (pityriasis folliculorum or rosacea-like erythematous follicular papules and pustules with a background of erythema on the face. Etiology: *Demodex folliculorum.*

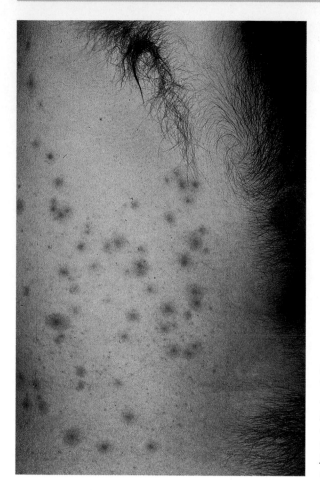

**FIGURE 29-23    Infectious folliculitis: *P. aeruginosa* or "hot tub"** *Multiple follicular pustules are present on the trunk, appearing 3 days after bathing in a hot tub. P. aeruginosa was isolated on culture from a lesion. The lesions resolved spontaneously within a week.*

## DIFFERENTIAL DIAGNOSIS

**Follicular Inflammatory Disorders** Acneiform disorders (acne vulgaris, rosacea, perioral dermatitis), HIV-associated eosinophilic folliculitis, chemical irritants (chloracne), acneiform adverse cutaneous drug reactions (halogens, glucocorticoids, lithium), keloidal folliculitis, pseudofolliculitis barbae.

**Regional Differential Diagnosis** *Face*: acne, rosacea, perioral dermatitis, keratosis pilaris, pseudofolliculitis barbae (ingrowing hairs). *Scalp*: folliculitis necrotica. *Trunk*: acne vulgaris, pustular miliaria, transient acantholytic disease (Grover's disease). *Axillae and groins*: hidradenitis suppurativa.

## LABORATORY FINDINGS

**Direct Microscopy** *Gram's Stain S. aureus:* gram-positive cocci. Also visualizes fungi.
***KOH Preparation*** Dermatophytes: hyphae, spores. *M. furfur:* multiple yeast forms; *Candida*: mycelial forms.
**Culture** *Bacterial S. aureus, P. aeruginosa*; gram-negative folliculitis: *Proteus, Klebsiella, Escherichia coli.* In cases of chronic relapsing folliculitis, culture nares and perianal region for *S. aureus* carriage.
***Fungal*** Dermatophytes; *C. albicans.*
***Viral*** Herpes simplex virus (HSV).
**Dermatopathology** The following features should be evaluated: Are microorganisms

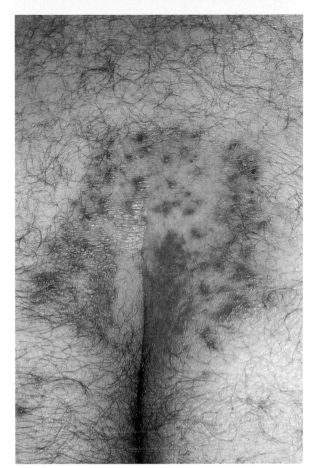

**FIGURE 29-24    Infectious folliculitis: dermatophytic**  *Multiple follicular papules on the sacral area; similar eruptions were present on the thighs. The patient was an HIV-infected male, who had been treated with topical glucocorticoids and antifungal agents without response. The lesions resolved with oral terbinafine therapy.*

present? Is the inflammatory infiltrate predominantly follicular or perifollicular? What region of the pilosebaceous structure is involved? Is the inflammatory process acute suppurative (neutrophilic), chronic lymphocytic, or granulomatous (foreign-body response to keratin subsequent to rupture of follicle)? Is any portion of the pilosebaceous structure destroyed?

## DIAGNOSIS

Clinical findings confirmed by laboratory findings.

## COURSE AND PROGNOSIS

*S. aureus* folliculitis can progress to deeper follicular and perifollicular infection with abscess (furuncle, carbuncle) or cellulitis. Infection of multiple contiguous follicles results in a carbuncle. Many types of infectious folliculitis tend to recur or become chronic unless the predisposing conditions are corrected.

## MANAGEMENT

**Prophylaxis**  *Correct underlying predisposing condition.* Washing with antibacterial soap or

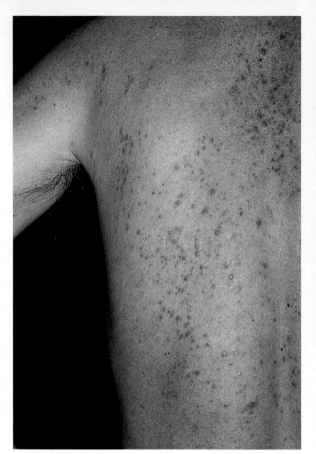

**FIGURE 29-25   Infectious folliculitis: Malassezia furfur** *Multiple, discrete, follicular papulopustules on the back, mimicking acne vulgaris. Lesional biopsy showed yeast forms of Malassezia furfur. The lesions resolved after treatment with oral itraconazole.*

benzoyl peroxide preparation or isopropyl/ethanol gel.

**Antimicrobial Therapy** *Bacterial Folliculitis* See Table 22-2.

*Gram-negative Folliculitis* Associated with systemic antibiotic therapy of acne vulgaris. Discontinue current antibiotics. Wash with benzoyl peroxide. In some cases, ampicillin (250 mg qid) or trimethoprim-sulfamethoxazole qid. Isotretinoin.

*Fungal Folliculitis* Various topical antifungal agents. For dermatophytic folliculitis: terbinafine, 250 mg PO for 14 days, or itraconazole, 100 mg bid for 14 days. For *Candida* folliculitis: fluconazole or itraconazole, 100 mg bid for 14 days.

*Herpetic Folliculitis* See "Herpes Simplex Virus Infections" (Section 25).

*Demodicidosis* Permethrin cream. Ivermectin, 200 μg/kg (usual range, 12 to 18 mg) stat.

*Pseudofolliculitis Barbae* Rule out secondary *S. aureus* infection. Discontinue shaving. Use beard clipper instead of safety razor. Destruction of hair follicle: electrolysis; laser hair removal.

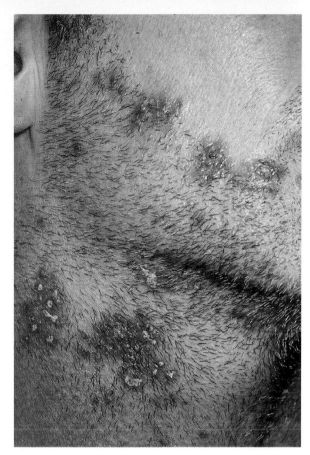

**FIGURE 29-26   Infectious folliculitis: herpes simplex virus**   *Discrete and grouped pustules and erosions in the beard area of an otherwise healthy 40-year-old male. HSV was isolated on culture. The initial diagnosis was* S. aureus *folliculitis; however, no pathogens were isolated on bacterial culture. There was no response to dicloxacillin, but lesions resolved with oral acyclovir.*

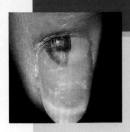

# DISORDERS OF THE NAIL APPARATUS

## NORMAL NAIL APPARATUS

The nail apparatus is made up of the nail plate and surrounding soft tissue structures. Fingernails add function to multiple uses of the hands and protect the terminal digits. Nail apparatus disorders can be traumatic, structural, primary, manifestations of cutaneous disease (e.g., psoriasis), neoplastic, infectious, or manifestations of systemic diseases (e.g., lupus erythematosus).

### COMPONENTS OF THE NAIL APPARATUS
(Fig. 30-1)

**Nail Plate** The hard protective tool, the product of the nail apparatus. Rests on and is firmly attached to nail bed, which is attached to underlying bone. Surrounded on three sides by nail folds. Made of three horizontal layers: thin dorsal lamina, thicker intermediate lamina, ventral layer from nail bed. Hardness of nail plate due to high sulfur matrix protein. Nail plate shape relates to shape of underlying phalangeal bone.

**Proximal Nail Fold (PNF)** Covers proximal one-quarter of the nail plate. Has two epithelial surfaces, dorsal and ventral. Devoid of dermatoglyphic markings and sebaceous glands.

**Cuticle** Junction of two epithelial surfaces of PNF, projects distally onto nail surface, sealing PNF and nail. Protects structures at base of nail (germinative matrix) from irritants, allergens, bacterial/fungal pathogens. Loss of cuticle produces potential space or pocket: inflammation of this pocket results in chronic paronychia.

**Lateral Folds** Usually cover lateral edges of plate.

**Lunula** Underlies proximal fold. Normally is white. Represents most distal region of the matrix.

**Free Margin** Distal nail. Natural shape same as contour of distal lunula.

**Nail Matrix** Proximal matrix underlies nail plate to distal border of lunula. Distal matrix is that portion distal to distal border of lunula. Produces the major part of nail plate. As in epidermis, possesses a dividing basal cell layer producing keratinocytes, which differentiate, harden, die, and contribute to nail plate—analogous to epidermal stratum corneum. Keratinocytes mature and keratinize without keratohyalin (granular layer) formation. Melanocytes are present in lower layers and produce melanin. Linear longitudinal pigmented bands may be seen in persons of darker skin phototypes.

**Nail Bed** Consists of epidermal part (ventral matrix) (no more than two to three cells thick) and underlying dermis closely apposed to periosteum of distal phalanx. Within connective tissue network lie blood vessels, lymphatics, a fine network of elastic fibers, and scattered fat cells. Subcutaneous fat layer is absent. Normally pink due to vasculature as seen through the translucent nail plate.

**Hyponychium** Space under free margin of nail plate, from point of separation of nail plate from nail bed to the distal end of the nail plate. Extension of hyponychium proximally is onycholysis.

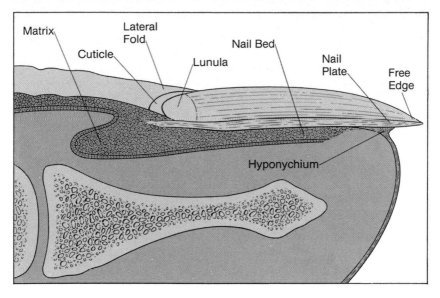

**FIGURE 30-1   Schematic drawing of normal nail.**

# ABNORMAL NAIL APPARATUS

## NOMENCLATURE

**Beau's Lines**   Transverse depression in nail plate. Single nail involvement is usually traumatic. Multiple nail involvement indicates systemic disease.

**Koilonychia**   Spoon nails; thinned concave nails. Physiologic in children; in adults, most commonly occupational.

**Leukonychia**   *True leukonychia*: White opaque discoloration of the nail plate associated with distal nail matrix damage; may be punctate, striate, or diffuse. *Single nail*: traumatic, psoriasis. *Punctate leukonychia*: small white opaque spots; commonly seen following trauma or as the only finding in psoriasis. *Transverse leukonychia*: multiple transverse opaque parallel bands; commonly associated with matrix trauma of manicure or tight shoes. *Diffuse leukonychia*: nail plate completely opaque and white. Fungal infections cause superficial white onychomycosis and proximal subungual onychomycosis.

*Apparent leukonychia*   White discoloration that fades with pressure; abnormalities of color of nailbed; nail transparency maintained. Occurs with chemotherapeutic drugs and systemic disease.

**Melanonychia**   Melanin hyperpigmentation of the nail, either partial (longitudinal) or complete.

**Onychauxis**   Nail plate appears to be thickened due to subungual hyperkeratosis of nailbed. Common in psoriasis, eczema, distal subungual onychomycosis.

**Onychia**   Inflammation of the matrix of the nail resulting in shedding of nail.

**Onychoclasis**   Breaking of the nail.

**Onychocryptosis**   Ingrowing nail.

**Onychogryphosis**   Hypertrophy of the nail(s), producing a hooked or incurved clawlike deformity.

**Onycholysis**   Separation of the nail plate from the nailbed, usually beginning at the free margin and progressing proximally. Common in psoriasis, trauma, distal subungual onychomycosis.

**Onychomadesis**   Periodic separation of the proximal portions of the nail plate from the matrix and bed with subsequent shedding of the nails. Single nail: usually traumatic. Multiple nails: systemic cause.

**Onychomalacia**    Softening of the nail(s).

**Onychomycosis**    Tinea unguium.

**Onychorrhexis**    Longitudinal ridging and fissuring of the nail plate with brittleness and breakage. Common with aging.

**Onychoschizia**    Splitting or lamination of the nail plate, usually in the horizontal plane at the free edge.

**Onychotillomania**    Compulsive picking or tearing at the nails.

**Pitting of Nail Plate**    Punctate depressions of the nail plate surface. Common in psoriasis, alopecia areata, eczema.

**Trachonychia**    Nails rough, often thinned. Twenty-nail dystrophy or sandpaper nails associated with proximal nail matrix damage: alopecia areata, lichen planus, psoriasis.

## LOCAL DISORDERS OF NAIL APPARATUS

Local disorders affecting the nail apparatus can result in a spectrum of chronic nail diseases.

### CHRONIC PARONYCHIA    ■    ◑

Chronic dermatitis: erythema/swelling with secondary retraction of periungual tissue; loss of cuticle, separation of nail plate from undersurface of PNF (Fig. 30-2). Predisposing factors: (1) irritant dermatitis (occupational), (2) allergic contact dermatitis, (3) drug (indinavir), (4) dermatosis (lichen planus), (5) *Candida*, (6) foreign body (hair, bristle, wood splinters). Intermittently, persistent low-grade inflammation may flare into subacute painful exacerbations, resulting in discolored transverse ridging of lateral edges. Secondary infection: *Candida* spp., *Pseudomonas aeruginosa*, or *Staphylococcus aureus*, that discolor nail plate. *Management*: (1) treat the dermatitis with glucocorticoid: topical, intralesional triamcinolone, short course of prednisone; (2) minimize irritants/water exposure; (3) treatment of secondary infection.

### ONYCHOLYSIS    ■    ○

Detachment of nail from its bed at distal and/or lateral attachments (Fig. 30-3). Onycholysis creates a subungual space that collects dirt and keratinous debris; grayish-white color due to presence of air under nail, but color varies from yellow to brown; area may be malodorous. In psoriasis, yellowish-brown margin is visible between pink normal nail and white separated areas. In "oil spot" or "salmon-patch" variety (Fig. 30-3), nail plate–nail bed separation may start in middle of nail. Colonization with *P. aeruginosa* results in a biofilm on the undersurface of the onycholytic nail plate, causing a brown or greenish discoloration (Fig. 30-4).

Other secondary pathogens that can colonize/infect the space are *Candida* spp., dermatophytes, and numerous environmental fungi. Underlying disorders in fingernail onycholysis: trauma (e.g., splinter), psoriasis, photoonycholysis (e.g., doxycycline), dermatosis adjacent to nail bed (e.g., psoriasis, dermatitis, chemical exposure), congenital/hereditary. Underlying toenail onycholysis: additional factors of onychomycosis (*Trichophyton rubrum*), shoe trauma. *Management*: debride all nail separated from nail bed (patient should continue weekly debridement); remove debris on nail bed; treat underlying disorders.

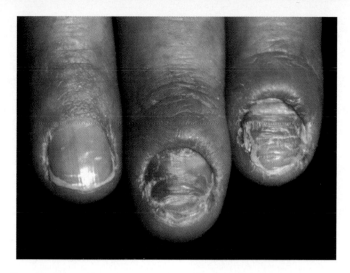

**FIGURE 30-2   Chronic paronychia**   *The index and middle fingers show chronic inflammation (edema, erythema, scaling) of the paronychial skin; inflammation of the nail matrix results in a roughened nail surface, transverse ridging. The normal ring fingernail shows punctate leukony-chia, a marker for psoriasis. Secondary* Candida *or* S. aureus *infections commonly complicate chronic paronychia.*

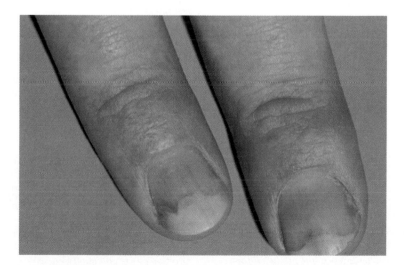

**FIGURE 30-3   Onycholysis**   *The distal nail bed is separated from the nail plate in two nails. In this case, the distal nail bed has a pink-tan color, a so-called "oil-stain," which is indicative of psoriasis. In onycholysis associated with psoriasis, the subungual space may or may not be filled with hyperkeratotic debris.*

## GREEN NAIL SYNDROME

Usually associated with onycholysis (see above). *P. aeruginosa*, the most common cause, produces the green pigment pyocyanin (Fig. 30-4). *Management*: debride "lytic" nail. See above.

## ONYCHAUXIS AND ONYCHOGRYPHOSIS

*Onychauxis*: Thickening of entire nail plate, seen in elderly. *Onychogryphosis*: Onychauxis with ram's horn–like deformity, most commonly of great toe. Nail is severely distorted, thickened, brownish, ±spiraled, without attachment to nail bed (Fig. 30-5). *Etiology*: pressure from footware in elderly; also, inherited autosomal dominant. Keratin produced by matrix at uneven rates, with faster-growing site determining direction of deformity.

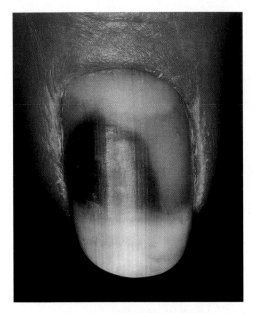

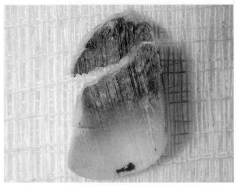

**FIGURE 30-4   Onycholysis with *Pseudomonas colonization*** *Psoriasis has resulted in distal onycholysis of the thumbnail. A biofilm of* Pseudomonas aeruginosa *has produced the green-black discoloration of the undersurface of the onycholytic nail. Onycholysis resolved following the debridement and treatment of the nail bed with glucocorticoid cream.*

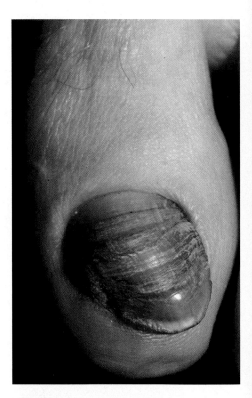

**FIGURE 30-5   Onychogryphosis** *The nail plate of the great toe is greatly thickened. Onycholysis is commonly present. The nail grows very slowly, requiring clipping infrequently. Pressure on the nail bed may compromise the circulation of those with reduced arterial blood flow.*

## PSYCHIATRIC DISORDERS  ▯ ▮  ○

Repeated manipulation of the nail apparatus can result in changes of the paronychial skin and the nail plate.

**Habit-tic Deformity**   *Synonyms*: central longitudinal grooved dystrophy, onychodystrophia mediana canaliformis. Washboard nail plate (Figs. 30-6 and 30-7). Caused by chronic, mechanical injury. Cuticle is pushed back with inflammation and thickening of proximal nail fold.

Occurs most commonly on thumbnail(s), as compulsive disorders (tic habit), caused by the index finger repeatedly picking at cuticle of thumbnail.

**Obsessive Compulsive Disorder**   Repeat picking at the paronychia skin can result in lichen simplex chronicus. *S. aureus* secondary infection is a common complication. In extreme cases, the nail plate can be destroyed (Fig. 30-8).

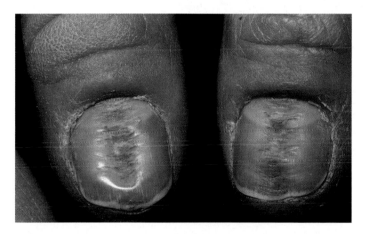

**FIGURE 30-6   Central longitudinal grooved dystrophy**   *A central groove is seen in the thumbnails bilaterally. The patient had picked at the proximal nail fold with the index fingernail of the same hand as a compulsive habit for many years. Once aware of the cause of the nail dystrophy, the patient stopped picking and both nails grew normally.*

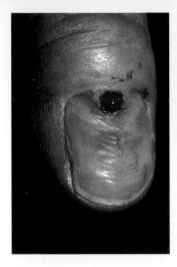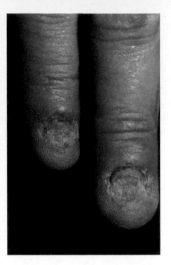

**FIGURE 30-7  (Left)    Central longitudinal grooved dystrophy with pyogenic granuloma**    *Pyogenic granuloma has occurred in the proximal nail fold following chronic trauma in an individual with obsessive-compulsive disorder.*

**FIGURE 30-8  (Right)    Onychotillomania**    *Obsessive compulsive behavior has resulted in removal of the nail plates of the index and middle fingers. The nail regrew normally when the nails were continually occluded with tape.*

## MYXOID PSEUDOCYSTS OF DIGITS    ◼ ○
### (See "Digital Myxoid Cyst," Section 9)

Pseudocyst or ganglion originates in distal interphalangeal joint, associated with osteoarthritis (Herberden's nodes). Lesions can present on the proximal nail fold, above and compressing the matrix, resulting in a longitudinal depressed groove in the nail plate. When cysts expand between the periosteum and matrix, nail becomes dystrophic with a dusky red lunula.

# NAIL APPARATUS INVOLVEMENT OF CUTANEOUS DISEASES

## PSORIASIS

Most common dermatosis affecting the nail apparatus; >50% of persons with psoriasis have nail involvement at one point in time, with lifetime involvement up to 80 to 90% See also Psoriasis, Section 3.

### LABORATORY EXAMINATION

KOH preparation and/or nail clipping to pathology for PAS stain to rule out fungal colonization/infection.

### PHYSICAL EXAMINATION

**Skin**

Typical psoriatic lesion on nail folds (Fig. 30-9).

**Matrix**

*Pitting*: Punctate depressions; small, shallow; vary in size, depth, shape (Fig. 30-9). Characteristically, isolated, deep. May occur as regular lines (transverse; long axis) or grid-like pattern. >20 fingernail pits suggests psoriasis. Uncommon on toenails.

*Trachyonychia*: Nail dull, rough, fragile.

*Elkonyxis*: Focal psoriasis produces a hole in nail plate.

*Serial transverse depressions*: May mimic "washboard" nails of tic habit (pushing back cuticle).

*Longitudinal ridging*: Resembles melted wax.

*Punctate leukonychia*: 1- to 2-mm white spots in nail plate. (mistakenly attributed to trauma).

*Leukonychia*: Proximal matrix involvement: surface rough and nail coarse.

**Nail Bed**

*"Oil" spots*: Oval, salmon-colored nail beds (Fig. 30-9).

*Onycholysis*: Secondary to "oil" spots affecting hyponychium medially or laterally (Fig. 30-9).

*Colonization of onycholytic nail*: May affect nail bed or undersurface of nail (biofilm). *Candida*, environmental fungi (e.g., *Aspergillus*), *Pseudomonas*. Predisposes to distal/lateral onychomycosis in toenail.

*Subungual hyperkeratosis*: Nail plate becomes raised off hyponychium.

*Splinter hemorrhages*

### MANAGEMENT

Often unsatisfactory. See "Psoriasis," Section 3.

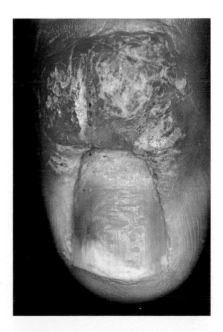

**FIGURE 30-9  Psoriasis vulgaris**  *All nail changes associated with psoriasis are seen in this finger. A psoriatic plaque is present on the periungual skin. The adjacent nail matrix is involved with transverse ridging and pits. There is distal onycholysis. "Oil staining" of the adjacent distal nail bed is present.*

## LICHEN PLANUS (LP)　　□　

Nail involvement occurs in 10% of individuals with disseminated LP. Nail apparatus involvement may be the only manifestation. One, several, or all 20 nails may be involved ("twenty-nail syndrome," where there is loss of all 20 nails without any other evidence of lichen planus elsewhere on the body). Similar changes are seen in lichenoid graft-versus-host disease See also lichen planus, Section 7.

### PHYSICAL EXAMINATION

#### Skin
Dorsum of PNF: swelling with blue/red discoloration of PNF.

#### Matrix
*Small focus in matrix*: Bulge under PNF (Fig. 30-10).
*Subsequent longitudinal red line*: Thinned nail plate evolving into distal split nail (onychorrhexis) (Fig. 30-10).
*Diffuse matrix involvement*: Selective atrophy of nail plate with onychorrhexis and/or transverse splitting (Fig. 30-10).
*Red lunula*: Focal or disseminated.
*Melanonychia, longitudinal*: Transitory.
*Complete nail split*
*Pterygium formation (scar, matrix destroyed)*: Partial loss of the central nail plate presents as a distal notch or entire split nail (Fig. 30-10).
*"Idiopathic atrophy of nails"*: Extreme pitting arising secondary to LP.

*Ulcerative LP*: Bulla formation, erosion, hemorrhage, scarring; cutaneous lesions usually present on palms/soles.

#### Nail bed
Onycholysis, distal subungual hyperkeratosis, bulla formation, permanent anonychia.

#### Variants
*20-nail dystrophy of childhood*: Resolves spontaneously.
*LP-like eruptions following bone marrow transplant*: Graft-versus-host disease.
*Drug-induced LP-like reaction.*
*Permanent anonychia*: May be only manifestation of LP.

### MANAGEMENT

See "Lichen Planus," Section 7.

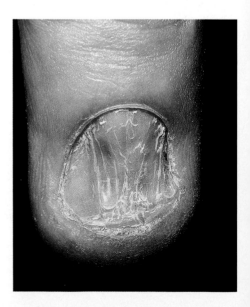

**FIGURE 30-10　Lichen planus**　*The nail bed is inflamed, affecting the matrix with resultant thinning of the nail plate and longitudinal ridging. Two other fingernails were similarly involved. Untreated, the matrix can be destroyed with pterygium formation where the skin of the cuticle grows over and merges with the thinned nail plate. Typically, the area of the lunula is more elevated than the more distal portion. Typical lichen planus was present on the buccal mucosa. All findings resolved with triamcinolone injection into the proximal nail fold.*

## ALOPECIA AREATA (AA)   □   ○

See "Nonscarring Alopecia," Section 29. *Findings*: geometric pitting (Fig. 30-11) (small, superficial, regularly distributed in geometric pattern); mottled erythema of lunulae; trachonychia (roughness caused by excessive longitudinal striations).

## DARIER'S DISEASE (DARIER-WHITE DISEASE, KERATOSIS FOLLICULARIS)   □   ○

A rare genodermatosis (autosomal dominant) characterized by keratotoic papules/plaques on scalp, forehead, face, neck, retoruricular, and trunkal areas. Nail changes are pathognomonic: longitudinal streaks (red and white); distal subungual hyperkeratosis with distal wedge-shaped fissuring of nail plate (Fig. 30-12).

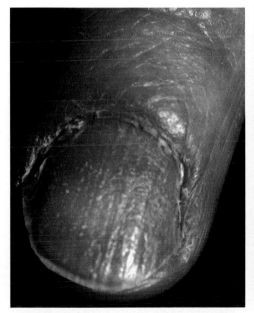

**FIGURE 30-11   Alopecia areata: trachonychia** *The nail plate is rough with a "hammered brass" appearance.*

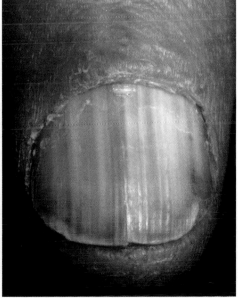

**FIGURE 30-12   Darier's disease** *Longitudinal red and white streaks with distal nail fissuring.*

## CHEMICAL IRRITANT OR ALLERGIC DAMAGE OR DERMATITIS    ▨  ○

Chemicals in nail polish and adhesive for pasteon nails can cause damage to the nail plate, i.e., discoloration, onychoschizia (Fig. 30-13). Irritant or allergic contact dermatitis can also occur on the paronychial skin.

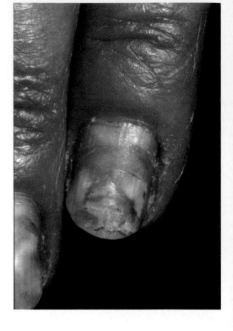

**FIGURE 30-13    Chemically damaged nail**  *False nail glued to the fingernail has chemically damage the nail plate with leukonychia and onychoschizia.*

# NEOPLASMS OF THE NAIL APPARATUS

Keratinocytes, melanocytes, and Merkel cells may give risk to primary squamous cell carcinoma (SCC), melanoma, and Merkel cell carcinoma of the nail apparatus.

## LONGITUDINAL MELANONYCHIA (LM)    ▨  ○

*Findings*: Tan, brown, or black longitudinal streak within nail plate (Fig. 30-14). *Pathogenesis*: (1) Increased melanin synthesis in normally nonfunctional matrix melanocytes, (2) increase in total number of melanocytes synthesizing melanin. *Onset*: Congenital or acquired. Most LM originate in distal matrix. *Differential diagnosis*: Focal activation of nail matrix (e.g., trauma), hyperplasia of nail matrix melanocytes, nevomelanocytic nevus (junctional), drug-induced [e.g., zidovudine (AZT)], or melanoma of nail matrix.

## ACROLENTIGINOUS MELANOMA (ALM)    ▨  ●

*Mean age*: 55 to 60 y. *Incidence*: 2 to 3% of melanomas in whites; 15 to 20% in blacks. Usually asymptomatic; most patients notice pigmented lesion, especially after trauma. *Findings*: Arises subungually or periungually, presenting with pigmentation and/or nail plate dystrophy (Fig. 30-15). Matrix lesions usually present as ALM in whites or broadening of an existing ALM in blacks. *Hutchinson's sign*: Periungual extension of brown-black pigmentation from ALM onto proximal and lateral nail folds (Fig. 30-16). 25% of ALM may be amelanotic (pigmentation not obvious or prominent). *Distribution*: Thumbs, great toes. Nail apparatus melanoma has a poor prognosis: 5-year survival rates from 35 to 50%.

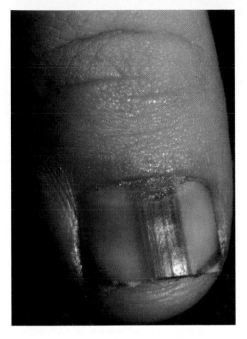

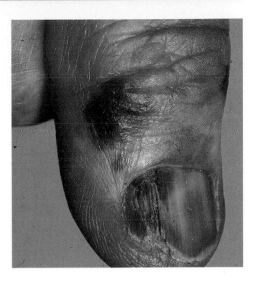

**FIGURE 30-15   Acrolentiginous melanoma**
*The melanoma arose in the nail matrix of the thumb with resultant nail plate dystrophy, sub-ungual melanosis, and extension into the proximal nail fold and beyond it (Hutchinson's sign).*

**FIGURE 30-14   Junctional nevomelanocytic nevus of the nail matrix**   *A junctional nevus is present in the nail matrix resulting in a longitudinal brown stripe in the nail bed. The proximal nail fold/cuticle are not pigmented.*

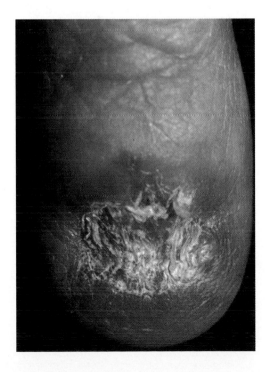

**FIGURE 30-16   Acrolentiginous amelanotic melanoma**   *The patient initially presented with worsening proximal nail dystrophy; the proximal nail fold subsequently became erythematous. The tan pigmentation is much more apparent in the image than at presentation. (See also Fig. 12-24.)*

## SQUAMOUS CELL CARCINOMA

SCC in situ (SCCIS) occurring periungually is usually caused by the oncogenic human papillomavirus (HPV) types 16 and 18. *Findings*: Skin-colored or hyperpigmented, keratotic, hyperkeratotic, or warty papules/plaques; onycholysis; failure of nail formation. *Distribution*: Proximal and lateral nails, matrix, hyponychium (Fig. 30-17).

*Invasive SCC* arises within SCCIS. *Symptoms*: Pain if periosteal invasion has occurred. *Findings*: Solitary nodule is most common, often destroying the nail. *Distribution*: Much more common on fingers (thumb and index finger most often) than toes; multiple fingers may be involved in the immunocompromised host. *Management*: Mohs' surgery or amputation of digit for more deeply invasive lesions involving periosteum.

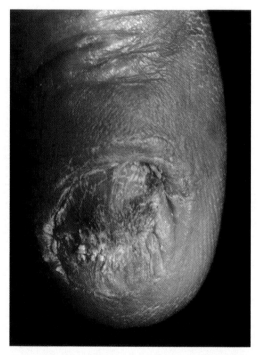

**FIGURE 30-17  HPV-induced in situ and invasive squamous cell carcinoma**  *A 46-year-old HIV-infected male presented with nail dystrophy. The nail plate is essentially absent. Sequential biopsy specimens showed progressive dysplasia to SCCIS. The lesion was removed by Mohs' micrographic surgery. HPV-induced dysplasia was also present on the glans penis with SCCIS of the perineum and anus. (See also Figs. 10-26 and 10-27.)*

# INFECTIONS OF THE NAIL APPARATUS

Dermatophytes are the most common pathogens infecting the nail apparatus. *S. aureus* and group A streptococcus cause soft tissue infection of the nail fold. *Candida* and *S. aureus* can cause secondary infection of chronic paronychia. Recurrent herpes simplex virus infection.

## BACTERIAL INFECTIONS

*S. aureus* is the most common cause of acute paronychia and felon.
*Management*: See "Antimicrobial Therapy," Section 22.

## ACUTE PARONYCHIA  ■  ◐

Acute infection of lateral or proximal nail fold. Usually associated with break in integrity of epidermis (e.g., hang nail), trauma. *Findings*: Throbbing pain, erythema, swelling, pain, ± abscess formation (Figs. 30-18 and 30-19). Infection may extend deeper, forming a felon.

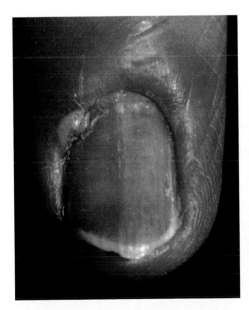

**FIGURE 30-18   Acute paronychia**   *The nail fold is erythematous, edematous, with early abscess formation, and is very painful. Portal of entry was via a small break in the lateral nail fold. Staphylococcus aureus was isolated on culture from dislodged nail.*

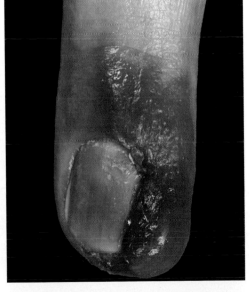

**FIGURE 30-19   Acute paronychia with pyogenic granuloma**   *Lateral and proximal nail folds are acutely inflamed; pyogenic granuloma has arisen on the lateral nail fold. Isotretinoin and acitretin therapy are associated with these findings.*

## FELON ☐ ◑

Soft tissue infecion of pulp space of distal phalanx (Fig. 30-20); closed space infection of multiple compartments created by fibrous septa passing between the skin and periosteum. *History*: Penetrating injury, splint, paronychia. *Findings*: Pain, erythema, swelling, abscess; abscess may break in center of pulp space and decompress spontaneously, with slough of necrotic skin over pulp space. *Distribution*: Thumb, index finger. *Complications*: Osteitis, osteomyelitis of distal phalanx, sequestration of diaphysis of the phalanx; rupture into distal interphalangeal joint with septic arthritis; extension into distal end of flexor tendon sheath, producing tenosynovitis. *Course*: May be rapid and severe; contained by unyielding skin of fingertip, infection creates tension with microvascular compromise, necrosis, and abscess formation.

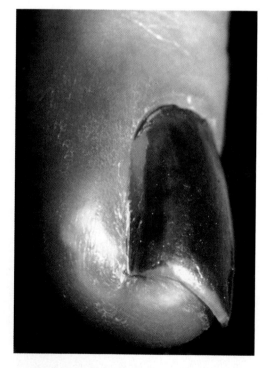

**FIGURE 30-20   Felon**   *Cellulitis on the fingertip arose following acute paronychia of lateral nail fold.* Staphylococcus aureus *was isolated on culture.*

# FUNGAL INFECTIONS AND ONYCHOMYCOSIS

*Candida* spp. usually cause "space" infections of chronic paronychia or onycholytic nail and can cause destruction of the nail in the immunocompromised host. Dermatophytes infect the skin around the nail apparatus and cause superficial destruction of nail. Environment fungi cause secondary colonization of diseased nail and are rarely primary pathogens.
*Onychomycosis*: Chronic progressive fungal infection of nail apparatus, most commonly caused by dermatophytes, less often by *Candida* spp.; molds can be cultured from diseased nails but are not primary pathogens. *Candida onychia*: Onychomycosis caused by *Candida* spp. *Tinea unguium*: Onychomycosis caused by dermatophytes.

## *CANDIDA* ONYCHIA

*Candida albicans* infections of the nail apparatus occur most often on fingers, most commonly as secondary infection of chronic paronychia. *Candida* can cause distal and lateral onycholysis, especially in diabetics. Invasion of nail usually occurs only in the immunocompromised host, i.e., chronic mucocutaneous candidiasis (CMC) or HIV disease.

## EPIDEMIOLOGY

**C. albicans and Other Species**   Normal flora, which causes infection if local ecology is changed in favor of yeast or in association with altered immune status. See "Candidiasis," Section 23.

### Classification

1. Subungual infection associated with onycholysis
2. Intermittent flares of chronic paronychia
3. Colonization in tinea unguium
4. Total nail dystrophy (TND) (Fig. 30-21): CMC and HIV disease

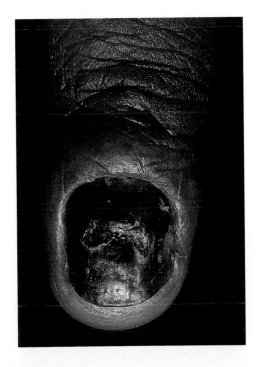

**FIGURE 30-21   *Candida* onychomycosis: total dystrophic type**   *The entire fingernail plate is thickened and dystrophic and is associated with a paronychial infection; both findings were caused by C. albicans in an individual with advanced HIV disease.*

**Chronic Mucocutaneous Candidiasis** See "Candidiasis," Section 23.

## HISTORY

See "Candidiasis," Section 23.

**HIV Disease** Candidal onychia and paronychia are common in children with HIV disease, often associated with mucosal candidiasis.

## PHYSICAL EXAMINATION

### Nail Apparatus

*Chronic Paronychia with Acute Candidal Flare* *Candida* spp. can cause intermittent painful infection of chronic paronychia with pain, tenderness, erythema, ± pus. Nail may become dystrophic with areas of opacification; white, yellow, green, or black discoloration; with transverse furrowing.

*Subungual Candidiasis ± Abscess* These occur in onycholytic space. Risk factor: diabetes.

*Colonization in Tinea Unguium* Secondary pathogen in distal/lateral onychomycosis.

*Total Nail Dystrophy* Proximal/lateral nail folds are inflamed and thickened. Fingertips appear bulbous. Nail is invaded and may eventually become totally dystrophic (Fig. 30-21). Nail apparatus thickens due to nail dystrophy and subungual hyperkeratosis. HIV disease: one nail may be involved. CMC: 20 nails may be involved in time.

**Other Findings CMC:** vitiligo, alopecia areata.

**Mucosal Findings** CMC and HIV disease: Oropharyngeal, esophageal, tracheobronchial, and vulvovaginal candidiasis.

**General Findings** CMC: polyglandular failure (hypoparathyroidism, hypoadrenalism, hypothyroidism, and diabetes mellitus).

## DIFFERENTIAL DIAGNOSIS

Tinea unguium, psoriasis, eczema, chronic paronychia, lichen planus.

## MANAGEMENT

See "Candidiasis," Section 23.

---

### TINEA UNGUIUM    ■  ◗

---

In addition to appearance, tinea unguium/onychomycosis of toenails can cause pain and predispose to secondary bacterial infections and ulcerations of the underling nail bed. These complications occur more commonly in the growing population of immunocompromised individuals and diabetics. See also Section 23.

---

## CLASSIFICATION BY ANATOMIC SITE INVOLVED

**Distal and Lateral Subungual Onychomycosis (DLSO)** (Figs. 30-22 and 30-23) Infection begins in stratum corneum of hyponychial area or nail fold, extending subungually, and progressively involves the nail centripetally and medially. May be either primary, i.e., involving a healthy nail apparatus, or secondary (e.g., psoriasis) associated with onycholysis. *Findings*: Onycholysis, subungual hyperkeratosis, yellow-brown discoloration of keratinaceous debris. Always associated with tinea pedis.

**Superficial White Onychomycosis (SWO)** Pathogen invades surface of dorsal nail (Fig. 30-24). *Etiology*: *Trichophyton mentagrophytes* or *T. rubrum* (children). Much less commonly, mold: *Acremonium*, *Fusarium*, *Aspergillus terreus*.

**Proximal Subungual Onychomycosis (PSO)** Pathogen enters by way of the posterior nail fold–cuticle area and then migrates along the

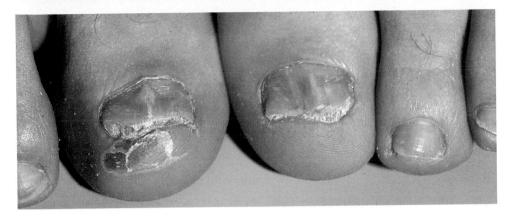

**FIGURE 30-22 Onychomycosis of toenails: distal and lateral subungual type (DLSO)** *Distal subungual hyperkeratosis and onycholysis involving most of the nail bed of the great toenails; these findings are usually associated with tinea pedis.*

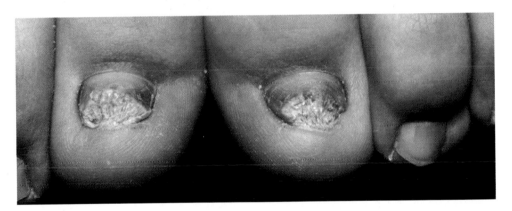

**FIGURE 30-23 Onychomycosis of toenails: distal and lateral subungual type (DLSO)** *A 13-year-old male with progressive distal onycholysis and subungual onychomycosis for 2 years. Tinea pedis was present. His mother also had DLSO.*

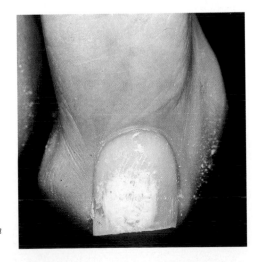

**FIGURE 30-24 Onychomycosis of toenails: superficial white type (SWO)** *The dorsal nail plate is chalky white. White nail dystrophy can easily be treated by curettage; KOH preparation of the curetting shows hyphae.*

proximal nail groove to involve the underlying matrix, proximal to the nail bed, and finally the underlying nail (Fig. 30-25). *Etiology*: *T. rubrum*. *Findings*: Leukonychia that extends distally from under proximal nail fold. Usually one or two nails involved. Always associated with immunocompromised states.

## EPIDEMIOLOGY AND ETIOLOGY

**Age of Onset** Children or adults. Once acquired, usually does not remit spontaneously. Therefore, the incidence increases with advancing age; 1% of individuals <18 years affected; almost 50% of those >70 years.

**Sex** Somewhat more common in men.

**Etiology** Between 95 and 97% caused by *T. rubrum* and *T. mentagrophytes*. *T. rubrum* imported into industrialized nations during the twentieth century, resulting in an epidemic of tinea unguium, tinea pedis, and other types of epidermal dermatophytoses. Much less common: *Epidermophyton floccosum, T. violaceum, T. schoenleinii, T. verrucosum* (usually infects only fingernails).

**Molds** Rarely, primary pathogens in onychomycosis, but rather secondarily colonize already dystrophic nails/nail apparatus. *Acremonium, Fusarium*, and *Aspergillus* spp. can rarely cause SWO. Dermatosis such as psoriasis, which results in onycholysis and subungual hyperkeratosis, or dermatophytic onychomycosis can be secondarily colonized/infected by molds. More than 40 mold species have been reported to be isolated from dystrophic nails, including *Scopulariopsis brevicaulis, Aspergillus* spp., *Alternaria* spp., *Acremonium* spp., *Fusarium* spp., *Scytalidium dimidiatum (Hendersonula toruloidea), S. hyalinum*.

*Etiology of Anatomic Types of Onychomycosis* DLSO: *T. rubrum, T. mentagrophytes*. PSO: *T. rubrum*. SWO: *T. mentagrophytes*.

**Geographic Distribution** Worldwide. Etiologic agent varies in different geographic areas. More common in urban than in rural areas (associated with wearing occlusive footwear).

**Prevalence** Incidence varies in different geographic regions. In the United States and Europe, up to 10% of adult population affected (related to occlusive footwear). In developing nations where open footwear is worn, uncommon.

**Transmission** *Dermatophytes* Anthropophilic dermatophyte infections are transmitted from one individual to another, by fomite or direct contact, commonly among family members. Some spore forms (arthroconidia) remain viable and infective in the environment for up to 5 years.

**Molds** Ubiquitous in environment; not transmitted between humans.

**Risk Factors** Atopics are at increased risk for *T. rubrum* infections. Diabetes mellitus, treatment with immunosuppressive drugs, HIV disease. For toenail onychomycosis, most important factor is wearing of occlusive footwear.

## PATHOGENESIS

**Primary Onychomycosis/Tinea Unguium** Invasion occurs in an otherwise healthy nail. The probability of nail invasion by fungi increases with defective vascular supply (i.e., with increasing age, chronic venous insufficiency, peripheral arterial disease), in posttraumatic states (lower leg fractures), or disturbance of innervation (e.g., injury to brachial plexus, trauma of spine).

**Secondary Onychomycosis** Infection occurs in already altered nail apparatus, such as psoriatic or traumatized nail. Toenail onychomycosis usually occurs after tinea pedis; fingernail involvement is usually secondary to tinea manuum, tinea corporis, or tinea capitis. Infection of first and fifth toenails probably occurs secondary to damage to these nails by footwear.

**DLSO** (Figs. 30-22 and 30-23) Nail bed produces soft keratin stimulated by fungal infection that accumulates under the nail plate, thereby raising it, a change that clinically gives involved nail an altered cream color rather than normal transparent appearance. Dense keratin of nail plate is not involved primarily. Accumulated subungual keratin promotes further fungal growth and keratin production. Matrix is usually not invaded, and production of normal nail plate remains unimpaired despite fungal infection. In time, dermatophytes create air-containing tunnels within the nail plate; where the network is sufficiently dense, nail is opaque. Often invasion follows longitudinal ridges of nail bed. Subungual location of infection prevents effective topical antifungal agents.

## HISTORY

**PSO** Previously a rare pattern, it occurs commonly on toenails in persons with HIV disease or other immunocompromised states.

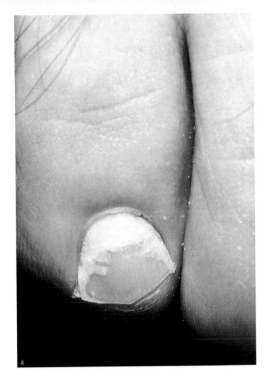

**FIGURE 30-25   Tinea unguium: proximal subungual onychomycosis type (PSO)**   *The proximal nail plate is a chalky white color due to invasion from the undersurface of the nail matrix. The patient had advanced HIV disease.*

## PHYSICAL EXAMINATION

### Skin Findings

Approximately 80% of onychomycosis occurs on the feet, especially on the big toes; simultaneous occurrence on toe- and fingernails is not common.

*DLSO* White patch is noted on the distal or lateral undersurface of the nail and nail bed, usually with sharply demarcated borders. In time, whitish color can become discolored to a brown or black hue. Progressive involvement of nail can occur in a matter of weeks, as in HIV disease, or more slowly over a period of months or years. With progressive infection, the nail becomes opaque, thickened cracked, friable, raised by underlying hyperkeratotic debris in hyponychium (Figs. 30-22 and 30-23). Sharply marginated white streaks beginning at the distal nail margin and extending proximally are filled with keratinaceous debris and air. Toenails are involved much more commonly than finger-

nails. First and fifth toenails are infected most frequently. Involvement of the fingernails is usually unilateral. When fingernails are involved, pattern is usually two feet and one hand.

*SWO* A white chalky plaque is seen on the proximal nail plate, which may become eroded with loss of the nail plate (Fig. 30-24). Diagnostically, the involved nail can be removed easily with a curette in comparison with a traumatized nail, which has white, air-containing areas. In some cases, the entire superficial nail plate may become involved. SWO may coexist with DLSO. Occurs almost exclusively on the toenails, rarely on the fingernails.

*PSO* (Fig. 30-25) A white spot appears from beneath proximal nail fold. In time, white discoloration fills lunula, eventually moving distally to involve much of undersurface of the nail. Patients treated with oral azoles show interruption of involved nail. Occurs more commonly on toenails.

## DIFFERENTIAL DIAGNOSIS

**DLSO**   Psoriatic nails ("oil drop" staining of the distal nail bed and nail pits is seen in psoriasis but not onychomycosis), paronychial psoriasis or eczema, Reiter's syndrome and keratoderma blennorrhagicum, onychogryphosis, pincer nails, congenital nail dystrophies.

**SWO**   Traumatic or chemical injury to nail, psoriasis with leukonychia.

## LABORATORY EXAMINATIONS

All clinical diagnoses of onychomycosis should be confirmed by laboratory testing (see "Dermatophytoses," Section 23).

**Nail Samples**   For DLSO: distal portion of involved nail bed; SWO: involved nail surface; PSO: punch biopsy through nail plate to involved nail bed.

**Direct Microscopy**   Direct microscopic examination of nail samples is used to confirm the clinical diagnosis. Keratinaceous material from involved nail scrapings is placed on glass slide, covered with glass coverslip, suspended in a solution of potassium hydroxide (KOH), and gently heated. Addition of dimethyl sulfoxide and/or Parker Quink ink to KOH solution may facilitate identification of fungal elements. Specific identification of pathogen is usually not possible by microscopy, but, in most cases, yeasts can be differentiated from dermatophytes by morphology.

**Fungal Culture**   Isolation of the pathogen permits better use of oral antifungal agents. Samples of infected nail are inoculated onto Sabouraud's agar with or without cycloheximide. Isolation of mold from psoriatic nail or tinea unguium is mostly colonizer and not primary pathogen.

**Histology of Nail Clipping**   Indicated if clinical findings suggest onychomycosis after negative KOH wet mounts. PAS stain is used to detect fungal elements in the nail. *Most reliable technique for diagnosing onychomycosis.*

## DIAGNOSIS

Clinical findings confirmed by finding fungal forms in KOH preparation and/or isolation of pathogenic fungus on culture.

## COURSE AND PROGNOSIS

Without effective therapy, onychomycosis does not resolve spontaneously; progressive involvement of multiple toenails is the rule. DLSO persists after topical treatment of tinea pedis and often results in repeated episodes of epidermal dermatophytosis of feet, groin, and other sites. Tinea pedis and/or DLSO provide portal of entry for recurrent bacterial infections (*S. aureus*, group A streptococcus), especially cellulitis of lower leg after venous harvesting. Prevalence in diabetics estimated to be 33%; DLSO contributes to severity of foot problems: superficial bacterial infection, ulceration, cellulitis, osteomyelitis, necrosis, amputation. *Diabetics need early intervention and should be screened regularly by a dermatologist.* Untreated HIV disease is associated with increased prevalence of dermatophytoses. Long-term relapse rate with newer oral agents such as terbinafine or itraconazole reported to be 15 to 21% two years after successful therapy; long-term follow-up studies not yet reported. Causes of relapse/reinfection uncertain: reinfection, immunologic incompetence, persistent trauma, unknown causes. Mycologic cultures may be positive without any clinically apparent disease. Nail/foot hygiene is important: benzoyl peroxide soap in shower or antifungal preparation or ethanol/isopropyl gel.

## MANAGEMENT See Table 30-1.

**Indications for Systemic Therapy**   Fingernail involvement, limitation of function, pain (thickened great toenails with pressure on nail bed, ingrowing toe nails), physical disability, potential for secondary bacterial infection, source of recurrent epidermal dermatophytosis, quality-of-life issues (poorer perceptions of general and mental health, social functioning, physical appearance, difficulty in trimming nails, discomfort in wearing shoes). Early onychomycosis easier to cure in younger, healthier individuals than in older individuals with more extensive involvement and associated medial conditions. *It is essential to prove (fungal) infection before starting systemic treatment; differentiate onychomycosis from other nail dystrophies.*

## TABLE 30-1  Management of Tinea Unguium

| | |
|---|---|
| **Debridement** | Debride dystrophic nails; patients should debride weekly. In DLSO, nail and hyperkeratotic nail bed should be removed. In SWO, abnormal nail can be debrided with curette. |
| **Topical agents** | Available as lotions and lacquer. *Usually not effective except for SWO.*<br>*Amorolfine nail lacquer:* reported to be effective when applied >12 months (available in Europe).<br>*Ciclopirox (Penlac) nail lacquer:* monthly professional nail debridement recommended. |
| **Systemic agents** | *Note:* In systemic treatment of onychomycosis, nails usually do not appear normal after the treatment times recommended because of slow growth of nail. If cultures and KOH preparations are negative after these time periods, medication can nonetheless be stopped and nails will usually regrow normally. |
| **Allylamines** | Most effective against dermatophyte infections; also efficacious against selected other fungi. |
| Terbinafine | 250 mg/d for 6 weeks for fingernails and 12–14 weeks for toenails. |
| **Azoles** | Drugs in this category are usually effective in treatment of nail infections caused by dermatophytes, yeasts, and molds. |
| Itraconazole: approved (USA) for onychomycosis. Effective in dermatophytes and *Candida* only. | 200 mg/d for 6 weeks (fingernails), 12 weeks (toenails) (continuous therapy). 200 mg bid for first 7 days of each month for 2 months (fingernails) (pulse dosing). Although not approved for toenail onychomycosis, pulse dosing is used, given for 3–4 months. |
| Fluconazole: not approved (USA) for onychomycosis. Effective in dermatophytes and *Candida.* | Reported effective at dosing of 150–400 mg 1 day per week or 100–200 mg/d until the nails grow back normally. Effective in yeasts and less so in dermatophytes. |
| Ketoconazole: not approved for onychomycosis. | Prolonged therapy as for onychomycosis has highest incidence of liver function abnormalities. Effective at 200 mg/d; more effective for *Candida* than dermatophytes; however, infrequently hepatotoxicity and antiandrogen effect have limited its long-term use for onychomycosis. |
| **Secondary prophylaxis** | Recommended for all patients. The entirety of both feet should be treated. Prophylaxis should be simple to use and inexpensive:<br>Benzoyl peroxide soap for washing feet when bathing.<br>Antifungal cream daily.<br>Miconazole lotion/powder on feet.<br>Antiseptic gels: ethanol or isopropyl alcohol.<br>Antifungal sprays or powders in shoes.<br>Discard old, moldy shoes.<br>Pedicures/manicures: make sure instruments are sterilized or individuals have their own. |

# NAILS AS CLUES TO MULTISYSTEM DISEASES

A wide spectrum of systemic disorders can affect the nail apparatus.

## LEUKONYCHIA   □   ○

**True Leukonychia**   Attributable to matrix dysfunction:

*Total leukonychia* (usually inherited)
*Subtotal leukonychia* Distal nail pink
*Transverse leukonychia* 1- to 2-mm wide arcuate bands
*Punctate leukonychia* Psoriasis, trauma
*Longitudinal leukonychia* Darier's disease (Fig. 30-12)

**Pseudoleukonychia**   Superficial white onychomycosis, chemical damage to nail keratin.

**Apparent Leukonychia**   Due to alteration of matrix and/or nail bed (e.g., apparent macrolunula):

*Terry's type leukonychia Association*: Cirrhosis. *Findings*: Opaque white plate obscuring lunula and extending to within 1 to 2 mm from distal edge of nail (Fig. 30-26). Involves all nails evenly.

*Uremic Half-and-Half Nail of Lindsay Association*: Uremia. *Findings*: Proximal nail dull white obscuring lunula (20 to 60% of nail); distal nail pink/reddish.

*Muehrcke's paired, narrow, white bands Association*: Hypoalbuminemia, cancer (antineoplastic) chemotherapy; unilateral following trauma. *Findings*: Bands are parallel to lunula, separated from one another, and from lunula, by strips of pink nail.

## YELLOW NAIL SYNDROME

*Association*: Lymphedema, respiratory tract disease (bronchiectasis, chronic bronchitis, malignant neoplasms). *Pathogenesis*: Arrest in nail growth. *Findings*: Nails hard, excessively curved from side to side; diffuse pale yellow to dark yellow-green discoloration (Fig. 30-27). Cuticles absent. Secondary onycholysis common. *Distribution*: 20 nails.

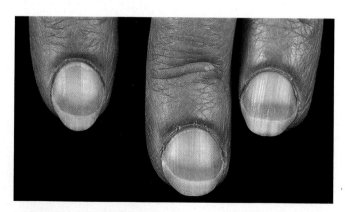

**FIGURE 30-26   Apparent leukonychia: Terry's nails**   *The proximal two-thirds of the nail plate is white, whereas the distal third shows the red color of the nail bed.*

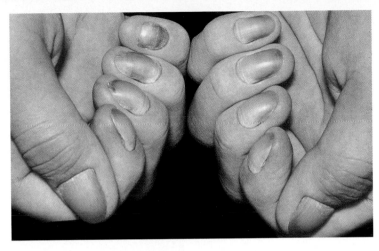

**FIGURE 30-27   Yellow nail syndrome**   *Diffuse yellow-to-green color of the fingernails, nail thickening, slowed growth, and excessive curvature from side to side of all ten fingernails.*

## PERIUNGUAL FIBROMA   □  ○

*Synonym:* Koenen tumors. *Association:* Tuberous sclerosis (see "Tuberous Sclerosis," Section 15) (Occur in 50% of individuals. *Onset:* Puberty. *Findings:* Usually multiple, small to large, elongated to nodular tumors; produce a longitudinal groove in nail plate due to matrix compression (Fig. 30-28).

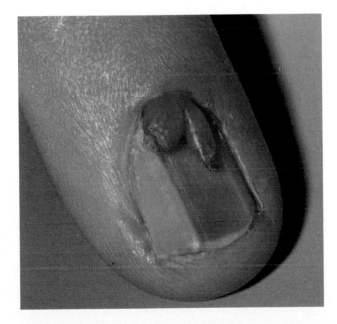

**FIGURE 30-28   Tuberous sclerosis: Periungual fibroma**   *A skin-colored tumor is seen emerging from beneath the proximal nail fold associated with a longitudinal groove in the nail plate.*

## SPLINTER HEMORRHAGES

Subungual epidermal ridges extend from lunula distally to hyponychium, fitting in a "tongue-and-groove" fashion between similarly arranged dermal ridges. Rupture of fine capillaries along these longitudinal dermal ridges results in splinter hemorrhages. *Etiology*: Trauma (most common cause, occurring in up to 20% of normal population) (Fig. 30-29); psoriasis, atopic dermatitis, systemic disorders (arterial emboli, antiphospholipid antibody syndrome, vasculitis, blood dyscrasias, scurvy), and systemic infections (trichinosis, endocarditis) (Fig. 30-30). *Findings*: Tiny linear structures, usually 2 to 3 mm long, arranged in the long axis of nail; plum-colored when formed, darkening to brown or black within 1 to 2 days; they subsequently move superficially and distally with nail growth.

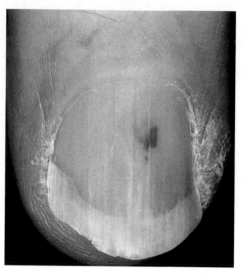

**FIGURE 30-30   Infective endocarditis: splinter hemorrhage**   *Subungual hemorrhage in the midportion of the fingernail bed in a 60-year-old female with enterococcal endocarditis; subconjunctival hemorrhage was also present.*

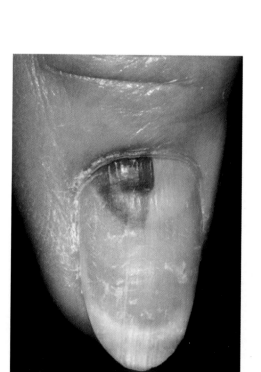

**FIGURE 30-29   Trauma: subungual hemorrhage**
*Trauma to the proximal nail resulted in hemorrhage and a tranverse depression across the nail plate.*

## NAIL FOLD/PERIUNGUAL ERYTHEMA AND TELANGIECTASIA  ☐ ○

Associated with connective tissue (collagen-vascular) disease.

**Erythema**  *Association*: Systemic lupus erythrmatosus (SLE), dermatomyositis (DM). *Findings*: Periungual erythema, edema, alterations of cuticle (Fig. 30-31), secondary nail changes.

**Telangiectasia**  *Association*:  Scleroderma, SLE, DM; rheumatoid arthritis. *Findings*: Linear wiry vessels perpendicular to nail base overlie proximal nail folds; usually bright red; may be black if thrombosed. In scleroderma, dilated vessels develop on normally colored skin; in SLE and DM, arise within erythema.

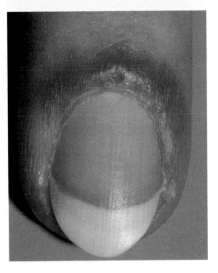

**FIGURE 30-31    Systemic lupus erythematosus: nail fold erythema**  *The proximal nail fold is inflamed (erythematous and edematous) in a patient with SLE.*

## TRANSVERSE OR BEAU'S LINES  ☐ ○

Systemic disease implicated if all 20 nails involved. *Pathogenesis*: Occur after any severe, sudden, acute, particularly febrile illness. *Etiology*: High fever, postnatal, cytotoxic drugs, severe adverse cutaneous drug reaction. *Findings*: Transverse, bandlike depressions in nail, extending from one lateral edge to the other, affecting all nails at corresponding levels (Fig. 30-32). If duration of disease completely inhibits matrix activity for 7 to 14 days, transverse depression results in total division of nail plate (onychomadesis). *Duration*: Thumbnails (lines present for 6 to 9 months) and big nails (lines present for up to 2 years) are most reliable markers.

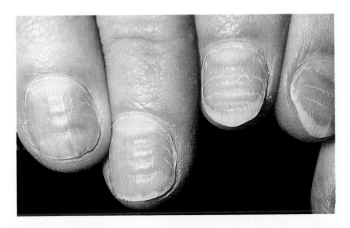

**FIGURE 30-32    Cancer chemotherapy: Beau's lines**  *Multiple transverse ridging of multiple fingernails was associated with chemotherapy for breast cancer.*

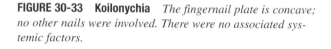

## KOILONYCHIA   □   ○

Spoon-shaped nails (Fig. 30-33). *Etiology* (more often due to local rather than systemic factors): physiologic (early childhood); thin nails (old age, peripheral vascular disease); soft nails (mainly occupational); hereditary and congenital; Plummer-Vinson syndrome (iron-deficiency anemia, dysphagia, glossitis). *Findings*: In early stages, nail plate becomes flattened; later, edges become everted upwards and nail appears concave.

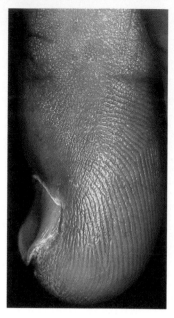

**FIGURE 30-33   Koilonychia**   *The fingernail plate is concave; no other nails were involved. There were no associated systemic factors.*

## CLUBBED NAILS   □   ○

*Pathogenesis*: Hypertrophy of soft tissue components of digital pulp; hyperplasia of fibrovascular tissue at base of nail (nail can be "rocked"); local cyanosis. *Etiology*: Congenital, familial, associated with edema of soft tissues; cardiovascular disorders; bronchopulmonary disorders (neoplasms, suppurative disease); GI disorders; chronic methemoglobinemia. *Findings*: Overcurvature of nails in proximal to distal and transverse planes with enlargement of periungual soft tissue structures confined to the tip of each digit (Fig. 30-34). Increased curvature usually affects all 20 nails.

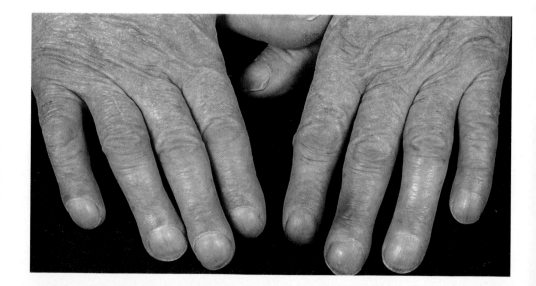

## DRUG-INDUCED NAIL CHANGES

See Table 30-2.
Adverse nail drug changes are similar to those
occurring in cutaneous and mucosal sites.

**TABLE 30-2   Drug-Induced Nail Changes**

| Nail findings | Causative drug |
|---|---|
| Discoloration (non-melanin) (Fig. 30–35) | Antimalarials: chloroquine, hydroxychloroquine, qunacrine<br>Minocycline<br>Gold |
| Melanonychia (Figs. 30–36 to 30–38) | Zidovudine (AZT)<br>Psoralens (Fig. 30–36)<br>Chemotherapeutic drugs: 5-fluorouracil (Fig. 30–37), daunorubicin, doxorubicin |
| Leukonychia: true | Chemotherapeutic drugs |
| Leukonychis: apparent | Chemotherapeutic drugs<br>Polypharmacy: anthracyclines, vincristine |
| Beau's lines, onychomadesis (Fig. 30–32) | Chemotherapeutic drugs |
| Paronychia; paronychial pyogenic granuloma (Fig. 30–19) | Retinoids: isotretinoin, acetretin<br>Indinavir<br>Methotrexate |
| Ischemic changes | β-Blockers |

**FIGURE 30-34  (Opposite page)   Lung cancer: clubbed fingers**  *Bulbous enlargement and broadening of the fingertips in a smoker with lung cancer. The tissue between the nail and underlying bone had a spongy quality giving a "floating" sensation when pressure is applied downward and forward at the junction between the plate and proximal fold. Cigarette smoke has stained the left middle finger.*

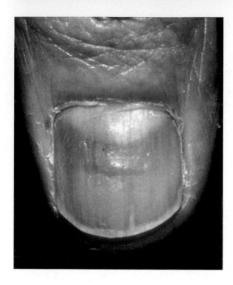

**FIGURE 30-35    Nail discoloration: quinacrine**    *Bluish discoloration of the nail in a patient with SLE treated with quinacrine.*

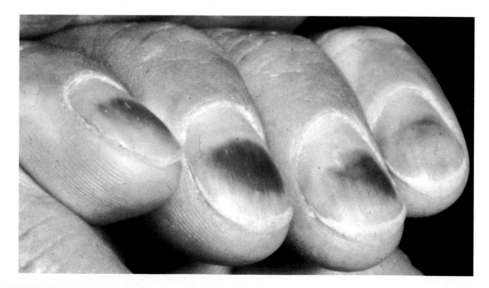

**FIGURE 30-36    Phototoxic onycholysis: psoralen**    *Phototoxic burn of nail bed with hemorrhage and onycholysis in a patient treated with oral psoralen and UVA phototherapy (PUVA).*

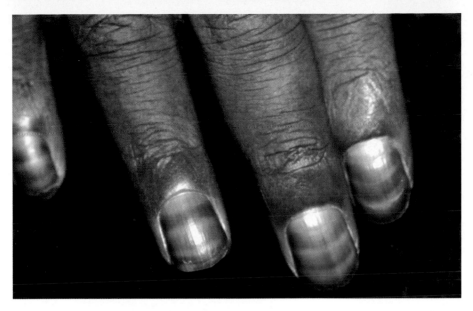

**FIGURE 30-37    Nail discoloration and transverse bands: chemotherapy**    *Period transverse bands on the fingernail in a patient with breast cancer being treated with chemotherapy (5-fluorouracil).*

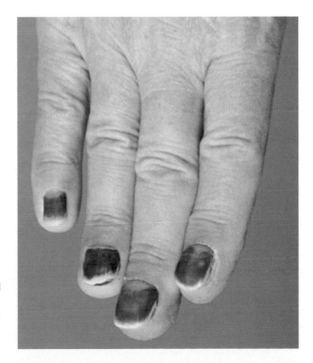

**FIGURE 30-38    Nail discoloration and onycholysis: capecitabine**    *Striking discoloration of the nails in a patient with breast cancer treated with capecitabine.*

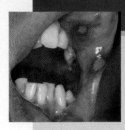

# DISORDERS OF OROPHARYNX

Oral mucosa covers and protects tissues beneath it and conveys sensory information from the surface. Normal function is required for mastication, deglutition, chemosensory function, phonation. Impaired oral mucosal health causes pain, malnutrition, infection, compromised immune function, and exacerbations of medical disorders.

## APHTHOUS ULCER ■ ◖

Aphthous ulcers (AUs) are painful mucosal ulcerations of idiopathic etiology occurring commonly in the oropharynx and less commonly in the esophagus, upper and lower GI tract, and anogenital epithelium, characterized clinically by pain and sharply marginated gray-based, red-rimmed ulcer(s). AU occurs in otherwise healthy people.

*Synonyms*: Aphthous (ancient Greek word for "ulcer") stomatitis, "canker sore." *Minor AU*: recurrent aphthae of Mikulicz. *Major AU*: Sutton's disease, periadenitis mucosa necrotica recurrens.

### EPIDEMIOLOGY

**Age of Onset**   Any age; often during second decade, persisting into adulthood, and becoming less frequent with advancing age.
**Sex**   Females > males.
**Incidence**   Extremely common; most adults experience AU at some time during their lives.
**Risk Factors**   Local trauma, heredity.
**Associated Disorders**   Behçet's disease (see Section 14), cyclic neutropenia, HIV disease.
**Classification**   Minor (MiAU), <1 cm in diameter; major (MaAu), up to 3 cm; herpetiform (HAU), up to 100 tiny erosions.

### ETIOLOGY AND PATHOGENESIS

Unknown

### HISTORY

AU may occur at the site of minor mucosal injury, such as a minor bite by teeth.

**Symptoms**   Even though small, AU can be quite painful, which may impair nutrition. A burning or tingling sensation may be felt before ulceration. In persons with severe AU, malaise: weight loss associated with persistent, painful AU.

### PHYSICAL EXAMINATION

#### Mucous Membranes
At times, small, painful red macule or papule before ulceration. More commonly, ulcer(s) <1 cm (Figs. 31-1 and 31-2), covered with fibrin (gray-white), with sharp, discrete, and at times edematous borders. White-gray base with an erythematous rim. Most commonly single; at times, multiple or numerous small, shallow, grouped—i.e., herpetiform. MaAU may heal with white, depressed scars.

*Distribution* Oropharyngeal, anogenital, any site in the GI tract. Oral lesions most commonly on the buccal and labial mucosae, less commonly on tongue, sulci, floor of mouth. MiAU rarely occur on the palate or gums. MaAU often occur on soft palate and pharynx.

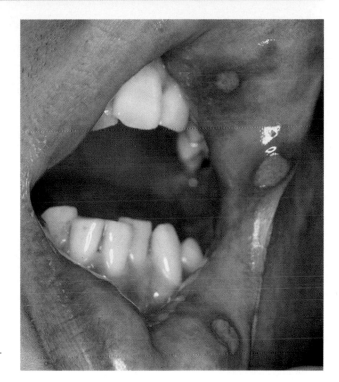

**FIGURE 31-1   Aphthous ulcers:
minor**   *Multiple, very painful,
gray-based ulcers with erythematous halos on the labial mucosa.*

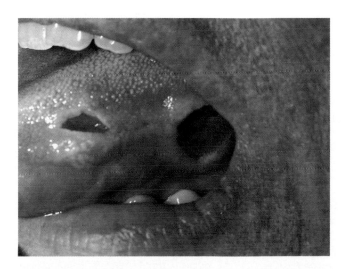

**FIGURE 31-2   Aphthous ulcers: major**   *Two huge painful deep ulcers on the lateral tongue, present for 5 months in a 52-year-old female with HIV disease. Ulcers resolved with intralesional triamcinolone injection.*

**Number** MiAU, 1 to 5; MaAU, 1 to 10; HAU up to 100.

**General Findings**   With MaAU, occasionally tender cervical lymphadenopathy. Findings of Behçet's disease, cyclic neutropenia, HIV disease.

## DIFFERENTIAL DIAGNOSIS

**Oropharyngeal Ulcer(s)**   Primary herpetic gingivostomatitis, herpangina, hand-foot-and-mouth disease, bullous diseases (erythema multiforme, pemphigus vulgaris, bullous pemphigoid, cicatricial pemphigoid), lichen planus, Reiter's syndrome, adverse drug reaction (fixed eruption, systemic chemotherapy, gold), squamous cell carcinoma (SCC), Behçet's disease.

## LABORATORY EXAMINATION

**Dermatopathology**   The findings are not diagnostic, showing varying degrees of epithelial ulceration and inflammatory response; specific causes of epithelial ulceration can be ruled out by histologic findings, including infection (syphilitic chancre, histoplasmosis), inflammatory disorders (lichen planus), or cancers (SCC).

## DIAGNOSIS

Usually by clinical findings.

## COURSE AND PROGNOSIS

In many persons, MiAU tend to recur during adulthood. Uncommonly, may be almost constant in the oropharynx or anogenitalia, referred to as *complex aphthosis*. MiAU heal spontaneously in 1 to 2 weeks. MaAU may persist for ≥6 weeks, healing with scarring. HAU usually heal in 1 to 2 weeks. Behçet's disease should be considered in patients with persistent oropharyngeal AU, with or without anogenital AU, associated with systemic findings (eye, nervous system). See Section 14.

## MANAGEMENT

**Topical Modalities**   Topical glucocorticoids in a base suited for mucous membranes. Topical anesthetics (diphenhydramine EMLA, viscous lidocaine).
**Intralesional Therapy**   Triamcinolone injection: 3 to 10 mg/mL.
**Systemic Therapy**   In persons with large, persistent, painful AU interfering with nutrition, a brief course of oral glucocorticoids is effective (70 mg, tapered by 10 or 5 mg/d) Thalidomide effective in HIV disease, Behçet's disease, large painful AU.

## LEUKOPLAKIA

Leukoplakia is a descriptive clinical term regarding morphology of a white plaque or lesion in the oropharynx; biologic behavior ranges from benign to malignant. *Findings:* a white plaque that cannot be wiped off and cannot be diagnosed as any other distinct lesion. When diagnosis is definitive histologically, "leukoplakia" is no longer appropriate. Leukoplakia may be premalignant or malignant, so a definitive diagnosis should be made on clinical findings and/or histology. The differential diagnosis of leukoplakia is shown in Table 31-1.

**FIGURE 31-3 (Opposite page, top)   Hairy tongue**   *Filiform hyperkeratoses of the papillae result in a brownish coating on the dorsum of the tongue in this 31-year-old cigarette smoker.*

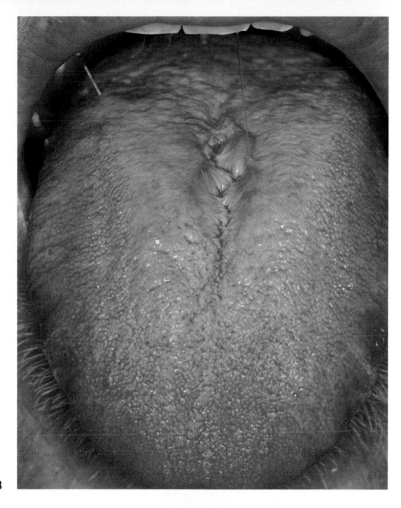

**FIGURE 31-3**

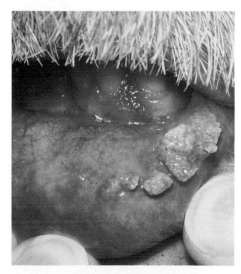

**FIGURE 31-4  Condyloma acuminatum**  *Cluster of white cauliflower-floret-like lesions on the mucosa of the lower lip in a 35-year-old male with HIV disease.*

## TABLE 31-1   Differential Diagnosis of Leukoplakia

| Lesion/Disorder | Characteristics |
| --- | --- |
| Leukoedema | Grayish-white opalescence of buccal mucosa; variant of normal. Histology: acanthosis. |
| Frictional keratosis | Acanthosis, hyperkeratosis secondary to friction (e.g., sharp tooth, rough or overextended denture border) |
| Chronic chewing: lip, tongue, cheek | Form of frictional keratosis. Surface white, rough. On buccal mucosa, wedge-shaped. |
| Linea alba | White raised line with epidermal hyperplasia and overlying hyperkeratosis. Occurs on buccal mucosa at edge of teeth (occlusal plane). Occurs normally or with teeth-clenching. |
| Nicotine stomatitis | Chemical irritation from smoking pipe, cigar, cigarette. Occurs on hard palate; obstructs minor salivary glands on palate; ducts become inflamed. Ducts appear raised, erythematous dots on posterior hard palate and soft palate. White appearance resolves with cessation of smoking. Not considered premalignant. |
| Tobacco chewer's white lesion | Develops where chewing tobacco is held. Mucosa granular or wrinkled. *Location*: mucobuccal fold. Lesion is premalignant. Usually resolves with discontinuation of habit. |
| Hairy tongue (HT) (Fig. 31-3) | Elongation of filiform papillae of dorsal tongue; color white, brown, or black. Brown HT associated with tobacco smoking; black HT, chromogenic bacteria. Etiology poorly understood: chemical mouth rinses, radiation-induced xerostomia, systemic antibiotic, systemic glucocorticoid. *Management*: debride with toothbrush or tongue scraper. |
| Aspirin/chemical burn | Occurs following placement of aspirin tablet on mucosal surface. Mucosal surface becomes necrotic; white/painful lesion loosely adherent, easily sloughs off. |
| Oral hairy leukoplakia (see Fig. 28-3) | See HIV disease (Section 28). White corduroy appearance on inferolateral aspect of tongue. Associated with low CD4 cell count. |
| HPV: condyloma acuminatum, verruca vulgaris (Fig. 31-4), squamous papilloma | *Findings*: white papules, plaques; small, sessile, papillated, exophytic. Solitary, multiple, mosaic. Common in HIV disease |
| Verrucous carcinoma | See below |
| Other white lesions | Keratoacanthoma, squamous acanthoma, submucous fibrosis (betel nut chewing), white sponge nevus |

# ERYTHEMATOUS LESIONS AND/OR LEUKOPLAKIA

Erythematous lesions ± leukoplakia appear red because of inflammation, hemorrhage, increased angiogenesis, epithelial atrophy, acantholysis, ulceration. The differential diagnosis is shown in Table 31-2.

**TABLE 31-2   Differential Diagnosis of Erythematous Lesions and/or Leukoplakia**

| Lesion/Disorder | Characteristics |
|---|---|
| Dysplasia, squamous cell carcinoma in situ (SCCIS) (Fig. 31-7) | Findings: white (leukoplakic, red/white; erythroleukoplakic), or red (erythroplakic). Suspicious lesions have erythroplakic components with poorly defined borders, nonhomogeneous colorations, ulcerations. |
| Invasive SCC (see Figs. 23-29 to 23-31, 31-8, and 31-9) | See below |
| Candidiasis | See Section 23, "Candidiasis." |
| Migratory glossitis (geographic tongue) | Findings: mixed red/white areas on dorsal tongue, depapillation, sharply marginated by whitish rim; maplike or "geographic" appearance. Course: intermittently remits and recurs, creating the appearance of migration lesions (Fig. 31-5) over days to weeks. Etiology: idiopathic; may be associated with psoriasis. About 40% of patients also have a fissured tongue. |
| Fissured (scrotal) tongue | Findings: surface morphology of the dorsum of tongue becomes convoluted; tongue has numerous linear "valleys," resulting in corrugated appearance. "Fissures" (Fig. 31-6), linear patterns are related to the deep valleys in the dorsal tongue that do not involve the mucosal epithelium and are therefore not painful. Persists and becomes more exaggerated throughout life. |
| Radiotherapy (XRT)-induced mucositis | Onset after XRT: 1–2 weeks. Findings: mucosal painful erythema, necrosis, ulceration. Salivary dysfunction. Stomatodynia, dysphagia. Dessicated lips and oral mucosa, dental caries, candidiasis, poorly fitting dentures. Healing begins after completion of XRT. |
| Chemotherapy-induced mucositis | Similar to those of XRT-induced mucositis |
| Oral lichen planus (see Figs. 31-16 to 31-18) | See "Lichen Planus," below. Lichenoid form: lacelike pattern on buccal mucosa, gingiva. Erosive, ulcerative form: buccal, labial, gingival, glossal mucosa. Lichenoid lesions occur as adverse mucosal drug reactions, graft-versus-host disease. |
| Lupus erythematosus (see Fig. 31-19) | See "Lupus Erythematosus," below. |

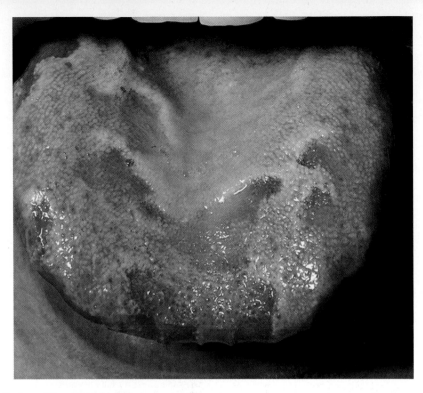

**FIGURE 31-5    Migratory glossitis**    *Areas of hyperkeratosis alternate with areas of normal pink epithelium, creating a geographic pattern in a female with psoriasis.*

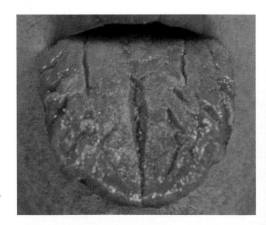

**FIGURE 31-6    Fissured (scrotal) tongue**
*Deep furrows on the dorsum of the tongue are asymptomatic.*

# PREMALIGNANT AND MALIGNANT NEOPLASMS

## DYSPLASIA AND SQUAMOUS CELL CARCINOMA IN SITU (SCCIS)
□  ◑ → ●

*Etiology*: Tobacco-related habits [smoking moist snuff, pan (betel nut)]; human papillomavirus (HPV). *Risk factors*: Tobacco use, alcohol use, oral lichen planus. *Oncogenesis*: Complex, multifocal process, multiclonal field carcinogenesis, and intraepithelial clonal spread; multifocal nature of early process reduces efficacy of local treatment. *Findings*: Chronic, ± solitary patch/plaque on oropharyngeal mucosa. ± Reddish velvety appearance with either stippled or patchy regions of leukoplakia (Fig. 31-7). ± Smooth patch with minimal or no leukoplakia. *Size*: Usually < 2 cm. *Location*: Floor of mouth (men); tongue and buccal surface (women). *Course*: Most dysplasia do not progress to invasive SCC; some do. Biopsy all lesions that persist for >3 weeks without definitive diagnosis.

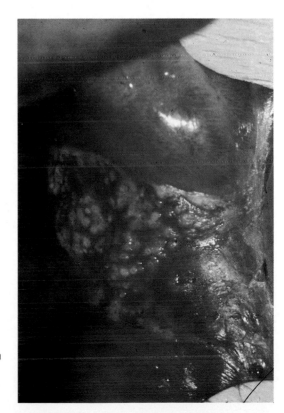

**FIGURE 31-7  Squamous cell carcinoma in situ: buccal mucosa**  *A well-demarcated white/red plaque in a 45-year-old tobacco smoker.*

## ORAL INVASIVE SQUAMOUS CELL CARCINOMA (See also Section 11)

This has high associated morbidity and mortality, accounting for about 5% of all neoplasms in men and 2% of those in women. *Findings*: Usually appears as a granulating, velvety plaque or nodule with stippled hyperkeratosis ± ulceration (Fig. 31-8) (lips, floor of the mouth, central and lateral sides of the tongue). Biopsy all lesions that persist for >3 weeks without definitive diagnosis. *Management*: Aggressive surgical intervention.

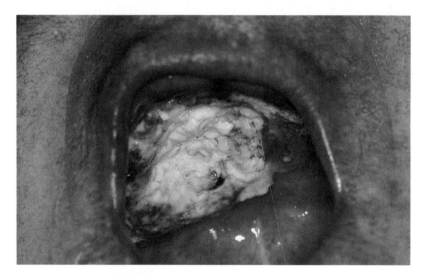

**FIGURE 31-8    Invasive squamous cell carcinoma: palate**    *An advanced leukoplakic tumor on the hard palate of a cigarette smoker.*

## VERRUCOUS CARCINOMA

*Etiology*: Oncogenic HPV type 16, 18. *Findings*: Extensive hyperkeratotic white leukoplakia (Fig. 31-9). *Course*: Metastasizes late. Biopsy all lesions that persist for >3 weeks without definitive diagnosis. *Management*: Aggressive surgical intervention.

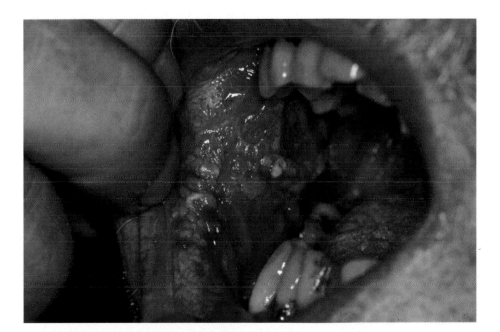

**FIGURE 31-9   Verrucous carcinoma: buccal mucosa**   *Extensive thick plaque arising on the buccal mucosa.*

## OROPHARYNGEAL MELANOMA
(See also Section 12)    □    ●

*Incidence*: 4% of primary oral malignancies. For the most part, lesions are asymptomatic; often advanced when first detected. *Findings*: Presents as pigmented lesion (Fig. 31-10), with variegation of color and irregular borders; rarely amelanotic. In situ lesions are macular; sites of invasion are usually raised within the in situ lesion. *Distribution*: 80% arise on pigmented mucosa of the palate and gingiva. *Risk factors*: More deeply pigmented individuals (Africans) have higher proportional incidence rates of mucosal melanoma than whites (because of the lower incidence of cutaneous melanoma).

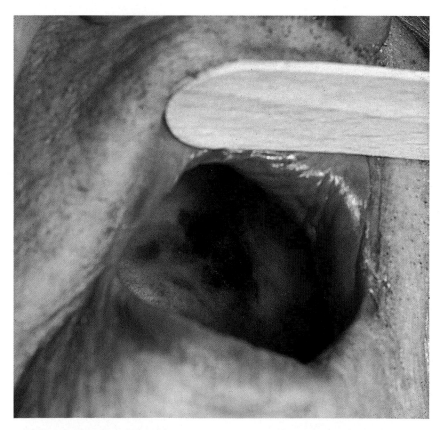

**FIGURE 31-10    Melanoma: hard palate**  *A large, highly variegated pigmented lesion in a 63-year-old male. Lesional biopsy of a raised part showed invasive acrolentiginous melanoma.*

## SUBMUCOSAL NODULES

### MUCOCELE  ☐ ○

These arise following traumatic rupture of minor salivary gland. *Findings*: Nodule with mucus-filled cavity, with a thick roof (Fig. 31-11). Chronic lesions are firm, inflamed, poorly circumscribed nodules; bluish, translucent; fluctuant. *Location*: Develops at sites where minor salivary glands are easily traumatized: mucous membranes of the lip and floor of the mouth. *Course*: Chronic, recurrent, and then it presents as a firm, inflamed nodule.
*Synonym*: ranula.

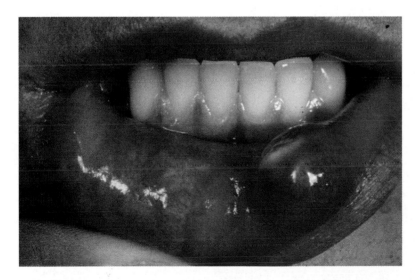

**FIGURE 31-11   Mucocele**   *A well-defined, soft bluish submucosal fluctuant nodule on the lip. Thick clear mucus drained when the lesion was incised.*

## IRRITATION FIBROMA   

This is a submucosal nodular scar, occurring at a site of recurrent trauma (Figs. 31-12 and 31-13). *Findings*: Sessile or pedunculated, well-demarcated nodule, usually 2 cm in diameter (may be large if neglected). Normal color of the mucous membrane to pink-red; firm to hard. *Location*: Buccal mucosa along bite line; tongue, gingiva, labial mucosa.

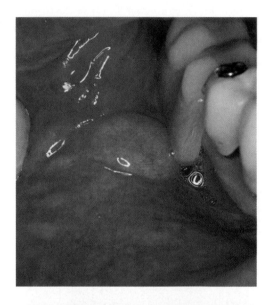

**FIGURE 31-12    Irritation fibroma: buccal**   *A rubbery pink nodule at the reflection of the buccal mucosa.*

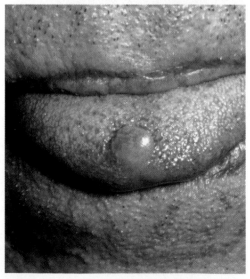

**FIGURE 31-13    Irritation (bite) fibroma: Tongue**   *Firm nodule on the tip of the tongue, repeatedly traumatized by biting.*

## PERIODONTAL DISEASES   ■   ◐

*Marginal gingivitis* is the most common periodontal disease, presenting as erythema and bleeding of the gingival margin. Untreated, the disease results in extreme bone loss, tooth mobility, and recurrent abscess formation, leading to tooth exfoliation or mandate tooth extraction. *Gingivitis and periodontitis* are infections associated with the accumulation of bacterial plaque, which may become mineralized (calculus). *Adult periodontitis* is an infection associated by various gram-negative organisms. *Acute necrotizing ulcerative gingivitis* (ANUG) involves sudden inflammation of the gingivae with necrosis, tissue loss, pain, bleeding, and halitosis (Fig. 31-14); associated with *Prevotella intermedia* infection and spirochetes; associated with HIV disease. *Drug-induced fibrous hyperplasia of gingivae,* which may cover the teeth, is associated with phenytoin, nifedipine, and cyclosporine treatment. Chronic myelomonocytic leukemia may infiltrate the gingivae.

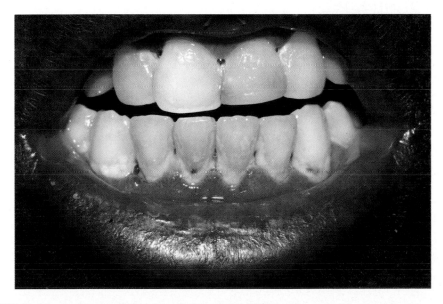

**FIGURE 31-14   Acute necrotizing ulcerative gingivitis (ANUG)**   *Very painful gingivitis with necrosis on marginal gingival, edema, purulence, and halitosis in a 35-year-old female with advanced HIV disease. ANUG resolved with oral clindamycin.*

# MUCOCUTANEOUS DISORDERS

## PEMPHIGUS VULGARIS (PV)
(See also Section 6)          □    ●

PV often presents in oral mucosa; may be confined to this site for months before cutaneous bullae occur. *Findings*: Blisters are very fragile, rupture easily, rarely seen. Sharply marginated erosions of the mouth (buccal mucosa, hard and soft palate, and gingiva) are presenting symptoms (Fig. 31-15). Erosions are extremely painful, interfering with nutrition. Biopsy confirms diagnosis (see "Pemphigus Vulgaris," Section 6, and "Paraneoplastic Pemphigus," Section 17).

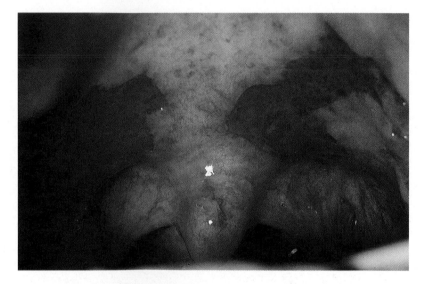

**FIGURE 31-15   Pemphigus vulgaris: erosions**   *Well-demarcated, painful erosions on the soft palate were the presenting complaint of this 55-year-old female.*

## BULLOUS PEMPHIGOID (BP)
(See also Section 6)          □    ◐
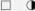

In contrast to PV, bullous pemphigoid rarely has mucosal involvment. *Findings*: Blisters, which initally are tense, erupt on the buccal mucosa and the palate, rupture, and leave sharply defined erosions that are practically indistinguishable from those of PV. However, erosions less painful and less extensive than in PV. Erosions also occur in cicatricial pemphigoid (see Section 6), where lesions occur only in the oropharynx. Diagnosis, see "Bullous Pemphigoid," Section 6.

## LICHEN PLANUS (LP)
(See also Section 7)

*Incidence*: 40 to 60% of individuals with LP have oropharyngeal involvement. *Findings*: (1) milky-white papules; (2) reticulate (netlike) patterns of lacy-white hyperkeratosis [buccal mucosa (Fig. 31-16), lips, tongue, and gingiva]; (3) hypertrophic LP—leukoplakia with Wickham's striae usually on the buccal mucosa; (4) atrophic LP—shiny plaque often with Wickham's striae in surrounding mucosa; (5) erosive/ulcerative LP—superficial erosions with overlying fibrin clots that are seen on the tongue and buccal mucosa (Fig. 31-17); (6) bullous LP—intact blisters (rupture and result in erosive LP); (7) desquamative gingivitis—bright red gingiva (Fig. 31-18). Erosive and ulcerative LP is painful.

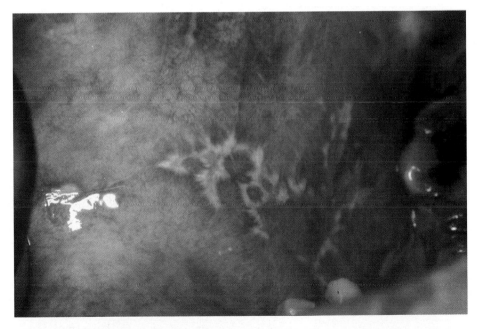

**FIGURE 31-16   Lichen planus: Wickham's striae**   *Poorly defined violaceous plaque with lacy-white pattern on the buccal mucosa.*

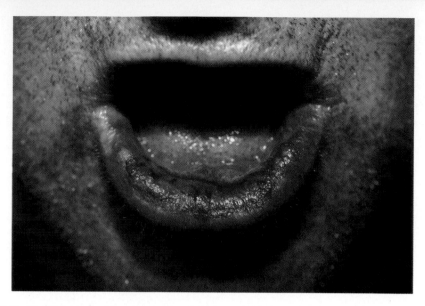

**FIGURE 31-17   Lichen planus: erosive**   *Eroded very painful lower lip in a 45-year-old male with hepatitis C virus and cirrhosis. Lesion and pain resolved several days following intralesional triamcinolone injection.*

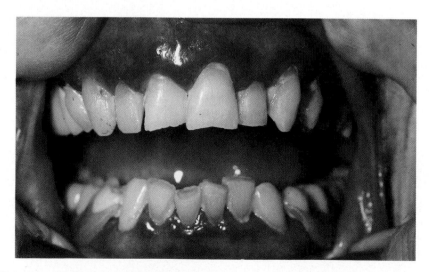

**FIGURE 31-18   Lichen planus: desquamative gingivitis**   *The gingival margins are erythematous, edematous, and retracted in a 72-year-old female. The lesions were painful, making dental hygiene difficult, resulting in plaque formation of the teeth.*

# SYSTEMIC DISEASES WITH ORAL MANIFESTATIONS

## LUPUS ERYTHEMATOSUS
(See also Section 14)

Mucosal involvement occurs in approximately 25% of those with chronic cutaneous lupus erythematosus (CCLE). *Findings*: Lesions: painless erythematous patches to chronic plaques, sharply marginated, irregularly scalloped white borders, radiating white striae, and telangiectasia. In older lesions: central depression, painful ulceration. Distribution: buccal mucosa; palate (Fig. 31-19), alveolar process, tongue. Chronic plaques may also appear on the vermilion border of the lips.

In acute systemic lupus erythematosus (SLE), ulcers arise in purpuric necrotic lesions of the palate (80%), buccal mucosa, or gums.

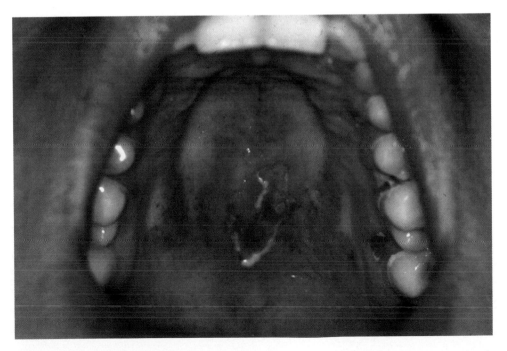

**FIGURE 31-19  Lupus erythematosus: hard palate**  *Erythematous eroded plaques were associated with chronic cutaneous LE.*

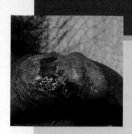

# DISORDERS OF THE GENITALIA, PERINEUM, AND ANUS

Anogenital skin and mucosa are subject to unique disorders because of their special anatomy. Dermatologic and systemic disorders occur in the anogenital region, often with associated extragenital involvement. Primary neoplasms arise in these areas, most commonly associated with chronic human papillomavirus (HPV) infection. Sexually transmitted as well as other infections also occur commonly in these sites.

## DISORDERS SPECIFIC TO GENITAL ANATOMY

### PEARLY PENILE PAPULES

Normal anatomic structures. *Incidence*: up to 19%. *Symptoms*: asymptomatic; may arouse some anxiety when first noted. *Clinical findings*: skin-colored 1- to 2-mm, discrete, domed papules evenly distributed circumferentially around the corona (Fig. 32-1), giving a cobblestone pattern. *Differential diagnosis*: condylomata acuminatum, molluscum contagiosum, *Histology*: angiofibromas. *Management*: reassurance: normal anatomic structures.

### SCLEROSING LYMPHANGITIS OF PENIS

*Pathogenesis*: thrombosed or sclerosed lymphatic vessel. *Etiology*: unknown; may follow trauma, i.e., vigorous sexual activity. *Clinical findings*: painless, firm, at times nodular, translucent cord appears suddenly, usually parallel to corona; not attached to overlying epidermis. *Histology*: walls of lymphatic vessels edematous, thickened with minimal lymphocytic infiltrates. *Course*: resolves spontaneously in weeks to months.

### PHIMOSIS, PARAPHIMOSIS, BALANITIS XEROTICA OBLITERANS

*Phimosis:* inability to retract foreskin over corona of glans penis. Etiology: chronic low-grade balanoposthitis; lichen sclerosus. Risk factor: diabetes mellitus (<2 years). *Paraphimosis*: inability to replace the prepuce over the glans once it has been retracted. *Balanitis xerotica obliterans*: characterized by foreskin (prepuce) that is thickened, contracted, fissured, fixed over glans and cannot be retracted over glans; commonly caused by lichen sclerosus.

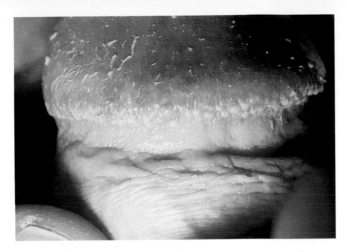

**FIGURE 32-1   Pearly penile papules**   *Pink (skin-colored), 1- to 2-mm papules are seen regularly spaced along the corona of the glans penis. These structures, which are part of the normal anatomy of the glans, are commonly mistaken for condylomata or molluscum contagiosum.*

## MUCOCUTANEOUS DISORDERS

### GENITAL (PENILE/VULVAR/ANAL) LENTIGINOSES (GL)

*Synonyms*: Penile lentigo, vulvar melanosis. *Onset*: adulthood. *Clinical findings*: tan, brown, intense blue-black; usually variegated, 5- to 15-mm macules occurring in clusters on vulva (labia minora, Fig. 32-2), penis (glans, shaft) (Fig. 32-3), and perianal areas. *Course*: persist for years without change in size. *Histology:* no significant melanocytic hyperplasia; nevus cells are not present; pigmentation due to increased melanin in basal cell layer. *Differential diagnosis*: melanoma in situ, PUVA lentigo, fixed drug reaction, blue nevus, HPV-induced intraepithelial neoplasia (IN). *Diagnosis*: dermoscopy rules out in situ melanoma; histology confirms diagnosis. Extensive lesions that cannot be easily removed should be followed photographically; areas that show significant change should be biopsied.

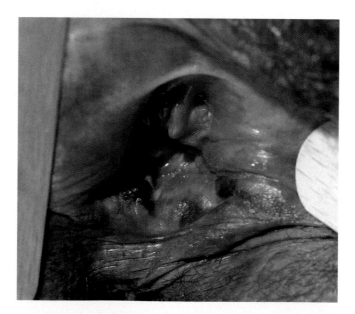

**FIGURE 32-2   Genital lentiginoses: vulva**   *Multiple, variegated dark brown macules, bilateral on the labia minora. Lesions had been present for >5 years and are multifocal in origin. Acrolentiginous melanoma in situ must be ruled out.*

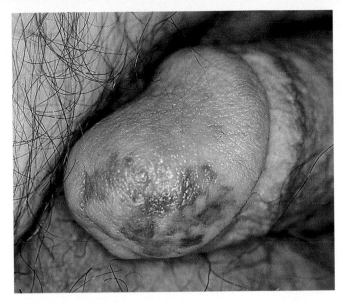

**FIGURE 32-3    Genital lentiginoses: penis**  *Variegated tan-brown macules on the glans of a 70-year-old male; lesions were present for many years. With these clinical findings, acrolentiginous melanoma in situ must be ruled out.*

## VITILIGO AND LEUKODERMA
(See also Section 13)

*Etiology*: (1) vitiligo is an idiopathic autoimmune disorder, (2) chemically induced leukoderma. Isomorphic or Koebner phenomenon (depigmenta-tion at sites of injury): genital herpes, cryosurgery, imiquimod therapy. Wood's lamp: differentiate from depigmentation from hypopigmentation. *Clinical findings*: sharply dermarcated, depigmented, white macules (Fig. 32-4); examine skin for other depigmented areas. *Differential diagnosis*: lichen sclerosus, old genital herpes; iatrogenic after cryo-, electro-, or laser surgery.

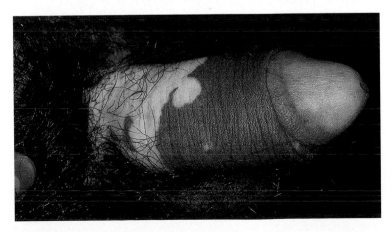

**FIGURE 32-4    Vitiligo: penis**  *Depigmentation of the proximal penile shaft. Multiple macules have become confluent. The lesions were an isolated finding.*

## PSORIASIS VULGARIS (See also Section 3)

*Incidence*: most common noninfectious dermatosis occurring on the glans penis and vulva. *Onset*: may be initial presentation of psoriasis. *Clinical findings*: (1) erythematous scaling plaques on nonoccluded skin (Fig. 32-5): (2) inverse-pattern psoriasis, well-demarcated erythematous plaques without scale in naturally occluded skin (Fig. 32-6). *Distribution* (inverse psoriasis): penis, vulva, intergluteal cleft, inguinal folds. *Differential diagnosis*: lichen planus (LP), fixed drug eruption, condyloma acuminata, HPV-induced IN, squamous cell carcinoma (SCC) in situ, invasive SCC.

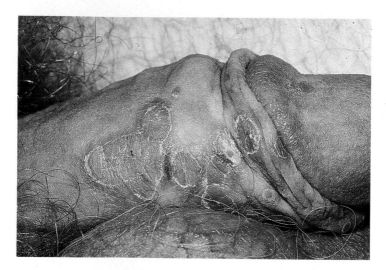

**FIGURE 32-5    Psoriasis vulgaris: penis**   *Well-demarcated scaling plaques on the penile shaft of a 25-year-old male. "Pinking" of the intergluteal cleft and nail findings of psoriasis were also present. The patient presented to a clinic for sexually transmitted diseases.*

## LICHEN PLANUS (See also Section 7)

Commonly associated with LP at other sites: however, may occur as initial or sole manifestation. *Symptoms*: not pruritic; pain in eroded lesions, anxiety about sexually transmitted disease (STD). *Clinical findings*: violaceous flat-topped papules, discrete or confluent (Fig. 32-7). Lacy white surface pattern most commonly on glans. Older lesions may have grayish hue with melanin incontinence. Annular lesions occur on glans and shaft (Fig. 32-8). Bullous and/or erosive LP on glans, vulva. *Distribution*: glans, penile shaft; vulva (Fig. 32-9). *Course*: spontaneous remission; erosive LP may persist for decades; SCC rarely.

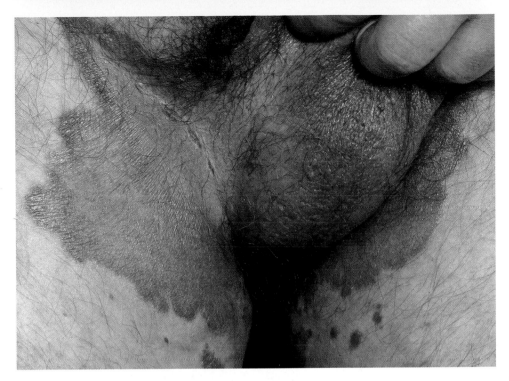

**FIGURE 32-6    Psoriasis vulgaris: inverse pattern**   *Well-demarcated erythematous plaques on the intertriginous skin at the junction of the scrotum and the medial thigh. Candidiasis at this site always has satellite pustules. Tinea cruris usually has marginal scaling and often, central clearing.*

## LICHEN SCLEROSUS (See also Section 7)

*Symptoms*: pruritus, burning; pain with ulceration. *Clinical findings*: Early: erythema ± hypopigmentation. Later: typical ivory- or porcelain-white macules and plaques; white due to loss of dermal vasculature (Figs. 32-10 and 32-11). Ecchymosis, bullae, and/or erosions may occur in involved sites. May obstruct urethral orifice. *Endstage*: balanitis xerotica obliterans (BXO). Labia minora and clitoral hood may be reabsorbed. Chronic LS predisposes to SCC. *Management*: clobetasol ointment; monitor for steroid-induced atrophy.

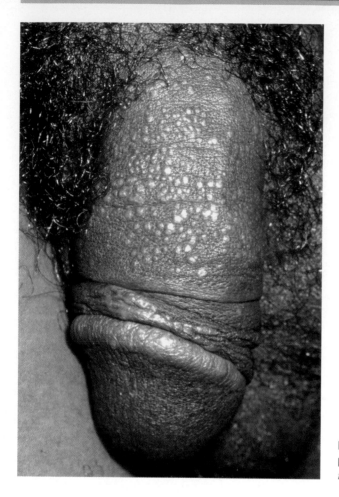

**FIGURE 32-7   Lichen planus: penis**   *Flat-topped papules on the shaft of the penis.*

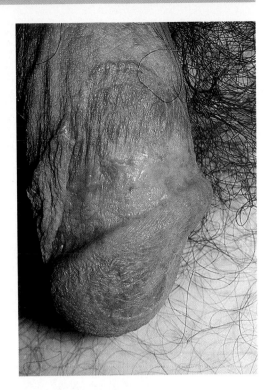

**FIGURE 32-8   Lichen planus: penis**   *Violaceous annular plaques on the distal shaft and glans of a 26-year-old patient, present for >1 year. White lace-like plaques were also present on the buccal mucosa.*

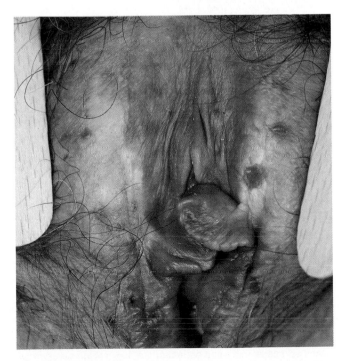

**FIGURE 32-9   Lichen planus: vulva**   *White bilateral hyperkeratotic plaques with areas of painful erosion. Vulvar lentiginosis is also present, posteriorly.*

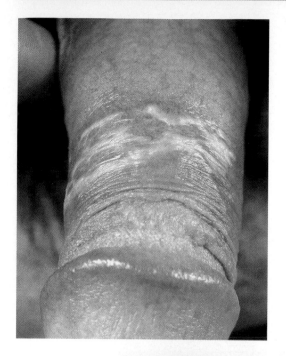

**FIGURE 32-10　Lichen sclerosus: penis**
*Early involvement with shiny white plaques on the prepuce of a 40-year-old patient.*

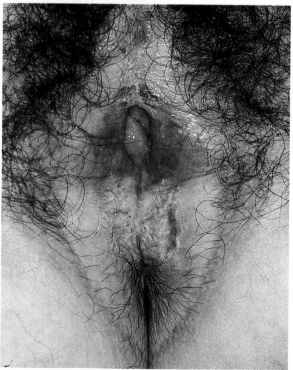

**FIGURE 32-11　Lichen sclerosus: vulva and perineum**　*A larger white sclerotic plaque extensively involving the anogenital region. The clitoral region is completely atrophic (agglutination). Ecchymoses are noted in association with atrophy. Ulcerations can occur and are painful. Sclerosis was improved with clobetasol ointment therapy.*

## ECZEMATOUS DERMATITIS

### ALLERGIC CONTACT DERMATITIS (ACD)
(See also Section 2)

ACD occurring on genitalia is often more florid and symptomatic than at other sites. *Allergens*: topically apply agents (medications, lubricants); haptens blotted onto genitals by hands (e.g., poison ivy sap). *Symptoms*: intense pruritus, burning sensation; edema. *Clinical findings*: erythema, microvesicles; edema; exudation of genitals (Fig. 32-12). With phytodermatitis (e.g., poison ivy or oak), lesions are usually present at other sites. *Differential diagnosis*: genital herpes.

### ATOPIC DERMATITIS (AD), LICHEN SIMPLEX CHRONICUS (LSC), PRURITUS ANI

AD usally occurs associated with more widespread involvement but can be isolated to genitalia. Chronic rubbing/scratching result in a single plaque of LSC on scrotum (Fig. 32-13) or vulva, persisting for years or decades. In dark skin, hypo- and hyperpigmentation occurs.

Pruritus ani can occur in the absence of any identifiable dermatologic disorder. Chronic pruritus and rubbing often produces some lichenification (Fig. 32-14). *Risk factors*: atopic

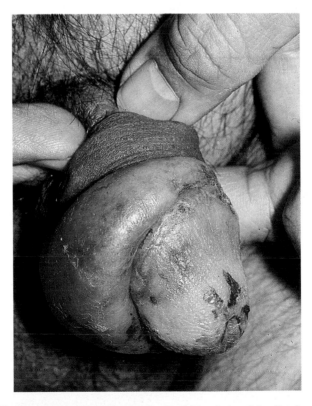

**FIGURE 32-12   Allergic contact dermatitis: penis**   *Striking edema of the distal penile shaft associated with severe pruritus in a 21-year-old patient. He had touched poison ivy with his hands, transferring the resin to his penis while urinating; pruritus and then edema occurred within 24 h of exposure. The magenta-colored pigment is Castellani's paint. The patient was initially seen in an urgent care unit where a diagnosis of cellulitis was made. Pruritus is the distinguishing feature of allergic contact dermatitis.*

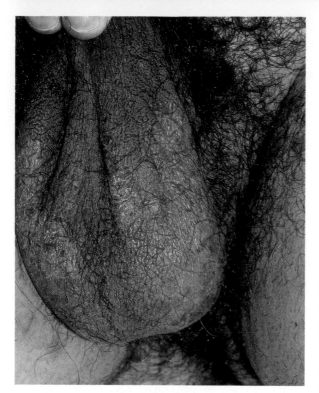

**FIGURE 32-13   Lichen simplex chronicus: scrotum**   *Pruritic bilateral erythematous hyperpigmented plaques in a 46-year-old Hispanic male. Lesions had been present for >20 years. Lesions resolved following an injection of intralesional triamcinolone (3 mg/mL).*

diathesis; multifactorial. *Secondary infection:* *Staphylococcus aureus*, group A and B streptococci, *Candida albicans*, and herpes simplex virus. *Management*: discontinue compulsive rubbing/scratching; maintenance of perianal hygiene.

**FIXED DRUG ERUPTION** See Section 20. (Fig. 32-15)

**FIGURE 32-15 (Opposite page, bottom)   Fixed drug eruption: trimethoprim-sulfamethoxazole**   *Violaceous bulla that had ruptured, occurring on the dorsum of the penis (glans and shaft), recurring after treatment with trimethoprim-sulfamethoxazole in a male with HIV infection.*

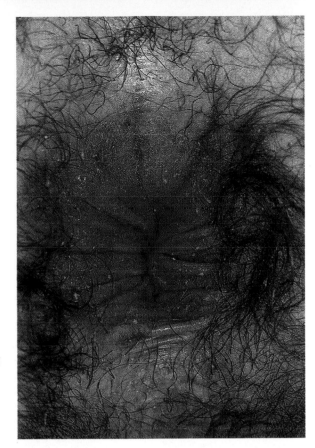

**FIGURE 32-14    Pruritus ani: lichen simplex chronicus**   *The patient had experienced intense anal pruritus for many years. Perianal erythema with mild lichen simplex chronicus and fissure is associated with chronic rubbing of the skin.*

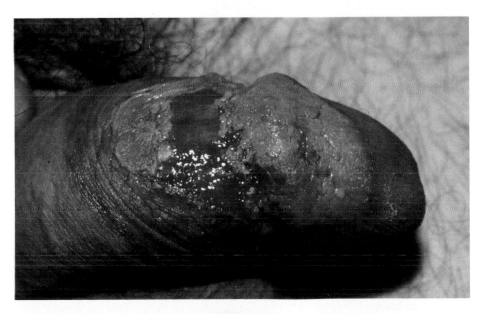

**FIGURE 32-15**

## PRECANCEROUS AND CANCEROUS LESIONS

## SQUAMOUS CELL CARCINOMA

### SQUAMOUS CELL CARCINOMA IN SITU

*Terminology*: Squamous cell carcinoma in situ (SCCIS) is specific; intraepithelial neoplasia (IN) is HPV-induced SCCIS. Older/archaic terminology: erythroplasia of Queyrat on glans; Bowen's disease, on penile shaft. *Etiology*: HPV infection, chronic low-grade balanoposthitis (poor hygeine, LS) in older individuals; chronic dermatoses (ulcerative lichen planus, lichen sclerosus).

Clinical findings: solitary, well-defined, irregularly bordered, red patch with a glazed-to-velvety surface hyperkeratosis on the glans (Fig. 32-16) or vulva (Fig. 32-17); associated dermatoses. HPV-associated lesions are usually multifocal, occurring at any sites of the anogenital region. *Diagnosis*: lesional biopsy. *Course*: Appearance of a nodule or ulcer suggests progression to invasive SCC. In HPV-associated SCCIS, rate of transformation to invasive SCC is relatively low; rate is higher for vulvar SCCIS: Rate of invasiveness and metastasis higher when associated with poor hygiene/chronic balanoposthitis. (See also Sections 11 and 27.)

### HPV-INDUCED INTRAEPITHELIAL NEOPLASIA (IN) AND SQUAMOUS CELL CARCINOMA IN SITU
(See also Section 27)

*Etiology*: HPV types 16, 18, 31, 33. *Risk factors*: immunosuppression, occurring in HIV disease, iatrogenically induced immunosuppression in solid organ transplant recipients. *Clinical findings*: erythematous patches (Fig. 32-18); papules (flattopped), pigmented papules. *Arrangement*: solitary, clustering, confluence, plaque(s) formation. *Distribution*: mucosa and anogenital and inguinocrural skin. *Course*: spontaneous resolution; persist for years; multiple new lesions appear; progress to invasive SCC. Progression to invasive SCC highest in cervix, anus. Monitor cervix/anus by periodic Pap testing (cytology) to detect dysplastic changes.

Vulvar, penile, anal IN nomenclature:

- IN I: mild dysplasia
- IN II: moderate dysplasia
- IN III: neoplastic cells penetrate into upper third of epithelial layers; SCCIS
- Invasive SCC: neoplastic cells penetrate stromal layer of epithelium

### INVASIVE ANOGENITAL SQUAMOUS CELL CARCINOMA

#### Invasive SCC of Penis
*Risk factors*: lack of circumcision, poor penile hygiene, phimosis (25 to 75%), low socioeconomic status, HPV infection (15 to 80%), UV-radiation exposure, tobacco use. *Demography*: more common in developing nations (up to 10% of cancers in men; rare in industrialized nations. *Precancerous lesion/disorders*: cutaneous horn, phimosis, chronic balanoposthitis, pseudoepitheliomatous keratotic and micaceous balanitis, lichen planus, lichen sclerosus, giant condyloma, HPV-induced IN.

*Symptoms*: precursor lesion, itching/burning under foreskin, ulceration of glans or prepuce. *Clinical findings*: subtle induration; small excrescence; small papule; warty growth (Figs. 32-18 and 32-19; see Fig. 11-9) to an obvious extensive carcinoma with sloughing. Necrosis and/or secondary infection in phimotic foreskin. Extends along the penile shaft and involves corpora cavernosa. Rarely, bleeding, urinary fistula, and urinary retention occur. Metastasis: inguinal lymph node metastases; distant sites rare. *Distribution*: glans (48%), prepuce (21%), glans and prepuce (9%), prepuce glans and shaft (14%), coronal sulcus (6%), shaft (<2%).

#### Invasive SCC of Vulva
*Risk factors*: HPV infection, abnormal cervical Pap test, immunosuppression, HIV disease, advanced age, increased number of sexual partners, younger age at first episode of intercourse, tobacco use, lichen planus, lichen sclerosus (Fig. 32-17). *Symptoms*: vulvar pruritus, localized pain, discharge, dysuria, bleeding, ulceration. *Clinical findings*: IN, bulky whitish or pigmented lesion

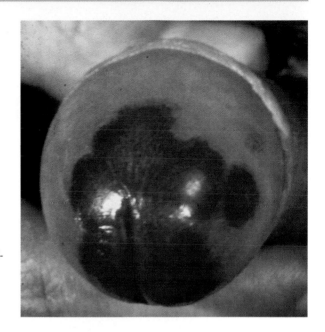

**FIGURE 32-16   Squamous cell carcinoma in situ: glans penis** *A well-demarcated, erythematous, glistening plaque of an elderly male, which had been present for >5 years.*

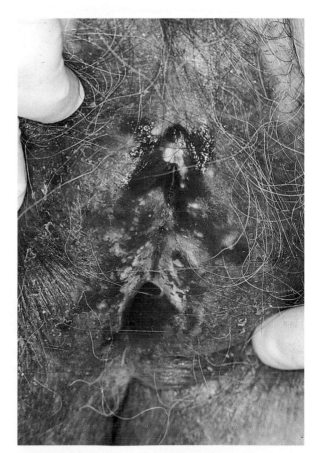

**FIGURE 32-17   Squamous cell carcinoma in situ arising in lichen sclerosus: vulva** *A 60-year-old patient with longstanding genital lichen sclerosus, characterized by erythema and erosions with marked atrophy of the labia minora and clitoris. Lesional biopsy of a white hyperkeratotic area shows associated SCC in situ arising in lichen sclerosus.*

of thickened or hard skin; verrucoid, polypoid, papular. *Location*: 65% arise on labia majora.

## Invasive Anal SCC

*Etiology*: Oncogenic HPV infection. *Risk factors*: chronic immunosuppression, HIV disease. *Location*: (1) cutaneous, (2) junction of columnar and squamous epithelium. *Precursor lesion*: anal IN. *Clinical findings*: papule, nodule, ulcerated nodule (Fig. 32-20).

## Genital Verrucous Carcinoma

*Etiology*: HPV infection. *Clinical findings*: large, cauliflower-like, warty tumors. *Distribution*: vulva, penis, anus.
*Course*: slow-growing; rarely metastasize.

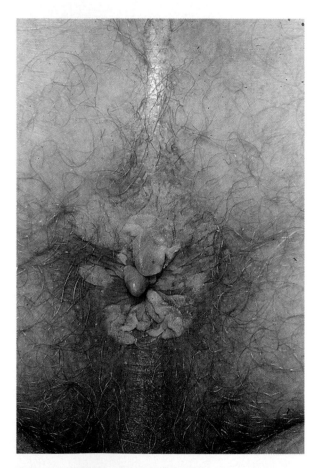

**FIGURE 32-18   HPV-induced squamous cell carcinoma in situ: perianal**   *A well-demarcated pink perianal plaque in a 35-year-old HIV-infected male. Anal Pap test showed low-grade squamous intraepithelial lesion (LSIL). All clinical findings resolved with 5% imiquimod cream applied three times a week followed by weekly applications.*

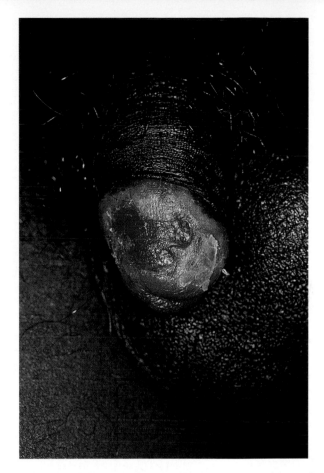

**FIGURE 32-19  Invasive squamous cell carcinoma: glans penis**  *An eroded indurated plaque on the glans in a 45-year-old black male. The patient had a history of chronic balanoposthitis for >5 years; circumcision had been performed 1 year previously. Treatment was amputation.*

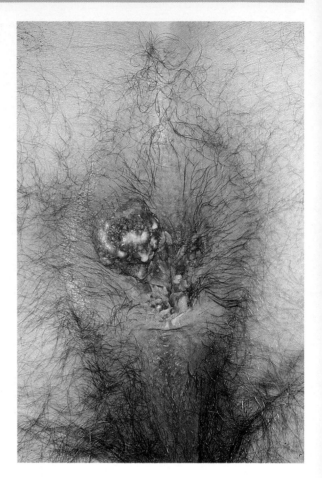

**FIGURE 32-20   HPV-induced invasive squamous cell carcinoma: perineum**   *A 32-year-old HIV-infected male presented with a perineal tumor of several months' duration. Histology of the excised specimen showed invasive SCC.*

## MALIGNANT MELANOMA OF THE ANOGENITAL REGION
(See also Section 12)

Incidence: rare. *Precursor lesions*: preexisting pigmented lesion or de novo from epidermal melanocytes. *Clinical findings*: macules or papules with variegation of brown-black color, irregular borders, and often with papular elevation (Fig. 32-21) or ulceration. *Distribution*: males: glans (67%), prepuce (13%), urethral meatus (10%), penile shaft (7%), and coronal sulcus (3%) (Fig. 32-21); females: labia minora, clitoris (Fig. 32-22) . *Differential diagnosis*: genital lentiginosis, old fixed drug eruption, SCC, hemangioma, intraepithelial neoplasia (Bowenoid papulosis). *Histologic types*: acral lentiginous melanoma; rarely, desmoplastic melanoma. *Prognosis*: poor because of early metastases via lymphatic vessels; most patients die within 1 to 3 years.

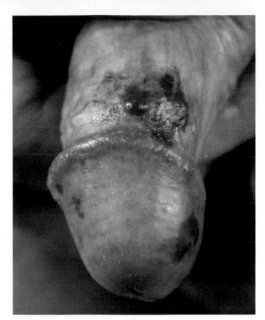

**FIGURE 32-21    Melanoma, invasive: penis**   *A violaceous nodule arising in an area of macular variegated hyperpigmentation in a 60-year-old male. The macular lesions had been present for 5 years and resembled genital lentiginosis. The most common histologic type of genital melanoma is the acrolentiginous melanoma.*

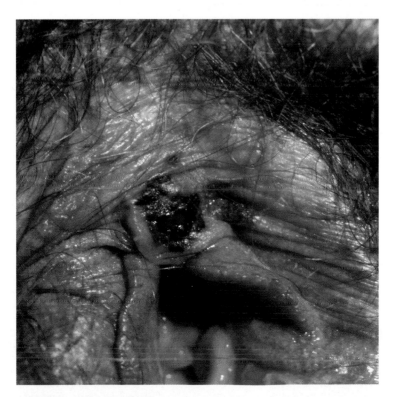

**FIGURE 32-22    Melanoma, invasive: vulva**   *A violaceous nodule in a black plaque in a 52-year-old female.*

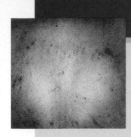

# GENERALIZED PRURITUS WITHOUT SKIN LESIONS (Pruritus sine materia)

Persistent severe pruritus, like pain, is a dominating factor in existence; from day to day it takes over one's life. Intense pruritus may, in fact, be more maddening for the patient than pain because there may not be an effective medication to control the pruritus, whereas pain can usually be controlled with analgesics. The physician, therefore, often feels somewhat helpless in the management of these unfortunate patients. Pruritus leads to sleepless nights; a state of permanent fatigue ensues that precludes work and confounds family relationships. Most skin eruptions and rashes are more or less pruritic, but there are states where there is severe pruritus in the absence of skin lesions, except for scratch marks (Fig. 33-1). This is called *pruritus sine materia* (from Latin, "itch without physical substance"). The diagnostic approach to the patient with generalized pruritus without identifiable skin lesions is a *diagnosis of exclusion:* all organic causes must be excluded within reasonable limits.

This pruritus may be intrinsic to the skin but not due to a skin disease with specific lesions; it may be a symptom of a skin disease that at the time of examination does not manifest with specific lesions; it may be due to an internal organ disease, metabolic and endocrine conditions, or hematologic disease; it may be a manifestation of malignant tumors, psychogenic states, or HIV-1 infection; or it may be related to injected or ingested drugs. The various causes of pruritus sine materia are listed in Table 33-1, and an algorithm of how to approach a patient with pruritus sine materia is shown in Table 33-2. A careful history and physical examination are essential and should take into account the different types of itching and their duration, the quality of itching, and its distribution and timing. It is understood that any patient referred with generalized pruritus without skin lesions should be assumed to have minimal or latent disease of the skin until proven otherwise. Skin signs may be clinically inapparent, perhaps confined to only circumscribed areas, and this is particularly important with regard to the exclusion of scabies, pediculosis, or conditions such as urticaria factitia.

## MOST IMPORTANT CAUSES

*Chronic renal disease:* Pruritus is one of the most important and distressing problems of chronic renal failure, affecting up to 50% of patients. Secondary skin lesions may develop due to intense scratching, such as nummular eczema, prurigo nodularis, or lichenified plaques.

*Cholestasis:* Distressing persistent pruritus accompanying biliary obstruction starts with an acral distribution and becomes generalized. It may be due to both bile salts in the skin and elevated levels of opioid peptides.

*Endocrine disease:* Intractable itching occurs in thyrotoxicosis, probably due to increased blood flow, and in hypothyroidism, where it is probably due to excessive skin dryness. In contrast to previous beliefs, pruritus is not a feature of diabetes mellitus but can be a manifestation of diabetic neuropathy.

*Hematologic disease:* Pruritus occurs in about 50% of patients with polycythemia vera, often after contact with water ("bath-itch"), and may be associated with raised blood histamine levels. In Hodgkin's disease it is a presenting symptom, and it occurs in leukemias; in cutaneous masto-

**FIGURE 33-1   Pruritus without diagnostic skin lesions** *This patient had multiple scratch marks due to compulsive scratching because of severe pruritus. There were no other, and in particular, diagnostic lesions. Workup revealed biliary cirrhosis without jaundice.*

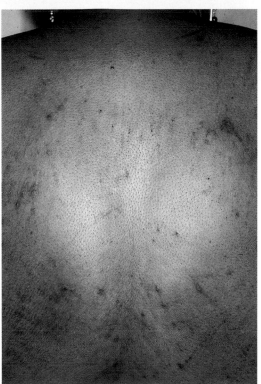

cytosis (without visible skin lesions), it usually occurs locally following rubbing of the skin.

*HIV infection:* Pruritus may occur as a primary symptom of HIV infection and may be pruritus sine materia or be associated with infestations; xerosis; or hepatic disease, renal disease, lymphoma, or adverse drug reactions.

*Senile pruritus:* This is common in persons aged ≥70 years and in many patients. No causes found. Desiccation of the skin may be one reason, but sometimes pruritus may also be provoked by water contact mimicking aquagenic pruritus (see below).

*Psychiatric disease:* Localized pruritus is often a common manifestation of chronic anxiety, and persistent rubbing of the localized area will result in lichenification. Parasitophobia is a more serious problem (see Section 21).

*Aquagenic pruritus:* This pruritus, usually in the middle aged and elderly, is provoked by contact with water of any temperature; it lasts up to 1 h, and there are no visible signs on the skin. Elevated levels of histamine have been found in the blood and skin of such patients, and this condition must be distinguished from "bath-itch" in polycythemia vera or water-induced senile pruritus. The causes are unknown; since no lesions can be found, such patients are often labeled as neurotic.

*Notalgia paresthetica:* This is a common localized itch usually in the interscapular area, sometimes more widespread. The sensations are part itch/part paresthesia. It

is probably a neuropathic itch due to the entrapment of spinal nerves as they emerge through the muscle fascias of the back.

*Brachioradial pruritus:* This is a localized pruritus on the outer surface of the upper arm, elbow, and forearm, often associated with clinical evidence of chronic sun damage and xerosis (hence "golfer's itch").

## MANAGEMENT

1. Identify and treat underlying disease.
2. Treat xerosis with baths and emollients.
3. UVB and narrow-band (311 nm) phototherapy or PUVA (in renal-, biliary-, aquagenic-, and polycythemia vera–related pruritus).
4. Nolaxone, naltrexone, or odansetron; cholestyramine in cholestatic itch (but ineffective in total biliary obstruction).

**TABLE 33-1   Causes of Pruritus Sine Materia**

| | |
|---|---|
| **Metabolic, endocrine conditions** | **Hepatic disease** |
|   Hyperthyroidism |   Obstructive biliary disease |
|   Hypothyroidism |   Pregnancy (intrahepatic cholestasis) |
|   Pregnancy related | **Psychogenic states** |
| **Malignant neoplasms** |   Transitory: |
|   Lymphoma, myeloid and lymphatic |     Periods of emotional stress |
|     leukemia, myelodysplasia |   Persistent: |
|   Multiple myeloma |     Delusions of parasitosis |
|   Hodgkin's disease |     Psychogenic pruritus |
|   Other cancer (rare) |     Neurotic excoriations |
| **Drug ingestion** |     Anorexia nervosa |
|   Subclinical drug sensitivities | **Latent dermatoses and miscellaneous** |
|   Aspirin, alcohol, dextran, polymyxin B, |   **conditions** |
|     morphine, codeine, scopolamine, |   Xerosis (dry skin, "winter itch") |
|     D-tubocurarine, IV hydroxyethyl starch |   Senile pruritus[†] |
| **Infestations** |   Bullous pemphigoid (without skin |
|   Scabies[*] |     lesions) |
|   Pediculosis corporis, capitis, pubis |   Dermatitis herpetiformis (without skin |
|   Hookworm (ancylostomiasis) |     lesions) |
|   Onchocerciasis |   Atopic dermatitis (without skin |
|   Ascariasis |     lesions) |
| **Renal disease** |   Factitious urticaria (dermographism) |
|   Renal failure |   Fiber glass exposure |
| **Other hematologic disease** |   Aquagenic pruritus |
|   Polycythemia vera |   Notalgia paresthetica |
|   Paraproteinemia, iron deficiency |   Brachioradial pruritus |

[*]Diagnostic lesions may or may not present.
[†]Unexplained intense pruritus in patients >70 years without obvious "dry skin" and with no apparent emotional stress.

## PRURITUS ANI

Many patients, in desperation, become resigned to accepting pruritus ani as part of their lives and endure the embarrassment and the sleepless nights.

*Pruritus ani* is pruritus of the anal skin without evidence of a primary dermatologic disorder sometimes seen in this region, e.g., dermatophytosis, candidiasis, psoriasis, or seborrheic dermatitis. Pinworms are a rare cause and are seen usually only in children. The major factor in the pathogenesis of pruritus ani is irritation from the presence of fecal soiling on the anal skin; this is most often the result of incomplete cleansing of the area after defecation but also results in some persons from the weakness of the anal sphincter, which allows for fecal soiling when the rectum is distended by the arrival of feces or with flatus. The vicious cycle is irritation → itching → rubbing with the development of lichenification → more pruritus.

When lichenification is present, control begins with a *very limited* course of potent topical glucocorticoids to reduce lichenification. The main thrust of management, however, must be directed at two provoking factors:

1. *Paroxysmal compulsive rubbing and scratching of the anal sphincter and skin around it.* Anxiety and stress appear to contribute to the itching. The "fits" of rubbing or scratching occur most often after defecation and at night, when the patient is often awakened by the itching. These bouts of pruritus can be somewhat relieved by menthol-camphor lotions.

**TABLE 33-2   Approach to the Diagnosis of Generalized Pruritus Without Diagnostic Skin Lesions**

It is critical to recognize that nonspecific skin changes can be induced by rubbing and scratching. The false conclusion that a dermatologic cause for itching is necessarily present just because a rash can be seen is a trap that must be avoided. The approach to the patient with persistent generalized pruritus begins with careful history and meticulous examination of the (entire) skin, followed by additional attention to the general history, review of systems, general physical examination, and investigations as outlined below.

*Initial Visit*

1. Detailed history of pruritus:
   - Are there any skin lesions that precede the itching?
   - Is the itching continuous or does it occur in waves?
   - Is the itching related to certain times of the day, does it occur at night, and does it keep the patient awake?
   - Is the itching related to environmental conditions (heat, cold); is it related to emotional stress, physical exertion, sweating; contact with water?
2. Examine carefully for subtle primary skin disorders as a cause of the pruritus; xerosis or asteatosis, scabies, pediculosis (nits?). Discrete papules on elbows, scalp (dermatitis herpetiformis), on scrotum or shaft of penis (scabies).
3. Check for dermographism, rub skin for Darier's sign (see "Mastocytosis Syndromes," Section 18).
4. Repeat history related to pruritus. Obtain history of constitutional symptoms, weight loss, fatigue, fever, malaise. History of oral or parenteral medication that can be a cause of generalized pruritus without a rash.
5. General physical examination including *all* the lymph nodes; rectal examination and stool guaiac in adult patients (depending on the individual clinical situation, may be deferred to second or later visit).
6. If dry skin or winter itch is a reasonable possible explanation, give the patient bath oil, followed by an emollient ointment. No soap; the bath is therapeutic, not for cleansing the skin; shower to clean.
7. Follow-up appointment in 2 weeks.

*Subsequent Visit(s)*

If no relief from symptomatic treatment given on the first visit, proceed as follows:

1. Detailed review of systems.
2. Laboratory tests: complete blood tests including erythrocyte sedimentation rate, fasting blood sugar, renal function tests, liver function tests, hepatitis antigens, thyroid tests, stool and serologic examination for parasites.
3. If the diagnosis has not been established at this point, the patient should be referred for complete workup including pelvic examination and Pap smear.

SOURCE: Adapted from JD Bernhard (ed): *Itch Mechanisms and Management of Pruritus.* New York, McGraw-Hill, 1994, pp. 211–215.

2. *Poor anal hygiene.* Strict, "squeaky" clean cleansing with cotton pledgets soaked in water is ideal. "Baby wipes" available in any supermarket/drugstore will also do the job. Whenever possible, a shower or tub bath is the best method of cleansing; a more convenient method is with a bidet. After cleansing the area, liberal application of talcum powder helps absorb the fecal soiling that can occur during the day; ointments and oily lotions may actually aggravate the pruritus.

# APPENDICES

## APPENDIX A: "TRAVEL" DERMATOLOGY

With the marked increase in international travel in the past decades among persons of all walks of life and all ages, it is necessary to ask patients with skin lesions where they have lived and traveled. This is particularly true for infectious skin disease or infectious systemic disease with skin manifestations. Website *http://www.cdc.gov/travel/index.com* gives information on diseases endemic in different parts of the world and on modes of acquisition. Links provide updated information relevant to diagnosis and thus appropriate treatment.

It is important to keep in mind that a patient with an infection acquired in one geographic location may undergo medical evaluation in another location where the infection is not endemic. Also, many infections may be rare or sporadically acquired in regions outside of endemic areas. An example is anthrax. Sporadic infection may be acquired in any geographic location by way of contact with imported contaminated animal products.

Equally important to note is that infections that require a specific vector for transmission have a distribution limited by the vector distribution. However, presence of the vector is not sufficient for disease to occur. For example, a mosquito competent to transmit dengue is found in many states in the southern United States. However, in recent years, transmission of dengue has been documented only rarely within the United States (Texas).

# APPENDIX B: DERMATOLOGIC MANIFESTATIONS OF DISEASES INFLICTED BY BIOLOGIC WARFARE/BIOTERRORISM

The use of microbial pathogens as potential or actual weapons of terrorism and warfare dates from antiquity. In 2001, the anthrax attacks via the U.S. postal system resulted in 12 cutaneous and 10 inhalational cases of anthrax with 4 deaths. These caused a tremendous amount of anxiety, had an impact on the U.S. postal system, and led to a functional interruption of the activities of the legislative branch of the U.S. government. The Working Group for Civilian Biodefense has compiled a list of characteristics of biologic agents that can be used as bioweapons (Table B-1), and the U.S. Centers for Disease Control and Prevention (CDC) has classified potential biologic agents into three categories: A, B, and C (Table B-2). Category A agents are the priority pathogens requiring special attention for public health preparedness. Many of these lead to skin signs and symptoms and are therefore of major concern to dermatologists. The potential bioterrorism diseases with dermatologic manifestations are

- Anthrax (page 630)
- Plague
- Smallpox (page 769)
- Smallpox vaccine (vaccinia) (page 773)
- Tularemia (page 650)
- Viral hemorrhagic Fevers

Full information on plague and the viral hemorrhagic fevers as well as infections with anthrax by inhalation can be obtained at the CDC website *http://www.bt.cdc.gov/agent/agentlist.asp.*

Also, information on all of these agents and related links can be obtained at the following websites:

- *www.bt.cdc.gov/agent/smallpox/diagnosis/pdf/spox-poster-full.pdf*
- *http://www.cdc.gov/ncidod/dvrd/spb/mnpages/disinfo.htm*
- *http://jama.ama-assn.org/cgi/content/full/287/18/2391*

---

**TABLE B-1  Key Features of Biologic Agents Used as Bioweapons**

1. High morbidity and mortality
2. Potential for person-to-person spread
3. Low infective dose and highly infectious by aerosol
4. Lack of rapid diagnostic capability
5. Lack of universally available effective vaccine
6. Potential to cause anxiety
7. Availability of pathogen and feasibility of production
8. Environmental stability
9. Database of prior research and development
10. Potential to be "weaponized"

*Source:* From L Borio et al: JAMA 287:2391, 2002, with permission.

## TABLE B-2   CDC Category A, B, and C Agents

### Category A
Anthrax (*Bacillus anthracis*)
Botulism (*Clostridium botulinum* toxin)
Plague (*Yersinia pestis*)
Smallpox (*Variola major*)
Tularemia (*Francisella tularensis*)
Viral hemorrhagic fevers
    Arenaviruses: Lassa, New World (Machupo, Junin, Guanarito, and Sabia)
    Bunyaviridae: Crimean Congo, Rift Valley
    Filoviridae: Ebola, Marburg
    Flaviviridae: Yellow fever, Omsk fever, Kyasanur Forest

### Category B
Brucellosis (*Brucella* spp.)
Epsilon toxin of *Closteridium perfringens*
Food safety threats (e.g., *Salmonella* spp., *Escherichia coli* 0157:H7, Shigella
Glanders (*Burkholderia mallei*)
Melioidosis (*B. pseudomallei*)
Psittacosis (*Chlamydia psittaci*)
Q fever (*Coxiella burnettii*)
Ricin toxin from *Ricinus communis* (castor beans)
Staphylococcal enterotoxin B
Typhus fever (*Rickettsia prowazekii*)
Viral encephalitis [alphaviruses (e.g., Venezuelan, eastern, and western equine encephalitis)]
Water safety threats (e.g., *Vibrio cholerae, Cryptosporidium parvum*)

### Category C
Emerging infectious disease threats such as Nipah, hantavirus, and SARS coronavirus.

*Source:* Centers for Disease Control and Prevention and the National Institute of Allergy and Infectious Diseases.

# APPENDIX C: CHEMICAL BIOTERRORISM

Chemical agents have been used as weapons on a large scale in World War I, in the Iraq-Iran War, by Iraq against Kurdish civilians, and in the Sarin attacks in Japan. Industrial hazardous materials (HAZMATs), produced in chemical plants, could also be used as weapons in chemical terrorism.

Table C-1 lists potential agents for such attacks and the symptoms they elicit. Of these, the blistering agent sulfur mustard is one of the most likely agents to be used in a terrorist attack scenario, and it also induces skin lesions (see website http://www.bt.cdc.gov/agent/agentlist.asp).

Following exposure and an asymptomatic latent period, erythema, pruritus, burning, and pain may present; initial blistering of the skin will start on the second day after exposure and will progress for up to 2 weeks. Vesicles coalesce, forming large blisters, and wound healing is considerably slower than for a comparable thermal burn. Differential diagnoses are thermal burn or scalding, toxic epidermal necrolysis, and staphylococcal scalded skin syndrome. (See also W.R. Heymann: Threats of biological and chemical warfare on civilian populations. J Am Acad Dermatol 2004, 51:452.)

**TABLE C-1  Recognizing and Diagnosing Health Effects of Chemical Terrorism**

| Agent | Agent Name | Unique Characteristics | Initial Effects |
|---|---|---|---|
| Nerve | Cyclohexyl sarin (GF)<br>Sarin (GB)<br>Soman (GD)<br>Tabun (GA)<br>VX | Miosis (pinpoint pupils)<br>Copious secretions<br>Muscle twitching/ fasciculations | Miosis (pinpoint pupils)<br>Blurred/dim vision<br>Headache<br>Nausea, vomiting, diarrhea<br>Copious secretions/sweating<br>Muscle twitching/ fasciculations<br>Breathing difficulty<br>Seizures |
| Asphyxiant/blood | Arsine<br>Cyanogen chloride<br>Hydrogen cyanide | Possible cherry red skin<br>Possible cyanosis<br>Possible frostbite[*] | Confusion<br>Nausea<br>Patients may gasp for air, similar to asphyxiation but more abrupt onset<br>Seizures prior to death |
| Choking/pulmonary- damage | Chlorine<br>Hydrogen chloride<br>Nitrogen oxides<br>Phosgene | Chlorine is a greenish-yellow gas with pungent odor<br>Phosgene gas smells like newly mown hay or grass<br>Possible frostbite[*] | Eye and skin irritation<br>Airway irritation<br>Dyspnea, cough<br>Sore throat<br>Chest tightness |

*continued*

**TABLE C-1   Continued**

| Agent | Agent Name | Unique Characteristics | Initial Effects |
|---|---|---|---|
| Blistering/vesicant | Mustard/Sulfur mustard (HD, H) Mustard gas (H) Nitrogen mustard (HN-1, HN-2, HN-3) Lewisite (L) Phosgene oxime (CX) | Mustard (HD) has an odor like burning garlic or horseradish Lewisite (L) has an odor like penetrating geranium Phosgene oxime (CX) has a pepperish or pungent odor | Severe irritation Redness and blisters of the skin Tearing, conjunctivitis, corneal damage Mild respiratory distress to marked airway damage May cause death |
| Incapacitating/ behavior-altering | Agent 15/BZ | May appear as mass drug intoxication with erratic behaviors, shared realistic and distinct hallucinations, disrobing and confusion Hyperthermia Mydriasis (dilated pupils) | Dry mouth and skin Initial tachycardia Altered consciousness, delusions, denial of illness, belligerence Hyperthermia Ataxia (lack of coordination) Hallucinations Mydriasis (dilated pupils) |

* Frostbite may occur from skin contact with liquid arsine, cyanogen chloride, or phosgene.

*Source:* State of New York, Department of Health.

# INDEX

*Page numbers followed by an "f" indicate figures and images; page numbers followed by "t" indicate tables.*